This book is due for ret

TREATMENT of SKIN DISEASE

Comprehensive therapeutic strategies

SECOND EDITION

Commissioning Editor: Karen Bowler
Project Development Manager: Joanne Scott
Editorial Assistant: Amy Head and Katie McCormack
Project Manager: Glenys Norquay
Design Manager: Andy Chapman
Marketing Manager (UK): Amy Hey
Marketing Manager (USA): Megan Carr

TREATMENT of SKIN DISEASE

Comprehensive therapeutic strategies

SECOND EDITION

Mark G Lebwohl MD
Professor and Chairman
Department of Dermatology
The Mount Sinai School of Medicine
New York, NY, USA

Warren R Heymann MD
Head, Division of Dermatology
Professor of Medicine
UMDNJ – Robert Wood Johnson Medical School at Camden
Clinical Associate Professor of Dermatology
University of Pennsylvania School of Medicine
Marlton, NJ, USA

John Berth-Jones FRCP
Consultant Dermatologist
Department of Dermatology
University Hospitals Coventry and Warwickshire NHS Trust
Walsgrave Hospital
Coventry, UK

Ian Coulson BSc MB FRCP
Consultant Dermatologist
Dermatology Unit
Burnley General Hospital
Burnley, UK

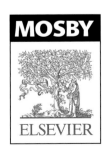

MOSBY

ELSEVIER

MOSBY

Mosby is an affiliate of Elsevier Limited

First edition published 2002
   Reprinted 2002 (twice), 2003 (twice), 2004
Second edition 2006
   Reprinted 2007

ISBN 0 323 03603 1
EAN 9780323036030

This book is also available as a package of book and PDA software:
ISBN 0 323 03598 1
EAN 9780323035989

A PDA software version of this book is also available:
ISBN 0 323 03615 5
EAN 9780323036153

British Library Cataloguing in Publication Data
A catalogue record for this book is available from the British Library

Library of Congress Cataloguing in Publication Data
A catalogue record for this book is available from the Library of Congress

ELSEVIER your source for books, journals and multimedia in the health sciences

www.elsevierhealth.com

Working together to grow libraries in developing countries
www.elsevier.com | www.bookaid.org | www.sabre.org

ELSEVIER   BOOK AID International   Sabre Foundation

The publisher's policy is to use **paper manufactured from sustainable forests**

Printed in China
Last digit is the print number: 9 8 7 6 5 4 3 2

Contents

Contents

Contents

Contents

Contents

Contents

List of Contributors

Anthony Abdullah BSc (Hons) MBChB (Hons) FRCP DTM&H
Consultant Dermatologist
The Birmingham Skin Centre
City Hospital
Birmingham, UK

Beverley Adriaans MD
Consultant Dermatologist
Department of Dermatology
Gloucestershire Royal Hospital
Gloucester, UK

Sanjay Agarwal MBBS MD MRCP
Dermatologist
Department of Dermatology
Royal Hallamshire Hospital
Sheffield, UK

Imtiaz Ahmed MRCP
Consultant Dermatologist
Dermatology Department
University Hospitals Coventry and
Warwickshire
Coventry, UK

Arash Akhavan MD
Dermatologist
Department of Dermatology
The Mount Sinai Medical Center
New York, NY, USA

Haitham Al-Qari MD
Dermatology Fellow
Department of Dermatology
The Mount Sinai Medical Center
New York, NY, USA

Sandra Albert MBBS MD DNB
Visiting Fellow
St John's Institute of Dermatology
St Thomas' Hospital
London, UK

Robert A Allen MD
Clinical Assistant Professor of
Dermatology
Drexel University College of Medicine
Philadelphia, PA, USA

Grant J Anhalt MD
Professor of Dermatology and
Pathology
Department of Dermatology
Johns Hopkins University Hospital
Baltimore, MD, USA

Neda Ashourian MD
Dermatologist
Department of Dermatology
Indiana University School of Medicine
Indianapolis, IN, USA

Richard Ashton MA MD FRCP
Consultant Dermatologist
Dermatology Department
Royal Hospital Haslar
Gosport, UK

Donald J Baker MD
Clinical Assistant Professor of
Dermatology
Department of Medicine
UMDNJ – Robert Wood Johnson Medical
School at Camden
Gibbsboro, NJ, USA

**Periasamy Balasubramaniam
MD MRCP (UK)**
Dermatologist
Department of Dermatology
Selly Oak Hospital
University Hospital of Birmingham NHS
Foundation Trust
Birmingham, UK

Robert Baran MD
Head
Nail Disease Center
Cannes, France

Melissa C Barkham MBChB MRCP
Dermatologist
Department of Dermatology
University Hospital of North
Staffordshire
Stoke-on-Trent, UK

Ysabel M Bello MD
Voluntary Instructor of Dermatology
Department of Dermatology and
Cutaneous Surgery
University of Miami School of Medicine
Miami, FL, USA

E Claire Benton BSc MBChB FRCPE
Consultant Dermatologist
Honorary Clinical Senior Lecturer
Department of Dermatology
The Royal Infirmary
Edinburgh, UK

Philippe Berbis MD
Professor
Service de Dermatologie
Hopital Nord
Marseille, France

Eric Berkowitz MD
Fellow
Department of Dermatology
The Mount Sinai School of Medicine
New York, NY, USA

Brian Berman MD PhD
Professor of Dermatology and
Internal Medicine
Department of Dermatology
University of Miami
Miami, FL, USA

Jeffrey D Bernhard MD
Professor of Medicine
Department of Dermatology
University of Massachusetts Medical
School
Worcester, MA, USA

John Berth-Jones FRCP
Consultant Dermatologist
Department of Dermatology
University Hospitals Coventry and
Warwickshire NHS Trust
Walsgrave Hospital
Coventry, UK

**Monica Bhushan BSc (Hons) MBChB
FRCP**
Consultant Dermatologist
Department of Dermatology
Hope Hospital
Manchester, UK

David J Bilsland MBChB FRCP DCH
Consultant Dermatologist
Department of Dermatology
South Glasgow University Hospitals NHS
Trust
Glasgow, UK

Verity Blackwell MRCP MD
Consultant Dermatologist
Department of Dermatology
Hemel Hempstead and St Albans Hospital
Hemel Hempstead, UK

Jonathan E Blume MD
Dermatologist
Department of Dermatology
State University of New York at Buffalo
Buffalo, NY, USA

Jan D Bos MD PhD FRCP
Professor and Chairman
Department of Dermatology
Academic Medical Center
University of Amsterdam
Amsterdam, The Netherlands

Paul H Bowman MD
Director
The Bowman Institute for Dermatologic
Surgery
Tampa, FL, USA

Gary J Brauner MD
Associate Clinical Professor
Department of Dermatology
Mount Sinai School of Medicine
New York, NY, USA

Robert T Brodell MD
Professor of Internal Medicine
Clinical Professor of Dermatopathology in
Pathology
Permanent Master Teacher
Northeastern Ohio Universities College of
Medicine
Rootstown, OH, USA
Associate Clinical Professor of
Dermatology
Department of Dermatology
Case Western Reserve University School of
Medicine
Cleveland, OH, USA

Rebecca C C Brooke MBChB MRCP
Consultant Dermatologist
Dermatology Centre
University of Manchester School of
Medicine
Manchester, UK

Alison J Bruce MBChB
Consultant, Department of Dermatology
Assistant Professor of Dermatology
Mayo Graduate School of Medicine
Mayo Clinic
Rochester, MN, USA

Robin Buchholz MD
Assistant Professor of Medicine
Department of Dermatology
Albert Einstein College of Medicine
New York, NY, USA

Robert Burd MBChB MRCP
Consultant Dermatologist
Department of Dermatology
Leicester Royal Infirmary
Leicester, UK

Anne E Burdick MD MPh
Professor of Dermatology
Department of Dermatology and
Cutaneous Surgery
University of Miami
Miami, FL, USA

Susan M Burge DM FRCP
Consultant Dermatologist
Department of Dermatology
The Churchill Hospital
Oxford, UK

Katina Byrd-Miles MD
Dermatologist
Department of Dermatology
Washington Hospital Center
Washington, DC, USA

Jeffrey P Callen MD
Professor of Medicine (Dermatology)
Chief, Division of Dermatology
University of Louisville
Louisville, KY, USA

Mitchell S Cappell MD PhD
Director, Gastroenterology Fellowship
Training Program
Division of Gastroenterology
Albert Einstein Medical Center
Philadelphia, PA, USA

Robert Carruthers BA
Research Assistant
Department of Dermatology
The Mount Sinai School of Medicine
New York, NY, USA

John A Carucci MD PhD
Chief, Mohs Micrographic and
Dermatologic Surgery
Assistant Professor of Dermatology
Department of Dermatology
Weill Medical College of Cornell
New York, NY, USA

Bridgette Cave BM MRCP
Dermatologist
Department of Dermatology
North Staffordshire Hospital
Stoke-On-Trent, UK

Santiago A Centurión MD
Dermatology Fellow
Department of Dermatopathology
UMDNJ – New Jersey Medical School
Newark, NJ, USA

Robert J G Chalmers MB FRCP
Consultant Dermatologist
Dermatology Centre
University of Manchester School of
Medicine
Manchester, UK

Lawrence S Chan MD
Professor and Head
Department of Dermatology
University of Illinois College of Medicine
Chicago, IL, USA

**Loi Yuen Chan FHKCP(HK)
FHKAM(Med)**
Dermatologist
Tuen Mun Social Hygiene Clinic
Tuen Mun, New Territories, Hong Kong

Yuchi C Chang MD
Department of Internal Medicine
University of Texas Medical School –
Houston
Houston, TX, USA

Fiona J Child MD FRCP
Consultant Dermatologist
Department of Dermatology
Royal Free Hospital
London, UK

Alvin H Chong MBBS MMED FACD
Consultant Dermatologist and Lecturer in
Dermatology
Department of Dermatology
St Vincent's Hospital
Melbourne, VIC, Australia

Anthony Chu FRCP
Senior Lecturer/Consultant Dermatologist
Unit of Dermatology
Hammersmith Hospital
London, UK

Sheila M Clark MBChB FRCP
Consultant Dermatologist
Department of Dermatology
Leeds General Infirmary
Leeds, UK

**Timothy H Clayton MB ChB MRCPCH
(UK)**
Dermatologist
Department of Dermatology
Leeds General Infirmary
Leeds, UK

Sandeep H Cliff FRCP BSc
Consultant Dermatologist
Department of Dermatology
East Surrey Hospital
Redhill, Surrey, UK

Clay J Cockerell MD
Clinical Professor of Dermatology and
Pathology
Director of Dermatopathology
University of Texas Southwestern Medical
Center
Dallas, TX, USA

Susan M Cooper MRCP
Locum Consultant Dermatologist
Department of Dermatology
Churchill Hospital
Oxford, UK

Ian Coulson BSc MB FRCP
Consultant Dermatologist
Dermatology Unit
Burnley General Hospital
Burnley, UK

Neil H Cox BSc (Hons) MB ChB FRCP
Consultant Dermatologist
Department of Dermatology
Cumberland Infirmary
Carlisle, UK

Nicholas M Craven BM BCh MA FRCP
Consultant Dermatologist
Department of Dermatology
Burnley General Hospital
Burnley, UK

Ponciano D Cruz Jr MD
JB Shelmire Professor and Vice Chairman
Department of Dermatology
The University of Texas Southwestern
Medical Center
Dallas, TX, USA

Mary L Curry MD
Department of Dermatology
The University of Texas Southwestern
Medical Center
Dallas, TX, USA

List of Contributors

Jack F Dalton MD
Professor
Department of Radiation Oncology
The Mount Sinai School of Medicine
New York, NY, USA

Bahar Dasgeb MD
Dermatology Fellow
Department of Dermatology
Boston University School of Medicine
Boston, MA, USA

Mark D P Davis MD
Consultant, Department of Dermatology,
Mayo Clinic
Associate Professor of Dermatology
Mayo Clinic College of Medicine
Rochester, MN, USA

Rosie Davis MRCP
Dermatologist
Department of Dermatology
Leicester Royal Infirmary
Leicester, UK

Robert S Dawe MBChB MD FRCP
Consultant Dermatologist
Department of Dermatology
Ninewells Hospital and Medical School
Dundee, UK

David de Berker BA MBBS MRCP
Consultant Dermatologist
Bristol Dermatology Centre
Bristol Royal Infirmary
Bristol, UK

Avani D Desai MD
Dermatologist
Department of Internal Medicine
Pennsylvania Hospital
Philadelphia, PA, USA

Stephanie A Diamantis BA
Research Assistant
Department of Dermatology
Mount Sinai School of Medicine
New York, NY, USA

Sarah E Dick MD
Resident Physician
Department of Dermatology
Hospital of the University of
Pennsylvania
Philadelphia, PA, USA

John J DiGiovanna MD
Director, Division of
Dermatopharmacology
Professor, Department of Dermatology
Brown Medical School
Providence, RI, USA
DNA Repair Section
Basic Research Laboratory
Center for Cancer Research
National Cancer Institute
National Institutes of Health
Bethesda, MD, USA

Lori M DiRusso MD
Pediatrician
Department of Pediatrics
Colorado Permanente Medical Group
Denver, CO, USA

Alexander Doctoroff DO MS
Dermatologist
Clinical Assistant Professor of Medicine
University of Medicine and Dentistry of
New Jersey
School of Osteopathic Medicine
Clark, NJ, USA

Pauline Dowd BSc (Hons) MD FRCP
Professor of Dermatology
University College London Hospitals Trust
London, UK

Lisa A Drage MD
Assistant Professor of Dermatology
Department of Dermatology
Mayo Clinic College of Medicine
Rochester, MN, USA

**Jacqueline A Dyche MBChB MRCP
DTM&H**
Consultant Dermatologist
Department of Dermatology
Royal Free Hospital
London, UK

Lawrence F Eichenfield MD
Clinical Professor of Pediatrics and
Medicine (Dermatology)
Division of Pediatrics & Adolescent
Dermatology
Children's Hospital and Health Center
San Diego, CA, USA

Natalie N Ellis MD
General Medical Officer
Medical Corps
United States Navy
Key West, FL, USA

Dirk M Elston MD
Teaching Faculty
Departments of Dermatology and
Laboratory Medicine
Geisinger Medical Center
Danville, PA, USA

Jan Faergemann MD PhD
Professor of Dermatology
Department of Dermatology
Sahlgrenska University Hospital
Gothenburg, Sweden

Anna F Falabella MD CWS
Voluntary Associate Professor
Department of Dermatology and
Cutaneous Surgery
University of Miami School of Medicine
Miami, FL, USA

Alyssa M Feiner MD
Dermatologist
Department of Dermatology
SUNY Downstate University
Brooklyn, NY, USA

James Ferguson MD FRCP
Professor of Dermatology
Photobiology Unit
Ninewells Hospital and Medical School
Dundee, Scotland

Geover Fernandez MD
Dermatologist
Department of Dermatology
New Jersey Medical School
Newark, NJ, USA

Andrew Y Finlay MBBS FRCP
Professor of Dermatology
Department of Dermatology
Cardiff University
Wales College of Medicine
Cardiff, UK

Michael Fisher MD
Professor of Medicine, Head
Division of Dermatology
Albert Einstein College of Medicine
New York, NY, USA

Richard G Fried MD PhD
Clinical Director
Yardley Dermatology Associates
Yardley, PA, USA

Brian S Fuchs BA
Research Associate
Department of Dermatology
The Mount Sinai School of Medicine
New York, NY, USA

Claude E Gagna PhD
Assistant Professor of Pathology
Department of Life Sciences
New York Institute of Technology
Old Westbury, NY, USA

Joel M Gelfand MD MSCE
Assistant Professor of Dermatology
Department of Dermatology
Hospital of the University of Pennsylvania
Philadelphia, PA, USA

Carlo Gelmetti MD
Full Professor and Head, Unit of Pediatric
Dermatology
Clinica Dermatologica
IRCCS "Ospedale Maggiore Policlinico,
Mangiagalli e Regina Elena" di Milano
University of Milan
Milan, Italy

Sam Gibbs MA MB BChir FRCP
Consultant Dermatologist
Department of Dermatology
Ipswich Hospital NHS Trust
Ipswich, UK

Gillian E Gibson MD MRCPI
Consultant Dermatologist
Shanakiel Hospital
Cork, Ireland

Gary Goldenberg MD
Dermatologist
Department of Dermatology
Wake Forest University School of
Medicine
Winston-Salem, NC, USA

Darrell W Gonzales MD
Dermatologist
Department of Dermatology
Rush Medical University
Chicago, IL, USA

**Mark J D Goodfield MA MB BChir MD
FRCP**
Consultant Dermatologist
Department of Dermatology
Leeds General Infirmary
Leeds, UK

Marsha L Gordon MD
Associate Clinical Professor
Department of Dermatology
The Mount Sinai School of Medicine
New York, NY, USA

**Robin A C Graham-Brown BSc
MB FRCP**
Consultant and Honorary Senior Lecturer
in Dermatology
University Hospitals of Leicester
NHS Trust
Leicester, UK

Clive E H Grattan MA MD FRCP
Consultant Dermatologist
St John's Institute of Dermatology,
London
Norfolk and Norwich University Hospital
Norwich, UK

**Malcolm W Greaves MD PhD FRCP
FAMS**
Emeritus Professor of Dermatology
Senior Consultant Dermatologist
National Skin Centre
Singapore

Charlot Grech MD MRCP
Consultant Dermatologist
Sir Paul Boffa Hospital
Floriana, Malta

Justin J Green MD
Assistant Professor of Dermatology
Department of Dermatology
University of Medicine and Dentistry of
New Jersey
Robert Wood Johnson School of Medicine
Marlton, NJ, USA

**Christopher E M Griffiths BSc MD FRCP
FRCPath**
Professor of Dermatology
Dermatology Centre
Hope Hospital
University of Manchester
Manchester, UK

Alejandra Gurtman MD
Associate Professor
Department of Medicine
Division of Infectious Diseases
The Mount Sinai School of Medicine
New York, NY, USA

Suhail M Hadi MBChB M Phil FAAD
Assistant Professor of Dermatology
Department of Dermatology
The Mount Sinai Medical Center
New York, NY, USA

Abdul Hafejee MBChB MRCP (UK)
Dermatologist
Department of Dermatology
Hope Hospital
Manchester, UK

Joanne Hague MBBS MRCP
Dermatologist
Department of Dermatology
University Hospitals Coventry and
Warwick
Walsgrave Hospital
Coventry, UK

Julia E Haimowitz MD
Dermatologist
Department of Dermatology
Kaiser Permanente Medical Center
San Rafael, CA, USA

Bethany R Hairston MD
Dermatologist
Mayo School of Graduate Medical
Education
Mayo Clinic College of Medicine
Rochester, MN, USA

Analisa Vincent Halpern MD
Resident Physician
Division of Dermatology
Department of Medicine
UMDNJ – Robert Wood Johnson Medical
School
Cooper University Hospital
Camden, NJ, USA

Susan E Handfield-Jones BM FRCP
Consultant Dermatologist
Department of Dermatology
West Suffolk Hospital
Bury St Edmunds, UK

John Harper MD FRCP FRCPCH
Professor of Paediatric Dermatology
Department of Dermatology
Great Ormond Street Hospital
London, UK

Ronald M Harris MD MBA
Assistant Professor of Dermatology and
Pathology
Department of Dermatology
University of Utah Health Sciences Center
Salt Lake City, UT, USA

John L M Hawk BSc MD FRCP
Professor of Dermatological Photobiology
Photobiology Unit
St John's Institute of Dermatology
London, UK

Adrian H M Heagerty BSc MD FRCP
Consultant Dermatologist
Department of Dermatology
Heart of England Trust
Solihull, UK

Adelaide A Hebert MD
Professor of Dermatology and Pediatrics
Department of Dermatology
University of Texas Medical School
Houston, TX, USA

Stephen E Helms MD
Associate Professor of Internal Medicine
Northeastern Ohio University College of
Medicine
Assistant Clinical Professor of Dermatology
Case Western Reserve University College
of Medicine
Warren, OH, USA

Catriona A Henderson FRCP
Consultant Dermatologist
Department of Dermatology
Royal South Hants Hospital
Southampton, UK

Doris M Hexsel MD
Former Professor of Dermatology
School of Medicine
University of Passo Fundo
Passo Fundo, Brazil

Warren R Heymann MD
Head, Division of Dermatology
Professor of Medicine
UMDNJ – Robert Wood Johnson Medical
School at Camden
Clinical Associate Professor of
Dermatology
University of Pennsylvania School of
Medicine
Marlton, NJ, USA

Sarah Hodulik BA
Research Assistant
Department of Dermatology
The Mount Sinai School of Medicine
New York, NY, USA

Herbert Hönigsmann MD
Professor and Chairman
Department of Dermatology
Division of Special and Environmental
Dermatology
Medical University of Vienna
Vienna, Austria

Marcelo G Horenstein MD
Director of Dermatopathology
The Dermatology Group
Verona, NJ, USA

List of Contributors

Karen R Houpt MD
Associate Professor
Department of Dermatology
The University of Texas Southwestern
Medical Center
Dallas, TX, USA

Frances Humphreys MB BS FRCP
Consultant Dermatologist, Warwick
Hospital
Honorary Senior Lecturer, University of
Warwick
Department of Dermatology
Warwick Hospital
Warwick, UK

**Walayat Hussain BSc (Hons) MBChB
MRCP**
Dermatologist
The Dermatology Unit
Burnley General Hospital
Burnley, UK

Linda Y Hwang MD
Dermatologist
Department of Dermatology
Kaiser Permanente Medical Center
San Rafael, CA, USA

Andrew Ilchyshyn MB ChB FRCP
Consultant Dermatologist
Walsgrave Hospital
Coventry, UK

Erum N Ilyas MD
Dermatologist
Dermatology Division
Cooper University Hospital
Camden, NJ, USA

Stefania Jablonska MD
Professor of Medicine
Department of Dermatology
Warsaw School of Medicine
Warsaw, Poland

William D James MD
The Paul R Gross Professor of
Dermatology
Department of Dermatology
University of Pennsylvania Health System
Philadelphia, PA, USA

Gregor B E Jemec MD DMedSci
Associate Professor of Dermatology
Department of Dermatology
Roskilde Hospital, University of
Copenhagen
Roskilde, Denmark

Graham Johnston MBChB MRCP
Consultant Dermatologist
Department of Dermatology
Leicester Royal Infirmary
Leicester, UK

Siân Jones MD
Clinical Assistant Professor of Medicine
Division of Infectious Diseases
Mount Sinai School of Medicine
New York, NY, USA

**Stephen K Jones BM BS BMedSci MD
FRCP**
Consultant Dermatologist
Department of Dermatology
Clatterbridge Hospital
Wirral, UK

Joseph L Jorizzo MD
Professor, Former and Founding Chair
Department of Dermatology
Wake Forest University School of Medicine
Winston-Salem, NC, USA

Jacqueline M Junkins-Hopkins MD
Assistant Professor of Dermatology
Department of Dermatology
University of Pennsylvania
Philadelphia, PA, USA

Wolfgang Jurecka MD
Professor of Dermatology and Head
Department of Dermatology
Wilhelminenspital
Vienna, Austria

Aleksey Kamenshchikov BA
Research Assistant
Department of Dermatology
The Mount Sinai School of Medicine
New York, NY, USA

Carmen E Kannee MD
Dermatologist
Department of Dermatology
Instituto de Biomedicina
Caracas, Venezuela

Jonathan Kantor MD MSCE
Department of Dermatology
University of Pennsylvania
Philadelphia, PA, USA

Ruwani P Katugampola BM MRCP (UK)
Dermatologist
Department of Dermatology
Cardiff University
Wales College of Medicine
Cardiff, UK

Bruce E Katz MD
Clinical Professor
Mount Sinai School of Medicine
Director, JUVA Skin & Laser Center
Director, Cosmetic Surgery & Laser Clinic
Mount Sinai Medical Center
New York, NY, USA

Martin Keefe DM FRCP
Consultant Dermatologist
Department of Dermatology
Royal South Hants Hospital
Southampton, UK

Sam Kim MD
Dermatologist
Private Practice
New York City, NY, USA and Hatboro, PA,
USA

Brian Kirby MB FRCPI
Consultant Dermatologist
Adelaide and Meath Hospital
Incorporating National Children's Hospital
Honorary Lecturer in Medicine
Trinity College
University of Dublin
Dublin, Ireland

John Koo MD FAAD
Professor and Vice Chairman
Department of Dermatology
University of California San Francisco
Medical Center
San Francisco, CA, USA

Alfred W Kopf MD
Clinical Professor of Dermatology
Department of Dermatology
New York University School of Medicine
New York, NY, USA

Neil J Korman MD PhD
Associate Professor of Dermatology
Department of Dermatology
Case Western Reserve University
Cleveland, OH, USA

Bernice R Krafchik MB ChB FRCPC
Professor Emeritus
Department of Medicine and Pediatrics
University of Toronto
Toronto, ON, Canada

Anjeli Krishnan MD
Internal Medicine
UCSF Psoriasis Treatment Center
University of California San Francisco
Medical Center
San Francisco, CA, USA

Erine A Kupetsky DO
School of Osteopathic Medicine
University of Medicine and Dentistry of
New Jersey
Stratford, NJ, USA

Knut Kvernebo MD PhD FRCS
Professor of Cardiothoracic Surgery
Department of Thoracic Surgery
University of Oslo
Oslo, Norway

**Wing Yin Lam MBBS FRCPath FHKAM
(Path)**
Consultant Pathologist
Institute of Pathology
Tuen Mun Hospital
Tuen Mun, New Territories, Hong Kong

W Clark Lambert MD PhD
Professor of Pathology
Professor of Medicine (Dermatology)
UMDNJ – New Jersey Medical School
Newark, NJ, USA

List of Contributors

James A A Langtry MBBS FRCP
Consultant Dermatologist
Department of Dermatology
Sunderland Royal Hospital
Sunderland, UK

Frances Lawlor MD FRCP FRCPI DCH
D Obst RCOG
Consultant Dermatologist
Newham University Hospital Dermatology
Unit
St Andrew's Hospital
Urticaria Unit
St John's Institute of Dermatology
St Thomas' Hospital
London, UK

Clifford M Lawrence MD FRCP
Consultant Dermatologist
Department of Dermatology
Royal Victoria Infirmary
Newcastle upon Tyne, UK

Naomi Lawrence MD
Head of Procedural Dermatology
Associate Professor
Center for Dermatologic Surgery
Marlton, NJ, USA

Alison Lazinsky BA
Research Assistant
Department of Dermatology
The Mount Sinai School of Medicine
New York, NY, USA

Mark G Lebwohl MD
Professor and Chairman
Department of Dermatology
The Mount Sinai School of Medicine
New York, NY, USA

Oscar Lebwohl MD
Clinical Professor of Medicine
Department of Medicine
Division of Digestive and Liver Diseases
Columbia University College of Physicians
and Surgeons
New York, NY, USA

Joshua M Levin MD
Dermatologist
Department of Dermatology
University of Pennsylvania
Philadelphia, PA, USA

Robin M Levin MD
Assistant Professor of Dermatology
Department of Family Medicine
Division of Dermatology
University of Medicine and Dentistry of
New Jersey
School of Osteopathic Medicine
Stratford, NJ, USA

Erika Gaines Levine MD
Dermatologist
Dermatology Center of Washington
Township
Sewell, NJ, USA

Tsui Chin Ling MRCP
Dermatologist
Department of Dermatology
Hope Hospital
Manchester, UK

Thomas A Luger MD
Professor and Chairman
Department of Dermatology
University of Münster
Münster, Germany

Slawomir Majewski MD
Professor of Dermatology
Department of Dermatology and
Venereology
Warsaw School of Medicine
Warsaw, Poland

Richard B Mallett MB FRCP
Consultant Dermatologist
Department of Dermatology
Peterborough District Hospital
Peterborough, UK

Steven M Manders MD
Associate Professor of Medicine
Division of Dermatology
UMDNJ – Robert Wood Johnson Medical
School at Camden
Marlton, NJ, USA

Ranon Mann MD
Instructor of Medicine
Department of Dermatology
Albert Einstein College of Medicine
New York, NY, USA

David J Margolis MD PhD
Associate Professor of Dermatology
Department of Biostatistics and
Epidemiology
University of Pennsylvania
Philadelphia, PA, USA

Jeremy R Marsden FRCP
Consultant Dermatologist
University Hospital Birmingham
Birmingham, UK

Agustin Martin-Clavijo LSM PhD MRCP
Dermatologist
University Hospitals of Coventry and
Warwickshire
Walsgrave Hospital
Coventry, UK

Anna Martinez MBBS MRCP MRCPCH
Consultant Paediatrician
Paediatric Dermatology
Great Ormond Street Hospital
London, UK

Susan Coutinho McAllister MD
Clinical Instructor of Medicine
Cooper Hospital University Medical Center
Camden, NJ, USA

Andrew J G McDonagh MB ChB FRCP
MRCP
Consultant Dermatologist
Department of Dermatology
Royal Hallamshire Hospital
Sheffield, UK

Karen S McGinnis MD
Dermatologist
Department of Dermatology
University of Pennsylvania
Philadelphia, PA, USA

Dermot B McKenna MD MRCPI DCH
Consultant Dermatologist
Department of Dermatology
Sligo General Hospital
Sligo, Ireland

Manjeet Mehmi MBChB (Hons) MRCP
Dermatologist
Department of Dermatology
University Hospital Coventry and
Warwickshire NHS Trust
Coventry, UK

Corinna Mendonca MBChB MRCP
Dermatologist
Dermatology Department
Hope Hospital
Manchester, UK

Giuseppe Micali MD
Professor and Chairman
Clinica Dermatologica
Universita' di Catania
Catania, Italy

Leslie G Millard MD FRCP
Consultant Dermatologist
Queens Medical Centre
University Hospitals NHS Trust
Nottingham, UK

Alex Milligan FRCP
Consultant Dermatologist
Department of Dermatology
Leicester Royal Infirmary
Leicester, UK

Ginat Mirowski DMD MD
Adjunct Associate Professor
Indiana University School of Dentistry
Indianapolis, IN, USA

Dwayne Montie DO
Dermatologist
Department of Dermatology
Columbia Hospital
Palm Beach, FL, USA

Patrice Morel MD
Professor of Dermatology
Department of Dermatology
Hopital St Louis
Paris, France

List of Contributors

Warwick L Morison MB BS MD FRCP
Professor
Department of Dermatology
Johns Hopkins Hospital
Lutherville, MD, USA

Cato Mørk MD PhD
Consultant Dermatologist
Department of Dermatology
Rikshospitalet University Hospital
Oslo, Norway

Peter S Mortimer MD FRCP
Professor of Dermatological Medicine
St George's, University of London
Consultant Skin Physician
St George's Hospital and Royal Marsden
Hospital
London, UK

Richard J Motley MA MD FRCP
Consultant in Dermatology and
Cutaneous Surgery
Welsh Institute of Dermatology
University Hospital of Wales
Cardiff, UK

Anna E Muncaster MBChB FRCP
Consultant Dermatologist
Department of Dermatology
Rotherham General Hospital
Rotherham, UK

George J Murakawa MD PhD
President, Somerset Skin Center
Troy, MI, USA
Clinical Professor
Department of Internal Medicine
Michigan State University
East Lansing, MI, USA

Michele E Murdoch BSc FRCP
Consultant Dermatologist
Dermatology Center
Watford General Hospital
Watford, UK

Stuart C Murray BM BS BSc BEc FACD
Consultant Dermatologist
Department of Dermatology
Flinders Medical Centre
Adelaide, SA, Australia

Farzana Nayeemuddin MB BS MRCP
Dermatologist
Department of Dermatology
Burnley General Hospital,
Burnley, UK

Rachel Nazarian BS
Research Assistant
Department of Dermatology
The Mount Sinai School of Medicine
New York, NY, USA

Sallie Neill MB ChB FRCP
Consultant Dermatologist
St John's Institute of Dermatology
St Thomas' Hospital
London, UK

Kenneth H Neldner MD
Professor and Chairman Emeritus
Department of Dermatology
Texas Tech University Health Sciences
Center
Lubbock, TX, USA

Glenn C Newell MD FACP
Division Head of Medical Education
Associate Professor of Medicine
Cooper Hospital
Camden, NJ, USA

**Rosemary Nixon BSc (Hons) MBBS MPH
FACD FAFOM**
Dermatologist and Director
Occupational Dermatology Research and
Education Centre
Melbourne, VIC, Australia

Carlos H Nousari MD
Director
Institute for Immunofluorescence
Dermpath Diagnostics
Pompano Beach, FL, USA

Nuala O'Donoghue MB ChB MRCPI
Locum Consultant Dermatologist
St John's Institute of Dermatology
Guy's Hospital
London, UK

John B O'Driscoll FRCP
Consultant Dermatologist
Hope Hospital
University of Manchester School of
Medicine
Manchester, UK

Malobi Ogboli MBBS MRCP UK
Consultant Dermatologist
Department of Dermatology
City Hospital
Birmingham, UK

**Stephanie Ogden MB ChB (Hons)
MRCP (UK)**
Dermatologist
Department of Dermatology
Macclesfield District General Hospital
Macclesfield, UK

Caroline M Owen MBChB MRCP
Consultant Dermatologist
Department of Dermatology
Burnley General Hospital
Burnley, UK

Roy A Palmer MA MRCP
Fellow in Photodermatology
Photobiology Unit
St John's Institute of Dermatology
London, UK

Jennifer L Parish MD
Clinical Assistant Professor of Dermatology
and Cutaneous Biology
Jefferson Medical College
Thomas Jefferson University
Philadelphia, PA, USA

Lawrence Charles Parish MD
Clinical Professor of Dermatology and
Cutaneous Biology
Jefferson Medical College
Thomas Jefferson University
Philadelphia, PA, USA

Gary L Peck MD
Director, Melanoma Center
Cancer Institute
Washington Hospital Center
Washington, DC, USA

William Perkins MBBS FRCP
Consultant Dermatologist
Department of Dermatology
Queens Hospital NHS Trust
Queens Medical Centre
Nottingham, UK

Robert G Phelps MD
Director of Dermatopathology
Associate Professor of Dermatology and
Pathology
Mount Sinai School of Medicine
New York, NY, USA

Tania J Phillips MD FRCPC
Professor of Dermatology
Department of Dermatology
Boston University School of Medicine
Boston, MA, USA

Maureen B Poh-Fitzpatrick MD
Professor of Medicine (Dermatology)
University of Tennessee College of
Medicine
Professor Emerita of Dermatology and
Special Lecturer
Columbia University College of Physicians
and Surgeons
Memphis, TN, USA

Sajjad F Rajpar MBChB (Hons) MRCP
Dermatologist
Department of Dermatology
Selly Oak Hospital
Birmingham, UK

Claudia C Ramirez MD
Clinical Research Fellow
Department of Dermatology
University of Miami
Miami, FL, USA

Ronald P Rapini MD
Professor and Chair
Department of Dermatology
University of Texas Medical School and
MD Anderson Cancer Center
Houston, TX, USA

Ravi Ratnavel DM (Oxon) FRCP (UK)
Consultant Dermatologist
Buckingham NHS Trust
Stoke Mandeville Hospital
Aylesbury, UK

List of Contributors

Larisa Ravitskiy MD
Dermatologist
Division of Dermatology
Cooper University Hospital
Camden, NJ, USA

Jean Revuz MD
Professor of Dermatology
Chairman, Department of
Dermatology
Hopital Henri Mondor
Creteil, France

Gabriele Richard MD FACMG
Associate Scientific Director
Gene Dx Inc
Gaithersburg, MD, USA

Darrell S Rigel MD
Clinical Professor
Department of Dermatology
New York University Medical Centre
New York, NY, USA

Brandie J Roberts MD
Assistant Clinical Professor of Pediatrics
and Medicine (Dermatology)
Pediatric and Adolescent Dermatology
Children's Hospital and Health Center
San Diego, CA, USA

David T Roberts MB ChB FRCP
(Glasgow)
Consultant Dermatologist
Department of Dermatology
South Glasgow University Hospitals NHS
Trust
Glasgow, UK

Wanda Sonia Robles MD PhD
Consultant Dermatologist
Department of Dermatology
Chase Farm Hospital
Enfield, UK

Roy S Rogers III MD
Professor of Dermatology
Department of Dermatology
Mayo Clinic College of Medicine
Rochester, MN, USA

Ricardo Romagosa MD
Voluntary Instructor
Department of Dermatology and
Cutaneous Surgery
University of Miami, Miller School of
Medicine
Miami, FL, USA

Alain H Rook MD
Professor of Dermatology
Department of Dermatology
University of Pennsylvania Hospital
Philadelphia, PA, USA

Donald Rudikoff MD
Chief of Dermatology
Bronx Lebanon Medical Center
Bronx, NY, USA
Associate Professor
Department of Dermatology
The Mount Sinai Medical Center
New York, NY, USA

Malcolm Rustin BSc MD FRCP
Consultant Dermatologist
Dermatology Department
The Royal Free Hospital
London, UK

Thomas Ruzicka MD
Professor of Dermatology
Department of Dermatology
Heinrich-Heine University
Düsseldorf, Germany

Miguel R Sanchez MD
Associate Professor of Clinical
Dermatology
Department of Dermatology
NYU School of Medicine
New York, NY, USA

Lawrence A Schachner MD
Chairman and Harvey Blank Professor
Dermatology and Cutaneous Surgery
University of Miami Miller Medical School
Miami, FL, USA

Rhonda E Schnur MD FACMG
Head, Division of Genetics
Associate Professor of Pediatrics
Cooper University Hospital
Robert Wood Johnson Medical School
Camden, NJ, USA

Olivia M V Schofield MBBS MRCP(UK)
FRCP(Edin)
Consultant Dermatologist
Department of Dermatology
Royal Infirmary of Edinburgh
Edinburgh, UK

Robert A Schwartz MD MPH
Professor and Head, Dermatology
Professor of Pathology, Medicine,
Pediatrics, Preventive Medicine and
Community Health
UMDNJ – New Jersey Medical School
Newark, NJ, USA

Elana T Segal MD
Dermatologist
Dermatology Center of Washington
Township
Sewell, NJ, USA

Bryan A Selkin MD
Instructor in Dermatology
Beth Israel Deaconess Medical
Center
Boston, MA, USA

Christopher R Shea MD
Professor of Medicine
Chief, Section of Dermatology
University of Chicago
Chicago, IL, USA

Neil H Shear MD FRCPC FACP
Helen and Paul Phelan Professor of
Dermatology
Department of Dermatology
University of Toronto
Toronto, ON, Canada

Bav Shergill MRCP
Dermatologist
Dermatology Department
The Royal Free Hospital
London, UK

Hiroshi Shimizu MD PhD
Professor and Chairman
Department of Dermatology
Hokkaido University Graduate School of
Medicine
Sapporo, Japan

Rodney Sinclair MBBS MD FACD
Director of Dermatology
Department of Dermatology
St Vincent's Hospital
Melbourne, VIC, Australia

Michael Sladden MBChB MAE MRCP
Dermatologist
Department of Dermatology
Leicester Royal Infirmary
Leicester, UK

Andrew G Smith MA MD FRCP
Consultant Dermatologist
Department of Dermatology
University Hospital of North Staffordshire
Stoke-on-Trent, UK

Christine Soon MRCP
Dermatologist
Department of Dermatology
Walsgrave Hospital
Coventry, UK

Nicholas A Soter MD
Professor of Dermatology
Ronald. O Perelman Department of
Dermatology
New York University Medical Center
New York, New York, USA

James M Spencer MD MS
Clinical Professor of Dermatology
Department of Dermatology
The Mount Sinai School of Medicine
New York, NY, USA

Richard L Spielvogel MD
Clinical Professor of Dermatology and
Pathology
Drexel University College of Medicine
Institute for Dermatopathology
Conshohocken, PA, USA

List of Contributors

Jennifer R Stalkup MD
Dermatologist
Department of Dermatology
The University of Texas Southwestern
Medical Center
Dallas, TX, USA

Richard C D Staughton MA BChir FRCP
Consultant Dermatologist
Daniel Turner Skin Clinic
Chelsea and Westminster Hospital
London, UK

Helger Stege MD
Senior Lecturer
Department of Dermatology
Heinrich-Heine University
Düsseldorf, Germany

Jane C Sterling MB BChir FRCP PhD
Clinical Lecturer and Honorary Consultant
Dermatologist
Department of Dermatology
Addenbrooke's Hospital
Cambridge, UK

Adam S Stibich MD
Fellow in Dermatology
Department of Dermatology
Stough Clinic
Hot Springs, AR, USA

Cord Sunderkötter MD
Associate Professor
Department of Dermatology
University of Ulm
Ulm, Germany

Anita Takwale MD MRCP
Dermatologist
Bristol Dermatology Center
United Bristol Healthcare NHS Trust
Bristol, UK

Carolina Talhari MD
Dermatologist
Department of Dermatology
Heinrich-Heine University
Düsseldorf, Germany

Eunice Tan MRCP
Research Fellow
Department of Dermatology
University Hospitals of Coventry and
Warwickshire NHS Trust
The George Eliot Hospital
Nuneaton, UK

Jianyou Tan MD PhD
Director of Anatomic Pathology
Chair of Dermatopathology
GenPath/Bio-Reference Laboratories
Elmwood Park, NJ, USA

**William Yuk Ming Tang FRCP(Edin)
FHKAM(Med)**
Dermatologist
Tuen Mun Social Hygiene Clinic
Tuen Mun, New Territories, Hong Kong

Mordechai M Tarlow MD
Dermatologist
Department of Dermatology
New Jersey Medical School
Newark, NJ, USA

Nicholas R Telfer FRCP
Consultant Dermatological and Mohs
Micrographic Surgeon
Department of Dermatology
Hope Hospital
Manchester, UK

Maryanna C Ter Poorten MD
Private Practice
Dermatology Group of the Carolinas
Concord, NC, USA

Keng-Ee Thai MBBS BMedSci
Dermatologist
Department of Dermatology
Prince of Wales Hospital
Sydney, NSW, Australia

Bruce H Thiers MD
Professor and Chairman
Department of Dermatology
Medical University of South Carolina
Charleston, SC, USA

Michelle A Thomson MRCP
Dermatologist
Department of Dermatology
Walsgrave Hospital
Coventry, UK

Anne-Marie Tobin MB BSc MRCPI
Dermatologist
Adelaide and Meath Hospital
Dublin, Ireland

Jackie M Tripp MD
Dermatologist
Division of Dermatology
University of British Columbia
Vancouver, BC, Canada

Yukiko Tsuji-Abe MD
Department of Dermatology
Hokkaido University Graduate School of
Medicine
Sapporo, Japan

William F G Tucker MB FRCP
Consultant Dermatologist
Department of Dermatology
Alexandra Hospital
Worcester Acute Hospitals Trust
Redditch, UK

Peter van de Kerkhof MD PhD
Professor and Chairman
Department of Dermatology
University Medical Centre Nijmegen
Nijmegen, The Netherlands

Abby S Van Voorhees MD
Assistant Professor
Department of Dermatology
University of Pennsylvania
Philadelphia, PA, USA

Carmela C Vittorio MD
The Sandra J Lazarus Associate Professor
of Dermatology
Department of Dermatology
University of Pennsylvania School of
Medicine
Philadelphia, PA, USA

Heidi A Waldorf MD
Assistant Clinical Professor
Department of Dermatology
Mount Sinai School of Medicine
New York, NY, USA

Fran Wallach MD
Associate Professor of Medicine
Mount Sinai Hospital
New York, NY, USA

Jon R Ward MD
Private Practice of Dermatology
Brentwood, TN, USA

Gabriele Weichert MD PhD
Dermatologist
Nanaimo, BC, Canada

Victoria P Werth MD
Professor of Dermatology
Department of Dermatology
University of Pennsylvania and
Philadelphia VA Medical Center
Philadelphia, PA, USA

James R Wharton MD
Dermatopathology Fellow
University of Texas Southwestern Medical
Center
Dallas, TX, USA

Lucile E White MD
Assistant Professor of Medicine
Department of Dermatology
Northwestern University
Chicago, IL, USA

Sean J Whittaker MD FRCP
Consultant Dermatologist
Skin Tumor Unit
St John's Institute of Dermatology
London, UK

Adam H Wiener DO
Physician
Somerset Skin Center
Troy, MI, USA

Jonathan K Wilkin MD
Director
Division of Dermatologic Drugs
FDA
Rockville, MD, USA

List of Contributors

Nathaniel K Wilkin MD
Associate Physician
Division of Dermatology
University of Tennessee Health Science
Center
Memphis, TN, USA

Sandra M Winhoven MRCP
Dermatologist
The Dermatology Centre
Hope Hospital
Manchester, UK

Karen Wiss MD
Associate Professor of Medicine
(Dermatology) and Pediatrics
Dermatology Division
UMass Memorial – Hahnemann Campus
Worcester, MA, USA

Joseph A Witkowski MD
Clinical Professor of Dermatology
University of Pennsylvania School of
Medicine
Philadelphia, PA, USA

Andrew L Wright MBChB FRCP
Consultant Dermatologist
Department of Dermatology
St Luke's Hospital
Bradford, UK

Victoria M Yates MBChB FRCP
Consultant Dermatologist
Department of Dermatology
Royal Bolton Hospital
Bolton, UK

Helen S Young MB ChB MRCP
Dermatologist
Department of Dermatology
Hope Hospital
Manchester, UK

**Irshad Zaki BMed Sci (Hons) BM BS
FRCP**
Consultant Dermatologist
Department of Dermatology
Solihull Hospital
Solihull, UK

Joshua A Zeichner MD
Fellow
Department of Dermatology
The Mount Sinai School of Medicine
New York, NY, USA

Deborah Zell MD
Senior Clinical Research Fellow
Department of Dermatology
University of Miami
Miami, FL, USA

John J Zone MD
Professor and Chair
Department of Dermatology
University of Utah Health Sciences Center
Salt Lake City, UT, USA

Evidence Levels

Each therapy covered has been assigned a letter from A (most evidence) to E (least evidence) signifying the amount of published evidence available to support its use. The following table shows the criteria used in making this classification.

A DOUBLE-BLIND STUDY
At least one prospective randomized, double-blind, controlled trial without major design flaws (in the author's view)

B CLINICAL TRIAL ≥20 SUBJECTS
Prospective clinical trials with 20 or more subjects; trials lacking adequate controls or another key facet of design, which would normally be considered desirable (in the author's opinion)

C CLINICAL TRIAL <20 SUBJECTS
Small trials with less than 20 subjects with significant design limitations, very large numbers of case reports (at least 20 cases in the literature), retrospective analyses of data

D SERIES ≥5 SUBJECTS
Series of patients reported to respond (at least 5 cases in the literature)

E ANECDOTAL CASE REPORTS
Individual case reports amounting to published experience of less than 5 cases

Preface

"Now what do I do?" The latter question confronts every dermatologist caring for patients with difficult-to-treat diseases, and with that question we launched the first edition of *Treatment of Skin Disease*. A PDA version and Portuguese edition quickly followed, and many dermatologists now turn to our book for their answers.

Why publish a second edition only four years after the first? Dramatic changes have occurred in dermatologic therapy. Biologics have changed the treatment of psoriasis and are used in many other diseases like sarcoid and graft versus host disease. Topical immunomodulators, newly introduced only a few years ago, successfully treat many off-label indications that weren't considered four years ago. The dermatologic literature and non-dermatologic literature contain volumes of information about new treatments and new off-label uses of old treatments.

Our second edition contains 23 entirely new chapters on disorders such as bioterrorism, that weren't current issues when the first edition was written, or conditions like capillaritis that simply weren't covered in the first edition. Chapters on a number of common disorders like drug eruptions and leg ulcers were suggested by readers. Rare disorders such as calciphylaxis, acute generalized exanthematous pustulosis, and livedoid vasculitis are also added because they are so therapeutically challenging. The addition of cosmetically important disorders like cellulite and striae highlights the growing importance of cosmetic aspects of dermatology to our specialty. We have included over 200 new photographs and there are updates and changes in nearly all of the book's chapters. In many cases the chapters have been completely rewritten.

We have retained the evidence-based ratings which are measured on a 5 point scale: A rating of *A* is the highest level of evidence and can be achieved by those drugs which have been studied in well-done, double-blind, placebo-controlled trials that are adequately powered. A rating of *B* is given to those drugs studied in clinical trials with 20 or more subjects but lacking some of the components of a perfect double-blind, randomized, placebo-controlled study. Those clinical trials with fewer than 20 subjects (or at least 20 published cases in the literature) are given an evidence-based rating of *C*. Treatments used in five to nineteen subjects in the literature are rated *D*, while fewer than five anecdotal case reports are given a score of *E*. The current text also retains the first line, second line and third line therapy model used in our first edition to enable busy clinicians to quickly look up treatments without having to search books or computers for hours.

As in our first edition, many of the studies reported are not double-blind, placebo-controlled trials, yet there has been substantial progress in achieving higher levels of evidence for many of the treatments offered to our patients. Unfortunately, many disorders in dermatology are sufficiently uncommon that they will never be studied in large double-blind, placebo-controlled trials. We can, nevertheless, glean substantial useful information from published anecdotes and small series, and we hope that the information presented in this edition will help physicians and, ultimately, patients around the world.

Mark G Lebwohl MD
Warren R Heymann MD
John Berth-Jones FRCP
Ian Coulson BSc MB FRCP
2005

Acknowledgments

The editors want to thank their families for devotion, support, and patience, and several of their children for computer assistance. We are also grateful to Sue Hodgson, Karen Bowler, Glenys Norquay, Shuet-Kei Cheung, and Joanne Scott of Elsevier, for their steadfast support and encouragement throughout the many months of writing and editing. Special thanks go to our assistants and secretaries, Marion Rodriguez and Victoria White, for their hard work and dedication. Thanks also to Abdul Hafejee, Walayat Hussain, Corinna Mendonca, and Emma Benton for their work on the PDA and formulary. We are grateful to the many authors who put their best efforts into this unique textbook. Most of all, we thank our patients, who we hope will be the ultimate beneficiaries of this book.

Dedication

Dedicated to our families:
Rebecca Berth-Jones
Susan, Christopher, and Chloe Coulson
Ronnie, Andrea, and Deborah Heymann
Madeleine, Andy, and Eve Lebwohl

Acanthosis nigricans

Mary L Curry, Jennifer R Stalkup,
Karen R Houpt, Ponciano D Cruz Jr

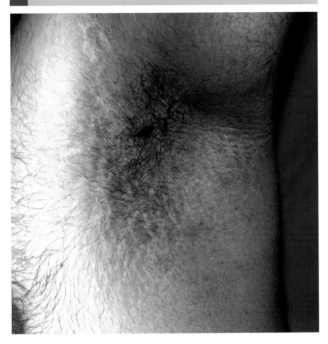

Acanthosis nigricans is characterized by hyperpigmented, verrucous or velvety plaques, which usually appear in flexural surfaces and intertriginous regions. It is most commonly seen in individuals with insulin resistance states, especially obesity, and less frequently in association with other metabolic disorders, drugs, and malignancy. Although hyperinsulinemia, hyperandrogenemia, and activating mutations in fibroblast growth factor receptor (especially for syndromes associated with skeletal dysplasia) have been implicated as causal factors, the precise pathogenesis is not yet known.

MANAGEMENT STRATEGY

Management of patients with acanthosis nigricans depends on the underlying cause, the identification of which requires a salient history, a targeted physical examination, and a finite set of laboratory tests.

Relevant historical information includes age of onset, presence or absence of a family history, medications, and presence or absence of symptoms related to hyperinsulinemia (with or without diabetes mellitus), hyperandrogenemia (with or without virilism) and internal malignancy (with or without weight loss).

Drugs reported in association with acanthosis nigricans include nicotinic acid, corticosteroids, estrogens, insulin, fusidic acid, protease inhibitors, and recombinant growth hormone.

Physical examination should document obesity, masculinization, lymphadenopathy, and organomegaly. Initial laboratory screening should include fasting blood glucose and insulin tested concurrently to confirm or exclude insulin resistance (insulin value inappropriately high for the glucose level).

Because obesity is the most common cause of both insulin resistance and acanthosis nigricans, it is reasonable to assume that it is the cause of acanthosis nigricans in obese patients with no historical and physical examination evidence of malignancy or of suspect drugs.

Rare causes of insulin resistance and acanthosis nigricans include the type A and B syndromes, the former characterized by defective insulin receptors and manifested typically in young girls with masculinized features, and the latter reported mostly in women with circulating anti-insulin receptor antibodies in association with autoimmune disorders such as lupus erythematosus. Other causes of insulin resistance and acanthosis nigricans are polycystic ovarian disease, HAIR-AN syndrome (hyperandrogenism, insulin resistance and acanthosis nigricans), familial lipodystrophies, and various endocrinopathies. If insulin resistance is present, then the possibility of malignancy becomes unlikely.

The most common malignancy associated with acanthosis nigricans is gastric adenocarcinoma. Less frequently reported are endocrine, genitourinary and lung carcinomas, and melanoma. Malignant acanthosis nigricans may coexist with other cutaneous markers of internal malignancy such as tripe palms, the sign of Leser-Trelat, florid cutaneous papillomatosis, and hyperkeratosis of the palms and soles (tylosis). If malignancy-associated acanthosis nigricans is suspected, the initial laboratory screen may include a complete blood count, stool test for occult blood, chest and gastrointestinal radiographs, as well as gastrointestinal endoscopy. Pelvic and rectal examinations, including pelvic ultrasonography, may be warranted in women and men depending on their age.

In the absence of objective evidence for a specific cause, the acanthosis nigricans may be labeled as idiopathic, which may or may not be familial. *Treatment of the underlying cause* often leads to resolution of the acanthosis nigricans. Otherwise, most published modes of treatment are *symptomatic* and/or *cosmetic*, and testimony to their efficacy has been anecdotal.

SPECIFIC INVESTIGATIONS

- Document obesity based on ideal body weight
- Determine fasting blood glucose and insulin levels in parallel
- Depending on historical clues, screen for other endocrine disease
- Consider malignancy; if suspected refer to appropriate specialist for the best diagnostic procedure
- Consider drugs as a cause

Prevalence and significance of acanthosis nigricans in an adult population. Hud J, Cohen J, Wagner J, Cruz P. Arch Dermatol 1992;128:941–4.

Up to 74% of obese adult patients seen at the Parkland Memorial Hospital Adult Obesity Clinic in Dallas, Texas had acanthosis nigricans. The skin disorder predicted the existence of hyperinsulinemia.

Prevalence of acanthosis nigricans in an unselected (pediatric) population. Stuart C, Pate C, Peters E. Am J Med 1989;87:269–72.

Among primary school children in Galveston, Texas with greater than 120% of ideal body weight 28% had acanthosis nigricans.

Acanthosis nigricans associated with insulin resistance: pathophysiology and management. Hermanns-Le T, Scheen A, Pierard G. Am J Clin Dermatol 2004:5:199–203.

An up-to-date review of the pathogenesis and treatment of acanthosis nigricans.

Genes, growth factors and acanthosis nigricans. Torleyu D, Bellus G, Munro C. Br J Dermatol 2002;147:1096–101.

Craniosynostosis and skeletal dysplasia syndromes with acanthosis nigricans are associated with activating mutations in fibroblast growth factor receptors, particularly FGFR3.

Characterization of groups of hyperandrogenic women with acanthosis nigricans, impaired glucose tolerance and/or hyperinsulinemia. Dunaif A, Gra M, Mandeli J, et al. J Clin Endocrinol Metab 1987;65:499–507.

Among obese women with polycystic ovaries 50% had acanthosis nigricans.

Malignant acanthosis nigricans: a review. Rigel D, Jacobe M. J Dermatol Surg Oncol 1980;6:923–7.

Gastric carcinoma was reported in 55% of 227 cases of acanthosis nigricans associated with an internal malignancy. Other intra-abdominal malignancies accounted for 18% of cases and the remaining 27% had extra-abdominal sites of malignancy.

Acanthosis nigricans: a new manifestation of insulin resistance in patients receiving treatment with protease inhibitors. Mellor-Pita S, Yebra-Bango M, Alfaro-Martinez J, Suarez E. Clin Infect Dis 2002;34:716–7.

A man with HIV infection developed insulin resistance, diabetes mellitus and acanthosis nigricans soon after starting treatment with protease inhibitors.

Acanthosis nigricans-like lesions from nicotinic acid. Tromovitch T, Jacobs P, Kern S. Arch Dermatol 1964;89:222–3.

A man treated with nicotinic acid (4 g/day) developed acanthosis nigricans, which cleared after discontinuance of the drug.

Somatotrophin-induced acanthosis nigricans. Downs A, Kennedy C. Br J Dermatol 1999;141:390–1.

A boy with achondroplasia treated long-term with recombinant growth hormone (3–4 units of subcutaneous somatotrophin weekly for 7 years) developed acanthosis nigricans in the groin and axilla.

FIRST LINE THERAPY

■ Treat the underlying cause	D

Acanthosis nigricans: a cutaneous marker of tissue resistant to insulin. Rendon M, Cruz P, Sontheimer R, Bergstresser P. J Am Acad Dermatol 1989;21:461–9.

In a woman with systemic lupus erythematosus and the type B syndrome of insulin resistance, the acanthosis nigricans cleared after treatment with oral corticosteroids and subcutaneous injection of insulin. Her circulating anti-insulin antibodies also disappeared with treatment of the autoimmune disease.

Clearance of acanthosis nigricans associated with the HAIR-AN syndrome after partial pancreatectomy: an 11-year follow up. Pfeifer SL, Wilson RM, Gawkrodger DJ. Postgrad Med J 1999;75:421–2.

An obese woman with HAIR-AN syndrome was diagnosed a year later with insulinoma. One year after resection of the tumor, the patient's virilism resolved, and 9 years after the surgery the acanthosis nigricans was much improved.

SECOND LINE THERAPY

■ Topical tretinoin and ammonium lactate	D
■ Oral metformin	E
■ Topical vitamin A	E
■ Topical tazarotene	E
■ Topical calcipotriol	E

Topical therapy with tretinoin and ammonium lactate for acanthosis nigricans associated with obesity. Blobstein SH. Cutis 2003;71:33–4.

Five obese patients with acanthosis nigricans were successfully treated with 12% ammonium lactate cream twice daily and tretinoin 0.05% cream nightly to one side of the neck (the other side serving as control).

There was no mention of whether the obese patients lost weight during the treatment period, which could have contributed to improvement.

Acanthosis nigricans and hypovitaminosis A. Response to topical vitamin A acid. Montes L, Hirschowitz B, Krumdieck C. J Cutan Pathol 1974;1:88–94.

A teenage girl had acanthosis nigricans, deafness, steatorrhea, peripheral sensory nerve demyelination, and hypovitaminosis A. The skin condition improved within 2 weeks of applying retinoic acid ointment (0.1% twice daily).

Successful symptomatic tazarotene treatment of juvenile acanthosis nigricans of the familial obesity-associated type in insulin resistance. Weisshaar E, Bonnekoh B, Franke I, Gollnick H. Hautarzt 2001;52:499–503. [Article in German]

A single report of a boy suffering from morbid obesity since infancy. In a right–left comparison the affected skin of one body side was treated with tazarotene 0.05% versus urea 10%, once daily each. A great benefit for the tazarotene-treated side over the opposite side was seen after 3 weeks.

Treatment of mixed-type acanthosis nigricans with topical calcipotriol. Bohm M, Luger T, Metze D. Br J Dermatol 1998;139:932–3.

An obese patient with metastatic transitional cell carcinoma of the bladder, insulin resistance and acanthosis nigricans was treated with topical calcipotriol (0.005% twice daily for 3 months), which led to improvement of her skin condition.

Evidence levels A Double-blind study **B** Clinical trial ≥ 20 subjects **C** Clinical trial < 20 subjects **D** Series ≥ 5 subjects **E** Anecdotal case reports

Therapeutic approach in insulin resistance with acanthosis nigricans. Tankova T, Koev D, Dakovska L, Kirilov G. Int J Clin Pract 2002;56:578–81.

Five obese patients (two children and three adults with diabetes mellitus) were treated with metformin daily for 6 months, resulting in significant reduction in plasma insulin, body weight, and body fat mass. Both children and one adult showed improvement of acanthosis nigricans.

THIRD LINE THERAPY

■ Oral isotretinoin	E
■ Oral ketoconazole	E
■ Palliative chemotherapy	E
■ Cyproheptadine	E
■ Dietary fish oil	E
■ Oral contraceptives	E
■ Dermabrasion	E
■ Long-pulsed alexandrite laser	E
■ Continuous wave carbon dioxide laser	E

Treatment of acanthosis nigricans with oral isotretinoin. Katz R. Arch Dermatol 1980;116:110–1.

An obese, hirsute, diabetic woman with acanthosis nigricans was treated with oral isotretinoin (2–3 mg/kg/day for 4 months), producing clearance of the skin problem. However, long-term treatment was required to maintain clearance because the acanthosis nigricans recurred when the retinoid was discontinued.

Because of the side-effects of isotretinoin, long-term use for a benign condition may not be practical.

Improvement of acanthosis nigricans on isotretinoin and metformin. Walling HW, Messingham M, Myers LM, et al. J Drugs Dermatol 2003;2:677–81.

An obese man developed acanthosis nigricans, tripe palms and laryngeal papillomatosis, with no evidence of malignancy after 6 years of follow-up. Isotretinoin (80 mg/day) led to improvement after 2 months of therapy. Addition of metformin produced added improvement.

Effect of ketoconazole in the hyperandrogenism, insulin resistance and acanthosis nigricans (HAIR-AN) syndrome. Tercedor J, Rodenas JM. J Am Acad Dermatol 1992;27:786.

Ketoconazole improved acanthosis nigricans in a patient with HAIR-AN syndrome.

Because of its hepatotoxic effects, oral ketoconazole, which has antiandrogenic effects is largely avoided now.

Malignant acanthosis nigricans: potential role of chemotherapy. Anderson SH, Hudson-Peacock M, Muller AF. Br J Dermatol 1999;141:714–6.

A man with metastatic gastric adenocarcinoma and disseminated acanthosis nigricans was treated with palliative chemotherapy, leading to significant improvement.

Treatment of acanthosis nigricans with cyproheptadine. Greenwood R, Tring F. Br J Dermatol 1982;106:697–8.

A man with gastric adenocarcinoma and acanthosis nigricans showed clearance of the skin disease following treatment with cyproheptadine (4 mg three times daily for 3 weeks).

Because the patient underwent palliative gastrectomy 4 months earlier, it is not clear whether removal of the adenocarcinoma or the cyproheptadine was responsible for clearing the acanthosis nigricans.

Acanthosis nigricans. Schwartz RA. J Am Acad Dermatol 1994;31:1.

A white woman with lipodystrophic diabetes mellitus and acanthosis nigricans was treated with dietary fish oil supplementation, leading to improvement of the skin condition despite continued elevation of triglyceride levels.

Remission of acanthosis nigricans associated with polycystic ovarian disease and stromal luteoma. Givens J, Kerber I, Wise W, et al. J Clin Endocrinol Metab 1974;38:347–55.

A girl with acanthosis nigricans and polycystic ovaries showed complete clearance of acanthosis nigricans and hyperandrogenism after treatment with OrthoNovum (2 mg/day).

Treatment of acanthosis nigricans of the axillae using a long-pulsed (5-msec) alexandrite laser. Rosenback A, Ram R. Dermatol Surg 2004;30:1158–60.

A woman with axillary acanthosis nigricans was treated with long-pulsed alexandrite laser (5 ms) on one axilla (with the other axilla as untreated control). The treated axilla showed significant improvement.

Continuous-wave carbon dioxide laser therapy of pseudoacanthosis nigricans. Bredlich R, Krahn G, Kunzi-Rapp K, et al. Br J Dermatol 1998;139:937–8.

An obese man with acanthosis nigricans who had failed previous treatments with topical retinoids and salicylic acid was then treated with continuous-wave carbon dioxide laser (three sessions at 4–6 week intervals). His acanthosis nigricans improved after 6 months of treatment.

Acne keloidalis nuchae

William Perkins

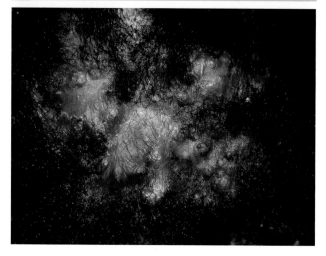

Acne keloidalis nuchae (AKN) is an idiopathic chronic inflammatory process affecting the nape of the neck and occipital scalp, occurring predominantly in black males. Initial features consist of papules and pustules on the occiput and posterior neck, which subsequently coalesce into plaques of dense scar tissue with central scarring alopecia. Although the etiology is unknown, the histology of early cases shows evidence of acute and chronic folliculitis with ruptured follicles, perifolliculitis, and a foreign body granulomatous response. Later cases may show similar features, but additionally there may be hypertrophic scar formation. Close shaving of the hair has been postulated as a cause for AKN, however during the 1960s and 1970s, with its fashion for longer hair, AKN was still seen. Physical trauma by collars rubbing and picking by patients have all been suggested as precipitants, but none of these has been investigated in any systematic way. Whether folliculitis leading to ruptured follicles and the subsequent foreign body reaction or the development of ingrowing hairs is the primary event, the term 'acne keloidalis' is a misnomer. Keloids at other sites or a family history of keloids are not features of AKN, and excision of the area does not result in keloid formation. Pseudofolliculitis barbae has been associated with AKN in five of six cases in one series, but clinical or histologic evidence of superficial hair penetration is lacking. Lesions resembling AKN have been reported in those receiving long-term cyclosporine, and sarcoid papules may occasionally mimic the condition.

MANAGEMENT STRATEGY

A clear diagnosis is a prerequisite for the management of AKN. The presence of inflammatory papules, pustules and hypertrophic scar formation on the occipital scalp and posterior neck in a black male is pathognomonic, but cases have been described in Caucasians, and occasionally in females. Biopsy of the area is not usually required, but concerns over keloidal scarring should not inhibit obtaining histologic con-

firmation. Folliculitis secondary to bacterial infections, particularly staphylococcal, needs to be excluded. In staphylococcal folliculitis the pustules and papules tend to be more widely distributed across the scalp, especially over the crown. Culture will yield heavy growths of staphylococci, and the condition usually responds well to treatment with *oral antibiotics*, but may recur and require long-term treatment.

In view of the suggested associations with close cropped hair and picking, it may be worthwhile enquiring about these factors. If present, these practices should be avoided.

Treatment depends upon the stage of presentation. Unfortunately the evidence base for many of the management recommendations is weak, but many patients will prefer no treatment or conservative treatment in the early stages of the disease. This is demonstrated by the fact that only 30% of patients identified in one survey had tried any treatment at all. Early disease with papules and pustules scattered across the posterior neck and occipital scalp may well be best managed by *topical antiseptics, antibiotics,* or *potent topical corticosteroids* topically.

With the development of hypertrophic scar formation, *topical or intralesional corticosteroids* may well be of benefit. Once scarring alopecia, hypertrophic scars and symptoms related to itch, pain and discharging sinuses are present, treatment directed at the removal of the follicles from the affected area in their entirety is to be recommended.

Excisional surgery is the only treatment reported in any significant case series. The factors influencing the use of excision will be the severity of symptoms the patient is experiencing and the confidence the patient and surgeon have in the process of surgery. Scattered papules and pustules across the occipital scalp without any confluent areas of hypertrophic scar formation and limited symptoms may lead patients to seek a more conservative treatment option.

The prioritization of the following treatments is not meant to be a strict hierarchy; for a well-developed case of AKN, the treatment of choice in the author's mind is excision. When this is not acceptable some of the following nonsurgical approaches may be appropriate. Advice to *reduce the picking* (a consistently reported association) *and close cropping* of the hair is the first measure one should employ. This may be aided by the anti-inflammatory effect of potent topical corticosteroids. In mild early cases treatment with topical antibiotic such as 1% *clindamycin* or *erythromycin* may be helpful. Oral antistaphylococcal antibiotics, such as *flucloxacillin* or *erythromycin* may be helpful, but this is not a recommendation supported by trial evidence. A very good response to flucloxacillin or erythromycin in the early stages when no scarring is present may suggest staphylococcal folliculitis rather than AKN. Long-term oral *tetracycline* antibiotics may be of help in some cases of early disease. Limited hypertrophic scars may respond to intralesional *triamcinolone*. *Isotretinoin* has been used with success.

SPECIFIC INVESTIGATIONS

- ■ Pustule swab
- ■ Deep biopsy

Investigations are not particularly helpful in AKN and even histology tends to be a byproduct of excisional treatment. If

Evidence levels A Double-blind study B Clinical trial ≥ 20 subjects C Clinical trial < 20 subjects D Series ≥ 5 subjects E Anecdotal case reports

the diagnosis is in doubt, a deep biopsy to below the level of the scar tissue and follicular bulbs will confirm the diagnosis. Folliculitis secondary to *Staphylococcus aureus* is worth excluding, largely based on clinical features such as the distribution and the lack of hypertrophic scar formation, but positive cultures from pustules may direct topical and systemic antibiotic therapy. Pustular lesions of AKN may well grow *S. aureus* but the response to treatment in the context of a simple bacterial folliculitis will be much greater than that seen in AKN.

FIRST LINE THERAPIES

■ Dissuade picking, close hair cutting	E
■ Topical clindamycin	E
■ Oral antistaphylococcal antibiotics – erythromycin or flucloxacillin	E
■ Oral tetracycline	E

Pseudofolliculitis barbae. Chu T. Practitioner 1989;233: 307–9.

In a limited open study, 1% topical clindamycin was found anecdotally effective for pseudofolliculitis and acne keloidalis.

Acne keloidalis is a form of scarring alopecia. Sperling LC, Homoky C, Pratt L, Sau P. Arch Dermatol 2000;136:479–84.

Medical treatment for early papular lesions includes intralesional injections of corticosteroids, topical steroids, and topical or oral antibiotics (usually tetracycline).

SECOND LINE THERAPIES

■ 13 *cis*-retinoic acid	E
■ Intralesional triamcinolone	E

Folliculitis nuchae scleroticans – successful treatment with 13-cis-retinoic acid (isotretinoin). Stieler W, Senff H, Janner M. Hautarzt 1988;39:739–42.

Oral therapy with 13-*cis*-retinoic acid (isotretinoin) in a 23-year-old white man resulted in remarkable improvement within a few weeks.

If antibiotic treatment fails, oral isotretinoin may be helpful in selected cases. Once hypertrophic scarring has developed, treatment with oral or topical antibiotics is less successful and measures to control the formation of hypertrophic scar need to be employed. Potent topical corticosteroid creams may help, but intralesional injections of corticosteroids such as triamcinolone can reduce the bulk of the scar tissue. Despite these injections the process tends to continue and the treatment will need to be repeated at intervals.

THIRD LINE THERAPIES

■ Excision to deep fat or fascia below follicles. Fusiform excision along posterior hairline where possible. Heal by second intention or primary closure as a staged procedure	C

The surgical management of extensive cases of acne keloidalis nuchae. Gloster HM. Arch Dermatol 2000;136:1376–9.

Of 25 young African-Caribbean men with extensive AKN who underwent surgical excision of AKN, 20 underwent excision with layered closure in one stage. Four patients underwent two-stage excisions with layered closure. One patient underwent excision with second-intention healing. All rated the cosmetic result of surgery as good to excellent. No patient experienced complete recurrence of acne keloidis; 15 patients developed tiny pustules and papules within the surgical scar; five patients developed hypertrophic scars, all of which were successfully treated with high-potency topical and intralesional corticosteroids. Extremely large lesions should be excised in multiple stages.

Anesthesia can be achieved simply with either 0.5 or 1% lidocaine plus epinephrine (adrenaline) 1:200 000 or even 0.1% with epinephrine 1:1 000 000. The advantage of the latter type of anesthesia is that it gives excellent longer term control of bleeding, which can be a problem with large scalp excisions. The use of electrosurgical excision can thus be avoided because this is associated with increased levels of pain postoperatively and an increased risk of wound dehiscence.

Acne vulgaris

Anthony Chu

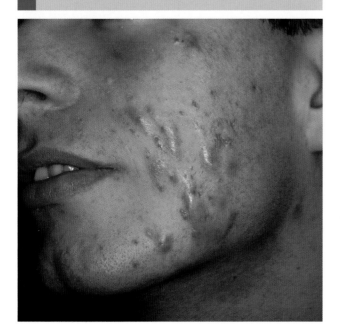

Acne is the commonest skin condition to affect man. It is a chronic inflammatory condition of the pilosebaceous follicle and thus can occur anywhere on the body, apart from the palms and soles, but most frequently affects the face, back, chest, neck and upper arms. The severity of acne differs from patient to patient and treatment must therefore be tailored to the individual patient, with the goal of preventing physical and/or psychological scarring.

MANAGEMENT STRATEGY

Acne represents a spectrum of disease severity from a couple of blackheads and a pustule to severe nodulocystic, fulminant acne. Management of acne will thus depend on the type of acne present, the clinical severity of the disease, the effects the acne has on the patient's quality of life and response to previous treatment. To understand the treatment of acne it is essential that the physician comprehends the pathophysiology of the disease.

With the onset of acne, the sebaceous gland increases its excretion rate, despite normal androgen levels in all men and most women. The composition of the sebum alters, with a reduction of linoleic acid. Sebum excretion is mainly driven by androgens. 30% of women with acne have a raised free testosterone, but this does not generally affect treatment.

The first morphological change to occur in the follicle is a growth change of keratinocytes within the follicular ostium resulting in follicular hypercornification and the development of the microcomedone, the primary lesion of both non-inflammatory and inflammatory acne. Follicular hypercornification may be the result of reduced sebum linoleic acid concentrations or may be immunologically mediated by interleukin 1. The microcomedone restricts sebum passage to the skin surface and eventually sebum solidifies to leave the waxy substance expressed when squeezing blackheads. As the microcomedone enlarges it becomes an open or closed comedone (blackhead or whitehead). With follicular occlusion, sebum pools in the follicle with proliferation of the anaerobic bacterium, *Propionibacterium acnes*, generating a T cell response, which results in inflammation. Recruitment of polymorphs into the follicle, mediated by the inflammatory process or release of *P. acnes* generated chemokines, leads to pus formation. The pus eventually bursts onto the surface with resolution of the inflammation, or into the dermis with deep inflammation resulting in nodule formation and possible scarring.

The most critical target for treatment is the microcomedone because without the follicular occlusion the whole cascade of acne is arrested. The major agents for this are the *topical retinoids*, and all patients with acne should be treated with one of these drugs. The newer topical retinoids – *isotretinoin* and *adapalene* – are the least irritating. Combination preparations containing 0.05% isotretinoin with 2% *erythromycin* or 0.025% *tretinoin* with 4% erythromycin are better tolerated because the antibiotic has anti-inflammatory properties. Some patients, particularly phototype V patients, are very sensitive to the irritant effects of the topical retinoids. In these patients, short contact using the preparation for 2–3 h at night may allow them to use the preparations. In patients who are intolerant to the retinoids, *topical salicylic acid* as a 2% wash or 20% *azelaic acid* are possible substitutes.

In patients with inflammatory lesions, antibiotics, either topical or systemic, are the mainstay of treatment. Topical antibiotics have the advantage of achieving high local concentrations of the drug in the skin while avoiding systemic side effects such as vaginal thrush and gastrointestinal upset. The advent of topical antibiotics, however, has been paralleled by a rapid increase in antibiotic resistance in *P. acnes* populations. Antibiotic resistance is highest to erythromycin, cross-reacting to *clindamycin*, but resistance is now growing to include systemic antibiotics such as the *tetracyclines* and *minocycline*. The clinical relevance of antibiotic drug resistance is still unknown, but recent studies suggest that it is of little relevance to the response rate in patients who have acne. Antibiotics have additional anti-inflammatory activity, which seems to be of importance in the response of acne to antibiotic treatment.

A worrying feature of antibiotic drug resistance, however, is the emergence of antibiotic-resistant *Staphylococcus epidermidis*. Antibiotic drug resistance can be transferred from these coagulase-negative staphylococci to *Staphylococcus aureus*, with increasing multiple drug resistance. Combination preparations containing antibiotic and benzoyl peroxide (*3% erythromycin and 5% benzoyl peroxide gel* and *1% clindamycin with 5% benzoyl peroxide gel*) prevent this drug resistance from developing, suggesting that these preparations should be used in preference to monotherapy with antibiotics. Benzoyl peroxide works by killing *P. acnes* by release of oxygen into the anaerobic follicular microenvironment. Bacteria cannot develop resistance to this mode of action. Benzoyl peroxide preparations should thus be seen as the first line treatment for mild to moderate acne. Benzoyl peroxide is a bleaching agent that can cause skin irritation, potentially limiting its use. In patients who cannot tolerate benzoyl peroxide, or who do not respond to it, a topical antibiotic should be tried. 3% erythromycin with 5% benzoyl peroxide or 1% clindamycin with 5% benzoyl peroxide are appropriate agents.

Evidence levels A Double-blind study   B Clinical trial ≥ 20 subjects   C Clinical trial < 20 subjects   D Series ≥ 5 subjects   E Anecdotal case reports

In patients who fail on topical antibiotics or who have moderate to severe acne, most physicians would use a *systemic antibiotic*. The most commonly used systemic antibiotics are *oxytetracycline* and *erythromycin*, but patient's compliance to these drugs may be poor. The half life of oxytetracycline is 8.5 h and that of erythromycin is 2.5 h. The absorption of tetracyclines is inhibited by fat or iron in the stomach, and absorption of erythromycin is inhibited by carbohydrates. Both antibiotics should thus be taken on an empty stomach, with no subsequent food intake for 1 h. Patient compliance is understandably low. *Lymecycline* is a relatively cheap new tetracycline with a long half life, so it can be taken once daily. Its absorption is not affected by food in the stomach. This drug should be seen as first line treatment, apart from for women who are trying to conceive, for whom erythromycin is the safest option. Other tetracyclines such as *minocycline* and *doxycycline*, as well as *trimethoprim*, are used as first line or second line therapies.

There is limited evidence to suggest whether topical antibiotic therapy combined with oral antibiotic therapy really does add any benefit to oral therapy alone, however, many physicians do use *combined therapy*. Suggestions that it is best to avoid dissimilar oral and topical antibiotics because this may encourage *P. acnes* resistance are not realistic because most topical antibiotics are erythromycin-based and most oral antibiotics are tetracycline-based.

In female patients who have severe or recalcitrant acne, or need control of their menstrual cycle, *ethinylestradiol* 35 μg and 2 mg *cyproterone acetate* , combined with topical therapy, is a useful choice. This drug is only successful as monotherapy in about 40% of women and has the problem of recurrence of acne when the drug is stopped, even if it has been used for a number of years. It is generally overutilized and should not be seen as an option for women who have mild acne and want the oral contraceptive. Oral *spironolactone* blocks 5-α-reductase and thus has antiandrogen effects. It can be used in older women at a dose of 100–200 mg a day, and may be valuable for patients with coexisting hirsutism and androgenic alopecia. It may produce menstrual irregularity and serum electrolytes will require monitoring, and it is essential that pregnancy be avoided during therapy to prevent feminization of a male fetus.

For severe acne, however defined, serious consideration should be given to prescribing *oral isotretinoin,* but *oral antibiotics in higher doses* may be worthy of a trial (i.e. minocycline 200 mg/day or trimethoprim 600 mg/day). In some patients, oral isotretinoin would be appropriate, and even necessary, as first line therapy. A risk–benefit evaluation should be conducted for each patient before starting oral isotretinoin. Patients must be informed of the potential side effects of the drug, including its teratogenic potential, and the possible induction of depression and psychosis. The new European directive means that all women of childbearing age should be pregnancy tested before oral isotretinoin is started. Prescriptions of not more than 4 weeks should be given, ensuring close monitoring. Due to the teratogenic nature of the drug, pregnancy should be avoided while the drug is taken, and for at least 1 month after the course has been completed. Oral contraception should be advised in all women of childbearing age.

Oral isotretinoin should be considered for severe acne, moderate acne that has failed to respond to at least two courses of different antibiotics with topical retinoids, significant scarring psychologically or physically, and Gram-negative folliculitis.

Patients must be counseled about the side effects of oral isotretinoin before the drug is started. They need to be informed that relapse can occur when the drug is stopped, although it may be delayed by months or years. Baseline blood tests should be conducted for fasting lipids, liver function tests, glucose level and hematology. Oral isotretinoin will increase blood sugar levels and there have been reports of blood dyscrasias occurring with the drug. Blood tests should be repeated, where indicated, every month while the patient is on the drug.

Oral isotretinoin should be started at a dose of 0.5 mg/kg/day for the first month and then increased to 1 mg/kg/day. The rationale for using a low dose to begin with is to limit the worsening of acne that is frequently seen when the drug is first started. In patients with highly inflammatory acne, a severe flare of acne may occur with the initiation of oral isotretinoin, and, in such patients, oral antibiotics (non-tetracyclines without the risk of benign intracranial hypertension, see page 8) should be given for 1 month, or oral *prednisolone* starting at 40 mg/day and tapering down quickly over 1 month.

Repeated courses of isotretinoin can be given. There does not seem to be any drug tolerance and side effects are usually similar in the same patient when the drug is represcribed. In some patients, relapse will occur, even with subsequent courses. Many physicians use lower doses of oral isotretinoin in mature adults who have had acne for 20 or 30 years and no longer desire further antibiotics. Low-dose oral isotretinoin can be given in variable regimens, such as 40 mg, 7 days out of 28, or 40 mg on Monday and Friday of each week. Such therapy may be given for up to 6 to 12 months, and repeat courses given, if necessary.

Mucocutaneous side effects of isotretinoin are well known and include cheilitis, facial dermatitis, dermatitis elsewhere, blepharoconjunctivitis, and nasal dryness, which can be associated with troublesome nosebleeds. Rare mucocutaneous side effects include discoid eczema, follicular eczema, fingertip eczema, sticky palms, curly hair, alopecia, paronychia and staphylococcal infection (more commonly if there is active dermatitis). Treatment of mucocutaneous side effects involves the liberal use of moisturizers, topical corticosteroids, and occasionally, dose reduction or cessation of the drug. Always suspect secondary infection with *S. aureus* if the dermatitis is extensive or significantly inflammatory. In these circumstances consider a topical antibiotic such as fusidic acid, oral flucloxacillin, or erythromycin 250 mg four times a day for 5–7 days.

Mood swings and depression are the most important though uncommon systemic side effects of isotretinoin. It is important to stress to patients and their families and partners the uncommon side effects of mood swings and depression, and the potential risk of suicide. This can be best achieved by providing patients with a personalized abbreviated summary of the data sheet, which is also provided by the manufacturers.

Diffuse interstitial skeletal hyperostosis (DISH) is a recognized, but very uncommon problem in patients receiving oral isotretinoin. Even in patients receiving several courses it is not usually a significant clinical problem. Routine radiographs of the appropriate joints, such as the lumbar/sacral spine and calcaneum, are not recommended unless there are related symptoms. Retinoid osteoporosis has been recently described, but further work is necessary before embarking on regular scans for patients taking oral isotretinoin.

Duration of therapy

The duration of therapy relates to the natural history of the patient's acne, and clearly in an individual patient it is impossible to predict. Acne trials rarely last longer than 4 months but a patient's acne may persist for years. Mild acne may last a few years, whereas more significant disease is likely to last longer, but again precise evidence is lacking. We inform our patients that they will need to use topical therapy for many years. In 7% of patients, acne may persist well into the fourth decade, though development of the disease after the age of 25 years is unusual.

Oral antibiotics should probably be prescribed for courses of 6–8 months, using high doses until the disease is under control and with gradual reduction of the dosage to avoid rebound. Dianette® can be prescribed for up to 4 years, but recurrence is frequently seen on withdrawal. Oral isotretinoin is usually given in courses of 4–6 months but the drug should be continued until the patient is clinically clear, which may take up to 9 months. Achieving a cumulative dose of at least 120 mg/kg reduces the risk of relapse. Even so, relapse rates of about 50% are usually seen from 6 weeks to 6 years after completion of the course. Repeat courses of all drugs can be prescribed as required.

It is important to give an expectation of response. There is usually little improvement in the first 4 weeks of therapy, and indeed the acne may flare on therapy introduction (e.g. if therapy is given prior to a premenstrual flare). To prevent disillusion, stress that acne is a slowly responding disorder, but at 2–3 months, 50% improvement is expected. It is important not to continue treatment if the regimen is not working. Patients should be regularly reviewed and treatment modified depending on clinical response.

Side effects

Physicians should be aware of the common and less common side effects of the drugs they frequently use. It is important to recognize the uncommon or rare side effects of drugs because these are often the more important ones.

Uncommon side effects include a fixed drug eruption with tetracyclines, and a maculopapular rash in 5% of patients receiving trimethoprim. Doxycycline induces a dose-dependent phototoxic eruption in 4% of patients, and rarely painful photo-onycholysis.

All tetracyclines and oral isotretinoin may cause benign intracranial hypertension with headache, dizziness, nausea, and visual disturbances. The symptoms usually stop within a few days of stopping therapy.

Minocycline pigmentation presents usually as gray-black discoloration, particularly in acne and other scars. It occasionally affects the mucosae and sclerae. It is dose and duration dependent. In younger patients the pigmentation usually clears in 18 months, but in older patients it takes longer. The Q-switched ruby laser may help to clear the pigmentation.

Minocycline may cause drug-induced lupus erythematosus (LE). Drug-induced lupus is dose and duration dependent. It usually presents with arthritis, hepatitis and an LE rash, not typically on the face. It may be prudent to check the autoantibodies, especially perinuclear antineutrophil cytoplasmic antibodies (pANCA) and liver function tests, approximately every 8 months in patients receiving regular minocycline.

The sudden onset of many pustules, particularly in the perioral and perinasal areas, should suggest Gram-negative folliculitis. A simple deterioration of ordinary acne occasionally may mimic Gram-negative folliculitis. Swabbing of the nares and skin for relevant organisms is necessary. Treatment includes stopping the current antibiotic therapy and prescribing trimethoprim 300 mg twice daily, or oral isotretinoin 0.5 mg/kg/day. Relapse is much greater with antibiotics (80% compared to about 20% with isotretinoin).

Resistance to *P. acnes* was unknown until 1975, but it has now been demonstrated with an incidence of 65% in many countries (US, UK, New Zealand, Japan, France, Germany). In 60% of such patients the resistance is to erythromycin and/or clindamycin. Mixed resistances are also frequent (35%) and for tetracycline and doxycycline the resistance is in the order of 20%. Resistance to minocycline is rare in most countries, except in the US where it is currently 20%. The precise clinical significance of microbiologically detected *P. acnes* resistance is unknown.

Light and laser treatment

The use of ultraviolet light in acne has now been shown to have no therapeutic benefit.

Blue light at 440 nm has been shown to target protoporphyrins present in *P. acnes*, leading to the release of oxygen and killing of the anaerobic bacteria. A high-intensity, narrow band (407–420 nm) blue light source has been shown to be effective in treating acne. The treatment is office based and used twice weekly, which can be problematic for patients. Clinical studies have demonstrated efficacy and improvements that lasted over a month after treatment was stopped. A commercially available home-use lamp producing blue light at 440 nm and red light at 660 nm has been shown to be an effective treatment for acne when used daily. Such treatment avoids medication that could cause side effects.

The NLite® laser, a pulsed dye laser at 585 nm with a very short pulse duration of 350 μs, when used at subpurpuric energy levels, has been shown to be an effective treatment for acne. A single treatment with the laser will give persistent improvement for up to 3 months. We have been using this laser as monotherapy or in combination with topical retinoids and/or oral antibiotics for the past 2 years with a success rate of about 80%.

Physical treatment of acne

Significant nodular acne producing the so-called 'cysts' can be a therapeutic challenge (the term 'cyst' is a misnomer because such lesions are not lined with epithelium – the term nodule is preferred). Some patients appreciate the use of a *topical corticosteroid* such as *clobetasol* cream twice daily for 5–7 days during the development of a nodule. Larger nodules can be aspirated with a wide bore needle and then instilled with *intralesional triamcinolone* 2.5 mg/mL; 0.1 mL is injected into the top of the lesion with the drainage being performed from the bottom. More persistent indolent nodules (i.e. older than 2–3 weeks) can be treated with *cryotherapy*, two cycles each of 20 s. The aim of such treatment is to trigger off a local inflammatory response to help break down the fibrosing wall that develops around the inflammation.

Evidence levels A Double-blind study B Clinical trial ≥ 20 subjects C Clinical trial < 20 subjects D Series ≥ 5 subjects E Anecdotal case reports

The simple removal of blackheads with a *comedone extractor* must not be forgotten, especially in those patients with multiple blackheads.

Some whiteheads can be particularly large, and these so-called microcysts or macrocomedones can be a cosmetic problem and can flare into significant, potentially scarring, inflamed lesions, particularly in patients receiving oral isotretinoin. These are best treated using very gentle *cautery* after the application of a topical anesthetic such as a lidocaine–prilocaine mixture. It is best to treat a small number of lesions first, and treat the remaining lesions on two or three subsequent visits. Scarring and pigmentation is unusual from this technique. Such treatment for these macrocomedones is far superior to topical retinoids.

Scars

We now have adequate treatments to prevent scarring, but sadly we still have many patients scarred from acne. It is beyond the scope of this chapter to discuss in detail the treatment of acne scarring, however, keloids and hypertrophic scars can be treated with *intralesional triamcinolone*, *cryotherapy*, *topical corticosteroids* and *silicone sheeting* (see Keloids, page 314).

Atrophic scars, such as icepick scars and atrophic macular scars, can be treated by laser resurfacing using *carbon dioxide* or *erbium:YAG lasers*. Laser subsurfacing using nonablative pulsed dye laser or intense pulsed light has gained considerable support because these techniques can be used in skin phototypes V and VI without causing pigmentary changes. Such facilities are not available in all countries. Laser therapy is expensive and should be performed by well-trained physicians. Complications are not uncommon, but some patients do benefit from the procedure. Other surgical procedures such as *excision of scars, augmentation of scars with fat* or *collagen, chemical peels, subcision and the injection of autologous fibroblasts (Isolagen®)* are among therapeutic options.

SPECIFIC INVESTIGATIONS

- Acne grade and assessment of disability
- Sex hormones – when an abnormality is suspected (i.e. poor response, very irregular periods, significant hirsutism and female pattern alopecia) check levels of testosterone, sex hormone binding globulin (SHBG), prolactin, follicular hormone/lutein stimulating hormone (FH/LSH), and dehydroepiandrosterone; a scan of the ovaries may also be necessary
- In poorly responding male and female patients check 9.00 a.m levels of cortisol and 17-α-hydroxyprogesterone to exclude late-onset congenital adrenal hyperplasia
- Skin and nasal swabs to exclude Gram-negative folliculitis
- Pre oral isotretinoin tests – pregnancy test; liver function tests, fasting lipids, glucose, full blood count
- Minocycline monitoring – antinuclear antibodies (ANA), DNA binding, pANCA, and liver function tests at 6–8 months

The Leeds Revised Acne Grading System. O'Brien S, Lewis J, Cunliffe WJ. J Derm Treat 1998;9:215–20.

An easy to use comparative photographic severity scoring system.

Practical use of a disability index in the routine management of acne. Motley RJ, Finlay AY. Clin Exp Dermatol 1992;17:1–3.

A brief questionnaire that highlights disability caused by acne.

FIRST LINE THERAPIES

■ Topical benzoyl peroxide	A
■ Topical azelaic acid	A
■ Topical antibiotics	A
■ Topical retinoids	A
■ Oral antibiotics – lymecycline, oxytetracycline	A

Local treatment of acne. A double blind study and evaluation of the effect of different concentrations of benzoyl peroxide gel. Lassus A. Curr Med Res Opin 1987;1:370–3.

There appears to be little difference in response between 2.5 and 10% benzoyl peroxide.

Benzoyl peroxide versus topical erythromycin in the treatment of acne vulgaris. Burke B, Eady EA, Cunliffe WJ. Br J Dermatol 1983;108:199–204.

1.5% (w/v) erythromycin lotion was as effective as 5% (w/v) benzoyl peroxide gel in significantly reducing the number of small inflamed lesions and the overall acne severity. However, benzoyl peroxide also significantly reduced the number of noninflamed lesions whereas erythromycin had no effect on these.

Topical azelaic acid and the treatment of acne: a clinical and laboratory comparison with oral tetracycline. Bladon PT, Burke BM, Cunliffe WJ, et al. Br J Dermatol 1986;114: 493–9.

Topical azelaic acid and oral tetracycline were compared in a 6-month double-blind study for treatment of acne vulgaris in 45 male subjects with clinical acne. Both treatments were of benefit and produced only a few minor side effects. Although oral tetracycline was more effective than azelaic acid, the differences were only just significant.

Efficacy of topical isotretinoin 0.05% gel in acne vulgaris: results of a multicenter, double-blind investigation. Chalker DK, Lesher JL, Smith JG, et al. J Am Acad Dermatol 1987;17:251–4.

Of 268 patients using the gel twice a day, only two dropped out due to irritation. Isotretinoin fared significantly better at 12 weeks than vehicle for inflammatory and non-inflammatory lesions.

Efficacy and safety of CD 271 alcoholic gels in the topical treatment of acne vulgaris. Verschoore M, Langner A, Wolska H, et al. Br J Dermatol 1991;124:368–71.

0.1% CD 271 gel (adapalene) was as effective as 0.025% tretinoin gel in reducing total comedone counts (83% reduction for both products after 12 weeks' treatment), but the number of inflammatory lesions and the total number of acne lesions were significantly greater with 0.1% CD 271 gel than with tretinoin gel. Seventy-two male patients participated in this double-blind trial.

A comparison of the efficacy and safety of adapalene gel 0.1% and tretinoin gel 0.025% in the treatment of acne vulgaris: a multicenter trial. Shalita A, Weiss JS, Chalker DK, et al. J Am Acad Dermatol 1996;34:482–5.

Adapalene gel 0.1% applied once daily was significantly more effective in reducing acne lesions and was better tolerated than tretinoin gel 0.025% in the treatment of acne vulgaris.

Evaluation of a therapeutic strategy for the treatment of acne vulgaris with conventional therapy. Greenwood R, Burke B, Cunliffe WJ. Br J Dermatol 1986;114:353–8.

A large study demonstrating the improved response and reduced relapse rate of erythromycin or tetracycline 1 g a day compared to 0.5 g/day dosage.

Lymecycline in the treatment of acne: an efficacious, safe and cost-effective alternative to minocycline. Bossuyt L, Bosschaert J, Richert B, et al. Eur J Dermatol 2003;13:130–5.

Multicenter, randomized, investigator-masked, parallel group study in 136 patients, comparing the efficacy, safety and cost-effectiveness of lymecycline with minocycline. Lymecycline was found to be as effective, but four times more cost-effective than minocycline.

SECOND LINE THERAPIES

■ Oral antibiotics – minocycline, doxycycline, trimethoprim	B
■ Combined antiandrogen estrogen oral contraceptive	A
■ Spironolactone	B
■ Red and blue light	B
■ Subpurpuric pulsed dye laser	B

Doxycycline versus minocycline in the treatment of acne vulgaris: a double-blind study. Olafsson JH, Gudgeirsson J, Eggertsdottir GE, Kristjansson F. J Dermatol Treat 1989; 1:15–17.

This study demonstrated no significant difference between doxycycline and minocycline.

Minocycline for acne vulgaris: efficacy and safety. Garner SE, Eady EA, Popescu C, et al. Cochrane Database Syst Rev 2003 (1):CD002086.

This report demonstrates that minocycline is an effective treatment for acne but only two studies showed that it was superior to other tetracyclines. The authors concluded that there was no good evidence to justify its use as first line treatment, particularly given the price differential and possible side effects. It remains a good second line treatment for acne.

Oral trimethoprim as a third-line antibiotic in the management of acne vulgaris. Bottomley WW, Cunliffe WJ. Dermatology 1993;187:193–6.

An open retrospective study of the efficacy of trimethoprim in the treatment of patients whose acne vulgaris failed to respond to at least two courses of first or second line antibiotics – 56 patients received trimethoprim in a dosage of 300 mg twice daily for at least 4 months, unless it had been withdrawn due to side effects. Topically they were given 1% clindamycin lotion twice daily to the affected areas. At 4 months there were significant improvements from the grades at initiation of facial, chest and back acne. Twenty-one patients remained on the treatment for 8 months, and a significant improvement in the changes of the acne grades remained. Two patients had the trimethoprim stopped due to side effects.

The role of oral minocycline and erythromycin in tetracycline therapy-resistant acne – a retrospective study and a review. Knaggs HE, Layton AM, Cunliffe WJ. J Dermatol Treat 1993;4:53–6.

The failing of this paper is that it was retrospective; nevertheless the data clearly showed a benefit for minocycline in tetracycline-resistant acne. Although erythromycin showed some benefit, minocycline was superior in its efficacy.

Anti-androgen treatment in women with acne; a controlled trial. Miller JA, Wojnarowska FT, Dowd PM, Ashton RE, et al. Br J Dermatol 1986;114:705–16.

Ninety female patients with acne were allocated randomly to one of three groups and treated either with Diane® (2 mg cyproterone and 50 µg estrogen), a high-dose cyproterone acetate (CPA 50 mg) regimen with ethinylestradiol, or Minovlar®. The same dose of estrogen was common to all three treatment groups. The results showed a clinical improvement in all three treatment groups, but a more rapid and complete response was seen in those groups who received CPA. There was also a consistent trend suggesting a more favorable response in those in the high-dose CPA group.

Acne: double-blind clinical and laboratory trial of tetracycline, oestrogen, cyproterone acetate and combined treatment. Greenwood R, Brummitt L, Burke B, Cunliffe WJ. Br Med J 1985;291:1231–5.

Double-blind studies of 62 patients with moderate or moderately severe acne for 6 months comparing tetracycline alone, estrogen–cyproterone acetate alone (as Diane®), and a combination of these agents. At 6 months the acne had improved by 68% in the antibiotic treated group and by 74% in the estrogen–cyproterone treated group. The group given a combination of both agents improved by 82%, which was significantly better than the improvement in the tetracycline treated patients, but no significant difference was found between the groups given estrogen–cyproterone alone and the combined treatment.

Oral spironolactone therapy for female patients with acne, hirsutism or androgenic alopecia. Burke BM, Cunliffe WJ. Br J Dermatol 1985;112:124–5.

For the hirsute woman with acne, spironolactone 100–200 mg daily is a possible approach. Ten of 12 patients who were unresponsive to antibiotics and benzoyl peroxide had a gratifying response. The authors suggest avoiding in patients under 30 years of age; pregnancy must be avoided.

Phototherapy with blue (415nm) and red (660nm) light in the treatment of acne vulgaris. Papageorgiuo P, Katsambas A, Chu A. Br J Dermatol 2000;142:973–8.

Randomized, controlled, single-blind study of red and blue light, blue light, white light and 5% benzoyl peroxide in 140 patients, demonstrating the superiority of red and blue light over white light and 5% benzoyl peroxide in treating acne.

A good home treatment that can avoid medications and the side effects associated with them.

Pulsed-dye laser treatment for inflammatory acne vulgaris: randomised controlled trial. Seaton ED, Charikida A, Mouser P, et al. Lancet 2003;362:1347–52.

Double-blind, placebo-controlled study in 41 patients. Actively treated patients showed significant improvement of inflammatory acne and acne grading which lasted up to 3 months following a single treatment with the NLite laser. Subsequent experience with the NLite has shown about 80% success in improving acne with the laser as monotherapy or in addition to conventional therapy.

THIRD LINE THERAPIES

■ High dose systemic antibiotics	B
■ Systemic isotretinoin	A

Isotretinoin therapy for acne: results of a multicenter dose-response study. Strauss JA, Rapini RP, Shalita AR, et al. J Am Acad Dermatol 1984;10:490–6.

One hundred and fifty patients with treatment-resistant nodulocystic acne were entered into a double-blind clinical study. Three different dosing levels (0.1, 0.5, 1.0 mg/kg/day) were used in equal sized groups. There was a highly significant clinical response to treatment with all three dosages of isotretinoin, but relapses were more frequent at the lower dose.

Roaccutane treatment guidelines: results of an international survey. Cunliffe WJ, Van de Kerkhof P, Caputo R, et al. Dermatology 1997;194:351–7.

Oral isotretinoin should be prescribed not only to patients with severe disease, but also to patients with less severe acne, especially if there is scarring and significant psychological stress associated with the disease. Patients with acne should, where appropriate, be prescribed isotretinoin sooner rather than later. Treatment is usually initiated at daily doses of 0.5 mg/kg (but may be higher) and is increased to 1.0 mg/kg. Most of the physicians aimed to achieve a cumulative dose of over 100–120 mg/kg. Mucocutaneous side effects occur frequently, but are manageable, while severe systemic side-effects are rarely problematic (2%).

Treatment of adult acne with low dose intermittent isotretinoin. Goulden V, Clark SM, McGeown C, Cunliffe WJ. Br J Dermatol 1998;137:106–8.

Eighty adults over 25 years of age received isotretinoin 0.5 mg/kg per day for 1 week in every 4 weeks for a total period of 6 months. Seventy-five patients completed the study. Side effects were minimal. The acne had resolved in 68 (85%) patients. Twelve months after treatment, acne grades and inflamed lesion counts remained significantly improved in the responders, but 29 (39%) patients had relapsed (particularly those with truncal acne). Patients who relapsed also had a significantly higher total acne grade, lesion count, and sebum excretion rate. The authors suggest this regimen for predominantly facial acne, total acne grade less than 1, inflamed lesion count less than 20, and sebum excretion rate less than 1.25 $\mu g/cm^2/min$.

Isotretinoin use and risk of depression, psychotic symptoms, suicide, and attempted suicide. Jick SS, Kremers HM, Vasilakis-Scaramozza C. Arch Dermatol 2000;136:1231–6.

A large study comparing psychological symptoms in acne sufferers taking antibiotics compared to those receiving isotretinoin, and also a smaller number of patients before and during isotretinoin. They found no increase in psychological morbidity with isotretinoin.

Depression and suicide in patients treated with isotretinoin. Wysowski D, Pitts D, Beitz J. N Engl J Med 2001;344:460.

A review from the FDA of 37 patients who committed suicide, 24 of them while using isotretinoin and 13 after ceasing to use it during an 18-year period in the US. A history of psychiatric illness was reported for 8 of the 37 patients. It also reports on 110 US patients who had been hospitalized for depression, suicidal ideation, or suicide attempts while using isotretinoin (85 patients) or after stopping its use (25 patients). A history of psychiatric illness was reported for 48. In many patients, there was improvement after discontinuation of the drug and psychiatric treatment, but others had persistent depression after the drug was discontinued. Four patients were rechallenged with isotretinoin; symptoms developed again in one, and the other three were able to continue using the drug at a reduced dose while abstaining from alcohol, or while continuing to take an antidepressant. There were an additional 284 reports of patients with depression who were not hospitalized, of whom 149 (52%) had accompanying physical side effects. Of these patients, 24 were rechallenged with isotretinoin, with return of depression. The number of suicides reported among users of isotretinoin does not exceed the number that would be predicted on the basis of the suicide rate in the US and the estimated number of patients exposed to the drug.

PHYSICAL AND SCAR THERAPY

■ Comedone cautery	C
■ Cryotherapy and intralesional corticosteroids to keloids	C
■ Laser resurfacing	B
■ Chemical peels	B

Treatment of closed comedones – comparison of fulguration with topical tretinoin and electrocautery. Bottomley WW, Knaggs H, Cunliffe WJ. Dermatology 1993;186:253–7.

Fulguration was superior to topical retinoids, but electrocautery was better than fulguration for macrocomedones.

Ablation of whiteheads by cautery under topical anaesthetic. Peppall L, Cosgrove M, Cunliffe WJ. Br J Dermatol 1991;125:256–9.

A description of the technique for dealing with macrocomedones. Their ablation prior to isotretinoin may prevent some of the retinoid-induced flares.

A comparison of intralesional triamcinolone and cryosurgery in the treatment of acne keloids. Layton AM, Yip J, Cunliffe WJ. Br J Dermatol 1994;130:498–501.

A double-blind study in which intralesional triamcinolone or cryosurgery was used as treatment for keloids. Treatment with intralesional triamcinolone was beneficial, but the response to cryosurgery was significantly better in early vascular lesions.

Postacne scarring: a review of its pathophysiology and treatment. Goodman GJ. Dermatol Surg 2000;26:857–71.

A description of therapies available, including newer resurfacing tools such as the resurfacing CO_2 and infrared lasers, dermasanding, and others in their infancy such as nonablative resurfacing and radiofrequency methods. *Multiple methods are often required to ensure the best results.*

Chemical peeling: how, when, why? Ghersetich I, Teofoll P, Gantcheva M, et al. J Eur Acad Dermatol Venereol 1997;8:1–11.

A review of the indications for and execution of peels.

Acrodermatitis enteropathica

Kenneth H Neldner

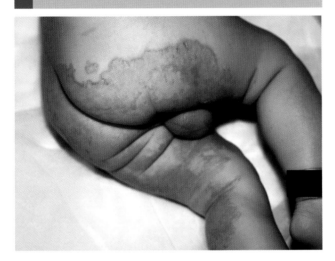

Acrodermatitis enteropathica (AE) is an autosomal dominant hereditary disorder of zinc absorption, characterized by severe dermatitis in the acral areas (face, anogenital area, feet and hands). Additional symptoms include diarrhea and irritability in infants. Growth retardation and gonadal underdevelopment occur in older children. Most cases begin in bottle-fed infants because zinc is very poorly absorbed from cow's milk compared with human breast milk.

MANAGEMENT STRATEGY

Chronic dermatitis in an acral area should always raise the possibility of zinc deficiency. As soon as the diagnosis of zinc deficiency is suspected and confirmed, the management becomes simple. *Dietary supplementation with oral zinc* produces rapid and dramatic resolution of all areas, including mental status. Dermatitis clears rapidly without the need for antibiotics. A major remaining problem is to rule out other non-hereditary causes for zinc deficiency.

The potential life-long need for zinc supplementation and medical supervision must be discussed. Discuss foods rich in zinc, such as seafood and meat. With age and more varied diet, the dose of daily zinc supplementation will decrease. Cereal grains should be avoided because of their phytate content. Phytates are known chelators of zinc.

Genetic counseling is required. Create a family tree to detect relatives who might have had AE during childhood but managed to survive with varying degrees of disability and may need supplemental zinc. It may also be possible to predict future family members as candidates for having children with AE.

SPECIFIC INVESTIGATIONS

- Blood zinc levels
- Urinary zinc
- Serum copper levels
- Genetic studies

The normal plasma zinc level is 70–110 µg/dL and serum is 80–120 µg/dL. Zinc contamination during blood drawing and laboratory testing is common. For example, rubber stoppers contain zinc. Anticoagulants and laboratory solutions may not be zinc-free. Reported results may therefore be somewhat higher than the true values. Urinary zinc can be measured but is unreliable for diagnosis or follow-up. Routine laboratory studies should include serum copper levels, which can be depressed by hypozincemia.

Homozygosity mapping places the acrodermatitis enteropathica gene on chromosomal region 8q24.3. Wang K, Pugh EW, Griffen S, et al. Am J Hum Genet 2001;68:1055–60.

The genetic locus for AE is known. Genetic studies can therefore be done if desired.

Transient symptomatic zinc deficiency in a full-term, breast-fed infant. Lee MG, Hong KT, Kim JJ. J Am Acad Dermatol 1990;23:375–9.

Maternal breast milk zinc may be low in the absence of hereditary AE and create a clinical situation resembling hereditary AE.

Acrodermatitis enteropathica and other zinc deficiency disorders. Neldner KH. In: Freedberg IM, Eisen AZ, Wolff K, et al, eds. Fitzpatrick's Dermatology in General Medicine, 6th edn. New York: McGraw-Hill; 2003:412–8.

There is a long list of chronic disorders with nutrient deficiencies that can result in signs of marginal zinc deficiency which are seldom recognized as being related to zinc.

FIRST LINE THERAPIES

■ Oral zinc supplementation	C

The normal recommended daily allowance (RDA) for zinc is 15 mg daily. In AE, the starting dose should be ~50 mg daily until all signs and symptoms clear. Dosage is then determined by follow-up blood zinc values. Available zinc preparations include zinc sulfate, zinc acetate, zinc gluconate, zinc propionate, and amino acid chelates of zinc. It is important to know the amount of elemental zinc in each preparation used. For example, one commercial preparation (Zincate® 220 mg) has a formula of $ZnSO_4 \cdot 7H_2O$ but has 55 mg of elemental zinc per tablet. If other commercial preparations are used, it is important to know the amount of elemental zinc in a tablet in order to determine the correct daily dose.

Zinc therapy of acrodermatitis enteropathica. Neldner KH, Hambridge KM. N Engl J Med 1975;292:879–81.

Actinic keratoses

Alvin H Chong, Rodney Sinclair

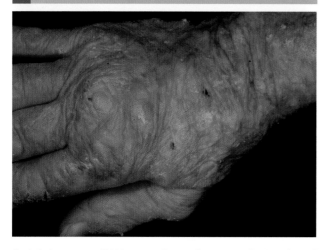

Actinic keratoses (AKs) are scaly, erythematous lesions found on sun-damaged skin on pale-skinned individuals and are often associated with signs of UV damage including solar elastosis and pigmentary change. The prevalence rate varies from 11–25% in the Northern hemisphere to 60% in Australians. Although many of these lesions may spontaneously regress, a small proportion may progress to squamous cell carcinoma (SCC).

MANAGEMENT STRATEGY

Actinic keratoses show keratinocyte atypia histologically. Although up to 70% of SCCs demonstrate adjacent AKs, the actual transformation rate is unknown. Reports vary from 25% to 1/1000 per year. The principle rationale for the treatment of AKs is to prevent the development of SCCs, however, there are no randomized controlled studies demonstrating that treatment of AKs reduces the frequency of SCCs. Nevertheless, where there is an increased risk of metastasis from SCCs it seems prudent to treat AKs. This would apply to patients with drug-induced immunosuppression, such as solid organ transplant recipients, and to AKs on high-risk sites such as the lip and ear. Signs of transformation into SCCs include thickening, rapid growth, hyperkeratosis, bleeding and tenderness. It is important to biopsy suspicious lesions to exclude malignancy. The other treatment indications are for cosmesis and symptomatic relief because AKs can be itchy or painful.

Fundamental to the management of AKs is *sun avoidance* and the use of *high sun protection factor (SPF) sunscreens*. These measures prevent the formation of new AKs and increase the likelihood of remission of existing lesions. For patients with few AKs, *liquid nitrogen cryotherapy* is the most frequently used treatment option because it is cheap, effective and convenient. Patients with 'field-change' and multiple AKs may benefit from the use of topical *5-fluorouracil (5-FU)*. The consequent skin irritation and inflammation needs to be explained when this method is used to treat AKs. *Topical imiquimod* has been shown to be effective as topical therapy and a number of different regimens have been described. Photodynamic therapy with *aminolevulinic acid* is also helpful for the management of multiple AKs, but its use

may be limited by availability. *Salicylic acid* may reduce associated hyperkeratosis, while *topical retinoids* may be helpful for early lesions and in patients with coexistent photodamage. *Laser resurfacing*, *chemical peels* and *dermabrasion* are techniques that may be considered where extensive coexistent photodamage is present or for lesions less likely to respond to topical 5-FU, for example, on the dorsum of the hands. For lesions that are hyperkeratotic or recalcitrant, *excision* or *curettage* may be appropriate.

SPECIFIC INVESTIGATIONS

■ Biopsy	

Actinic keratoses are usually diagnosed clinically. However, tender, hyperkeratotic and recalcitrant lesions should be biopsied to exclude malignancy.

High rate of malignant transformation in hyperkeratotic actinic keratoses. Suchniak JM, Baer S, Goldberg LH. J Am Acad Dermatol 1997;37:392–4.

Fifty hyperkeratotic AKs measuring at least 1 cm on the upper limbs of 42 white patients were biopsied. Eighteen lesions (36%) demonstrated invasive SCC. Due to the high incidence of SCC in these lesions, skin biopsy is recommended for hyperkeratotic AKs.

FIRST LINE THERAPIES

■ Sunscreens	A
■ Cryosurgery	B
■ Topical 5-FU	A

Reduction of solar keratoses by regular sunscreen use. Thompson SC, Jolley D, Marks R. N Engl J Med 1993;14:1147–51.

In a 6-month randomized, placebo-controlled trial of 588 patients in Australia, SPF 17 sunscreen applied daily was found to both reduce the development of new AKs and increase the remission of pre-existing AKs when compared to a vehicle cream.

High sun protection factor sunscreens in the suppression of actinic neoplasia. Naylor MF, Boyd A, Smith DW, et al. Arch Dermatol 1995;131:170–5.

In a 2-year randomized, placebo-controlled trial of 53 patients in North America, SPF 29 sunscreen applied daily was found to reduce the development of new AKs compared to a vehicle cream.

A prospective study of the use of cryosurgery for the treatment of actinic keratoses. Thai K, Fergin P, Freeman M, et al. Int J Dermatol 2004;43:687–92.

In this prospective multi-center study, 90 patients with 421 AKs on the face and scalp were treated with cryotherapy with a single freeze–thaw cycle with different freeze times. The patients were reviewed 3 months later. Overall, the complete response (CR) rate was 67.2%, varying from 39% for freeze times less than 5 s to 83% for freeze times longer than 20 s. The authors also found that hypopigmentation was present in 29% of CR lesions. Patients rated

Evidence levels A Double-blind study B Clinical trial ≥ 20 subjects C Clinical trial < 20 subjects D Series ≥ 5 subjects E Anecdotal case reports

cosmetic outcomes as good to excellent for 94% of CR lesions.

Effect of a 1 week treatment with 0.5% topical fluorouracil on occurrence of actinic keratosis after cryosurgery. Jorizzo J, Weiss J, Furst K, et al. Arch Dermatol 2004; 140:813–6.

This study demonstrates that there is a role for the combination of therapeutic modalities in the treatment of AKs. In this prospective, double-blind, randomized controlled trial, 144 patients, each with at least five AKs on the face, were randomized to receive 1 week of treatment with 0.5% 5-FU cream daily for 7 days or placebo cream. Patients were then treated with single freeze–thaw cycle cryotherapy using liquid nitrogen, with a thaw time of 10 s. These patients were then followed up at 4 weeks and 6 months. The authors found that at 4 weeks, 16.7% of patients in the 5-FU group were completely clear of lesions compared with 0% in the vehicle group (p<0.001). At 6 months post-treatment, 30% of patients in the 5-FU group were clear of lesions compared to 7.7% of patients in the vehicle group (p<0.001).

Effective treatment of actinic keratosis with 0.5% fluorouracil cream for 1, 2 or 4 weeks. Weiss J, Menter A, Hevia O, et al. Cutis 2002;70:22–29.

In this randomized, double-blind, parallel group, vehicle-controlled study, 177 patients with at least five AKs were treated with topical 0.5% 5-fluorouracil cream daily for 1, 2 or 4 weeks. In patients who were treated for 4 weeks, complete clearance of lesions was observed in 47.5% of patients (p<0.001 vs vehicle). Moderate-to-severe irritation of the skin was noted in 90% of these patients. This was compared to complete clearance in 26.3% of patients who were treated for 1 week.

Does intermittent pulse topical 5-fluorouracil therapy allow destruction of actinic keratoses without significant inflammation? Epstein E. J Am Acad Dermatol 1998;38:77–80.

Eight of 13 patients who were treated with once or twice weekly dosing with 5% 5-FU did not show discernible improvement. The author concluded that although pulse treatment with 5-FU causes less inflammation, the effectiveness is significantly less.

SECOND LINE THERAPIES

■ Topical imiquimod	A
■ Photodynamic therapy	A
■ Topical adapalene gel	A
■ Topical diclofenac	A

Imiquimod 5% cream for the treatment of actinic keratosis: results from two phase III, randomized, double-blind, parallel group, vehicle-controlled trials. Lebwohl M, Dinehart S, Whiting D, et al. J Am Acad Dermatol 2004; 50:714–21.

In this study, 436 patients were randomized to either receive 5% topical imiquimod cream or vehicle cream on two days per week for 16 weeks. The cream was applied to between four and eight AKs within a contiguous 25 cm² area on the face or scalp. The complete clearance rate was 45.1% in imiquimod-treated patients compared to 3.2% for the vehicle group (p<0.001). Severe erythema was reported by 17.7% of imiquimod-treated patients, and crusting was noted in 8.4%, with erosion and ulceration in 2.3% of patients.

Short-course therapy with imiquimod 5% cream for solar keratoses: a randomized controlled trial. Chen K, Yap LM, Marks R, Shumack S. Australas J Dermatol 2003;44:250–5.

In this randomized, double-blind, vehicle-controlled study, 44 patients with a mean of ten AKs on a treatment area on the face or scalp were treated with topical 5% imiquimod cream three times per week for 3 weeks, then assessed at week 4. Patients who had less than 75% clearance of lesions were treated with a second 3-week course of imiquimod. Of the 29 patients randomized to receive imiquimod cream, 16 patients needed a second course of imiquimod. All patients were then assessed 14 weeks after initiation of treatment – in 21 of 29 imiquimod-treated patients over 75% of lesions cleared, compared with three of ten subjects using the vehicle cream (p=0.027). A short course of topical imiquimod may be effective in treating AKs.

A comparison of photodynamic therapy using topical methyl aminolevulinate (Metvix®) with single cycle cryotherapy in patients with actinic keratosis: a prospective randomized study. Freeman M, Vinciullo C, Francis D, et al. J Dermatol Treat 2003;14:99–106.

In this randomized, reference and placebo-controlled, parallel group study, 204 patients with a total of 855 AKs on the face and scalp were treated with two cycles of photodynamic therapy (PDT) with methyl aminolevulinate, two cycles of PDT with a placebo cream or single freeze–thaw cycle cryotherapy with liquid nitrogen spray. The lesions were assessed after 3 months. The authors found 91% of lesions treated with methyl aminolevulinate PDT cleared completely, compared with 68% in the cryotherapy group and 30% in the placebo PDT group. The main adverse events with methyl aminolevulinate PDT were burning, stinging and skin pain during treatment, which occurred in 46% of patients.

Photodynamic therapy using topical methyl 5-aminolevulinate compared with cyotherapy for actinic keratosis: a prospective, randomized study. Szeimies RM, Karrer S, Radakovic-Fijan S, et al. J Am Acad Dermatol 2002; 47:258–62.

In this randomized prospective study, 193 patients with 699 clinical AKs received either methyl aminolevulinate PDT (repeated 1 week later for lesions not on the scalp and face) or a single treatment with a double freeze–thaw cycle of liquid nitrogen cryotherapy. Patients were assessed in 3 months. The authors found that methyl aminolevulinate PDT treatment resulted in complete clearance of 69% of AKs, compared with 75% for cryotherapy. The difference was not statistically significant, but patient satisfaction and cosmetic outcome was rated higher for PDT-treated patients.

Assessment of adapalene gel for the treatment of actinic keratoses and lentigines: a randomized trial. Kang S, Goldfarb MT, Weiss JS, et al. J Am Acad Dermatol 2003; 49:83–90.

In this prospective randomized, vehicle-controlled study, 90 patients received either 0.1% adapalene gel, 0.3% adapalene gel or vehicle gel, initially daily for 4 weeks, then twice daily for up to 9 months. Overall, 62% (p<0.01) of those who received 0.1% adapalene gel and 66% (p<0.01) of those who received 0.3% adapalene gel showed at least a moderate improvement of their AKs compared to 34% of patients receiving a vehicle cream. Adapalene gel recipients reported a higher level of mild erythema, peeling and dryness compared to control groups.

Topical 3.0% diclofenac in 2.5% hyaluronan gel in the treatment of actinic keratoses. Wolf JE, Taylor JR, Tschen E, Kang S. Int J Dermatol 2001;40:709–13.

Both these studies were randomized, double-blind, placebo-controlled, trials demonstrating that topical diclofenac applied twice daily was more effective than placebo in clearing AKs from selected areas on the body. There was a difference detected after 30 days of treatment. Mild-to-moderate skin irritation was reported in the majority of diclofenac-treated patients.

Topical treatment of actinic keratoses with 3.0% diclofenac in 2.5% hyaluronan gel. Rivers JK, Arlette J, Shear N, et al. Br J Dermatol 2002;146:94–100.

THIRD LINE THERAPIES

■ Curettage	E
■ Excision	E
■ Ablative lasers	C
■ Chemical peels	D
■ Dermabrasion	D

Guidelines of care of actinic keratoses. Committee on Guidelines of Care. Drake LA, Ceilley RI, Cornelison RL, et al. J Am Acad Dermatol 1995;32:95–8.

Recalcitrant, treatment-resistant AKs may be treated with curettage or surgical excision. Both techniques enable tissue to be obtained for the purposes of histological analysis. Curettage can be used alone or in conjunction with electrosurgery, cryotherapy or chemical applications. Surgical excision is particularly useful in lesions suspected of being SCCs because this technique enables the clinician to treat the lesion and establish the diagnosis.

Widespread, extensive AKs may benefit from field treatments of a physical nature. These include ablative laser resurfacing, dermabrasion and chemical peels. Photodynamic therapy utilizing an intense pulsed light source has also been used in this manner.

Full face laser resurfacing: Therapy and prophylaxis for actinic keratoses and non-melanoma skin cancer. Iyer S, Friedli A, Bowes L, Kricorian G, Fitzpatrick RE. Lasers Surg Med 2004;34:114–9.

In this retrospective study of 24 patients with over 30 AKs on the face treated with full face ultrapulse CO_2 laser or erbium: Er:YAG laser resurfacing, the authors found that 21 patients remained lesion free for at least 1 year.

Long-term efficacy and safety of Jessner's solution and 35% trichloroacetic acid vs 5% fluorouracil in the treatment of widespread facial actinic keratoses. Witheiler DD, Lawrence N, Cox SE, et al. Dermatol Surg 1997;23:191–6.

In this prospective study, 15 patients with severe facial AKs were treated on one side of the face with a single application of Jessner's solution, a medium-depth chemical peel, and the other side with twice daily applications of topical 5-FU 5% for 3 weeks. The authors found that both treatments resulted in a similar reduction of AKs at 12 months, with an increase in the number of AKs in both groups from 12–32 months. The authors concluded that both treatments were similarly efficacious in the treatment of AKs, and re-treatment may need to be performed after 12 months for recurrences.

Dermabrasion for prophylaxis and treatment of actinic keratoses. Coleman WP, Yardborough JM, Mandy SH. Dermatol Surg 1996;22:17–21.

In this retrospective study, 23 patients who had undergone dermabrasion for facial AKs were followed up for 2–5 years. The authors found that the benefits of dermabrasion diminished with time: 1 year post-dermabrasion, 22 patients remained clear of AKs. Of 13 patients who were followed up for 5 years, seven remained clear. The authors concluded that dermabrasion provided long-term clearance of AKs in some patients.

Evidence levels   **A** Double-blind study   **B** Clinical trial ≥ 20 subjects   **C** Clinical trial < 20 subjects   **D** Series ≥ 5 subjects   **E** Anecdotal case reports

Actinic prurigo

Robert S Dawe, James Ferguson

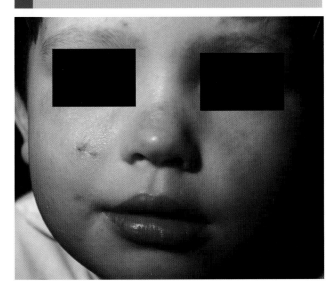

Actinic prurigo is a distinct photodermatosis diagnosed on the basis of characteristic clinical features including perennial nature (although tending to be worse in summer), vesiculopapular eruption during acute flares, persistent eroded nodules and/or dermatitic patches (sometimes affecting covered sites), dorsal nose involvement, scarring, cheilitis and conjunctivitis. Abnormal photosensitivity (UVA, UVB) is frequently severe, but generally gradually improves, especially when (as is usual) it presents before the age of 10 years.

MANAGEMENT STRATEGY

Diagnosis is normally straightforward, but the differential diagnosis can include severe polymorphic light eruption or photoaggravated atopic dermatitis. Although differences between European and Amerindian forms of actinic prurigo have been noted, these appear to be closely related conditions. Phototesting and human leukocyte antigen (HLA)-typing may be helpful in cases of diagnostic uncertainty. Possible coexistent conditions such as sunscreen allergic contact dermatitis or photocontact reactions should be considered because their presence will affect the recommended treatments.

Once the diagnosis is established, initial treatment consists of advice on *sunlight avoidance* (behavioral, clothing and topical sunscreen) measures, and the use of *potent or very potent topical corticosteroids*. This approach alone is often insufficient, and many patients require the addition of a *springtime course of TL-01 UVB or psoralen and UVA (PUVA)*. When phototherapy is administered for this indication, only normally sunlight-exposed sites should be treated. It is helpful to apply a potent topical corticosteroid to the treated areas immediately after each exposure to reduce the risk of actinic prurigo flares.

In Scotland systemic treatment is rarely required, but is more often necessary where availability of phototherapy is limited and in countries with more intense year-round sunlight exposure. *Antimalarials* and *betacarotene* are sometimes tried, but it remains uncertain whether they are of true value. *Thalidomide* may be more useful, but its value is restricted by teratogenicity and the risk of irreversible peripheral neuropathy. *Pentoxifylline* has anti-tumor necrosis factor (TNF)-α effects and, although listed as a third line therapy here, may be worth considering before thalidomide because of its more attractive safety profile.

SPECIFIC INVESTIGATIONS

- Phototesting
- HLA typing
- Histopathology of cheilitis

Actinic prurigo – a specific photodermatosis? Addo HA, Frain-Bell W. Photodermatol 1984;1:119–28.

This study showed that almost 60% of patients with actinic prurigo have abnormal delayed erythemal responses on monochromator phototesting.

Phototest abnormalities tend to more severe in actinic prurigo than in polymorphic light eruption.

Actinic prurigo among the Chimila Indians in Colombia: HLA studies. Bernal JE, Duran de Rueda MM, Ordonez CP, et al. J Am Acad Dermatol 1990;22:1049–51.

In this population, the HLA class 1 antigen Cw4 was more frequent in actinic prurigo patients than in controls.

Actinic prurigo: an update. Hojyo-Tomoka T, Vega-Memije E, Granados J, et al. Int J Dermatol 1995;34:380–4.

HLA-DR4 may determine expression of actinic prurigo in British patients. Menage H du P, Vaughan RW, Baker CS, et al. J Invest Dermatol 1996;106:362–7.

Actinic prurigo and HLA-DR4. Dawe RS, Collins P, O'Sullivan A, Ferguson J. J Invest Dermatol 1997;108:233–4.

An even stronger association was shown with the HLA class 2 antigen HLA-DR4 and, more specifically, HLA-DRB1*0407. These associations are not a feature of polymorphic light eruption.

*The absence of HLA-DR4 can help to rule out the diagnosis of actinic prurigo, whereas the presence of HLA-DRB1*0407 helps to rule in the diagnosis.*

Actinic prurigo: clinical features and HLA associations in a Canadian Inuit population. Wiseman MC, Orr PH, MacDonald SM, et al. J Am Acad Dermatol 2001;44:952–6.

No statistically significant association of actinic prurigo with HLA-DR4 (frequent in the studied population) or HLA-DRB1*0407 was detected, and another HLA type (DRB1*14) was found more commonly than expected, although it was only present in 19 of 37 subjects with actinic prurigo.

The authors acknowledge the possibility that they were studying a different condition from actinic prurigo in other populations. Nevertheless, these findings suggest caution in attempting to use HLA typing as a diagnostic test, especially in populations in which strong HLA associations have not been confirmed.

Actinic prurigo of the lower lip – review of the literature and report of five cases. Mounsdon T, Kratochvil F, Auclair P, et al. Oral Surg Oral Med Oral Pathol 1988; 65:327–32.

Follicular cheilitis – a distinctive histopathologic finding in actinic prurigo. Herrera-Geopfert R, Magana M. Am J Dermatopathol 1995;17:357–61.

Actinic prurigo cheilitis: clinicopathologic analysis and therapeutic results in 116 cases. Vega-Memije ME, Mosqueda-Taylor A, Irigoyen-Camacho ME, et al. Oral Surg Oral Med Oral Pathol Oral Radiol Endod 2002;94:83–91.

A 'follicular cheilitis' has been reported to be characteristic of actinic prurigo. Thirty-two of 116 patients attending a dermatology clinic in Mexico City had cheilitis as their sole manifestation of disease.

Lip histopathology may be helpful diagnostically, especially in patients presenting with cheilitis without cutaneous features at presentation. Where other typical features (skin, eyes) are present, it is arguable how much lip histopathology will contribute to diagnosis.

Augmentation of ultraviolet erythema by indomethacin in actinic prurigo: evidence of mechanism of photosensitivity. Farr PM, Diffey BL. Photochem Photobiol 1988;47:413–7.

Topical indomethacin was found to augment the erythemal response on phototesting.

This study has not been replicated in the literature, and has not developed into a routine diagnostic test.

FIRST LINE THERAPIES

■ Sunlight avoidance – behavioral, clothing, topical sunscreen	C
■ Potent/very potent topical corticosteroids	C
■ Narrow-band (TL-01 lamp) UVB phototherapy	C

Topical photoprotection for hereditary polymorphic light eruption of American Indians. Fusaro RM, Johnson JA. J Am Acad Dermatol 1991;24:744–6.

The authors of this open study found 18 of 30 patients with hereditary polymorphic light eruption of American Indians (with described features indistinguishable from actinic prurigo) to show 'good to excellent results' with use of a broad-spectrum sunscreen.

Although broad-spectrum sunscreens are useful, advice on other sunlight avoidance measures, including appropriate clothing and behavioral avoidance, is equally important.

Treatment of actinic prurigo with intermittent short-course topical 0.05% clobetasol 17-propionate – a preliminary report. Lane PR, Moreland AA, Hogan DJ. Arch Dermatol 1990;126:1211–3.

Seven of eight patients treated with intermittent 3–14 day courses of topical 0.05% clobetasol 17-propionate cream or ointment cleared or markedly improved. All had previously found less potent topical corticosteroids ineffective.

Narrow-band UVB (TL-01) phototherapy: an effective preventative treatment for the photodermatoses. Collins P, Ferguson J. Br J Dermatol 1995;132:956–63.

Six patients with actinic prurigo were included in this open study. All six reported an increase of at least sixfold in tolerable sunlight exposure duration, which was sustained 4 months after treatment. In one patient, whose phototesting (severely abnormal before treatment) was repeated after treatment, the test results normalized.

SECOND LINE THERAPIES

■ Psoralen-UVA photochemotherapy	C
■ Thalidomide	C

Controlled trial of methoxsalen in solar dermatitis of Chippewa Indians. Schenck RR. JAMA 1960;172:1134–7.

This small (13 patients recruited, eight completed) placebo-controlled, crossover study showed no benefit. However, the psoralen dose was low (10 mg), the irradiation source was uncontrollable (the sun), and the study was conducted during summer.

Treatment of actinic prurigo with PUVA: mechanism of action. Farr PM, Diffey BL. Br J Dermatol 1989;120:411–8.

Five patients were treated in this open study. Clinical improvement was accompanied by an increase of UVA minimal erythemal doses to within the normal range on phototesting. Corroboration that PUVA worked through a local effect was provided by before and after phototesting of areas kept covered during treatment. The UVA minimal erythema dose did not increase in these areas.

In the absence of any controlled study comparisons of PUVA and TL-01 phototherapy for this condition, PUVA should generally be reserved for those who fail to benefit from TL-01.

Thalidomide in the treatment of actinic prurigo. Londoño F. Int J Dermatol 1973;12:326–8.

Thirty-four patients were treated, with a starting dose of 300 mg, gradually reduced to a minimum of 15 mg, thalidomide daily; 32 had good results while on the drug, but relapsed on stopping.

Thalidomide in actinic prurigo. Lovell CR, Hawk JL, Calnan CD, Magnus IA. Br J Dermatol 1983;108:467–71.

Of 14 patients treated with thalidomide (adult starting dose 100–200 mg daily), 13 (one could not tolerate the drug due to dizziness) reported improvement. This benefit was sustained in 11, of whom eight required maintenance doses of between 50 mg weekly and 100 mg daily. This paper includes a review of earlier open studies reporting the use of thalidomide in actinic prurigo.

THIRD LINE THERAPIES

■ β-carotene	C
■ Pentoxifylline	C
■ Tetracycline and vitamin E	C
■ Oral corticosteroids	E
■ Azathioprine	E
■ Chloroquine	E
■ Topical cyclosporine	E

Hereditary polymorphic light eruption in American Indians – photoprotection and prevention of streptococcal pyoderma and glomerulonephritis. Fusaro RM, Johnson JA. JAMA 1980;244:1456–9.

Of 54 patients who participated in this open study, 17 were reported to have achieved complete photoprotection, and 16 'marked improvement.' The plasma carotene level tended to be higher in those who benefited. The authors also comment on their use of dihydroxyacetone and lawsone cream, with apparent benefit. The clinical features of the study patients were not reported, but the authors' introductory description of hereditary polymorphic light eruption suggests that they probably included actinic prurigo.

Pentoxifylline in the treatment of actinic prurigo: a preliminary report of 10 patients. Torres-Alvarez B, Castanedo-Cazares JP, Moncada B. Dermatology 2004; 208:198–201.

Clinical improvement was reported in all ten participants in this 6-month open-label uncontrolled study.

Treatment of actinic prurigo in Chimila Indians. Duran MM, Ordonez CP, Prieto JC, Bernal J. Int J Dermatol 1996;35:413–6.

One group of eight patients was treated with tetracycline (1.5 g daily), and another eight patients with vitamin E (100 IU daily). On follow-up analysis, comparing signs and itch, no difference was found between the groups. Both treatments were considered promising, and the possibility of using tetracycline–vitamin E combination therapy was raised.

These treatments need further investigation, but may be worth considering if first line therapies are inadequate and thalidomide is contraindicated or not tolerated.

The clinical features and management of actinic prurigo: a retrospective study. Lestarini D, Khoo LS, Goh CL. Photodermatol Photoimmunol Photomed 1999;15:183–7.

This was a review of the features and clinical course of 11 patients. Of three patients treated with systemic corticosteroids, one improved slightly. Intralesional corticosteroids helped one. Three patients were treated with azathioprine; two appeared to benefit.

Actinic prurigo: clinico-pathological correlation. Hojyo-Tomoka MT, Dominguez-Soto L, Vargasocamp F. Int J Dermatol 1978;17:706–10.

In this review, the authors comment that chloroquine 'seems to give temporary relief', and also suggest that antihistamines and tranquilizers may also be of some benefit.

Use of topical cyclosporin for conjunctival manifestations of actinic prurigo. McCoombes JA, Hirst LW, Green WR. Am J Ophthalmol 2000;130:830–1.

Topical 2% cyclosporine in olive oil eye drops three times daily for 3 months was associated with resolution of chronic actinic prurigo conjunctivitis in a 12-year-old girl, and drops continued once daily over 3 years maintained the improvement.

Actinomycosis

Jonathan E Blume

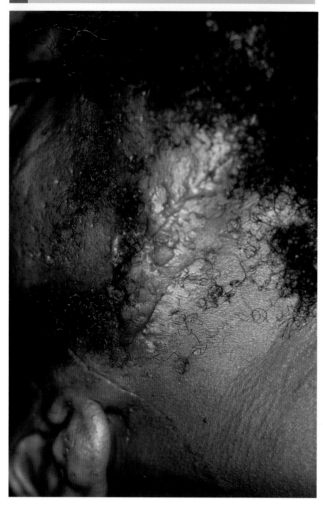

Actinomycosis is an infection caused by *Actinomyces* spp., anaerobic or microaerophilic, gram positive, filamentous bacteria that reside in the human oropharynx and gastro-intestinal tract. The infection typically affects immuno-competent patients and has multiple forms (e.g. cervicofacial, thoracic, abdominopelvic, primary cuta-neous). 'Lumpy jaw', the cervicofacial variant, often pres-ents as 'wooden' induration with draining sinuses at the angle of the jaw or submandibular region. This is the most common form of the disease, and is likely the most common type to be seen by dermatologists.

MANAGEMENT STRATEGY

Mild disease can usually be fully cured with antibiotics, whereas more extensive disease often requires a combina-tion of antibiotics and surgery. Except for minor cases, most patients are initially treated with parenteral antibiotics, fol-lowed by a course of oral therapy. Although recently many antibiotics have shown in-vitro and in-vivo activity against *Actinomyces* spp., *penicillin* has remained the drug of choice since the 1940s.

Historically, actinomycosis was treated with long courses of antibiotics. However, there is mounting evidence that actinomycosis, if diagnosed in an early stage, can be suc-cessfully treated with brief courses (less that 6 months) of therapy. Ultimately, the patient's condition and response to therapy will dictate the duration of treatment.

Treatment failures with penicillin are extremely rare; but when they occur, they are likely due to β-lactamase pro-ducing bacteria that accompany *Actinomyces* spp. and help initiate infection. When faced with such a case, modifying the antibiotic regimen to cover these accomplices is war-ranted (e.g. switching to *imipenem* or *clindamycin*).

Short-term treatment of actinomycosis: two cases and a review. Sudhakar SS, Ross JJ. Clin Infect Dis 2004;38:444–7.

Susceptibility of pathogenic actinomycetes to antimicro-bial compounds. Lerner PI. Antimicrob Agents Chemother 1974;5:302–9.

SPECIFIC INVESTIGATIONS

- Gram stain
- Biopsy with special stains
- Culture and measurement of physiological and biochemical characteristics
- Immunofluorescent staining
- Direct immunoperoxidase technique
- Ribosomal RNA gene sequencing
- Computed tomography (CT) and magnetic resonance imaging (MRI)

Diagnostic methods for human actinomycosis. Holmberg K. Microbiol Sci 1987;4:72–8.

An excellent review of the diagnosis of actinomycosis.

The most accurate way to diagnose actinomycosis is via culture – a usually difficult task, which requires thioglycolate or brain-heart enriched agar at 37°C under anaerobic or microaerophilic conditions. 'Molar-tooth' and 'bread-crumb' colonies may take up to 3 weeks to grow. Unfortunately, definitive identification cannot be based on colony morphology and requires the measurement of physiological and biochemical characteristics (e.g. sensitivity to oxygen, presence of preformed enzymes).

Because cultures of Actinomyces *spp. are often unsuccessful, observation of 'sulfur granules' on a peripheral smear or histology often helps make the diagnosis. The granules are bacterial colonies that on hematoxylin and eosin staining have a basophilic central area surrounded by a zone of eosinophilic 'clubs'. Other typical histologic findings include extensive fibrosis, chronic granulation tissue, sinus tracts, and scattered microabscesses.*

Immunofluorescent staining of Actinomyces *spp. is available and can be used on clinical material, granules and formalin-fixed tissues. The direct immunoperoxidase technique can specifically show* Actinomyces *spp. in formalin-fixed sections via light microscopy. These techniques, as well as gene sequencing (see below), are promising diagnostic modalities given the difficulty of culture and histologic identification.*

Diagnosis of pelvic actinomycosis by 16s ribosomal RNA gene sequencing and its clinical significance. Woo PCY, Fung AMY, Lau SKP, et al. Diagn Microbiol Infect Dis 2002;43:113–8.

Actinomyces odontolyticus *was identified by rRNA gene sequencing. Because the 16S ribosomal RNA gene is* conserved within a species, it can be used to identify a specific species of bacteria.

Cervicofacial actinomycosis: CT and MR imaging findings in seven patients. Park JK, Lee HK, Ha HK, et al. AJNR Am J Neuroradiol 2003;24:331–5.

Findings on CT and MRI may be helpful in distinguishing cervicofacial actinomycosis from malignant neoplasms, tuberculosis and fungal infections.

FIRST LINE THERAPIES

■ Penicillin	C

Actinomycosis. Smego RA, Foglia G. Clin Infect Dis 1998;26:1255–63.

The authors recommend 2 months of oral penicillin V or a tetracycline (e.g. oral doxycycline 100 mg twice a day) for mild cervicofacial disease. For more complicated infections, parenteral penicillin G (10–20 million U/day divided every 6 h) for 4–6 weeks followed by 6–12 months of oral penicillin V (2–4 g/day divided every 6 h) is suggested. A tetracycline, erythromycin, clindamycin or cephalosporins are advocated for patients allergic to penicillin.

Actinomycosis and nocardiosis. A review of basic differences in therapy. Peabody JW, Seabury JH. Am J Med 1960;28:99–115.

The authors review the treatment of actinomycosis and state that penicillin is the drug of choice.

SECOND LINE THERAPIES

■ Amoxicillin	C
■ Ceftriaxone	D
■ Clindamycin	C
■ Doxycycline	D
■ Erythromycin	D
■ Imipenem	C
■ Minocycline	C
■ Tetracycline	D

The use of oral amoxycillin for the treatment of actinomycosis: a clinical and in vitro study. Martin MV. Br Dent J 1984;156:252–4.

Ten patients with cervicofacial actinomycosis were cured in less than 6 weeks with a combination of amoxicillin (500 mg four times daily) and surgery.

Actinomycosis abscess of the thyroid gland. Cevera JJ, Butehorn HF, Shapiro J, Setzen G. Laryngoscope 2003; 113:2108–11.

A 39-year-old female patient who developed actinomycosis of the thyroid gland after tooth extraction was cured with thyroidectomy and 6 months of ceftriaxone.

Successful treatment of thoracic actinomycosis with ceftriaxone. Skoutelis A, Petrochilos J, Bassaris H. Clin Infect Dis 1994;19:161–2.

A 38-year-old patient with pulmonary actinomycosis was successfully treated with a 3-week course of daily ceftriaxone followed by 3 months of daily oral ampicillin.

Mandibular actinomycosis treated with oral clindamycin. Badgett JT, Adams G. Pediatr Infect Dis J 1987;6:221–2.

Clindamycin in the treatment of cervicofacial actinomycosis. de Vries J, Bentley KC. Int J Clin Pharmacol 1974;9:46–8.

A 60-year-old man with cervicofacial actinomycosis that was resistant to penicillin and tetracycline responded fully to a 1 month course of clindamycin (150 mg four times a day).

Clindamycin in the treatment of serious anaerobic infections. Fass RJ, Scholand JF, Hodges GR, Saslaw S. Ann Intern Med 1973;78:853–9.

Four patients with cervicofacial actinomycosis and one patient with thoracic actinomycosis were successfully treated with a combination of intravenous and oral clindamycin.

Primary actinomycosis of the hand: a case report and literature review. Mert A, Bilir M, Bahar H, et al. Int J Infect Dis 2001;5:112–4.

A 35-year-old man with primary actinomycosis of the hand was cured with one month of intravenous ampicillin (12 g/day) followed by 11 months of oral doxycycline (200 mg/day).

Actinomycosis of the prostate. de Souza E, Katz DA, Dworzack DL, Longo G. J Urol 1985;133:290–1.

A case of acute prostatitis due to *Actinomyces* spp. was cured with long-term erythromycin, chosen because of its excellent penetration into prostatic secretions.

Actinomycosis of the temporomandibular joint. Bradley P. Br J Oral Surg 1971;9:54–6.

A 58-year-old man with actinomycosis of the temporomandibular joint was cured with a 12 week course of erythromycin (500 mg six times a day).

Use of imipenem in the treatment of thoracic actinomycosis. Yew WW, Wong PC, Wong CF, Chau CH. Clin Infect Dis 1994;19:983–4.

Report of eight cases of pulmonary actinomycosis and their treatment with imipenem–cilastatin. Yew WW, Wong PC, Lee J, et al. Monaldi Arch Chest Dis 1994;54:126–9.

Seven of eight patients with pulmonary actinomycosis were successfully treated with a 4-week course of parenteral imipenem–cilastatin.

Cutaneous disseminated actinomycosis in a patient with acute lymphocytic leukemia. Takeda H, Mitsuhashi Y, Kondo S. J Dermatol 1998;25:37–40.

A patient with primary cutaneous disseminated actinomycosis was cured with a 3-month course of intravenous minocycline (2 mg/kg/day).

Antibiotic treatment of cervicofacial actinomycosis for patients allergic to penicillin: a clinical and in vitro study. Martin MV. Br J Oral Maxillofac Surg 1985;23:428–34.

Six patients with cervicofacial actinomycosis were cured with 8–16 weeks of oral minocycline (250 mg four times a day). There were no recurrences after 1 year.

Primary actinomycosis of the quadriceps. Langloh JT, Lauerman WC. J Pediatr Orthop 1987;7:222–3.

Surgical drainage followed by a 6-week course of oral tetracycline cured a case of actinomycosis of the quadriceps.

THIRD LINE THERAPIES

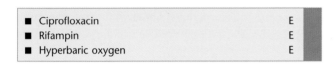

■ Ciprofloxacin	E
■ Rifampin	E
■ Hyperbaric oxygen	E

Treatment of recalcitrant actinomycosis with ciprofloxacin. Macfarlane DJ, Tucker LG, Kemp RJ. J Infect 1993;27:177–80.

Treatment of pulmonary actinomycosis with rifampin. Morrone N, De Castro Pereira CA, Saito M, et al. G Ital Chemioter 1982;29:121–4.

Pulmonary actinomycosis. Rapid improvement with isoniazid and rifampin. King JW, White MC. Arch Intern Med 1981;141:1234–5.

Adjunctive hyperbaric oxygen therapy for actinomycotic lacrimal canaliculitis. Shauly Y, Nachum Z, Gdal-On M, et al. Graefes Arch Clin Exp Ophthalmol 1993;231:429–31.

A 52-year-old patient with treatment resistant lacrimal canaliculitis due to *A. israelii* was cured with hyperbaric oxygen.

Hyperbaric oxygen in the treatment of actinomycosis. Manheim SD, Voleti C, Ludwig A, Jacobson JH. J Am Med Assoc 1969;210:552–3.

After failing to respond to surgery and intravenous penicillin, a 63-year-old patient with perirectal actinomycosis was cured with hyperbaric oxygen.

Acute generalized exanthematous pustulosis

Walayat Hussain, Ian Coulson

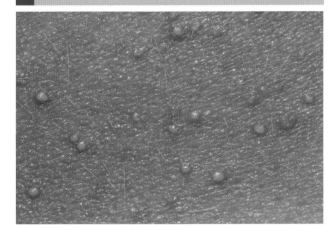

Acute generalized exanthematous pustulosis (AGEP) is characterized by the acute onset of numerous small, non-follicular, sterile pustules arising on a diffuse erythematous base in a febrile patient with an accompanying blood neutrophilia. The majority of cases occur in the context of drug ingestion (commonly within 24 hours). Rapid resolution following drug withdrawal is the usual outcome.

MANAGEMENT STRATEGY

Treatment of AGEP involves establishing the correct diagnosis coupled with the *withdrawal of any implicated medication* (Table 1). Pustular psoriasis is its main differential diagnosis. A comprehensive drug history and personal or family history of psoriasis is therefore required.

Intraepidermal or subcorneal pustules in conjunction with a leukocytoclastic vasculitis, focal necrosis of keratinocytes, marked edema of the papillary dermis and an infiltrate of eosinophils are histological features that help distinguish AGEP from pustular psoriasis: biopsy is thus an integral facet of management.

Differentiation of AGEP from other inflammatory, toxic or infectious conditions such as Sneddon-Wilkinson disease (subcorneal pustular dermatosis) or, in severe cases, toxic epidermal necrolysis, is often readily apparent both clinically and histologically. The clinician should, however, be aware that erythema multiforme-like targetoid lesions, mucous membrane involvement, facial edema, purpura and vesicobullous lesions have all been documented within the context of AGEP.

Antibiotics (primarily penicillin or macrolide-based) are the most frequently implicated medications. Numerous case reports have cited various other causative agents including calcium channel blockers, nonsteroidal anti-inflammatory drugs (NSAIDs), angiotensin-converting enzyme (ACE)-inhibitors and anticonvulsants (Table 1). Acute enterovirus infection and mercury exposure have also been reported as possible causes.

Table 1 Drugs reported to cause AGEP

Acetaminophen	Hydroxychloroquine
Acetazolamide	Imipenem/cilastatin
Allopurinol	Isoniazid
Amoxapine	Itraconazole
Amoxicillin	Lansoprazole
Ampicillin	Metronidazole
Aspirin	Minocycline
Azithromycin	Naproxen
Bacampicillin	Nifedipine
Captopril	Nimodipine
Carbamazepine	Nitrazepam
Cefaclor	Norfloxacin
Cefazolin	Nystatin
Cefuroxime	Ofloxacin
Cephalexin	Penicillins
Cephradine	Phenobarbital
Chloramphenicol	Phenytoin
Chloroquine	Piperazine
Chlorpromazine	Progestins
Clindamycin	Propicillin
Clozapine	Protease inhibitors
Co-trimoxazole	Pyrimethamine
Codeine	Quinidine
Corticosteroids	Ranitidine
Diltiazem	Streptomycin
Doxycycline	Sulfamethoxazole
Enalapril	Sulfasalazine
Eprazinone	Terbinafine
Erythromycin	Ticlopidine
Furosemide	Vancomycin

There is no specific therapy for AGEP. A skin swab establishes the sterile nature of the pustules and drug withdrawal, if feasible, results in rapid spontaneous resolution. *Supportive therapy* is all that is required. A superficial desquamation often occurs during this time and may be treated with *simple emollients*. Only a single case report supports the use of *systemic corticosteroids* for this self limiting condition.

SPECIFIC INVESTIGATIONS

- Detailed history
- Full blood count
- Skin swab of pustule – microscopy, culture, Gram stain
- Skin biopsy

FIRST LINE THERAPIES

■ Drug withdrawal	E

Acute generalized exanthematous pustulosis. Roujeau JC, Bioulac-Sage P, Bourseau C, et al. Analysis of 63 cases. Arch Dermatol 1991;127:1333–8.

A thorough retrospective review of cases which remains the largest series of AGEP to date. Almost 90% of cases were attributable to drugs with 50% of reactions occurring within 24 hours of ingestion.

AGEP is distinct from pustular psoriasis based upon histological differences, drug induction in most cases, a more acute course of fever and pustulosis, blood neutrophilia and rapid spontaneous healing (within 15 days).

Acute generalized exanthematous pustulosis. Manders SM, Heymann WR. Cutis 1994;54:194–6.

Two of the three cases reported in this series were attributable to penicillin. This succinct overview of AGEP also provides the reader with useful clinicopathological features that may help distinguish AGEP from pustular psoriasis.

Pustular eruption after drug exposure: is it pustular psoriasis or a pustular drug eruption? Spencer JM, Silvers DN, Grossman ME. Br J Dermatol 1994;130:514–519.

Another series highlighting the diagnostic challenge when confronted with a patient with pustulosis and fever. One of the four cases of AGEP occurred in a patient with known psoriasis who was given trimethoprim for a urinary tract infection. An awareness of the condition, eosinophils in the biopsy and rapid resolution following drug withdrawal prevented unnecessary treatment for pustular psoriasis.

Generalized pustular psoriasis or drug-induced toxic pustuloderma? The use of patch testing. Whittam LR, Wakelin SH, Barker JNWN. Clin Exp Dermatol 2000;25:122–4.

Patch testing to a 1% and 5% amoxicillin preparation confirmed a type 4 hypersensitivity reaction in a patient with longstanding plaque psoriasis who developed a generalized pustular eruption when treated with amoxicillin for an episode of epididymo-orchitis.

SECOND LINE THERAPIES

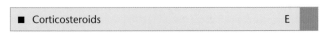

■ Corticosteroids	E

Acute generalised exanthematous pustulosis. Criton S, Sofia B. Indian J Dermatol Venereol Leprol 2001;67:93–5.

A case report in which the authors claim that parental corticosteroids hastened the resolution of AGEP presumptively caused by benzylpenicillin.

Evidence levels A Double-blind study **B** Clinical trial ≥ 20 subjects **C** Clinical trial < 20 subjects **D** Series ≥ 5 subjects **E** Anecdotal case reports

Allergic contact dermatitis and photoallergy

Rosemary L Nixon

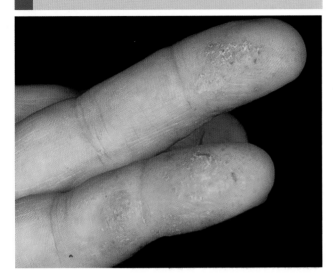

Allergic contact dermatitis (ACD) is a delayed hypersensitivity reaction, usually to the topical application of an allergen to which the sufferer is sensitized. At first, the rash is localized to the site of contact with the causative allergen, but it may spread to other areas, either from transfer of the allergen to other sites or because of an 'id' or hypersensitivity eruption. Spread of the rash to other areas is very characteristic of ACD and may help clinically to differentiate it from an irritant contact dermatitis.

In photoallergy, a substance does not become allergenic until exposed to UV light. The most important photoallergens are currently sunscreens, and perhaps some pesticides, but in the past fragrances (especially musk ambrette), halogenated salicylanilides and topical nonsteroidal agents (such as ketoprofen) were common photoallergens.

Some patients with an airborne contact dermatitis to sesquiterpene lactones, found in the Compositae group of plants, will develop photosensitivity, as evidenced by abnormal results on monochromator testing. This condition is generally termed chronic actinic dermatitis (CAD).

Localization may give clues to the causative allergen, for example involvement of the hands in cases of ACD caused by rubber accelerators in gloves, the ears and neck caused by nickel in costume jewelry, eyelid and neck dermatitis from preservatives or perfumes in moisturizing creams.

Determinants of whether sensitization will occur include the nature of the allergen involved, the duration and concentration of skin contact with the allergen, and individual susceptibility.

MANAGEMENT STRATEGY

The primary responsibility is to *identify and avoid further contact* with the offending allergen as well as any poten-

tially cross-reacting agents. *Patch testing* is required to elucidate this. From a public health perspective, it is important to decrease exposure to known allergens. In parts of Europe, legislation has been enacted to decrease the nickel content of jewelry in contact with the skin. The addition of ferrous sulfate to cement, initially in Denmark, effectively decreases the available chromate through chemical reduction. Higher molecular weight epoxy resins are preferred to lower weight resins because of their decreased allergenicity.

In the workplace other measures should be undertaken to reduce exposure to known allergens, such as substitution of known allergens, changing the design of an engineering process to limit skin contact with chemicals, installation of appropriate ventilation to reduce airborne exposure to substances, and by the use of personal protective equipment.

It is most important to wear gloves that are appropriate for handling a particular chemical. In addition, it is often suggested that cotton gloves be worn underneath rubber or leather outer gloves to prevent sensitization to rubber accelerators and chromate, respectively. This is especially important in the context of work in hot environments where sweating and leaching of allergens is likely.

The initial treatments utilize the general principles of eczema therapy, including *avoidance of skin irritants*, such as water, soap, solvents, oils, heat, sweating, dust, and friction. Use of *soap substitutes* and *moisturizing creams*, together with *topical corticosteroids* are recommended.

Use of *barrier creams* to prevent dermatitis has been of limited success, however the development of *topical skin protectant* in the US has had encouraging results when used experimentally to prevent allergic reactions caused by poison ivy. Use of chelating agents in skin creams may be helpful. Short courses of *oral corticosteroids*, such as prednisolone 25–50 mg daily for 1 week, are sometimes required in severe cases. Occasionally the dermatitis may become secondarily infected, so a course of *antibiotics*, such as *cephalosporin*, *erythromycin* or *flucloxacillin* may be required. *Topical antibiotics* such as *mupirocin* or *fusidic acid* are often helpful, particularly for the treatment of persistently cracked or fissured skin that becomes infected.

Once the cause of ACD has been identified, long-term treatments other than avoidance of the allergen(s) are usually not required. Desensitization, commonly used in the treatment of allergies caused by immediate hypersensitivity reactions, has been of extremely limited value when employed in delayed hypersensitivity.

Occasionally, severe episodes of dermatitis may precipitate a recurring eczematous condition, termed persisting post-occupational dermatitis.

In persistent cases, *ultraviolet light therapy* may be considered, such as with hand UVB or PUVA (psoralen plus UVA).

Systemic immunosuppression utilizing *azathioprine or cyclosporine* may be considered. Other agents such as *methotrexate or acitretin* (particularly if the hands are hyperkeratotic) are less often used. Newer topical treatments include *tacrolimus* and *pimecrolimus*. *Disulfiram* has been used in the treatment of nickel dermatitis with equivocal success. Chelation of nickel topically with *clioquinol* may be a more useful approach, but has been little studied. *Superficial X-ray* and *Grenz ray* treatment have been successfully used in some cases.

In photoallergy, identification and avoidance of the photoallergen is of major importance. In the case of allergy to chemical sunscreening agents, this may involve substitution with physical sunscreening agents such as titanium dioxide.

In CAD, treatments have centered on reduction of UV exposure, including hospitalization and use of *plastic films* for windows to decrease UV transmission. The use of *topical tacrolimus* has recently been reported. Systemic therapies include *azathioprine, prednisolone, hydroxychloroquine, cyclosporine, PUVA or UVB, and combinations of UV with prednisolone.*

SPECIFIC INVESTIGATIONS

- Patch testing to appropriately diluted allergens
- Photopatch testing if photoallergic dermatitis is suspected – duplicate sets of allergens are applied, and after 48 h one set is exposed to 5 J/cm UVA; results are read after a further 48 h

Contact dermatitis: Allergic. Beck MH, Wilkinson SM. Chapter 20. In: Rook's Textbook of Dermatology. Burns DA, Breathnach SM, Cox N, Griffiths C, Eds, 7th edition: Blackwell Science; 2004.

This comprehensive chapter from a major dermatology text is a great source of information.

FIRST LINE THERAPIES

Contact dermatitis	
■ Topical corticosteroids	B
■ Emollients and soap substitutes	C
■ Barrier creams	B
■ Tacrolimus	B
■ Pimecrolimus	B
■ Topical clioquinol (nickel dermatitis)	D
■ Prednisolone	D
■ Antibiotics – topical and systemic	D
Photoallergy/CAD	
■ Reduction of ultraviolet light	C
■ Sunscreens – physical agents	E
■ Tacrolimus	D

Efficacy of topical corticosteroids in nickel-induced contact allergy Hachem JP, De Paepe K, Vanpe'e E, et al. Clin Exp Derm 2002;27:47–50.

Twenty female volunteers with known nickel allergy had patch tests applied with nickel on one forearm and control saline on the other. Topical corticosteroid was applied twice daily after day 4. Transepidermal water loss values were significantly decreased on the topical corticosteroid-treated sites in the early phase of ACD.

The effect of two moisturisers on skin barrier damage in allergic contact dermatitis Hachem J-P, De Paepe K, Vanpee E, et al. Eur J Dermatol 2002;12:136–8.

Fifteen female volunteers with known nickel allergy had two different moisturizers, with both highly and poorly hydrating formulations, applied to nickel-induced ACD on their forearms. Transepidermal water loss measurements were significantly increased on the sites pre-treated with the poorly hydrating moisturizer.

A cream containing the chelator DTPA (diethylenetri-aminepenta-acetic acid) can prevent contact allergic reactions to metals. Wohrl S, Kriechbaumer N, Hemmer W, et al. Contact Derm 2001;44:224–8.

Patients with known allergies to nickel, cobalt and copper had abrogation of their patch test reactions with pretreatment with DTPA cream.

Assessment of the ability of the topical skin protectant (TSP) to protect against contact dermatitis to urushiol (Rhus) antigen. Vidmar DA, Iwane MK. Am J Contact Dermatol 1999;10:190–7.

Fifty Rhus-sensitive subjects underwent paired open patch tests to urushiol, with and without prior skin application of TSP. TSP-protected sites were associated with significantly less dermatitis. TSP is composed of polytetrafluoroethylene resins mixed in a perfluorinated polyether oil (similar to Teflon®).

Prevention of poison ivy and poison oak allergic contact dermatitis by quaternium-18 bentonite. Marks JG, Fowler JF, Sheretz EF. J Am Acad Dermatol 1995;33:212–6.

5% quaternium-18 bentonite lotion was applied to the skin 1 h before patch testing to urushiol in a large group of poison ivy allergic individuals. Non-pretreated sites were used as controls. Pretreated sites had absent or significantly reduced reactions to the urushiol compared with controls.

Treatment of chronic actinic dermatitis with tacrolimus ointment. Uetsu N, Okamoto H, Fujii K, et al. J Am Acad Dermatol 2002;47:881–4.

Six patients with CAD unresponsive to other topical agents including topical corticosteroids and sunscreens, and also oral antihistamines, improved with application of 0.1% tacrolimus ointment applied twice daily. Improvement was moderate after 2 weeks, and greater after 4 weeks.

Tacrolimus ointment in the treatment of nickel-induced allergic contact dermatitis. Saripelli YV, Gadzia JE, Belsito DV. J Am Acad Dermatol 2003;49:477–82

Of 19 volunteers with known nickel sensitivity, 18 had improvement in signs and symptoms of ACD with topical tacrolimus compared to ten using vehicle.

Topical tacrolimus 0.1% ointment (Protopic®) reverses nickel contact dermatitis elicited by allergen challenge to a similar degree to mometasone furoate 0.1% with greater suppression of late erythema. Alomar A, Puig L, Gallardo CM, Valenzuela N. Contact Derm 2003;49:185–8.

Twenty eight female volunteers who were allergic to nickel had patch tests removed at day 2 and then applied either tacrolimus or mometasone furoate under occlusion for 48 h. The reactions were assessed with visual scores and measurement of erythema.

SDZ ASM 981 is the first non-steroid that suppresses established nickel contact dermatitis elicited by allergen challenge. Queille-Roussel C, Graeber M, Thurston M, et al. Contact Derm 2000;42:349–50.

Evidence levels A Double-blind study **B** Clinical trial ≥ 20 subjects **C** Clinical trial < 20 subjects **D** Series ≥ 5 subjects **E** Anecdotal case reports

Sixty six nickel sensitive subjects were exposed to nickel and the ensuing dermatitis was treated twice daily with SDZ ASM 981 (pimecrolimus) at 0.2% and 0.6%. This was significantly more effective than treatment with the corresponding vehicle, and similar in effectiveness of treatment to use of 0.1% betamethasone-17-valerate cream.

The inhibitory effects of topical chelating agents and antioxidants on nickel-induced hypersensitivity reactions. Memon AA, Molokhia MM, Friedmann PS. J Am Acad Dermatol 1994;30:560–5.

3% clioquinol ointment applied to a coin completely abolished the allergic reaction to it in all 29 nickel-sensitive subjects. In clinical use, sites treated with a cream containing 3% clioquinol and 1% hydrocortisone showed marked clinical improvement in all ten subjects. Clioquinol is a potent inhibitor of nickel-induced hypersensitivity reactions and it is feasible to use it as a barrier ointment to block the allergenic effects of nickel in sensitive patients.

SECOND LINE THERAPIES

Contact dermatitis	
■ Ultraviolet light	B
■ Azathioprine	C
■ Cyclosporine	D
■ Methotrexate	D
■ Acitretin	E
■ Superficial X-ray and Grenz ray therapy	C
■ Low nickel diet	C
Photoallergy/chronic actinic dermatitis	
■ Azathioprine	C
■ Prednisolone	D
■ Hydroxychloroquine	D
■ Cyclosporine	B
■ PUVA/UVB	D
■ PUVA/UVB and prednisolone	D

Chronic eczematous dermatitis of the hands: a comparison of PUVA and UVB treatment. Rosen K, Mobacken H, Swanbeck G. Acta Derm Venereol 1987;67:48–54.

Thirty five patients were randomly allocated to PUVA or UVB, with one hand acting as untreated control. While there was statistically significant improvement in both groups, treatment with PUVA was superior to UVB.

Azathioprine in the treatment of Parthenium dermatitis. Sharma VK, Chakrabarti A, Mahajan V. Int J Dermatol 1998;37:299–302.

Avoidance of this allergen is almost impossible. Twenty patients with chronic Parthenium dermatitis, with relative contraindications to systemic corticosteroids or their side effects, were treated with oral azathioprine (100–150 mg daily) for 6 months. Ten showed near-total clearance, three showed more than 50% eczema reduction.

Oral cyclosporin inhibits the expression of contact hypersensitivity in man. Higgins EM, McLelland J, Friedmann PS, Matthews JN, Shuster S. J Dermatol Sci 1991; 2:79–83.

The expression of delayed contact hypersensitivity was studied in 6 patients with chronic contact dermatitis treated with cyclosporine 5 mg/kg/day. Quantitative patch test reactions were diminished in all six patients; responses were reduced over the whole range of allergen concentrations. In addition, the clinical manifestations of ACD underwent complete resolution within 2–3 weeks of cyclosporine therapy.

Low-dose oral methotrexate treatment for recalcitrant palmoplantar pompholyx. Egan CA, Rallis TM, Meadows KP, Krueger GG. J Am Acad Dermatol 1999;40:612–4.

Five patients with severe pompholyx who did not respond to conventional therapy or who had debilitating side effects from corticosteroids responded to low-dose methotrexate with clearing of their dermatitis and reduction in their need for oral corticosteroid therapy.

A double-blind study of Grenz ray therapy in chronic eczema of the hands. Lidelof B, Wrangso K, Liden S. Br J Dermatol 1987;117:77–80.

Three Gy of Grenz rays were applied on six occasions at intervals of 1 week, with significant improvement in the treated hand eczema compared to the sham treated control hand.

Low nickel diet: an open prospective trial. Veien NK, Hattel T, Laurberg G. J Am Acad Dermatol 1993;29:1002–7.

Ninety nickel-sensitive patients who had previously flared with oral nickel challenge were treated with a nickel-free diet. Fifty eight improved, and 40 had had long-term benefit when followed 1–2 years later. Those with moderately positive patch test reactions rather than strong positive appeared to benefit more from the diet.

Chronic actinic dermatitis: An analysis of 51 patients evaluated in the United States and Japan. Lim HW, Morison WL, Kamide R, et al. Arch Dermatol 1994;130: 1284–9.

The clinical features of 51 patients were detailed. Topical corticosteroids were helpful for minor eruptions. Nine patients were treated with hydroxychloroquine sulfate (200 mg once to twice daily) with a partial to good response in some patients.

Azathioprine treatment in chronic actinic dermatitis: a double-blind controlled trial with monitoring of exposure to ultraviolet radiation. Murphy GM, Maurice PD, Norris PG, et al. Br J Dermatol 1989;121:639–46.

Azathioprine 150 mg/day was compared with placebo in 18 severely affected patients. Five of eight patients treated with azathioprine, but none of ten patients on placebo achieved remission within 6 months.

Successful treatment of musk ketone-induced chronic actinic dermatitis with cyclosporine and PUVA. Gardeazabal J, Arregui MA, Gil N, et al. J Am Acad Dermatol 1992;27:838–42.

A single case of musk ambrette persistent light reaction responding to cyclosporine and PUVA.

Actinic reticuloid: response to cyclosporin. Norris P, Camp RDR, Hawk JLM. J Am Acad Dermatol 1989;21:307–9.

Two patients responded to treatment with cyclosporine after failure of azathioprine.

Psoralen plus UVA protocol for Compositae photosensitivity. Burke DA, Corey G, Storrs FJ. Am J Contact Dermat 1996;7:171–6.

Two elderly men received prednisolone-assisted PUVA for their chronic photodistributed dermatitis associated with Compositae sensitivity, which resolved with this treatment and in one instance remained clear for 18 months without needing further PUVA therapy.

THIRD LINE THERAPIES

- Pentoxifylline

Prevention of nickel-induced contact reactions with pentoxifylline. Saricaoglu H, Tunali S, Bulbul E, et al. Contact Derm 1998;39:244–7.

A guinea pig study showing that oral pentoxifylline inhibits nickel contact dermatitis elicitation. *Others have questioned the effects in humans.*

Evidence levels A Double-blind study   B Clinical trial ≥ 20 subjects   C Clinical trial < 20 subjects   D Series ≥ 5 subjects   E Anecdotal case reports

Alopecia areata

*Joanne Hague, Manjeet Mehmi,
John Berth-Jones*

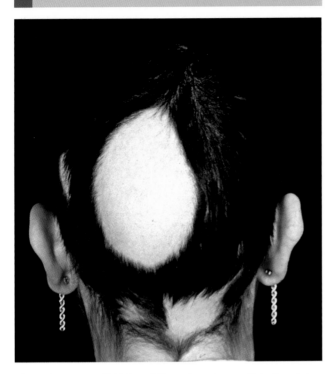

Alopecia areata (AA) is a T-lymphocyte mediated autoimmune disease of the hair follicle. It is characterized by patchy hair loss developing in otherwise normal skin, with exclamation mark hairs around margins of expanding areas. Most cases are limited to one or more coin-sized patches, but in severe cases there may be complete baldness of the scalp (alopecia totalis, AT) or of the entire body (alopecia universalis, AU). The alopecia is noncicatrizing, and in most cases resolves spontaneously after a few months.

MANAGEMENT STRATEGY

Leaving AA untreated is a reasonable option for many patients because spontaneous remission often occurs. Treatment can be time consuming, uncomfortable, and potentially toxic, and relapse after treatment may be difficult to cope with. On the other hand some patients find the condition so embarrassing that they require psychological support and counseling. Contact with other sufferers and patient support groups may help.

Patients should receive a thorough explanation of the natural history of the disease, and a realistic expectation of treatment outcome.

The treatments listed as first line are the most consistently effective and safe, but the response to any treatment is variable and depends largely on the extent and duration of the alopecia. This is one reason why the results of trials are often conflicting. Trials involving recent-onset patchy alopecia may have a high rate of spontaneous remission, whereas trials limited to severe longstanding disease that is resistant to treatment do not exclude efficacy in mild alopecia.

Intralesional corticosteroid injections are considered first line treatment for adult patients when only one or two small patches of alopecia are present, but can be used on up to 50% of the scalp if patients can tolerate the discomfort. The authors most frequently use triamcinolone acetonide aqueous suspension (2.5–10 mg/mL) injected just beneath the dermis in 0.05–0.1 mL doses, and repeated on a monthly basis. At a concentration of 5 mg/mL a maximum of 3 mL can be used on the scalp in one visit. A concentration of 2.5 mg/mL should be used on the beard and eyebrow area. The main side effect is minimal, often transient, pitting atrophy.

Topical immunotherapy is the induction of contact allergy on the scalp. Contact sensitizers include dinitrochlorobenzene (DNCB, now considered potentially carcinogenic and therefore no longer used), squaric acid dibutyl ester (SADBE, this has limited stability), primula leaves, nickel (as nickel sulfate 0.1–1% in petrolatum, in sensitized individuals) and diphencyprone (DPCP, diphenylcyclopropenone). The latter compound combines established efficacy and safety with a practical shelf-life and has become the most widely used sensitizer.

Diphencyprone is initially applied as 2% lotion to a small area (2–4 cm²) of scalp until the site of application becomes pruritic and erythematous. Treatment can then be continued over a larger area with weekly applications of lower concentrations, typically ranging from 0.001% to 0.1%. The lowest concentration that maintains mild erythema or pruritus should be used. Our patients usually have half of their scalp treated initially, until a favorable result means treatment can then be extended to the contralateral scalp. This is one of the best documented therapies for AA, and is the treatment most likely to be effective in extensive longstanding disease. The timing of the response is quite unpredictable, however, so the authors treat patients for as long as they wish to continue. Relapse rates may be high. Side effects include regional lymphadenopathy and the contact allergic dermatitis very rarely causes autosensitization, resulting in generalized eczema or even an eruption resembling erythema multiforme. Vitiligo may develop during application of DPCP, and this is usually but not always confined to the treated areas. For this reason, sensitization is best avoided in patients with pigmented skin types.

Topical corticosteroids have demonstrated efficacy in some studies of patchy AA, particularly those using potent corticosteroids or occlusion. They are fairly inexpensive and practical to use, and the main side effect is transient folliculitis. Results are variable however, and in particular they do not appear effective in AT or AU.

Psoralen plus UVA treatment (PUVA) has been studied in several uncontrolled trials with variable results. The relapse rate following treatment is high, and continued treatment with high cumulative UVA doses appears to be necessary for maintenance of hair growth.

Irritants, including *anthralin (dithranol), retinoic acid, croton oil* and *phenol* have been used to induce a mild irritant dermatitis, though the evidence for their efficacy is weak. Anthralin and retinoic acid are safe and practical to use. For patients with dark hair, anthralin has the advantage of camouflaging a pale area of scalp by staining it brown. Application needs to be frequent and at a fairly high concentration because it needs to induce brisk irritation in order to be effective. Retinoic acid is more practical for patients with fair hair.

Topical minoxidil is a safe treatment and seems to demonstrate biological effect, but most studies have failed to demonstrate a good cosmetic result.

Systemic corticosteroids are effective in most cases if high enough doses are employed, but prolonged treatment is often required to maintain a response. Attempts have been made to use pulsed regimens with some limited success. AT, AU and ophiasiform AA do not appear to respond well, and high relapse rates make this potentially toxic treatment hard to justify. This is particularly an issue in patients who are already emotionally distressed.

Systemic cyclosporine also appears effective if given in high dosage, but the response is not maintained on cessation of therapy, so again it is difficult to justify the use of this potentially toxic drug in this 'harmless' disease.

Topical tacrolimus (FK506) trials have shown encouraging results in rats and mice, but to date there are no double-blind, placebo-controlled trials, or indeed anecdotal evidence to suggest it is an effective treatment in humans.

By way of *camouflage*, many patients feel much happier wearing a wig. Both acrylic and real hair wigs are available. Tattooing (dermatography) of the eyebrows may lead to a more socially acceptable image for some patients.

SPECIFIC INVESTIGATIONS

- Consider complete blood count, thyroid function tests, serum vitamin B12 and autoantibodies as a screen for associated autoimmune conditions.

No routine investigation is normally necessary and the diagnosis is essentially clinical. However, in patients with symptoms or a family history of autoimmune diseases such as thyroiditis, pernicious anemia or Addison's disease, autoantibody screening and further investigation may be indicated.

FIRST LINE THERAPIES

■ Intralesional corticosteroids	A
■ Topical immunotherapy	A

A comparison of intralesional triamcinolone hexacetonide and triamcinolone acetonide in alopecia areata. Porter D, Burton J. Br J Dermatol 1971;85:272–3.

Tufts of hair grew in 33 of 34 sites injected with triamcinolone hexacetonide in 11 patients with AA, and in 16 of 25 sites injected with triamcinolone acetonide in 17 patients. Growth continued for 18 months, even in two patients in whom the alopecia had progressed over the rest of the scalp to AT.

Intralesional treatment of alopecia areata with triamcinolone acetonide by jet injector. Abell E, Munro DD. Br J Dermatol 1973;88:55–9.

A report of 84 patients treated with 0.1 mL needleless injections of triamcinolone acetonide 5 mg/mL and normal saline controls. After 6 weeks regrowth was observed in 86% of patients treated with triamcinolone and 7% of controls. Mild transient atrophy was frequently observed.

Diphencyprone in the treatment of alopecia areata. Happle R, Hausen BM, Weisner-Menzel L. Acta Derm Venereol 1983;63:49–52.

Twenty seven patients with AA (five patients) or AT (22 patients) were treated with DPCP on half of their scalp. Unilateral hair growth occurred in 23 cases.

Prognostic factors in the treatment of alopecia areata with diphenylcyclopropenone. Van der Steen PHM, Van Baar HMJ, Happle R, et al. J Am Acad Dermatol 1991;24:227–30.

A study with DPCP involving 139 patients, 85 of whom had greater than 90% scalp involvement, and 54 had 40–90% scalp involvement. Those with scalp involvement of 40–90% had a response rate of 75%, compared to a response rate of 40% for those with more extensive disease. Long duration of AA and nail changes also adversely affected prognosis. Atopy, age of onset, and sex did not influence the response rate.

The use of topical diphenylcyclopropenone for the treatment of extensive alopecia areata. Cotellessa C, Peris K, Caracciolo E, et al. J Am Acad Dermatol 2001;44:73–6.

Fifty six patients with chronic alopecia (mean duration 6 years) were treated on half of their scalp with DPCP – 42 had greater than 90% hair loss, 14 had 30–90% patchy alopecia. Of these, 52 completed the study, while four atopic patients withdrew due to development of widespread eczema; 25 (48%) achieved total regrowth at 6 months. An additional three (6%) responded after extending the treatment to 12 months. Fifteen maintained the regrowth after 6–18 months of follow-up. Five of the ten patients who relapsed achieved complete regrowth with a second course.

Predictive model for immunotherapy of alopecia areata with diphencyprone. Wiseman M, Shapiro J, MacDonald N, et al. Arch Dermatol 2001;137:1063–8.

A retrospective review of 148 patients with alopecia for a mean duration of 9.6 years (range 0.5 months to 55 years). Patients were treated on half of their scalp, and a response was defined as greater than 75% regrowth or a cosmetically acceptable result. Response rates were 22.5% at 6 months, 52.0% at 12 months, and 77.9% after 32 months. Disease severity was important, such that response rates were 100% in those with AA affecting 25–49% of their scalp, but only 17.8% in AT/AU. A relapse (defined as more than 25% hair loss) occurred in 62.9% of patients after 37 months of follow-up.

The response rates with severe alopecia are not ideal, and treatment may need to be prolonged before a response is seen. DPCP, however, still offers the best chance of success compared to other therapies, and has a good safety profile.

SECOND LINE THERAPIES

■ Topical corticosteroids	B
■ Topical minoxidil	B
■ Phototherapy	B
■ Anthralin/dithranol	C
■ Retinoic acid	E

Assay of 0.2% fluocinolone acetonide cream for alopecia areata and totalis. Pascher F, Kurtin S, Andrade R. Dermatologica 1970;141:193–202.

A placebo-controlled trial of 0.2% fluocinolone acetonide cream applied twice daily with night-time occlusion in 47 patients with AA and AT. Thirteen of these patients participated in a double-blind trial, which showed that the corticosteroid was superior to its vehicle in seven cases, but not in the other six. Continuous treatment for 3–4 months was necessary for hair regrowth to become evident. A satisfactory to excellent therapeutic response was obtained in 17 (61%) of 28 patients who completed 6 months of treatment and observation. Children (including those with AT) between ages 3 and 10 years showed a 100% response, those between 11 and 15 showed a 44% response, and patients between 16 and 50 years showed a 33% response. Duration of 1 year or less was associated with a 100% response, while a duration of 1.5–2 years was associated with a 57% response, 3–7 years with a 25% response and 8 years or greater with no response.

Randomized double-blind placebo-controlled trial in the treatment of alopecia areata with 0.25% desoximetasone cream. Charuwichitratana S, Wattanakrai P, Tanrattanakorn S. Arch Dermatol 2000;136:1276–7.

Seventy patients with patchy alopecia were enrolled in this placebo-controlled trial and 54 completed the study, with twice daily application of either active cream or placebo for 12 weeks. Fifteen of 26 in the active group, and 11 of 28 in the placebo group achieved a complete regrowth, which was not statistically significant. Nineteen nonresponders were then treated with intralesional triamcinolone, and 13 achieved complete regrowth.

Clobetasol propionate 0.05% under occlusion in the treatment of alopecia totalis/universalis. Tosti A, Piraccini B, Pazzaglia M, et al. J Am Acad Dermatol 2003;49:96–8.

Twenty eight patients with AT/AU of 3–12 years' duration, who had not responded to immunotherapy, were treated on half of their scalp with 2.5 g of clobetasol propionate under plastic film on six nights per week for 6 months. Regrowth started at 6–14 weeks, and eight patients (28.5%) achieved greater than 75% regrowth, which was then extended to the other side of the scalp. Eleven patients developed painful folliculitis, including five of the six patients who withdrew from the study. Serum and urine cortisol did not change. Three patients relapsed over the next 6 months despite further treatment.

Efficacy of betamethasone valerate foam formulation in comparison with betamethasone dipropionate lotion in the treatment of mild–moderate alopecia areata; a multicenter, prospective, randomized, controlled, investigator-blinded trial. Mancuso G, Balducci A, Casadio C, et al. Int J Dermatol 2003;42:572–5.

In this investigator-blinded study 61 patients with mild–moderate hair loss (<26%) were treated in parallel groups with twice daily application of foam or lotion for 12 weeks; 57 completed the trial. At week 20 more than 75% regrowth was achieved in 19 of the 31 patients treated with betamethasone valerate foam (61%), compared to eight out of 30 treated with betamethasone dipropionate lotion (27%), which was statistically significant. This study suggests foam may be preferable to lotion as a vehicle for corticosteroid application in scalp AA.

Alopecia areata treated with topical minoxidil. Fenton DA, Wilkinson JD. Br Med J 1983;287:1015–7.

A double-blind, crossover trial in which 30 subjects applied 1% minoxidil (lotion or ointment) and placebo twice daily, each for 3 months. By the end of the study 16 patients had grown cosmetically acceptable terminal hair, only one of them while on placebo.

Topical minoxidil for extended areate alopecia. Frentz G. Acta Derm Venereol 1985;65:172–5.

This was a double-blind, placebo-controlled, crossover trial in which 23 patients with severe alopecia applied 1% minoxidil lotion and placebo twice daily, each for 3 months. Thirteen subjects demonstrated some degree of regrowth on the active medication while none did so on placebo. The result was cosmetically satisfactory in only one case.

A trial of 1% minoxidil used topically for severe alopecia areata. Vesty JP, Savin JA. Acta Derm Venereol 1986;66: 179–80.

In this double-blind, placebo-controlled trial, 48 patients with severe AA, AT and AU were treated for 32 weeks. There was no significant difference in response between the minoxidil and placebo groups.

Topical minoxidil solution (1% and 5%) in the treatment of alopecia areata. Fiedler-Weiss VC. J Am Acad Dermatol 1987;16:745–8.

A total of 66 patients with greater than 75% scalp hair loss applied treatments twice daily. Terminal hair growth was seen in 38% of cases using 1% minoxidil versus 81% with 5% minoxidil. However, even in the high-dose group, only 6% showed a cosmetically acceptable response. Occlusion of the treated area with white petrolatum at night was necessary to achieve and maintain maximum results.

Alopecia areata: current therapy. Fiedler VC. J Invest Dermatol 1991;96(suppl):69S.

A double-blind study of 5% minoxidil, 0.05% betamethasone dipropionate, both treatments and placebo. After 16 weeks, terminal hair growth was present in 33% of patients on placebo, 55% on betamethasone dipropionate, 64% on minoxidil and 74% on the combined treatment. Quality of response was fair to good in 13, 22, 27 and 56%, respectively. (Subject numbers and statistical analysis were not reported.)

These results indicate a possible role for combination therapies in severe, recalcitrant AA. However a small study examining the combination of minoxidil with DPCP was less promising.

Treatment of chronic severe alopecia areata with topical diphenylcyclopropenone and 5% minoxidil: a clinical and immunopathologic evaluation. Shapiro J, Tan J, Ho V, Abbott F, Tron V. J Am Acad Dermatol 1993;29:729–35.

A group of 15 patients with severe AA was treated with DPCP and either 5% minoxidil lotion or vehicle. Although five patients responded to the DPCP, only two of these were receiving the minoxidil so the addition of the latter conferred no clear advantage.

PUVA treatment of alopecia totalis. Larko O, Swanbeck G. Acta Derm Venereol 1983;63:546–9.

Forty patients with AT were treated twice weekly with oral 8-MOP and whole body or local irradiation. Fourteen patients responded, of whom eight experienced complete remission. This latter group required a mean of 44.5 sessions and 431 J to achieve complete remission, which lasted for a median time of 10 weeks before relapse. Whole body treatment was not considered superior to local irradiation.

Treatment of alopecia areata with three different PUVA modalities. Lassus A, Eskelinen A, Johansson E. Photodermatol 1984;1:141–4.

Seventy six patients with severe AA were treated with local or oral 8-methoxypsoralen (8-MOP) and local or whole body UVA irradiations. In 43 cases (57%) a good-to-excellent result was obtained, with 20–40 treatments being sufficient in most cases. No particular treatment method was significantly superior. Patients with circumscribed or ophiasic alopecia responded better than patients with AT or AU. Disease duration, onset before the age of 20 years, and atopy were poor prognostic factors. A family history of AA did not affect the outcome. During a follow-up period of 6–68 months, 22 patients had a relapse.

The PUVA-turban as a new option of applying a dilute psoralen solution selectively to the scalp of patients with alopecia areata. Behrens-Williams SC, Leiter U, Schiener R, et al. J Am Acad Dermatol 2001;44:248–52.

Nine patients with severe, rapidly progressing, treatment-resistant AA were studied. Two had less than 30% scalp involvement, while the rest had greater than 30% involvement, including one with AT, and one with AU. Disease duration ranged from 5 weeks to 15 years. A cotton towel was soaked with an 8-MOP solution, and wrapped around the patient's head in a turban fashion for 20 minutes. This was directly followed by UVA radiation using a small UVA source with a curvilinear surface. Treatment sessions were 3 to 4 times per week for up to 24 weeks, with cumulative UVA doses of 60.9 to 178.2 J/cm^2, with single doses ranging from 0.3 to 8.0 J/cm^2. After 10 weeks there was greater than 75% regrowth in bald areas in six of the nine patients.

PUVA treatment of alopecia areata totalis and universalis: a retrospective study. Whitmont KJ, Cooper AJ. Australas J Dermatol 2003;44:106–9.

Patients were treated with oral (24 patients) or topical (two patients) 8-MOP and whole body irradiations. Eight of 15 patients with AT (53%), and six of 11 patients with AU (55%) achieved a complete response (>90% hair regrowth). Patients with a family history of AA were significantly less likely to have a positive response to PUVA than those with no family history. Sex, age at diagnosis and treatment, interval between diagnosis and treatment, and background of atopy were not significant determinants of outcome. The relapse rate was 21% within a long period of follow up (mean 5.2 years). Mean cumulative doses were high at 444 J/cm^2 for AT (average 88 sessions), and 593 J/cm^2 for AU (average 125 sessions).

Treatment of alopecia areata by anthralin-induced dermatitis. Schmoeckel C, Weissmann I, Plewig G, Braun-Falco O. Arch Dermatol 1979;115:1254–5.

Anthralin 0.2–0.8% was applied daily to maintain dermatitis over involved areas of the scalp. A cosmetically good result was seen in 18 of 24 cases of AA and two of eight patients with AT. Untreated 'control' sites did not regrow. Regrowth was first visible after 5–8 weeks.

Evaluation of anthralin in the treatment of alopecia areata. Fiedler-Weiss VC, Buys CM. Arch Dermatol 1987;123:1491–3.

In this study using 0.5% and 1.0% concentrations of anthralin, the mean time to response was 11 weeks and the mean time to cosmetic response was 23 weeks (range, 8–60 weeks). Cosmetic response was achieved in 29% (11/38) of patients with less than 75% scalp hair loss and in 20% (6/30) of patients with greater than 75% scalp hair loss. Even some patients with 100% scalp hair loss did obtain cosmetic results in this study. Approximately 75% of patients with cosmetic results maintained adequate hair growth with continued treatment.

Topical tretinoin as an adjunctive therapy with intralesional triamcinolone acetonide for alopecia areata. Clinical experience in northern Saudi Arabia. Kubeyinje EP, C'Mathur M. Int J Dermatol 1997;36:320.

In this open study 58 patients with mainly patchy alopecia were treated with monthly triamcinolone injections, and 28 patients also had daily application of 0.05% tretinoin cream. More than 90% regrowth was achieved in 66.7% of patients with triamcinolone alone, and in 85.7% of patients with both treatments. This was statistically significant.

Allergic and irritant contact dermatitis compared in the treatment of alopecia totalis and universalis. A comparison of the value of topical diphencyprone and tretinoin gel. Ashworth J, Tuyp E, Mackie RM. Br J Dermatol 1989;120:397–401.

Seventeen patients (eight with AT, nine with AU) were treated by maintaining on one side of the scalp an allergic contact dermatitis induced by DPCP, and on the other side an irritant contact dermatitis using tretinoin gel. After 20 weeks, treatment with tretinoin was stopped and DPCP was applied bilaterally for a further 10 weeks. Some patients improved on DPCP, but there was no response to the tretinoin.

THIRD LINE THERAPIES

■ Systemic corticosteroids	B
■ Systemic cyclosporine	C
■ Topical cyclosporine	E
■ Oral minoxidil	B
■ Inosine pranobex	B
■ Nitrogen mustard	C
■ Dermatography	B
■ Cryotherapy	B
■ Sulfasalazine	C
■ Photodynamic therapy	E
■ Excimer laser	E
■ Polarized infrared irradiation	D
■ Aromatherapy	B
■ Onion juice	C

Pulsed administration of corticosteroids in the treatment of alopecia areata. Sharma VK. Int J Dermatol 1996;35:133–6.

Thirty two patients with alopecia for a mean duration of 2.8 years were studied. Twenty seven patients (21 with extensive AA, one with AT, five with AU) received 300 mg prednisolone in one dose each month for up to 4 months, and eight patients were treated in the same way with pulses of 1 g. Fourteen patients out of 24 of those evaluated after 300 mg pulses showed complete or cosmetically acceptable hair growth. Response was evident on average after 2.4 months and was cosmetically acceptable at 4 months. Three out of 7 patients assessed after 1 g pulses had cosmetically acceptable hair growth at 6–9 months. Side effects were rare and mild.

Twice weekly 5 mg dexamethasone oral pulse in the treatment of extensive alopecia areata. Sharma VK, Gupta S. J Dermatol 1999;26:562–5.

Thirty two patients with AA, mean duration 4.2 years, were studied. Those above age 12 years received 5 mg dexamethasone oral pulses on 2 consecutive days every week. Three children received 2.5–3.5 mg. Patients who received treatment for a minimum of 12 weeks were evaluated for terminal hair growth – 75–95% regrowth was observed in 16 (63.3%) patients and 50–74% regrowth occurred in two cases. Less than 50% regrowth occurred in three cases, and six (20%) patients had no growth. Side effects were seen in eight patients, but were mild.

High-dose pulse corticosteroid therapy in the treatment of severe alopecia areata. Seiter S, Ugurel S, Tilgen W, et al. Dermatology 2001;202:230–4.

In this prospective open study 30 patients with greater than 30% hair loss were treated with intravenous methylprednisolone (8 mg/kg) on 3 consecutive days at 4 week intervals for three courses. Twelve of 18 AA patients achieved greater than 50% regrowth. None of four patients with AT, five with AU, or three with ophiasic AA responded. Ten patients retained the growth at 10 months' follow-up.

Oral cyclosporine for the treatment of alopecia areata. Gupta AK, Ellis CN, Cooper KD, et al. J Am Acad Dermatol 1990;22:242–50.

Six patients with alopecia were treated with oral cyclosporine, 6 mg/kg/day for 12 weeks. Two had AA, one had AT and three had AU. Hair regrowth in the scalp of all patients occurred within the second and fourth weeks of therapy, followed by hair regrowth of the face and other sites. Cosmetically acceptable terminal hair regrowth of the scalp occurred in three of six patients. In no case did this persist 3 months after stopping the drug.

Systemic cyclosporine and low dose prednisolone in the treatment of chronic severe alopecia areata: a clinical and immunopathologic evaluation. Shapiro J, Lui H, Tron V, Ho V. J Am Acad Dermatol 1997;36:114–7.

Eight patients with alopecia involving at least 95% of the scalp were treated with a combination of cyclosporine 5 mg/kg/day and prednisolone 5 mg/day. Only two patients demonstrated a cosmetically satisfactory response. The addition of low-dose prednisolone did not produce any obvious benefit.

Placebo-controlled trial of topical cyclosporin in alopecia areata. deProst Y, Teillac D, Paquez F, Carrugi L, et al. Lancet 1986;2:803–4.

Forty three patients with severe alopecia applied cyclosporine solution 100 mg/mL or placebo to their scalp once daily for 6 months. Small tufts of terminal hairs developed in seven patients using cyclosporine, but in none of the controls. Regrowth was 'mild' and never complete.

Topical cyclosporine A in alopecia areata. Gilhar A, Pillar T, Etzioni A. Acta Derm Venereol 1989;69:252–3.

Ten patients with severe alopecia showed no useful response to twice daily application of an oily solution of 10% cyclosporine for 12 months.

Is topical tacrolimus effective in alopecia areata universalis? Feldmann KA, Kunte C, Wollenberg A, Wolff H. Br J Dermatol 2002;147:1031–2.

None of five patients treated with 0.1% tacrolimus topically showed evidence of hair regrowth.

This study involved patients with extensive AA who had failed to respond to other therapies including DPCP. Trials are ongoing, but most anecdotal evidence suggests that topical tacrolimus is ineffective.

Evaluation of oral minoxidil in the treatment of alopecia areata. Fiedler-Weiss VC, Rumsfield J, Buys CM, et al. Arch Dermatol 1987;123:1488–90.

Sixty five patients with severe AA were treated with oral minoxidil, 5 mg twice daily. Cosmetic response was reported in 18% of the patients. The drug was well tolerated at this dose, provided that the recommended restriction on sodium intake (2 g daily) was observed. Higher sodium intake increased the risk of fluid retention.

A randomized double-blind study of inosiplex (Isoprinosine) therapy in patients with alopecia totalis. Galbraith GMP, Thiers BH, Jensen J, Hoeder F. J Am Acad Dermatol 1987;16:977–83.

Thirty-four patients were studied in this trial of crossover design comparing inosiplex 50 mg/kg/day for 20 weeks with placebo. Eleven were reported to develop some hair regrowth during the treatment phase although this was statistically of only marginal significance.

A parallel study of inosine pranobex, diphencyprone and both treatments combined in the treatment of alopecia totalis. Berth-Jones J, Hutchinson PE. Clin Exp Dermatol 1991;16:172–5.

Thirty three subjects with AT were randomized into three groups and treated with inosine pranobex 50 mg/kg/day, topical DPCP or both. There was no response to inosine pranobex in the 22 subjects who received this treatment.

Treatment of alopecia areata with topical nitrogen mustard. Arrazola JM, Sendagorta E, Harto A, Ledo A. Int J Dermatol 1985;9:608–10.

Cosmetically acceptable hair regrowth was seen in seven of 11 patients (including two of six with AT), after 4–8 weeks of self-treatment with mechlorethamine hydrochloride (nitrogen mustard) 0.2 mg/mL once daily. Two patients became sensitized and treatment was discontinued

Topical nitrogen mustard in the treatment of alopecia areata: a bilateral comparison study. Bernardo O, Tang L, Lui H, Shapiro J. J Am Acad Dermatol 2003;49:291–4.

In this half-head controlled study ten patients with AA for at least 1 year, and greater than 50% head involvement, applied nitrogen mustard three times weekly for 16 weeks. A significant change was seen in only in one patient, and another four patients did not complete the trial.

Dermatography as a new treatment for alopecia areata of the eyebrows. Van der Velden EM, Drost RHIM, Ijsselmuiden OE, et al. Int J Dermatol 1998;37:617–21.

Thirty three patients with AA of the eyebrows were treated with dermatography. The eyebrow areas were covered with a halftone pattern of tiny dots of color pigments, using a Van der Velden Derma-injector, without anesthesia. On average, two or three dermatography sessions of 1 h were required. The follow-up was 4 years. The results were excellent in 30 patients and good in three patients.

Effect of superficial hypothermic cryotherapy with liquid nitrogen on alopecia areata. Lei Y, Nie Y, Zhang JM, et al. Arch Dermatol 1991;127:1851–2.

Seventy two patients with AA involving greater than 25% of their scalp (disease duration 3 days to 15 years) were treated with liquid nitrogen on a cotton swab for 2–3 s on a double freeze–thaw cycle. This was repeated weekly for 4 weeks. Forty comparable controls were treated with glacial acetic acid in a bland emollient vehicle three times a day for 4 weeks. More than 60% regrowth occurred in 70 (97.2%) of the active group, compared to 14 (35%) of the controls.

Sulfasalazine for alopecia areata. Ellis CN, Brown MF, Voorhees JJ. J Am Acad Dermatol 2002;46:541–4.

In this series of 39 patients treated with sulfasalazine, 11 withdrew from treatment due to side effects and nine were lost to follow-up. Seven patients had cosmetically acceptable results. Based on the authors' experience, starting doses of 500 mg daily were suggested, increasing the dose steadily to achieve a dose of 3 g daily for at least 4 months. For an adequate trial of sulfasalazine, nonresponding patients should receive 4 g daily for at least 3 additional months.

Topical hematoporphyrin plus UVA for the treatment of alopecia areata. Monfrecola G, D'Anna F, Delfino M. Photodermatol 1987;4:305–6.

The authors reported coarse terminal hair regrowth in two patients with AA when 0.5% hematoporphyrin was applied three times a week for 2 h and followed by irradiation with light of 360–365 nm, 4 J/cm². The cumulative dose of UVA ranged from 96 to 120 J/cm². After 8–10 weeks, treated areas showed growth of fine vellus hair, and by 3–4 months they were replaced by coarse terminal hair. Control sites treated with placebo did not grow hair.

Topical photodynamic therapy with 5-aminolaevulinic acid does not induce hair regrowth in patients with extensive alopecia areata. Bissonnette R, Shapiro J, Zeng H, McLean DI, Lui H. Br J Dermatol 2000;143:1032–5.

This was a double-blind study of six patients with extensive AA. Topical 5-aminolevulinic acid (ALA) lotion at 5, 10 and 20%, as well as the vehicle lotion alone were applied separately to different scalp areas, followed 3 h later by exposure to red light. No significant hair growth was observed after 20 twice-weekly treatment sessions. A significant increase in erythema and pigmentation was observed for the three concentrations of ALA lotion versus the vehicle, implying that a phototoxic photodynamic therapy (PDT) effect was achieved in the skin.

Treatment of alopecia areata with the 308-nm xenon chloride excimer laser: case report of two successful treatments with the excimer laser. Gundogan C, Greve B, Raulin C. Lasers Surg Med 2004;34:86–90.

Two patients with a solitary patch of alopecia less than 3.5 cm² were treated with a 308 nm xenon chloride excimer laser (dosage 300–2300 mJ/cm² per session). After 11 and 12 sessions within a 9-week and 11-week period, the entire affected focus showed homogenous and thick regrowth. No relapse was observed during the follow-up period of 5 and 18 months.

Linear polarized infrared irradiation using Super Lizer is an effective treatment for multiple-type alopecia areata. Yamazaki M, Miura Y, Tsuboi R, Ogawa H. Int J Dermatol 2003;42:738–40.

Using a linear polarized light instrument 15 patients with patchy hair loss were topically irradiated with infrared radiation using the Super Lizer® for 3 min once every week or every 2 weeks. In seven cases regrowth occurred earlier in irradiated areas than in nonirradiated areas, while in the other eight regrowth was simultaneous.

Randomized trial of aromatherapy. Successful treatment for alopecia areata. Hay IC, Jamieson M, Ormerod AD. Arch Dermatol 1998;134:1349–52.

This is a randomized, double-blind, controlled trial. Eighty six patients were randomized into two groups. The active group massaged essential oils (thyme, rosemary, lavender and cedarwood) in a mixture of carrier oils (jojoba and grapeseed) into their scalp daily. The control group used only carrier oils for their massage, also daily. The results indicated that 19 (44%) of 43 patients in the active group showed improvement compared with six (15%) of 41 patients in the control group.

Perhaps the nicest smelling treatment!

Onion juice (*Allium cepa* L.), a new topical treatment for alopecia areata. Sharquie KE, Al-Obaidi HK. J Dermatol 2002;29:343–6.

Sixty two patients with patchy alopecia were randomized to either topical onion juice or tap water twice daily for 2 months. Mean duration of disease was 3 weeks and 2.7 weeks, respectively, and 43.4% and 73.3% in each group had a single patch. Twenty three of the 45 in the onion juice group completed the trial, with full regrowth occurring in 20.

In the tap-water treated-control group, two patients defaulted, and hair regrowth was apparent in only two of the remaining 15 patients at 8 weeks of treatment. Mild erythema occurred in 14 of the onion juice group.

Probably the worst smelling treatment!

Amyloidosis

Joshua M Levin, William D James

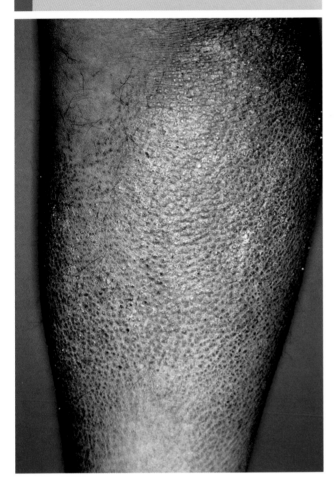

Amyloid is an altered, insoluble protein that can accumulate in one or many organs causing dysfunction. Amyloidosis encompasses several clinical subtypes, which are divided into systemic and localized forms. Systemic amyloidosis can be further subdivided into primary (AL), secondary (AA), or familial (AF). Cutaneous amyloidosis is one of the many localized forms of the disease.

MANAGEMENT STRATEGY

Of the systemic amyloidoses, AL most frequently involves the skin. Forty percent of patients present with skin lesions, the most common being purpura, which occurs in 15% of patients. It localizes preferentially to the orbital, umbilical, and anogenital regions, but may occur in any location as a result of minor trauma (i.e. pinch purpura). With systemic disease, amyloid deposition in the gastrointestinal, cardiac, neural, and renal tissues may lead to their dysfunction, necessitating treatment. AF and AA typically do not produce skin disease and are beyond the scope of this chapter.

Patients seek treatment for localized cutaneous amyloidosis to alleviate associated pruritus and the undesirable appearance of the lesions. Currently there are no accepted standard treatments that manage the various subtypes of cutaneous amyloidosis successfully. Although some small trials have been reported, many of the treatments discussed below are based on case reports.

Primary systemic amyloidosis

The prognosis for AL is very poor, with an overall median survival of approximately 2 years. Therapy is suboptimal and often mainly supportive. Cytotoxic chemotherapy is the first line of treatment, with the combination of *melphalan* and *prednisone* being the most common regimen. Other agents used include *vincristine, carmustine, cyclophosphamide, dexamethasone* and *interferon. Thalidomide, 4'-iodo-4'-deoxydoxorubicin* and *etanercept* are newer agents under investigation. Alternatives to chemotherapy, such as *colchicine* and *dimethylsulfoxide (DMSO)*, were used in the past but are now infrequently part of the management of AL. *Hematopoietic stem cell transplantation* has been associated with longer survival times than conventional chemotherapy, but those eligible for transplant are inherently low-risk patients, and the procedure carries significant morbidity and mortality.

Localized cutaneous amyloidosis

The purely cutaneous forms of amyloidosis are lichen, macular and nodular, with some being biphasic (combined lichen and macular). Lesions of localized cutaneous amyloidosis can produce considerable pruritus. *Intralesional* and *high-potency topical corticosteroids* may provide temporary relief to patients who suffer from this symptom.

Ultraviolet B light therapy (broadband) has been shown to be effective in treating the roughness and pruritus experienced in cutaneous amyloidosis. Remissions have been reported to last up to 6 months following therapy. Best results are reported with treatments three times per week. Treatments may be restarted, with the expectation of response, when symptoms recur.

An alternative approach to alleviate pruritus associated with localized disease is *naltrexone* at a dose of 50 mg once daily. A response may be seen within days of beginning the treatment, but recurrences are common after cessation of therapy.

Tacrolimus has been successful in resolving pruritus and decreasing plaque thickness in lichen amyloidosis. Results were seen after 2 weeks of 0.1% ointment twice daily.

Dermabrasion has been successful in patients with lichen and nodular amyloidosis. This treatment has been reported to alleviate pruritus and remove cosmetically undesirable lesions. For nodular amyloidosis, positive results have been reported for the CO_2 laser, the *pulsed dye laser* and the *neodymium:yttrium aluminum garnet (Nd:YAG) laser*.

Oral retinoids are another alternative treatment for lichen amyloidosis. Disappearance of pruritus has been noted after 2 weeks of acitretin therapy at 35 mg once daily.

Topical *psoralen plus UVA (PUVA)* has recently been shown to be beneficial in patients with lichen amyloidosis. Treatments three times per week improved pruritus and roughness over an 18-week trial period.

Topical DMSO has been reported to be beneficial for lichen and macular amyloidosis, but more recent data suggests a lack of effect.

SPECIFIC INVESTIGATIONS

- Skin biopsy
- Staining for amyloid deposits
- Demonstration of monoclonal light chain and immunohistochemical amyloid typing
- Cardiac, renal, gastrointestinal, neurological and liver evaluation
- Coagulopathy evaluation

All forms of amyloidosis have similar histological findings. On light microscopy, amyloid is characteristically a pink, amorphous material. Special stains, such as Congored and crystal violet, further support the diagnosis. Demonstration of monoclonal light chain by serum protein electrophoresis and immunofixation, and amyloid typing by immunohistochemical staining of tissues are valuable in the diagnosis and subclassification of systemic amyloidosis.

For systemic disease, cardiac evaluation is critical because the most common cause of death is from congestive heart failure or sudden cardiac death. In renal amyloidosis, glomerular pathology may lead to proteinuria, nephrotic syndrome and renal failure. Gastrointestinal deposition can lead to alternating diarrhea and obstruction; more proximal involvement manifests as macroglossia and decreased esophageal motility. Deposition of amyloid around nerves may cause autonomic or peripheral neuropathy. Coagulopathies may result from clotting factor deficiencies and impaired platelet function, and contribute to purpura formation.

The classification and typing of amyloid deposits. Gertz MA. Am J Clin Pathol 2004;121:787–9.

Immunohistochemical staining of tissues with κ and λ immunoglobulin light chains is specific for AL.

Primary systemic amyloidosis. Gertz MA, Rajkumar SV. Curr Treat Options Oncol 2002;3:261–71.

Echocardiography is routine in evaluating a patient with AL. Electrophysiological studies may also be warranted for possible implantable defibrillator insertion.

FIRST LINE THERAPIES

Primary systemic amyloidosis	
■ Melphalan and prednisone	B
Localized cutaneous amyloidosis	
Lichen and macular amyloidosis	
■ Topical high-strength corticosteroids with occlusion	E
Nodular amyloidosis	
■ Intralesional corticosteroids	E

Therapy for immunoglobulin light chain amyloidosis: the new and the old. Gertz MA, Lacy MQ, Dispenzieri A. Blood Rev 2004;18:17–37.

A crossover study, three-armed study, and randomized clinical trial are reviewed comparing melphalan, pred-

nisone, and colchicine in the treatment of primary systemic amyloidosis. All three studies demonstrate improved survival in melphalan-based therapy.

Intralesional, topical and occluded corticosteroids

No specific studies have been done to investigate the efficacy of intralesional and topical corticosteroids in cutaneous amyloidosis. However, it is a common practice to use corticosteroids in an attempt to decrease pruritus associated with various types of lesions.

SECOND LINE THERAPIES

Primary systemic amyloidosis	
■ Dexamethasone and interferon	D
Localized cutaneous amyloidosis	
Macular amyloidosis	
■ UVB	E
Lichen amyloidosis	
■ Dermabrasion	E
■ Tacrolimus	E
Nodular amyloidosis	
■ Excision, dermabrasion and laser (pulsed dye, Nd:YAG and CO_2)	E

Therapy for immunoglobulin light chain amyloidosis: the new and the old. Gertz MA, Lacy MQ, Dispenzieri A. Blood Rev 2004; 18:17–37.

Two case series are described with dexamethasone. Of nine patients treated with dexamethasone and interferon, eight showed improvement. Three of 25 patients who did not respond to melphalan and prednisone showed objective disease regression when treated with high-dose dexamethasone.

Macular amyloidosis: treatment with ultraviolet B. Hudson LD. Cutis 1986;38:61–2.

This case report demonstrates the ability of UVB to successfully decrease pruritus, with remission for 6 months following the cessation of therapy.

Dermabrasion for lichen amyloidosis: report of a long-term study. Wong CK, Li MW. Arch Dermatol 1982; 118:302–4.

Pruritus was fully alleviated in seven of seven patients.

Lichen amyloidosis improved by 0.1% topical tacrolimus. Castanedo-Cazares JP, Lepe V, Moncada B. Dermatology 2002;205:420–1.

One patient with clinical lichen amyloidosis was treated with tacrolimus 0.1% ointment twice daily. Resolution of pruritus was noted after 2 weeks of tacrolimus therapy, and marked improvement of plaque thickness was observed after 2 months.

The efficacy of dermabrasion in the treatment of nodular amyloidosis. Lien MH, Railan D, Nelson BR. J Am Acad Dermatol 1997;36:315–6.

One patient responded with no recurrence at 26 months of follow-up.

Evidence levels A Double-blind study **B** Clinical trial ≥ 20 subjects **C** Clinical trial < 20 subjects **D** Series ≥ 5 subjects **E** Anecdotal case reports

Nodular primary localized cutaneous amyloidosis: immunohistochemical evaluation and treatment with the carbon dioxide laser. Truhan AP, Garden JM, Roenigk HH. J Am Acad Dermatol 1986;14:1058–62.

A patient received two separate treatments at 3-month intervals. There was no recurrence in the treated area; however, an adjacent site showed a new nodular lesion 9 months following treatment.

Nodular amyloidosis treated with a pulsed dye laser. Alster TS, Manaloto RM. Dermatol Surg 1999;25:133–5.

The patient's nodules showed marked clinical improvement in size, color and pliability after pulsed dye laser therapy. This response continued for 6 months following cessation of treatment.

Treatment of lichen amyloidosis and disseminated superficial porokeratosis with frequency-doubled Q-switched Nd:YAG laser. Liu HT. Dermatol Surg 2000;10:958–62.

One patient with lichen amyloidosis treated with Nd:YAG laser achieved a long-term response.

THIRD LINE THERAPIES

Primary systemic amyloidosis	
■ 4'-Iodo-4'deoxydoxorubicin	B
Localized cutaneous amyloidosis	
Macular amyloidosis	
■ Naltrexone	E
Lichen amyloidosis	
■ Oral retinoids	E
■ UVB or PUVA	E
Lichen and macular amyloidosis	
■ Topical DMSO	D

Therapy for immunoglobulin light chain amyloidosis: the new and the old. Gertz MA, Lacy MQ, Dispenzieri A. Blood Rev 2004; 18:17–37.

A response rate of 15% was achieved in a study of 45 patients with AL given 4'-iodo-4' deoxydoxorubicin.

Efficacy and safety of naltrexone, an oral opiate receptor antagonist, in the treatment of pruritus in internal and dermatological diseases. Metze D, Reimann S, Beissert S, Luger T. J Am Acad Dermatol 1999;41:533–9.

One patient with macular amyloid was treated with naltrexone for 10 months and experienced alleviation of pruritus. Relapse occurred 4 months after cessation of therapy.

Widespread biphasic amyloidosis: response to acitretin. Hernander-Nunez A, Dauden E, Moreno de Vega MJ, et al. Clin Exp Dermatol 2001;26:256–9.

One patient with macular and lichen amyloidosis was treated with acitretin at 35 mg once daily. Pruritus completely resolved after 2 weeks of treatment, which was continued for 6 months. There was no recurrence during 6 months of follow-up.

Comparative study of phototherapy (UVB) vs. photochemotherapy (PUVA) vs. topical steroids in the treatment of primary cutaneous lichen amyloidosis. Jin AG, Ang P, Wee LK, et al. Photodermatol Photoimmunol Photomed 2001;17:42–3.

Prospective trial of 14 patients with lichen amyloidosis. Patients were treated with either UVB (n=9) or PUVA (n=5) to half of the body, applying potent topical corticosteroids to the other half as a control. After 8 weeks of treatment, patients treated with UVB had a significant improvement in average roughness of lesions compared to those treated with topical corticosteroids. UVB- and PUVA-treated lesions had a slightly greater improvement in pruritus when compared to those treated with topical corticosteroids, but this was not significantly different.

Lack of effect of dimethylsulphoxide in cutaneous amyloidosis. Pandhi R, Kaur I, Kumar B. J Dermatol Treat 2002; 13:11–14.

Twenty-five patients with lichen, macular, or biphasic amyloidosis were treated with topical DMSO in an open, prospective trial. A 27% decrease in the average severity of pruritus was noted – considerably less than in previous studies.

Androgenetic alopecia

Rodney Sinclair, Keng-Ee Thai

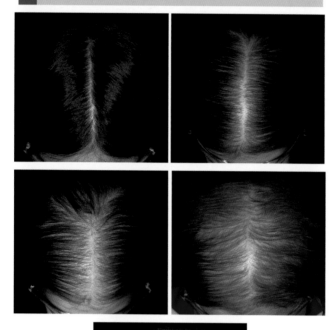

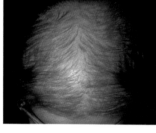

Androgenetic alopecia is a progressive patterned hair loss of the scalp that is sufficiently common to be considered a secondary sexual characteristic. Bitemporal hair loss occurs to some degree in almost all men, usually by the mid to late twenties. Patterned hair loss may also occur over the vertex and mid-frontal scalp. Women never develop vertex hair loss. Patterned hair loss in women occurs as a diffuse thinning over the mid-frontal scalp. Bitemporal hair loss also occurs in many women, but does not correlate in presence and severity with mid-frontal hair loss. A *polygenetically* inherited susceptibility is a prerequisite, and androgens initiate and perpetuate the hair loss. The key androgen in men appears to be dihydrotestosterone (DHT), and this is possibly also the key androgen in women. The effect of DHT on susceptible scalp follicles is to shorten the duration of the anagen growth phase and to miniaturize the dermal papilla and subsequently the entire follicle.

The images above show stages in the development of female pattern hair loss.

MANAGEMENT STRATEGY

Once an accurate diagnosis has been made, the primary aim of treatment of androgenetic alopecia is to *prevent further hair loss* and where possible, *stimulate hair regrowth*. Provision of emotional and social support is important while awaiting regrowth and when hair regrowth cannot be achieved.

For men the diagnosis is usually made clinically, but scalp biopsy may be useful in difficult cases, for example in a prepubertal boy who presents with a Ludwig pattern of hair loss. Women may present with increased hair shedding, or a diffuse reduction in hair volume most marked over the mid-frontal scalp or a combination of both. When women present with increased hair shedding and little or no reduction in hair volume, other differential diagnoses may need to be considered. Screening investigations including a scalp biopsy may be required to exclude other possible causes of hair loss, including chronic telogen effluvium.

Topical minoxidil acts by recruiting hairs into the anagen growth phase and by prolonging the duration of anagen – 1 mL is applied twice daily to the scalp; 2 and 5% solutions are available. The principle advantage of the 5% formulation is a more rapid onset of action. Treatment may be initiated with the 5% formulation and then changed to 2% after 6 months. Cessation of treatment results in loss of all new hairs.

Finasteride (1 mg daily) inhibits the synthesis of DHT. It has demonstrated efficacy only in men, and is a teratogen. In clinical trials, global scalp photography at 2 years indicates that one-third of men will have moderate or marked hair regrowth, one-third will have minimal regrowth, and one-third will have remained unchanged. Progression can only be seen in 1% with global photography, but hair count data show that 13% show some ongoing hair loss. Cessation of treatment will result in the resumption of hair loss.

Women may benefit from the androgen receptor antagonists *spironolactone* 200 mg daily or *cyproterone acetate*. Premenopausal women take 100 mg of cyproterone acetate daily for 10 days of each menstrual cycle, while postmenopausal women may use a continuous dose of cyproterone 50 mg daily. Both medications will prevent further hair loss in up to 90% of women. Regrowth may be seen in up to 40% after 1–2 years of treatment. Extreme caution should be taken with women of childbearing potential because spironolactone and cyproterone acetate are contraindicated in pregnancy because of the risk of feminizing a male fetus and hypospadias. These drugs should be ceased a few months prior to planned conception. As testosterone and DHT share a common androgen receptor, the receptor antagonists induce a chemical castration in men and are therefore not used.

Flutamide has been used for hirsutism, but liver toxicity and lack of demonstrated efficacy in androgenetic alopecia make it undesirable. *Scalp surgery* can be considered for advanced cases. *Excision of bald scalp with or without tissue expansion, scalp flaps,* and *various hair transplantation techniques* have all been used. For women, a diffuse pattern of loss as well as a poor donor population of unaffected hairs may make transplantation less rewarding, but newer techniques have improved the situation.

The effect of a combination of oral and topical therapies have not been formally studied, but appear to be additive. At all stages, *camouflage sprays* and *wigs* may be useful while awaiting adequate regrowth.

Standardized scalp photography 6–12-monthly is advantageous where available, in view of the slow natural history of androgenetic alopecia, the slow response to treatment, and the difficulty many patients experience with monitoring their treatment progress.

SPECIFIC INVESTIGATIONS

- Often none required
- Scalp biopsy
- Fe (iron) studies
- Serum electrolytes, urea and creatinine
- Thyroid function tests
- Androgen profile (if suspicious of virilization)
- Testosterone
- DHT (dihydrotestosterone)
- Sex hormone binding globulin
- Leuteinizing hormone
- Follicle stimulating hormone
- Antinuclear antibody
- Scalp photography

Scalp biopsy as a diagnostic and prognostic tool in androgenetic alopecia. Whiting DA. Dermatol Ther 1998; 8:24–33.

Scalp biopsy is useful in doubtful and undiagnosed cases of hair loss. Biopsies are also useful as predictors of possible regrowth in severe hair loss. A standardized 4 mm punch to the level of subcutaneous fat is required. Both horizontal and vertical sections are required for accurate diagnosis.

The reliability of horizontally sectioned scalp biopsies in the diagnosis of chronic diffuse telogen hair loss in women. Sinclair R, Jolley D, Mallari R, Magee J. J Am Acad Dermatol 2004;51:189–99.

Multiple scalp biopsy increases diagnostic accuracy. Androgenetic alopecia can be demonstrated in 60% of women who present with increased hair shedding, but little or no reduction in scalp hair volume. Biopsy is not required in women with diffuse loss of hair volume over the midfrontal scalp.

There is no clear association between low serum ferritin and chronic diffuse telogen hair loss. Sinclair R. Br J Dermatol 2002;147:982–4.

The role of routine measurement of serum iron and ferritin is controversial, as is the role of iron replacement therapy in the management of hair loss

Diffuse hair loss. Sinclair RD. Int J Dermatol 1999;38 (supp1):8–18.

Routinely investigating men is unnecessary. Routinely screening for thyroid abnormalities in women may be considered. Androgen assays should be reserved for those with clinical signs of hyperandrogenism. A drug history is important.

FIRST LINE THERAPIES

■ Topical minoxidil	A
■ Finasteride	A
■ Dutasteride	C
■ Spironolactone	B
■ Cyproterone acetate	B
■ Camouflage	D

Use of topical minoxidil in the treatment of male pattern baldness. Savin RC. J Am Acad Dermatol 1987;16:696–704.

Topical minoxidil arrested hair loss and promoted regrowth of hair in 90% of men; 60% had a medium to dense regrowth of hair.

A large placebo response here may indicate less than perfect tools for assessing hair loss and regrowth, and may lead to an overestimation of beneficial effect of topical minoxidil.

A randomized placebo-controlled trial of 5% and 2% topical minoxidil solutions in the treatment of female pattern hair loss. Lucky AW, Piacquadio DJ, Ditre CM, et al. J Am Acad Dermatol 2004;50:541–53.

Both 5% and 2% minoxidil solutions were superior to placebo after 48 weeks of treatment and were well tolerated. Minoxidil 5% solution was superior to 2% solution in terms of patient perception, but not in terms of nonvellus hair count or investigator-rated hair density.

Even though minoxidil was clearly superior to placebo a clear dose–response relationship was not found.

Use of finasteride in the treatment of men with androgenetic alopecia (male pattern hair loss). Shapiro J, Kaufman KD. J Investig Dermatol Symp Proc 2003;8:20–3.

Finasteride, a type-2 selective 5-α-reductase inhibitor decreases tissue and circulating levels of DHT by approximately 70%. Vertex hair loss is arrested in over 90% and around 66% experience regrowth to some degree after 2 years of continuous use, which is maintained over 5 years of use. In comparison, placebo patients were characterized by significant and progressive hair loss. In men with hair loss in the anterior/mid area of the scalp, finasteride 1 mg/day slowed hair loss and increased hair growth. After 1 year, about 50% of men noted improvement in the appearance of their hair, and 70% reported slowing of hair loss. Less than 2% reported sexual adverse effects in both groups.

The influence of finasteride on the development of prostate cancer. Thompson IM, Goodman PJ, Tangen CM, et al. N Engl J Med 2003;349:215–24.

The Prostate Cancer Prevention Trial was the first clinical trial to show that a direct intervention (5 mg of finasteride daily for 7 years) could reduce a man's risk of developing prostate cancer. Initial results also suggested that men taking finasteride had an increased risk of developing what appeared to be higher-grade disease (Gleason score 7–10). The person-years saved model shows that the administration of finasteride is likely to result in a net positive impact of finasteride on population mortality rates, even with an increase in the rate of high-grade prostate cancers.

Finasteride prevents or delays the appearance of prostate cancer, but this possible benefit and a reduced risk of urinary problems must be weighed against sexual side effects and the increased risk of high-grade prostate cancer.

Lack of efficacy of finasteride in postmenopausal women with androgenetic alopecia. Price VH, Roberts JL, Hordinsky M, et al. J Am Acad Dermatol. 2000;43:768–76.

After 1 year of therapy, there was no significant difference in the change in hair count between the finasteride and placebo groups. Both treatment groups had significant decreases in hair count in the frontal/parietal (anterior/mid) scalp during the 1-year study period. In postmenopausal women with androgenetic alopecia, finasteride 1 mg/day taken for 12 months did not increase hair growth or slow the progression of hair thinning.

Subsequent case series have shown anecdotal benefit in premenopausal women with hyperandrogenism

Marked suppression of dihydrotestosterone in men with benign prostatic hyperplasia by dutasteride, a dual 5-alpha-reductase inhibitor. Clark RV, Hermann DJ, Cunningham GR, et al. J Clin Endocrinol Metab 2004;89: 2179–84

5-α-reductase exists in two isoenzyme forms (types 1 and 2). DHT is associated with development of benign prostatic hyperplasia (BPH) as well as androgenetic alopecia, and reduction in its level with 5α-reductase inhibitors also improves the symptoms associated with BPH and reduces the risk of acute urinary retention and prostate surgery. Finasteride has been shown to decrease serum DHT by about 70%, while dutasteride, a combined type 1 and type 2 inhibitor decreases DHT by $98.4 \pm 1.2\%$ with 5 mg dutasteride and $94.7 \pm 3.3\%$ with 0.5 mg dutasteride ($p < 0.001$). Mean testosterone levels increased, but remained in the normal range for all treatment groups. Dutasteride appeared to be well tolerated with an adverse event profile similar to finasteride.

As the percentage reduction in DHT closely corresponds to clinical improvement in androgenetic alopecia, dutasteride is likely to be superior to finasteride, but phase III studies have not been performed to confirm this.

Treatment of female pattern hair loss with oral antiandrogens. Sinclair R, Wewerinke M, Jolley D. Br J Dermatol 2005; 152:466–73.

In this pilot study 80 women received either spironolactone 200 mg daily or cyproterone acetate 100 mg daily for 10 days per month for a minimum of 12 months. Hair loss was arrested in over 90%, and 40% demonstrated some degree of improved hair density as assessed by serial photography. No difference in response was seen between these two agents.

SECOND LINE THERAPIES

■ Scalp surgery or transplantation	C

Surgical approach to hair loss. Unger WP. In: Olsen EA, ed. Disorders of hair growth. Diagnosis and treatment. New York: McGraw-Hill; 1994:353–74.

A review of surgical treatments of androgenetic alopecia.

The interview: patient selection. Unger WP. In: Unger WP, ed. Hair transplantation. 3rd edn. New York: Marcel Bekker, Inc.; 1995:91–105.

Women with diffuse hair loss tend to lack adequate donor sites, and thus are unsuitable for hair transplantation.

Hair transplanting: an important but often forgotten treatment for female pattern hair loss. Unger WP, Unger RH. J Am Acad Dermatol 2003;49:853–60.

Grafting follicular units has resulted in improved outcome for women.

Evidence levels **A** Double-blind study **B** Clinical trial ≥ 20 subjects **C** Clinical trial < 20 subjects **D** Series ≥ 5 subjects **E** Anecdotal case reports

Angiokeratoma corporis diffusum

Analisa Vincent Halpern, Rhonda E Schnur

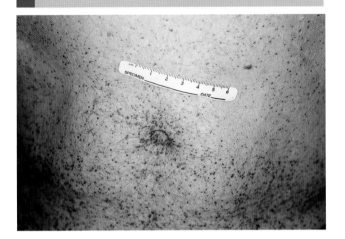

Angiokeratomas are hyperkeratotic, dark red to blue-black telangiectatic papules commonly associated with lysosomal storage diseases including Fabry disease, fucosidosis, sialidosis, aspartylglucosaminuria and β-galactosidase deficiency. This chapter focuses specifically on the treatment of angiokeratomas in the context of Fabry disease, an X-linked disorder caused by the deficiency or absence of the lysosomal enzyme α-galactosidase A (GLA). Systemic complications of Fabry disease include renal failure, cardiomyopathy, corneal opacities, hearing loss, gastrointestinal symptoms, and central nervous system manifestations secondary to deposition of glycosphingolipids in the vascular endothelia and perineural cells. Males are more severely affected, but female carriers may exhibit symptoms depending upon the pattern of X-inactivation. Single organ variants, with more residual enzyme activity than the classic disease have also been described. To date, more than 300 GLA mutations have been reported.

MANAGEMENT STRATEGY

Cutaneous manifestations of Fabry disease include angiokeratomas, hypohidrosis, pain crises, acroparesthesias, and lymphedema. Angiokeratomas increase in number and size over time. They cluster around the umbilicus, hips, thighs, buttocks and scrotum; mucosal involvement may also be seen. Lesions are usually bilateral and symmetric. The differential diagnosis of angiokeratoma includes malignant melanoma, angiokeratoma of Fordyce, angiokeratoma of Mibelli, and angiokeratoma circumscriptum. One should also consider blue rubber bleb nevus syndrome, hereditary hemorrhagic telangiectasia, cherry angiomas, and other lysosomal storage diseases.

Pain is the most debilitating cutaneous symptom of Fabry disease, typified by severe, burning, episodic pain crises of the palms and soles, and acroparesthesias, a constant tingling discomfort in the extremities. Pain crises are felt to result from glycolipid accumulation in the autonomic nervous system and vascular endothelium. A similar mech-

anism underlies Fabry-associated hypohidrosis, which is seen early in the disease process. *Carbamazepine, gabapentin, lamotrigine, tricyclic antidepressants,* and *diphenylhydantoin* are effective for analgesia. Gastrointestinal complications (diarrhea, abdominal discomfort, nausea and vomiting) have been treated with *metoclopramide* and *pancrealipase* with some success.

Traditionally, angiokeratomas have been treated with *surgical excision, electrocoagulation,* and *cryosurgery.* These procedures can be associated with pain, bleeding and scarring. Laser therapy is the treatment of choice for multiple angiokeratomas. Various lasers have been utilized, including the CO₂, argon, copper vapor, and flashlamp-pumped dye lasers. Copper vapor lasers are superior to argon because of their wavelength specificity for hemoglobin. However, the flashlamp-pumped dye laser may produce less pain and bleeding, a shorter healing time, and decreased risk of pigment changes and scarring. Local anesthetics are used when treating sensitive areas (e.g. penile skin). Because angiokeratomas are progressive, repeated treatments are often necessary.

Renal transplantation produces marked improvement of angiokeratomas, arrests the development of new lesions, relieves acroparesthesias, and may improve sweating ability. However, the long-term improvement of cutaneous lesions in these patients is unclear.

Enzyme replacement therapy (ERT) has revolutionized the treatment of Fabry disease. In 2003, the FDA approved *recombinant human α-galactosidase A (agalsidase beta).* Stage III clinical trials have proved that ERT not only halts progression of disease and pain crises, but may also reverse renal, cardiac, and cutaneous disease, including angiokeratomas. A second recombinant enzyme, *agalsidase alpha* shows similar efficacy in clinical trials and was approved in Europe in 2001.

Future options for treating Fabry disease include infusion therapy with chemical 'chaperones' such as galactose (which stabilizes residual GLA enzyme activity) and somatic gene therapy.

SPECIFIC INVESTIGATIONS

Diagnostic work-up
- Obtain family history
- Enzymatic assay of α-galactosidase A (males only; test not reliable in females)
- GLA DNA analysis (highest sensitivity)

Systemic work-up of patients with Fabry disease
- Renal function studies
- Cardiac evaluation including electrocardiogram, echocardiography
- Audiologic testing
- Periodic skin biopsy to monitor clearance of globotriaosylceramide during therapy
- Ophthalmologic evaluation (slit-lamp examination to screen for corneal opacity, lenticular changes)

The expanding clinical spectrum of Anderson-Fabry disease: a challenge to diagnosis in the novel era of enzyme replacement therapy. Hauser AC, Lorenz M, Sunder-Plassmann G. J Int Med 2004;255:629–36.

Review of the clinical manifestations in affected males and heterozygous females and atypical variants.

Fabry disease, an under-recognized multisystemic disorder: expert recommendations for diagnosis, management, and enzyme replacement therapy. Desnick RJ, Brady R, Barranger J, et al. Ann Intern Med 2003;138:338–46.

An expert panel reviews the signs and symptoms of the disease and offers recommendations for diagnosis, management and treatment.

Human Gene Mutation Database (HGMD): 2003 update. Stenson PD, Ball EV, Mort M, et al. Hum Mutat 2003; 21:577–81.

Over 300 mutations in the *GLA* gene have been identified. Mutation information is used for diagnosis, particularly in heterozygotes, prenatal testing, and correlation with clinical phenotypes.

Fabry disease. Desnick RJ, Astrin KH. GeneReviews@www.genetests.org. 2004.

An up-to-date review of Fabry disease.

FIRST LINE THERAPIES

■ Enzyme replacement therapy	A
■ Laser therapy	C
■ Surgical excision	D
■ Diphenylhydantoin	C
■ Gabapentin	C
■ Carbamazepine	C

Long-term safety and efficacy of enzyme replacement therapy for Fabry disease. Wilcox WR, Banikazemi M, Guffon N, et al. Am J Hum Genet 2004;75:65–74.

Latest data from phase III clinical trials of ERT after 30–36 months of treatment. ERT resulted in decreased plasma globotriaosylceramide (GL-3) levels and sustained endothelial GL-3 clearance with few adverse reactions and stabilized renal function.

Monitoring the 3-year efficacy of enzyme replacement therapy in Fabry disease by repeated skin biopsies. Thurberg BL, Randolph Byers H, Granter SR, et al. J Invest Dermatol 2004;122:900–8.

Long-term treatment with recombinant enzyme replacement may halt the progression of the cutaneous lesions in patients with Fabry disease. Periodic skin biopsy to assess the clearance of globotriaosylceramide in dermal tissues may serve as a reliable indicator of the efficacy of ERT.

Enzyme replacement therapy with agalsidase beta improves cardiac involvement in Fabry's disease. Spinelli L, Pisani A, Sabbatini M, et al. Clin Genet 2004;66:158–65.

Statistically significant reduction of left ventricular (LV) mass and amelioration of LV stiffness was seen in nine patients.

Enzyme replacement therapy with agalsidase beta in kidney transplant patients with Fabry disease: a pilot study. Mignani R, Panichi V, Giudicissi A, et al. Kidney Int 2004;65:1381–5.

In patients who were already treated with renal transplants, ERT was effective in treating extrarenal manifestations of Fabry disease while renal function remained stable.

Hearing loss in Fabry disease: the effect of agalsidase alfa replacement therapy. Hajioff D, Enever Y, Quiney R, et al. J Inherit Metab Dis 2003;26:787–94.

ERT given for 30 months resulted in significant improvement in high frequency sensorineural hearing loss.

Angiokeratomas in Fabry's disease and Fordyce's disease: successful treatment with copper vapour laser. Lapins J, Emtestam L, Marcusson JA. Acta Derm Venereol 1993; 73:133–5.

Angiokeratomas were undetected at 3-month follow-up; treated skin was smooth with minimal pigmentary alteration.

Successful treatment of angiokeratoma with potassium titanyl phosphate laser. Gorse SJ, James W, Murison MSC. Br J Derm 2004;150:620–1.

Excellent results were seen in two subjects with angiokeratomas.

Pathophysiology and assessment of neuropathic pain in Fabry disease. Schiffmann R, Scott LJC. Acta Paediatr Suppl 2002;439:48–52.

An excellent review of neuropathic pain and hypohidrosis in Fabry disease.

Use of gabapentin to reduce chronic neuropathic pain in Fabry disease. Ries M, Mengel E, Kutschke G, et al. J Inherit Metab Dis 2003;26:413–4.

Six patients with Fabry disease experienced decreased pain compared to baseline with few side effects after 4 weeks of treatment.

SECOND LINE THERAPIES

■ Renal transplantation/dialysis	C

Excellent outcome of renal transplantation in patients with Fabry's disease. Ojo A, Meier-Kriesche HU, Friedman G, et al. Transplantation 2000 15;69:2337–9.

Equivalent 5-year patient and graft survival in Fabry patients compared with 'controls' (non-Fabry patients with renal failure).

Chronic renal failure, dialysis, and renal transplantation in Anderson-Fabry disease. Sessa A, Meroni M, Battini G, et al. Semin Nephrol 2004;24:532–6.

Patients with Fabry disease who received dialysis had a better prognosis than diabetics, but clearly fared worse than uremic patients with other nephropathies. The outcome of renal transplantation is similar to that in other patients with end-stage renal disease. The recurrence of glycosphingolipid deposition in newly grafted kidney was previously reported by the authors.

THIRD LINE AND FUTURE THERAPIES

■ Galactose infusion therapy	E
■ Gene transfer	E

Evidence levels A Double-blind study **B** Clinical trial ≥ 20 subjects **C** Clinical trial < 20 subjects **D** Series ≥ 5 subjects **E** Anecdotal case reports

Improvement in cardiac function in the cardiac variant of Fabry's disease with galactose-infusion therapy. Frustaci A, Chimenti C, Ricci R, et al. N Engl J Med 2001 5;345:25–32.

A patient with severe cardiac-variant Fabry disease showed marked improvement in cardiac function at 2 years after galactose infusions. Galactose is thought to act as a reversible competitive inhibitor, a 'chemical chaperone', enhancing the stability of residual enzyme.

Long-term correction of globotriaosylceramide storage in Fabry mice by recombinant adeno-associated virus-mediated gene transfer. Park J, Murray GJ, Limaye A, et al. Proc Natl Acad Sci USA 2003;100:3450–4.

Enzyme expression, activity and levels of glycosphingo-lipid were measured in transgenic mice. Accumulation of globotriaosylceramide in hepatic, cardiac and splenic tissues was greatly reduced.

Angiolymphoid hyperplasia with eosinophilia

William Y M Tang, Loi Yuen Chan, Wing Yin Lam

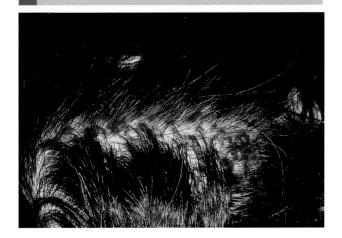

Angiolymphoid hyperplasia with eosinophilia (ALHE) is a benign vascular proliferation of unknown etiology with a characteristic component of epithelioid endothelial cells. It is a rare disease and data on its natural course, clinical outcome and treatment response are based on a small number of patients.

MANAGEMENT STRATEGY

ALHE commonly affects women in their third decade. It presents as cutaneous papules or subcutaneous nodules, sometimes with inflammatory features, on the head, neck and periauricular region. Involvement elsewhere is rare. Malignant transformation has not been observed. Although benign in nature, there may be disfigurement, bleeding and pain. Whether ALHE is a neoplastic or reactive condition is still in dispute. The coexistence of ALHE and lichen amyloidosis in a recent report implied that ALHE is an inflammatory disorder. The previous alleged overlap with Kimura's disease is incorrect: ALHE and Kimura's disease are separate clinicopathological entities.

Spontaneous resolution of ALHE has been reported by some authors. As ALHE has a benign and slow growing nature, initially conservative treatments and *clinical observation* may be appropriate. *Complete surgical excision* is preferred for persistent lesions. Recurrence may occur if excision is incomplete. *Electrosurgery* and *cryotherapy* are alternative surgical options. *Laser ablation* has successfully treated ALHE with minimal adverse effects. *Pulsed dye, argon, copper vapor* and *CO_2 lasers* each has its advocates. Other agents that have positive therapeutic effects include *topical and intralesional corticosteroids, pentoxifylline* (400 mg three times a day), *indomethacin farnesil* (400 mg twice a day), *interferon α-2b* and *oral retinoids*. *Oral corticosteroids, cancer chemotherapeutic drugs* and *radiotherapy* would seem appropriate only for severely disabling disease unresponsive to less toxic therapies.

SPECIFIC INVESTIGATIONS

- Histology
- Digital subtraction angiography
- Mast cell interleukin 5 (IL-5), vascular endothelial growth factor (VEGF)
- Renin, eosinophil cationic protein, IL-5
- Estrogen receptors and sex hormones

Angiolymphoid hyperplasia with eosinophilia associated with anomalous dilatation of occipital artery: IL-5 and VEGF expression of lesional mast cells. Aoki M, Kimura Y, Kusunoki T, et al. Arch Dermatol 2002;138:982–4.

There was an increased number of mast cells in ALHE lesions of a 30-year-old Japanese female. The mast cells also expressed IL-5 and VEGF. The authors suggested the possibility of mast cells influencing the angiogenic response and the eosinophilic infiltration in the skin lesion of ALHE.

Angiolymphoid hyperplasia with eosinophilia associated with arteriovenous malformation: a clinicopathological correlation with angiography and serial estimation of serum levels of renin, eosinophil cationic protein and interleukin 5. Onishi Y, Ohara K. Br J Dermatol 1999; 140:1153–6.

Digital subtraction angiography was used to evaluate the auricular lesion in a 31-year-old man. It showed feeding arteries, nidus, early venous filling and late-phase contrast pooling, features of an arteriovenous malformation. The serum levels of renin, eosinophil cationic protein and IL-5 are closely correlated with the clinical course. These findings, together with other reports revealing histological evidence of arteriovenous shunts and renin-containing cells in ALHE lesions, led to the suggestion that renin, through angiotensin II, contributed to endothelial proliferation in ALHE.

Estrogen receptors and the response to sex hormones in angiolymphoid hyperplasia with eosinophilia. Moy RL, Luftman DB, Nguyen QH, Amenta JS. Arch Dermatol 1992;128:825–8.

Two female patients showed lesion regression, one following cessation of oral contraception and the other after parturition. An increased level of estrogen and progesterone receptors was demonstrated in tumor specimens of the first patient, suggesting a hormone-responsive feature for ALHE.

FIRST LINE THERAPIES

■ Surgery	E
■ Corticosteroid, topical or intralesional	E
■ Cryotherapy	E
■ Electrosurgery	E

Angiolymphoid hyperplasia with eosinophilia and vascular tumors of the head and neck. Don DM, Ishiyama A, Johnstone AK, Fu YS, Abemayor E. Am J Otolaryngol 1996; 17:240–5.

A review of eight patients with confirmed ALHE showed that low-dose irradiation, intralesional corticosteroid and cryotherapy were not successful. The authors suggested that the preferred treatment is complete surgical extirpation. Recurrence is common when the lesions are inadequately excised.

Evidence levels A Double-blind study   B Clinical trial ≥ 20 subjects   C Clinical trial < 20 subjects   D Series ≥ 5 subjects   E Anecdotal case reports

Therapeutic problem. Angiolymphoid hyperplasia with eosinophilia. Bunse T, Kuhn A, Groth W, Mahrle G. Hautarzt 1993;44:225–8.

A 35-year-old female patient failed to respond to systemic treatment with γ-interferon and corticosteroids, intralesional injections of corticosteroids and argon laser therapy, but responded to electrocautery and remained symptom free for 1 year.

Angiolymphoid hyperplasia with eosinophilia. The disease and a comparison of treatment modalities. Baum EW, Sams WM Jr, Monheit GD. J Dermatol Surg Oncol 1982;8:966–70.

Three treatment modalities given to a patient with multiple scalp lesions were compared: intralesional injections of 5-fluorouracil, vinblastine or bleomycin; superficial excision and cryotherapy; and deep surgical excision. Intralesional injections gave no sign of improvement; superficial excision and cryotherapy produced temporary regression, but lesions recurred after 3 months; deep surgical excision resulted in complete resolution with no recurrence during the study period.

Treatment for multiple lesions of ALHE is difficult and recurrence is common. Radical surgical excision for a solitary lesion provides a high chance of cure.

SECOND LINE THERAPIES

■ Laser therapy	E
■ Pentoxifylline	E
■ Indomethacin farnesil	E
■ Isotretinoin	E

Eradication of angiolymphoid hyperplasia with eosinophilia by copper vapor laser. Fosko SW, Glaser DA, Rogers CJ. Arch Dermatol 2001;137: 863–5.

Two patients with ALHE were treated with copper vapor laser (578 nm) successfully. One showed gross clearing of lesions after five treatments and the other had improvement after three treatments.

Angiolymphoid hyperplasia with eosinophilia responsive to pulsed dye laser. Abrahamson TG, Davis DA. J Am Acad Dermatol 2003;49:S195–6.

A 41-year-old woman with ALHE over her right ear received four treatments with a 585 nm pulsed dye laser with a 5 mm spot size at energy densities 6.5–7.25 J/cm² at 6-week intervals showed clearing of lesions. There was no clinical recurrence at 7 months after the fourth treatment.

Angiolymphoid hyperplasia with eosinophilia successfully treated with the flash-lamp pulsed-dye laser. Papadavid E, Krausz T, Chu AC, Walker NP. Br J Dermatol 2000; 142:192–4.

Treatment with a 585 nm flashlamp pulsed dye laser with a spot size of 5 mm at energy densities 5–6 J/cm² was given at monthly intervals to an 8-year-old girl with lesions on her cheeks and periorbital areas. After two treatments over 70% clearance was obtained. There was mild treatment pain, bruising and postinflammatory hyperpigmentation. No recurrence was noted 2 years after completion of treatment.

Angiolymphoid hyperplasia with eosinophilia successfully treated with a long-pulsed tunable dye laser. Rohrer TE, Allan AE. Dermatol Surg 2000;26:211–4.

Long-pulsed tunable dye laser can be employed successfully to treat superficial lesions of ALHE, particularly in cosmetically sensitive areas. The lesions on the right temporal hairline of a 46-year-old female were treated with a single pass using a 7 mm spot size with a 1500 µs pulse duration, 595 nm, and 8.5 J/cm². The lesions flattened after the initial treatment and resolved after the second treatment given 2 months later. There was no scarring or recurrence noted in follow-up after 1 year.

Treatment using pulsed-dye laser is based on the principle of selective photothermolysis, causing destruction of blood vessels in the lesions. It appears that long-pulsed tunable dye laser, which can deliver a longer target wavelength with wider pulse duration, enables destruction of deeper and larger vessels and provides a higher chance of cure. Carbon dioxide and argon laser have also been used with success in treating ALHE. As the number of patients treated with laser is still small, further studies are required to clarify its therapeutic role in ALHE.

Angiolymphoid hyperplasia with eosinophilia may respond to pentoxifylline. Person JR. J Am Acad Dermatol 1994;31:117–8.

A 35-year-old female treated with pentoxifylline 400 mg three times a day improved after one week of commencing therapy but lesions recurred upon drug cessation. The proposed mechanism of action included inhibition of platelet aggregation causing decreased cytokine release and vascular proliferation.

Angiolymphoid hyperplasia with eosinophilia: successful treatment with indomethacin farnesil. Nomura K, Sasaki C, Murai T, et al. Br J Dermatol 1996;134:189–90.

Indomethacin farnesil, a prodrug of indomethacin given 400 mg twice a day, was reported to be effective in a 32-year-old pregnant female presenting with nodules on her right pre- and postauricular areas. Subjective reduction of itch was noted on the second day of therapy; this was followed by reduction of size and redness, and flattening of nodules. The mechanism of action is unknown, but may be related to prostaglandin metabolism.

Is angiolymphoid hyperplasia with eosinophilia a benign vascular tumor? A case improved with oral isotretinoin. Oh CW, Kim KH. Dermatology 1998;197:189–91.

The authors reported marked reduction of size and number of lesions in a 48-year-old woman treated with oral isotretinoin; however, lesions recurred after cessation of treatment.

THIRD LINE THERAPIES

■ Radiotherapy	E
■ Systemic corticosteroid	E
■ Chemotherapy	E
■ Cessation of estrogen	E

Angiolymphoid hyperplasia with eosinophilia of the nail bed and bone: successful treatment with radiation therapy. Conill C, Toscas I, Mascaro J Jr, et al. J Eur Acad Dermatol Venereol 2004;18:584–5.

The authors reported a 32-year-old Caucasian woman with multiple ALHE nodules involving the skin, subcutaneous tissue and bone of the distal phalanx of the fingers treated successfully with orthovoltage radiation therapy (40 Gy/20 fractions) and without any side effects after 9 years of follow-up.

Considering the benign nature of ALHE and potential carcinogenicity of radiotherapy, the latter should only be given when other treatment modalities have failed.

Angiolymphoid hyperplasia with eosinophilia associated with arteriovenous malformation: a clinicopathological correlation with angiography and serial estimation of serum levels of renin, eosinophil cationic protein and interleukin 5. Onishi Y, Ohara K. Br J Dermatol 1999; 140:1153–6.

The authors reported that systemic corticosteroids and local irradiation therapy produced only a temporary effect on the inflammatory changes of ALHE and recommended surgical resection as a curative treatment.

Treatment of angiolymphoid hyperplasia with eosinophilia. Bonnetblanc JM, Bernard P, Malinvaud G. J Am Acad Dermatol 1985;13:668–9.

Vincristine given in a weekly injection dose of 2 mg for a 59-year-old woman with ALHE and concurrent thrombocytopenic purpura produced flattening of lesions and a rise of platelet count. At one time, she was treated with prednisolone with an initial dose of 1 mg/kg per day; this resulted in normalization of platelet count but did not prevent the appearance of new lesions.

Systemic corticosteroids could be tried, but abrupt withdrawal could precipitate recurrence.

Estrogen receptors and the response to sex hormones in angiolymphoid hyperplasia with eosinophilia. Moy RL, Luftman DB, Nguyen QH, Amenta JS. Arch Dermatol 1992; 128:825–8.

Observation of two female patients with ALHE suggested a role for hyperestrogen states with the presence of hormonal receptors.

However, experience of successful treatment of ALHE using direct hormonal therapy on patients with ALHE has not yet been reported.

Evidence levels A Double-blind study **B** Clinical trial ≥ 20 subjects **C** Clinical trial < 20 subjects **D** Series ≥ 5 subjects **E** Anecdotal case reports

Anogenital warts

Brian Berman, Claudia C Ramirez

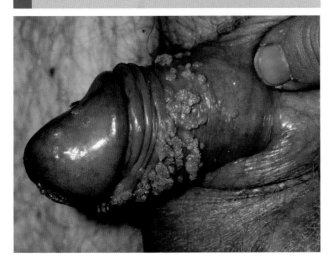

External anogenital warts develop on the skin and mucosal surfaces of the genitalia and perianal areas. They are caused by the human papillomavirus (HPV). At least 30 types of HPV can infect the genital tract. Condyloma acuminata, the classic form of anogenital warts, as well as the more difficult to detect anogenital flat condylomata, are most frequently associated with 'benign' HPV types 6 and 11, but may be caused by oncogenic HPV types.

MANAGEMENT STRATEGY

In most cases, genital warts are not life-threatening and may be asymptomatic. They are, however, cosmetically disfiguring, may be associated with physical discomfort, and can lead to psychological suffering from guilt, anger and doubts. If left untreated, genital warts may remain unchanged, increase in size or number, or resolve on their own.

Although many therapies used to treat genital warts have been available for decades, currently available treatments do not target the viral components of HPV during replication, but some may affect viral replication via cellular targets (*5-fluorouracil*). It appears that control of HPV is most likely mediated by the host's immunological reaction. The treatment of external genital warts should be guided by the preference of the patient, the available resources, and the experience of the healthcare provider.

The available treatments for external genital warts can be divided into two categories: patient applied and provider administered. The patient applied therapies include *podofilox 0.5% solution or gel* and *imiquimod 5% cream*. Podophyllotoxin requires twice daily application for 3 days, no treatment for 4 days, then repeat of this cycle 4–6 times as necessary. The total wart area should not exceed 10 cm², and the total volume of podofilox should not exceed 0.5 mL daily.

Imiquimod 5% cream stimulates the host's own immune response via cytokine induction (interferons, interleukin [IL]-1, IL-6, IL-8 and IL-12) and Langerhans cell activation to resolve genital HPV infection. Imiquimod is applied overnight, three times a week, for as long as 16 weeks. The treatment area should be washed with mild soap and water 6–10 h after the application.

The provider applied therapies for external genital warts include *cryotherapy, podophyllin resin 10–25%, podophyllotoxin, bichloroacetic acid (BCA)* or *trichloroacetic acid (TCA)*, and *surgical removal* either by tangential excision using a cold knife or scissors, curettage, or electrosurgery. CO₂ laser removal and intralesional interferon-α have also been reported as safe and effective therapies.

Cryotherapy kills the epidermal or epithelial cells capable of hosting HPV replication. Freezing with refrigerants like liquid nitrogen is usually continued until a frozen area larger than the diameter of the wart is formed, and often requires two to three sessions. However, HPV DNA is detectable up to 1 cm from the periphery of the visible wart, which may limit the practicality of destructive modalities.

Podophyllin resin is applied directly to affected areas in the office and is left on for 1–6 h. The strong resulting irritation means that the patient must wash the compound off after no more than 6 h. In addition, podophyllin is ineffective on relatively dry anogenital areas, including the penile shaft, scrotum and labia majora. Concerns over variability of potency from batch to batch of resin, stability of potency, and possible mutagenicity have led to reduced use of the resin and increased reliance upon purified podophyllotoxin.

A small amount of TCA or BCA can be applied to warts and allowed to dry. The application of these acids may be repeated weekly.

The CO₂ laser and surgery may be useful in the management of extensive warts or intraurethral warts and particularly in the treatment of recalcitrant warts. Phase III clinical trials are being conducted to determine the efficacy and tolerability of an HPV quadrivalent vaccine which includes 6, 11, 16 and 18 HPV strains.

Estimates of clearance and recurrence rates with various therapies are difficult due to differences in method of analysis, patient population, and duration of follow-up. Over the years many treatment modalities have emerged, but no single treatment has proved superior to the others. No available therapy can be guaranteed to clear genital warts without any recurrence. Combination therapy using an immunomodulator after a physical ablative therapy has shown to reduce the recurrence rates; however, the possibility of additive adverse events should be taken in consideration.

SPECIFIC INVESTIGATIONS

- Papanicolaou (Pap) smear
- Anoscopy with Pap smear for perianal warts
- HPV typing (not standard of care)

Carcinoma of the anal canal. Ryan DP, Compton CC, Mayer RJ. N Engl J Med 2000;342:792–800.

A good article delineating why anal squamous cell carcinoma is a sexually transmitted disease.

Papillomavirus and HPV typing. de Villiers EM. Clin Dermatol 1997;15:199–206.

Describes methods available for HPV identification as well as localization and type of lesion related to the identified HPV types.

Common association of HPV 2 with anogenital warts in prepubertal children. Handley J, Hanks E, Armstrong K, et al. Pediatr Dermatol 1997;14:339–43.

HPV typing was performed among 31 prepubertal children with anogenital warts. Data on mode of transmission were also collected. The most commonly detected strains were HPV 2 (42%), HPV 6 (22.6%), and HPV 11 (16.1%). Sexual abuse was found in two of 31 children (6.5%). HPV typing did not provide helpful information regarding actual mode of transmission of anogenital warts.

FIRST LINE THERAPIES

■ Imiquimod 5% cream	A
■ Podophyllotoxin (solution, cream or gel)	A
■ Podophyllin	B
■ Cryotherapy	B

Imiquimod, a patient-applied immune response modifier for treatment of external genital warts. Beutner KR, Tyring SK, Trofatter KF, et al. Antimicrob Agents Chemother 1998;42:789–94.

A prospective, multicenter, double-blind, randomized, vehicle controlled trial that evaluated the efficacy and safety of daily patient-applied imiquimod for up to 16 weeks. Baseline warts cleared from 52% of patients treated with 5% imiquimod cream, 14% of patients treated with 1% imiquimod cream, and 4% of vehicle-treated patients (p< 0.0001). The recurrence rate after a complete response was 19% in the 5% imiquimod cream group.

Patient-applied 5% imiquimod cream has a favorable safety profile and is effective for the treatment of external genital warts.

Self-administered topical 5% imiquimod cream for external anogenital warts. Edwards L, Ferenczy A, Eron L, et al. Arch Dermatol 1998;134:25–30.

A randomized, double-blind, placebo-controlled comparison that evaluated patients for clearance of their warts. Baseline warts cleared from 50% of patients treated with 5% imiquimod cream, 21% of those who received 1% imiquimod cream, and 11% of patients treated with vehicle cream. Of patients who received 5% imiquimod cream, 13% experienced a recurrence of at least one wart. Imiquimod 5% cream is a safe and effective self-administered therapy for external anogenital warts with a low recurrence rate when applied three times a week overnight for up to 16 weeks.

Patient-applied podofilox for treatment of genital warts. Beutner KR, Conant MA, Friedman-Kien AE, at al. Lancet 1989;1:831–4.

At the end of treatment, 73.6% of the original warts in podofilox-treated patients had resolved compared with only 8.3% of those in the placebo group. The recurrence rate of previously resolved warts was 34%. The safety of podofilox (class C) and imiquimod 5% (class B) during pregnancy has not been established.

Treatment of external genital warts: a randomized clinical trial comparing podophyllin, cryotherapy, and electrodesiccation. Stone KM, Becker TM, Hadgu A, Kraus SJ. Genitourin Med 1990;66:16–19.

Four hundred and fifty patients received up to six weekly treatments. Complete clearance was observed in 41% of patients treated with podophyllin, 79% of patients treated with cryotherapy, and 94% of patients treated with electrodesiccation. The 3-month clearance rates were 17, 55,

and 71% for podophyllin, cryotherapy, and electrodesiccation, respectively. Cryotherapy with liquid nitrogen or cryoprobe is used for patients who do not have extensive disease.

Cryotherapy is safe to use during pregnancy. Podophyllin, however, has been demonstrated to have systemic toxicity and may not be used in pregnant women. Additionally, unlike podofilox, podophyllin is not a standardized compound, and therefore the efficacy of different batches may vary greatly.

Cryotherapy versus podophyllin in the treatment of genital warts. Bashi SA. Int J Dermatol 1985;24:535–6.

Five hundred and seventy two patients were allocated to either podophyllin or cryotherapy for the treatment of their warts. At follow-up examination, the complete clearance rate was lower in the podophyllin-treated group versus the cryotherapy-treated group – 51 versus 79%. In addition, on the average, those treated with podophyllin required a greater number of treatments over a longer period of time than those treated with cryotherapy.

SECOND LINE THERAPIES

■ Surgical excision (with cold knife or scissors)	B
■ Electrodesiccation (see above)	B
■ Loop electrosurgical excisional procedure	B
■ CO$_2$ laser	C
■ TCA	B

Podophyllin versus scissor excision in the treatment of perianal condyloma acuminata. Khawaja HT. Br J Surg 1989;76:1067–8.

In this study of 37 patients, complete clearance of warts by scissor excision and podophyllin was comparable – 89 and 79%, respectively. At 42 weeks, however, 32% of patients were free of disease in the podophyllin group compared with 72% in the scissor excision group.

Comparison of podophyllin application with simple surgical excision in clearance and recurrence of perianal condyloma acuminata. Jensen SL. Lancet 1985;2:1146–8.

A randomized clinical study of 60 patients documenting complete clearance in 76.6% of podophyllin-treated patients compared with 93.3% of surgically treated patients. At 3 months, the cumulative recurrence rates were 43% for podophyllin and 18% for surgical excision.

The CO$_2$ laser for recurrent and therapy resistant condyloma acuminata. Kerbs HB, Wheelock JB. J Reprod Med 1985;30:489–92.

Of 48 patients, 79% were treated successfully with one-time laser ablation of the lesions.

Treating vaginal and external anogenital condylomas with electrosurgery vs. CO$_2$ laser ablation. Ferenczy A, Behelak Y, Haber G, et al. J Gynecol Surg 1995;148:9–12.

The efficacy and adverse effects of loop electrosurgical excision procedure (LEEP) are similar to those associated with laser ablation. If the loop electrode penetrates deep into the dermis bleeding and scarring may result.

Scarring of the penis can result in dysfunction, therefore most physicians prefer CO$_2$ laser ablation or cryotherapy for penile warts.

Evidence levels A Double-blind study B Clinical trial ≥ 20 subjects C Clinical trial < 20 subjects D Series ≥ 5 subjects E Anecdotal case reports

Treatment of external genital warts comparing cryotherapy and trichloroacetic acid. Abdullah AN, Walzman M, Wade A. Sex Transm Dis 1993;20:344–5.

A randomized clinical trial of 86 patients. After up to six treatments, complete clearance was noted in 86% of the cryotherapy-treated patients compared with 70% of the TCA-treated patients. Ulcerations at the site of application developed in 30% of the TCA-treated patients.

THIRD LINE THERAPIES

■ Intralesional interferon-α	A
■ Interferon gel	D
■ Oral isotretinoin	D
■ Intralesional fluorouracil/epinephrine gel	D
■ Cidofovir	D

Interferon therapy for condyloma acuminata. Eron LJ, Judson F, Tucker S, et al. N Engl J Med 1986;315:1059–64.

A randomized, double-blind trial to compare interferon α-2b with placebo in the treatment of condyloma acuminata. Interferon was an effective and fairly well tolerated therapy (complete clearance in 36% of warts treated with interferon).

Natural interferon alpha for treatment of condyloma acuminata. Friedman-Kien AE, Eron LJ, Conant M, et al. JAMA 1988;259:533–8.

Complete clearance was experienced by 62% of patients in the treatment group compared with 21% of patients in the placebo group. The results of combining interferon treatment with cryosurgery, podophyllin, or laser ablation have been promising.

Recombinant interferon beta gel as an adjuvant in the treatment of recurrent genital warts: results of a placebo-controlled double-blind study in 120 patients. Gross G, Rogozinski T, Schöfer H, et al. J Dermatology 1998;196: 330–4.

Topical application of recombinant interferon-β gel is safe and appeared to reduce recurrence of condyloma acuminata after surgical treatment.

Treatment of condyloma acuminata with oral isotretinoin. Tsambaos D, Georgiou S, Monastirli A, et al. J Urol 1997;158: 1810–2.

Oral isotretinoin may be considered an effective and fairly well tolerated alternative treatment for immature and small condyloma acuminata.

Intralesional fluorouracil/epinephrine injectable gel for the treatment of condyloma acuminata. A phase 3 clinical study. Swinehart JM, Sperling M, Phillips S, et al. Arch Dermatol 1997;133:67–73.

A randomized, double-blind, placebo controlled study to evaluate the safety and efficacy of this intralesional treatment; 401 patients were treated with either fluorouracil/ epinephrine (adrenaline) gel, fluorouracil gel alone, or placebo. Complete response rates were 61, 43, and 5%, respectively. Recurrence rates were between 50 and 60% for both treatment groups.

Intralesional or topical cidofovir (HPMPC, VISTIDE) for the treatment of recurrent genital warts in HIV-1-infected patients. Orlando G, Fasolo MM, Beretta R, et al. AIDS 1999; 13:1978–80.

Twelve HIV-positive patients with very extensive or relapsing warts were treated with either topical gel cidofovir alone or a combination of topical gel and intralesional cidofovir. Although the addition of intralesional cidofovir did not seem to affect the extent of the lesions, topical gel cidofovir appeared to flatten lesions in the ten evaluable patients. Four of the ten patients were completely cured. The effectiveness of the therapy seemed to be independent of the stage of HIV disease.

Antiphospholipid syndrome

Gillian E Gibson

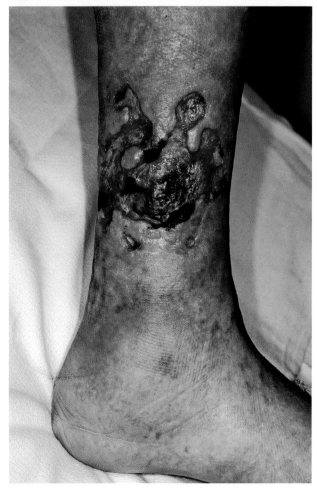

The antiphospholipid syndrome (APS) is an acquired multisystem disorder of hypercoagulation which may be primary or secondary to underlying disease (e.g. autoimmune disease, malignancy, infection, drugs). Clinical features include recurrent thrombotic events (arterial or venous), repeated fetal loss, and thrombocytopenia. Cutaneous manifestations may occur as the first sign of APS, and non-inflammatory thrombosis of dermal vessels is a common histopathologic finding.

MANAGEMENT STRATEGY

Asymptomatic patients with antiphospholipid antibodies and no history of thrombosis should be counselled like those with a history of thrombosis, to reduce other risk factors such as smoking, hypertension, hypercholesterolemia, and estrogen-containing contraceptive pills. At the present time, prophylactic anticoagulation is not recommended except at times of high risk, e.g. surgery. *Hydroxychloroquine* may be considered in patients with systemic lupus erythematosus (SLE) (may have intrinsic antithrombotic properties).

Treatment of a **thrombotic event** in patients with APS is the same as in patients without APS. *Intravenous monitored unfractionated or subcutaneous low-molecular-weight heparin* (LMWH) is followed by *warfarin* therapy, with a target international normalized ratio (INR) of 2.5 (optimal range 2.0–3.0). There is controversy over the need for more intensive anticoagulant therapy and the duration of anticoagulation. Three retrospective studies suggest an ongoing risk of thrombosis with an INR of less than 3.0. In one study, treatment with high-intensity warfarin (INR > 3.0) was more effective than low-intensity warfarin. However, bleeding risk was also increased. A more recent double-blind randomized trial showed that high-intensity warfarin therapy (INR 3.1–4.0) was not superior to moderate-intensity warfarin therapy (INR 2.0–3.0) for preventing recurrence of thrombosis. Intensity and duration of anticoagulation should be determined on an individual basis, taking into account other remediable risk factors, the severity of thrombosis (e.g. small or large vessel, venous or arterial, organ affected) and the risk of bleeding on warfarin, especially in the elderly patient. It is not known whether additional therapy with *aspirin* is efficacious in cerebral arterial thrombosis but the risk of hemorrhage is increased when used with oral anticoagulant therapy. *Thrombolytic therapy* (e.g. streptokinase, tissue plasminogen activator [tPA]) has been successfully used in some patients with APS.

The use of the activated partial thromboplastin time (APTT) to monitor unfractionated heparin may be difficult in the presence of a lupus anticoagulant (LAC). This can be circumvented by the use of an anti-Xa assay. There have also been concerns that the INR may be misleading due to the effect of the LAC on the prothrombin time. Current evidence suggests that the INR is reliable when thromboplastin with a low international sensitivity index and calibrated for the method and equipment utilized is used in the determination of the prothrombin time.

The risk of **recurrent thrombosis** in patients with APS is high. Recurrent thrombosis should be treated by *long-term anticoagulation*. Moderate-intensity warfarin therapy (INR 2.0–3.0) is appropriate. LMWH is an option for the secondary prevention of thrombosis in patients who have failed adequate warfarin doses. Some authors recommend long-term self-administration of subcutaneous porcine heparin or LMWH from the beginning. However, bone loss, which is related to duration of treatment, is a serious concern with long-term heparin use. In the Hopkins Lupus Cohort, SLE patients on *hydroxychloroquine* have been protected against future thrombotic events.

Antiphospholipid antibodies are associated with **recurrent miscarriage** in the first trimester and pregnancy loss during the second and third trimesters. Treatment with *low-dose aspirin* and *subcutaneous heparin* is recommended for women with a history of recurrent pregnancy loss. *Intravenous gammaglobulin* (IVIG) has a limited role but may sometimes be useful, especially if there is another indication, e.g. immune thrombocytopenia. The use of *corticosteroids* in pregnancy is associated with significant maternal and fetal morbidity, is usually ineffective, and is currently not recommended. Warfarin is avoided in pregnancy.

The **catastrophic antiphospholipid syndrome (CAPS)** is a rare, widespread, multiorgan failure due to small vessel vasculopathy, sometimes associated with large vessel occlusions. Mortality is 50%, usually due to cardiorespiratory failure. The most common precipitating factor is infection and this should be energetically treated. Treatments have included *intravenous heparin, fibrinolytics, plasmapheresis, fresh frozen plasma, high-dose intravenous corticosteroids, prostacyclin, cyclophosphamide,*

Evidence levels A Double-blind study B Clinical trial ≥ 20 subjects C Clinical trial < 20 subjects D Series ≥ 5 subjects E Anecdotal case reports

antibiotics, and *defibrotide*, a metallic salt of DNA with marked antithrombotic and fibrinolytic properties.

SPECIFIC INVESTIGATIONS

- Medication history
- Lupus anticoagulant and anticardiolipin antibodies
- Full thrombosis screen (activated protein C resistance, deficiencies of antithrombin III, protein C and protein S, prothrombin 20210 gene mutation, anti-prothrombin antibodies, homocysteine level)
- Connective tissue serology
- Hepatitis and HIV serology
- Complete blood count (CBC) and blood smear

Serologic markers for this syndrome are the LAC and anti-cardiolipin antibodies (ACA), one of which should be positive on more than one occasion at least 6 weeks apart. In a patient in whom clinical APS is suspected but LAC and ACA are negative, consider testing for antibodies to β_2-glycoprotein-1 and other related antibodies (to phosphatidylserine, phosphatidylcholine, phosphatidylglycerol, and phosphatidylinositol). In a patient with proteinuria, antibody testing in blood may be negative, but urine testing may be positive. Antibodies may not be detectable at the time of a thrombotic episode. Thus, if the clinical suspicion is high, retesting several weeks later is recommended.

In patients with APS, the other known causes of thrombophilia, congenital and acquired, are additional risk factors for thrombosis, and a full thrombosis screen (to include activated protein C resistance, deficiencies of antithrombin III, protein C, and protein S, prothrombin 20210 gene mutation, anti-prothrombin antibodies, and homocysteine level) is desirable.

Underlying disease associations should be sought (secondary APS) to facilitate appropriate treatment. An initial screen may include connective tissue serology, hepatitis and HIV serology, and CBC and blood smear.

The anti-phospholipid antibody syndrome: clinical and serological aspects. Alarcon-Segovia D, Cabral AR. Baillières Best Pract Res Clin Rheumatol 2000;14:139–50.

Good discussion on the various subgroups of antiphospholipid antibodies which may be important in the pathogenesis of APS.

Antiphospholipid antibodies and thrombosis. Greaves M. Lancet 1999;353:1348–53.

APS has protean clinical manifestations and associations, and this, along with the limitations of existing laboratory tests for antiphospholipids, can make diagnosis difficult.

Drugs associated with APS include hydralazine, procainimide, phenytoin, interferon, chlorpromazine, and quinidine.

Laboratory investigation of hypercoagulability. Francis JL. Semin Thromb Hemost 1998;24:111–26

An excellent review of the laboratory investigation of patients with thrombophilia.

FIRST LINE THERAPIES

- Address other modifiable risk factors for thrombosis   C
- Heparin followed by warfarin for acute thrombosis   C
- Thrombolytic therapy for acute thrombosis   E
- Long-term warfarin for recurrent thrombosis   A
- Low-dose aspirin and subcutaneous heparin for pregnant women with a history of recurrent miscarriage   B
- Corticosteroids for underlying autoimmune disease or associated autoimmune thrombocytopenia   D

Guidelines on the investigation and management of the antiphospholipid syndrome. Greaves M, Cohen H, Machin SJ, Mackie I. Br J Haematol 2000;109:704–15.

Guidelines prepared against a background of an improved understanding of the nature of antiphospholipid antibodies and the clinical course of APS.

A comparison of two intensities of warfarin for the prevention of recurrent thrombosis in patients with the antiphospholipid antibody syndrome. Crowther MA, Ginsberg JS, Julian J, et al. N Engl J Med 2003;349:1133–8.

A randomized double-blind trial with 114 patients followed for a mean of 2.7 years demonstrated a low rate of recurrent thrombosis in patients in whom the target INR was 2.0–3.0.

Randomised controlled trial of aspirin and aspirin plus heparin in pregnant women with recurrent miscarriage associated with phospholipid antibodies (or antiphospholipid antibodies). Rai R, Cohen H, Dave M, Regan L. BMJ 1997;314:253–7.

The rate of live births with low-dose aspirin and heparin was 71% (32/45 pregnancies) and 42% (19/45 pregnancies) with low-dose aspirin alone. Women randomly allocated aspirin and heparin had a median decrease in lumbar spine bone density of 5.4% (range 1.7–8.6%). The authors discuss that this degree of bone density loss is equivalent to that lost after 6 months of lactation and that osteopenia is reversible when heparin is stopped.

Systemic therapy with fibrinolytic agents and heparin for recalcitrant nonhealing cutaneous ulcers in the antiphospholipid syndrome. Gertner E, Lie JT. J Rheumatol 1994;21:2159–61.

One patient with a non-healing ulcer responded to heparin and low-dose tPA. Another patient responded to urokinase and heparin followed by tPA alone. When the latter patient's ulcer recurred, tPA plus heparin led to complete resolution.

The antiphospholipid syndrome: immunologic and clinical aspects. Clinical spectrum and treatment. Myones BL, McCurdy D. J Rheumatol Suppl 2000;58:20–8.

Corticosteroids are the treatment of choice for patients with autoimmune thrombocytopenia and APS. Other therapeutic interventions that have been used include IVIG, dapsone, chloroquine, cyclosporine, low-dose aspirin, and splenectomy.

SECOND LINE THERAPIES

■ Long-term LMWH for recurrent thrombosis	D
■ IVIG in APS pregnancy	C
■ IVIG for autoimmune thrombocytopenia	E
■ Hydroxychloroquine to prevent thrombosis in SLE	D

Antiphospholipid syndrome and thrombosis. Bick RL, Baker WF. Semin Thromb Hemost 1999;25:333–50.

These authors feel that LMWH and unfractionated heparin are the most effective therapies for secondary prevention of thrombosis in APS. They caution patients about heparin-induced thrombocytopenia, mild alopecia, mild allergic reactions, osteoporosis, benign transaminasemia, and benign eosinophilia. They monitor patients with weekly heparin levels (anti-Xa method) and CBC/platelet counts for the first month of therapy and monthly thereafter.

Intravenous immunoglobulin therapy of antiphospholipid syndrome. Sherer Y, Levy Y, Shoenfeld Y. Rheumatology (Oxford) 2000;39:421–6.

In several series, the use of IVIG, either solely or in combination with aspirin/heparin, resulted in a successful pregnancy outcome in the vast majority of patients with recurrent miscarriage. IVIG was also beneficial in antiphospholipid antibody-positive patients undergoing in-vitro fertilization.

Recurrent cerebral infarction and the antiphospholipid syndrome: effect of intravenous gammaglobulin in a patient with systemic lupus erythematosus. Sturfelt G, Mousa F, Jonsson H, et al. Ann Rheum Dis 1990;49:939–41.

Successful treatment of thrombocytopenia with IVIG after treatment failure with corticosteroids and cytostatic drugs.

Pathogenesis and treatment of the antiphospholipid antibody syndrome. Petri M. Med Clin North Am 1997;81: 151–77.

Hydroxychloroquine has been shown to decrease the titers of antiphospholipid antibodies and may protect against future thrombosis in patients with SLE.

CATASTROPHIC ANTIPHOSPHOLIPID SYNDROME

■ Plasmapheresis/fresh frozen plasma	D
■ High-dose intravenous corticosteroids	D
■ Cyclophosphamide	D
■ IVIG	D
■ Prostacyclin	E
■ Defibrotide	E

The catastrophic antiphospholipid syndrome: a review of pathogenesis, clinical features and treatment. Asherson RA, Cervera R. Isr Med Assoc J 2000;2:268–73.

The number of published (and unpublished cases) to date is almost 100.

Good review of hypotheses for pathogenesis, clinical manifestations, and treatments.

Catastrophic antiphospholipid syndrome. Clinical and laboratory features of 50 patients. Asherson RA, Cervera R, Piette JC, et al. Medicine (Baltimore) 1998;77:195–207.

A detailed review of 50 patients with CAPS, their clinical presentations and responses to varying treatments. Anticoagulation was used in 70%, steroids in 70%, plasmapheresis in 40%, cyclophosphamide in 34%, IVIG in 16%, and splenectomy in 4%. Most patients received a combination of nonsurgical therapies. Death occurred in 50%. Among the 20 patients who received the combination of anticoagulation, steroids, and plasmapheresis or IVIG, recovery occurred in 14 (70%).

Aphthous stomatitis

*Larisa Ravitskiy, Justin J Green,
Gary Goldenberg, Joseph L Jorizzo*

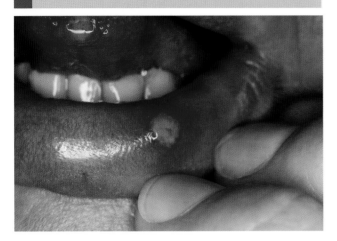

Recurrent aphthous stomatitis (RAS) is the most common cause of oral ulceration. It is characterized by the recurrence of one or more painful, sharply marginated ulcers with a fibrinous coating and an erythematous halo on non-keratinized, mobile oral mucosa. The three main types are minor, major, and herpetiform aphthae.

MANAGEMENT STRATEGY

The therapeutic approach to aphthae is dependent upon frequency of recurrence, duration and severity of symptoms. In addition, hematologic, viral and systemic factors may direct appropriate therapy.

Because there is no definitive treatment, the emphasis is on measures that may afford symptomatic relief. These include application of *topical anesthetics* such as *lidocaine*, *dyclonine* or *benzocaine*. Patients must avoid desensitization of the entire oral vault, which may lead to self-induced trauma. A compounded *anesthetic mouthwash* (aluminum hydroxide-magnesium hydroxide, diphenhydramine, and lidocaine) has better mucosal adhesiveness. *Systemic non-steroidal anti-inflammatory drugs (NSAIDs)*, narcotics, sucralfate suspension, 0.2% *chlorhexidine gluconate* mouthwash, *tetracycline* suspension 250 mg/5 mL, and *amlexanox* 5% oral paste may reduce healing time and provide pain relief, although these are less effective than potent topical corticosteroids. Bioadhesive *2-octyl cyanoacrylate* forms a protective film and decreases healing time.

Topical corticosteroids are the mainstay of therapy. For milder disease, intermediate strength corticosteroids such as *fluocinonide* are used. Potent corticosteroids such as *clobetasol* or *halobetasol* are appropriate for more severe episodes. Applications can be as frequent as five to ten times daily. Gel or ointment formulations are preferable. These can be applied in equal parts with an occlusive dressing such as Orabase® for better adherence. Drug delivery can be enhanced with cotton-tip applications for 30 s and avoidance of eating and drinking for 30 min after application. Initial concentrations of 5–10 mg/mL and up to 40 mg/mL

of *intralesional triamcinolone acetonide* are helpful for major aphthae. Repeat injections over 2–4-week intervals are advised. *Dexamethasone elixir* 0.5 mg/5 mL three times daily used as a mouthwash or *beclomethasone dipropionate* aerosol spray can target ulcers on the soft palate or oropharynx.

RAS that elicits severe pain may require intermittent *systemic corticosteroid therapy*. Prednisone can be given 40–60 mg daily with a 2-week taper or as 'burst therapy' for shorter periods. Concomitant therapy with topical corticosteroids may be helpful. *Colchicine* 0.6 mg two to three times daily and *thalidomide* 100–200 mg daily are the most effective steroid-sparing agents. *Dapsone* 100 mg daily, *pentoxifylline* 400 mg three times daily, and *levamisole* 50 mg three times daily for 3 days every 2 weeks may also lead to suppression of aphthae. *Anti-tumor necrosis factor (TNF)-α* therapies are efficacious in recalcitrant cases. Those patients who require suppressive therapy, but cannot tolerate the side effects of systemic agents can try medications such as *topical cyclosporine* rinse 500 mg/5 mL three times daily or *interferon-alfa-2a* 1200 IU daily as a 1 min rinse and swallow.

Trigger avoidance is key. Predisposing factors include food (nuts, chocolate, tomatoes, and spices), trauma, menstruation or stress. A *food diary* may be of value in identification of an offending agent. *Hormonal therapy* may alleviate RAS associated with menstruation.

SPECIFIC INVESTIGATIONS

- Complete blood count
- Vitamin B1, B2, B6 and B12, folate, zinc, and iron levels
- Culture/polymerase chain reaction of aphthae to exclude herpes simplex virus (HSV)

Recurrent aphthous stomatitis: an update. Ship JA. Oral Surg Oral Med Oral Pathol Oral Radiol Endod 1996; 81:141–7.

Systemic factors associated with recurrent aphthae include Behçet's disease, cyclic neutropenia, mouth and genital ulcers with inflamed cartilage (MAGIC syndrome), inflammatory bowel disease, celiac disease, and HIV infection. Local factors such as trauma and food allergies may also cause aphthae.

HSV infection may simulate recurrent aphthous stomatitis, but frequently involves keratinized attached mucosa. In patients with HIV infection, one should consider other viruses, fungi, acid-fast bacilli, and neoplasia in the differential diagnosis.

Recurrent aphthous stomatitis. Ship JA, Chavez EM, Doerr PA, et al. Quintessence Int 2000;31:95–112.

Causes of RAS are unknown, but local and systemic conditions, genetic, immunologic, and infectious microbial factors all have been identified as potential etiopathogenic agents.

Effects of zinc treatment in patients with recurrent aphthous stomatitis. Orbak R, Cicek Y, Tezel A, Dogru Y. Dent Materials J 2003;22:21–9.

Of 40 patients, 42.5% had reduced serum zinc levels. An open trial of 220 mg zinc sulfate daily for 1 month resulted in an 80–100% reduction in the frequency of episodes.

Celiac disease in patients having recurrent aphthous stomatitis. Aydemir S, Tekin NS, Aktunc E, et al. Gastroenterol 2004;15:192–5.

Of the forty-one patients with RAS studied, two (4.8%) were diagnosed with celiac disease. In serum samples of both patients, antibodies to gliadin IgA and antibodies to endomysium were found to be positive. Antibodies to gliadin IgG were positive in only one of these two patients. None of the 49 patients in the control group were diagnosed as having celiac disease.

Serum iron, ferritin, folic acid, and vitamin B12 levels in recurrent aphthous stomatitis. Piskin S, Sayan C, Durukan N, Senol M. J Eur Acad Dermatol Venereol 2002; 16:66–7.

Serum iron, ferritin, folic acid and vitamin B12 levels were investigated in 35 patients with RAS and in 26 healthy controls. Vitamin B12 levels were found significantly lower in subjects with RAS than in controls. No significant differences were found in other parameters.

In another study, vitamin B12, iron and folate were deficient in 17.7% of patients with RAS.

Oxidant/antioxidant status in patients with recurrent aphthous stomatitis. Cimen MY, Kaya TI, Eskandari G, et al. Clin Exp Dermatol 2003;28:647–50.

In twenty-two patients with RAS and 23 healthy controls, superoxide dismutase, glutathione peroxidase (GSHPx), and catalase (CAT) activities, and malondialdehyde (MDA) and antioxidant potential (AOP) levels were measured in plasma and erythrocytes. Decreased CAT and GSHPx activities and AOP levels in the erythrocytes, and decreased AOP and increased MDA plasma levels were found in patients with RAS in comparison with control subjects.

Recurrent aphthous ulceration: vitamin B1, B2, and B6 status and response to replacement therapy. Nolan A, McIntosh WB, Allam BF, Lamey P-J. J Oral Pathol Med 1991;20:389–91.

Seventeen of 60 (28.2%) patients with RAS were deficient in one or more of these B vitamins. Significant sustained improvement occurred in those patients with vitamin B deficiencies who received replacement compared to patients without documented deficiencies.

FIRST LINE THERAPIES

■ Vitamin and mineral deficiency replacement	B
■ Topical corticosteroids	A
■ Intralesional corticosteroids	B
■ Amlexanox	A
■ Tetracycline	A
■ Antimicrobial mouth rinses	A
■ Sucralfate	A
■ Hydroxypropyl cellulose/carboxymethylcellulose	C

The treatment of oral aphthous ulcerations or erosive lichen planus with topical clobetasol propionate in three preparations: a clinical and pilot study on 54 patients. Muzio LL, della Valle A, Mignogna MD, et al. J Oral Pathol Med 2001;30:611–7.

In this double-blind study, topical clobetasol in adhesive denture paste significantly reduced healing time vs clobetasol in Orabase® or clobetasol alone.

A controlled clinical trial of the efficacy of topically applied fluocinonide in the treatment of recurrent aphthous ulceration. Pimlott SJ, Walker DM. Br Dent J 1983; 154:174–7.

In a single-blind clinical trial fluocinonide 0.05% ointment in Orabase® applied up to 5 times daily was more effective than Orabase® alone in reducing the duration of ulcers and increasing the number of ulcer-free days.

In some countries, triamcinolone in Orabase® is more readily available.

Topical triamcinolone acetonide in recurrent aphthous stomatitis. Browne RM, Fox EC, Anderson RJ. Lancet 1968; 1:565–7.

Twenty-six patients underwent a double blind study in which triamcinolone acetonide 0.1% in Orabase was compared to Orabase alone and aqueous triamcinolone alone. Subjective and objective improvement was best in the triamcinolone with Orabase group.

Treatment of aphthous ulcers in AIDS patients. Friedman M, Brenski A, Taylor L. Laryngoscope 1994; 104:566–70.

Intralesional triamcinolone acetonide 40 mg/mL was used in patients with AIDS with major aphthae that were present for at least 2 weeks and culture-negative for bacteria, viruses, fungi or acid-fast bacilli. Quantities of 0.5–1.0 mL were administered every 2 weeks. Pain relief was achieved within 2 days in 94% patients. One half of affected patients had complete resolution after one injection.

5% Amlexanox oral paste, a new treatment for recurrent minor aphthous ulcers. Khandwala A, Van Inwegan RG, Alfano MC. Oral Surg Oral Med Oral Pathol 1997;83: 222–30.

Amlexanox 5% oral paste applied four times daily was studied in four randomized, controlled, double-blind trials involving 1335 patients with minor aphthae. Significant acceleration in healing of ulcers and reduction in pain were achieved with amlexanox therapy.

Amlexanox oral paste: a novel treatment that accelerates the healing of aphthous ulcers. Binnie WH, Curro FA, Khandwala A, Van Inwegan RG. Compend Contin Educ Dent 1997;18:1116–8, 1120–2, 1124 passim.

In 3 controlled clinical studies that evaluated 1124 immunocompetent patients with mild to moderate aphthous ulcers, 5% amlexanox oral paste was shown to accelerate healing of these ulcers.

Double-blind trial of tetracycline in recurrent aphthous ulceration. Graykowski EA, Kingman A. J Oral Pathol 1978; 7:376–82.

A combined use of tetracycline suspension 250 mg/5 mL was used four times daily in patients with RAS. The suspension was held in the mouth for 2 min then swallowed. This study found that tetracycline therapy significantly reduced ulcer duration, size and pain, but did not alter the recurrence rate.

Other studies using tetracycline or its derivatives (topically or orally) have drawn similar conclusions.

Chlorhexidine gluconate mouthwash in the management of minor aphthous ulceration: a double-blind, placebo controlled cross-over trial. Hunter L, Addy M. Br Dent J 1987;162:106–10.

This crossover study included 38 patients who used 0.2% chlorhexidine gluconate mouthwash three times daily for 6 weeks. The total number of days with ulcers was significantly reduced, and the interval between successive ulcers was increased.

Gel and mouthwash formulations of 0.1% chlorhexidine have also been efficacious. Chlorhexidine mouthwash is not associated with systemic side effects.

Effect of an antimicrobial mouthrinse on recurrent aphthous ulcerations. Meiller TF, Kutcher MJ, Overholser CD, et al. Oral Surg Oral Med Oral Pathol 1991;72:425–9.

A 6-month double-blind study compared Listerine® antiseptic and a hydroalcoholic control used as a vigorous mouthrinse twice daily. The duration of ulcers and pain severity were significantly reduced in the Listerine® group. Both the Listerine® and the control group experienced a decreased incidence of ulcers.

Use of proprietary agents to relieve recurrent aphthous stomatitis. Edres MAG, Scully C, Gelbier M. Br Dent J 1997;182:144–6.

Retrospective, subjective opinions were taken from 50 patients with aphthae. Of the ten most frequently used products in this patient population, benzydamine hydrochloride and chlorhexidine gluconate were the most effective.

No significant differences in efficacy have been shown in a trial comparing 0.15% benzydamine hydrochloride, 0.2% aqueous chlorhexidine gluconate, and an alcohol placebo used as mouthwashes.

Sucralfate suspension as a treatment of recurrent aphthous stomatitis. Rattan J, Schneider M, Arber N, et al. J Int Med 1994;236:341–3.

Sucralfate applied four times daily to ulcers was found to be superior to antacid (aluminum hydroxide and magnesium hydroxide) and placebo with regard to duration of pain, reduction in healing time, response to first treatment, and duration of remission. The 2-year prospective, randomized, double-blind, placebo-controlled, crossover trial included 21 patients unresponsive to conventional therapy.

A randomized, placebo-controlled, double-blind study of sucralfate applied four times daily to oral and genital ulcerations of Behçet's disease resulted in decreased frequency, healing time and pain in oral ulcerations, and decreased healing time and pain in genital ulcerations.

Performance of a hydroxypropyl cellulose film former in normal and ulcerated mucosa. Rodu B, Russell CM. Oral Surg Oral Med Oral Pathol 1988;65:699–703.

Zilactin, which contains hydroxypropyl cellulose, led to pain relief after an acidic challenge followed by rechallenge.

Orabase®, which contains carboxymethylcellulose, has been beneficial in trials when combined with topical corticosteroids, possibly due to its adhesive properties.

SECOND LINE THERAPIES

■ Oral corticosteroids	C
■ Colchicine	B
■ Thalidomide	A

Clinical, historic, and therapeutic features of aphthous stomatitis: literature review and open trial employing steroids. Vincent SD, Lilly GE. Oral Surg Oral Med Oral Pathol 1992;74:79–86.

'Burst therapy' with prednisone 40 mg once daily for 5 days, followed by 20 mg every other day for 1 week in addition to topical triamcinolone acetonide 0.1% or 0.2% four times daily led to complete or partial control of aphthae in 12 of 13 patients.

Prevention of recurrent aphthous stomatitis with colchicine: an open trial. Katz J, Langevitz P, Shemer J, et al. J Am Acad Dermatol 1994;31:459–61.

Twenty patients with RAS were studied in a 4 month open, prospective trial. During therapy with colchicine 0.5 mg three times daily, the mean aphthae count and the mean pain score decreased by 71 and 77%, respectively.

Colchicine has demonstrated efficacy in a double-blinded trial in Behçet's disease, and some clinicians regard recurrent aphthous stomatitis as an incomplete form of Behçet's disease.

Crossover study of thalidomide vs placebo in severe recurrent aphthous stomatitis. Revuz J, Guillaume JC, Janier M, et al. Arch Dermatol 1990;126:923–7.

A multicenter crossover randomized, double-blind trial of thalidomide 100 mg daily versus placebo led to complete remissions in 32 of 67 (48%) patients treated with thalidomide and in 6 of 67 (9%) patients treated with placebo. Side effects, which included drowsiness, constipation, headache, vertigo and neuropathy, resulted in treatment interruptions in 11 patients.

Similar complete remission rates were seen in a double-blind, placebo-controlled study involving patients with HIV infection and oral aphthous ulcers treated with thalidomide 200 mg daily.

Thalidomide for the treatment of oral aphthous ulcers in patients with human immunodeficiency virus infection. National Institute of Allergy and Infectious Diseases AIDS Clinical Trials Group. Jacobson JM, Greenspan JS, Spritzler J, et al. N Engl J Med 1997;336:1487–93.

Fifty-seven HIV positive patients were included in this double-blind, randomized, placebo-controlled study of thalidomide 200 mg daily vs placebo as therapy for oral aphthous ulcers in HIV-infected patients. Sixteen of 29 patients in the thalidomide group (55%) had complete healing of their aphthous ulcers after four weeks, as compared with only 2 of 28 patients in the placebo group (7%; p < 0.001).

Recurrent aphthous stomatitis unresponsive to topical corticosteroids: a study of the comparative therapeutic effects of systemic prednisone and systemic sulodexide. Femiano F, Gombos F, Scully C. Int J Dermatol 2003;42: 394–7.

Thirty patients with RAS were randomly assigned to one of three study groups: blind therapy with systemic sulodexide or systemic prednisone and control. Systemic prednisone was slightly more effective than sulodexide and both were more effective than placebo.

THIRD LINE THERAPIES

■ Dapsone	D
■ Pentoxifylline	C
■ Levamisole	A
■ Topical cyclosporine	C
■ Oral interferon α-2a	A
■ Disodium cromoglycate	A
■ Azathioprine	E
■ Topical 5-aminosalicylic acid	A
■ Topical diclofenac in hyaluronan	A
■ Topical prostaglandin E2	A
■ Triclosan	A
■ Azelastine	B
■ Longo Vital®	A
■ Phenelzine	E
■ Acyclovir	C
■ Etretinate	E
■ Low-intensity ultrasound	B
■ CO_2 laser	C
■ Potassium nitrate/dimethyl isosorbide	C
■ Penicillin G potassium troches	A
■ Sulodexide	C
■ Etanercept	E

Dapsone use with oral-genital ulcers. Handfield-Jones S, Allen BR, Littlewood SM. Br J Dermatol 1985;113:501.

Complete or partial clearing of aphthae was achieved in 11 of 19 patients with previously resistant oral aphthae, oral and genital aphthae, or Behçet's disease with dapsone 100 mg daily. The average duration of treatment was 19 days. Concomitant therapy consisted of zinc sulfate and co-trimoxazole.

Treatment of recurrent aphthous stomatitis with pentoxifylline. Pizarro A, Navarro A, Fonseca E, et al. Br J Dermatol 1995;133:659–60.

In patients with minor RAS receiving pentoxifylline 400 mg three times daily over a 6-month period, 50% did not experience a recurrence and 27% experienced a reduced number and duration of ulcers.

In other studies, over 50% of patients noted either complete resolution or a decrease in number and/or duration of ulcers during the treatment period. However, these are open-label trials involving small numbers of patients.

Oxypentifylline in the management of recurrent aphthous oral ulcers: an open clinical trial. Chandrasekhar J, Liem AA, Cox NH, Paterson AW. Oral Surg Oral Med Oral Pathol Oral Radiol Endod 1999;87:564–7.

Twenty-four patients were included in this open label trial and were given oxypentifylline 400 mg orally three times daily for 4 weeks. A positive response was seen in 63.6% of male patients and 61.5% of female patients.

A randomized double-blind trial of levamisole in the therapy of recurrent aphthous stomatitis. De Cree J, Verhaegen H, De Cock W, Verbruggen F. Oral Surg Oral Med Oral Pathol 1978;45:378–84.

Eighteen patients with RAS underwent a placebo-controlled, double-blind study in which they were given placebo or levamisole 50 mg three times daily for three consecutive days at the start of an aphthous lesion. Statistical evaluation showed decreased frequency of lesions, shorter duration, and diminished pain of lesions in the group receiving levamisole.

Levamisole in aphthous stomatitis: evaluation of three regimens. De Meyer J, Degraeve M, Clarysse J, et al. Br Med J 1977;1:671–4.

Levamisole 50 mg three times daily for three consecutive days every 2 weeks resulted in significant improvements in aphthae in this double-blind trial.

However, other double-blind studies do not demonstrate a beneficial effect on incidence or severity of ulcers.

Topical cyclosporine for oral mucosal disorders. Eisen D, Ellis CN. J Am Acad Dermatol 1990;23:1259–64.

Four of eight patients with severe aphthous stomatitis obtained nearly complete suppression of ulcers during an 8-week course of topical cyclosporine 500 mg/5 mL swish and rinse three times daily.

Chronic recurrent aphthous stomatitis: oral treatment with low-dose interferon alpha. Hutchinson VA, Angenend JL, Mok WL, et al. Mol Biother 1990;2:160–4.

Oral administration of interferon-alfa 1200 IU daily resulted in remissions of aphthae within 2 weeks of initiating therapy compared to no improvement in the placebo group.

Di-sodium cromoglycate in the treatment of recurrent aphthous ulceration. Kowolik MJ, Muir KF, MacPhee IT. Br Dent J 1978;144:384.

Disodium cromoglycate lozenges, 20 mg four times daily, resulted in an increase in ulcer free days after a 6-week treatment period in this double-blind crossover trial.

An earlier study found only pain relief was achieved with cromoglycic acid.

Combination immunosuppressant and topical steroid therapy for treatment of recurrent major aphthae. Brown RS, Bottomley WK. Oral Surg Oral Med Oral Pathol 1990;69:42–4.

A 32-year-old female with recurrent major aphthae was successfully treated with azathioprine 50 mg twice daily, ibuprofen 600 mg four times daily and dexamethasone elixir 0.5 mg/5 mL swish and rinse.

The patient had not used topical corticosteroids prior to azathioprine, thus it is difficult to assess either drug's individual merit.

Topical 5-aminosalicylic acid: a treatment for aphthous ulcers. Collier PM, Neill SM, Copeman PWM. Br J Dermatol 1992;126:185–8.

Decreased discomfort and pain, shortened healing time, and reduced difficulty with eating were found with 5-aminosalicylic cream three times daily compared to placebo.

Although this trial was double blinded and placebo controlled, the duration of treatment was brief – 14 days or until ulcer clearance.

Sustained relief of oral aphthous ulcer pain from topical diclofenac in hyaluronan: a randomized, double-blind clinical trial. Saxen MA, Ambrosius WT, Rehemtula AF, et al. Oral Surg Oral Med Oral Pathol Oral Radiol Endod 1997;84:356–61.

Gels containing 3% diclofenac in 2.5% hyaluronan, 2.5% hyaluronan, and 2% viscous lidocaine resulted in similar pain relief after application of noxious stimuli. A significant

Evidence levels **A** Double-blind study **B** Clinical trial ≥ 20 subjects **C** Clinical trial < 20 subjects **D** Series ≥ 5 subjects **E** Anecdotal case reports

treatment effect was observed with the combination diclofenac and hyaluronan gel 2–6 h after application with respect to pain relief following food/drink consumption.

NSAIDs can be used systemically for analgesia. However, change in ulcer size or suppression of recurrence has not been documented with topical or oral NSAIDs.

A clinical trial of prostaglandin E2 in recurrent aphthous ulceration. Taylor LJ, Walker DM, Bagg J. Br Dent J 1993; 175:125.

Topical prostaglandin E2 (PGE2) gel may exert a prophylactic effect for aphthae.

Treatment time in this randomized, double-blind, placebo-controlled study was only 10 days, and patients experienced fewer new lesions despite applying PGE2 to active aphthae. No significant differences in speed of healing or pain relief were found. PGE2 may produce myotonic effects on the uterus, thus pregnancy tests were checked in female patients in this study.

Mouthrinses containing triclosan reduce the incidence of recurrent aphthous ulcers (RAU). Skaare AB, Herlofson BB, Barkvoll P. J Clin Periodontol 1996;23:778–81.

In a double-blind crossover study, 0.15% triclosan mouthrinse caused a significant decrease in the number of ulcers during the experimental period. Compared to the 7.8% ethanol and triclosan formulation, the efficacy of the mouthrinses was reduced when propylene glycol or a higher concentration of ethanol (15.6%) were used as solubilizing agents.

A clinical trial of azelastine in recurrent aphthous ulceration with an analysis of its actions on leukocytes. Ueta E, Osaki T, Yoneda K, et al. J Oral Pathol Med 1994;23:123–9.

Azelastine hydrochloride was administered orally to 43 patients with RAS. During 6 months after treatment no oral lesions occurred in seven patients, and improvement was exhibited in all but four patients.

Longo Vital® in the prevention of recurrent aphthous ulceration. Pedersen A, Hougen HP, Klausen B, Winther K. J Oral Pathol Med 1990;19:371–5.

Longo Vital® is a herbal tablet composed of numerous vitamins (including B1, B2, and B6) and herbs (pumpkin seeds, rosemary leaves, paprika, milfoil flowers, and arnica flowers). This double-blind study found a reduced number of ulcer recurrences with the herbal tablet compared to placebo.

Although the patients had some vitamin levels assessed prior to therapy, vitamins B1, B2, and B6 were not checked despite the fact that their deficiencies have been associated with aphthae.

Does phenelzine relieve aphthous ulcers of the mouth? Rosenthal SH. N Engl J Med 1984;311:1442.

In two patients, use of phenelzine resulted in remissions of aphthae, and periodic withdrawal led to exacerbations.

Acyclovir in the prevention of severe aphthous ulcers. Pederson A. Arch Dermatol 1992;128:119–20.

Acyclovir 800 mg twice daily led to milder or no recurrences in six of eight patients over 10 weeks.

A double-blind trial using acyclovir 400 mg twice daily in 25 patients over 1 year failed to demonstrate a similar prophylactic benefit.

Aphthous ulcers responding to etretinate – a case report. Murphy GM, Griffiths AD. Clin Exp Dermatol 1989;14: 330–1.

A 34-year-old woman was treated with etretinate 25 mg daily for plantar pustular psoriasis. Two month remissions of her minor aphthae occurred with two courses of etretinate.

Clinical evaluation of the use of low-intensity ultrasound in the treatment of recurrent aphthous stomatitis. Brice SL. Oral Surg Oral Med Oral Pathol Oral Radiol Endod 1997; 83:14–20.

An ultrasonic toothbrush used twice daily showed modest efficacy in reducing ulcer activity over a standard toothbrush in one part of a crossover trial.

Managing aphthous ulcers: laser treatment applied. Colvard M, Kuo P. J Am Dent Assoc 1991;122:51–3.

Pain alleviation was observed in 16 of 18 patients following CO_2 laser therapy of minor aphthae.

Treatment of aphthous stomatitis with saturated potassium nitrate/dimethyl isosorbide. Hodosh M, Hodosh SH, Hodosh AJ. Quintessence Int 2004;35:137–41.

Eighteen patients treated with 35% potassium nitrate with dimethyl isosorbide experienced complete pain relief for 4–8 h and significantly shortened ulcer healing time compared to 35% potassium nitrate or vehicle alone.

The efficacy and safety of 50 mg penicillin G potassium troches for recurrent aphthous ulcers. Kerr AR, Drexel CA, Speilman AI. Oral Surg Oral Med Oral Pathol Oral Radiol Endod 2003;96:685–94.

Topical application of 50 mg penicillin G troches in 31 patients with minor RAS resulted in a reduction in healing time and earlier pain relief.

The difference between the treatment group and placebo group was borderline in both healing time and pain relief.

Recurrent aphthous stomatitis unresponsive to topical corticosteroids: a study of the comparative therapeutic effects of systemic prednisone and systemic sulodexide. Femiano F, Gombos F, Scully C. Int J Derm 2003;42:394–7.

Double-blind trial systemic sulodexide 250 mg twice daily for month 1, then once daily for month 2 vs prednisone taper vs placebo showed reduction in days to aphthae re-epithelialization that was superior to placebo yet inferior to prednisone.

Recalcitrant, recurrent aphthous stomatitis treated with etanercept. Robinson ND, Guitart J. Arch Dermatol 2003; 139:1259–62.

A case report of treatment of recalcitrant RAS with subcutaneous etanercept 25 mg twice weekly with a resultant decrease in frequency, severity and duration of flares during the 7 months of therapy.

Arthropod bites and stings

Dirk M Elston

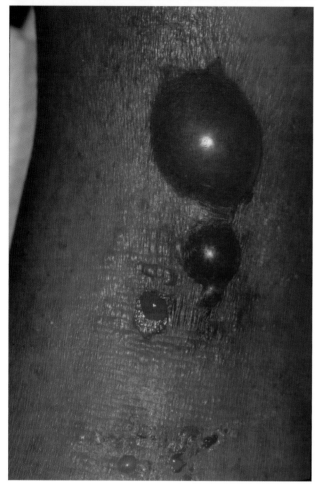

Bites and stings produce papular urticaria, pruritic bullae, pseudolymphomatous reactions and anaphylaxis. Exaggerated bite reactions occur in patients with lymphoma and chronic lymphocytic leukemia. Brown recluse spider bites can produce large areas of dermal necrosis. Vector-borne disease remains a worldwide problem. This chapter presents strategies for the prevention and management of bites and stings.

MANAGEMENT STRATEGY

Bite reactions

First line management for bites is prevention. *N,N-diethyl-3-methylbenzamide* (DEET) is effective against a broad range of arthropods. *Permethrin-treated fabric* is beneficial, especially for crawling arthropods. *Picaridin* has been available in Europe and is a recent addition to the marketplace in the US. A veterinarian should be consulted about the best regimens currently available to prevent flea infestation in pets. *Antivenin* is available for many arachnid toxins.

If prevention fails, second line treatments aim to improve pruritus. Delayed-type hypersensitivity to bites often results in maddening pruritus. *Topical antipruritics*, such as 1/4% camphor and menthol in cream, lotion or gel formulations can provide symptomatic relief. *Topical anesthetics* such as *pramoxine* and *lidocaine* may be helpful. *Benzocaine* products are also marketed, but these products have greater potential to cause allergic contact dermatitis. For limited areas of severe pruritus, a eutectic mixture of lidocaine and prilocaine can be very helpful.

For persistent bite reactions, *topical corticosteroid* preparations are generally helpful. For young children, mild to mid-strength corticosteroid preparations often suffice. In adults, the author generally recommends superpotent or potent corticosteroids. They must often be applied under occlusion to achieve rapid results. Superpotent corticosteroid preparations typically carry a warning that occlusion may result in cutaneous atrophy and striae. Certainly, these agents should not be occluded for more than a few applications. Long-term use of these products is generally unnecessary. In the author's experience, one to three applications of a sufficiently potent agent is generally sufficient to control symptoms.

When topical agents fail, *intralesional injection of a corticosteroid* may be helpful. *Triamcinolone*, in doses from 3 to 10 mg/mL, is useful. In the setting of insect bites, the author generally does not use doses in excess of 10 mg/mL. The risk of cutaneous atrophy is greater with higher doses, or if the agent is injected superficially. Some severe and persistent bite reactions respond only to excision.

Anaphylaxis

Individuals who experience anaphylaxis in response to stings should be referred to an allergist for desensitization. They should also carry *epinephrine (adrenaline) in the form of an autoinjector* (EpiPen®). Injectors require training, and patients should be properly instructed regarding the use of the device before leaving the physician's office. Individuals who demonstrate hypersensitivity to stings should avoid bright clothing and perfume when outdoors. *Avoidance of beehives, wasp nests and outdoor garbage cans* can prevent many stings.

Vector-borne disease

Most tick-borne illness responds to *doxycycline*. For early Lyme disease, evidence suggests that a 10-day course is as effective as longer courses of antibiotic. Babesiosis responds to *clindamycin* and *quinine*, but *azithromycin* and *atovaquone* may be as effective with a lower incidence of side effects. *Malaria prophylaxis* and treatment is highly variable depending on the region. Guidelines are updated continuously.

SPECIFIC INVESTIGATIONS

- Hematology and fibrin split products after brown recluse spider bite
- Rickettsial serologic tests
- Lyme serologic tests
- Skin biopsy with appropriate stains or immunofluorescence

Severe intravascular hemolysis associated with brown recluse spider envenomation. A report of two cases and

Evidence levels A Double-blind study B Clinical trial ≥ 20 subjects C Clinical trial < 20 subjects D Series ≥ 5 subjects E Anecdotal case reports

review of the literature. Williams ST, Khare VK, Johnston GA, Blackall DP. Am J Clin Pathol 1995;104:463–7.

A report of two women with severe hemolysis following brown recluse spider bites.

Patients with brown recluse spider envenomation can develop disseminated intravascular coagulation. This may be more common with minor appearing wounds.

Diagnoses of brown recluse spider bites (loxoscelism) greatly outnumber actual verifications of the spider in four western American states. Vetter RS, Cushing PE, Crawford RL, Royce LA. Toxicon 2003;42:413–8.

Over a period of 41 months, 216 cases of loxoscelism were diagnosed in California, Oregon, Washington and Colorado. In contrast, historical evidence of only 35 brown recluse or Mediterranean recluse spiders were found in these four states.

Brown spider bites are overdiagnosed. Physicians in non-endemic areas often make a diagnosis of loxoscelism solely on the basis of dermonecrotic lesions. Loxosceles *spiders are often rare or nonexistent in these areas.*

An infestation of 2,055 brown recluse spiders (Araneae: Sicariidae) and no envenomations in a Kansas home: implications for bite diagnoses in nonendemic areas. Vetter RS, Barger DK. J Med Entomol 2002;39:948–51.

At least 400 of 2055 brown recluse spiders recovered from a single occupied home during a 6-month period were large enough to cause envenomation, yet no bites occurred.

Brown recluse spiders are nonaggressive and reclusive, as the name suggests. Even in the face of heavy infestation, bites are rare. In nonendemic areas, brown recluse bites are likely to be extremely rare occurrences.

A new assay for the detection of *Loxosceles* **species (brown recluse) spider venom.** Gomez HF, Krywko DM, Stoecker WV. Ann Emerg Med 2002;39:469–74.

A sensitive *Loxosceles* venom enzyme-linked immunosorbent assay (ELISA) assay was tested with inoculations of as little as 40 ng of venom. At this concentration, the assay only detected *Loxosceles* spp. venom. At very high concentrations, the assay also detected other arachnid venoms.

This assay shows excellent sensitivity and specificity in the range of venom concentration that would actually be found in tissue after a bite. It can identify those necrotic reactions really caused by brown recluse spiders.

Rickettsia parkeri: **a newly recognized cause of spotted fever rickettsiosis in the United States.** Paddock CD, Sumner JW, Comer JA, et al. Clin Infect Dis 2004;38:805–11.

A spotted fever organism other than *Rickettsia rickettsii* was shown to cause human disease in North America.

Rocky Mountain spotted fever (RMSF) is not the only tick-borne spotted fever to occur in North America. Fortunately, they all respond to doxycycline.

Evaluation of a PCR assay for quantitation of *Rickettsia rickettsii* **and closely related spotted fever group rickettsiae.** Eremeeva ME, Dasch GA, Silverman DJ. J Clin Microbiol 2003;41:5466–72.

A quantitative polymerase chain reaction assay was developed for the detection of *Rickettsia rickettsii.*

Fluorescent antibody testing has most commonly been used to detect RMSF. This PCR assay has the potential to improve surveillance.

Consequences of delayed diagnosis of Rocky Mountain spotted fever in children—West Virginia, Michigan, Tennessee, and Oklahoma, May–July 2000. MMWR Morb Mortal Wkly Rep 2000;49:885–8.

A report of severe illness and death related to delays in diagnosis of RMSF in children from four different regions of the US. Young children have the highest age-specific incidence of RMSF. Most cases occur between April and September.

Delays in therapy may be fatal in patients with RMSF. In endemic areas, any child with fever accompanied by rash or headache should be suspected of having RMSF. Treatment should never be delayed for serologic confirmation.

Intralaboratory reliability of serologic and urine testing for Lyme disease. Klempner MS, Schmid CH, Hu L, et al. Am J Med 2001;110:217–9.

Conventional Lyme titers are widely available, but are of limited value. Better laboratory tests are needed for the diagnosis of Lyme disease.

C6 test as an indicator of therapy outcome for patients with localized or disseminated lyme borreliosis. Philipp MT, Marques AR, Fawcett PT, et al. J Clin Microbiol 2003; 41:4955–60.

The antibody level to the *Borrelia burgdorferi* C(6) peptide declines by at least fourfold after successful antibiotic treatment of early or late disease.

This improved test could prove to be useful in the management of patients with Lyme disease.

FIRST LINE THERAPIES

Prevention	
■ DEET	A
■ Permethrin	A
■ Picaridin	B
Flea treatments for pets (consult a veterinarian)	
■ Lufenuron	A
■ Fipronil	A
■ Imidacloprid	A
Anaphylaxis	
■ Epinephrine	A
■ Immunotherapy	A

Does anything beat DEET? Roberts JR, Reigart JR. Pediatr Ann 2004;33:443–53.

In field comparison trials, DEET consistently performs well against a wide range of disease vectors. Overall, it has a good safety record, although serious reactions can occur. The appropriate concentration to use on children remains unclear.

The American Academy of Pediatrics has revised its statement about DEET. In the past, they advised no more than 10% DEET in children. They now cite evidence about a plateau of efficacy at 30%. In general, the minimal effective concentration should be used. Because ethanol in the vehicle of some preparations may increase absorption, new formulations should be studied.

In vitro repellency of N,N-diethyl-3-methylbenzamide and N,N-diethylphenylacetamide analogs against *Aedes* *aegypti* and *Anopheles stephensi* (Diptera: Culicidae). Debboun M, Wagman J. J Med Entomol 2004;41:430–4.

Seventeen analogs of DEET and N,N-diethylphenylacetamide (DEPA) were evaluated in vitro against *Ae. aegypti* and *An. stephensi*. Two DEPA analogs and a single DEET analog were superior to DEET and warrant field evaluation.

DEET's supremacy among repellents is being challenged. Field evaluations remain the gold standard for determination of efficacy.

Comparative resistance of *Anopheles albimanus* and *Aedes aegypti* to N,N-diethyl-3-methylbenzamide (Deet) and 2-methylpiperidinyl-3-cyclohexen-1-carboxamide (AI3-37220) in laboratory human-volunteer repellent assays. Klun JA, Strickman D, Rowton E, et al. J Med Entomol 2004; 41:418–22.

DEET and racemic AI3-37220 were tested against *Ae. aegypti* and *An. albimanus*. *Anopheles albimanus* is resistant to the usual skin doses of DEET, higher doses offer reasonable protection. The racemic mix was highly effective against *Ae. aegypti*, but not against *An. albimanus*.

The minimal effective dose varies by species.

Field evaluation of repellent formulations containing deet and picaridin against mosquitoes in Northern Territory, Australia. Frances SP, Waterson DG, Beebe NW, Cooper RD. J Med Entomol 2004;41:414–7.

Field testing of picaridin (1-methyl-propyl 2-(2-hydroxyethyl)-1-piperidinecarboxylate) (Autan Repel Army 20) and DEET against *Culex annulirostris*, *Anopheles merankensis* and *Anopheles bancroftii* showed protection against *Anopheles* spp. The repellents provided good protection against *Cx annulirostris* (an important vector of arboviruses in Australia).

Some species of mosquito remain highly resistant to available repellents. Picaridin has recently been licensed in the US and provides an alternative to DEET.

In vitro human metabolism and interactions of repellent N,N-diethyl-m-toluamide. Usmani KA, Rose RL, Goldstein JA, et al. Drug Metab Dispos 2002;30:289–94.

Preincubation of human or rodent microsomes with chlorpyrifos, permethrin and pyridostigmine bromide alone or in combination can stimulate or inhibit DEET metabolism.

After the first Gulf War, questions were raised about the safety of DEET in combination with other products, and a possible link to Gulf War syndrome was suggested by some. This study provides evidence that some agents may interact with DEET, but does not prove any causal association with Gulf War syndrome.

Control of fleas on naturally infested dogs and cats and in private residences with topical spot applications of fipronil or imidacloprid. Dryden MW, Denenberg TM, Bunch S. Systemic Vet Parasitol 2000;93:69–75.

Field trial demonstrating that imidacloprid and fipronil reduced flea burdens on pets by 99.5 and 96.5%, respectively.

Control of flea populations in a simulated home environment model using lufenuron, imidacloprid or fipronil. Jacobs DE, Hutchinson MJ, Ryan WG. Med Vet Entomol 2001;15:73–7.

In a home simulation model imidacloprid and fipronil provided virtually complete control. Lufenuron was somewhat less effective.

Control of fleas on pets and in homes by use of imidacloprid or lufenuron and a pyrethrin spray. Dryden MW, Perez HR, Ulitchny DM. J Am Vet Med Assoc 1999;215:36–9.

Field trial. Imidacloprid reduced flea burdens on pets by 96 and 93.5% on days 7 and 28. Lufenuron and pyrethrin spray reduced flea numbers on pets by 48.9 and 91.1% on days 7 and 28, respectively.

Comparison of flea control strategies using imidacloprid or lufenuron on cats in a controlled simulated home environment. Jacobs DE, Hutchinson MJ, Fox MT, Krieger KJ. Am J Vet Res 1997;58:1260–2.

Imidacloprid maintained flea burdens below the limit of detection, whereas clinically important flea populations developed in the lufenuron treatment pen.

Venom immunotherapy improves health-related quality of life in patients allergic to yellow jacket venom. Oude Elberink JN, De Monchy JG, Van Der Heide S, et al. J Allergy Clin Immunol 2002;110:174–82.

Compared with epinephrine treatment, immunotherapy improved health-related quality of life.

Venom immunotherapy is effective in preventing anaphylactic reactions after insect stings and improves the quality of life. Patients should be evaluated by an allergist.

Discontinuing venom immunotherapy: extended observations. Golden DB, Kwiterovich KA, Kagey-Sobotka A, Lichtenstein LM. J Allergy Clin Immunol 1998;101:298–305.

In adults, venom immunotherapy can be discontinued after 5–6 years with a 5–10% risk of a systemic reaction. Risk factors include a history of a systemic reaction during venom immunotherapy, persistent strongly positive skin tests, and the severity of the pretreatment reaction.

Outcomes of allergy to insect stings in children, with and without venom immunotherapy. Golden DB, Kagey-Sobotka A, Norman PS, et al. N Engl J Med 2004;351:668–74.

Venom immunotherapy in children reduces the risk of systemic reaction even 10–20 years after treatment is stopped.

The prolonged benefit from immunotherapy may be greater in children than in adults.

Safety of rush insect venom immunotherapy. The results of a retrospective study in 178 patients. Wenzel J, Meissner-Kraemer M, Bauer R, et al. Allergy 2003;58:1176–9.

In a 7-day protocol of rush immunotherapy, there was a 17.9% rate of systemic adverse reactions Mueller grade I–IV.

This compares favorably with historical data.

Comparison of colchicine, dapsone, triamcinolone, and diphenhydramine therapy for the treatment of brown recluse spider envenomation: a double-blind, controlled study in a rabbit model. Elston DM, Miller SD, Young RJ, et al. Arch Dermatol 2005;141:595–7.

In this animal model, none of the treatment regimens (including dapsone) prevented necrosis. Only intralesional triamcinolone showed any trend towards efficacy.

Scorpion envenomations in young children in central Arizona. LoVecchio F, McBride C. J Toxicol Clin Toxicol 2003;41:937–40.

Poison center data from Arizona showed that of 491 patients, 133 (27.5%) presented to an emergency department. 86 (17.8%) received antivenin and 25 (5.2%) were admitted. The mean time of abatement of symptoms following antivenin was 31 min vs 22.2 h. There was one acute rash to antivenin and 49 cases (57%) of serum sickness.

Hospital admission was less common among those receiving antivenin.

Use of antivenin to treat priapism after a black widow spider bite. Hoover NG, Fortenberry JD. Pediatrics 2004; 114:e128–9.

Priapism is a rare complication of black widow envenomation. In this report, priapism responded to antivenin within hours. Pain abated and opiates were discontinued.

Treatment for black widow envenomation is primarily symptomatic with the use of opiates and benzodiazepines. Antivenin is effective for refractory symptoms, including priapism.

Antivenom treatment in arachnidism. Isbister GK, Graudins A, White J, Warrell D. J Toxicol Clin Toxicol 2003;41:291–300.

There are four widow spider antivenins available, including American black widow antivenin and Australian redback spider antivenin. They are associated with a relatively low rate of adverse reactions.

SECOND LINE THERAPIES

Relief of pruritus	
■ Camphor and menthol	E
■ Pramoxine	E
■ Lidocaine	E
■ Benzocaine	E
■ Lidocaine/prilocaine	E
Treatment of bite reactions	
■ Superpotent and potent topical corticosteroids	E
■ For young children: mild to moderate strength topical corticosteroids	E

THIRD LINE THERAPIES

Prevention	
Repellents	
■ Soybean oil-based products	C
■ Botanicals	C
Vector-borne illness	
■ Host-targeted bait	B
Fleas (consult a veterinarian)	
■ Pyriproxyfen for fleas	B
Treatment of bites	
■ Intralesional corticosteroids	E
■ Excision	E
■ Desensitization for mosquito bites	B

Evaluation of botanicals as repellents against mosquitoes. Das NG, Baruah I, Talukdar PK, Das SC. J Vector Borne Dis 2003;40:49–53.

Three plant extracts (*Zanthoxylum limonella* and *Citrus aurantifolia* distillates and petroleum ether extract of *Z. limonella*) were evaluated against *Aedes albopictus* under laboratory conditions. At 30% concentration, 296–304 min protection time was achieved by the test repellents in mustard oil base.

Comparative efficacy of insect repellents against mosquito bites. Fradin MS, Day JF. N Engl J Med 2002;347:13–8.

DEET performed better than IR3535 (ethyl butylacetylaminopropionate) and repellent-impregnated wristbands. A soybean-oil-based repellent provided 94.6 min of protection compared to only 22.9 min for the IR3535-based repellent.

This was not a field trial.

Use of liquid deltamethrin in modified, host-targeted bait tubes for control of fleas on sciurid rodents in northern California. Bronson LR, Smith CR. J Vector Ecol 2002; 27:55–62.

A host-targeted bait tube delivering liquid deltamethrin controlled vector fleas on rodent hosts in plague-endemic regions.

Field efficacy of a 10 per cent pyriproxyfen spot-on for the prevention of flea infestations on cats. Maynard L, Houffschmitt P, Lebreux B. J Small Anim Pract 2001;42:491–4.

The insect growth regulator pyriproxyfen was evaluated for spot-on application. The comparison group received lufenuron suspension orally. Flea counts were significantly lower in the pyriproxyfen group.

Potential to become a first line treatment.

Efficacy and safety of specific immunotherapy to mosquito bites. Ariano R, Panzani RC. Allerg Immunol (Paris) 2004; 36:131–8.

Immunotherapy with an extract of whole body *Aedes communis* produced a significant improvement of symptoms.

Atopic dermatitis

Donald Rudikoff, Jan D Bos

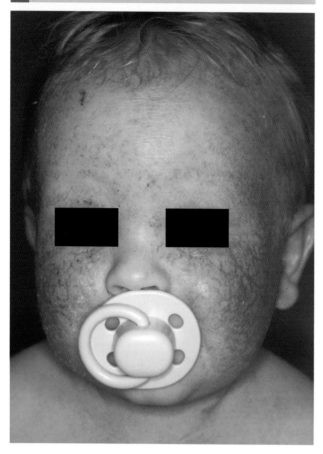

Atopic dermatitis (AD) is a chronic, relapsing, intensely pruritic dermatosis which usually affects infants, children, and young adults and in most cases is associated with a personal or family history of atopy (seasonal rhinitis, asthma, or eczema). Skin involvement ranges from acute, weeping and crusted areas of eczema to papular lesions or lichenified plaques. Although there is no consensus, atopy is defined by many as a syndrome primarily characterized by the presence of allergen-specific IgE. For those cases in which atopy cannot be demonstrated, a diagnosis of atopiform dermatitis has been proposed.

MANAGEMENT STRATEGY

The treatment of AD entails an individualized regimen that depends on the age of the patient, the stage and variety of lesions present (acute, subacute, chronic lichenified, or a mixture of these), the sites and extent of involvement, the presence of infection, and the previous response to treatment. While a superpotent corticosteroid ointment might be useful in an adult with chronic, recalcitrant, lichenified plaques, such treatment would be inappropriate in an infant with weeping, eczematous facial lesions.

The therapy regimen should be carefully explained to the patient and/or his parents and should outline instructions regarding bathing, skin hydration, avoidance of disease triggers, local and systemic treatments, stress reduction, and

possible complications of the disease or its therapy. Factors that are known to exacerbate eczema include sweating, irritants such as detergents and solvents, inappropriate bathing habits, infection, emotional stress, in some cases contact allergens or environmental aeroallergens, and, in some very young children, food allergy. It is helpful at the start of treatment to identify the particular triggers that might be relevant in each patient.

Bathing habits should be carefully investigated and recommendations made to assure adequate hydration of the skin. Although 'dry lesions' of AD might theoretically be worsened by evaporation after bathing, application of an *emollient* such as petrolatum to damp skin right after a bath or shower will maintain adequate skin moisture. Older children and adults may object to greasy ointments, but they are usually tolerated by young children and infants. *Balneotherapy, wet-wrap dressings*, with or without topical corticosteroids, and wet pyjamas soaked in *chlorhexidine* have been advocated. *Burrow's solution* soaks or compresses at a dilution of 1 : 40 are helpful for exudative lesions.

In 10–20% of children, usually those below 2 years of age, relevant food allergies can contribute to eczema. The foods most often implicated are eggs, milk, wheat, peanuts, and soy. It is important to avoid non-supervised overly restrictive elimination diets as these may result in malnutrition and reintroduction of eliminated food occasionally causes anaphylaxis. Exposure to the house dust mite *Dermatophagoides pteronyssinus* exacerbates eczema in some patients. Measures to decrease exposure to dust mites, such as frequent vacuuming and special mattress covers, are recommended. In general, avoidance of aeroallergens should become part of a lifestyle, as eczema patients may later develop allergic rhinitis or asthma, or they may have children with these atopy-related diseases. Such advice cannot be given in patients with atopiform dermatitis, where allergen-specific IgE is absent.

Topical corticosteroid preparations are the cornerstone of therapy for inflammation and pruritus, and are best applied immediately after bathing. They are considered the 'standard of care'. An adequate supply of a mid-potency corticosteroid such as fluocinolone or triamcinolone acetonide ointment should be prescribed. Lower potency preparations such as hydrocortisone 2% or clobetasone butyrate are used sparingly on the face and intertriginous areas. Once inflammation is controlled, a milder corticosteroid may be substituted or the original corticosteroid can be used less frequently. Intermittent short bursts of a potent corticosteroid ointment followed by emollient are equivalent to continuous use of a milder corticosteroid ointment in mild to moderate disease. In general, application of corticosteroids more than once daily is not necessary.

Two *topical immunomodulators* are available for the treatment of AD, tacrolimus (FK506) and pimecrolimus. Tacrolimus ointment is available as 0.1% and 0.03%; pimecrolimus is available as a 1% cream. Both are effective and well tolerated for the treatment of children and adults with moderate to severe AD. Neither agent causes cutaneous atrophy. Systemic absorption of these compounds is minimal. Recent reports to the US Food and Drug Administration linking topical immunomodulators to lymphoma and skin cancer are currently under investigation. Neither drug is approved in the USA for use in patients less than 2 years of age. The main side effect is a sensation of burning in the skin, which is less prominent as the skin improves. Since most patients with AD are children who are

Evidence levels **A** Double-blind study **B** Clinical trial ≥ 20 subjects **C** Clinical trial < 20 subjects **D** Series ≥ 5 subjects **E** Anecdotal case reports

at risk for corticosteroid-induced adverse effects, topical immunomodulators seem likely to be considered as first line agents in future.

Systemic corticosteroids are effective for severe flares of AD. Their use should be limited to one or two courses per year, except in extremely recalcitrant cases resistant to other therapies. Prednisone is initiated at doses of 60–80 mg daily in adults. Once improvement occurs, the dose is tapered over 1 to 2 weeks. Intralesional triamcinolone acetonide may be useful for thick lichenified plaques such as in the chronic AD variant 'prurigo of Besnier'.

Phototherapy is helpful in cases that are unresponsive to topical treatment or that are so widespread that topical treatment is impractical. Combined UVA and UVB is more effective than UVB alone. Therapy is initiated using 3–5 J/cm² UVA and 30–50 mJ/cm² UVB, and increased slowly up to 10 J/cm² UVA and 100 mJ/cm² UVB. Narrowband UVB (311 nm) is superior to broadband UVB, but is less readily available. Recently, high-dose UVA1 (340–400 nm) has been shown to be highly efficacious for acute flares of AD. It reduces pruritus and results in clearing of difficult areas, like the face, that are especially sensitive to the deleterious effects of topical corticosteroids.

Oral and bath PUVA are also effective, but since flares can occur at the initiation of therapy, concomitant oral corticosteroids are given at first and then tapered rapidly. Extracorporeal photopheresis has been suggested to be effective in severe cases.

Topical antibiotic ointments such as mupirocin or fusidic acid are used by many practitioners. If secondary staphylococcal infection is present, oral antibiotics such as dicloxacillin or cefalexin are used. *Topical coal tar preparations* in an ointment base, though messy, are helpful to some patients, but can sometimes cause irritation. Their use should be limited to subacute or chronic lichenified lesions.

In general, *antihistamines* have limited effectiveness for the pruritus of AD. We sometimes use sedating antihistamines at bedtime to provide some respite from itching during the night, since sleep deprivation can adversely affect outcome. Topical doxepin may be helpful in reducing pruritus, but occasionally causes sensitization, and, if used on large areas, can induce drowsiness.

Systemic immunosuppressant therapy is reserved for severe recalcitrant AD. Before such therapy is initiated, long-term side effects, including the development of lymphoma, should be discussed. Cyclosporine dramatically clears AD in adults and children at doses of 2.5 to 5.0 mg/kg daily. Patients typically relapse within 2 to 6 weeks after discontinuation of cyclosporine therapy, but usually not to baseline levels. Periodic short courses of cyclosporine can control disease and reduce overall exposure to the drug.

Other options include a variety of treatments for which evidence is limited. Azathioprine at doses of 100 to 200 mg daily is an effective treatment for AD but has a slow onset of action, usually 4–6 weeks, and can cause bone marrow suppression.

Mycophenolate mofetil in doses of 1–2 g daily and low-dose methotrexate (2.5 mg daily) given 4 days per week have been reported anecdotally to be effective in the treatment of atopic eczema. UVB therapy may be given with methotrexate and the drug may be reduced and then discontinued.

Intravenous immunoglobulin has been reported by some investigators, but not others, to be effective in the treatment of severe corticosteroid-dependent and corticosteroid-resistant AD. Other agents that have shown some promise in anecdotal reports are *propyl thiouracil* (100 mg every 8 h for 12 weeks) and the *leukotriene antagonists* zafirlukast and zileuton. Several dietary manipulations have been suggested as possibly helpful in the treatment of AD. Studies on the use of oils containing γ-*linolenic acid*, such as evening oil of primrose and borage oil, have yielded conflicting results. Dramatic improvements reported mainly in small early trials have not been confirmed by more recent, larger, placebo-controlled trials. However, since this treatment is harmless and may be helpful in a subgroup of patients, it is possibly worth trying in some cases. Oral and topical *sodium cromoglycate* have been reported to be efficacious in some studies.

Chinese herbal therapy has shown some promise in the treatment of AD, but liver toxicity and lack of standardization have limited its use.

Several new treatments are under investigation for the treatment of AD, including *phosphodiesterase inhibitors*, *interleukin-11*, *thalidomide*, and *thymopentin*, but, so far, experience with these drugs is limited. *Probiotics* form another new avenue in the treatment of AD.

SPECIFIC INVESTIGATIONS

In selected cases only:

- Skin biopsy
- IgE, IgA, IgM, and IgG levels
- RAST or intracutaneous allergen testing and oral food challenges
- HIV ELISA

Atopic dermatitis. Leung DYM, Bieber T. Lancet 2003; 361:151–60.

An overview of the epidemiology, diagnosis, pathophysiology, genetics, and management of AD.

Guidelines of care for atopic dermatitis. Hanifin JM, Cooper KD, Ho VC, et al. J Am Acad Dermatol 2004;50: 391–404.

A recent overview of the management of AD, reflecting a consensus meeting by a working group. Nine clinical questions related to diagnosis and management were handled using the principles of evidence-based medicine.

Atopiform dermatitis. Bos JD. Br J Dermatol 2002;147:415–7.

The definition of AD is lacking consensus. A diagnosis of atopiform dermatitis has been suggested to be applicable in cases with clinical AD but without the major sign of atopy, the presence of allergen-specific IgE. To make such a distinction is important in view of advice to be given about avoidance of allergens.

Tumor stage mycosis fungoides in a patient treated with long-term corticosteroids for asthma and atopic-like dermatitis. Abel EA, Nickoloff BJ, Shelby DM, et al. J Dermatol Surg Oncol 1986;12:1089–93.

A 53-year-old woman developed asthma and an atopic-like dermatitis at age 42. Treated with oral and topical corticosteroids for presumed atopic eczema, she developed tumor stage mycosis fungoides 11 years later.

The onset of AD late in life is unusual and should suggest other diagnoses such as cutaneous T cell lymphoma.

Food hypersensitivity and atopic dermatitis: pathophysiology, epidemiology, diagnosis, and management. Sicherer SH, Sampson HA. J Allergy Clin Immunol 1999; 104:S114–22.

Food allergy plays a pathogenic role in a subset of patients, primarily infants and children, with AD. Identifying this subset of patients and determining the relevant food necessitate appropriate laboratory tests and, in some cases, physician-supervised oral food challenges. Most food allergies resolve in early childhood, and food allergy is rarely of importance in older children and adults.

Laboratory evaluation of the child with recalcitrant eczema. Hebert AA. Dermatol Clin 1994;12:109–21.

Although the diagnosis of AD is usually straightforward, several conditions, including Wiskott–Aldrich syndrome, selective IgA deficiency, hyper IgE syndrome, Netherton syndrome, and Letterer Siwe disease, should be considered during infancy.

Seborrheic dermatitis-like and atopic dermatitis-like eruptions in HIV-infected patients. Cockerell CJ. Clin Dermatol 1991;9:49–51.

Patients with advanced HIV infection may develop a dermatitis that is 'AD-like', with crusting and lichenification in the flexural areas or in a more widespread distribution.

FIRST LINE THERAPIES

■ Emollients	B
■ Topical corticosteroids	A
■ Topical immunomodulators	A

Improvement in skin barrier function in patients with atopic dermatitis after treatment with a moisturizing cream (Canoderm). Loden M, Andersson AC, Lindberg M. Br J Dermatol 1999;140:264–7.

A urea-containing moisturizer improved barrier function in AD patients and decreased sensitivity to irritants.

Use of an emollient as a steroid-sparing agent in the treatment of mild to moderate atopic dermatitis in children. Lucky AW, Leach AD, Laskarzewski P, Wenck H. Pediatr Dermatol 1997;14:321–4.

The adjunctive use of a water-in-oil emulsion with once-daily hydrocortisone 2.5% cream was equivalent in efficacy to twice-daily applications of hydrocortisone 2.5% cream in 25 children studied for 3 weeks.

The management of moderate to severe atopic dermatitis in adults with topical fluticasone propionate. The Netherlands Adult Atopic Dermatitis Study Group. Van Der Meer JB, Glazenburg EJ, Mulder PG, et al. Br J Dermatol 1999;140:1114–21.

Intermittent dosing of fluticasone propionate cream for reducing the risk of relapse in atopic dermatitis patients. Hanifin J, Gupta AK, Rajagopalan R. Br J Dermatol 2002; 147:528–37.

Twice weekly fluticasone propionate added to emollient maintenance treatment to reduce risk of relapse in atopic dermatitis: randomised, double blind, parallel group study. Berth-Jones J, Damstra RJ, Golsch S, et al. BMJ 2003;326:1367–70.

In these studies, twice-weekly maintenance therapy with fluticasone propionate ointment maintained improvements achieved in patients who had initially cleared with this therapy, increasing duration of remission, and reducing risk of relapse.

Topical corticosteroids for atopic eczema: clinical and cost effectiveness of once-daily vs. more frequent use. Green C, Colquitt JL, Kirby J, Davidson P. Br J Dermatol 2005; 152:130–41.

Differences in outcomes between once-daily and more frequent application of corticosteroids could not be identified in this systematic review, which includes one other systematic review and 10 randomized controlled trials.

A short-term trial of tacrolimus ointment for atopic dermatitis. European Tacrolimus Multicenter Atopic Dermatitis Study Group. Ruzicka T, Bieber T, Schopf E, et al. N Engl J Med 1997;337:816–21.

In this randomized, multicenter, double-blind study, 3 weeks of treatment resulted in a median percentage decrease in the summary score for dermatitis on the trunk and extremities of 66.7% for patients receiving 0.03% tacrolimus and 83.3% for patients receiving 0.1% tacrolimus. Results for the face and neck were similar.

Safety and efficacy of 1 year of tacrolimus ointment monotherapy in adults with atopic dermatitis. The European Tacrolimus Ointment Study Group. Reitamo S, Wollenberg A, Schopf E, et al. Arch Dermatol 2000; 136:999–1006.

Tacrolimus ointment 0.1% applied twice daily to affected skin of patients with moderate to severe AD resulted in marked or excellent improvement or clearance of disease in 54%, 81%, and 86% of patients at week 1, month 6, and month 12, respectively.

0.03% Tacrolimus ointment applied once or twice daily is more efficacious than 1% hydrocortisone acetate in children with moderate to severe atopic dermatitis: results of a randomized double-blind controlled trial. Reitamo S, Harper J, Bos JD, et al; European Tacrolimus Ointment Group. Br J Dermatol 2004;150:554–62.

Once- or twice-daily tacrolimus ointment 0.03% was significantly more effective than hydrocortisone acetate 1% in treating moderate to severe AD in children. Twice-daily application was particularly effective in patients with severe baseline disease compared with once-daily application.

Efficacy and safety of tacrolimus ointment compared with hydrocortisone butyrate ointment in adult patients with atopic dermatitis. Reitamo S, Rustin M, Ruzicka T, et al. J Allergy Clin Immunol 2002;109:547–55.

Phase III comparative study of FK506 ointment versus betamethasone valerate ointment in atopic dermatitis of the trunk and extremities. FK506 Ointment Study Group. Nishinihon J Dermatol 1997;59:870–9.

In these studies, 0.1% tacrolimus ointment was equivalent in efficacy to potent topical corticosteroids, hydrocortisone butyrate and betamethasone valerate.

Effectiveness of the ascomycin macrolactam SDZ ASM 981 in the topical treatment of atopic dermatitis. Van Leent EJ, Graber M, Thurston M, Wagenaar A, et al. Arch Dermatol 1998;134:805–9.

Evidence levels A Double-blind study B Clinical trial ≥ 20 subjects C Clinical trial < 20 subjects D Series ≥ 5 subjects E Anecdotal case reports

Application of topical 1% SDZ ASM 981 (pimecrolimus) cream twice daily resulted in significant improvement after 2 days in 34 adults with moderate AD. Within 3 weeks, there was a mean reduction in the AD Severity Index of 71.9% at the SDZ ASM treated sites, compared with a 10.3% reduction at placebo treated sites.

SDZ ASM 981: an emerging safe and effective treatment for atopic dermatitis. Luger T, Van Leent EJM, Graeber M, et al. Br J Dermatol 2001;144:788–94.

A placebo-controlled, dose-ranging trial with 260 subjects, comparing the response to pimecrolimus cream (0.05%, 0.2%, 0.6%, and 1.0%), placebo, and 0.1% betamethasone valerate. The most effective concentration of pimecrolimus was the highest and the most effective treatment of all was the betamethasone.

Efficacy and safety of pimecrolimus cream in the long-term management of atopic dermatitis in children. Wahn U, Bos JD, Goodfield M, et al. Pediatrics 2002;110:e2.

Pimecrolimus prevented progression to flares in more than 50% of patients and reduced or eliminated the need for topical corticosteroids. Benefits were consistently seen at 6 months and were sustained for 12 months.

SECOND LINE THERAPIES

■ UVB and UVA/UVB phototherapy	A
■ Systemic corticosteroids	E
■ Antihistamines	C
■ Antibiotics	D

A UVB phototherapy protocol with very low dose increments as a treatment of atopic dermatitis. Wulf HC, Bech-Thomsen N. Photodermatol Photoimmunol Photomed 1998; 14:1–6.

This study based on skin reflectance measurements used very low dose increments in the treatment of AD. Although the median cumulative dose increment during therapy was only 20% and cumulative UV exposure was four times lower with the new regimen, it was more effective than standard UVB treatment.

Combined UVB and UVA phototherapy of atopic eczema. Midelfart K, Stenvold SE, Volden G. Dermatologica 1985; 171:95–8.

Combined UVA–UVB therapy of severe AD (n = 23) was compared with UVB alone (n = 22). Combined UVA–UVB therapy resulted in 48% complete resolution and 48% good improvement, compared with 27% resolution and 58% improvement in the UVB group. A few treatment failures occurred in the UVB group.

Phototherapy for atopic eczema with narrow-band UVB. Grundmann-Kollmann M, Behrens S, Podda M, et al. J Am Acad Dermatol 1999;40:995–7.

Five patients with moderate to severe AD were treated with narrowband UVB for a cumulative dose of 9.2 J/cm^2 over a mean of 19 treatments. Narrowband UVB was effective after 3 weeks in all patients.

Do some patients with atopic dermatitis require long term oral steroid therapy? Sonenthal KR, Grammer LC, Patterson R. J Allergy Clin Immunol 1993;91:971–3.

Three patients with recalcitrant, disabling AD successfully maintained on oral corticosteroids are presented.

Combined oral and nasal beclomethasone diproprionate in children with atopic eczema: a randomised controlled trial. Heddle RJ, Soothill JF, Bulpitt CJ, Atherton DJ. BMJ (Clin Res Ed) 1984;289:651–4.

Twenty-six children, aged 3–14 years, with severe AD receiving combined oral plus nasal beclomethasone diproprionate (total dose 1200 μg daily) improved significantly more than patients receiving placebo after 4 weeks of treatment, with minimal adrenal suppression.

An evidence-based review of the efficacy of antihistamines in relieving pruritus in atopic dermatitis. Klein PA, Clark RA. Arch Dermatol 1999;135:1522–5.

This excellent review examines clinical trials of antihistamines for AD and concludes that the efficacy of nonsedating antihistamines remains to be adequately investigated.

Sedating antihistamines are thought by many clinicians to be useful at bedtime by virtue of their soporific effect.

Staphylococcal colonization in atopic dermatitis and the effect of topical mupirocin therapy. Lever R, Hadley K, Downey D, MacKie R. Br J Dermatol 1988;119:189–98.

In this double-blind, placebo-controlled, crossover study, 49 patients with AD used mupirocin ointment or vehicle in conjunction with a topical steroid. A significant reduction in clinical severity was observed after treatment with mupirocin, which was maintained over 4 weeks.

Flucloxacillin in the treatment of atopic dermatitis. Ewing CI, Ashcroft C, Gibbs AC, et al. Br J Dermatol 1998; 138:1022–9.

In 50 children with AD, treatment with oral flucloxacillin for 4 weeks reduced bacterial colonization, but, 2 weeks following discontinuation of antibiotics, there was no difference in bacterial counts between treated patients and controls. Flucloxacillin did not improve the symptoms or clinical appearance of AD.

THIRD LINE THERAPIES

■ Oral PUVA	A
■ Bath PUVA	B
■ UVA1 phototherapy	A
■ Photopheresis	D
■ Elimination diets	A
■ Dust mite reduction	A
■ Azathioprine	A
■ Cyclosporine	A
■ Mycophenolate mofetil	D
■ Leflunomide	E
■ Wet dressings	D
■ Oral γ-linolenic acid	C
■ Crude coal tar	D
■ Leukotriene antagonists	D
■ Interferon-γ (IFNγ)	A
■ Sodium cromoglicate	B
■ Hydroxychloroquine, chloroquine	E
■ Intravenous immunoglobulin	E
■ Propylthiouracil	C
■ Topical dinitrochlorobenzene (DNCB)	D
■ Probiotics	C

The role of psoralen photochemotherapy (PUVA) in the treatment of severe atopic eczema in adolescents.

Atherton DJ, Carabott F, Glover MT, Hawk JL. Br J Dermatol 1988;118:791–5.

Oral PUVA resulted in initial clearance of eczema in 14 of 15 children, nine of whom achieved complete remission. This was associated with resumption of normal growth in children who were previously growing poorly.

Oral psoralen photochemotherapy in severe childhood atopic eczema: an update. Sheehan MP, Atherton DJ, Norris P, Hawk J. Br J Dermatol 1993;129:431–6.

Twice-weekly treatment of 53 children (mean age 11.2 years) resulted in clearance or near-clearance of disease in 39 (74%) after a mean of 9 weeks.

Bath psoralen-ultraviolet A therapy in atopic eczema. De Kort WJ, van Weelden H. J Eur Acad Dermatol Venereol 2000;14:172–4.

In this study, 35 adults with severe AD underwent bath PUVA, one to three times weekly, for a maximum of 30 sessions. Six patients dropped out, three due to aggravation of symptoms. After completion of treatment, the remaining 29 patients had marked improvement in the severity of lesions, itching, and nighttime rest.

Half-side comparison study on the efficacy of 8-methoxypsoralen bath-PUVA versus narrow-band ultra-violet B phototherapy in patients with severe chronic atopic dermatitis. Der-Petrossian M, Seeber A, Honigsmann H, Tanew A. Br J Dermatol 2000;142:39–43.

In this randomized, investigator-blinded, half-side comparison study in 12 patients with severe chronic AD, half-side irradiation with threshold erythemogenic doses of 8-methoxypsoralen bath-PUVA and narrowband UVB was performed three times weekly over a period of 6 weeks. The two modalities were equally effective in equi-erythemogenic doses.

High-dose UVA1 therapy for atopic dermatitis: results of a multicenter trial. Krutmann J, Diepgen TL, Luger TA, et al. J Am Acad Dermatol 1998;38:589–93.

In this randomized multicenter trial, high-dose UVA1 phototherapy (130 J/cm^2 daily) was compared with topical glucocorticoid therapy and UVA–UVB therapy for acute, severe AD. Significant differences in favor of high-dose UVA1 radiation and fluocortolone therapy were observed, as compared with UVA–UVB therapy. At day 10, high-dose UVA1 radiation was superior to fluocortolone therapy.

Long-term efficacy of medium-dose UVA1 phototherapy in atopic dermatitis. Abeck D, Schmidt T, Fesq H, et al. J Am Acad Dermatol 2000;42:254–7.

Thirty-two patients with acute exacerbated AD underwent medium-dose UVA1 therapy consisting of 15 treatments over 3 weeks (cumulative dose 750 J/cm^2). There was a significant improvement in the skin condition at the end of the treatment period; this was still present 1 month later, but by 3 months the skin condition had returned to pretreatment levels.

Successful monotherapy of severe and intractable atopic dermatitis by photopheresis. Richter HI, Billmann-Eberwein C, Grewe M, et al. J Am Acad Dermatol 1998;38:585–8.

Photopheresis at 2-week intervals induced improvement in three patients previously resistant to glucocorticosteroids, cyclosporine, phototherapy, or photochemotherapy.

Diet and atopic eczema. Atherton DJ. Clin Allergy 1988;18:215–28.

A balanced review of the role of diet in eczema. Occasional children do show dramatic long-lasting response to dietary management.

Elimination diet in cow's milk allergy: risk for impaired growth in young children. Isolauri E, Sutas Y, Salo MK, et al. J Pediatr 1998;132:1004–9.

In 100 children (mean age 7 months) with AD and cow's milk allergy, treatment with a cow's milk elimination diet resulted in growth delay, a low weight-for-length index, low serum albumin, and an abnormal urea concentration.

Double-blind controlled trial of effect of housedust-mite allergen avoidance on atopic dermatitis. Tan BB, Weald D, Strickland I, Friedmann PS. Lancet 1996;347:15–8.

Measures to reduce house dust mites using a combination of Goretex bedcovers, benzyltannate spray, and a high-filtration vacuum cleaner were compared with cotton bedcovers, water spray, and a conventional vacuum cleaner in the households of 48 children and adults with AD. Both active and placebo treatments caused significant reductions in house dust mite antigen concentrations. The severity of eczema decreased in both groups, but the active group showed significantly greater improvement.

Retrospective review of the use of azathioprine in severe atopic dermatitis. Lear JT, English JS, Jones P, Smith AG. J Am Acad Dermatol 1996;35:642–3.

A retrospective study of 35 patients who had received azathioprine for severe AD showed a decrease in antibiotic use, fewer outpatient visits and hospital admissions, and decreased use of similar or higher potency topical steroids in the year after treatment.

Azathioprine in severe adult atopic dermatitis: a double-blind, placebo-controlled, crossover trial. Berth-Jones J, Takwale A, Tan E, et al. Br J Dermatol 2002;147:324–30.

In this double-blind crossover trial, adult patients with severe AD were treated with azathioprine (2.5 mg/kg daily) and placebo for 3 months each. There was a significant difference in favour of azathioprine in the improvement of the Six Area, Six Sign Atopic Dermatitis (SASSAD) sign score, which was the primary endpoint. This decreased by 26% during treatment with azathioprine versus 3% on placebo. Pruritus, sleep disturbance, and disruption of work/daytime activity all improved significantly on active treatment, but the difference in mean improvement between azathioprine and placebo was statistically significant only for disruption of work/daytime activity. The authors suggested that a longer period of treatment may have further improved the eczema. Gastrointestinal disturbances and deranged liver enzymes were common. Of the 37 patients enrolled, 12 prematurely terminated treatment with azathioprine and four with placebo.

Parallel-group randomized controlled trial of azathioprine in moderate to severe atopic eczema, using a thiopurine methyltransferase-based dose regimen. Meggitt SJ, Gray JC, Reynolds NJ. Br J Dermatol 2003;149(suppl 64):3.

In this study of parallel-group design, 63 patients were randomized. There was again a significant improvement in sign score on azathioprine (39%) relative to placebo (24%).

Evidence levels **A** Double-blind study **B** Clinical trial ≥ 20 subjects **C** Clinical trial < 20 subjects **D** Series ≥ 5 subjects **E** Anecdotal case reports

In contrast to the previous study, there was a marked placebo effect. However, pruritus and the physician's global assessment also improved significantly better in the azathioprine group. Six patients withdrew from azathioprine treatment due to nausea or hypersensitivity.

Double-blind, controlled, crossover study of cyclosporin in adults with severe refractory atopic dermatitis. Sowden JM, Berth-Jones J, Ross J, et al. Lancet 1991; 338:137–40.

Cyclosporin greatly improves the quality of life of adults with severe atopic dermatitis. Salek MS, Finlay AY, Luscombe DK, et al. Br J Dermatol 1993;129:422–30.

In this study, both sign score and quality of life improved rapidly on cyclosporine 5 mg/kg daily. While the sign score rapidly deteriorated on stopping treatment, the improvement in quality of life was more persistent.

Cyclosporin in atopic dermatitis: time to relapse and effect of intermittent therapy. Granlund H, Erkko P, Sinisalo M, Reitamo S. Br J Dermatol 1994;132:106–12.

Forty-three patients with severe AD were treated with a 6-week course of cyclosporine 5 mg/kg daily and were then retreated after a follow-up of 6–26 weeks (depending on the time to relapse) with an identical course of cyclosporine. A significant reduction in disease activity was observed after 2 weeks of cyclosporine treatment. After both treatment periods, approximately half of the patients relapsed after 2 weeks; after 6 weeks follow-up, the relapse rates were 71% and 90%, respectively, for the two treatment periods. Notably, after the first treatment period, five patients did not relapse during the 26-week follow-up, and for the second treatment period, two did not relapse. All of these seven patients were still in remission at 1 year.

Long-term efficacy and safety of cyclosporin in severe adult atopic dermatitis. Berth-Jones J, Graham-Brown RAC, Marks R, et al. Br J Dermatol 1997;136:76–81.

An open study of 48 weeks' duration in which 100 patients were enrolled. Improvements in sign score, itch, and sleep disturbance were maintained throughout treatment. Sixty-five subjects completed the trial and only seven were withdrawn due to adverse events considered likely to have been related to treatment.

Cyclosporin in atopic dermatitis: review of the literature and outline of a Belgian consensus. Naeyaert JM, Lachapelle JM, Degreef H, et al. Dermatology 1999;198: 145–52.

This excellent review summarizes all the major trials of cyclosporine for AD and gives practical recommendations for the clinician.

These authors recommend that cyclosporine be reserved for adults with severe AD and only be used in children with recalcitrant disease for short periods. A starting dosage of 2.5 mg/kg daily can be adjusted up after 2 weeks depending on response, to a maximum dose of 5 mg/kg daily. Screening for gynecologic or prostate malignancy, and skin biopsy to exclude cutaneous T cell lymphoma, as well as close monitoring of renal function and blood pressure, are recommended.

Treatment of atopic eczema with oral mycophenolate mofetil. Neuber K, Schwartz I, Itschert G, Dieck AT. Br J Dermatol 2000;143:385–91.

Ten patients with severe AD were treated with oral mycophenolate mofetil at an initial dose of 1 g daily during the first week and then 2 g daily for a further 11 weeks. Median scores for disease severity improved by 68% (100% in one patient, >75% in three patients, and >50% in the remainder).

Leflunomide as a novel treatment option in severe atopic dermatitis. Schmitt J, Wozel G, Pfeiffer C. Br J Dermatol 2004;150:1182–5.

Two patients with severe, almost erythrodermic AD achieved partial remission within 4 and 7 weeks, respectively, which was maintained over 20 months.

Diluted steroid facial wet wraps for childhood atopic eczema. Tang WYM. Dermatology 2000;200:338–9.

A short period of diluted steroid wet-wrap dressings, e.g. mometasone 0.1% diluted to 0.01% (one part mometasone cream or ointment to nine parts diluent cream or ointment), is useful in selected children with dry eczematous facial lesions.

Efficacy and safety of wet-wrap dressings in children with severe atopic dermatitis: influence of corticosteroid dilution. Wolkerstorfer A, Visser RL, De Waard, et al. Br J Dermatol 2000;143:999–1004.

In children with severe refractory AD, 5%, 10%, and 25% dilutions of fluticasone propionate 0.05% cream proved highly efficacious, irrespective of dilution, when applied under wet-wrap dressings. Improvement occurred mainly during the first week and the only significant adverse effect was folliculitis.

Double-blind, multicentre analysis of the efficacy of borage oil in patients with atopic eczema. Henz BM, Jablonska S, van de Kerkhof PC, et al. Br J Dermatol 1999; 140:685–8.

This study looked at the effect of borage oil on AD. Although the overall improvement in study patients over controls did not reach statistical significance, improvement of individual symptoms over placebo were observed for erythema, vesiculation, crusting, excoriation, lichenification, and insomnia, but not for pruritus.

Atopic eczema unresponsive to evening primrose oil (linoleic and gamma-linolenic acids). Bamford JT, Gibson RW, Renier CM. J Am Acad Dermatol 1985;13:959–65.

Essential fatty acid supplementation in atopic dermatitis: a placebo-controlled trial. Berth-Jones J, Graham-Brown RAC. Lancet 1993;341:1557–60.

Efficacy and tolerability of borage oil in adults and children with atopic eczema: randomized, double-blind, placebo-controlled, parallel-group trial. Takwale A, Tan E, Agarwal S, et al. BMJ 2003;327:1385–7.

Clinical studies of oils containing γ-linolenic acid, such as evening primrose oil and borage oil, have had conflicting results in patients with AD. Some initial small studies showed remarkable improvements and steroid-sparing effects. However, these three large placebo-controlled trials have shown no benefit.

Out-patient treatment of atopic dermatitis with crude coal tar. Van der Valk PG, Snater E, Verbeek-Gijsbers W, et al. Dermatology 1996;193:41–4.

Outpatient treatment with crude coal tar 1.5% to 5% three times a week compared favorably with inpatient daily tar therapy in the treatment of AD, with improvements in score being 29.5% for the outpatient group and 35.0% for the inpatient group. The outpatient treatment period was longer, however, and there was significant impairment of life activities.

Clinical evaluation of ketotifen syrup on atopic dermatitis: a comparative multicenter double-blind study of ketotifen and clemastine. Yoshida H, Niimura M, Ueda H, et al. Ann Allergy 1989;62:507–12.

Ketotifen, a compound with effects on histamine, slow-reacting substance of anaphylaxis (SRS-A), and platelet-activating factor (PAF), was superior to clemastine, a typical antihistamine, in reduction of itch and other dermatologic parameters.

A pilot study examing the role of zileuton in atopic dermatitis. Woodmansee DP, Simon RA. Ann Allergy Asthma Immunol 1999;83:548–52.

Zileuton, 600 mg four times daily, decreased erythema and patient-reported dissatisfaction with disease. Pruritus scores showed a trend toward improvement.

Leukotriene receptor antagonists are ineffective for severe atopic dermatitis. Silverberg NB, Paller AS. J Am Acad Dermatol 2004;50:485–6.

Among five children and two adults with severe widespread AD, two patients had temporary improvement with the leukotriene inhibitors montelukast or zafirlukast, but results were not sustained. Three patients had no response at all.

Topical sodium cromoglycate in the treatment of moderate-to-severe atopic dermatitis. Moore C, Ehlayel MS, Junprasert J, Sorensen RU. Ann Allergy Asthma Immunol 1998;81:452–8.

In this study, patients treated with cromolyn sodium inhalation solution mixed in a water-based emollient cream to a final concentration of 0.21% improved to a greater extent than did the placebo group.

Topical cromoglycate has yielded conflicting results in several studies.

Oral sodium cromoglycate in the management of atopic dermatitis in children. Businco L, Cantani A. Allergy Proc 1991;12:333–8.

This is a review of 12 papers on the use of oral sodium cromoglycate in pediatric AD including 281 children aged 0.5 to 15 years. Four out of five open trials found oral sodium cromoglycate effective in the management of AD. The double-blind studies were positive in three cases and negative in three.

Recombinant interferon gamma therapy for atopic dermatitis. Hanifin JM, Schneider LC, Leung DY, et al. J Am Acad Dermatol 1993;28:189–97.

In this randomized, double-blind study, patients with moderate to severe AD received recombinant human IFNγ (rIFNγ; 50 μg/m²) or placebo by daily subcutaneous injection for 12 weeks. Significant decreases in erythema, pruritus, and excoriation occurred in rIFNγ treated patients. Edema, papulation, induration, scaling, dryness, and lichenification showed greater improvement for the rIFNγ group, but differences were not statistically significant.

Long-term effectiveness and safety of recombinant human interferon gamma therapy for atopic dermatitis despite unchanged serum IgE levels. Stevens SR, Hanifin JM, Hamilton T, et al. Arch Dermatol 1998;134:799–804.

Twenty-four of 32 eligible patients who participated in a previously reported, 12-week, double-blind, placebo-controlled study, self-administered rIFNγ, 50 μg/m², by daily subcutaneous injection. The initial efficacy and adverse effects reported for rIFNγ treatment of patients with AD were maintained after 2 years of long-term use.

Hydroxychloroquine is useful in the management of atopic dermatitis. Smith KC. Br J Dermatol 1992;126:93–4.

A 21-year-old woman with severe AD responded to hydroxychloroquine 200 mg daily, which was subsequently tapered to 200 mg every second or third day.

The treatment of atopic dermatitis with adjunctive high-dose intravenous immunoglobulin: a report of three patients and review of the literature. Jolles S, Hughes J, Rustin M. Br J Dermatol 2000;142:551–4.

Intravenous immunoglobulin 2 g/kg monthly, added to the patients' usual treatment of oral corticosteroid and/or hydroxychloroquine, resulted in marked improvement and allowed reduction or discontinuation of oral corticosteroid.

Propylthiouracil therapy reduces the clinical severity of atopic dermatitis: results of an open trial. Chung JH, Bang HD, Moon SH, et al. Clin Exp Dermatol 1998;23:290–1.

Of 13 patients treated with propylthiouracil 100 mg every 8 h, eight showed greater than 50% improvement and two showed slight improvement in itching and skin texture.

Topical dinitrochlorobenzene therapy in the treatment of refractory atopic dermatitis: systemic immunotherapy. Yoshizawa Y, Matsui H, Izaki S, et al. J Am Acad Dermatol 2000;42:258–62.

Six of eight patients with refractory AD treated weekly with 0.2% to 1% DNCB showed improvement.

Probiotics in primary prevention of atopic disease: a randomised placebo-controlled trial. Kalliomäki M, Salminen S, Arvilommi H, et al. Lancet 2001;357:1076–9.

Lactobacillus was given orally to mothers predisposed to giving birth to a possible atopic child, and postnatally for 6 months to the child. The frequency of atopic eczema in the treated group was half of that in the placebo group.

Bacillary angiomatosis

Jacqueline A Dyche, Richard C D Staughton

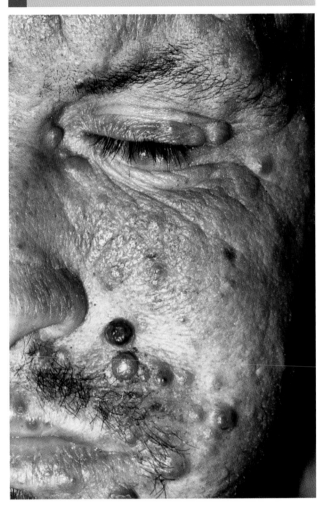

Bacillary angiomatosis was first described in 1983 and typically presents in patients with profound immunocompromise (e.g. in advanced HIV infection, or post transplant or cytotoxic chemotherapy). Angioproliferative papules, nodules, or plaques can arise in the skin or internally, involving the viscera, bone, and the liver, where the condition is termed peliosis hepatis. Lesions are now known to be due to the cat scratch disease infectious agents Bartonella (previously Rochalimaea, see Cat scratch disease, page 113), which are also the agents for trench fever, culture-negative endocarditis, neuroretinitis and verruga peruana, a localized cutaneous form of the disease that occurs in South America. The latter disease continues to plague those in endemic regions and poses a significant threat to travelers in these areas.

MANAGEMENT STRATEGY

Bacillary angiomatosis can present in an indolent manner over several months and adequate treatment is essential to prevent dissemination, which can be fatal. Clinical suspicion should be aroused in the context of a low CD4 lymphocyte

count (<100) especially if there is a history of exposure to cats, the reservoir of infection for *Bartonella henselae*, the cat scratch agent, or the human body louse, the vector for *Bartonella quintana,* the trench fever agent. Lesions can be predominantly cutaneous or subcutaneous and present as multiple brick or cherry red round papules and nodules. They can be mistaken for Kaposi sarcoma (dull, dark red cutaneous swellings that are often oval and expanding between tissue planes) and pyogenic granuloma (usually single proud lesions with a hemorrhagic surface and collarette). In-transit metastatic amelanotic melanoma and other malignancies can be hard to differentiate because of the highly vascular and erosive nature of the lesions in skin, bones, and soft tissues. Histology allows easy differentiation and shows a lobular proliferation of small blood vessels, with swollen endothelial cells containing clumps of bacteria.

The response of bacillary angiomatosis to *antibiotic treatment* is usually dramatic, in contrast to the response of cat scratch disease in the immunocompetent. Our drugs of first choice are the macrolides (e.g. azithromycin 500 mg daily, clarithromycin 500 mg twice daily, erythromycin 500 mg four times daily), with doxycycline 100 mg twice daily as an alternative. Their use is based on anecdotal experience in the absence of systematic trials. Current recommendations are that treatment should be continued for 2 months where there is skin disease only and 4 months where there is bone/visceral involvement or peliosis hepatis. Should relapse occur on the above regimens, then long-term prophylaxis with erythromycin or doxycycline may be indicated. In practice, however, the introduction of highly active anti-retroviral therapy (HAART) should reverse immunocompromise and thus alter the response to treatment, making long-term antibiotic less necessary. The patient should be evaluated for parenchymal and osseous disease prior to treatment and warned that a Jarisch–Herxheimer reaction may occur after the first few doses of antibiotic.

A wide variety of therapeutic agents is described in the literature, but there is a lack of correlation between the in-vitro and in-vivo drug susceptibility of *Bartonella* spp., which reduces the usefulness of laboratory data. The picture is clouded further by the different response of *Bartonella* sp. to drugs in each of the diseases it causes.

SPECIFIC INVESTIGATIONS

- Full blood count, liver function tests, and CD4 lymphocyte count
- Biopsy and Warthin–Starry stains/electron microscopy
- Prolonged culture of blood and biopsy tissue
- Polymerase chain reaction (PCR) of biopsy material
- Serology – indirect fluorescence assay (IFA)

Culture of the fastidious Gram-negative rods of *Bartonella* spp. is extremely difficult, requiring specialist media and prolonged incubation of up to 45 days; it is invariably negative if antibiotics have been given. Skin biopsy is the essential diagnostic tool and shows characteristic appearances on histology and Warthin–Starry silver stains, which shows the organism, as can electron microscopy. Species confirmation can be obtained by PCR. The role of serology is reduced by the poor immune response often mounted in these patients.

The Centers for Disease Control (CDC) definition of a positive test is an indirect fluorescence assay (IFA) titer of over 1 : 64.

Laboratory diagnosis of *Bartonella* infections. Agan BK, Dolan MJ. Clin Lab Med 2002;22:937–62.

Culture methods have improved, but are still prolonged. Serologic testing for *B. henselae* has become the cornerstone for diagnosis. Ideal antigens for enzyme immunoassays have yet to be clearly identified. PCR currently offers the ability to establish the diagnosis when other tests fail.

Bacillary angiomatosis and bacillary peliosis in patients infected with human immunodeficiency virus: clinical characteristics in a case–control study. Mohle-Boetani JC, Koehler JE, Berger TG, et al. Clin Infect Dis 1996;22:794–800.

Forty two cases were compared to 84 matched controls and the distinguishing clinical characteristics were evaluated. Significant differences included the presence of anemia (hematocrit <0.36), raised alkaline phosphatase and aspartate aminotransferase levels, and a low CD4 lymphocyte count (median being 21/mm^3 compared to 186/mm^3 in controls). There was no difference in the white blood cell count, creatinine, bilirubin, and alanine aminotransferase levels. Clinical signs included fever, abdominal pain, and lymphadenopathy.

Bacillary angiomatosis in immunocompromised patients. Gasquet S, Maurin M, Brouqui P, et al. AIDS 1998;12:1793–803.

Diagnosis remains mainly based on histological appearance. On hematoxylin and eosin stains the appearance can be highly variable and so Warthin–Starry stains are essential to visualize the bacillus and confirm the diagnosis.

Culture of *Bartonella quintana* and *Bartonella henselae* from human samples: a 5-year experience (1993 to 1998). La Scola B, Raoult D. J Clin Microbiol 1999;37:1899–905.

In the large number of samples cultured, seven patients were diagnosed with bacillary angiomatosis. PCR was 100% sensitive in diagnosing these cases, in contrast to culture, which isolated *Bartonella* spp. from only three specimens. Serology was of no value, being positive in only one patient.

Rapid identification and differentiation of *Bartonella* species using a single step PCR assay. Jensen WA, Fall MZ, Rooney J, et al. J Clin Microbiol 2000;38:1717–22.

The single step assay described provided a simple and rapid means of identifying *Bartonella* spp.

FIRST LINE THERAPIES

■ Azithromycin	C
■ Clarithromycin	C
■ Erythromycin	C

Molecular epidemiology of *Bartonella* infections in patients with bacillary angiomatosis-peliosis. Koehler JE, Sanchez MA, Garrido CS, et al. N Engl J Med 1997;337:1876–83.

A case–control study of 49 patients (92% HIV positive) in whom macrolides, doxycycline, tetracycline, and rifampin were found to be effective. This was in contrast to patients treated with trimethoprim–sulfamethoxazole, ciprofloxacin, penicillins, and cephalosporins in whom *Bartonella* spp. could be isolated on PCR or culture.

MICs of 28 antibiotic compounds for 14 *Bartonella* (formerly *Rochalimaea*) isolates. Maurin M, Gasquet S, Ducco C, Raoult D. Antimicrob Agents Chemother 1995;39:2387–91.

The newer macrolides were highly effective in preventing bacterial growth with MIC 90s of 0.03 µg/mL for azithromycin and clarithromycin. Erythromycin, doxycycline, and rifampin all had MIC 90s of 0.25 µg/mL.

AIDS commentary: bacillary angiomatosis and bacillary peliosis in patients infected with human immunodeficiency virus. Koehler JE, Tappero JW. Clin Infect Dis 1993;17:612–4.

This review article refers to 50 patients whose lesions and symptoms responded to erythromycin or doxycycline therapy.

Rapid response of AIDS-related bacillary angiomatosis to azithromycin. Guerra LG, Neira CJ, Boman D, et al. Clin Infect Dis 1993;17:264–6.

This documents successful treatment with azithromycin.

Molecular diagnosis of deep nodular bacillary angiomatosis and monitoring of therapeutic success. Schlupen E-M, Schirren CG, Hoegl L, et al. Br J Dermatol 1997;136:747–51.

An HIV-positive man presented with a 10-month history of bacillary angiomatosis on his ankle and was treated with erythromycin 500 mg four times daily. The swabs became negative on PCR at 12 weeks, at which point treatment was successfully stopped.

***Bartonella*-associated infections.** Spach DH, Koehler JE. Infect Dis Clin North Am 1998;12:137–55.

A good review article.

Although azithromycin, clarithromycin, and erythromycin are the authors' first line treatments for bacillary angiomatosis, their use has been based on anecdotal case reports rather than on controlled clinical trials. Azithromycin has emerged as the first line treatment for cat scratch disease for which there are formal trial data (see page 114).

SECOND LINE THERAPIES

■ Doxycycline	C
■ Tetracycline	D
■ Rifampin	D

Clarithromycin therapy for bacillary peliosis did not prevent bacillary angiomatosis. Mukunda BN, West BC, Shekar R. Clin Infect Dis 1998;27:658.

A patient with AIDS presented with bacillary peliosis and was initially treated for a presumed *Mycobacterium avium intracellulare* complex infection with clarithromycin, ciprofloxacin, and rifabutin. He continued to be febrile and re-presented 15 days later with bacillary angiomatosis. This swiftly responded to doxycycline, which was continued for 6 weeks.

Evidence levels **A** Double-blind study **B** Clinical trial ≥ 20 subjects **C** Clinical trial < 20 subjects **D** Series ≥ 5 subjects **E** Anecdotal case reports

Bacillary angiomatosis: presentation of six patients, some with unusual features. Schwartz RA, Nychay SG, Janniger CK, Lambert WC. Br J Dermatol 1997;136:60–5.

This describes a variety of successful treatment regimens, including tetracycline and ciprofloxacin.

Although rifampin has activity in vitro, its efficacy when used alone has not yet been established and so it is recommended as a second line drug in combination with either erythromycin or doxycycline for severely ill patients or where there is neurological involvement. It is, however, effective in the treatment of verruga peruana (Bartonella bacilliformis) and cat scratch disease.

THIRD LINE THERAPIES

■ Gentamicin	E
■ Third and fourth generation cephalosporins	E

Bacillary angiomatosis in a pregnant patient with acquired immunodeficiency syndrome. Riley LE, Tuomala RE. Obstet Gynecol 1992;79:818–9.

A pregnant patient was treated with a third generation cephalosporin, ceftizoxime. However, there are inadequate data to recommend its use at present.

Lack of bactericidal effect of antibiotics except aminoglycosides on *Bartonella (Rochalimaea) henselae*. Musso D, Drancourt M, Raoult D. J Antimicrob Chemother 1995;36:101–8.

Aminoglycosides display in-vitro bactericidal activity against *Bartonella* spp. and as such warrant further clinical investigation.

Balanitis

Neda Ashourian, Ginat Mirowski

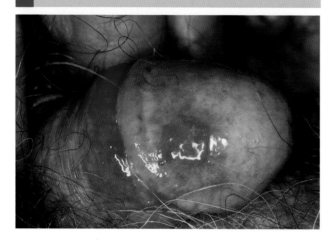

Balanitis is defined as inflammation of the glans penis, and occasionally, the prepuce. Most commonly it is of multifactorial etiology. Potential causes include infection, trauma, poor hygiene, contact allergy, dermatoses, cicatricial disorder, malignancy, rheumatologic disease and fixed drug eruption. This chapter will focus on the treatment of non-specific balanitis, balanitis xerotica obliterans (BXO, see also page 353) , and Zoon's balanitis.

MANAGEMENT STRATEGY

Patients with balanitis commonly complain of itching and irritation of the glans penis. This condition is seen more frequently in uncircumcised men. Clinical manifestations vary from erythematous shiny plaques to white papules or erosions. Complications include phimosis, meatal stenosis, fissures and involvement of the urethra requiring surgical treatment.

Evaluation of a patient with balanitis should begin with a thorough history. Patients should be asked specifically about sexual practices, use of condoms or spermatocidal agents, and symptoms in any partners. The patient's hygiene regimen should be discussed in detail. It is also important to identify potential irritants or allergens and determine oral and topical medications. A comprehensive physical examination with special attention to mucosal membranes may reveal an underlying dermatosis. Underlying infections should be sought and treated aggressively. Any lesion that is not of an obvious infectious or irritant etiology or not responding to topical therapy should be biopsied.

The initial treatment for balanitis revolves around *hygiene, emollient creams* and *topical corticosteroids*. The patient should be instructed to retract the foreskin and clean the glans penis with a weak saline solution twice a day. Soap, an irritant, should be avoided. All topical agents should be used with caution, as they may be irritants or allergens, thus worsening the condition. Ointments are preferable because they contain fewer preservatives. An emollient applied twice a day after cleaning with clean water will both lubricate and protect the area. A low potency topical steroid such as 1% hydrocortisone ointment applied twice daily can help to decrease inflammation. If symptoms persist, a higher potency corticosteroid should be used once or twice daily for 3 weeks. *Carbenoxolone gel*, *topical testosterone propionate*, *topical tacrolimus* and *intralesional corticosteroids* may be used judiciously.

Other options for recalcitrant cases are *CO₂* or *erbium: YAG laser ablation* and *long-term systemic antibiotics*. The definitive treatment for balanitis of any etiology is *circumcision*. Circumcision is a very effective therapy and is a reasonable option to offer patients early in the treatment of balanitis. It will usually result in complete relief of symptoms, even in refractory cases.

SPECIFIC INVESTIGATIONS

- Microscopy for fungi and Tzanck smear
- Subpreputial swab for Candida spp., and viral/bacterial cultures
- Fasting blood glucose
- Serological tests for syphilis
- Biopsy
- Patch testing

Mild balanoposthitis. Fornasa CV, Calabro A, Miglietta A, et al. Genitourin Med 1994;70:345–6.

Three hundred and twenty one patients with balanoposthitis were evaluated. An infectious etiology was identified in 185 patients. Organisms isolated included *Candida albicans, Chlamydia trachomatis, Trichomonas vaginalis, Neisseria gonorrhoeae* and β-hemolytic streptococcus. Traumatic/irritant contact dermatitis was the etiology in 17 cases. Allergic contact dermatitis was found in three cases. Neoplasia was found in eight cases. Other etiologies included psoriasis, lichen planus, BXO, Zoon's balanitis, and fixed drug eruption.

Balanitis xerotica obliterans and its differential diagnosis. Neuhaus IM, Skidmore RA. J Am Board Fam Pract 1999; 12:473–6.

Review of the medical literature showed that BXO was distinguishable from other genital dermatoses through patient history, clinical findings and laboratory evaluation. Tzanck smear, viral and fungal cultures, a rapid protein reagin test and cutaneous biopsy provided a definitive diagnosis.

FIRST LINE THERAPIES

■ Attention to hygiene	C
■ Emollients	C
■ Topical tacrolimus	E
■ Low-potency topical corticosteroids	A

Clinical features and management of recurrent balanitis; association with atopy and genital washing. Birley HD, Walker MM, Luzzi GA, et al. Genitourin Med 1990;69:400–3.

Eighteen patients with a histologic diagnosis of nonspecific balanitis were treated with emollient cream and restriction of soap use. Fifteen had resolution of symptoms. The remaining three responded to 1% hydrocortisone, but two relapsed.

Plasma cell balanitis and vulvitis (of Zoon). Yoganathan S, Bohl T, Mason G. J Reprod Med 1994;39:939–44.

Evidence levels   A Double-blind study   **B** Clinical trial ≥ 20 subjects   **C** Clinical trial < 20 subjects   **D** Series ≥ 5 subjects   **E** Anecdotal case reports

Attention to hygiene combined with topical corticosteroids resulted in improvement of symptoms and signs in six cases of plasma cell balanitis.

Treatment of balanitis xerotica obliterans with topical tacrolimus. Pandher BS, Rustin MHA, Kaisary AV. J Urol 2003;170:923.

In a single case, 0.1% tacrolimus ointment applied twice daily to the glans after circumcision decreased the severity and extent of the inflammation and resulted in total resolution of symptoms.

National guidelines for the management of balanitis. Anonymous. Sex Trans Infect 1999;75(suppl.1):S85–8.

Saline baths and avoidance of soap are recommended for the general management of nonspecific balanitis.

Excellent review.

SECOND LINE THERAPIES

■ High-potency topical corticosteroids	A
■ Moderate-potency topical corticosteroid plus antimicrobials	E
■ Intralesional corticosteroids	E
■ Carbenoxolone gel	A
■ Testosterone propionate	E

The response of balanitis xerotica obliterans to local steroid application compared with placebo in children. Kiss A, Csontai A, Pirot L, et al. J Urol 2001;165:219–20.

This double-blind, placebo controlled, randomized study of 40 boys with clinical BXO showed that the application of a potent topical corticosteroid improves BXO in the histologically early and intermediate stages of disease, and may inhibit progression in the late stage.

Plasma cell balanitis of Zoon; response to Trimovate cream. Tang A, David N, Horton LW. Int J STD AIDS 2001;12:216–20.

Ten patients with biopsy proven plasma balanitis applied a topical mixture comprising of oxytetracycline 3%, nystatin 100 000 U/g, and clobetasone butyrate 0.05% (Trimovate) for 3–12 weeks until complete clinical resolution was observed. Three had recurrence within 3 months after cessation of therapy and responded to a second course of treatment. A fourth patient had three recurrences within 12 months and each time responded to re-treatment within a few days.

Balanitis xerotica obliterans and its differential diagnosis. Neuhaus IM, Skidmore RA. J Am Board Fam Pract 1999;12:473–6.

Report of a case of BXO treated with topical 0.05% clobetasol ointment. Symptomatic relief was achieved.

Clinical evaluation of carbenoxolone in balanitis. Csonka GW, Murray M. Br J Vener Dis 1971;47:179–81.

A controlled double-blind study of 50 patients with non-infectious balanitis showed that carbenoxolone gel was as effective as hydrocortisone cream in treating balanitis. Of patients treated with carbenoxolone gel 73% were fully satisfied, as opposed to 58% treated with hydrocortisone.

The treatment of balanitis xerotica obliterans with testosterone propionate ointment. Pasieczny T. Acta Derm Venereol 1977;57:275–7.

A report of four cases of BXO treated with 2.5% testosterone propionate ointment. Marked improvement was observed after 3–4 months of treatment.

THIRD LINE THERAPIES

■ Circumcision	B
■ CO$_2$ laser	E
■ Erbium: YAG laser	E
■ Copper vapor laser	E
■ Long-term systemic antibiotics	E

Zoon's balanitis treated with erbium: YAG laser ablation. Albertini JG, Holck DE, Farley MF. Lasers Surg Med 2002;30:123–6.

Single case of 67-year-old male who failed prior treatment with 5-fluorouracil, CO$_2$ laser, and 5 months of topical therapy with potent corticosteroids plus mupirocin ointment, responded to 3–6 overlapping passes of laser ablation using the lowest power setting (0.5 J/cm^2; 3 mm spot size; 5 Hz). The lesion healed in a week, but recurred and the patient required two more passes of ablation. He remained disease free at 2 year follow-up.

Plasma cell balanitis: clinical and histopathological features – response to circumcision. Kumar B, Sharma R, Rajagopalan M, Radotra BD. Genitourin Med 1995;71: 32–4.

Twenty seven patients with plasma cell balanitis were cured with circumcision. There were no recurrences at 3-year follow-up.

Zoon's balanitis treated by circumcision. Ferrandez C, Ribera M. J Dermatol Surg Oncol 1984;10:622–5.

Six of seven patients with Zoon's balanitis treated with circumcision were cured. No recurrences were reported at up to 3 years of follow-up. The seventh patient had a small lesion that persisted under an area of residual foreskin.

Surgical treatment of balanitis xerotica obliterans. Campus GV, Ena P, Scuderi N. Plast Reconstr Surg 1984;73:652–7.

Nineteen patients underwent surgical treatment for BXO. The exact procedure performed was determined by the extent of the disease. All patients experienced relief of symptoms. No relapse was reported in up to 4 years of follow-up.

The treatment of Zoon's balanitis with the carbon dioxide laser. Baldwin HE, Geronemus RG. Dermatol Surg Oncol 1989;15:491–4.

A case of Zoon's balanitis successfully treated with carbon dioxide laser. The patient was symptom free for 2 years of follow-up.

Plasma cell balanitis treated with a copper vapour laser. Haedersdal M, Wulf HC. Scand J Plast Reconstr Hand Surg 1995;29:357–8.

Report of an uncircumcised male with plasma cell balanitis treated with copper vapor laser. The lesion resolved, but the patient had a minor relapse. No further treatment was required.

Carbon dioxide laser treatment of external genital lesions. Rosemberg SK. Urology 1985;25:555–8.

Three cases of BXO were treated with CO_2 laser. Complete eradication was achieved after one treatment in two patients. The third patient required a repeat treatment with the laser to achieve cure.

Long-term antibiotic therapy for balanitis xerotica obliterans. Shelley WB, Shelley ED, Grunenwald MA, et al. J Am Acad Dermatol 1999;40:69–71.

Three patients with BXO were treated with various antibacterial regimens. All showed significant improvement after long-term therapy. The antibiotics used included oral and intramuscular penicillin and dirithromycin.

Evidence levels **A** Double-blind study   **B** Clinical trial ≥ 20 subjects   **C** Clinical trial < 20 subjects   **D** Series ≥ 5 subjects   **E** Anecdotal case reports

Basal cell carcinoma

James M Spencer

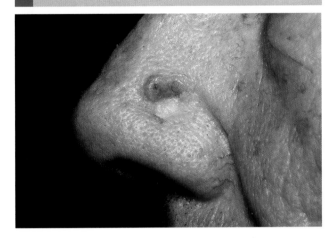

Basal cell carcinoma is a slow-growing malignancy originating in the epidermis. It most commonly arises in areas chronically exposed to UV light, especially the head and neck. Although it is very rare for BCC to metastasize, it can produce significant local tissue destruction, including cartilage and bony invasion.

MANAGEMENT STRATEGY

Basal cell carcinoma slowly but relentlessly grows larger and deeper, and therefore therapeutic intervention is geared towards complete eradication of all malignant cells. Local recurrence is the consequence of inadequate therapy. Complete eradication is especially important because recurrent tumors are often larger and more aggressive than the original incompletely treated primary tumor. Although complete eradication is the primary goal, the therapy chosen should achieve this with the maximal preservation of function and the optimal cosmetic result. Most often, therapy utilizes destructive techniques such as *cryotherapy* or *curettage and electrodesiccation (C&D)*, and more complex tumors may be treated by *excisional surgery, Mohs surgery*, or *radiation therapy (RT)*. The decision about which therapy to use is best made by considering four factors: tumor size; location; histology; history (recurrent vs primary). When assessing a tumor, the clinician may wish to consider each of these four factors and decide whether the patient is high risk or low risk for each, to determine whether to use a simple or complex therapeutic strategy.

Most BCCs are discovered as primary tumors, when they are still less than 1 cm in diameter. Generally tumors smaller than 1 cm on the face and 2 cm on the body are low risk.

Histologic growth pattern is a separate risk factor. The cytology of BCC does not vary, that is all BCCs have well-differentiated, relatively monomorphic cell populations, and these tumors are not graded the way other malignancies are. However, the pattern of growth is variable, and makes a large difference in choosing therapy. One must consider whether the tumor has a circumscribed growth pattern or a diffuse growth pattern. Basal cell carcinoma most typically exhibits a circumscribed, cohesive growth pattern known as

nodular. Nodular BCCs may show partial differentiation towards other structures, such as a cystic or keratotic, but these variants are without therapeutic significance, because the growth pattern is still nodular. Morpheaform, micronodular, infiltrating and superficial BCCs are all variants that exhibit a diffuse growth pattern. These lesions are more likely to recur due to subclinical extension or more aggressive tumor behavior, or both. Unfortunately, all too often biopsy reports come back to the clinician and simply state 'BCC' with no information about the growth pattern. Inadequately treated nodular BCC often recurs with a more aggressive diffuse growth pattern, such as infiltrating or micronodular.

Location is also an important variable to consider when choosing which therapy to use. Basal cell carcinoma tends to occur in chronically sun-exposed sites, especially the head and neck. Approximately 80% of BCCs occur on the head and neck, and fully 25% occur on the nose. The central portion of the face, with the highest incidence of BCC, contains the eyes, nose and mouth, structures of functional and cosmetic importance highly vulnerable to the destructive effects of BCC. These same structures are also highly vulnerable to the destructive effects of therapy directed against BCC. The center of the face extending onto the area around the ears defines a roughly H shaped area known as the H zone. Tumors in this zone have the highest recurrence rate and thus deserve special therapeutic attention. This zone also contains the most vulnerable structures and has the highest rate of BCC occurrence. Tumors near the ear canal, in the H-zone, are of special concern. Extension down the ear canal provides tumor with access to the brain and other intracranial structures, and when there is evidence of ear canal invasion particularly aggressive therapy is warranted.

Lastly, tumor history is important to consider. Recurrent tumors are more difficult to treat than primary tumors and require more aggressive methods.

When confronted with a BCC, the clinician may wish to consider these four variables in the context of the individual patient. The patient's overall medical status, medical history and age may influence the therapeutic decision making.

SPECIFIC INVESTIGATIONS

- Biopsy with adequate dermal component

An adequate biopsy is critical in assessing the tumor. The tumor growth pattern is important information that is impossible to determine if only a superficial fragment is submitted to the lab. Deep shave, punch, incisional or excisional biopsy can all give sufficient dermis for such an evaluation. Because metastasis is so rare, no further evaluation is warranted.

A number of noninvasive imaging technologies are being investigated to delineate tumor depth and extent preoperatively and thus guide treatment. These include confocal microscopy, infrared spectroscopy and ultrasound, but these all remain experimental and are not part of routine care.

Rarely, a BCC may have been neglected and reached a size such that direct bony invasion has occurred. If strongly suspected, a preoperative CT scan should be considered.

The possibility that patients with a BCC have an increased risk of developing subsequent internal malignancies has been suggested over the years, and remains controversial. At present, there is no recommendation for extraordinary evaluation for internal malignancies beyond routine medical care in patients with a history of BCC.

Subsequent primary cancers after basal-cell carcinoma: a nationwide study in Finland from 1953 to 1995. Milan T, Pukkala E, Verkasalo PK, et al. Int J Cancer 2000;87:283–8.

A total of 71 924 patients with a diagnosis of BCC were followed during the study period. There was a statistically significant increased risk in developing non-cutaneous malignancies in patients who had had a BCC.

Basal cell carcinoma and risk of subsequent malignancies: a cancer registry-based study in southwest England. Bower CP, Lear JT, Bygrave S, et al. J Am Acad Dermatol 2000;42:988–91.

A cohort of 13 961 patients diagnosed with a BCC between 1981 and 1988 were followed for additional malignancies. There was a significant increased risk of subsequent melanoma, but no increased risk for internal malignancies.

FIRST LINE THERAPIES

■ Curettage and electrodesiccation	B
■ Cryosurgery	B
■ Excisional surgery	B
■ Mohs micrographic surgery	B

Recurrence rates of treated basal cell carcinomas. Part 2: curettage–electrodesiccation. Silverman MK, Kopf AW, Grin CM, et al. J Dermatol Surg Oncol 1991;17:720–6.

Retrospective study of 2314 primary BCCs treated by C&D at a university dermatology clinic reports a 13.2% 5-year recurrence rate following C&D. Further analysis showed size and location were important variables, with 5-year recurrence rates varying from 9.5% in low-risk locations to over 16.3% in high-risk sites. Similarly, 5-year recurrence rates ranged from 8.5% for tumors 0–5 mm in diameter to 19.8% for tumors 20 mm or more.

Long term recurrence rates in previously untreated (primary) basal cell carcinoma: implications for patient follow-up. Rowe DE, Carroll RJ, Day CL. J Dermatol Surg Oncol 1989;15:315–28.

Reviewed literature since 1947, and reported a weighed average 5-year recurrence rate of 7.7% of primary BCCs treated with C&D.

Mohs surgery is the treatment of choice for recurrent (previously treated) basal cell carcinoma. Rowe DE, Carroll RJ, Day CL. J Dermatol Surg Oncol 1989;15:424–31.

Reports a nearly 40% 5-year recurrence rate of recurrent tumors treated by C&D, emphasizing that this modality is not appropriate for recurrent tumors.

Extensive retrospective studies exist supporting the utility of this simple, rapid and inexpensive method to treat BCC. However, prospective studies directly comparing C&D and other therapeutic modalities are lacking, and drawing conclusions from retrospective studies not controlled for size, histology, location and history make comparisons impossible.

Cryosurgery of basal cell carcinoma: a study of 358 patients. Bernardeau K, Derancourt C, Cambie M, et al. Ann Dermatol Venereol 2000;127:175–9.

A retrospective study of 395 BCCs in 358 patients reports a 5-year recurrence rate of 9%, which is in line with other reports, but that the use of a cryoprobe or other temperature sensing device made no difference in outcome.

A systematic review of treatment modalities for primary basal cell carcinomas. Thissen MR, Neumann MH, Schouten LJ. Arch Dermatol 1999;135:1177–83.

Meta-analysis of published studies evaluating therapeutic methods for treating BCC. Inclusion criteria were prospective studies of at least 50 patients with at least 5-year follow-up with primary BCC. Four studies of cryosurgery filled these criteria, with recurrence rates ranging from 0 to 20.4%

Several large retrospective reports indicate a greater than 95% cure rate with cryotherapy. However, once again size, histology, location and history of the tumors are not defined, and thus such reports are difficult to interpret in a clinically useful way. The authors of such series generally recommend two freeze–thaw cycles to maximize cell death and the use of a cryoprobe to assess tissue temperature achieved; –50°C is generally regarded as sufficiently cytotoxic.

Surgical margins for basal cell carcinoma. Wolf DJ, Zitelli JA. Arch Dermatol 1987;123:340–4.

Detailed histologic examination following excision with various margins revealed that for BCC less than 1 cm in diameter in low-risk areas, a surgical margin of 4 mm of normal appearing skin around the tumor gave a 98% histologic cure rate.

Morpheaform basal-cell epitheliomas: a study of sub-clinical extensions in a series of 51 cases. Salasche SJ, Amonette RA. J Dermatol Surg Oncol 1981;7:387–94.

The average subclinical extension of morpheaform BCC is 7 mm, so a 4 mm margin would be inadequate.

Use the 4 mm margin for primary nodular BCC less than 1 cm in diameter. Larger tumors, diffuse growth pattern tumors and recurrent tumors require larger margins or intraoperative histologic control.

Efficacy of curettage before excision in clearing surgical margins of nonmelanoma skin cancer. Chiller K, Passaro D, McCalmont T, Vin-Christian K. Arch Dermatol 2000;136:1327–32.

Preoperative curettage to better delineate surgical margins produced a statistically significant decrease in positive margins following surgical excision, suggesting the utility of curettage immediately prior to surgical excision.

Long-term recurrence rates in previously untreated (primary) basal cell carcinoma: implications for patient follow-up. Rowe DE, Carroll RJ, Day CL. J Dermatol Surg Oncol 1989;15:315–28.

Retrospective analysis of literature since 1947 reports a weighed average 5-year recurrence rate of 1% when primary BCCs are treated using the Mohs technique

Mohs surgery is the treatment of choice for recurrent (previously treated) basal cell carcinoma. Rowe DE, Carroll RJ, Day CL. J Dermatol Surg Oncol 1989;15: 424–31.

Evidence levels **A** Double-blind study **B** Clinical trial ≥ 20 subjects **C** Clinical trial < 20 subjects **D** Series ≥ 5 subjects **E** Anecdotal case reports

Retrospective analysis of literature since 1947 reports weighed average 5-year recurrence rate of 5.6% when recurrent BCC are treated using the Mohs technique.

Both this and the previous study are retrospective rather than prospective, and thus direct comparison with other therapeutic modalities is difficult. However, it is most likely that the Mohs technique was utilized for higher risk tumors while simple methods such as C&D or cryosurgery are used for low-risk lesions, so the superior results utilizing the Mohs technique may be greater than these numbers would indicate.

Surgical excision vs Mohs' micrographic surgery for basal-cell carcinoma of the face: randomized controlled trial. Smeets NW, Krekels GA, Ostertag JU, et al. Lancet 2004;364: 1766–72.

A randomized, prospective trial comparing Mohs surgery vs conventional surgical excision has been initiated. In this preliminary report, 408 primary and 204 recurrent facial BCCs were randomized to surgical excision with 3 mm margins or Mohs surgery. At 18-month follow-up the recurrence rate of primary BCC in the surgical excision group available for analysis was 2.9% (5/171) and 1.9% (3/160) in the Mohs group. The patients with recurrent tumor were seen at 30-month follow-up, and the recurrence rate of patients actually seen for follow-up was 3.2% (3/93) for the surgical excision group and 0% (0/95) for the Mohs group.

This preliminary report gives the suggestion that Mohs surgery has a lower recurrence rate than conventional surgical excision, but does not reach statistical significance. It is the intention of the authors to continue this study to 5 years of follow-up, at which time any differences may be more obvious.

Mohs micrographic surgery: a cost analysis. Cook J, Zitelli JA. J Am Acad Dermatol 1998;39:698–703.

Cost analysis showing the Mohs technique is economically comparable to excisional surgery, and thus not an unreasonable expense. This report does not take into account the additional savings of preventing recurrences.

SECOND LINE THERAPIES

■ Radiation therapy	B

Basal cell carcinoma of the face: surgery or radiotherapy? Results of a randomized study. Avril MF, Auperin A, Margulis A, et al. Br J Cancer 1997;76:100–6.

A randomized trial in which 347 primary BCC less than 4 cm in size were assigned to surgical excision or radiotherapy (RT). The 4-year recurrence rate was 0.7% for surgical excision and 7.5% for RT. More significantly, cosmesis as judged by the patient and blinded judges was significantly better in the surgery group than in the RT group.

This is a significant result because RT is often recommended as an option for those patients who wish to avoid a scar.

Therapeutic ionizing radiation and the incidence of basal cell carcinoma and squamous cell carcinoma. The New Hampshire Skin Cancer Study Group. Lichter MD, Karagas MR, Mott LA, et al. Arch Dermatol 2000;136: 1007–11.

There is a statistically significant increased risk of the development of BCC within the exposure window follow-

ing therapeutic RT. The development of subsequent tumors is a significant possible side effect.

Radiation therapy is an effective, though expensive and time consuming option for patients unable or unwilling to undergo surgery. Generally, 3000–5000 cGy is given in six to 20 fractionated doses, so therapy may take weeks. Cure rates have repeatedly been reported to be in excess of 90%. BCCs with perineural invasion have a very high local recurrence rate, and postoperative radiation is a wise precaution.

THIRD LINE THERAPIES

■ Intralesional interferon	B
■ Retinoids	D
■ Topical imiquimod	C
■ Photodynamic therapy	A
■ Topical 5-fluorouracil (5-FU)	A
■ Electrochemotherapy	B
■ CO_2 laser	D
■ Intralesional interleukin	D
■ Systemic chemotherapy	D

Intralesional interferon therapy for basal cell carcinoma. Cornell RC, Greenway HT, Tucker SB, et al. J Am Acad Dermatol 1990;23:694–700.

One hundred and seventy two patients with nodular or superficial BCC received 1.5 million units of interferon-α three times a week for 3 weeks and had an 80% histologic cure rate 1 year after treatment.

The injection produces transient flu like symptoms, which are improved with preinjection or oral acetaminophen (paracetamol). An 80% cure rate is not comparable to the greater than 90% cure rate attainable with other modalities, but this may be an option for some patients unable to undergo surgery or RT.

Intralesional recombinant interferon beta-1a in the treatment of basal cell carcinoma: results of an open-label multicentre study. Kowalzick L, Rogozinski T, Wimheuer R, et al. Eur J Dermatol 2002;12:558–61.

One hundred and thirty three BCCs treated with intralesional interferon-β-1a, 1 million units three times a week for 3 weeks. At 16-week follow-up, 66.9% were clinically and biopsy clear. At 2-year follow-up, 4.5% of those that had cleared had recurred.

Alternative preparations of interferons have not been as successful as the α-2a preparation

Treatment and prevention of basal cell carcinoma with oral isotretinoin. Peck GL, DiGiovanna JJ, Sarnoff DS, et al. J Am Acad Dermatol 1988;19:176–85.

Twelve patients with multiple BCCs resulting from varying causes were treated with high-dose oral isotretinoin (mean daily dosage 3.1 mg/kg per day) for a mean of 8 months. Of the 270 tumors monitored in these patients, only 8% underwent complete clinical and histologic regression.

Topical tretinoin treatment in basal cell carcinoma. Brenner S, Wolf R, Dascalu DI. J Dermatol Surg Oncol 1993; 19:264–66.

Case report of patient with multiple superficial BCCs. Four lesions were treated with 0.05% topical tretinoin twice a day for 3 weeks, followed by a 3 week rest. This cycle was repeated two more times. Short-term clinical and histologic evaluation showed clearance in all four lesions, but all four lesions recurred within 9 months.

Topical treatment of basal cell carcinoma with tazarotene: a clinicopathological study on a large series of cases. Bianchi L, Orlandi A, Campione E, et al. Br J Dermatol 2004; 151:148–56.

One hundred and fifty four small superficial and nodular BCCs were treated daily for 24 weeks with topical tazarotene. At the end of the treatment period, 70.8% of the lesions showed evidence of regression, but only 30.5% actually resolved clinically.

Retinoids, either systemically or topically have not shown great efficacy in the treatment of BCC. However, retinoids definitely have an effective role in the chemoprevention of future BCCs in high-risk patients.

Imiquimod 5% cream for the treatment of superficial basal cell carcinoma: results from two phase III, randomized, vehicle-controlled studies. Geisse J, Caro I, Lindholm J, et al. J Am Acad Dermatol 2004;50:722–33.

Multicenter trials of topical imiquimod for superficial BCC with 724 subjects. Patients applied the cream daily five or seven times a week for 6 weeks. Twelve weeks after the treatment period, the area of the tumor was excised and examined histologically. The excised area was tumor free in 82% of the five times a week group and 79% of the seven times a week group.

Open study of the efficacy and mechanism of action of topical imiquimod in basal cell carcinoma. Vidal D, Matias-Guiu X, Alomar A. Clin Exp Dermatol 2004;29:518–25.

Fifty five BCCs measuring greater than 8 mm in diameter with superficial, nodular, or infiltrative histologic growth patterns were treated daily either three times a week for 8 weeks or five times a week for 5 weeks. Punch biopsies were taken 6 weeks after therapy, and patients were followed clinically for 2 years – 4/4 (100%) superficial BCCs, 7/8 (88%) of nodular BCCs, and 30/43 (70%) of infiltrating BCCs were tumor-free following therapy.

This product upregulates interferons α and γ and interleukin 12, among other cytokines. It seems to be reasonably effective for superficial BCCs, but less so for other histologic growth patterns

Photodynamic therapy for the treatment of basal cell carcinoma. Wilson BD, Mang TS, Stoll H, et al. Arch Dermatol 1992;128:1597–1601.

One hundred and fifty one BCCs in 37 patients were treated utilizing photofrin, a systemic photosensitizer that preferentially accumulates in tumors, followed by exposure to 630 nm laser light. Overall, complete response rate by clinical observation at 3 months was 88%.

These authors noted failures tended to be in high-risk areas such as the nose and high-risk histologic variants (morpheaform). Photofrin is a systemic photosensitizer, and some degree of cutaneous and ocular photosensitivity may last up to 4–6 weeks. A variety of other systemic photosensitizers are currently under investigation.

Photodynamic therapy of multiple nonmelanoma skin cancers with verteporfin and red light-emitting diodes: two year results evaluating tumor response and cosmetic outcomes. Lui H, Hobbs L, Tope WD, et al. Arch Dermatol 2004;140:26–32.

Fifty four patients with 421 nonmelanoma skin cancers, including superficial BCC, nodular BCC and SCC in situ, were treated with intravenous verteporfin followed by varying doses of red light. Treated areas were biopsied 6 months after treatment, and patients were followed clinically for 2 years. At the highest light dose, 93% of treated tumors were clear on biopsy, and 95% were clinically clear at 2-year follow-up

Like Photofrin, verteporfin is an intravenous medication, but has the advantage that patients are photosensitive for only 3–5 days.

Photodynamic therapy utilizing topical delta-aminolevulinic acid in non-melanoma skin malignancies of the eyelids and the periocular skin. Wang I, Bauer B, Andersson-Engels S, et al. Acta Ophthalmol Scand 1999;77:182–88.

Nineteen BCCs of the periocular region were treated with topical 20% δ-aminolevulinic acid, a photosensitizer that preferentially accumulates in malignant cells, followed by illumination with 635 nm laser light. Clinically, 42% had a complete response, 42% had a partial response, and 16% had no response.

Topical therapy avoids systemic photosensitivity, but penetration into the skin remains a problem. The eyelid skin is particularly thin, so if penetration were to be effective anywhere, it would be in this area.

Photodynamic therapy by topical aminolevulinic acid, dimethylsulphoxide, and curettage in nodular basal cell carcinoma: a one year follow up study. Soler AM, Warloe T, Tausjo J, Berner A. Acta Derm Venereol 1999;79:204–6.

One hundred and nineteen nodular BCC were first debulked by curettage, then treated topically with dimethyl sulfoxide (DMSO) then 20% topical δ-aminolevulinic acid. Clinically, there was a 5% recurrence rate at mean follow-up of 17 months.

The curettage and DMSO are to help the topical aminolevulinic acid (ALA) penetrate better. However, the point of PDT is to avoid surgery, so if a curettage has been performed, it is not clear how this technique offers an improvement over conventional C&D. Also, we will need to evaluate the 5-year recurrence rate when it becomes available.

Treatment of basal cell carcinoma of the skin with 5-fluorouracil ointment. A 10 year follow-up study. Reymann F. Dermatologica 1979;158:368–72.

Ninety five BCCs were treated with 5% 5-FU ointment. At 10-year follow-up, there was a 21.4% recurrence rate.

Fluorouracil paste treatment of thin basal cell carcinomas. Epstein E. Arch Dermatol 1985;121:207–13.

Forty four thin BCCs were treated with 25% 5-FU in petrolatum under occlusion for 3 weeks with weekly dressing changes. The 5-year recurrence rate was 21%.

Topical 5 FU is not an effective treatment even for thin BCCs. Furthermore, topical 5-FU can mask the deeper component by treating the superficial component and lead to disastrous recurrences.

A pilot study to evaluate the treatment of basal cell carcinoma with 5-flurouracil using phosphatidyl choline as a transepidermal carrier. Romagosa R, Saap L, Givens M, et al. Dermatol Surg 2000;26:338–40.

Ten moderately thick BCCs were treated with 5% 5-FU in a phosphatidyl choline carrier ointment, while seven similar

BCCs were treated with 5% 5-FU in a petrolatum base. The histologic cure rate was 90% in the phosphatidyl choline carrier, but only 57% in the petrolatum vehicle group.

This very small study does not have enough subjects to reach statistical significance, but points out that penetration is the problem with topical 5-FU, and future more penetrant vehicles may solve this problem.

Effective treatment of cutaneous and subcutaneous malignant tumors by electrochemotherapy. Mir LM, Glass LF, Sersa G, et al. Br J Cancer 1998;77:2336–42.

A variety of cutaneous and subcutaneous tumors including BCC (32), malignant melanoma (142), adenocarcinoma (30) and squamous cell carcinomas (87) were treated with a novel drug delivery system. Short and intense electrical pulses were applied directly to the tumors shortly after intravenous or intralesional administration of bleomycin. The electrical pulses are thought to increase intracellular drug uptake by altering cell membrane permeability, thus leading to higher intracellular concentrations of the chemotherapeutic agent bleomycin. Complete clinical resolution was observed in 56.4% of the tumors and a partial response in an additional 28.9%.

Can the carbon dioxide laser completely ablate basal cell carcinomas? A histological study. Horlock N, Grobbelaar AO, Gault DT. Br J Plastic Surg 2000;53:286–93.

Use of the continuous wave CO_2 laser to destroy BCCs was examined by post-laser excision and histologic check. Superficial BCCs of the trunk could be reliably ablated, but nodular and infiltrating (a diffuse growth pattern) could not reliably be treated by this method.

Effect of perilesional injections of PEG-interleukin-2 from ne dose a week to four doses a week. Kaplan B, Moy RL. Dermatol Surg 2000;26:1037–40.

Intralesional injection of interleukin-2 in varying doses from one dose a week to four doses a week was given to eight patients with 12 BCCs. A complete response was seen in eight of the 12 (66%) tumors.

Preoperative treatment of advanced skin carcinoma with cisplatin and bleomycin. Denic S. Am J Clin Oncol 1999;22:32–4.

Five patients with advanced skin cancer of the head and neck were treated with systemic cisplatin and bleomycin before definitive excision to decrease the size of the tumor. Three patients had squamous cell carcinoma, and two had BCC. One patient had clinical, but not pathologic resolution, three had a partial response and one progressed. The surgical resection was decreased from that predicted prior to chemotherapy only in the one patient with a dramatic response.

Systemic chemotherapy has not been extensively investigated for BCC because metastatic disease is so rare. For metastatic disease the response to chemotherapy is generally poor, and there is little reason to believe preoperative systemic chemotherapy for advanced primary BCC would reduce the extent of excisional surgery necessary to achieve a cure.

Becker's nevus

Warren R Heymann, Graham Johnston, Robert Burd

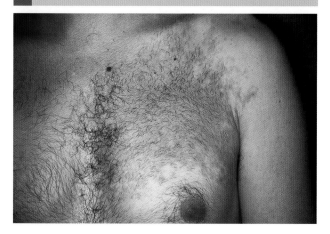

Becker's nevus is a unilateral, irregularly pigmented, macular lesion, with associated hypertrichosis. It is most commonly seen in males, situated over the shoulder, scapula, or anterior chest wall. It is not usually present at birth, but develops slowly during puberty.

MANAGEMENT STRATEGY

Becker's nevus is an organoid nevus with hamartomatous elements and not a melanocytic nevus. The lesion is usually asymptomatic and patients present either requesting a diagnosis or treatment for cosmetic reasons.

In assessing the patient with Becker's nevus it is important to look for any other associated abnormalities. Those most commonly reported are as follows:

- unilateral breast hypoplasia;
- unilateral hypoplasia of the shoulder girdle, pectoralis major, or upper limb;
- vertebral defects;
- acne;
- accessory mammary tissue (polythelia);
- multiple leiomyomas;
- localized lipoatrophy;
- acanthosis nigricans;
- Bowen's disease;
- congenital adrenal hypoplasia;
- accessory scrotum.

The risk of malignant melanoma in a Becker's nevus was previously thought to be nil, but a handful of cases have been reported. As the nevus itself is common (prevalence approximately 1 in 200 [0.52%] of postpubertal males) the risk of malignant transformation appears to be very low. Therefore, regular follow-up screening for melanoma is unnecessary and the patient can be reassured accordingly.

Management of the asymptomatic, benign lesion should be based on confirming the diagnosis and fully documenting any associated pathology.

Traditional *surgical* approaches to remove these lesions are either unsuccessful or result in significant and cosmeti-

cally unjustifiable scarring. *Laser* technology now offers the clinician a means to reduce both the pigmentation and the hypertrichosis seen in Becker's nevus and so may improve the cosmetic appearance of this lesion.

Becker's nevus syndrome revisited. Danarti R, König A, Salhi A, et al. J Am Acad Dermatol 2004;51:965–9.

This is an outstanding review of the ipsilateral breast hypoplasia, other cutaneous anomalies, musculoskeletal abnormalities, and maxillofacial findings that may be observed in the Becker nevus syndrome. The authors present the concept of paradominant inheritance that could explain why there may be occasional familial aggregation in this syndrome that typically presents sporadically.

Becker nevus syndrome. Happle R, Koopman RJJ. Am J Med Gen 1997;68:357–61.

The term 'Becker nevus syndrome' has been suggested because a proportion of patients have unilateral breast hypoplasia or other cutaneous, muscular, or skeletal defects, not always on the ipsilateral side.

Acne in a Becker's naevus: an androgen mediated link? Downs AMR, Mehta R, Lear JT, Peachey RDG. Clin Exp Dermatol 1998;23:191–2.

One of five reports of acne localizing to a Becker's nevus. An increase in androgen receptor protein and mRNA has previously been demonstrated in Becker's nevus compared to normal skin.

Becker's nevus and malignant melanoma. Fehr B, Panizzon RG, Schnyder UW. Dermatologica 1991;182:77–80.

A series of nine patients with Becker's nevus who subsequently developed malignant melanoma; five of these were in the same body site, but only one actually arose within the nevus itself.

SPECIFIC INVESTIGATIONS

The diagnosis can usually be made on clinical examination. A skin biopsy is diagnostic, but is often unnecessary.

Where clinically indicated, investigation and management of associated pathology such as musculoskeletal abnormalities should be considered. This should be discussed with a diagnostic radiologist and the relevant specialist where appropriate. Associated symptomatic cutaneous lesions such as leiomyomas should be excised. Familial Becker's nevus has been regularly reported and it would be prudent to enquire about other family members at presentation.

Familial Becker's nevus. Panizzon RG. Int J Dermatol 1990;29:158.

A review of 16 patients, most commonly same-sex siblings, with Becker's nevi.

FIRST LINE THERAPIES

Treatment requested by patients can be divided into two components:

- reduction of the hyperpigmentation;
- removal of excess hair.

Evidence levels A Double-blind study **B** Clinical trial ≥ 20 subjects **C** Clinical trial < 20 subjects **D** Series ≥ 5 subjects **E** Anecdotal case reports

Some patients will have both significant pigment and excess hair.

Reduction of hyperpigmentation

■ Erbium:YAG laser	C
■ Q-switched ruby laser (QSRL)	D

Becker's naevus: a comparative study between erbium : YAG and Q-switched neodynium : YAG; clinical and histopathological findings. Trelles MA, Allones I, Moreno-Arias GA, Velez M. Br J Dermatol 2005;152:308–13.

Twenty two patients with Becker's nevi were studied – 11 with each laser. Both erbium:YAG and Nd:YAG safely treated the lesions. In terms of pigment removal, one pass with erbium:YAG is a superior technique to three treatment sessions with the Nd:YAG.

Q-switched ruby laser treatment of tattoos and benign pigmented skin lesions: a critical review. Raulin C, Schonermark MP, Greve B, Werner S. Ann Plast Surg 1998; 41:555–65.

A review article that recommends three to ten treatments at monthly intervals with the QSRL at fluences between 7 and 20 J/cm² for pigmentation. The authors do not recommend the QSRL for long-term removal of associated hypertrichosis, but add that the long-pulsed (755 nm) alexandrite laser has produced promising results.

Quality-switched ruby laser treatment of solar lentigines and Becker's nevus: a histopathological and immunohistochemical study. Kopera D, Hohenleutner U, Landthaler M. Dermatology 1997;194:338–43.

A single case of a Becker's nevus treated with a single 8 J/cm² pulse that resulted in clinical fading within 2 weeks, but reactive patchy hyperpigmentation after 4 weeks.

The removal of cutaneous pigmented lesions with the Q-switched ruby laser and the Q-switched neodymium: yttrium-aluminum-garnet laser. A comparative study. Tse Y, Levine VJ, McClain SA, Ashinoff R. J Dermatol Surg Oncol 1994;20:795–800.

An area of Becker's nevus was anesthetized and bisected, and each half treated with the QSRL or QSNd:YAG laser at 532 nm. The results were a clinical lightening of 63 and 43% at fluences of 8.4 and 2.8 J/cm², respectively. Although the QSRL was more painful intraoperatively, the QSNd:YAG caused more postoperative discomfort.

Reduction of excess hair

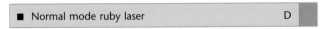

■ Normal mode ruby laser	D

The ruby laser in the normal or 'long-pulsed' mode has been used for laser epilation. A common side effect is hypopigmentation of adjacent skin. This 'side effect' can be used to advantage when treating hypertrichosis associated with a Becker's nevus.

Treatment of a Becker's nevus using a 694-nm long-pulsed ruby laser. Nanni CA, Alster TS. Dermatol Surg 1998;24: 1032–4.

A single case report that showed a 90% reduction in hair growth and also reduction in pigmentation after three treatments with the long pulsed ruby laser. This improvement was maintained for 10 months after the final treatment.

SECOND LINE THERAPIES

Reduction of hyperpigmentation

■ Frequency-doubled QSNd : YAG	D

The QSNd : YAG laser operating at 532 nm has been shown to reduce the pigmentation in a Becker's nevus, but does not appear to be as successful as the ruby laser.

Reduction of excess hair

■ Electrolysis	E

Electrolysis is a well-established method of epilation, but its use in removing hair from a Becker's nevus has not been described.

THIRD LINE THERAPIES

■ Spironolactone	E

Becker's nevus with ipsilateral breast hypoplasia: improvement with spironolactone. Hoon Jung J, Chan Kim Y, Joon Park H, Woo Cinn Y. J Dermatol 2003;30:154–6.

The pathogenesis of breast hypoplasia associated with Becker's nevi is not understood, but increased levels of androgen receptor in the affected area may play a role. Spironolactone, an anti-androgenic agent, was administered for the treatment of the hypoplasia, and 1 month later, breast enlargement was seen only in the hypoplastic breast with Becker's nevus.

The authors believe that this finding supports the theory that breast hypoplasia in Becker's nevi is related to the androgenic receptor.

Behçet's disease

Larisa Ravitskiy, Justin J Green,
Gary Goldenberg, Joseph L Jorizzo

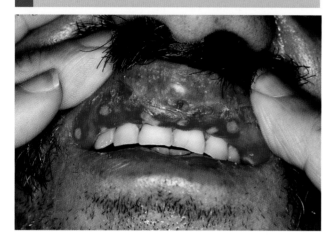

Behçet's disease is a chronic systemic vasculitis characterized by oral and genital aphthae, arthritis, cutaneous lesions (erythema nodosum-like lesions, pyoderma gangrenosum-like lesions, Sweet's syndrome-like lesions, and papulopustular eruptions) and ocular, gastrointestinal, and neurologic manifestations. Many regimens effective for recurrent aphthous stomatitis are used to treat the aphthae of Behçet's disease (see Aphthous stomatitis, page 53).

MANAGEMENT STRATEGY

In the absence of the multisystem disease, the severity and extent of the mucocutaneous manifestations direct the treatment. First line therapy for oral and genital aphthae is a *high-potency topical corticosteroid* in a gel or ointment formulation. Alternatively, *intralesional corticosteroid* (triamcinolone 5 mg/mL) can be used for major aphthae and severe minor aphthae. Other topical therapies accelerate healing or diminish pain associated with oral aphthae and include viscous *lidocaine* 2–5% applied directly to lesions, *chlorhexidine* 1–2%, *amlexanox* 5% oral paste, *sucralfate*, *tetracycline suspension* and *topical tacrolimus*.

Colchicine 0.6 mg three times daily combined with topical corticosteroid therapy is efficacious in mucocutaneous disease. *Dapsone* 100–200 mg daily is also effective, but requires a more rigorous follow-up.

Those patients who fail the more conservative approaches or have severe mucocutaneous disease may require aggressive therapy. *Thalidomide* 100–300 mg daily (pediatric dose varies from 1 mg/kg per week to 1 mg/kg daily) is more effective then low-dose *methotrexate* 7.5–20 mg per week for severe disease. *Prednisone* taper begun at 1 mg/kg daily can be used for severe mucocutaneous flares, but rebound is a possible complication.

Systemic *interferon (IFN)-α-2a* and *anti-tumor necrosis factor (TNF)-α* therapies may be best suited for those with severe mucocutaneous lesions and ocular or articular manifestations. Patients with certain extracutaneous signs (e.g. uveitis, aneurysms) may warrant combination therapy with *prednisone* and an immunosuppressive agent, such as *cyclosporine*, *azathioprine*, *chlorambucil* or *cyclophosphamide*.

Mucocutaneous disease alone rarely warrants this therapy. However, these agents have a beneficial effect on skin and mucous membrane lesions.

SPECIFIC INVESTIGATIONS

- Pathergy test
- Culture/polymerase chain reaction of aphthae to exclude herpes simplex virus (HSV)
- Vitamin B1, B2, B6 and B12, folate, zinc and iron levels
- Anti-streptolysin O (ASO) titer
- Urinalysis
- HLA-B27
- Exclude inflammatory bowel disease

Behçet's syndrome: immunopathological and histopathological assessment of pathergy lesions is useful in diagnosis and follow-up. Jorizzo JL, Soloman AR, Cavallo T. Arch Pathol Lab Med 1985;109:747–51.

This method of pathergy testing may be more sensitive than standard techniques devoid of histologic study.

Behçet's disease and complex aphthosis. Ghate JV, Jorizzo JL. J Am Acad Dermatol 1999;40:1–18.

A review of investigations that should be carried out in a patient with complex aphthosis is presented.

HSV, nutritional deficiencies, neutropenia, lymphopenia, reactive arthritis, inflammatory bowel disease may simulate the oral aphthae of Behçet's disease.

FIRST LINE THERAPIES

■ Topical/intralesional corticosteroid	B
■ Topical tacrolimus	D
■ Chlorhexidine gluconate	D
■ Amlexanox 5% paste	D
■ Sucralfate	A
■ Tetracycline suspension	D
■ Colchicine	A
■ Zinc sulfate	E

A double-blind trial of colchicine in Behçet's syndrome. Yurdakul S, Mat C, Tuzun Y, Ozyazgan Y, et al. Arthritis Rheum 2001;44:2686–92.

A prospective, double-blind, controlled trial of 116 patients treated with colchicine vs placebo. Therapy with colchicine 1–2 mg daily was effective for arthritis and erythema nodosum. Orogenital aphthae were more responsive to treatment in females.

Recurrent aphthous stomatitis: treatment with colchicine. An open trial of 54 cases. Fontes V, Machet L, Huttenberger B, et al. Ann Dermatol Venereol 2002; 129:1365–9.

Fifty-four patients were treated with 1–1.5 mg colchicine for at least three months. Twelve patients no longer had aphthae and were in complete remission; 22 patients were significantly improved, since the frequency and duration of the lesions had decreased by at least 50%. Treatment failed or tolerance was poor in 20 patients.

Evidence levels A Double-blind study B Clinical trial ≥ 20 subjects C Clinical trial < 20 subjects D Series ≥ 5 subjects E Anecdotal case reports

SECOND LINE THERAPIES

■ Dapsone	A
■ Thalidomide	A
■ Methotrexate	E
■ Systemic corticosteroid	B

Dapsone in Behçet's disease: a double-blind, placebo-controlled, cross-over study. Sharquie KE, Najim RA, Abu-Raghif AR. J Dermatol 2002;29:267–79.

Randomized, double-blind, placebo-controlled, cross-over trial of 20 patients treated with either dapsone 100 mg or placebo. There was a significant reduction of orogenital ulcers and other cutaneous manifestations in the dapsone group.

Vitamin E 800 IU daily may reduce the hemolysis induced by dapsone. Other studies confirmed the utility of dapsone for mucocutaneous Behçet's disease.

Thalidomide in the treatment of the mucocutaneous lesions of Behçet syndrome: a randomized, double-blind, placebo-controlled trial. Hamuryudan V, Mat C, Saip S, et al. Ann Intern Med 1998;128:443–50.

Randomized, double-blind, controlled trial of 96 males evaluated thalidomide 100 mg daily vs 300 mg daily vs placebo for 24 weeks. Both thalidomide dosages led to a significant suppression of oral ulcers at 4 weeks, and genital ulcers and follicular lesions at 8 weeks. Complete responses were observed in 11% of patients treated with thalidomide.

Thalidomide effects in Behçet's syndrome and pustular vasculitis. Jorizzo JL, Schmalstieg FC, Solomon AR Jr, et al. Arch Intern Med 1986;146:878–81.

Four patients with Behçet's syndrome who were given thalidomide in sequential four-week 'on' and 'off' cycle showed significant clinical benefit.

Treatment of Behçet's disease with thalidomide. Hamza MH. Clin Rheumatol 1986;5:365–71.

Thirty male patients were treated with thalidomide. Twenty-six patients with orogenital ulcerations responded (20 completely and 6 partially), all patients with arthritis responded (13 completely and 1 partially), and uveitis improved in 3 patients.

Low-dose weekly methotrexate for unusual neutrophilic vascular reactions: cutaneous polyarteritis nodosa and Behçet's disease. Jorizzo JL, White WL, Wise CM, et al. J Am Acad Dermatol 1991;24:973–8.

Two female patients with oral and genital aphthae, pyoderma gangrenosum-like lesions and cutaneous pustular vasculitic lesions cleared with methotrexate 15–20 mg/week.

Practical treatment recommendations for pharmacotherapy of Behçet's syndrome. Yazici H, Barnes CG. Drugs 1991;42:796–804.

Intravenous pulse methylprednisolone 1 g on three alternate days or 1 mg/kg daily of prednisone for several weeks with subsequent taper are recommended for severe or life-threatening major ulcerations.

Combined therapy with other immunosuppressives while on maintenance prednisone is found in multiple trials, but prednisone alone vs placebo has not been studied.

THIRD LINE THERAPIES

■ IFN-α-2a	B
■ Penicillin	B
■ Indomethacin	B
■ Etretinate	E
■ Cyclosporine	A
■ Azathioprine	A
■ Cyclophosphamide	E
■ Chlorambucil	B
■ Minocycline	C
■ Plasmapheresis	E
■ Prostaglandin E1	C
■ IVIG	D
■ Plasma exchange	E
■ Rebamipide	B
■ Anti-TNF-α agents	C
■ Peptide 336-351 linked to cholera toxin B	C
■ Levamisole	C
■ Adsorption apheresis	E

Differential efficacy of human recombinant interferon-alpha2a on ocular and extraocular manifestations of Behçet disease: results of an open 4-center trial. Kötter I, Grimbacher B, Eckstein AK, et al. Semin Arthritis Rheum 2004;33:311–9.

Open, uncontrolled study of 50 patients treated with subcutaneous 6×10^6 U rhIFN-α-2a daily resulted in 92% response rate of ocular manifestations, remission of genital ulcerations and skin lesions, and 36% response of oral aphthae.

There are additional reports substantiating benefits of IFN-α-2a in mucocutaneous Behçet's disease.

Interferon-alpha treatment of Behçet's disease. O'Duffy JD, Calamia K, Cohen S, et al. J Rheumatol 1998;25:1938–44.

Seven patients underwent daily subcutaneous injections of 3 million units of interferon 2-α. This open trial reported a substantial reduction in mucocutaneous lesions and joint disease. Flu-like symptoms, leukopenia, psoriasis, seizure, hyperthyroidism, and psychosis were side effects reported.

Effect of prophylactic benzathine penicillin on mucocutaneous symptoms of Behçet's disease. Calguneri M, Ertenli I, Kiraz S, et al. Dermatology 1996;192:125–8.

A prospective, randomized trial with 60 patients revealed statistically significant decrements in frequency and duration of oral aphthae and erythema nodosum-like lesions and the frequency of genital aphthae with addition of benzathine penicillin 1.2 million units every 3 weeks to colchicine vs colchicine monotherapy.

This study was apparently non-blinded and not placebo controlled.

Treatment of Behçet disease with indomethacin. Simsek H, Dundar S, Telatar H. Int J Dermatol 1991;30:54–7.

An open-label study used indomethacin 25 mg four times daily in 30 patients with articular and skin manifestations. Improvements were seen in reduction of aphthae, erythema nodosum-like lesions, pustular lesions and joint involvement.

A double-blind, randomized, placebo-controlled study of azapropazone and a few case reports describe unsuccessful treat-

ment of arthritis and leg ulcers with various nonsteroidal anti-inflammatory drugs (NSAIDs). When added to colchicine therapy, NSAIDs have been reported to cause an increase in ocular attacks.

Evidence for anti-inflammatory activities of oral synthetic retinoids: experimental findings and clinical experience. Orfanos CE, Bauer R. Br J Dermatol 1983;109:55–60.

Anecdotal report of Behçet's disease responding to etretinate (possibly with addition of prednisolone).

Double-masked trial of cyclosporin versus colchicine and long-term open study of cyclosporin in Behçet's disease. Masuda K, Nakajima A, Urayama A, et al. Lancet 1989;1:1093–6.

Cyclosporine was more effective than colchicine in reducing the number and frequency of oral aphthae and cutaneous lesions (erythema nodosum-like, subcutaneous thrombophlebitis and folliculitis-like lesions).
Several case reports and open studies corroborate these findings.

Cyclosporine in Behçet's disease: results in 16 patients after 24 months of therapy. Pacor ML, Biasi D, Lunardi C, et al. Clin Rheumatol 1994;13:224–7.

Sixteen subjects with Behçet's syndrome received 5 mg/kg daily of cyclosporine for 24 months. A marked improvement of the symptoms was observed after three months of therapy and 14 out of 16 patients obtained a complete clinical remission. Two patients dropped out of the study because of anemia and renal dysfunction, which returned to normal when cyclosporine was withdrawn.

Efficacy of cyclosporine on mucocutaneous manifestations of Behçet's disease. Avci O, Gurler N, Gunes AT. J Am Acad Dermatol 1997;36:796–7.

Mucocutaneous lesions were markedly suppressed in an open trial involving 24 patients treated for greater than 6 months with cyclosporine 5 mg/kg daily. Most responsive to therapy were genital ulcerations, thrombophlebitis, erythema nodosum-like lesions and acneiform lesions.

A controlled trial of azathioprine in Behçet's syndrome. Yazici H, Pazarli H, Barnes CG, et al. N Engl J Med 1990;322:281–5.

A randomized, controlled, double-blind trial of azathioprine 2.5 mg/kg daily vs placebo in patients with Behçet's disease resulted in prevention and decreased frequency of ocular disease. The prevalence of oral ulcers and the incidence of genital ulcers were diminished in the azathioprine group.

Cyclophosphamide therapy of Behçet's disease. Buckley CE III, Gillis JP Jr. J Allergy 1969;64:105–12.

A single report of oral aphthae and ocular manifestations responding to cyclophosphamide when it was added to prednisone therapy.

Long-lasting remission of Behçet's disease after chlorambucil therapy. Abdalla MI, Bahgat NE. Br J Ophthalmol 1973;57:706–11.

Remission of aphthae was achieved in all seven patients treated with oral chlorambucil and corticosteroids, but in a minority of patients treated with corticosteroids alone.

Chlorambucil in the treatment of uveitis and meningo-encephalitis of Behçet's disease. O'Duffy JD, Robertson DM, Goldstein NP. Am J Med 1984;76:75–84.

In ten patients treated with either chlorambucil 0.1 mg/kg daily or corticosteroids, uveitis and visual acuities improved in five of seven eyes when the patients were treated with chlorambucil and in only four of 13 eyes when treatment consisted of corticosteroids. Eight of nine patients with meningoencephalitis were treated with chlorambucil and had remission of their disease.
In one controlled study, chlorambucil, when used with corticosteroids, was superior to corticosteroids alone.

Streptococcal infection in the pathogenesis of Behçet's disease and clinical effects of minocycline on the disease symptoms. Kaneko F, Oyama N, Nishibu A. Yonsei Med J 1997;38:444–54.

In 11 patients treated with minocycline 100 mg daily, frequency of cutaneous symptoms was reduced by 10% for oral aphthae and by 100% for perifolliculitis.

Behçet's disease with severe cutaneous necrotizing vasculitis: response to plasma exchange – report of a case. Cornelis F, Sigal-Nahum M, Gaulier A, et al. J Am Acad Dermatol 1989;21:576–9.

Oral prostaglandin E1 as a therapeutic modality for leg ulcers in Behçet's disease. Takeuchi A, Hashimoto T. Int J Clin Pharm Res 1987;7:283–9.

In five patients, leg ulcers began to regranulate within 2 weeks of using oral prostaglandin E1 15–30 μg daily.

Intravenous immunoglobulin therapy for resistant ocular Behçet's disease. Seider N, Beiran I, Scharf J, Miller B. Br J Ophthalmol 2001;85:1287–8.

Four patients with ocular disease refractory to steroids and cyclosporine were treated with a course of IVIG. Six eyes showed good response to IVIG therapy.

Behçet's syndrome: response to infliximab after failure of etanercept. Estrach C, Mpofu S, Moots RJ. Rheumatology (Oxford) 2002;41:1213–4.

One patient with orogenital ulcerations, arthralgias, severe iritis, positive pathergy test and many episodes of erythema nodosum responded to infliximab therapy.

Efficacy of rebamipide as adjunctive therapy in the treatment of recurrent oral aphthous ulcers in patients with Behçet's disease. Matsuda T, Ohno S, Hirohata S, et al. Drugs R D 2003;4:19–28.

Multicenter, randomized, double-blind, placebo-controlled prospective study of rebamipide 300 mg/kg plus usual therapy (n = 19) vs placebo plus usual therapy (n = 16) showed moderate to marked improvement of oral aphthae in 65% of treatment group vs 36% in placebo group.

Behçet's disease: a new target for anti-tumor necrosis factor treatment. Sfikakis PP. Ann Rheum Dis 2002;61 (suppl):ii51–ii53.

A review of anti-TNF-α agents in Behçet's disease. Orogenital and cutaneous manifestations resolved in five patients (case reports) with therapy-resistant Behçet's disease treated with infliximab (3 mg/kg–10 mg/kg single or multiple infusions) and in two patients (double-blind, placebo-controlled study of four male patients) treated with etanercept 25 mg subcutaneously twice a week.

Evidence levels   A Double-blind study   **B** Clinical trial ≥ 20 subjects   **C** Clinical trial < 20 subjects   **D** Series ≥ 5 subjects   **E** Anecdotal case reports

Efficacy, safety, and pharmacokinetics of multiple administrations of infliximab in Behçet's disease with refractory uveoretinitis. Ohno S, Nakamura S, Hori S, et al. J Rheum 2004;31–7.

Thirteen patients with refractory uveoretinitis were randomized into 5 mg/kg and 10 mg/kg treatment groups. Five of the patients remained on cyclosporine during the study. After four infusions, the frequency of ocular attacks (ocular attack disappearance rate 71–83%) and improvement of mucocutaneous symptoms was similar in both groups.

A double blind placebo controlled trial of etanercept on the mucocutaneous lesions of Behçet's syndrome. Melikoglu M, Fresko I, Mat C, et al. Book of Abstracts. Berlin: 10th International Congress on Behçet's disease; 2002:Abs.48.

Etanercept was beneficial in suppressing oral aphthae, nodular lesions, arthritis and papulopustular lesions in short term follow-up.

Oral tolerization with peptide 336-351 linked to cholera toxin B subunit in preventing relapses of uveitis in Behçet's disease. Stanford M, Whittall T, Bergmeier LA, et al. Clin Exp Immunol 2004 ;137:201–8.

Phase I/II clinical trial of oral administration of peptide 336-351 linked to cholera toxin B, three times weekly, followed by gradual withdrawal of all immunosuppressive drugs can be used to control uveitis and extraocular manifestations of Behçet's disease.

Treatment of Behçet's syndrome with levamisole. De Merieux P, Spitler LE, Paulus HE. Arthritis Rheum 1981;24:64–70.

Open study of 11 patients led to complete resolution of orogenital lesions in three patients and a partial response in six patients.

Other studies confirm the benefits of levamisole treatment in Behçet's disease.

Remission induction in Behçet's disease following lymphocyte depletion by the anti-CD52 antibody CAMPATH 1-H. Lockwood CM, Hale G, Waldman H, Jayne DR. Rheumatology (Oxford) 2003;42:1539–44.

Open prospective study of 18 patients (skin involvement in 67%) treated with lymphocyte-depleting anti-CD52 antibody (total of 134 mg administered by intravenous infusion). Three months after treatment, eight patients were in complete remission, seven in partial remission, and two worsened. Of 13 patients in remission, seven relapsed after an average of 25 months.

Hypothyroidism and prolonged lymphopenia complicated treatment. There was routine prophylaxis against HSV and fungi.

Treatment of Behçet's disease with granulocyte and monocyte adsorption apheresis. Kanekura T, Gushi A, Fukumaru S, et al. J Am Acad Dermatol 2004;51:S83–7.

A report of successful treatment of orogenital ulceration in two patients who underwent five and eight treatments each.

Bioterrorism

Donald Rudikoff, Alejandra Gurtman

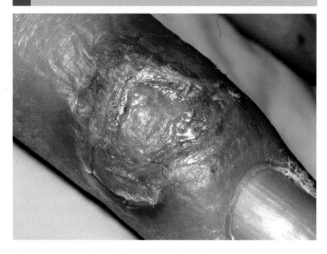

Cutaneous anthrax (illustrated above) starts as a papule at the site of inoculation and evolves into a vesicle and ultimately into an eschar. The events of September 11, 2001 and subsequent dissemination of anthrax through the US Postal Service have heightened concern among public health authorities and physicians about the specter of bioterrorist attack on populated areas. The diseases that are of greatest concern are smallpox, anthrax, tularemia, plague, the hemorrhagic fevers, and botulism. Some of these have prominent cutaneous manifestations in their natural setting but may be less likely to show typical skin lesions when spread by aerosol, which favors pulmonary disease. Dermatologists should familiarize themselves with these disorders, their recognition and treatment, and the measures that can be undertaken to limit spread of disease. Several of the conditions discussed including smallpox, pneumonic plague, and viral hemorrhagic fevers are contagious to caregivers, so appropriate care must be taken to prevent caregivers contracting disease.

Smallpox

Naturally occurring smallpox was eradicated in the 1970s and routine vaccination ceased after 1980 so most physicians alive today have never seen an active case of the disease. Smallpox presents with a febrile prodrome with headache, back pain, and prostration followed by a drop in temperature and apparent subjective improvement. The enanthem and characteristic exanthem ensue. Hoarseness may occur and the eyes can be swollen shut. The deep-seated lesions are firm and umbilicated, and may become multilocular. Around the tenth day of the rash, lesions start to dry, and sticky yellow pus from ruptured blisters forms a crust, imparting a sickening odor. The severe burning in the skin is replaced by itching, which the patient is too weak to scratch.

The diagnosis of smallpox is relatively straightforward. Major criteria for diagnosis are: 1. a prodrome of fever for 1–4 days before the onset of rash; 2. classic smallpox lesions – firm, deep-seated papules and pustules that are 3. all in the same stage of development. The minor criteria are: 1.

centrifugal distribution of skin lesions; 2. toxic or moribund appearance; 3. slow evolution of lesions (1–2 days per stage); and 4. palmoplantar lesions.

The conditions most likely to be confused with smallpox are varicella or disseminated herpes zoster, especially if severe as in immunocompromised individuals. The febrile prodrome is not a usual feature of chickenpox and the patient is not nearly as toxic. Varicella skin lesions are superficial vesicles appearing in crops (in different stages of development) compared to the deep-seated pearly pustules of variola, which are in the same stage of development in any given area of the body. Varicella spares the palms and soles, which are typically involved in variola. Patients with disseminated herpes zoster are often immunosuppressed from chemotherapy, underlying malignancy, or retroviral disease, and typically have concurrent dermatomal lesions. Other conditions that are less likely to be confused with variola are infected molluscum contagiosum in a febrile patient with AIDS, erythema multiforme, pustular drug eruption, purpura fulminans, and hand, foot, and mouth disease. Monkeypox can closely mimic variola.

Smallpox vaccination can cause a wide array of complications in those vaccinated and their close family contacts. Dermatologists are in a unique position to evaluate contraindications to vaccination, such as atopic dermatitis, pemphigus, or Darier's disease in potential vaccinees or their family members. Documented vaccinia transmission to close contacts of vaccinees occurred in recent military vaccination campaigns. Various self-limited side effects include headache, fatigue, muscle ache, fever, chills, local skin reactions, nonspecific rashes, erythema multiforme, lymphadenopathy, and pain at the inoculation site.

Inoculation vaccinia can occur from inadvertent spread to the eyelids, genitals, or other sites in vaccinees and their close contacts. Eczema vaccinatum, analogous to eczema herpeticum, occurs in vaccinees or contacts with atopic dermatitis or other disturbances of skin integrity. Progressive vaccinia extending from the vaccination site in patients with defective cell-mediated immunity is a relentless, often fatal complication with progressive necrosis and metastatic spread. Other adverse reactions of vaccination include post-vaccinial encephalopathy and encephalomyelitis, fetal vaccinia, and myocarditis.

MANAGEMENT STRATEGY

The management of a smallpox attack would involve *recognition of index cases, notification of appropriate government authorities, isolation, treatment, and appropriate public health measures to prevent spread of disease.* Anyone exposed to the patient, if not recently vaccinated, would require immediate vaccination and isolation. So-called *'ring vaccination'* – that is, vaccination and isolation of contacts (those with face-to-face exposure with a true case within 2 m) and contacts of contacts, would be instituted. Suspected cases of smallpox should be managed in a negative-pressure isolation room. If there were multiple suspected cases, an 'isolation hospital' or other facility would be designated by public health officials. Strict respiratory and contact isolation and universal precautions are mandatory.

Because *postexposure vaccination* is part of the currently recommended management, dermatologists must be familiar with the technique now in use, contraindications to

Evidence levels **A** Double-blind study **B** Clinical trial ≥ 20 subjects **C** Clinical trial < 20 subjects **D** Series ≥ 5 subjects **E** Anecdotal case reports

vaccination, recognition, and management of vaccine side effects. Treatment of smallpox cases involves *supportive care, management of cutaneous and oral lesions, antibiotic treatment of secondary bacterial infection and sepsis,* and *perhaps use of antiviral medications.*

SPECIFIC INVESTIGATIONS

- Tzanck smear
- Direct fluorescent antibody testing for varicella zoster virus (VZV) and herpes simplex virus (HSV)
- Polymerase chain reaction (PCR) for VZV, vaccinia, variola, other orthopox viruses (monkeypox)
- Electron microscopy
- Orthopox virus culture
- Serology

Laboratory diagnosis to differentiate smallpox, vaccinia, and other vesicular/pustular illnesses. Besser JM, Crouch NA, Sullivan M. J Lab Clin Med 2003;142:246–51.

Laboratory testing of low-risk patients can be carried out at standard reference laboratories according with local institutional guidelines. Laboratory testing of moderate- or high-risk patients should be done at a government-designated laboratory. In addition to Tzanck smears for low-risk patients, 'real-time' PCR assays for HSV and VZV can be done locally. Electron microscopy, PCR, orthopox virus culture, and variola serology are carried out at government reference laboratories.

Diagnosis and management of smallpox. Breman JG, Henderson DA. N Engl J Med 2002;346:1300–8.

A comprehensive review of the diagnosis and management of smallpox. Postexposure vaccination is crucial, especially if the disease is at an early stage.

Development and experience with an algorithm to evaluate suspected smallpox cases in the United States, 2002–2004. Seward JF, Galil K, Damon I, et al. Clin Infect Dis 2004;39:1477–83.

Diagnostic criteria and Centers for Disease Control and Prevention (CDC) algorithm to evaluate and manage suspected cases of smallpox. Three categories (i.e. those with low, moderate, or high risk of actually having smallpox) dictate subsequent diagnostic strategies. Specific variola laboratory testing is reserved for high-risk persons. An interactive version of the algorithm is available online at http://www.bt.cdc.gov/agent/smallpox/diagnosis/riskal gorithm/index.asp.

FIRST LINE THERAPIES

Suspected cases

- Isolation – negative pressure room
- Respiratory and contact isolation
- Vaccination of early stage patients
- Maintenance of hydration and adequate nutrition

Large-scale quarantine following biological terrorism in the United States: scientific examination, logistic and legal limits, and possible consequences. Barbera J, Macintyre A, Gostin L, et al. JAMA 2001;286:2711–7.

The scientific principles, logistics, and legal issues relevant to quarantine are discussed.

Vaccination reactions

■ Vaccinia immune globulin	D
■ Idoxuridine for corneal lesions	D

Smallpox vaccination and adverse reactions. Guidance for clinicians. Cono J, Casey CG, Bell DM. MMWR Recomm Rep 2003;52(RR-4):1–28.

The following people should not be vaccinated unless actually exposed to smallpox – those with a personal history of, or direct household contact with, persons with: 1. a history of atopic dermatitis; 2. active exfoliative skin conditions; 3. pregnant women or women planning to become pregnant in the next month; and 4. persons with systemic immunosuppression.

Outbreak-specific guidance will be disseminated by the CDC regarding populations to be vaccinated and specific contraindications to vaccination

Smallpox vaccination and patients with human immunodeficiency virus infection or acquired immunodeficiency syndrome. Bartlett JG. Clin Infect Dis 2003;36:468–71.

The risks associated with both smallpox and vaccinia viruses probably correlate with absolute CD4 cell count. People with HIV infection are advised to decline preemptive vaccination, but in the event of an actual smallpox attack, HIV-infected patients exposed to the disease would be advised to be vaccinated.

Smallpox and live-virus vaccination in transplant recipients. Fishman JA. Am J Transplant 2003;3:786–93.

Immunocompromised patients and family members, social contacts, and sexual consorts of immunocompromised persons must not be vaccinated unless actually exposed to smallpox. Should they be vaccinated, they should consider living apart for 3 weeks to avoid transmission to the at-risk individual.

Clinical efficacy of intramuscular vaccinia immune globulin: a literature review. Hopkins RJ, Lane JM. Clin Infect Dis 2004;39:819–26.

Vaccinia immune globulin (VIG) reduces morbidity and mortality associated with progressive vaccinia (vaccinia necrosum) and eczema vaccinatum. Indications for treatment include generalized vaccinia, progressive vaccinia, eczema vaccinatum, and some accidental implantations. The use of intramuscular administration of VIG to prevent smallpox in contacts of patients with documented cases of smallpox is also discussed.

Progressive vaccinia. Bray M, Wright ME. Clin Infect Dis 2003;36:766–74.

This rare complication (one person per million vaccinees) is characterized by the relentless outward spread of vaccinia from the inoculation site and later spread to other areas on the body. Defective cell-mediated immunity predisposes to this complication, which is lethal in infants with absent cellular immune function. Although one army recruit infected with HIV developed severe vaccinia, it appears that multiple HIV-infected enlistees with asymptomatic HIV infection have been vaccinated without developing the complication.

Ocular complications in the Department of Defense Smallpox Vaccination Program. Fillmore GL, Ward TP, Bower KS, et al. Ophthalmology 2004;111:2086–93.

In recent vaccination campaigns, cases of eyelid pustules, blepharitis, periorbital cellulitis, conjunctivitis, conjunctival ulcers, conjunctival membranes, limbal pustules, corneal infiltrates, and iritis occurred 3–24 days after inoculation or contact. Treatment for most cases was topical trifluridine 1%. VIG was used in one case. In all patients, recovery occurred without significant visual sequelae.

Myopericarditis following smallpox vaccination among vaccinia-naive US military personnel. Halsell JS, Riddle JR, Atwood JE, et al. JAMA 2003;289:3283–9.

Myopericarditis occurred at a rate of slightly less than one in 10 000 military personnel who underwent primary vaccination. Clinicians should consider this diagnosis in patients presenting with chest pain 4–30 days following smallpox vaccination.

Pregnancy discovered after smallpox vaccination: is vaccinia immune globulin appropriate? Napolitano PG, Ryan MA, Grabenstein JD. Am J Obstet Gynecol 2004; 191:1863–7.

Fetal vaccinia is a rare complication of smallpox vaccination during pregnancy. Although some have suggested that therapeutic treatment with VIG can prevent fetal vaccinia, VIG is currently not approved for such use and a conceivable risk of teratogenicity from mercury in the thimerosal preservative has been cited. VIG should only be given if a pregnant woman develops a condition in which VIG is indicated (e.g. eczema vaccinatum, progressive vaccinia, or serious generalized vaccinia).

SECOND LINE THERAPIES

■ Penicillinase-resistant antibiotics for secondary skin infection	E
■ Local treatments – manage like a 'burn patient'	E
■ Idoxuridine (topical) treatment of corneal lesions Efficacy is probable in view of use in vaccinia (see above)	

THIRD LINE THERAPIES

■ Cidofovir Experimental evidence only	
■ Cidofovir plus VIG Experimental evidence only	

Cidofovir in the treatment of poxvirus infections. De Clercq E. Antiviral Res 2002;55:1–13.

Excellent review of the experimental use of cidofovir in poxvirus infections.

Cutaneous infections of mice with vaccinia or cowpox viruses and efficacy of cidofovir. Quenelle DC, Collins DJ, Kern ER. Antiviral Res 2004;63:33–40.

In hairless mice, 5% topical cidofovir was more effective than systemic treatment at reducing virus titers in skin, lung, kidney, and spleen.

Anthrax

Anthrax typically causes disease in sheep and cattle, but uncommonly affects humans. The 2001 bioterrorist dissemination of anthrax spores in a white powder form through the US Postal Service caused the disease in 22 people and resulted in five fatalities. *Bacillus anthracis* can exist as a stable spore form for years. Human disease usually results from cutaneous inoculation, inhalation of spores, or gastrointestinal ingestion of infected material.

Cutaneous anthrax is generally the most common presentation and follows direct inoculation of material from infected animals into human skin, often in an occupational setting. A painless or itchy papule evolves into a vesicle with surrounding edema, and then into the classic black eschar. Fever and malaise may be present. Numerous cases of inhalational anthrax, the most dangerous form, would most likely follow a bioterrorist attack. Inhaled spores are taken up from alveoli by macrophages and transported via lymphatics to regional lymph nodes, resulting in a hemorrhagic mediastinitis. Initial symptoms are nonspecific or flu-like: fever, malaise, nonproductive cough, and myalgia. Within a few days, the bacteria disseminate and without treatment, hypotension, respiratory failure, obtundation, and death ensue. A gastrointestinal or oropharyngeal form may result from ingestion of inadequately cooked infected meat or meat products.

MANAGEMENT STRATEGY

Diagnosis of anthrax in an urban setting requires a high index of suspicion. The broad differential diagnosis of cutaneous anthrax includes insect bite, brown recluse spider bite, tularemia, the tache noir of rickettsialpox, ecthyma gangrenosum, staphylococcal or streptococcal ecthyma, cat scratch disease, orf, and other conditions with eschar or ulceroglandular presentation. Differentiation of pulmonary anthrax from other community-acquired pneumonias rests mostly on mediastinal widening or pleural effusion on chest radiography.

Universal precautions should be maintained in evaluating a patient with suspected cutaneous anthrax, but a face mask is not necessary. In the absence of spores there is no risk of contracting pulmonary anthrax. Material is obtained for culture using a Dacron® or rayon swab and skin biopsy is performed.

Prophylaxis

The need for prophylaxis is determined by public health officials on the basis of epidemiologic investigation. *Prophylaxis* is indicated for persons exposed to an air space contaminated with aerosolized *B. anthracis*. The optimal duration of prophylaxis is uncertain; however, 60 days has been recommended, primarily on the basis of animal studies of anthrax deaths and spore clearance after exposure.

Vaccine

The currently recommended regimen consists of *three subcutaneous injections at 0, 2, and 4 weeks, followed by three booster doses at 6, 12, and 18 months.* Routine vaccination is indicated for at-risk laboratory workers, workers who handle potentially infected hide or animals, and military personnel. In combination with *antibiotics*, postexposure vaccination may be effective at preventing disease after exposure to *B. anthracis* spores. Mild local reactions are common (20–30%), but severe adverse events have been rare.

SPECIFIC INVESTIGATIONS

- Culture and Gram stain of tissue, blood, or other fluids
- For cutaneous anthrax, use a Dacron® or rayon swab (not cotton) to swab the vesicle, ulcer, or eschar edge
- Punch biopsy fixed in formalin from a papule or vesicular lesion and including adjacent skin
- Biopsies should be taken from both vesicle and eschar, if present
- A photograph, digital image, or diagram indicating the site of each biopsy in relation to the lesion
- Immunohistochemical assays
- Serology (available through CDC)
- PCR assay

Recognition and management of anthrax – an update. Swartz MN. N Engl J Med 2001;345:1621–6.

Superb overall review of anthrax diagnosis and management.

Cutaneous anthrax management algorithm. Carucci JA, McGovern TW, Norton SA, et al. J Am Acad Dermatol 2002; 47:766–9.

Provides concise summary of the differential diagnosis and treatment of cutaneous anthrax.

Clinical predictors of bioterrorism-related inhalational anthrax. Kyriacou DN, Stein AC, Yarnold PR, et al. Lancet 2004;364:449–52.

In differentiating anthrax from community-acquired pneumonia, the most accurate predictor of anthrax is mediastinal widening or pleural effusion on chest radiography.

The critical role of pathology in the investigation of bioterrorism-related cutaneous anthrax. Shieh WJ, Guarner J, Paddock C, et al; Anthrax Bioterrorism Investigation Team. Am J Pathol 2003;163:1901–10.

Two novel immunohistochemical assays have been developed that can detect *B. anthracis* antigens in skin biopsy samples, even after prolonged antibiotic treatment. They are a highly sensitive and specific method for the diagnosis of cutaneous anthrax.

A two-component direct fluorescent-antibody assay for rapid identification of *Bacillus anthracis*. De BK, Bragg SL, Sanden GN, et al. Emerg Infect Dis 2002;8:1060–5.

Direct fluorescent antibody assay, using monoclonal antibodies to *B. anthracis* cell wall and capsule antigens is sensitive and specific and provides a quick confirmatory test for *B. anthracis* in cultures and may be useful directly on clinical specimens.

Real-time PCR assay for a unique chromosomal sequence of *Bacillus anthracis*. Bode E, Hurtle W, Norwood D. J Clin Microbiol 2004;42:5825–31.

Most real-time PCR assays for *B. anthracis* have been developed to detect virulence genes located on plasmids. This chromosomal assay can verify the presence of *B. anthracis* independently of plasmid occurrence.

FIRST LINE THERAPIES

■ Ciprofloxacin	E
■ Doxycycline	E

Oral antibiotics are used for cutaneous anthrax below the head and neck if systemic symptoms and malignant edema are absent. If they are present, intravenous antibiotics are used.

Update: investigation of bioterrorism-related anthrax and interim guidelines for exposure management and antimicrobial therapy, October 2001. MMWR Morb Mortal Wkly Rep 2001;50:962.

Anthrax as a biological weapon, 2002: updated recommendations for management. Inglesby TV, O'Toole T, Henderson DA, et al; Working Group on Civilian Biodefense. JAMA 2002;287:2236–52.

These two references provide comprehensive recommendations for managing exposure to anthrax and treating the various forms of the illness.

Anthrax: safe treatment for children. Benavides S, Nahata MC. Ann Pharmacother 2002;36:334–7.

Pediatric perspective on the management of anthrax.

Update: interim recommendations for antimicrobial prophylaxis for children and breastfeeding mothers and treatment of children with anthrax. MMWR Morb Mortal Wkly Rep 2001;50:1014–6.

Ciprofloxacin or doxycycline is recommended for antimicrobial prophylaxis and treatment of adults and children with *B. anthracis* infection. Amoxicillin is an option for antimicrobial prophylaxis for children and pregnant women and to complete treatment of cutaneous disease when *B. anthracis* is susceptible to penicillin.

SECOND LINE THERAPIES

■ Amoxicillin	E
■ Penicillin	D
■ Chloramphenicol	D
■ Clindamycin	E
■ Systemic corticosteroids for treatment of edema	E

THIRD LINE THERAPIES

■ Macrolides	E
■ Aminoglycosides	E
■ Chloroquine – experimental	E

Chloroquine enhances survival in *Bacillus anthracis* intoxication. Artenstein AW, Opal SM, Cristofaro P, et al. J Infect Dis 2004;190:1655–60.

Antibiotics target only replicating organisms, thus allowing bacterial toxins to cause severe physiological derangements in patients with inhalational anthrax. Chloroquine decreased tissue damage and enhanced survival in mice exposed to anthrax.

PROPHYLAXIS

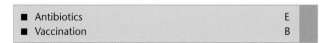

■ Antibiotics	E
■ Vaccination	B

Clinical issues in the prophylaxis, diagnosis, and treatment of anthrax. Bell DM, Kozarsky PE, Stephens DS. Emerg Infect Dis 2002;8:222–5.

Management of asymptomatic pregnant or lactating women exposed to anthrax. Committee on Obstetric Practice. Int J Gynaecol Obstet 2002;77:293–5.

Asymptomatic pregnant and lactating women who have been exposed to a confirmed environmental contamination or a high-risk source receive prophylactic treatment. Although some of the drugs may pose a risk to the developing fetus, this risk is clearly outweighed by the potential consequences of acquiring anthrax.

Use of anthrax vaccine in the United States. Advisory Committee on Immunization Practices. MMWR Recomm Rep 2000;49(RR-15):1–20.

Use of anthrax vaccine in response to terrorism: supplemental recommendations of the Advisory Committee on Immunization Practices. MMWR Morb Mortal Wkly Rep 2002;51:1024–6.

Recommendations for pre- and postexposure prophylaxis are provided and updated in these two references.

Recurrent, localized urticaria and erythema multiforme: a review and management of cutaneous anthrax vaccine-related events. Gilson RT, Schissel DJ. Cutis 2004;73:319–25.

This article reviews the latest recommended evaluation and management of anthrax vaccine adverse events.

Tularemia

Tularemia is caused by a highly infectious Gram-negative coccobacillus, *Francisella tularensis*. Seven clinical syndromes are described that correspond to the route of inoculation (i.e. respiratory tract, gastrointestinal tract, skin, eye, or other mucous membrane exposure). Because tularemia has no stable spore form, it is a less suitable bioterrorist agent than anthrax. It does not cause person-to-person spread.

Respiratory tularemia, as would occur after a bioterrorist attack, starts as a flu-like illness or atypical pneumonia with fever, chills, myalgia, and cephalalgia. Pulmonary symptoms such as nonproductive cough and pleuritic chest pain may not be prominent, but if treatment is not initiated, severe pneumonia, hemoptysis, respiratory failure, sepsis, and death can result. There is no specific skin rash with respiratory tularemia, but all of the clinical syndromes can cause bacteremia or tularemia sepsis with shock, acute respiratory distress syndrome (ARDS), organ failure, disseminated intravascular coagulation, and purpura. Nonspecific eruptions, described below, can occur in a minority of cases, usually on the face and extremities.

Ulceroglandular tularemia, the presentation most familiar to dermatologists, is not likely to occur after a bioterrorist attack. It usually presents with tender localized lymphadenitis. An erythematous, painful papule that then undergoes necrosis develops before, simultaneous with or shortly after the tender swollen lymph node.

Another form, oculoglandular tularemia could occur after an aerosol attack. It presents with purulent conjunctivitis, periorbital edema, ulceration and nodules of the conjunctivae, along with tender preauricular or cervical lymphadenopathy.

Water or food contaminated with *F. tularensis* can cause oropharyngeal disease, including stomatitis and exudative pharyngitis. Typhoidal tularemia presents as a febrile illness with chills, abdominal pain, nausea, vomiting, and diarrhea and can be rapidly fatal.

Exanthems have been described in all forms of tularemia. They may be macular, papular, papulovesicular, pustular, or petechial, and are most prominent on the face and extremities. Erythema nodosum occurs most commonly with pulmonary tularemia. Erythema multiforme and Sweet's syndrome have also been described.

MANAGEMENT STRATEGY

A high index of suspicion is necessary for the diagnosis of tularemia outside the natural setting. Ulceroglandular or oculoglandular disease have a rather straightforward presentation, but respiratory tularemia has variable pulmonary symptoms, though subspecies used in a bioterrorist attack would likely cause severe toxicity and cough. *F. tularensis* can be grown in the laboratory, but has stringent growth characteristics. Because laboratory workers are at risk of contracting the disease and routine reference laboratories are not experienced at growing the organism, government health department laboratories should be used. Antibody testing is highly specific, but not useful early on in the disease.

The organism can be detected in clinical specimens (secretions or biopsies) by direct fluorescent antibody or immunohistochemical techniques. PCR is likely to become the diagnostic test of choice in the future.

Although *streptomycin* has been used successfully for many years for tularemia, it is not widely available and has been replaced by *gentamicin*. *Oral ciprofloxacin* has proved effective in tularemia and is the drug of choice for uncomplicated disease. *Doxycycline* is a useful second line agent for uncomplicated disease. For severe disease, parenteral therapy is indicated. Gentamicin, ciprofloxacin, or doxycycline are the preferred agents in pregnancy.

SPECIFIC INVESTIGATIONS

- Gram stain
- Culture
- Serology – agglutination and enzyme-linked immunosorbent assay (ELISA) testing
- Direct fluorescent antibody and immunohistochemistry
- PCR

The development of tools for diagnosis of tularaemia and typing of *Francisella tularensis*. Johansson A, Forsman M, Sjostedt A. APMIS 2004;112:898–907.

Detailed description of laboratory diagnostic procedures useful for tularemia.

Methods for enhanced culture recovery of *Francisella tularensis*. Petersen JM, Schriefer ME, Gage KL, et al. Appl Environ Microbiol 2004;70:3733–5.

Antibiotic supplementation of enriched cysteine heart agar blood culture medium improved recovery of *F. tularensis* from contaminated specimens. Immediate freezing is useful for transport of tissue for enhanced recovery rates.

FIRST LINE THERAPIES

■ Streptomycin	D
■ Gentamicin	D
■ Ciprofloxacin for uncomplicated disease	D

SECOND LINE THERAPIES

■ Doxycycline	D
■ Chloramphenicol	D

Tularaemia: bioterrorism defence renews interest in *Francisella tularensis*. Oyston PC, Sjostedt A, Titball RW. Nat Rev Microbiol 2004;2:967–78.

Superb review of the epidemiology, pathophysiology, diagnosis, and treatment of tularemia.

Plague

Plague, caused by *Yersinia pestis* is a disease of rats that historically has spread to humans by the bite of a flea that has fed on an infected rat. A diversity of mammals and fleas can serve as vectors. Respiratory droplet infection occurs, following exposure to infected humans or to cats with plague pneumonia. An aerosol attack with plague would cause an abrupt outbreak of fatal pneumonia in an exposed community. Infected fleas could also be used to spread the disease. It is alleged that this was done by the Japanese in China during World War II.

The three main presentations are bubonic plague, a primary pulmonic form, and septicemia. Bubonic plague presents with fever and flu-like symptoms. A painful bubo develops near the site of the infected bite, most often in the cervical, axillary, femoral, or inguinal areas. There is overlying erythema and sometimes vesicles, pustules, eschars, or ulceration. Without antibiotic treatment, secondary pneumonia or septicemia may follow. Bubonic plague would only occur if fleas were used in a bioterrorist attack. Highly contagious pneumonic plague may be primary or may develop from bubonic or septicemic plague. The pneumonic form has no specific skin manifestations, but septicemic plague can cause vasculitis and disseminated intravascular coagulation with cyanosis, purpura, and gangrene of the nose, fingers, and toes.

MANAGEMENT STRATEGY

A bioterrorist attack with plague would most likely involve aerosol spread. The use of insect vectors would be much less likely. In the event that insect vectors were used, dermatologists would be called upon to evaluate patients with bubonic disease. Buboes, surrounded by edema, typically have adherent overlying erythematous skin. In a bioterrorist scenario, most cases would more likely be of the pneumonic type, many of which would progress to septicemic

plague with large areas of ecchymosis and peripheral gangrene. Cervical buboes might occur. High fever, tachycardia, and severe toxicity would be the rule. Pneumonic plague, early on, might be confused with inhalation anthrax; however chest radiography shows parenchymal disease. Gram-negative rods are evident on sputum Gram stain. Strict respiratory isolation is mandatory for the first 3 days of therapy of pneumonic plague. Prophylactic treatment of at-risk contacts is mandatory.

Skin biopsies of purpuric lesions of plague reveal subepidermal hemorrhage and capillary and venular fibrin thrombi. A diffuse papular eruption sometimes occurs, which on biopsy shows a mixed perivascular infiltrate.

Streptomycin has been the mainstay of treatment for plague, but has limited availability in the US. It is ototoxic and nephrotoxic to patients and if administered to pregnant women, can cause fetal hearing loss and kidney damage. *Gentamicin* is also used for plague and is favored in pregnancy. *Tetracyclines*, such as doxycycline, are adequate for uncomplicated plague alone or in combination with other agents. *Chloramphenicol, fluoroquinolones* (e.g. ciprofloxacin) and *sulfonamides* (e.g. sulfadiazine or trimethoprim–sulfamethoxazole) are alternatives.

Yersinia pestis (plague) vaccines. Titball RW, Williamson ED. Expert Opin Biol Ther 2004;4:965–73.

Reviews the current status of anti-plague vaccination.

SPECIFIC INVESTIGATIONS

■ Complete blood count and peripheral smear
■ Lactate dehydrogenase
■ Fibrin degradation products, fibrinogen
■ Gram stain and culture of sputum and fluid from buboes
■ Serology – anti-fraction 1 antibody ≥1:10
■ PCR

FIRST LINE THERAPIES

Aminoglycosides	
■ Intramuscular streptomycin	D
■ Intramuscular or intravenous gentamicin	D

SECOND LINE THERAPIES

■ Doxycycline	D
■ Ciprofloxacin	E

THIRD LINE THERAPIES

■ Chloramphenicol	D
■ Sulfonamides	E

Bacteria as agents of biowarfare. How to proceed when the worst is suspected. Tjaden JA, Lazarus AA, Martin GJ. Postgrad Med 2002;112:57–60,63–4,67–70.

This review covers the bacterial agents of anthrax, plague, and tularemia and their recognition and treatment.

Viral hemorrhagic fevers

The viral hemorrhagic fevers are a group of febrile illnesses associated with a bleeding diathesis that are caused by viruses belonging to one of the following families: Filoviridae, Arenaviridae, Bunyaviridae, and Flaviviridae. Ebola, Marburg, Lassa fever, New World arenaviruses, Rift Valley fever, yellow fever, Omsk hemorrhagic fever, and Kyasanur Forest disease have the greatest potential for weaponization. The diseases are usually transmitted to humans via contact with infected animal reservoirs or arthropod vectors. The mode of transmission, clinical course, and mortality of these illnesses vary with the specific virus involved, but each is capable of causing a hemorrhagic fever syndrome. Fever, severe toxicity, hemorrhagic manifestations; with at least two of the following – hemorrhagic or purple rash, epistaxis, hematemesis, hemoptysis, blood in stools – establish the diagnosis.

MANAGEMENT STRATEGY

A high index of suspicion should be maintained for patients presenting with a febrile illness and hemorrhagic manifestations. Cases should be *reported immediately to public health authorities*. Pending definitive diagnosis, patients with suspected hemorrhagic fevers should be classified as low, medium, or high risk. Because of the high risk of contagion to healthcare workers, *stringent universal precautions, appropriate barrier protection, and isolation should be instituted*. Contacts of suspected cases should be monitored closely and in the case of Lassa fever, *ribavirin* should be offered. Diagnostic test are only available through the CDC or the US Army Medical Research Institute of Infectious Diseases.

SPECIFIC INVESTIGATIONS

- Antigen detection by antigen-capture ELISA
- IgM antibody detection by antibody-capture ELISA
- Reverse transcriptase-PCR
- Viral isolation is of limited value because it requires a biosafety level 4 laboratory

Hemorrhagic fever viruses as biological weapons: medical and public health management. Borio L, Inglesby T, Peters CJ, et al; Working Group on Civilian Biodefense. JAMA 2002;287:2391–405.

Cutaneous manifestations of biological warfare and related threat agents. McGovern TW, Christopher GW, Eitzen EM. Arch Dermatol 1999;135:311–22.

Superb overview of the dermatologic manifestations of biowarfare agents.

Management of patients exposed to biologic weapons. Yetman RJ, Parks D, Taft E. J Pediatr Health Care 2002; 16:256–61.

This review of practice guidelines provides treatment recommendations for children as well as adults and also includes a comprehensive list of emergency contacts and educational resources.

Diagnosis and management of suspected cases of bioterrorism: a pediatric perspective. Patt HA, Feigin RD. Pediatrics 2002;109:685–92.

Review of bioterrorism from a pediatric perspective.

FIRST LINE THERAPIES

Supportive care

■ Intravenous ribavirin pending viral identification	D

SECOND LINE THERAPIES

■ Convalescent plasma	E

Update: management of patients with suspected viral hemorrhagic fever – United States. MMWR Morb Mortal Wkly Rep 1995;44:475–9.

CDC guidelines for the management of suspected cases of viral hemorrhagic fever.

Treatment of Ebola hemorrhagic fever with blood transfusions from convalescent patients. Mupapa K, Massamba M, Kibadi K, et al. J Infect Dis 1999;179(suppl 1):S18–23.

Eight patients who met the case definition for Ebola hemorrhagic fever, were transfused with blood donated by five convalescent patients. Only one transfused patient (12.5%) died compared to the overall case fatality rate of 80%. It is not entirely clear if the increased survival resulted from the transfusions or because of the better care received by transfusion recipients.

Evidence levels A Double-blind study B Clinical trial ≥ 20 subjects C Clinical trial < 20 subjects D Series ≥ 5 subjects E Anecdotal case reports

Blastomycosis (North American blastomycosis)

Wanda Sonia Robles

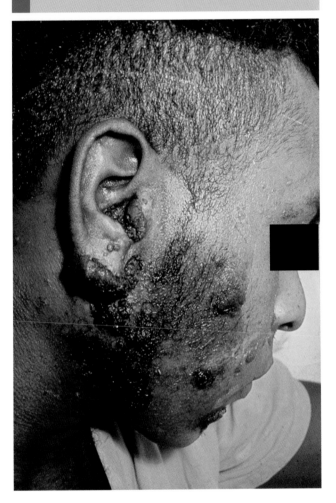

(Picture courtesy of Dr Fabio Barbosa.)

Blastomycosis is a primary, acute or suppurative granulomatous chronic infection caused by the thermally dimorphic fungus *Blastomyces dermatitidis*. Most cases are restricted to the respiratory system; however, in many instances, the disease manifests clinically with cutaneous lesions. The fungus may infect almost any organ. The condition is more prevalent in the North American continent, extending from Canada to the USA; cases have also been reported from Mexico, Central America, Africa, the Middle East, and India. The Mississippi Valley is considered one of the prevalent areas in the USA.

MANAGEMENT STRATEGY

The frequency and course of self-resolving forms of blastomycosis is not clearly established and therefore all active pulmonary cases, however mild, should be treated. The drugs most commonly used for treatment of blastomycosis are the *polyenes* and the *azoles*. *Amphotericin B* is the polyene used for the treatment of life-threatening blastomycosis. It is considered the gold standard of therapy for this condition and also for other systemic mycoses. The azole *ketoconazole*, however, often appears to be effective in cases of less severe disease, with the advantage that it can be given orally with less significant side effects. *Itraconazole* has now been established as the drug of choice for cases of progressive blastomycosis, either pulmonary or extrapulmonary disease, or both. It is also orally administered and less toxic than either amphotericin B or ketoconazole. *Fluconazole* has also been used to treat cases of blastomycosis. Alopecia has been reported in some patients treated with these agents. In immunocompromised patients, amphotericin B is the drug of choice.

SPECIFIC INVESTIGATIONS

- Direct examination
- Culture
- Serology for HIV infection (where relevant)

Preliminary diagnosis of blastomycosis is based on the observation of yeast cells in a clinical sample. The specimen varies according to the manifestation of the disease: skin scrapings, pus from skin lesions, sputum in cases of lung disease, and biopsy tissue from any lesion suspicious of infection. The material is mounted in a drop of 20% potassium hydroxide on a microscope slide. The organism on direct microscopy appears as a round cell with a double wall and quite often with a single broad-based bud.

Isolation and identification of the organism in culture is essential to confirm the diagnosis. The preferred medium is Emmons' modification of Sabouraud's glucose agar.

Blastomycosis and human immunodeficiency virus: three new cases and review. Witzig RS, Hoadley DJ, Greer DL, et al. South Med J 1994;87:715–19.

The authors report on three patients co-infected with HIV and blastomycosis and review the literature. The mortality rate from blastomycosis for patients with both HIV infection and blastomycosis is 54%, which is about five times the mortality rate of blastomycosis patients in the general population.

This is a good review.

Emerging disease issues and fungal pathogens associated with HIV infection. Ampel NM. Emerg Infect Dis 1996;2: 109–16.

Review article which reports that most cases of histoplasmosis, coccidioidomycosis, and blastomycosis in association with HIV infection occur in regions where their causative organisms are endemic.

Also a good review article.

Blastomycosis in the immunocompromised patient. Pappas P. Semin Respir Infect 1997;12:243–51.

Review article reporting mortality rates in excess of 30% in immunocompromised patients with blastomycosis.

Primary cutaneous North American blastomycosis in an immunosuppressed child. Zampogna JC, Hoy MJ, Ramos-Caro FA. Pediatr Dermatol 2003;20:128–30.

Case report of a 6-year-old immunosuppressed girl who developed a cutaneous lesion on the left lower leg and responded successfully to treatment with oral itraconazole.

An imported case of *Blastomyces dermatitidis* infection in Mexico. Velazques R, Munoz-Hernandez B, Arenas R, et al. Mycopathologia 2003;156:263–7.

Case report of a 3-year-old child in Mexico, who had been born in California and had lived in Chicago, who developed a skin ulcer proven to be cutaneous blastomycosis. Successful treatment was achieved with a combination of amphotericin B, oral ketaconazole, and itraconazole.

FIRST LINE THERAPIES

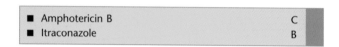

■ Amphotericin B	C
■ Itraconazole	B

Efficacy and safety of amphotericin B lipid complex injection (ABLC) in solid-organ transplant recipients with invasive fungal infections. Linden P, Williams P, Chan KM. Clin Transplant 2000;14(4 Pt 1):329–39.

Open-label study to assess the efficacy and safety of ABLC as treatment for severe life-threatening mycoses. This included 79 solid-organ transplant recipients. In this report, 46 of the 79 patients (58%) survived longer than 28 days after the last dose of ABLC. This medication is advocated particularly for patients with high risk of renal failure, in view of its renal-sparing properties.

Blastomycosis. Davies SF, Sarosi JA. Eur J Clin Microbiol Infect Dis 1989;8:474–9.

Review article with focus on disease progression. Treatment is advocated for patients with progressive lung infection and all cases of extrapulmonary disease. Systemic amphotericin is the drug of choice in cases of life-threatening infection or disease of the central nervous system (CNS).

Blastomycosis. Bradsher RW, Chapman SW, Pappas PG. Infect Dis Clin North Am 2003;17:21–40.

This very good review advocates the use of itraconazole as the drug of choice for either pulmonary or extrapulmonary infection, or both. Amphotericin B should be used for cases of life-threatening infection.

Self-limited blastomycosis: a report of 39 cases. Sarosi GA, Davies SF, Phillips JR. Semin Respir Infect 1986;1:40–4.

Report of 39 patients with pulmonary blastomycosis who did not have antifungal chemotherapy. Fourteen of those patients acquired the infection during an epidemic in 1972 with no mycology available. The remaining 25 patients had positive culture. The median observation period was 42 months. One patient relapsed 52 months after diagnosis.

This paper advocates that it may be safe for patients with blastomycosis restricted to the lungs to be followed without specific chemotherapy until clearance of clinical symptoms.

Itraconazole therapy for blastomycosis and histoplasmosis. NIAID Mycoses Study Group. Dismukes WE, Bradsher RW Jr, Cloud GC, et al. Am J Med 1992;93:489–97.

A prospective, nonrandomized, multicenter trial involving 85 patients (48 with blastomycosis and 37 with histoplasmosis). Patients were treated with itraconazole, 200–400 mg daily, for a median period of 6.2 months (blastomycosis) and 9.0 months (histoplasmosis). Among the 48 patients with blastomycosis, success was documented in 43

(90%). This study concludes that itraconazole is highly effective for nonmeningeal, non-life-threatening blastomycosis and histoplasmosis, with minimal toxicity.

Newer developments in therapy for endemic mycosis. Kauffman CA. Clin Infect Dis 1994;19:28–32.

Review article. It considers oral itraconazole the standard treatment for nonmeningeal, non-life-threatening blastomycosis and histoplasmosis.

Therapy of blastomycosis. Bradsher RW. Semin Respir Infect 1997;12:263–7.

Review article stating that amphotericin B achieves higher cure rates for blastomycosis, but because of its toxicity, the imidazoles and triazoles have been favored. Fluconazole is not considered as effective as itraconazole in the treatment of blastomycosis.

Disseminated blastomycosis. Assaly RA, Hammersley JR, Olson DE, et al. J Am Acad Dermatol 2003;48:123–7.

Case report of a 26-year-old female patient with both pulmonary and cutaneous blastomycosis, successfully treated with oral itraconazole. Both lung and skin lesions were reported to have improved within 6 weeks of treatment.

Cutaneous blastomycosis without evidence of pulmonary involvement. Clinton TS, Timko AL. Mil Med 2003;168:651–3.

Case report of a patient with cutaneous blastomycosis and no evidence of pulmonary or other systemic involvement. The patient responded to treatment with itraconazole for 6 months, with no evidence of recurrence after 1 year.

SECOND LINE THERAPIES

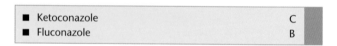

■ Ketoconazole	C
■ Fluconazole	B

The use of ketoconazole in the treatment of blastomycosis. MacManus EJ, Jones JM. Am Rev Resp Dis 1986;133:141–3.

Retrospective study of 11 patients with blastomycosis diagnosed over a 30-month period. Six of eight patients treated with ketoconazole 400 mg daily completed a 6-month course with good results. Medical follow-up is advocated for these patients.

Cutaneous blastomycosis presenting as non-healing ulcer and responding to oral ketoconazole. Balasaraswathy P, Theerthanath. Dermatol Online J 2003;9:19.

Case report of cutaneous blastomycosis diagnosed by histopathology which responded well to oral ketoconazole treatment.

Treatment of blastomycosis with fluconazole: a pilot study. The National Institute of Allergy and Infectious Disease Mycoses Study Group. Pappas PG, Bradsher RW, Chapman SW, et al. Clin Infect Dis 1995;20:267–71.

A multicenter, randomized, open-label pilot study comparing two daily doses of fluconazole, 200 and 400 mg, in the treatment of non-life-threatening blastomycosis. Twenty-four patients were included in this study and the analysis data included 23 patients. Successful treatment was achieved in 15 (65%) of 23 patients. This included eight (62%) of 15 patients who received the dose of 200 mg daily and seven (70%) of 10 patients who received the dose of 400 mg daily. The activity of the drug, given for a period of a minimum of 6 months, is considered moderate.

Treatment of blastomycosis with higher doses of fluconazole. The National Institute of Allergy and Infectious Disease Mycoses Study Group. Pappas PG, Bradsher RW, Kauffman CA, et al. Clin Infect Dis 1997;25:200–5.

Clinical trial designed to examine the usefulness of the higher dose of fluconazole in the treatment of non-life-threatening blastomycosis. This multicenter, randomized, open-label study included 39 patients. Of these, 34 (87%) were successfully treated; this included 89% and 85% of patients who received 400 and 800 mg of fluconazole, respectively. The duration of therapy is reported as 8.9 months for those successfully treated. The study concludes that fluconazole at the daily dose of 400–800 mg for a minimum period of 6 months is an effective therapy for non-life-threatening blastomycosis.

Recommendations for the treatment of fungal pneumonias. Yamada H, Kotaki H, Takahashi T. Expert Opin Pharmacother 2003;4:1241–58.

Echinocandines and second generation triazoles, e.g. voriconazole, are considered salvage therapy to overcome the limitations of the current therapy.

A very useful paper with practice guidelines for the use of anti-fungal drugs alone, or in combination.

Practice guidelines for the management of patients with blastomycosis. Infectious Diseases Society of America. Chapman SW, Bradsher RW Jr, Campbell GD Jr, et al. Clin Infect Dis 2000;30:679–83.

Guidelines for the treatment of blastomycosis are based on the clinical spectrum of the disease, which is varied and includes asymptomatic infection, acute or chronic pneumonia, and also extrapulmonary disease.

1. For immunocompetent patients with mild lung infection which is thought to have cleared spontaneously, close follow-up is necessary for evidence of progression or dissemination.
2. Immunocompromised patients with either pulmonary or extrapulmonary disease must be treated.
3. The treatment of choice for immunocompromised patients or individuals who have life-threatening blastomycosis or involvement of the CNS is amphotericin B.
4. Amphotericin B is also the drug of choice for patients who have failed to respond to azole treatment.
5. Amphotericin B is the only drug approved for the treatment of blastomycosis in pregnant women.
6. Immunocompetent patients with mild to moderate pulmonary or extrapulmonary disease, excluding CNS disease, can be treated with an azole, since this is equally effective as, and less toxic than, amphotericin B.
7. Itraconazole is the drug of choice for the treatment of non-life-threatening blastomycosis, excluding CNS disease, as this does appear more effective than either ketoconazole or fluconazole.

Blistering distal dactylitis

Irshad Zaki

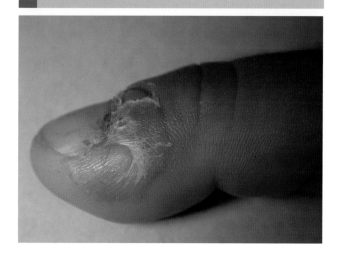

Blistering distal dactylitis (BDD) is a superficial, tender, blistering infection of childhood and the early teens. It is usually caused by group A β-hemolytic streptococci, although group B organisms and staphylococci have also been implicated. The distal volar fat pads of the fingers are the most common site of infection, but involvement of the nailfolds and toes can occasionally occur.

MANAGEMENT STRATEGY

Blistering distal dactylitis can cause considerable alarm to parents as large tense blisters rapidly develop. Despite the absence of constitutional symptoms, patients usually seek help soon after the onset of the infection. The condition does not resolve spontaneously, but prompt treatment results in rapid improvement. *Blisters should be incised to release fluid*, which can vary from clear and watery to frank pus. Subsequent application of topical antibiotics can be helpful, but systemic treatment is usually also required. *Penicillin V* is the treatment of choice for streptococcal infection, but *erythromycin* is an effective alternative for patients allergic to penicillin.

The differential diagnosis of the condition includes traumatic blisters, herpetic whitlow, staphylococcal bullous impetigo and the Weber-Cockayne variant of epidermolysis bullosa.

SPECIFIC INVESTIGATIONS

- Gram stain of blister fluid
- Culture of blister fluid
- Swab of nasopharynx for bacteriology

A clinically recognizable streptococcal infection. Hays GC, Mullard JE. Paediatrics 1975;56:129–31.

First large series report describing 13 patients with BDD. Streptococci were found on culture of blister fluid in all cases and Gram-positive cocci were usually found on Gram stain. This report suggests a link with infection of the nasopharynx, but this has not been confirmed in other case reports.

Staphylococcal blistering dactylitis: a case series in children under nine months of age. Lyon M, Doehring MC. J Emerg Med 2004;26:421–3.

Although uncommon under the age of 2, this paper reports three cases under 9 months of age.

These reports highlight the importance of initiating bacteriology prior to commencing treatment. Staphylococcal infection is a relatively rare but recognized cause of BDD.

FIRST LINE THERAPIES

■ Incision and drainage of blister	C
■ Topical antibiotics	C
■ Systemic penicillin	C

Blistering distal dactylitis. McCray MK, Easterly NB. J Am Acad Dermatol 1981;5:592–4.

Clear description of two children with this disorder. Both improved rapidly with incision and drainage in addition to a systemic 10-day course of penicillin V.

Group B streptococcal blistering distal dactylitis in an adult diabetic. Benson PM, Solivan G. J Am Acad Dermatol 1987;17:310–11.

Report of a diabetic patient who developed BDD as a result of group B β-hemolytic streptococci. Good response to treatment with topical antibiotic and oral dicloxacillin. Infection of skin with group B streptococci is uncommon, though diabetic patients appear to be more susceptible.

SECOND LINE THERAPIES

■ Systemic erythromycin	D

Blistering distal dactylitis: a manifestation of Group A beta-haemolytic streptococcal infection. Schneider JA, Parlette HL. Arch Dermatol 1982;118:879–80.

Short report of the authors' personal experience suggesting that this is a relatively common problem. Systemic penicillin and erythromycin were both found to be effective. It is likely that many cases of BDD are wrongly diagnosed as bullous impetigo by clinicians not familiar with this disorder.

THIRD LINE THERAPIES

■ Amoxicillin/clavulanic acid	D
■ Conservative measures for herpetic whitlow	D

Blistering distal dactylitis caused by *Staphylococcus aureus*. Norcross MC, Mitchell DF. Cutis 1993;51:353–4.

Staphylococcus aureus was found to be the etiologic agent in the patient described. The condition improved following treatment with a proprietary mixture of amoxicillin trihydrate and clavulanate potassium. The authors suggest that multiple digit involvement may be a predictor of staphylococcal rather than streptococcal etiology.

Coexistent infections on a child's distal phalanx: blistering dactylitis and herpetic whitlow. Ney AC, English JC 3rd, Greer KE. Cutis 2002;69:46–8.

Consider comorbidity if BDD does not respond to antibiotics.

Evidence levels **A** Double-blind study **B** Clinical trial ≥ 20 subjects **C** Clinical trial < 20 subjects **D** Series ≥ 5 subjects **E** Anecdotal case reports

Bowen's disease and Erythroplasia of Queyrat

Analisa Vincent Halpern, Naomi Lawrence

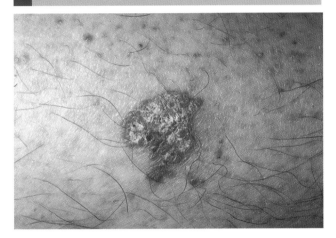

Bowen's disease (BD) is defined as intraepidermal squamous cell carcinoma. The clinical appearance is that of a sharply demarcated, erythematous, scaly patch up to several centimeters in diameter. Erythroplasia of Queyrat (EQ) is Bowen's disease of the glans penis and prepuce and may appear as a red, moist, velvety or smooth plaque. The development of Bowen's disease is frequently associated with excess sun exposure, but the human papillomavirus, prior radiation exposure and arsenic ingestion have also been implicated in its pathogenesis.

MANAGEMENT STRATEGY

Both Bowen's disease and EQ may progress to become invasive squamous cell carcinoma. Malignant transformation of EQ is more common (10%) and metastasizes earlier than that of Bowen's disease (3%). Ideal treatment options would focus on retaining form, function and cosmesis while achieving a high cure rate. Definitive treatment is *surgical excision* if the lesion is small and well-defined. *Mohs micrographic surgery (MMS)* is recommended over simple excision because the likelihood of recurrence is lower. MMS is also advised in the treatment of larger, ill-defined lesions, especially when preservation of normal tissue is crucial, as with EQ. Surgical ablation may be achieved with *electrodesiccation and curettage, cryotherapy,* or *laser.* Nonsurgical options include *imiquimod cream* (a topical immunomodulator), *topical 5-fluorouracil (5-FU), photodynamic therapy (PDT)* and *radiation therapy.*

Standard of care requires that a follow-up period of no less than 5 years be observed to claim clinical cure of Bowen's disease and EQ. Therefore, the extremely brief duration of follow-up for many studies addressing the treatment for Bowen's disease and EQ renders the data difficult to apply in the clinical setting.

SPECIFIC INVESTIGATIONS

- Skin biopsy
- Dermoscopy
- Immunoperoxidase studies for human papillomavirus

Dermoscopy of Bowen's disease. Zalaudek I, Argenziano G, Leinweber B, et al. Br J Dermatol 2004;150:1112–16.

The small sample size limits the application of this newly described diagnostic tool.

The prevalence of human papillomavirus genotypes in nonmelanoma skin cancers of nonimmunosuppressed individuals identifies high-risk genital types as possible risk factors. Iftner A, Klug SJ, Garbe C, Blum A, et al. Cancer Res 2003;63:7515–9.

Study found an odds ratio of 59 (95% confidence interval 5.4 to 645) for nonmelanoma skin cancer in patients who were DNA positive for the high-risk mucosal HPV types 16, 31, 35 and 51.

FIRST LINE THERAPIES

■ Surgical excision	C

Guidelines for management of Bowen's disease. Cox NH, Eedy DJ, Morton CA. Br J Dermatol 1999;141:633–41.

Literature review compares simple excision, MMS, cryotherapy, curettage, topical 5-FU, PDT and radiation therapy based on lesion size and location.

Extensive Bowen's disease of the penile shaft treated with fresh tissue Mohs micrographic surgery in two separate operations. Moritz DL, Lynch WS. J Dermatol Surg Oncol 1991;17:374–8.

MMS is the only therapy that allows for definitive demonstration of tumor-free margins. Appropriate surgical therapy should be based on lesion size, anatomic location, history of recurrence.

SECOND LINE THERAPIES

■ Cryosurgery	C
■ Electrodesiccation and curettage	C

Comparison of cryotherapy with curettage in the treatment of Bowen's disease: a prospective study. Ahmed I, Berth-Jones J, Charles-Holmes S, et al. Br J Dermatol 2000; 143:759–66.

Producing comparable cure rates, curettage resulted in more rapid healing, less pain and fewer complications than cryotherapy.

Curettage-cryosurgery for non-melanoma skin cancer of the external ear: excellent 5-year results. Nordin P. Br J Dermatol 1999;140:291–3.

Three lesions treated showed no recurrence at 5-year follow-up with good cosmetic result.

This therapy may be beneficial in areas such as the pinna that are prone to deformity after surgical excision.

THIRD LINE THERAPIES

■ 5-FU	B
■ 5-FU ± iontophoresis	C
■ PDT	B
■ Imiquimod 5% cream	C
■ Radiation therapy	C
■ Laser ablation	D
■ Isotretinoin and interferon-α	E

Topical treatment of Bowen's disease with 5-fluorouracil. Bargman H, Hochman J. J Cutan Med Surg 2003;7:101–5.

Only two of 26 biopsy-confirmed lesions recurred up to 10 years following treatment.

5-fluorouracil iontophoretic therapy for Bowen's disease. Welch ML, Grabski WJ, McCollough M, et al. J Am Acad Dermatol 1997;36:956–8.

One of twenty six patients showed recurrence of Bowen's disease at 3-month follow-up.

Recurrence after topical therapy has been attributed to deep follicular involvement. This study attempted to enhance the efficacy by utilizing iontophoresis for selective uptake of 5-FU by the follicles.

Guidelines for topical photodynamic therapy: report of a workshop of the British Photodermatology Group. Morton CA, Brown SB, Collins S, et al. Br J Dermatol 2002;146:552–67.

Evidence-based protocols for PDT and cost comparison information with standard therapies for Bowen's disease.

Photodynamic therapy for large or multiple patches of Bowen disease and basal cell carcinoma. Morton CA, Whitehurst C, McColl JH, et al. Arch Dermatol 2001;137: 319–24.

Clearance of lesions was 88% with a 10% recurrence rate in the 12-month follow-up period.

Comparison of photodynamic therapy with cryotherapy in the treatment of Bowen's disease. Morton CA, Whitehurst C, Moseley H, et al. Br J Dermatol 1996;135:766–71.

The clearance rates for PDT vs cryotherapy after one treatment was 75 and 50%, respectively, with 100% clearance after two treatments in the PDT group and three treatments in the cryotherapy group. There was no recurrence in the PDT group at 12-month follow-up.

Randomized comparison of photodynamic therapy with topical 5-fluorouracil in Bowen's disease. Salim A, Leman JA, McColl JH, et al. Br J Dermatol 2003;148:539–43.

The clearance rates at 12 months with PDT vs 5-FU were 82 and 48%, respectively.

Although the success rates in this study imply that PDT is a better therapy, a failure rate of almost 20% should alert the physician to question the true clinical utility of this approach.

Imiquimod 5% cream in the treatment of Bowen's disease. Mackenzie-Wood A, Kossard S, de Launey J, et al. J Am Acad Dermatol 2001;44:462–70.

Of 16 patients 93% had no residual tumor at 6-week post-treatment biopsy.

The small sample size and extremely short follow-up period of this study highly limits its usefulness.

Soft X-ray therapy in Bowen's disease and erythroplasia of Queyrat. Blank AA, Schnyder UW. Dermatologica 1985; 171:89–94.

Seventy three cases of Bowen's disease and four cases of EQ were treated with a cumulative dosage of 3200–5000 R.

At 3-year follow up, two cases of recurrent genital carcinoma in situ (50%) were noted.

Bowen's disease of the distal digit. Outcome of treatment with carbon dioxide laser vaporization. Gordon KB, Garden JM, Robinson JK. Dermatol Surg 1996;22:723–8.

Four of five patients had no sign of recurrence at follow-up of 6 months to 3 years.

Concomitant use of a high-energy pulsed CO_2 laser and a long-pulsed (810 nm) diode laser for squamous cell carcinoma in situ. Fader DJ, Lowe L. Dermatol Surg 2002;28:97–9

Three patients showed complete resolution at 4 months, with epidermal and follicular epithelium restored 2 weeks postoperatively.

Use of the diode laser for lesions in nonglabrous skin may enhance the efficacy of the CO_2 laser by targeting lesions that extend down the follicular infundibula.

Treatment of multiple lesions of Bowen's disease with isotretinoin and interferon alpha. Gordon KB, Roenigk HH, Gendleman M. Arch Dermatol 1997;133:691–3.

One patient was treated with oral isotretinoin and subcutaneous interferon-α-2a with no recurrence at 15 months.

Evidence levels A Double-blind study **B** Clinical trial ≥ 20 subjects **C** Clinical trial < 20 subjects **D** Series ≥ 5 subjects **E** Anecdotal case reports

Bullous pemphigoid

Darrell W Gonzales, Sam Kim, Victoria P Werth

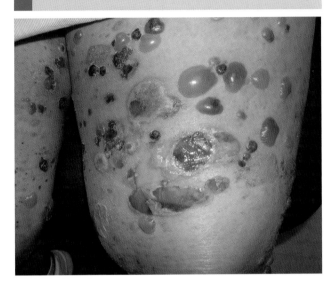

Bullous pemphigoid (BP) is an autoimmune subepidermal blistering disease that predominantly affects older patients. Mainly IgG autoantibodies bind to BP 230 and BP 180 antigens, components of the hemidesmosome adhesion complex, triggering activation of complement and release of tissue-destructive enzymes. Local or generalized tense blister formation on normal skin or on an erythematous base may be preceded by an urticarial or eczematous rash. Mucosal involvement with small blisters or erosions may exist in a minority of patients. Although there can be relapses and exacerbations, BP is generally self-limiting, with remission in most patients by 5 years.

MANAGEMENT STRATEGY

Patients with localized disease may be successfully treated with *potent topical or intralesional corticosteroids*. Those with generalized disease can be treated with *prednisone*, 40–80 mg daily, depending on disease severity and concomitant disorders. The risks of both short and long-term systemic corticosteroid therapy are well known and are heightened in the elderly patient population. Every effort should be made to find the minimum dosage of systemic corticosteroids required to suppress disease, and guidelines regarding osteoporosis prevention should be followed.

Tetracycline alone or in combination with nicotinamide, can be used for patients unable to tolerate, or with contraindications to corticosteroids. This treatment is also attractive for younger patients, who may otherwise need to be maintained on long-term immunosuppressive therapy. *Dapsone* is another alternative to systemic corticosteroids. It is particularly useful when histologic examination reveals a predominance of neutrophils.

Azathioprine may be used alone or as a corticosteroid-sparing agent in more severe disease. Thiopurine methyltransferase (TPMT) is an enzyme that metabolizes this agent. Due to genetic polymorphisms in expression of this enzyme, a TPMT level measurement prior to initiation of azathioprine may assist the physician in appropriate dosing. Azathioprine has a slow onset of action and corticosteroids should be started in tandem during the acute stage. Patients usually respond within 3–4 weeks of initiation.

Mycophenolate mofetil, an immunosuppressive agent, has recently been used as an effective corticosteroid-sparing agent in BP. It is generally well tolerated and does not carry the risk of liver toxicity seen with azathioprine. *Methotrexate* is another corticosteroid-sparing agent that may be useful in BP. It is given in a low-dosage weekly protocol in a similar manner as psoriasis therapy.

For severe and refractory BP, a variety of *immunosuppressive* and *immunomodulatory therapies* have demonstrated efficacy, including cyclophosphamide, cyclosporine, pulse intravenous corticosteroids, plasmapheresis and high-dose intravenous immunoglobulin.

SPECIFIC INVESTIGATIONS

- Thorough evaluation of medication history
- Thorough physical exam for internal malignancy
- Blood glucose screen
- Blister biopsy for hematoxylin and eosin histology
- Perilesional skin for immunofluorescence
- Blood (or blister fluid) for indirect immunofluorescence

Drug induced bullous pemphigoid. Fellner MJ. Clin Dermatol 1993;11:515–20.

Multiple drugs have been recognized to induce BP, including furosemide, phenacetin, penicillins, ibuprofen and UV light.

The association of bullous pemphigoid and malignant disease: a case control study. Venning VA, Wojnarowska F. Br J Derm 1990;123:439–45.

A retrospective review examining the rate of malignancy in 84 patients with BP versus 168 age- and sex-matched controls. Malignancy was found in 6% of BP patients within 8 weeks of diagnosis compared to an overall incidence of 5.3% in controls.

Although correlation between BP and malignancy remains obscure, a thorough review of systems and physical examination is recommended.

Increased frequency of diabetes mellitus in patients with bullous pemphigoid: a case–control study. Chuang TY, Korkij W, Soltani K, et al. J Am Acad Dermatol 1984;6: 1099–102.

The occurrence rate of primary diabetes mellitus prior to administration of systemic corticosteroids was significantly higher in patients with BP (20%) than in controls (2.5%).

FIRST LINE THERAPIES

■ Topical corticosteroids	B
■ Systemic corticosteroids	B
■ Tetracycline	C
■ Tetracycline and nicotinamide	C

Evaluation of the safety and efficacy of a potent topical corticosteroid in the treatment of bullous pemphigoid. Claudy A. Clin Dermatol 2001;19:778–80.

A review of the one hundred eleven patients with BP reported in the literature treated with topical clobetasol propionate cream as monotherapy, applied either to lesional skin or normal-appearing skin once or twice daily without occlusion. Absence of new blisters could be obtained within a few days in more than 80% of the patients with complete re-epithelialization of the affected skin in an average of 13.7 days. This therapy was effective in healing lesions in most of the patients with mild or moderate BP without adverse effects, but is not recommended for patients with severe forms of BP. The tapering off and discontinuation of topical corticosteroids should be performed over months.

A comparison of oral and topical corticosteroids in patients with bullous pemphigoid. Joly P, Roujeau JC, Benichou J, et al. N Engl J Med 2002;346:321–7.

A total of 341 patients with BP were enrolled in a randomized, multicenter trial and stratified according to the severity of their disease (moderate or extensive). Patients were randomly assigned to receive either topical clobetasol propionate cream or oral prednisone (0.5 mg/kg for moderate disease and 1 mg/kg for extensive disease). Overall, topical corticosteroid therapy was found to be effective for both moderate and severe BP and superior to oral corticosteroid therapy for extensive disease.

Treatment in bullous diseases with corticosteroid drugs and corticotrophin. Stevenson CJ. Br J Dermatol 1960; 72:11–21.

Sixty eight patients in an open study were treated with systemic corticosteroids with good response in all but six cases.

Generalized bullous pemphigoid controlled by tetracycline therapy alone. Pereyo NG, Loretta SD. J Am Acad Dermatol 1995;32:138–9.

A case report of an 82-year-old woman with generalized BP who completely responded to oral tetracycline (500 mg twice daily) in 2 weeks. The tetracycline was successfully tapered over 6 weeks.

Nicotinamide and tetracycline therapy of bullous pemphigoid. Fivenson DP, Breneman DL, Rosen GB, et al. Arch Dermatol 1994;130:753–8.

A randomized open-label trial of 20 patients with BP. The combination of nicotinamide (500 mg three times daily) and tetracycline (500 mg four times daily) was equally efficacious as systemic corticosteroids and resulted in less toxicity.

SECOND LINE THERAPIES

■ Azathioprine	B
■ Dapsone	C
■ Mycophenolate mofetil	D
■ Methotrexate	C

Azathioprine in the treatment of bullous pemphigoid. Greaves MW, Burton JL, Marks J. Br Med J 1971;1:144–5.

Of 11 patients on long-term maintenance therapy with systemic corticosteroids, nine remained symptom free on azathioprine alone and two were able to have a reduced dosage of prednisone.

Azathioprine plus prednisone in treatment of pemphigoid. Burton JL, Harman RMM, Peachey RDG, Warin RP. Br Med J 1978;2:1190–1.

A 3-year controlled trial of 25 patients comparing azathioprine (2.5 mg/kg daily) plus prednisone with prednisone alone showed that azathioprine greatly reduced the need for prednisone and improved outcome.

Dapsone as first line therapy for bullous pemphigoid. Venning VA, Millard PR, Wojnarowska F. Br J Dermatol 1989;120:83–92.

In an open trial of 13 patients placed on dapsone as initial treatment, six patients were completely controlled with dapsone (50–100 mg daily). Dapsone may be used to treat BP as initial treatment, particularly when there are contraindications to the use of corticosteroids or immunosuppressives.

Mycophenolate mofetil; a new therapeutic option in the treatment of blistering autoimmune diseases. Grundmann-Kollmann M, Korting HC, Behrens S, et al. J Am Acad Dermatol 1999;40:957–60.

Mycophenolate mofetil given in combination with prednisone in one patient and as monotherapy in two patients resulted in complete remission of symptoms within 8–11 weeks.

Low-dose methotrexate treatment in elderly patients with bullous pemphigoid. Paul MA, Hyg MS, Jorizzo JL, et al. J Am Acad Dermatol 1994;31:620–5.

In a retrospective chart review of 34 patients with BP, eight therapy-resistant patients received low-dose weekly methotrexate (average 5–10 mg) in combination with oral prednisone. Patients receiving combination therapy required significantly lower doses of prednisone to control their disease at 1 month compared with baseline dose.

Treatment of bullous pemphigoid by low-dose methotrexate associated with short-term potent topical steroids: an open prospective study of 18 cases. Dereure O. Arch Dermatol 2002;138:1255–6.

A prospective review of 18 patients with BP treated with a 2–3-week course of whole-body topical corticosteroid (clobetasol propionate) combined with oral or intramuscular methotrexate. Initial dosages of weekly methotrexate ranged from 7.5 to 10 mg. All 18 patients achieved a complete clinical response during the initial phase of intensive local corticosteroid treatment which was then maintained with methotrexate in monotherapy. Interruption of treatment was tolerated in 13 patients after 6–10 months with an uneventful follow-up for a mean period of 7.8 months.

Low-dose oral pulse methotrexate as monotherapy in elderly patients with bullous pemphigoid. Heilborn JD, Ståhle-Bäckdahl M, Albertioni F, et al. J Am Acad Dermatol 1999;40:741–9.

A prospective study of low-dose oral methotrexate (5–12.5 mg per week) in 11 elderly patients with generalized BP. Every patient demonstrated a rapid decrease in disease activity within 4–30 days.

THIRD LINE THERAPIES

■ Cyclophosphamide	D
■ Cyclosporine	D
■ Pulse intravenous corticosteroid	D
■ Plasmapheresis	C
■ Intravenous immunoglobulin (IVIG)	C
■ Minocycline	C
■ Erythromycin	D
■ Chlorambucil	C
■ Sulfapyridine	D

Severe bullous pemphigoid responsive to pulsed intravenous dexamethasone and oral cyclophosphamide. Dawe RS, Naidoo DK, Ferguson J. Br J Dermatol 1997; 137:826–7.

Refractory BP in a 59-year-old woman with diabetes mellitus cleared with pulsed intravenous dexamethasone therapy (100 mg dexamethasone in 500 mL 5% dextrose infused over 4 h, on three consecutive days, monthly) and low-dose oral cyclophosphamide (50 mg/day between pulses).

Successful treatment of bullous pemphigoid with pulsed intravenous cyclophosphamide. Itoh T, Hosokawa H, Shirai Y, Horio T. Br J Dermatol 1996;134:931–3.

Case report of a 67-year-old man with refractory BP who responded to monthly pulsed intravenous doses of cyclophosphamide (500–1000 mg) along with low-dose oral cyclophosphamide (50 mg/day).

Effects of cyclosporin on bullous pemphigoid and pemphigus. Thivolet J, Harthelemy H, Rigot-Muller G, Bendelac A. Lancet 1985;1:334–5.

Cyclosporine (6 mg/kg daily), adapted to obtain a plasma level of 80–180 μg/L, was successful in treating two patients with BP.

High-dose methylprednisolone in the treatment of bullous pemphigoid. Siegel J, Eaglstein WH. Arch Dermatol 1984;120:1157–65.

Seven of eight hospitalized patients with active BP responded within 24 h after methylprednisolone sodium succinate pulse therapy (15 mg/kg intravenously over a 1-h period daily for 3 days). Moderate doses of oral prednisone (0.4 mg/kg) were required for maintenance.

Plasmapheresis as a steroid sparing procedure in bullous pemphigoid. Egan CA, Meadows KP, Zone JJ. Int J Dermatol 2000;39:230–5.

A retrospective review of ten patients, all of whom went into remission with a lower daily dose of oral prednisone at 3 and 6 months after plasmapheresis. The drawbacks of plasmapheresis therapy include cost and procedural complications, such as line infection/sepsis and local thrombus formation.

Plasmapheresis therapy of pemphigus and bullous pemphigoid. Roujeau JC. Semin Dermatol 1988;7:195–200.

The potential value of plasma exchange is as an adjuvant to corticosteroids and immunosuppressive agents. It remains to be seen whether the corticosteroid-sparing effects reduce the incidence of side effects sufficiently to justify the cost.

Intravenous immunoglobulin therapy for patients with bullous pemphigoid unresponsive to conventional immunosuppressive treatment. Ahmed AR. J Am Acad Dermatol 2001;6:825–35.

Fifteen patients with recurrent BP who had experienced several significant side effects resulting from conventional therapy were treated with IVIG. In all 15 patients a rapid initial clinical response was observed along with a long-term remission. In all subjects oral prednisone and other immunosuppressives could be safely withdrawn without recurrence of disease shortly after initiating IVIG. A gradual withdrawal of IVIG was necessary to prevent relapses.

Consensus statement on the use of intravenous immunoglobulin therapy in the treatment of autoimmune mucocutaneous blistering diseases. Ahmed AR, Dahl MV. Arch Dermatol 2003;139:1051–9.

In 27 of 32 cases of BP reported in the literature as nonresponsive to conventional therapy, IVIG was of significant benefit and produced lasting clinical benefit with minimal adverse effects.

Minocycline as a therapeutic option in bullous pemphigoid. Loo WJ, Kirtschig G, Wojnarowska F. Clin Exp Dermatol 2001;26:376–9.

A retrospective analysis of 22 patients with BP treated with minocycline as an adjuvant therapy. A major response was seen in six patients, a minor response in 11, and no response was seen in five patients.

Erythromycin therapy in bullous pemphigoid: possible anti-inflammatory effects. Fox BJ, Odom RB, Findlay RF. J Am Acad Dermatol 1982;7:504–10.

Erythromycin was effective in both an 87-year-old woman (at a dosage of 250 mg four times a day) and a 4½-year-old girl with BP.

The use of chlorambucil in the treatment of bullous pemphigoid. Milligan A, Hutchinson PE. J Am Acad Dermatol 1990;22:796–801.

Twenty three patients treated with a combination of chlorambucil (40–60 mg/day) and systemic corticosteroids demonstrated a gradual response. Nine patients developed transient thrombocytopenia and one patient developed significant bone marrow suppression.

Bullous pemphigoid responding to sulfapyridine and the sulfones. Person JR, Rogers RS. Arch Dermatol 1977;113: 610–5.

Of 41 patients with BP, five completely responded to sulfapyridine (500–1000 mg four times daily) and one additional patient showed marked improvement. Histologic examination of skin biopsy specimens from these patients demonstrated a predominance of neutrophils.

Calcinosis cutis

F Nayeemuddin, Ian Coulson

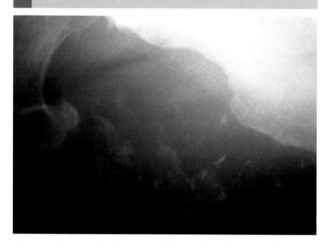

A rare disease of aberrant calcium deposition in the skin, calcinosis cutis can be congenital, idiopathic, dystrophic (secondary to tissue damage e.g. scleroderma and dermatomyositis), metastatic (secondary to abnormal calcium and phosphate metabolism e.g. renal failure, hyperparathyroidism) or iatrogenic (following application of calcium-containing paste for the electrodes in electro-encephalography and electromyography). Most cases present as nodules, which may extrude chalky white material. Calcinosis cutis may be isolated to a small area (circumscripta) or it may be diffuse (universalis). Ulceration with secondary infection can be a complication. In congenital calcinosis cutis lesions are usually seen on the head and extremities.

MANAGEMENT STRATEGY

The first step in management is to identify any underlying cause. Dystrophic calcification occurs in up to 10% of patients with scleroderma and 10–40% of patients with juvenile dermatomyositis, but is rare in systemic lupus erythematosus. Examination and investigations for connective tissue disease are, therefore, strongly recommended. Skin biopsy can help distinguish cutaneous calcification from ossification.

A number of malignancies have been implicated in metastatic calcification (e.g. leukemia and multiple myeloma). However, successful treatment of the underlying cause does not always have an impact on calcinosis cutis, which frequently requires other treatment modalities. There are no large studies for the treatment of calcinosis cutis, and most therapies are based on case reports. Spontaneous extrusion of calcium salts may occur; this may need *surgical* encouragement when calcification results in overlying ulceration (occasionally seen around chronic venous stasis ulcers). *Intralesional corticosteroids, aluminum hydroxide supplements, bisphosphonates, diltiazem, colchicine* and *probenecid* have shown success, mostly in calcinosis associated with dermatomyositis. *Warfarin* has been advocated in both dermatomyositis and systemic sclerosis-associated calcinosis.

SPECIFIC INVESTIGATIONS

- Full blood count
- Urea and creatinine
- Serum calcium and phosphate
- Serum electrophoresis
- Creatine kinase
- Autoantibodies (e.g. antinuclear antibody, Scl70)
- Parathyroid hormone levels
- Skin biopsy
- Soft tissue radiology

FIRST LINE THERAPIES

■ No treatment/self healing	E
■ Aluminum hydroxide	E
■ Intralesional corticosteroid	E

Self-healing dystrophic calcinosis following trauma with transepidermal elimination. Pitt AE, Ethington JE, Troy JL. Cutis 1990;45:28–32.

A case of dystrophic calcinosis following trauma which resolved over 8 weeks with spontaneous transepidermal elimination.

Calcinosis cutis and renal failure. Koltan B, Pederson J. Arch Dermatol 1974;110:256–7.

A 47-year-old man with metastatic calcinosis cutis secondary to chronic renal failure was successfully treated with oral aluminum hydroxide gel, 30 mL four times a day. After 8 weeks of treatment the patient had complete clearance of calcinosis cutis in all areas except the scrotum.

Calcinosis cutis in juvenile dermatomyositis: remarkable response to aluminum hydroxide therapy. Wang WJ, Lo WL, Wong CK. Arch Dermatol 1988;124:1721–2.

A 13-year-old girl with juvenile dermatomyositis complicated by calcinosis cutis was successfully treated with oral aluminum hydroxide and magnesium trisilicate administered four times a day. Clinical improvement of the calcification was observed within 8 months and near complete clearance by the end of 1 year's therapy.

Calcinosis cutis circumscripta. Treatment with an intralesional corticosteroid. Lee SS, Felsenstein J, Tanzer FR. Arch Dermatol 1978;114:1080–1.

A case report of a teenager with idiopathic calcinosis cutis over the knees, elbows, popliteal fossae and wrist, successfully treated with intralesional triamcinolone diacetate (25 mg/mL) administered at monthly intervals via Dermojet® injector and syringe and needle.

SECOND LINE THERAPIES

■ Bisphosphonates	E
■ Diltiazem	E
■ Probenecid	E
■ Colchicine	E

Disodium etidronate therapy for dystrophic cutaneous calcification. Rabens SF, Bethune JE. Arch Dermatol 1975;111:357–61.

A case report of a patient with extensive disabling dystrophic calcinosis cutis and possible scleroderma treated with oral disodium etidronate 10 mg/kg daily, showing arrest and partial reversal of the calcific process.

Regression of calcinosis associated with adult dermatomyositis following diltiazem therapy. Vinen CS, Patel S, Bruckner FE. Rheumatology 2000;39:333–40.

Case report of a patient with disabling calcinosis cutis secondary to dermatomyositis showing marked improvement following diltiazem therapy over 2.5 years. The dose was increased from 60 mg daily to 360 mg daily over 17 months.

Calcinosis in dermatomyositis treated with probenecid. Skuterud E, Sydnes OA, Haavik TK. Scand J Rheumatol 1981;10:92–4.

Case report of childhood dermatomyositis with calcinosis responding to treatment with probenecid 250 mg daily. Resorption of soft tissue calcification was observed soon after commencing therapy.

Ulcerated dystrophic calcinosis cutis secondary to localised linear scleroderma. Vereecken P, Stallenberg B, Tas S, et al. Int J Clin Pract 1998;52:593–4.

Case report of a 62-year-old lady with ulcerated dystrophic calcinosis cutis secondary to linear scleroderma. The ulceration healed after 4 months of treatment with colchicine 1 mg daily without modification of the calcinosis.

THIRD LINE THERAPIES

■ Warfarin	C
■ Surgery	C
■ Parathyroidectomy	E

Treatment of calcinosis universalis with low-dose warfarin. Berger RG, Featherstone GL, Raasch RH, et al. Am J Med 1987;83:72–6.

A randomized double-blind study of eight patients with subcutaneous calcification, secondary to either dermatomyositis or systemic sclerosis. Patients were treated with either warfarin 1 mg daily or placebo for 18 months. All patients had clinical assessment, plain radiographs and whole body bone scintigraphy to detect extraskeletal uptake. Two of the three patients in the warfarin-treated group had a reduction in extraskeletal uptake, as indicated by the bone scan scores, compared with none in the control group. No patient had a change in either clinical examination or plain radiographs.

Surgical treatment of calcinosis cutis in the upper extremity. Mendelson BC, Linsheid RL, Dobyns JH, Muller SA. J Hand Surg 1977;2:318–24.

A case series of surgical experience on 11 patients with calcinosis cutis in the upper extremity – seven with systemic scleroderma and four with dermatomyositis. Four patients healed without any complications and were not followed up. Of the seven follow-up patients, six found the procedure definitely beneficial.

Metastatic calcinosis cutis with renal hyperparathyroidism. Posey RE, Ritchie EB. Arch Dermatol 1967; 95:505–8.

A case report of a 28-year-old woman with metastatic calcinosis cutis secondary to renal failure, which showed rapid resolution following panparathyroidectomy.

Calciphylaxis

Alexander Doctoroff

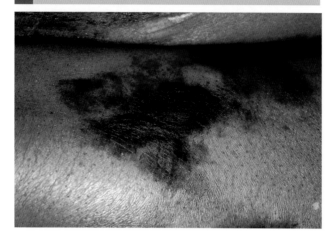

Calciphylaxis (calcific uremic arteriolopathy, uremic small-artery disease with medial calcification and intimal hyperplasia, vascular calcification-cutaneous necrosis syndrome, calcifying panniculitis) is a serious and often lethal condition of unknown pathogenesis affecting mostly patients with renal disease. It can present either with tender subcutaneous plaques, or skin ulcers reflecting various stages of the progression of the disease process.

MANAGEMENT STRATEGY

Calciphylaxis is a deadly disease with a mortality rate of up to 80%, so early diagnosis by skin biopsy and aggressive treatment are essential. Although various surgical and non-surgical methods may be tried, no effective therapy for calciphylaxis exists. This reflects lack of clarity in our understanding of this condition. Calciphylaxis is likely a multifactorial entity with calcium and phosphate abnormalities being only part of the pathogenesis.

Selye's theory of calciphylaxis is similar to the one of anaphylaxis. In anaphylaxis, the patient is exposed to the same antigen twice before reaction occurs. In calciphylaxis, the exposure occurs to two different antigens. First, a 'sensitizer', such as elevated parathyroid hormone or vitamin D supplement is encountered. Then a 'challenger,' such as a local injection is introduced, producing ulcerations. Further research will prove or disprove this theory. At this time however, *parathyroidectomy*, which removes a 'sensitizer', and improves calcium, phosphate, and parathyroid hormone levels, remains a first line therapy for those patients with high parathyroid hormone levels. Despite being a subject of controversy, for many patients it results in rapid healing of ulcerations.

Monitoring the patient's metabolic environment is of utmost importance. Hyperphosphatemia must be controlled with *non-calcium-containing phosphate binders*. A *phosphorus-restricted diet should be introduced*, and *vitamin D supplementation stopped*.

Aggressive *wound debridement* needs to be initiated without delay. Monitoring for infection and appropriate use of antibiotics are a mainstay of treatment because most patient deaths occur from sepsis.

If the patient's calciphylaxis is uncovered at an early stage (indurated plaques without ulcerations), *oral prednisone* appears to be helpful.

The use of *zero or low-calcium dialysate* with induction of hypocalcemia and calcium shift into the intravascular space appears to be a reasonable therapy. If *hyperbaric oxygen therapy* is available, it can be helpful to some patients.

The treatment of calciphylaxis should be a multidisciplinary effort with internists, critical care specialists, nephrologists, dermatologists, infectionists, surgeons, and pain specialists being involved.

SPECIFIC INVESTIGATIONS

- Skin biopsy
- Serum parathyroid hormone, calcium, phosphate
- Bone scan
- Measurements of transcutaneous oxygen saturation
- Radiography or xeroradiography

Calciphylaxis: emerging concepts in prevention, diagnosis, and treatment. Wilmer WA, Magro CM. Semin Dial 2002;15:172–86.

Excellent review of pathogenesis, histopathology, diagnosis and treatment.

FIRST LINE THERAPIES

- Parathyroidectomy (for patients with elevated parathyroid hormone)   C
- Discontinuation of calcium and vitamin D supplementation   C
- Decrease of serum phosphorus   C
- Treatment of low serum albumin   C
- Monitoring for infection   C
- Debridement of necrotic tissue and aggressive wound care   C
- Prednisone (for patients without ulcerations only)   C

Calciphylaxis: a syndrome of skin necrosis and acral gangrene in chronic renal failure. Hafner J, Keusch G, Wahl C, et al. Vasa 1998;27:137–43.

Meta-analysis of all case reports of calciphylaxis from 1936 to 1996 revealed that 70% of patients who were parathyroidectomized survived compared with 43% of those who did not receive the operation.

This study did not stratify patients into those with and without hyperparathyroidism.

Therapy for calciphylaxis: an outcome analysis. Arch-Ferrer JE, Beenken SW, Rue LW, et al. Surgery 2003;134: 941–4.

In this retrospective study of 35 patients, those who underwent parathyroidectomy showed improvement in serum calcium, phosphate, and parathyroid hormone values and had a longer median overall survival (80 months) than nonsurgical patients (35 months).

Most patients were African-American females.

Calcium use increases risk of calciphylaxis: a case–control study. Zacharias JM, Fontaine B, Fine A. Perit Dial Int 1999;19:248–52.

Retrospective case–control study of eight patients suggests increased risk of calciphylaxis with calcium ingestion.

Risk factors and mortality associated with calciphylaxis in end-stage renal disease. Mazhar AR, Johnson RJ, Gillen D, et al. Stehman-Breen CO. Kidney Int 2001;60:324–32.

Retrospective case–control study of 19 cases demonstrated female gender, hyperphosphatemia, high alkaline phosphatase, and low serum albumin to be risk factors for calciphylaxis.

The evolving pattern of calciphylaxis: therapeutic considerations. Llach F. Nephrol Dial Transplant 2001;16:448–51.

This and other reviews suggest aggressive lowering of serum phosphorus with non-calcium containing phosphate binders (such as sevelamer), dietary control of calcium and phosphorus intake, as well as aggressive wound debridement and monitoring for infection. Six of eight patients had significant improvement with zero calcium dialysate.

Calciphylaxis is usually non-ulcerating: risk factors, outcome and therapy. Fine A, Zacharias J. Kidney Int 2002; 61:2210–7.

Review of 36 patients who presented without ulcerations, but with subcutaneous indurated plaques in the legs demonstrated improvement from corticosteroid therapy (prednisone 30–50 mg orally daily for 3–8 weeks) in 80% of cases. Contraindications to corticosteroid therapy include ulceration anywhere (related to peripheral vascular disease or calciphylaxis) or high risk of infection.

SECOND LINE THERAPIES

■ Hyperbaric oxygen therapy	D
■ Low-calcium dialysate	D
■ Vitamin K supplementation in patients who are deficient	E
■ Pamidronate	E
■ Tissue plasminogen activator	E

Hyperbaric oxygen in the treatment of calciphylaxis: a case series. Podymow T, Wherrett C, Burns KD. Nephrol Dial Transplant 2001;16:2176.

In this retrospective study, two of five patients with calciphylaxis had complete resolution of their ulcers with hyperbaric oxygen therapy.

Low-calcium dialysis in calciphylaxis. Lipsker D, Chosidow O, Martinez F, Challier E, Frances C. Arch Dermatol 1997;133:798–9.

This is one of several case reports (such as the one by Llach 2001, referenced above) of successful calciphylaxis treatment with low-calcium dialysis.

Skin necrosis and protein C deficiency associated with vitamin K depletion in a patient with renal failure. Soundararajan R, Leehey DJ, Yu AW, Miller JB. Am J Med 1992;93:467–70.

Vitamin K replacement resulted in reversal of calciphylaxis in a vitamin K-deficient patient.

Rapid improvement of calciphylaxis after intravenous pamidronate therapy in a patient with chronic renal failure. Monney P, Nguyen QV, Perroud H, Descombes E. Nephrol Dial Transplant 2004;19:2130–2.

Five intravenous doses of 30 mg pamidronate resulted in healing of ulcerations in a patient whose clinical condition was worsening despite other medical therapy. When 6 weeks after discharge calciphylaxis returned, an additional 30 mg pamidronate dose aborted the recurrence.

Low-dose tissue plasminogen activator for calciphylaxis. Sewell LD, Weenig RH, Davis MD, et al. Arch Dermatol 2004;140:1045–8.

Tissue plasminogen activator (tPA; alteplase) in a 10 mg intravenous daily dose for 14 days followed by warfarin anticoagulation resulted in eventual healing of ulcerations.

THIRD LINE THERAPIES

■ Maggot therapy and pentoxyfillin	E
■ Ozone therapy	E
■ Cryofiltration apheresis (CFA)	E

Painful ulcers in calciphylaxis – combined treatment with maggot therapy and oral pentoxyfillin. Tittelbach J, Graefe T, Wollina U. J Dermatolog Treat 2001;12:211–4.

Maggot therapy and 800 mg daily of oral pentoxifylline were successful in healing of ulcers over a 6-month period.

Ozone therapy in a dialyzed patient with calcific uremic arteriolopathy. Biedunkiewicz B, Tylicki L, Lichodziejewska-Niemierko M, et al. Kidney Int 2003;64:367–8.

Fifteen sessions of treatment with ozonated auto-hemotherapy (O3-AHT) with ozone concentration of 50–70 μg/mL over 3 weeks, accompanied by local wound lavage with ozonated water led to healing of necrotic areas.

Intensive tandem cryofiltration apheresis and hemodialysis to treat a patient with severe calciphylaxis, cryoglobulinemia, and end-stage renal disease. Siami GA, Siami FS. ASAIO J 1999;45:229–33.

This is a report on tandem CFA and hemodialysis (HD) in a critically-ill patient with type II mixed cryoglobulinemia, hepatitis C virus, calciphylaxis, and end-stage renal disease. The patient received 18 tandem CFA/HD treatments, and four extra HD treatments in 1 month. His plasma cryoglobulin level dropped and his calciphylaxis also improved.

Candidiasis and chronic mucocutaneous candidiasis

Robin Buchholz, Michael Fisher, Ian Coulson

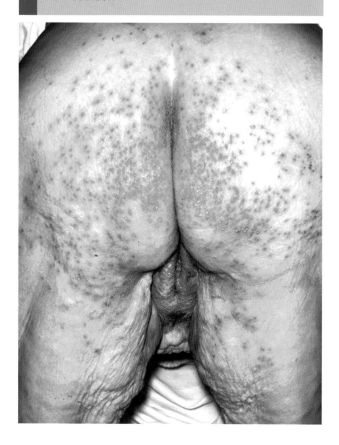

Candidiasis

Cutaneous candidiasis is a superficial mycotic infection of skin, usually caused by the yeast *Candida albicans*. Other *Candida* species are occasionally responsible. The intertriginous skin folds or other moist, occluded sites are most frequently affected, with satellite lesions often extending beyond the flexure. The diagnosis can easily be made with a potassium hydroxide (KOH) preparation by the presence of pseudohyphae and yeast forms, or by culture. Disseminated congenital cutaneous and systemic candidiasis is an important though rare disorder of low-birthweight infants. Disseminated cutaneous disease has been reported in intravenous drug abusers. Nipple candidiasis causes areolar redness, scaling, and lactation pain in nursing mothers.

MANAGEMENT STRATEGY

Candida yeasts are part of the normal flora of the skin. Colonization of the skin is supported by local factors, including heat, occlusion, loss of epithelial barrier function, and moisture. Superficial candidiasis occurs in these conditions. Infections are usually acute and self-limited when anti-yeast therapy is initiated in the normal host; however, chronic or relapsing infection should provoke the search for predisposing risk factors. The latter may include diabetes mellitus, tropical environment, obesity, use of systemic corticosteroids or antibiotics, neutropenia, primary and acquired immunodeficiency (including HIV), diseases which disturb the integument (e.g. psoriasis), occlusion (such as under diapers), and malignancy. Although numerous topical and systemic therapies are available, relapses and recurrences are common unless these predisposing factors are corrected.

Affected skin sites that are moist and/or occluded should be dried out with *wet-to-dry soaks* and *exposure of the sites to air*. In addition, various drying agents such as *Castellani's paint*, *potassium permanganate compresses*, *gentian violet*, *zinc oxide lotion*, and *talc powders* (not corn starch) are helpful. Promotion of good hygiene is important.

Topical antifungal products including but not limited to imidazole/triazoles, ciclopirox olamine, polyene antibiotics (including nystatin and amphotericin B lotion), and iodochlorhydroxyquin are applied to affected areas.

Topical corticosteroids may be used sparingly for short periods in conjunction with topical and/or systemic antifungals to reduce the inflammatory component.

Systemic therapy with *fluconazole, ketoconazole, terbinafine,* or *itraconazole* is occasionally indicated, particularly with extensive or recalcitrant disease, and in immunocompromised patients.

SPECIFIC INVESTIGATIONS

- KOH and culture
- Urinalysis for sugar
- Serum glucose*
- Serology for HIV*

*in recurrent cases

Incidence and distribution of *Candida* species isolated from human skin in Jordan. Abu-Elteen KH. Mycoses 1999;42:311–7.

The infected patients were divided into four categories: diabetics, those receiving steroids, those receiving antibiotics, and a non-risk group. Analysis of the data revealed that the incidence rate appears to be doubled in diabetes (49%), steroid therapy (33.8%), and antibiotic therapy (27.4%), compared with the control group (15.7%).

Factors affecting the adhesion of *Candida albicans* to epithelial cells of insulin-using diabetes mellitus patients. Willis AM, Coulter WA, Hayes JR, et al. J Med Microbiol 2000;49:291–3.

Palatal epithelial cells retained significantly more *C. albicans* in vivo and adhesion was influenced by the availability of sugars in the growth medium and the strain of *C. albicans*.

Guidelines of care for superficial mycotic infections of the skin: mucocutaneous candidiasis. Guidelines/Outcomes Committee. American Academy of Dermatology. [Anonymous]. J Am Acad Dermatol 1996;34:110–5.

Mentions HIV as one of the predisposing risk factors for recurrent or relapsing cutaneous candidiasis.

Evidence levels A Double-blind study **B** Clinical trial ≥ 20 subjects **C** Clinical trial < 20 subjects **D** Series ≥ 5 subjects **E** Anecdotal case reports

"White dots on the placenta and red dots on the baby": congenital cutaneous candidiasis – a rare disease of the neonate. Diana A, Epiney M, Ecoffey M, Pfister RE. Acta Paediatr 2004;93:996–9.

A rare important diagnosis that can progress to *Candida* pneumonia and meningitis.

Mammary candidosis in lactating women. Heinig MJ, Francis J, Pappagianis D. J Hum Lact 1999;15:281–8.

Both superficial (cutaneous) and localized (ductal) infection of the mammary gland occurs in lactating women. Severe pain during breastfeeding is characteristic.

FIRST LINE THERAPIES

■ Topical antifungals	A
■ Topical antifungals combined with topical corticosteroids	A, B

Cutaneous candidiasis: treatment with miconazole nitrate. Cullin SI. Cutis 1977;19:126–9.

A double-blind, randomized study in which 30 patients with cutaneous candidiasis were treated with 2% miconazole nitrate lotion or its placebo control. Both a clinical and mycologic cure was achieved in all patients receiving the active lotion.

Topical treatment of dermatophytosis and cutaneous candidosis with flutrimazole 1% cream: double-blind, randomized comparative trial with ketoconazole 2% cream. del Palacio A, Cuetara S, Perez A, et al. Mycoses 1999;42:649–55.

A double-blind, randomized study in which the efficacy and tolerance of flutrimazole 1% cream was compared with that of ketoconazole 2% cream in 60 patients with culturally proven dermatophytosis (47 patients) or cutaneous candidiasis (13 patients). The results showed that flutrimazole 1% cream is as effective and safe as ketoconazole 2% cream for candidal and dermatophyte skin infections.

Evaluation of a new antifungal cream, ciclopirox olamine 1%, in the treatment of cutaneous candidosis. [Anonymous]. Clin Ther 1985;8:41–8.

Two multicenter, randomized, double-blind trials in which ciclopirox olamine was compared with vehicle in one trial and with clotrimazole in the other. The results showed that ciclopirox olamine is a safe and effective treatment for cutaneous candidiasis. In addition, ciclopirox olamine has been shown to ameliorate the clinical manifestations of candidiasis more rapidly than clotrimazole.

A comparison of nystatin cream with nystatin/triamcinolone acetonide combination cream in the treatment of candidal inflammation of the flexures. Beveridge GW, Fairburn E, Finn OA, et al. Curr Med Res Opin 1977;4:584–7.

A multicenter double-blind trial in which 31 patients with bilateral candidal lesions of the flexures were treated for 14 days with nystatin cream on one side and with a combination of nystatin/triamcinolone acetonide on the other. Treatments proved equally effective in terms of mycologic cure and clinical improvement. There was a trend in favor of the combination preparation being preferred by both patients and physicians because of more rapid relief of symptoms.

SECOND LINE THERAPIES

■ Systemic antifungals	E

Persistent *Candida* intertrigo treated with fluconazole. Coldiron BM, Manders SM. Arch Dermatol 1991;127:165–6.

A case report of a 48-year-old woman with poorly controlled non-insulin-dependent diabetes and controlled schizophrenia treated for candidal intertrigo with various regimens.

Topical clotrimazole cream failed and this was followed by the administration of oral ketoconazole. Oral ketoconazole was discontinued because of hepatotoxicity, which was presumed to be due to the drug, although this was proven not to be the case. The regimen was changed to ketoconazole cream, which failed. The patient was noted to clear with oral fluconazole, 100 mg daily, for a period of 4 weeks. After a slight recurrence, she was maintained on a regimen of fluconazole 200 mg per month and remained clear on that schedule.

A search of the literature reveals a paucity of clinical trials and double-blind studies in the area of oral antifungal use for the treatment of cutaneous candidiasis. Most studies are done in the pursuit of treatment for systemic candidiasis, chronic mucocutaneous candidiasis (CMC), onychomycosis, oropharyngeal candidiasis, and vulvovaginal candidiasis.

THIRD LINE THERAPIES

■ Tea tree oils	E
■ Topical mupirocin	C

In-vitro activity of essential oils, in particular *Melaleuca alternifolia* (tea tree) oil and tea tree products, against *Candida* spp. Hammer KA, Carson CF, Riley TV. J Antimicrob Chemother 1998;42:591–5.

An in-vitro study that examined the activity of a range of essential oils, including tea tree oil, against *Candida*. The data presented indicate that some essential oils are active against *Candida* species, suggesting that they may be useful in the topical treatment of superficial candidal infections.

There are currently no clinical trials or double-blind studies examining the in-vivo activity of these oils against Candida *species.*

Perianal candidosis – a comparative study with mupirocin and nystatin. de Wet PM, Rode H, van Dyk A, Millar AJ. Int J Dermatol 1990;38:618–22.

A clinical trial to assess the efficacy and clinical outcome of 2% mupirocin in a polyethylene glycol base and nystatin cream as treatment regimens in diaper candidiasis. Both agents eradicated *Candida*, the major difference being in the marked response of the diaper dermatitis to mupirocin. Mupirocin should be applied topically three to four times daily or with each diaper change and is an excellent antifungal agent.

Chronic mucocutaneous candidiasis

CMC is a chronic recurring candidal infection of skin, nails, hair, and mucous membranes due to failure of the patient's T lymphocytes to produce cytokines that are essential for expression of cell-mediated immunity to *Candida*. This is a heterogeneous condition, occurring in the setting of auto-immune (alopecia areata, vitiligo, idiopathic thrombocytopenia), endocrinologic (hypothyroidism, hypoparathyroidism, Addison's disease), or immunologic (thymoma and myasthenia) disorders. Some variants are familial.

MANAGEMENT STRATEGY

A full assessment of the physical findings and the taking of appropriate nail, hair, and skin specimens for mycologic culture are mandatory. Assessment of the body mass index, and clinical evaluation for endocrine status, including pubertal stage if relevant, should be made, and blood taken for glucose and thyroid, parathyroid, and glucocorticoid hormone levels. Assessment of the humoral and cell-mediated immune function is advised. Associated abnormalities need treatment in their own right.

Management of the candidal infections involves both the use of specific *systemic antimycotic agents* such as amphotericin B, itraconazole, ketoconazole, fluconazole, and terbinafine (topical agents may augment the responses, but are seldom successful alone) and *immune stimulants*. Intermittent courses of systemic agents are advocated, but relapse on withdrawal is usual. *Candida* resistant to many of the systemic agents has been reported.

Maneuvers to help augment cell-mediated immune responses, such as *transfer factor* (TF) administered orally or parenterally and oral high-dose *cimetidine*, have been advocated. Iron deficiency complicates some variants and requires replacement.

SPECIAL INVESTIGATIONS

- Blood count, including platelets
- Serum calcium
- Blood glucose
- Blood cortisol
- Ferritin and serum iron
- Thyroid-stimulating hormone (TSH)
- Parathyroid hormone
- *Candida* intradermal test
- Immunoglobulins
- Chest X-ray

Chronic mucocutaneous candidiasis. Kirkpatrick CH. Pediatr Infect Dis J 2001;20:197–206.

The most recent review by the field leader.

FIRST LINE THERAPIES

■ Systemic azole antimycotics	C
■ Systemic amphotericin B	D
■ Systemic allylamine antimycotics	E

Long-term therapy of chronic mucocutaneous candidiasis with ketoconazole: experience with twenty-one patients. Horsburgh CR Jr, Kirkpatrick CH. Am J Med 1983;74:23–9.

Of 21 patients, 15 had evidence of deficient cellular immunity and eight had endocrine abnormalities. Six patients had concurrent dermatophytosis or chromomycosis. All patients responded to treatment. Mucosal lesions improved in 6.7 ± 0.5 days and cutaneous lesions responded in 22.7 ± 5.1 days. The responses by infected nails were more variable (mean response time 92.4 ± 14.4 days). Concurrent dermatophytoses did not prolong response times. Adverse effects were infrequent: one patient had drug-induced hepatitis and two patients became hypertensive. One patient was able to remain in remission after treatment was discontinued. Two patients had relapses while on treatment. *C. albicans* isolated from these patients was highly resistant to ketoconazole in vitro.

Although ketoconazole has the largest evidence base in CMC, its hepatotoxicity, as demonstrated in one of the above patients, mitigates against its use, and other azoles (itraconazole or fluconazole) are now preferred.

Itraconazole in the treatment of two young brothers with chronic mucocutaneous candidiasis. Tosti A, Piraccini BM, Vincenzi C, Cameli N. Pediatr Dermatol 1997;14:146–8.

Two children affected by CMC involving the mouth and all the nails who were successfully treated with itraconazole at 200 mg daily for 2 months. This therapy produced a rapid cure of both candidal nail and mouth infections. The drug was very well tolerated.

Fluconazole in the management of patients with chronic mucocutaneous candidosis. Hay RJ, Clayton YM. Br J Dermatol 1988;119:683–4.

Thirteen patients with oroesophageal candidiasis associated with CMC were treated with 50 or 200 mg of fluconazole daily, and clinical and mycologic remissions were achieved in a mean period of 10 days.

Terbinafine effectiveness in ketoconazole-resistant muco-cutaneous candidasis in polyglandular autoimmune syndrome type 1. Hassan G. J Assoc Physicians India 2003;51:323.

A useful approach using terbinafine if azole resistance occurs.

SECOND LINE THERAPIES

■ Transfer factor	B
■ Cimetidine	E
■ Zinc	E
■ Iron	E

Transfer factor in chronic mucocutaneous candidiasis. Masi M, De Vinci C, Baricordi OR. Biotherapy 1996;9:97–103.

Fifteen patients suffering from CMC were treated with an in-vitro produced TF specific for *C. albicans* antigens and/or with TF extracted from pooled buffy coats of blood donors: 400 million CEU per week for the first 2 weeks, followed by 100 million CEU per week for 6–12 months. (In this study, TF was encapsulated and administered orally.) Clinical observations were encouraging: all but one patient experienced significant improvement during treatment with specific TF.

Transfer factor in the treatment of chronic mucocutaneous candidiasis: a controlled study. Mobacken H, Hanson LA, Lindholm L, Ljunggren C. Acta Derm Venereol 1980;60:51–5.

A less encouraging report! A controlled crossover study with TF was carried out in seven patients suffering from CMC. Only one patient showed clinical improvement, which started during a period of pretreatment with 5-fluorocytosine given orally 14 days before the patient entered this trial. No conversion to a positive skin test with *Candida* antigen or purified protein derivative was demonstrated following TF in the six patients who were anergic to either of these antigens.

Case report: successful treatment with cimetidine and zinc sulphate in chronic mucocutaneous candidiasis. Polizzi B, Origgi L, Zuccaro G, et al. Am J Med Sci 1996;311:189–90.

The authors evaluated the clinical efficacy of treatment with cimetidine (400 mg three times daily) and zinc sulfate (200 mg a day, reduced later to maintain the blood zinc at the upper level of the normal range) for 16 months in a patient with CMC. An impressive and significant reduction of the infectious events and an increased CD4 (helper/inducer) cell count were observed.

Capillaritis

Cord Sunderkötter, Thomas A Luger

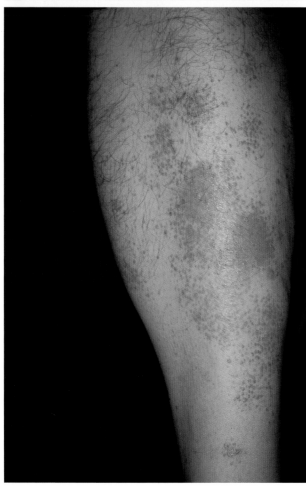

Capillaritis in the Anglo-American literature is the general term for pigmented purpuric dermatoses. These disorders present with the common feature of petechial macules or plaques (due to erythrocyte extravasation and perivascular infiltrates of T lymphocytes), subsequently taking a characteristic brown to orange color (due to hemosiderin deposits in macrophages). They may also present with additional, distinct or sometimes overlapping morphological patterns, which have given rise to several descriptive or eponymous names: papules in pigmented purpuric lichenoid dermatosis of Gougerot and Blum, eczematous spongiosis in epidermis with pruritus in eczematoid-like or itching purpura, annular forms with telangiectases in Majocchi's disease, and often solitary lichenoid lesions with bandlike infiltrates including a Grenz zone in lichen aureus. The etiology of capillaritis, including these variants, is not known. The reason for extravasation of erythrocytes is unclear, because inflammatory fibrinoid necrosis of vessels (vasculitis) can not be demonstrated.

MANAGEMENT STRATEGY

Diagnostic hallmarks are the yellow-brown or orange patches with superimposed pinpoint cayenne pepper spots,

which represent petechiae and persist with diascopy. The main differential diagnosis is leukocytoclastic vasculitis. The discerning criterion is the lack of a palpable infiltrate in capillaritis, but there are variants of vasculitis with petechial maculae (e.g. as part of Sjögren's syndrome). Thus, biopsies are warranted when in doubt.

In the differential diagnosis thrombocytopenia, hyper-gammaglobulinemic purpura of Waldenström, and rare cases of mycosis fungoides also need to be excluded.

Usually there is no need for treatment unless the patient has pruritus or suffers from cosmetic disfigurement.

Detection and *avoidance of possible eliciting agents* should always be attempted. Reported causes are:

- Drugs (14% in one series) – for example, thiamine, bromine-containing drugs, carbamazepine, furosemide, acetaminophen, nonsteroidal anti-inflammatory drugs (NSAIDs), interferon-α. As a rule, drug-induced capillaritis is more generalized and usually does not present with epidermal involvement or lichenoid infiltrate. When local agents are suspected (e.g. rubber) a hemorrhagic contact eczema needs to be excluded.
- (Chronic) infections such as viral hepatitis B or C or odontogenic infections, including their treatment. Drug- or infection-induced leukocytoclastic vasculitis would represent a different entity.

When no eliciting agent can be found, the etiology remains obscure. As there is also no fixed correlation with systemic disease, no causal therapy is available yet. However, immunohistochemical analyses suggested a cell-mediated immune response, so treatment with *local corticosteroids, calcineurin inhibitors,* and *psoralen plus UVA (PUVA)* may be reasonable. Increased venous pressure (particularly in the legs) or exercise are not a direct cause, but can sometimes aggravate capillaritis. In these cases compression stockings may be helpful.

There is some evidence for increased vascular permeability or vascular fragility due to subtle defects in the extracellular matrix. This may explain therapeutic effects reported for *bioflavonoids and ascorbic acid,* or *calcium dobesilate* (reduction of microvascular permeability in part by antioxidant properties). These agents are promising, but there are few published cases on therapy even with PUVA or local corticosteroids, though these two treatments have been much more widely in use for a longer period of time among dermatologists. Thus, there is awareness of their limitations, but also of their beneficial effect in some cases.

Purpura simplex (inflammatory purpura without vasculitis): a clinicopathologic study of 174 cases. Ratnam KV, Su WP, Peters MS. J Am Acad Dermatol 1991;25:642–7.

Retrospective review of 174 cases. A correlation between purpuric reaction and drugs was observed in 14%. Of the 87 patients who had follow-up, 67% appeared to eventually have clearing of lesions.

Drug-induced chronic pigmented purpura. Nishioka K, Katayama I, Masuzawa M, et al. J Dermatol 1989;16:220–2.

A close correlation between purpuric reaction and drugs was observed in seven cases of chronic pigmented purpura. The drugs included thiamine propyldisulfide and chlordiazepoxide. The purpuric lesions ceased after withdrawal of drug intake.

Evidence levels   A Double-blind study   **B** Clinical trial ≥ 20 subjects   **C** Clinical trial < 20 subjects   **D** Series ≥ 5 subjects   **E** Anecdotal case reports

Drug-induced purpura simplex: clinical and histological characteristics. Pang BK, Su D, Ratnam KV. Ann Acad Med Singapore 1993;22:870–2.

A prospective study of 183 patients with purpura simplex was carried out. Of these, 27 patients were confirmed to be drug induced, as the purpura cleared on withdrawal of medications within 4 months – NSAIDs, diuretics, meprobamate, and ampicillin were the commonest offenders.

Acetaminophen-induced progressive pigmentary purpura (Schamberg's disease). Abeck D, Gross GE, Kuwert C, et al. J Am Acad Dermatol 1992;27:123–4.

Schamberg's purpura: association with persistent hepatitis B surface antigenemia and treatment with pentoxifylline. Wahba-Yahav AV. Cutis 1994;54:205–6.

Chronic pigmented purpura associated with odontogenic infection. Satoh T, Yokozeki H, Nishioka K. J Am Acad Dermatol 2002;46:942–4.

Five patients with chronic pigmented purpura associated with odontogenic infection were resistant to topical corticosteroid treatment, but appearance of purpuric spots ceased after treatment for periodontitis, pulpitis, or both. No circulating immune complexes or perivascular deposits of immunoglobulins were detected.

Capillaritis associated with interferon-alfa treatment of chronic hepatitis C infection. Gupta G, Holmes SC, Spence E, Mills PR. J Am Acad Dermatol 2000;43:937–8.

SPECIFIC INVESTIGATIONS

- C-reactive protein, differential blood count (thrombocytopenia, leukemia, chronic infections)
- IgG, IgM, IgA in serum (in women with symmetrical petechial and slightly hemorrhagic macules to exclude monoclonal gammopathy; when raised → serum protein electrophoresis)
- Histology – whenever in doubt, to exclude vasculitis, mycosis fungoides
- Careful drug history
- Look for signs of chronic infection or rheumatoid arthritis
- Exclude contact eczema, chronic venous insufficiency

Capillaritis: a manifestation of rheumatoid disease. Wilkinson SM, Smith AG, Davis M, Dawes PT. Clin Rheumatol 1993;12:53–6.

Seven cases of capillaritis were described in patients with rheumatoid arthritis. In the majority, the rash resolved spontaneously with the use of a topical corticosteroid to treat the symptom of itch.

FIRST LINE THERAPIES

Local corticosteroids initially in case of pruritus/ eczematoid or itching purpura	D
PUVA	D
Calcium dobesilate	D
Oral bioflavonoids and ascorbic acid	E
Compression stocking when aggravated by increased venous pressure	E

Capillaritis: a manifestation of rheumatoid disease. Wilkinson SM, Smith AG, Davis M, Dawes PT. Clin Rheumatol 1993;12:53–6.

Seven cases of capillaritis were described in patients with rheumatoid arthritis. In the majority, the rash resolved spontaneously with the use of a topical corticosteroid to treat the symptom of itch.

PUVA therapy in lichen aureus. Ling TC, Goulden V, Goodfield MJ. J Am Acad Dermatol 2001;45:145–6.

One case of lichen aureus that responded dramatically to photochemotherapy (PUVA).

A report of two cases of pigmented purpuric dermatoses treated with PUVA therapy. Wong WK, Ratnam KV. Acta Derm Venereol 1991;71:68–70.

Successful treatment of two patients with PUVA.

Cell infiltrate in progressive pigmented purpura (Schamberg's disease): immunophenotype, adhesion receptors, and intercellular relationships. Ghersetich I, Lotti T, Bacci S, et al. Int J Dermatol 1995;34:846–50.

This immunohistochemical study suggested that a cell-mediated immune mechanism is important in progressive pigmented purpura. After PUVA (120 J/cm^2) and topical corticosteroid therapy of two patients who had a subsequent biopsy taken, the infiltrate disappeared completely.

Calcium dobesilate (Cd) in pigmented purpuric dermatosis (PPD): a pilot evaluation. Agrawal SK, Gandhi V, Bhattacharya SN. J Dermatol 2004;31:98–103.

Nine male patients (seven with Schamberg's and one each with lichenoid dermatosis of Gougerot and Blum and lichen aureus) were given calcium dobesilate 500 mg twice daily for two initial weeks and then 500 mg once daily for 3 months. No new lesions occurred within 2 weeks and itching ceased in all patients. Follow-up continued for 1 year after cessation of therapy. The improvement of existing lesions was moderate in 11.11% and mild in 66.67% of cases; 22.22% did not show any improvement.

Treatment of progressive pigmented purpura with oral bioflavonoids and ascorbic acid: an open pilot study in 3 patients. Reinhold U, Seiter S, Ugurel S, Tilgen W. J Am Acad Dermatol 1999;41:207–8.

Rutoside (50 mg twice daily) and ascorbic acid (500 mg twice daily) were administered orally to three patients with chronic progressive pigmented purpura in an open pilot study. Complete clearance of skin lesions was achieved after 4 weeks of treatment in all three patients and persisted for 3 months after treatment.

Since then, more than ten patients have been treated successfully (U. Reinhold, personal communication).

SECOND LINE THERAPIES

Pentoxifylline	E
Topical calcineurin inhibitors	E

Successful treatment of Schamberg's disease with pentoxifylline. Kano Y, Hirayama K, Orihara M, Shiohara T. J Am Acad Dermatol 1997;36:827–30.

111

Three patients with Schamberg's disease were treated with pentoxifylline 300 mg daily for 8 weeks. A significant response was observed within 2–3 weeks. One patient had recurrence after discontinuation of this treatment, but promptly responded to resumption of therapy.

Schamberg's purpura: association with persistent hepatitis B surface antigenemia and treatment with pentoxifylline. Wahba-Yahav AV. Cutis 1994;54:205–6.

A 54-year-old man experienced extensive Schamberg's purpura 3 months after an episode of hepatitis B. He was treated orally with pentoxifylline, 400 mg three times daily. After 3 months purpuric elements had disappeared and pigmentation had faded.

Resolution of lichen aureus in a 10-year-old child after topical pimecrolimus. Böhm M, Bonsmann G, Luger TA. Br J Dermatol 2004;150:519–20.

A 10-year-old boy presenting for 4 months with lichen aureus resistant to topical corticosteroids. A significant improvement was observed within 3 weeks with pimecrolimus cream twice daily.

Unlike topical corticosteroids, topical immunomodulators do not cause fragility of blood vessels, which is an advantage when *treating this group of diseases thought to be caused by vascular fragility and permeability.*

THIRD LINE THERAPIES

■ Colchicine	E
■ Griseofulvin	E
■ Cyclosporine	E

Benefit of colchicine in the treatment of Schamberg's disease. Geller M. Ann Allergy Asthma Immunol 2000;85:246.

Successful treatment of pigmented purpuric dermatosis with griseofulvin. Tamaki K, Yasaka N, Osada A, et al. Br J Dermatol 1995;132:159–60.

Only a solitary case report attests to the efficacy of griseofulvin.

Purpura pigmentosa chronica successfully treated with oral cyclosporin A. Okada K, Ishikawa O, Miyachi Y. Br J Dermatol 1996;134:180–1.

We do not recommend cyclosporine because of the severity of possible side effects

Cat scratch disease

Adam H Wiener, Bryan A Selkin,
George J Murakawa

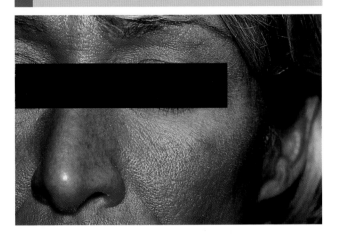

Cat scratch disease (CSD) is a benign, usually self-limited disease caused by *Bartonella henselae* (formerly *Rochalimaea henselae*), a Gram-negative pleomorphic rod. The primary lesion consists of a 0.5–1 cm papule or pustule, which may undergo ulceration, and adjacent unilateral lymphadenopathy is the hallmark of the disease. Systemic symptoms and complications include low-grade fever, malaise, nonspecific exanthem, hepatosplenomegaly, lytic bone lesions, oculoglandular syndrome of Parinaud (granulomatous conjunctivitis and preauricular adenopathy), and encephalopathy.

MANAGEMENT STRATEGY

Clear guidelines for the treatment of CSD do not exist. As there is a paucity of data showing a clear benefit of antimicrobial therapy in the treatment of patients with mild to moderate CSD, these patients should be managed with *conservative, symptomatic treatment*. The lymphadenopathy associated with CSD is self-limited and resolves in 2–4 months; therefore, most patients can be managed with *observation* until involution of the node.

For patients with systemic symptoms and/or complications, antibiotic therapy should be instituted. *Azithromycin* (500 mg day 1 followed by 250 mg days 2–5) is the only antibiotic that has been shown in a double-blind placebo controlled evaluation to be beneficial to immunocompetent patients with CSD. In a retrospective analysis of 202 patients with CSD who had been on at least 3 days of antimicrobial therapy, only four antibiotics *(rifampin, ciprofloxacin, gentamicin, and trimethoprim–sulfamethoxazole)* provided clinical benefit. Presumably, it is the paucity of organisms and the host inflammatory response that result in the poor efficacy of antibiotics.

In immunosuppressed patients, infection with the CSD bacillus can produce a spectrum of disease, from classic CSD to bacillary angiomatosis (BA), peliosis, or septicemia (see Bacillary angiomatosis, page 69). Antimicrobial treatment for such patients is beneficial and clearly indicated. Lesions and symptoms respond rapidly to *erythromycin* 500 mg four times daily or *doxycycline* 100 mg twice daily. Other antimicrobials used to successfully treat BA in immunocompromised patients include *tetracycline, minocycline, azithromycin,*

and *trimethoprim–sulfamethoxazole.* A Jarisch-Herxheimer reaction frequently occurs after the first dose. Patients with AIDS should be maintained on life-long antimicrobial therapy.

Of note, *B. henselae* has rarely been isolated from patients with CSD; however, patients who are immunosuppressed may be culture positive. A single dose of oral antibiotics will rapidly sterilize blood and lesional cultures.

SPECIFIC INVESTIGATIONS

- Histopathology
- Culture
- Serology
- Polymerase chain reaction (PCR)-based techniques

The agent of bacillary angiomatosis. Relman DA, Loutit JS, Schmidt TM, Falkow S, Tompkins LS. N Engl J Med 1990;323:153–80.

PCR was used to amplify, clone and sequence a portion of eubacterial 16S rRNA gene directly from tissue infected with the presumed agent of BA. Subsequent analysis of this sequence and study of infected tissues from other patients suggested that BA is caused by a rickettsia-like organism closely related to *Rochalimaea quintana.*

Bartonella-associated infections. Spach DH, Koehler JE. Infect Dis Clin North Am 1998;12:137–55.

Findings on lymph node biopsy specimens from immunocompetent patients with CSD depend on the stage of the infection. Early in the course, lymphoid hyperplasia and arteriolar proliferation are prominent. Subsequently, granulomas appear. Late in the disease, multiple stellate microabscesses are prominent. Warthin-Starry stains may show clumps of pleomorphic bacilli.

Cat scratch disease in Connecticut: epidemiology, risk factors and evaluation of a new diagnostic test. Zangwill KM, Hamilton DH, Perkins BA, et al. N Engl J Med 1993;320:8–13.

Serologic testing for the presence of antibodies to *B. henselae* is the most widely used test for laboratory confirmation of CSD. Indirect fluorescent antibody (IFA) assay has a sensitivity of 88% and a specificity of 97%. However, the IFA assay is not yet widely available and depends to some degree on subjective interpretation.

Cat-scratch disease. Midani S, Ayoub EM, Anderson B. Adv Pediatr 1996;43:397–422.

PCR is a powerful tool for the detection of *B. henselae,* but it is not widely available. Using PCR *B. henselae* can be detected in aspirates from lymph nodes or cutaneous lesions in 1–2 days. Currently, serologic and PCR-based analyses are considered definitive.

Detection by immunofluorescence assay of *Bartonella henselae* in lymph nodes from patients with cat scratch disease. Rolain JM, Gouriet F, Enea M, et al. Clin Diagn Lab Immunol 2003;10.4:686–91.

Immunofluorescence detection (IFD) in lymph node smears using a specific monoclonal antibody directed against *B. henselae* and a commercial serology assay (IFA) compared with PCR detection showed high specificity in diagnosis of *B. henselae* especially when associated with histological analysis and conventional bacterial culture.

FIRST LINE THERAPY

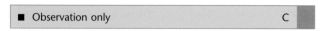
■ Observation only   C

Bartonellosis. Murakawa GJ, Berger T. In: Freedberg IM, Eisen AZ, Wolff K, Austen KF, et al., eds. Dermatology in general medicine, 5th edn. New York: McGraw-Hill; 1999:2249–56.

In the majority of patients with CSD, conservative management with careful observation over several months is sufficient. Spontaneous involution of lymphadenopathy should occur over 6 months.

SECOND LINE THERAPIES

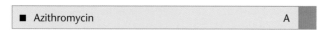
■ Azithromycin   A

Prospective randomized double blind placebo-controlled evaluation of azithromycin for treatment of cat-scratch disease. Bass JW, Freitas BC, Freitas AD, et al. Pediatr Infect Dis J 1998;17:447–52.

Seven of 14 azithromycin-treated patients (500 mg on day 1 followed by 250 mg days 2–5) showed an 80% decrease of initial lymph node volume compared to one of 15 placebo-treated controls during the first 30 days of observation.

This is the only controlled clinical trial of an antibiotic for the therapy of CSD; the use of all other antibiotics is based on anecdotal reports.

THIRD LINE THERAPIES

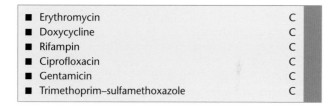
■ Erythromycin   C
■ Doxycycline   C
■ Rifampin   C
■ Ciprofloxacin   C
■ Gentamicin   C
■ Trimethoprim–sulfamethoxazole   C

Immunocompetent individuals

Antibiotic therapy for cat-scratch disease: clinical study of therapeutic outcome in 268 patients and a review of the literature. Margileth AM. Pediatr Infect Dis J 1992;11:474–8.

In 60 patients with CSD with systemic symptoms, one of four antibiotics was effective at least 72% of the time. Patients who received rifampin (10–20 mg/kg daily for 7–14 days), ciprofloxacin (20–30 mg/kg daily for 7–14 days), gentamicin (5 mg/kg daily intravenously in divided doses every 8 h for at least 3 days) or trimethoprim–sulfamethoxazole (6–8 mg/kg of trimethoprim component two to three times daily for 7 days) had a shorter mean duration of post-treatment illness than patients who received either no antibiotics or antibiotics thought to be ineffective.

Antimicrobial susceptibility of *Rochalimaea quintana*, *Rochalimaea vinsonii*, and the newly recognized *Rochalimaea henselae*. Maurin M, Raoult D. J Antimicrob Chemother 1993;32:587–94.

In-vitro testing revealed β-lactam drugs to be ineffective, tetracyclines to be intermediate, and erythromycin and rifampin to be most effective against *Rochalimaea* spp.

Hepatosplenic cat-scratch disease in children: selected clinical features and treatment. Arisoy ES, Correa AG, Wagner ML, Kaplan SL. Clin Infect Dis 1999;28:78–84.

Sixteen children with hepatosplenic CSD treated with rifampin (15–20 mg/kg daily), either alone or in combination with gentamicin (7.5 mg/kg daily) or trimethoprim–sulfamethoxazole (10–12 mg/kg daily), showed clinical improvement within 1–5 days.

Antibiotic therapy for cat-scratch disease? Bogue CW, Wise JD, Gray GF, Edwards KM. JAMA 1989;262:813–6.

Three patients with CSD treated with intravenous gentamicin (5 mg/kg daily) improved within 48 h.

Successful treatment of cat-scratch disease with ciprofloxacin. Holley HP. JAMA 1991;265:1563–5.

Five patients treated with oral ciprofloxacin, 500 mg twice daily, had dramatic improvement in symptoms within a few days with no relapse during follow-up. It should be noted that quinolones are not recommended for children or adolescents due to concerns about arthropathy. Moreover, in-vitro studies show only intermediate efficacy for ciprofloxacin.

Immunosuppressed individuals

Molecular epidemiology of *Bartonella* infections in patients with bacillary angiomatosis-peliosis. Koehler JE, Sanchez MA, Garrido MD, et al. N Engl J Med 1997;337:1876–83.

Treatment with macrolide antibiotics (e.g. erythromycin or clarithromycin) is protective for patients with *Bartonella* spp. infection.

Cat scratch disease, bacillary angiomatosis, and other infections due to *Rochalimaea*. Adal KA, Cockerell CJ, Petri WA. N Engl J Med 1994;330:1509–15.

For the treatment of BA, bacillary peliosis hepatis, and *Rochalimaea* spp. bacteremic syndrome, erythromycin 500 mg four times daily is the drug of choice on the basis of an excellent clinical response in virtually all patients treated to date.

Cutaneous vascular lesions and disseminated cat-scratch disease in patients with the acquired immunodeficiency syndrome (AIDS) and AIDS-related complex. Koehler JE, LeBoit PE, Egbert BM, Berger GT. Ann Intern Med 1988;109:449–55.

Erythromycin (500 mg four times daily), rifampin, and doxycycline (100 mg twice daily) were effective in the treatment of angiomatous skin nodules in three patients with HIV infection.

Cellulite

Bruce E Katz, Doris M Hexsel

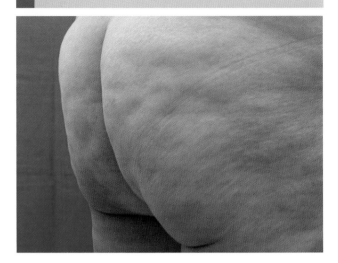

Cellulite may be defined as the surface relief alterations that give the skin an orange-peel or mattress-like appearance. The lesions tend to be asymptomatic and may be considered the anatomic expressions of the structures in the affected area, such as the fat and subcutaneous septa. Females are most frequently affected by this condition. Cellulite occurs mainly on the thighs and buttocks, but may also be found on the arms, abdomen, and legs.

MANAGEMENT STRATEGY

In managing cellulite, the aim is to obtain aesthetic improvement. This may be achieved by means of:

1. *Diet, weight control* (preferably maintaining a body mass index [BMI] between 19 and 24), and *physical exercise.*
2. Treatment of possible associated conditions such as circulatory alterations, edema, obesity, endocrine alterations, and flaccidity.
3. Specific treatments:
   - *subcision®*
   - *lasers* (TriActive®)
   - *mechanical treatments* (e.g. endermologie and massage)
   - topical treatment (e.g. many different compounds of doubtful value).

SPECIFIC INVESTIGATIONS

So called cellulite: an invented disease. Nurnberger F, Muller G. Dermatol Surg Oncol 1978;4:221–9.

This was the first study in which the anatomic basis for cellulite was demonstrated. The authors showed, by means of biopsies taken from the thighs and buttocks of 150 cadavers and 30 living women with cellulite, that the adipose tissue is projected into the dermis, forming the so-called 'papillae adipose' that are responsible for the mattress-like appearance on the skin surface.

An exploratory investigation of the morphology and biochemistry of cellulite. Rosenbaum M, Prieto V, Hellmer J, et al. Plast Reconstr Surg 1998;101:1934–9.

This study evaluated cellulite, by means of biopsies, sonographic examination, and physiologic examination, of the thighs of seven individuals. In those with cellulite, the studies showed a diffuse pattern of extrusion of underlying adipose tissue into the reticular dermis. This study also found differences between the sexes. Women had a diffuse pattern of irregular discontinuous connective tissue immediately below the dermis, but this same layer was smooth and continuous in men.

Anatomy and physiology of subcutaneous adipose tissue by in vivo magnetic resonance imaging and spectroscopy: relationships with sex and presence of cellulite. Querleux B, Cornillon C, Jolivet O, Bittoun J. Skin Res Tech 2002;8:118–24.

Using magnetic resonance imaging (MRI) and spectroscopy, this study evaluated the anatomy and physiology of subcutaneous tissue from the upper posterior region of the thighs in 67 individuals, according to sex and the presence of cellulite. It was shown that women with cellulite characteristically have a thicker dermis when compared to normal women and a thickened adipose layer when compared to normal women or men; the mean values of the adipose indentations into the dermis are significantly higher for women with cellulite; women with cellulite have a higher percentage of perpendicular fibrous septa than do normal women or men.

Pilot study of dermal and subcutaneous fat structures by MRI in individuals who differ in gender, BMI, and cellulite grading. Mirrashed F, Sharp JC, Krause V, et al. Skin Res Technol 2004;10:161–8.

A recent study used MRI to evaluate the architecture of the posterior lateral region of the thigh in both sexes. The subjects were divided according to their BMI and cellulite grade. It was shown that a diffuse pattern of adipose tissue extrusion into the dermis correlated with the degree of cellulite. In subjects with a high BMI, the percentile of fat inclusion into the dermis was found to be significantly higher in females with high cellulite than in men and low-cellulite females. In subjects with a low BMI, the hypodermis in women with high cellulite was thicker, when compared to women with unaffected skin, whereas in men the hypodermis was significantly thinner.

Body repair. Hexsel DM. In: Parish LC, Brenner S, Ramos-e-Silva M, eds. Women's Dermatology: From Infancy to Maturity. New York: Parthenon; 2001:586–95.

The discrete alterations on the surface of the quilted appearance corresponding to degree I cellulite should be treated by dietary and exercise measures with special emphasis on weight loss and treatment of the clinical conditions that may be the cause of weight gain and fluid retention.

FIRST LINE THERAPIES

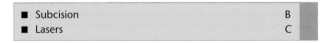

■ Subcision	B
■ Lasers	C

Subcision: uma alternativa cirúrgica para a lipodistrofia ginóide ("celulite") e outras alterações do relevo corporal. Hexsel DM, Mazzuco R. An Bras Dermatol 1997;72:27–32.

Subcision: a treatment for cellulite. Hexsel DM, Mazzuco R. Int J Dermatol 2000;39:539–44.

In this paper, the authors give a description of the subcision procedure and report the results based on a sample of 232 patients. Subcision® was shown to be efficient in the treatment of high-level cellulite, such as degrees II and III. This technique improves the major depressions on the skin surface of patients with cellulite through three mechanisms of action: sectioning the connective tissue septa responsible for the depressions, provoking the formation of new connective tissue from blood components, and redistributing the adipose tissue and the mechanical forces between the adipose lobules.

An innovative surgical technique that has generated scientific interest recently.

The efficacy of a diode laser with contact cooling and suction (Tri-Active® laser) in the treatment of cellulite. Frew K, Katz B. Dermatol Surg (in press).

In this single-blinded study, 10 female patients were evaluated. Half of the affected body areas were treated with the diode laser, contact cooling, and suction operational, while the contralateral side was treated with contact cooling and suction operational but with the laser diodes turned off. All patients were treated biweekly for a total of 16 treatments. Independent observer evaluation of photographs found an average of 83% improvement in cellulite on the laser treated side compared with a 17% improvement on the non-laser treated side.

A small pilot study evaluating new laser technology applied to the treatment of cellulite. Larger studies should be forthcoming to confirm these findings.

SECOND LINE THERAPIES

■ Iontophoresis	E
■ Ultrasound	E
■ Thermotherapy	E
■ Pressotherapy	E
■ Electrolipophoresis	E
■ Endermologie	E

Analysis of the effects of deep mechanical massage in the porcine model. Adcock D, Paulsen S, Jabour K, et al. Plast Reconstr Surg 2001;108:233–40.

This study evaluated the effects of deep mechanical massage in the dermis and hypodermis of pigs. Histologic examination of the areas submitted to the treatment showed a greater accumulation of dense longitudinal collagen.

THIRD LINE THERAPIES

■ Topical products	E
■ Oral supplements	E

A randomized, placebo-controlled trial of topical retinol in the treatment of cellulite. Franchimont CP, Piérard GE, Henry F, et al. Am J Clin Dermatol 2000;1:369–74.

A controlled study in 15 women who had requested liposuction for the improvement of cellulite assessed a topical product containing retinol versus a placebo formulation. Prior to liposuction, the women used topical retinol once a day on one leg and placebo on the other. After 6 months of treatment, the elasticity of the skin had increased 10.7% and the viscosity had diminished 15.8% on the side treated with the product containing retinol.

Modification of subcutaneous adipose tissue by a methylxanthine formulation: a double-blind controlled study. Lesser T, Ritvo E, Moy LS. Dermatol Surg 1999;25:455–62.

A placebo-controlled, double-blind study in 41 patients evaluated a product containing liposome-encapsulated caffeine in concentrations of 1% or 2%. The product was used on the thighs, arms, buttocks, and abdomen of the patients daily for 2 months. The final assessment of the treatment concluded that both concentrations of the cream significantly reduced the thickness of the adipose tissue in all treated areas.

Treating cellulite. Gasbarro V, Vettorello GF. Cosmetics & Toiletries 1992;107:64–6.

This study evaluated extract of *Aesculus hippocastanum* in the treatment of cellulite. The results showed that 80% of patients reduced one clinical stage of cellulite and in 4% of these there was a reduction in the circumference of the thigh.

[Venous constriction by local administration of ruscus extract]. Berg D. Fortschr Med 1990;108:473–6. In German.

The vasoconstrictive action of topically applied ruscus was evaluated in this placebo-controlled study. At 2.5 h after the application, the diameter of the femoral vein had decreased by an average of 1.25 mm in patients who had used the product containing ruscus extract, while in those who had used placebo there was an increase of 0.5 mm.

Addition of conjugated linoleic acid to a herbal anti-cellulite pill. Birnbaum L. Adv Ther 2001;18:225–9.

The treatment of cellulite with herbal anti-cellulite pills together with supplements of conjugated linoleic acid in 60 female volunteers showed that 75% of the patients who used the supplement obtained a beneficial effect.

A double-blind evaluation of the activity of an anti-cellulite product containing retinol, caffeine and ruscogenine by a combination of several non-invasive methods. Bertin C, Zunino H, Pittet JC, et al. J Cosmet Sci 2001;52:199–210.

This study assessed an anti-cellulite product containing retinol microcapsules, caffeine, Asian centella, ruscus and L-carnitine. The efficacy parameters included the appearance of the cellulite after treatment, histology, cutaneous flowmetry, and the mechanical characteristics of the skin. The results showed improvement in cellulite in the treated areas.

Cellulitis and erysipelas

Adrian H M Heagerty

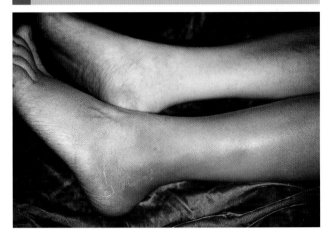

Cellulitis is strictly an acute, subacute, or chronic infection of the subcutaneous tissues, whereas erysipelas is an infection of the dermis and superficial subcutis. Infection of the more superficial layers gives rise to superficial edema and inflammation with the consequent development of a palpable, often advancing edge. The causative organism is usually regarded as *Streptococcus* sp., though many organisms have been isolated, including *Haemophilus influenzae*, and more rarely staphylococci, *Aeromonas hydrophilia*, and *Pseudomonas aeruginosa*, as well as Gram-negative rods and fungi. Fulminating and necrotic cellulitis and fasciitis may occur rarely, usually in relation to immune suppression or atypical organisms.

MANAGEMENT STRATEGY

Management of cellulitis and erysipelas should initially be directed to trying to *identify the organism responsible for the infection*, and then directing *appropriate antimicrobial therapy*. Any underlying and predisposing condition should be identified and treated to prevent subsequent recurrence. Perhaps the commonest condition that is not identified and treated is toe web tinea pedis, providing a portal of entry for infection.

Uncomplicated cellulitis and erysipelas may be managed without admission if the patient does not exhibit signs of systemic toxicity. In such cases *oral broad-spectrum antibiotics*, chosen to cover Group A streptococci and staphylococci, may be sufficient, supplemented with a single parenteral loading dose or long acting preparation. The drug of choice is *oral penicillin V (phenoxymethylpenicillin) with or without flucloxacillin*, or *erythromycin*, if the patient has known penicillin allergy.

Immunocompromised patients, those with signs of systemic toxicity, and otherwise debilitated patients should be treated as inpatients with *intravenous antimicrobials* (such as penicillin G (benzylpenicillin)) or *one of the newer antibiotics* (such as ciprofloxacin, ticarcillin, teicoplanin, or imipenem/cilastatin). If there is evidence of head and neck disease or sinus infection *amoxicillin combined with clavulanic acid* should be considered to cover *H. influenzae* infection.

Sites of entry for infection should be sought, such as excoriations in eczema or following trauma, and these should be treated.

SPECIFIC INVESTIGATIONS

- Blood cultures
- Cultures of aspirates and lesions
- Skin scrapings for mycology

Blood cultures may be positive and significant in only approximately 25% of cases. Swabs of wounds and broken skin may be helpful, but surface swabs of unbroken skin provide little or no useful information. If available, aspirate of bullae may yield positive cultures. Slightly better rates for isolation than that of needle aspirates have been achieved with punch skin biopsies. Rising titers of streptococcal antibodies may be helpful.

In the case of cellulitis or erysipelas of the lower leg, skin scrapings from toe webs should be taken for mycological examination. Facial erysipelas should warrant sinus radiographs to exclude underlying sinusitis. Crepitus should prompt the clinician to the presence of either clostridia or nonspore-forming anaerobes, either alone or mixed with other bacteria such as *Pseudomonas*, *Escherichia coli*, or *Klebsiella* spp.

FIRST LINE THERAPIES

■ Penicillin G	B
■ Penicillin G with flucloxacillin	B
■ Penicillin V	B
■ Amoxicillin with clavulanic acid	B
■ Oral versus parenteral antibiotics	B
■ Ceftriaxone versus flucloxacillin	A
■ Roxithromycin	B

The course, costs and complications of oral versus intravenous penicillin therapy of erysipelas. Jorup-Ronstrum C, Britton S, Gavlevik A, et al. Infection 1984:12;390–4.

In this study of 60 patients there appeared to be no appreciable benefit from intravenous therapy with penicillin over oral for erysipelas, and so recommend oral therapy if there are no associated complications with the infection.

Management and morbidity of cellulitis of the leg. Cox NH, Colver GB, Paterson WD. J Roy Soc Med 1998:91;634–7.

A case note review of 92 patients admitted for inpatient care for ascending cellulitis of the leg revealed a portal of entry, most commonly minor injury. The mean inpatient stay was 10 days. Bacteriology was seldom helpful, but group G streptococci was the most frequently identified pathogen. Benzylpenicillin was used in 43 cases (46%).

The authors emphasize the need for benzylpenicillin, treatment of tinea pedis, and retrospective diagnosis of streptococcal infection by serology.

Case survey of management of cellulitis in a tertiary teaching hospital. Aly AA, Roberts NM, Seipol KS, MacLellan DG. Med J Aust 1996:165;553–6.

This retrospective survey examined the management of 118 patients with lower limb cellulitis in a tertiary teaching hospital. In 79% of cases there was underlying disease, only 20% being investigated. Blood cultures were taken from 55%, all with negative results. A combination of flucloxacillin and penicillin was given intravenously for a mean of 6 days to 76% of patients, and where documented 94% responded within 5 days. However, 40% of patients had intravenous therapy for longer than this and 10% for 10 days or more. The length of inpatient stay averaged 13 days, prolonged stay being associated with surgical intervention or intercurrent problems, but 15% of patients had no clear indication for an extended stay. The authors concluded that excessive microbiological investigations, inadequate investigation, and treatment of underlying disease with prolonged use of intravenous antibiotics and questionable use of combination of antibiotic therapy were common.

Skin concentrations of phenoxymethylpenicillin in patients with erysipelas. Sjoblom AC, Bruchfeld J, Eriksson B, et al. Infection 1992;20:30–3.

Tissue and serum blood levels were measured in 45 patients with erysipelas after oral penicillin (phenoxymethylpenicillin), and the minimal inhibitory concentrations were exceeded for streptococci isolated, supporting the role of oral therapy.

A randomized comparative study of once-daily ceftriaxone and 6-hourly flucloxacillin in the treatment of moderate to severe cellulitis. Clinical efficacy, safety and pharmacoeconomic implications. Vinen J, Hudson B, Chan B, et al. Clin Drug Invest 1996;12:221–5.

A randomized comparative study in 58 patients with cellulitis; intravenous ceftriaxone cured 92%, but intravenous flucloxacillin cured only 64% after 4–6 days.

Roxithromycin versus penicillin in the treatment of erysipelas in adults: a comparative study. Plantin BP, Sassolas B, Villaret E, et al. Br J Dermatol 1992;127:155–9.

This prospective randomized multicenter trial compared oral roxithromycin with intravenous benzylpenicillin. Overall efficacy was similar.

Amoxicillin combined with clavulanic acid for the treatment of soft tissue infections in children. Fleischer GR, Wilmott CM, Capos JM. Antimicrob Agents Chemother 1983;24:679–81.

Amoxicillin with clavulanic acid was compared with cefaclor in children with impetigo and cellulitis due to staphylococci, streptococci, and *Haemophilus* sp. There was a 100% response to therapy with the combination, compared to 90% with the cephalosporin; the incidence of relapse and reinfection and side effects were small, but greater with the combination therapy.

SECOND LINE THERAPIES

■ Ciprofloxacin	B
■ Teicoplanin	B
■ Imipenem/cilastatin	B

Ciprofloxacin for soft tissue infections. Wood MJ, Logan MN. J Antimicrob Chemother 1986:18(Suppl D);159–64.

Twenty one patients with cellulitis or other soft tissue infection were treated with oral ciprofloxacin; 19 were clinically cured or improved and one was withdrawn from the study because of nausea and vomiting. Nine of the original 18 bacterial isolates were eradicated, but the majority of failures were due to staphylococci and streptococci.

Teicoplanin in the treatment of skin and soft tissue infections. Turpin PJ, Taylor GP, Logan MN, Wood MJ. J Antimicrob Chemother 1988:21(Suppl A);117–22.

Twenty four patients with cellulitis or other soft tissue infection were treated with once daily teicoplanin, resulting in clinical cure or improvement, without severe adverse reaction, but with a rise in the plasma platelet count.

Twice daily intramuscular imipenem/cilastatin in the treatment of skin and soft tissue infections. Sexton DJ, Wlodaver CG, Tobey LE, et al. Chemotherapy 1991:37(Suppl 2);26–30.

Of 102 patients enrolled in this study with mild to moderately severe skin and soft tissue infections, 74 were evaluable, with 20 having cellulitis, 23 wound infections, and 31 abscesses. Imipenem/cilastatin was given intramuscularly using doses of 500 or 750 mg 12-hourly. In this study there was no assessment by type of infection, but 82% were cured and 16% improved. Eight patients reported minor side effects.

THIRD LINE THERAPIES

■ Prednisolone as an adjunct to antibiotics	A
■ Granulocyte colony stimulating factor (G-CSF)	A
■ Hyperbaric oxygen	E

Antibiotic and prednisolone therapy of erysipelas: a randomized, double blind, placebo-controlled study. Bergkvist PI, Sjobeck K. Scand J Infect Dis 1997:29;377–82.

Although prednisolone may predispose to infection, its use in combination with intravenous antibiotics reduced the median time to cure by 1 day (5 vs 6 days), while at the 90th percentile healing time was 10 days vs 14.6 days, and median hospital stay was reduced from 6 to 5 days. The relapse rate within 3 weeks was approximately the same in both groups.

Randomized placebo controlled trial of granulocyte-colony stimulating factor in diabetic foot infection. Gough A, Clapperton M, Rolando N, Foster Foster A. Lancet 1997;350:855–9.

This randomized controlled trial compared the ability of G-CSF to improve clinical outcome in the treatment of cellulitis in diabetes mellitus, using resolution as the endpoint. The G-CSF stimulates the neutrophil response, which is impaired in diabetes mellitus, but is important for defense against infection. The risk is principally that of high white cell counts, which may predispose to coronary and cerebral vascular events.

Cellulitis owing to *Aeromonas hydrophilia*: treatment with hyperbaric oxygen. Mathur MN, Patrick WG, Unsworth IP, Bennett FM. Aust N Z J Surg. 1995:65;367–9.

This case report of *Aeromonas hydrophilia* cellulitis, unresponsive to antibiotics and surgical debridement, responded to hyperbaric oxygen therapy. Although there are few objective reports of similar treatment in streptococcal necrotizing fasciitis, it has been suggested that in all types of necrotizing fasciitis, hyperbaric oxygen reduces mortality.

PROPHYLAXIS

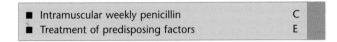

■ Intramuscular weekly penicillin	C
■ Treatment of predisposing factors	E

Prophylactic antibiotics in erysipelas. Duvanel T, Merot Y, Saurat JH. Lancet 1985;1:1401.

Sixteen cases who received weekly intramuscular penicillin as prophylaxis, were followed and assessed at 2 years. On cessation of prophylaxis the risk of recurrence rapidly returned to the non-treatment/no prophylaxis level.

Cellulitis and erysipelas. Morris A. Clin Evid 2004;12: 2268–74.

Although there is a consensus that successful treatment of predisposing factors such as leg edema, tinea pedis, and traumatic wounds reduces the risk of developing cellulitis, there are no randomized controlled trials or observational studies to support these.

Chancroid

Susan Coutinho McAllister, Glenn C Newell

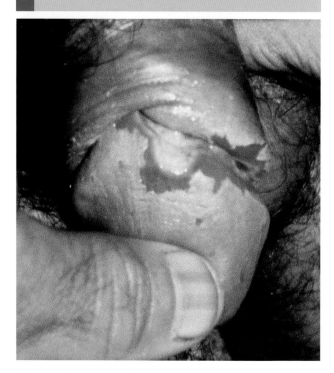

Chancroid is a genital ulcer disease caused by the Gram-negative facultative anaerobic bacillus *Haemophilus ducreyi*. It is common in many parts of the world including Africa, the Caribbean basin, and Southwest Asia. In more developed countries the incidence of chancroid appears to be decreasing; however, this may be due to underdiagnosis. Chancroid is typically described as a painful, ragged, deep genital ulcer 3–20 mm in diameter. There may be surrounding erythema and the base is often covered with a yellow gray exudate. The lesion may be single, but can be multiple from autoinoculation (kissing lesions). Painful lymphadenitis occurs in 30–60% of patients, and approximately 25% of patients with lymphadenopathy may develop a suppurating bubo.

MANAGEMENT STRATEGY

Diagnosis on clinical criteria alone is difficult. The painful ulcer of chancroid can be easily confused with herpes genitalis. Syphilis, especially if secondarily infected, can also mimic chancroid. The ulcer of chancroid may be transient and the disease may then present as painful lymphadenopathy, suggesting lymphogranuloma venereum. Coinfection with herpes simplex virus (HSV) or *Treponema pallidum* occurs in as many as 10% of patients, which may confuse the diagnosis. The combination of a painful genital ulcer with suppurative lymphadenopathy is the only clinical presentation that is nearly pathognomonic.

Gram stain of the ulcer base in chancroid may show Gram-negative coccobacilli in a 'school of fish' appearance. A definitive diagnosis may be made by culturing the exudate from the ulcer base or from aspiration of a bubo. Special culture media need to be used and specimens should

be handled by laboratories familiar with *H. ducreyi*. Polymerase chain reaction testing and indirect immunofluorescence hold promise, but are not yet widely available.

Chancroid is usually treated on a presumptive basis in endemic areas if clinical features are suggestive. Empiric therapy is also often used if patients fail to respond to treatment of syphilis and/or herpes genitalis.

SPECIFIC INVESTIGATIONS

- Gram stain of ulcer base or bubo aspirate
- Culture of ulcer base or bubo aspirate
- Syphilis serology

FIRST LINE THERAPIES

■ Azithromycin 1 g orally – one dose	B
■ Ceftriaxone 250 mg intramuscularly – one dose	B
■ Ciprofloxacin 500 mg twice a day for 3 days	A
■ Erythromycin 500 mg orally four times a day for 7 days	A

Treatment of chancroid with azithromycin. Ballard RC, Ye H, Matta A, Dangor Y, Radebe F. Int J STD AIDS 1996;7(suppl 1):9–12.

A single oral dose of azithromycin 1 g has been proven effective in the treatment of chancroid by a randomized, comparative study in Nairobi, Kenya, and a noncomparative study in Carletonville, South Africa, with cure rates of 89 and 92%, respectively.

A randomized, double-blind, placebo-controlled trial of single dose ciprofloxacin versus erythromycin for the treatment of chancroid in Nairobi, Kenya. Malonza IM, Tyndall MW, Ndinya-Achola JO, et al. J Infect Dis 1999;180:1886–93.

This clinical trial compared single-dose therapy with ciprofloxacin to a 7-day course of erythromycin for the treatment of chancroid. Cure rates of 92 and 91% were reported with ciprofloxacin and erythromycin, respectively, for the 111 participants with chancroid. The study, which included 208 men and 37 women, revealed a treatment failure rate of 15%. Failure rate was attributed to ulcer etiologies of HSV or syphilis.

Sexually transmitted diseases treatment guidelines 2002. Centers for Disease Control and Prevention. MMWR Recomm Rep 2002;51(RR-6):1–78.

The guidelines agree with the above choices for first line therapy in the treatment of chancroid. They also state that the safety of azithromycin has not been established for pregnant or lactating women. Quinolones are contraindicated in pregnancy. Chancroid itself has not been reported to have any adverse effects on pregnancy outcome or on the fetus.

Single-dose ceftriaxone for chancroid. Bowmer MI, Nsanze H, D'Costa LJ, et al. Antimicrob Agents Chemother 1987;31:67–9.

A randomized, non-blinded study in men of single-dose intramuscular ceftriaxone for chancroid demonstrated effectiveness. Doses of 1 g, 0.5 g and 0.25 g were equally effective.

SECOND LINE THERAPIES

■ Thiamphenicol 5 g orally – one dose	A
■ Fleroxacin 400 mg orally – one dose	B

Thiamphenicol in the treatment of chancroid. A study of 1,128 cases. Belda JW, Siqueira LF, Fagundes LJ. Rev Inst Med Trop Sao Paulo 2000;42:133–5.

Granulated thiamphenicol 5.0 g in a single oral dose was used to treat 1128 patients with chancroid. Only ten patients (0.89%) did not respond to therapy. Ulcers had healed in the majority of patients by post-treatment day 10.

Fleroxacin in the treatment of chancroid: an open study in men seropositive or seronegative for the human immunodeficiency virus type 1. Tyndall MW, Plourde PJ, Agoki E, et al. Am J Med 1993;94:85S–88S.

HIV-negative men were treated with a single 400 mg dose of fleroxacin, and HIV-positive men with 400 mg daily for 5 days. Three treatment failures occurred in 58 evaluable HIV-negative men and two in the 22 evaluable HIV-positive men. Fleroxacin was considered an acceptable alternative to existing treatment regimens for chancroid in men.

THIRD LINE THERAPIES

■ Trimethoprim–sulfamethoxazole (TMP–SMZ) 80/400 mg orally twice a day for 7 days	B
■ Spectinomycin 2 g intramuscularly – one dose	B

A comparison of single-dose spectinomycin with five days of trimethoprim–sulfamethoxazole for the treatment of chancroid. Fransen L, Nsanze H, Ndinya-Achola JO, et al. Sex Transm Dis 1987;14:98–101.

Thirty two patients were treated with a single 2 g dose of spectinomycin and 20 with a 5-day course of TMP–SMZ (160/800 mg) twice daily. Cure rates were 94% for spectinomycin and 95% for TMP–SMZ.

Treatment of chancroid with a single dose of spectinomycin. Guzman M, Guzman J, Bernal M. Sex Transm Dis 1992;19:291–4.

A prospective study on 50 patients treated with a single 2 g dose of spectinomycin intramuscularly. Only four patients (10%) required a second dose after 7 days to effect a cure; 98% of cases were cured at 14 days after treatment. No adverse reactions were reported.

Cheilitis

Alison J Bruce, Roy S Rogers III

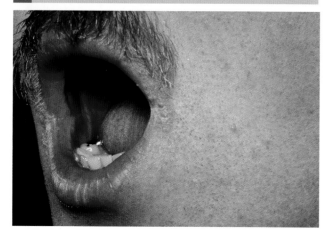

Angular cheilitis is a chronic inflammatory condition of the commissures of the lips characterized by atrophy, fissures, crusting, erythema, and scaling. Angular cheilitis is a reaction pattern with one or more causes including mechanical (intertrigo), infectious, nutritional, or inflammatory disease. It may be a sign of a systemic disease such as diabetes mellitus or HIV infection. It occurs commonly in Down syndrome.

MANAGEMENT STRATEGY

Successful therapy of cheilitis is based on *identifying and correcting each and all factors of this multifactorial condition.* The presence of dentures, and identification of palatal erythema and edema suggest denture stomatitis and candidiasis, respectively. A pale, depapillated, atrophic tongue suggests iron deficiency. A tender, glossy, depapillated tongue suggests folate or vitamin B12 deficiency. An eczematous dermatitis of the lower face suggests a staphylococcal infection.

Unilateral lesions are usually short-lived and induced by trauma. Bilateral lesions tend to be chronic and caused by infection or nutritional deficiency, and are more likely to be associated with an underlying disease process.

Maceration of the commissural epithelium and adjacent skin is a common, noninfectious cause of mechanical angular cheilitis. Trauma from dental flossing, habitual lip licking, and excessive salivation all contribute. Periods of oral hydration and then dryness disrupt epithelial integrity, with fissuring of the commissures. This provides an ideal environment for low-grade candidiasis and infectious eczematoid dermatitis.

Other traumatic factors are denture wearing, loss of vertical dimension of the jaws, sagging skin folds, xerostomia, orofacial granulomatosis, and perioral dermatitis.

Infectious causes must be sought. Angular cheilitis is frequently present in patients with HIV infection, and 10% may have a localized candidiasis. Both *Candida albicans* and *Staphylococcus aureus* organisms can colonize the fissures. Anemia, nutritional deficiencies, diabetes mellitus, Crohn's disease, and acrodermatitis enteropathica predispose to cheilitis and should be considered and sought.

Recurrence of angular cheilitis may be prevented by eliminating offending organisms from their reservoirs. Denture stomatitis, candidiasis, and nasal colonization of staphylococci should be sought. The organisms are treated with *topical miconazole cream* after meals and at bedtime. *Topical mupirocin* is valuable in treating staphylococcal colonization. Dentures should be removed from the mouth at night and cleansed well before reinserting in the morning. *New dentures* may restore facial contours, increasing the vertical dimension of the jaws and face. *Injection of collagen* in the commissures may alleviate causative mechanical factors.

SPECIFIC INVESTIGATIONS

- Culture for candidiasis
- Culture for bacteria
- Medical evaluation as for burning mouth syndrome (see page 241)
- HIV testing
- Patch testing

Diseases of the lips. Rogers RS III, Bekic M. Semin Cutan Med Surg 1997;16:325–36.

Discussion of multifactorial nature and evaluation of angular cheilitis.

Angular cheilosis: an analysis of 156 cases. Konstantinidis AB, Hatziotis JH. J Oral Med 1984;39: 199–205.

A careful analysis of the cause(s) of angular cheilitis in 156 patients.

Emphasizes that more than a single cause is often present.

Angular cheilitis. In: Scully C, Bagan J-V, Eisen D, et al., eds. Dermatology of the lips. Oxford, UK: Isis Medical; 2000:68–73.

Excellent clinical photographs and summary.

Nickel-induced angular cheilitis due to orthodontic braces. Yesudian PD, Memon A. Contact Derm 2003;48: 287–8.

Down syndrome: lip lesions (angular stomatitis and fissures) and *Candida albicans*. Scully C, van Bruggen W, Diz Dios P, et al. Br J Dermatol 2002;147:37–40.

Angular cheilitis was seen in 25% of patients with trisomy 21.

FIRST LINE THERAPIES

■ Topical miconazole cream	D
■ Topical fusidic acid, polymyxin B or mupirocin ointments	D
■ Remove dentures at night and cleanse before reinserting	D

Clinical management of oral and perioral candidiasis. Fotos PG, Lilly JP. Dermatol Clin 1996;14:273–80.

An excellent description of topical and systemic therapy of candidiasis.

Diseases of the lips. Rogers RS III, Bekic M. Semin Cutan Med Surg 1997;16:325–36.

Discussion of multifactorial nature, evaluation, and treatment of angular cheilitis.

Evidence levels **A** Double-blind study   **B** Clinical trial ≥ 20 subjects   **C** Clinical trial < 20 subjects   **D** Series ≥ 5 subjects   **E** Anecdotal case reports

Angular cheilitis. Schoenfeld RJ, Schoenfeld FI. Cutis 1977;19:213–6.

Discussion of the differential diagnosis, causes, and management of angular cheilitis.

SECOND LINE THERAPIES

| ■ Systemic antifungal therapy (fluconazole) | E |
| ■ Amphotericin B lozenges | E |

Treatment of oral Candida mucositis infections. Garber GE. Drugs 1994;47:734–40.

Reviews treatment of infections due to *Candida* spp., highlighting challenges in the immunocompromised patient.

THIRD LINE THERAPIES

| ■ Collagen injections | E |

Microlipoinjection and autologous collagen. Pinski KS, Coleman III WP. Dermatol Clin 1995;13:339–51.

Although these procedures may need to be repeated, mechanical correction of the deep furrows at the oral commissures can be very rewarding for the patient.

Chilblains

Pauline Dowd, Verity Blackwell

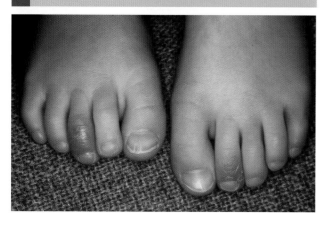

Chilblains (perniosis) are localized inflammatory, erythematous, itchy lesions that arise as an abnormal response to cold ambient temperatures above freezing, in combination with high humidity, which exacerbates conductive heat loss. The onset is usually in the autumn or winter. Individual lesions, which may ulcerate or blister, occur symmetrically on the fingers, toes, heels, lower legs, thighs, nose, and ears. A specific subset occurs on the thighs of patients wearing tight-fitting poorly insulating trousers (e.g. young horsewomen). A further subgroup with acral perniosis have had anorexia or bulimia and often indulged in vigorous exercise to maintain a low body weight; their perniosis may persist for several years after return to an acceptable body weight.

MANAGEMENT STRATEGY

Chilblains typically run a self-limiting course over a few weeks, but some severely affected individuals may have symptoms in the summer months. Underlying conditions should be sought with certain clinical presentations such as myelodysplastic disease, anorexia, and connective tissue diseases. The condition must be distinguished from chilblain lupus erythematosus, particularly if bullous lesions are present. In children, perniosis may be associated with cryoproteins. In elderly patients and those with ulcerative lesions, peripheral vascular insufficiency must be excluded. The initial management of chilblains involves stressing the importance of *prophylactic measures of wearing warm clothing and warm housing. Vasodilator calcium channel blockers* (nifedipine 20–60 mg daily, diltiazem 60–120 mg three times daily) have been shown to be an effective therapy and preventative measure in patients with idiopathic acral perniosis and in those patients with perniosis associated with low body weight. Patients who cannot tolerate the side effects of nifedipine or diltiazem may benefit from the *topical application of nicotinic acid derivatives or minoxidil* (5% lotion three times daily). UV light has traditionally been used for the treatment of chilblains, but a recent study has not demonstrated any benefit.

SPECIFIC INVESTIGATIONS

- Full blood count
- Autoimmune profile
- Cryoglobulins
- Cold agglutinins
- Consider vascular imaging in elderly patients
- Histology and immunofluorescence

Pernio. A possible association with chronic myelomonocytic leukaemia. Kelly JW, Dowling JP. Arch Dermatol 1985; 121:1048–52.

A series of four elderly male patients has been described in whom perniosis preceded the onset of chronic myelomonocytic leukemia.

Anorexia nervosa associated with acromegaloid features, onset of acrocyanosis and Raynaud's phenomenon and worsening of chilblains. Rustin MH, Foreman JC, Dowd PM. J R Soc Med 1990;83:495–6.

Two patients are reported who developed severe perniosis in association with anorexia nervosa.

Perniosis in association with anorexia nervosa. White KP, Rothe MJ, Milanese A, Grant-Kels JM. Paediatr Dermatol 1994;11:1–5.

Childhood pernio and cryoproteins. Weston WL, Morelli JG. Pediatr Dermatol 2000;17:97–9.

A 10-year retrospective study of a pediatric clinic identified eight patients with perniosis, four of whom had cryoglobulins or cold agglutinins and two had positive rheumatoid factor.

Equestrian perniosis associated with cold agglutinins: a novel finding. De Silva BD, McLaren K, Doherty VR. Clin Exp Dermatol 2000;25:285–8.

Two cases of equestrian perniosis associated with cold agglutinins.

FIRST LINE THERAPIES

Calcium channel blockers	D
Topical corticosteroids	E

The treatment of chilblains with nifedipine: the results of a pilot study, a double blind placebo-controlled randomized study and a long term open trial. Rustin MH, Newton JA, Smith NP, Dowd PM. Br J Dermatol 1989; 120:267–75.

Ten patients with severe recurrent acral perniosis were treated with 20 mg of nifedipine retard or placebo in a double-blind crossover trial for 12 weeks in total. No patients developed new lesions while on treatment and 70% were clear after a mean of 8 days. In the open study, 34 patients received up to 60 mg of nifedipine retard for 2 months; this was shown to be effective in reducing the healing time and symptoms of lesions.

Corticosteroid therapy for pernio. Gaynor S. J Am Acad Dermatol 1983;8:13.

Evidence levels **A** Double-blind study **B** Clinical trial > 20 subjects **C** Clinical trial < 20 subjects **D** Series ≤ 5 subjects **E** Anecdotal case reports

This author reports successful treatment of patients with perniosis using topical corticosteroids (0.025% fluocinolone cream) under occlusion nightly.

Topical corticosteroids are frequently used for the treatment of chilblains, but their use is not based on controlled trials.

SECOND LINE THERAPIES

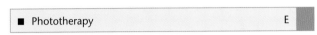

■ Topical 2% hexyl nicotinate cream	E
■ Minoxidil 5% lotion	E
■ Acidified nitrate cream	E
■ Tamoxifen	E

We have successfully used a 2% hexyl nicotinate in aqueous cream preparation and minoxidil 5% lotion applied three times a day, in a number of patients with chilblains and Raynaud's phenomenon, and acidified nitrite cream (3% salicylic acid and 3% potassium nitrate) three times daily in patients with chilblains intolerant of calcium channel blockers. Low-dose (5 mg daily) tamoxifen has also proved useful in anorexia-associated perniosis (PM Dowd, unpublished data).

Diltiazem hydrochloride 2% in a cream base is currently being assessed by the author in patients with anorexia-associated perniosis.

THIRD LINE THERAPIES

■ Phototherapy	E

A double blind study of ultraviolet phototherapy in the prophylaxis of chilblains. Langry JA, Diffey BL. Acta Derm Venereol 1989;69:320–2.

Anecdotally, UV light was used for the prophylactic treatment of chilblains, but this randomized double-blind study concluded that UV light was of no benefit.

Chondrodermatitis nodularis helicis

Clifford M Lawrence

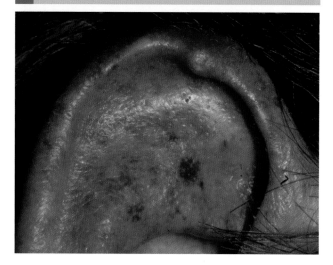

Chondrodermatitis nodularis helicis (CNH) is a benign condition. The only indication for treatment is pain causing sleep disturbance. Painless areas of chondrodermatitis can be ignored or managed conservatively. Lesions on the helix are easier to treat surgically than antihelix lesions. A pressure-relieving cushion is a good alternative to surgery for antihelix lesions.

MANAGEMENT STRATEGY

Chondrodermatitis almost always occurs on the lateral portion of the ear on the preferred sleeping side. It is caused by the pressure of the head crushing the ear into the pillow while sleeping. The most protuberant part of the ear is affected; this is generally the helix in men and the antihelix in women. Patients who can only adopt one sleeping position due to pain from for example arthritis, are particularly vulnerable. The incidence increases with age because ear cartilage becomes less flexible with time. Conservative or medical treatment, such as *lidocaine* gel, a potent *topical or intralesional corticosteroid* or *pressure relieving cushion* should be tried in all patients. Failing this, the treatment of choice is *excision* of the affected area of cartilage. There is no need to remove any skin or excise the ulcer. Other destructive therapies are less effective, but have the advantage of speed and simplicity.

SPECIFIC INVESTIGATIONS

- None required.
- Biopsy of a lesion only necessary if surgery is indicated. Lesions managed conservatively do not require biopsy

FIRST LINE THERAPIES

■ Reassurance that the lesion is not cancer	B
■ Conservative management	B
■ Topical corticosteroids	B
■ Intralesional corticosteroids	B

Treatment of chondrodermatitis nodularis helicis and conventional wisdom? Beck MH. Br J Dermatol 1985;113: 504–5.

Topical corticosteroids (betamethasone valerate cream 0.025%) used twice a day for 6 weeks and intralesional triamcinolone (0.2–0.5 mL 10 mg/mL) are effective in almost 25% of patients.

Intralesional triamcinolone for chondrodermatitis nodularis: a follow-up study of 60 patients. Cox NH, Denham PF. Br J Dermatol 2002;146:712–3.

A retrospective analysis of 60 patients with CNH treated with 0.1 mL intralesional triamcinolone acetonide 10 mg/ mL or triamcinolone hexacetonide 5 mg/mL showed a good response on 43% of helix and 31% of antihelix lesions.

Reassurance that CNH is not a tumor puts the patient's mind at rest. In many instances the symptoms are mild and can be tolerated without any major intervention. Initially, conservative therapy should be tried. Recommend a change in sleeping position and a soft pillow that can still be further compressed when the head is resting on it. 2% lidocaine gel applied 30 min before going to bed can also produce some symptomatic relief.

SECOND LINE THERAPIES

■ Surgical excision of affected cartilage without skin excision for helix lesions	B
■ Pressure relieving cushion for high-risk patients with antihelix lesions or if surgery contraindicated	B
■ Destructive therapies including CO₂ laser ablation, cryotherapy, curettage	B

The treatment of chondrodermatitis nodularis with cartilage removal alone. Lawrence CM. Arch Dermatol 1991;127:530–5.

Topical and intralesional corticosteroids were used in 44 patients preoperatively and were successful in 27%. Surgery was performed on symptomatic patients who did not respond to medical therapy. Surgical excision of the affected cartilage without removal of skin resulted in long-term cure rates of 84% for helix and 75% for antihelix lesions. Local anesthesia with lidocaine and epinephrine (adrenaline) reduced bleeding and improved the visibility and is not known to result in skin necrosis on the ear. A 3 mm punch biopsy was taken at the start of the procedure, but the core should only be removed at the same time as cartilage removal because the biopsy site helps to localize the target area. On the helix an incision was made along the helical rim and the skin reflected to expose the cartilage. A sliver of cartilage approximately 20 mm long was taken to include the 3 mm punch biopsy of the skin nodule. On the antihelix a flap of skin had to be raised over the affected area and the underlying cartilage excised. Care was taken to ensure that all remaining cartilage edges were smooth and gently shelving up to the uninvolved cartilage to prevent recurrences, which occur on rough or protuberant cartilage.

Evidence levels A Double-blind study B Clinical trial ≥ 20 subjects C Clinical trial < 20 subjects D Series ≥ 5 subjects E Anecdotal case reports

Cartilage excision alone is not disfiguring and further cartilage edges can be removed if recurrences occur after surgery, without producing a deformed ear.

The long-term results of cartilage removal alone for the treatment of chondrodermatitis nodularis. Hudson-Peacock MJ, Cox NH, Lawrence CM. Br J Dermatol 1999; 141:703–5.

Sixty two helix lesions were followed up for a mean of 52 months (range 8–99 months). There was recurrence in ten patients (all men; 16%). Twenty antihelix lesions were followed up for a mean of 55 months (range 8–93 months). There was recurrence in five patients (all women; 25%). This study confirms that only cartilage needs to be excised for the long-term effective treatment of CNH.

Simple elliptical excision involves the unnecessary removal of skin as well as cartilage; this inevitably makes the closure more difficult and results in higher reported recurrence rates of 31%. More extensive surgery such as wedge excision ignores the underlying cause and cannot be justified.

Treatment of chondrodermatitis nodularis with removal of the underlying cartilage alone: retrospective analysis of experience in 37 lesions. de Ru JA, Lohuis PJ, Saleh HA, Vuyk HD. J Laryngol Otol 2002;116:677–81.

Most otolaryngologists treat patients with CNH by wedge excision. Although the results of this technique are generally good, it can leave the patient with an asymmetric, deformed ear. The authors describe their results after changing to the technique described above. In a mean follow-up of 30 months, all 34 patients remained symptom-free and only one required surgical revision. The authors recommend this safe and simple technique to other physicians who treat patients with CNH.

Chondrodermatitis nodularis chronica helicis treated with curettage and electrocauterization: follow-up of a 15-year material. Kromann N, Hoyer H, Reymann F. Acta Derm Venereol 1983;63:85–7.

Curettage is simple and is reported to result in a 31% relapse rate.

Chondrodermatitis nodularis chronica helicis. Successful treatment with the carbon dioxide laser. Taylor MB. J Dermatol Surg Oncol 1991;17:862–4.

The CO_2 laser was used to vaporize the cutaneous nodules and involved cartilage. The wounds were allowed to heal with only minimal care using hydrogen peroxide cleansing and applications of topical antibiotic ointment. Twelve lesions have been treated with no recurrences after 2–15 months.

Cryotherapy has been advocated, but there are no published outcomes.

THIRD LINE THERAPIES

■ Pressure relieving cushion	B
■ Repeated surgical excision of affected cartilage without skin excision	B

Auricular pressure relieving cushions for chondrodermatitis nodularis helicis. Allen DL, Swinson PA, Arnstein PM. J Maxillofac Prosthet Technol 1998;2:5–10.

The ear cushion is custom-made by a maxillofacial laboratory technician and worn at night. Thirty-five of 46 patients treated in this way had complete resolution of their symptoms.

Effective treatment of chondrodermatitis nodularis chronica helicis using a conservative approach. Moncrieff M, Sassoon EM. Br J Dermatol 2004;150:892–4.

A simple to construct ear cushion design was used made of a bath sponge with the center removed, held in place with a head band. Thirteen of 15 patients followed for 1 month responded.

The aim of the device is to transfer the weight of the sleeping head from the ear to the surrounding scalp. This technique is very useful in patients in whom surgery has been unsuccessful, and particularly in older female patients with very thin skin and lesions on the antihelix, where recurrences are more common after surgery. Two different types of ear cushion have been described. The bath sponge method has the advantage of being simple and easily put together by the patient.

Chromoblastomycosis

Wanda Sonia Robles

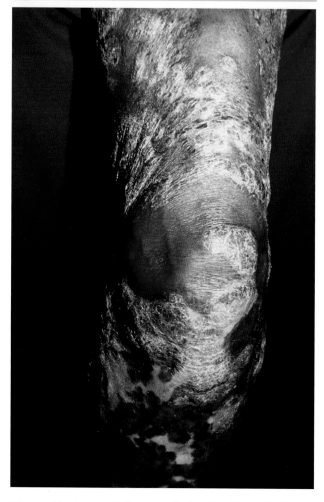

Chromoblastomycosis is a chronic, localized fungal infection of cutaneous and subcutaneous tissues caused by pigmented (dematiaceous) fungi. These are characterized by the production of thick-walled, single or multicell clusters in tissue, known as sclerotic or muriform bodies. Infection results from implantation of the organism into the skin by trauma and is encountered mainly in Central and South America, Africa, Australia, and Japan. Clinically, the lesions are characterized by the production of slow-growing warty exophytic lesions, most commonly affecting the lower legs and feet. Systemic involvement is a rare complication of this condition, and primary infection of the lung has been reported on two occasions.

MANAGEMENT STRATEGY

Treatment of chromoblastomycosis is mainly based on the use of *antifungal chemotherapy* but there is no treatment of choice in a condition well known for low cure rates and frequent relapses. *Surgical excision* has proved quite successful in patients with small areas of infection or localized disease, but there is a risk of local recurrence. There are also reports of equally successful treatment of localized infection with *cryosurgery using liquid nitrogen* and also with *carbon dioxide laser surgery*. Successful treatment of localized forms of chromoblastomycosis with *local application of heat* has been reported. A case of treatment with *Mohs' micrographic surgery* is also found in the literature. Antifungal chemotherapy with *itraconazole* has proven successful, used alone or in combination with flucytosine. Few clinical trials have been carried out with itraconazole and *terbinafine*, but there is evidence to indicate that good improvement and even cures can be achieved in many of the patients treated with these compounds. It does appear that itraconazole alone is more effective in the treatment of infections caused by the organism *Cladophialophora carrionii*.

Itraconazole and *flucytosine* (5-fluorocytosine), which is also an orally administered drug, have proved beneficial in cases where excision has not been possible. It is worth remembering, however, that toxicity from metabolites of flucytosine makes it mandatory to monitor the serum levels of this drug in patients during the course of treatment. The use of flucytosine alone is not recommended in view of the high possibility of development of resistance; however, it can be used in combination with *amphotericin B*. Another alternative is *thiabendazole*, with the limitation that it is not well tolerated by patients due to gastrointestinal side effects.

SPECIFIC INVESTIGATIONS

- Microscopy
- Culture

Chromoblastomycosis needs to be differentiated from many other conditions, including cutaneous blastomycosis, cutaneous tuberculosis, leishmaniasis, common warts, syphilis, and yaws. Isolation and identification of the pathogen is therefore mandatory. The infective organisms are seen in biopsy specimens as deeply pigmented, thick-walled, muriform or sclerotic cells, irrespective of species. The nomenclature varies according to the dominant form of condition of the pathogen, the most common being *Phialophora verrucosa*, *Fonsecaea pedrosoi*, and *Cladophialophora carrionii*.

Direct microscopy and culture are also highly sensitive techniques of diagnosis and relatively inexpensive. Serological testing is not widely available.

FIRST LINE THERAPIES

■ Itraconazole	B
■ Terbinafine	B

Itraconazole in the treatment of chromoblastomycosis due to *Fonsecaea pedrosoi*. Queiroz-Telles F, Purim KS, Fillus JN, et al. Int J Dermatol 1992;31:805–12.

This is a noncomparative open clinical trial in 19 patients who were classified according to severity and received itraconazole 200–400 mg daily. Clinical and mycologic cure was obtained in eight patients (42%) with a mean duration of therapy of 7.2 months (range 3.2–29.6 months).

Treatment of chromoblastomycosis with itraconazole, cryosurgery, and a combination of both. Bonifaz A, Martinez-Soto E, Carrasco-Gerard E, Peniche J. Int J Dermatol 1997;36:542–7.

This study included 12 patients assigned to three different groups. Group 1, with small lesions, was treated with itraconazole 300 mg daily. Group 2, also with small lesions, was treated with one or more sessions of cryosurgery. Group 3, with large lesions, started treatment with itraconazole 300 mg daily until reduction of lesions was achieved, followed by one or more sessions of cryosurgery. The results showed complete clinical and mycologic cure in two out of four patients in both groups 1 and 3. All four patients in group 2 achieved complete cure.

Both itraconazole and cryosurgery may have roles in the treatment of chromoblastomycosis.

Successful treatment of chromoblastomycosis with itraconazole. Yu R. Mycoses 1995;38:79–83.

A severe case of chromoblastomycosis unresponsive to flucytosine was treated with itraconazole 100 mg daily for 15 months, with full recovery.

A case of chromoblastomycosis responding to treatment with itraconazole. Smith CH, Barker JN, Hay RJ. Br J Dermatol 1993;128:436–9.

Case report of a patient with clinical and histologic features of chromoblastomycosis who also developed atypical dermal/subcutaneous nodules and was successfully treated with itraconazole.

Itraconazole pulse therapy in chromoblastomycosis. Kumarasinghe SP, Kumarasinghe MP. Eur J Dermatol 2000;10:220–2.

A 68-year-old female patient with chromoblastomycosis was treated with oral itraconazole 200 mg twice daily for 1 week followed by 3 weeks free of treatment. This cycle was carried out for 6 months (seven pulses). Clinical improvement was observed after 2 months. Follow-up 8 months after completion of treatment showed no recurrence.

This is the only case report of itraconazole pulse therapy in chromoblastomycosis. A larger study is needed to ascertain optimal dosage and duration of treatment.

Chromoblastomycosis imported from Malta. Ezughah FI, Orpin S, Finch TM, Colloby PS. Clin Exp Dermatol 2003;28:486–7.

Case report of a female patient who developed chromoblastomycosis on her right forearm after a visit to Malta. This was successfully treated with itraconazole for 6 months.

Therapeutic potential of terbinafine in subcutaneous and systemic mycoses. Hay RJ. Br J Dermatol 1999;141(suppl 56):36–40.

A review article on the potential of terbinafine, which exhibits a broad spectrum of activity against many pathogenic fungi, including those responsible for subcutaneous mycoses. Limited data show that terbinafine is effective as first line treatment in chromoblastomycosis.

A good review article.

Treatment of chromomycosis with terbinafine: preliminary results of an open pilot study. Esterre P, Inzan CK, Ramarcel ER, et al. Br J Dermatol 1996;134(suppl 46):33–6.

A multicenter study using long courses (6–12 months) of terbinafine at the dosage of 500 mg daily by oral administration to 43 patients. Sixteen individuals (37.2%) had previously relapsed after treatment with thiabendazole. Mycologic cure was reported in 41.4%, 74.1%, and 82.5% of patients infected with *Fonsecaea pedrosoi* after 4, 8, and 12

months of treatment, respectively. Total recovery is reported, even in cases unresponsive to treatment with imidazoles and those with chronic disease present for over 10 years.

A good clinical trial showing high efficacy of terbinafine in Cladophialophora carrionii-*infected patients.*

Case report. A case of chromoblastomycosis effectively treated with terbinafine. Characteristics of chromoblastomycosis in the Kitasato region, Japan. Tanuma H, Hiramatsu M, Mukai H. Mycoses 2000;43:79–83.

A longstanding (20 years' duration) case of chromoblastomycosis due to *Fonsecaea pedrosoi* in a 38-year-old male patient is described. The condition was unresponsive to flucytosine and local heat. The patient responded well to treatment with terbinafine combined with local heat therapy.

Treatment of chromoblastomycosis due to *Fonsecaea pedrosoi* with low-dose terbinafine. Sevigny GM, Ramos-Caro FA. Cutis 2000;66:45–6.

Report of a patient successfully treated with oral terbinafine 250 mg daily for a period of 8 months.

Alternate week and combination itraconazole and terbinafine therapy for chromoblastomycosis caused by *Fonsecaea pedrosoi* in Brazil. Gupta AK, Taborda PR, Sanzovo AD. Med Mycol 2002;40:529–34.

A small study, including four patients with longstanding chromoblastomycosis, which aimed to determine the potential of alternate-week and combination treatment with itraconazole and terbinafine for chromoblastomycosis poorly responsive or nonresponsive to standard therapies. The study concluded that combination therapy was effective in treating poorly responsive chromoblastomycosis.

Treating chromoblastomycosis with systemic antifungals. Bonifaz A, Paredes-Solis V, Saul A. Expert Opin Pharmacother 2004;5:247–54.

A review article which highlights the difficulties in treating this condition, as often there are several treatment options. It also states that the best results have been obtained with itraconazole and terbinafine at high doses for a minimum period of treatment of 6–12 months.

Chromoblastomycosis: a review of 100 cases in the state of Rio Grande do Sul, Brazil. Minotto R, Bernardi CD, Mallmann LF, et al. J Am Acad Dermatol 2001;44:585–92.

Review of 100 patients with chromoblastomycosis who were treated between 1963 and 1998. Patients showed different degrees of severity of the condition. Some of the severe cases showed eventual evidence of squamous cell carcinoma. Statistical analysis of all reviewed case records showed relapse of the disease in 43% of cases despite treatment.

A very good review.

SECOND LINE THERAPIES

■ Cryosurgery	C
■ Local heat	D
■ Surgical excision	D
■ Flucytosine	C
■ Thiabendazole	E

Treatment of chromomycosis by cryosurgery with liquid nitrogen: a report on eleven cases. Pimentel ER, Castro LG, Cuce LC, Sampaio SA. J Dermatol Surg Oncol 1989;15:72–7.

Cryosurgery was used to treat 11 patients with chromoblastomycosis, of whom five had localized infection and six had disseminated lesions. Freezing times varied from 30 s to 4 min and the number of cycles from 1 to more than 40. All patients with localized disease responded well, with complete clearance 53 months after treatment. Of the six patients with multiple lesions, three achieved complete remission after 26 months of treatment and the other three showed only partial improvement.

Treatment of chromomycosis by cryosurgery with liquid nitrogen: 15 years' experience. Castro LG, Pimentel ER, Lacaz CS. Int J Dermatol 2003;42:408–12.

This retrospective study included 22 patients with chromoblastomycosis treated by cryosurgery. The average number of treatments per patient was 6.7. Nine patients (40.9%) were considered cured after 3 years' follow-up; eight patients (36.4%) were clinically cured but relapsed in less than 3 years of follow-up; two patients (9.1%) still had active lesions; and three (13.6%) were considered unsuccessful.

Successful treatment of chromoblastomycosis with topical heat therapy. Tagami H, Ginoza M, Imaizumi S, Urano-Suehisa S. J Am Acad Dermatol 1984;10:615–9.

Four female patients with chromoblastomycosis are reported to have responded well to treatment with tolerable heat from pocket warmers. Three compliant patients responded after 2, 3 and 6 months, respectively, whereas a fourth patient, performing applications in an irregular manner, cleared only after a 12-month period.

Hyperthermic treatment of chromomycosis with disposable chemical pocket warmers. Report of a successfully treated case, with a review of the literature. Hiruma M, Kawada A, Yoshida M, Kouya M. Mycopathologia 1993; 122:107–14.

A 56-year-old male with a 7 cm × 10 cm infiltrated erythematous plaque on the extensor aspect of the left upper arm is described. Treatment with disposable chemical pocket warmers was carried out for 4 months. The devices were secured over the affected area with tight elastic bandage to retain warmth for 24 h.

A good review article.

Chromoblastomycosis treated by Mohs micrographic surgery. Pavlidakey GP, Snow SN, Mohs FE. J Dermatol Surg Oncol 1986;12:1073–5.

This surgical technique, which has been successfully used in the treatment of a variety of skin tumors, was used in the treatment of localized chromoblastomycosis, with no recurrence 1 year following surgery.

A different therapeutic approach.

Chromoblastomycosis. Vijaya D, Kumar BH. Mycoses 2005;48:82–4.

Report of a case of a 70-year-old male patient from a rural area who had an asymptomatic verrucous lesion on the left leg diagnosed as chromoblastomycosis. This failed to respond to treatment with itraconazole. Consequently, complete surgical resection was undertaken, with no relapse after 1-year follow-up.

Six years experience in treatment of chromomycosis with 5-fluorocytosine. Lopez CF, Alvarenga RJ, Cisalpino EO, et al. Int J Dermatol 1978;17:414–8.

Twenty-three patients with chromoblastomycosis were treated with oral flucytosine for 2–67 months. Sixteen were reported as cured after a 3-month period. Seven patients developed resistance. In these patients, subsequent treatment with amphotericin B, calciferol, or thiabendazole also failed.

THIRD LINE THERAPIES

■ Amphotericin	B
■ CO_2 laser	E
■ Ajoene	C

Treatment of chromomycosis with oral high-dose of amphotericin B. Iijima S, Takase T, Otsuka F. Arch Dermatol 1995;131:399–401.

Report of a 54-year-old male patient with chromoblastomycosis successfully treated with amphotericin B orally at an initial dose of 300 mg daily. The dose was increased every 2 weeks, up to the maximum dose of 2400 mg daily (24 tablets).

A case of chromomycosis treated by a combination of cryotherapy, shaving, oral 5-fluorocytosine, and oral amphotericin B. Poirriez J, Breuillard F, Francois N, et al. Am J Trop Med Hyg 2000;63:61–3.

A case report of a patient who failed to respond to high doses of amphotericin B and to oral itraconazole but responded to combination therapy with flucytosine and amphotericin B. The patient stopped this treatment after 6 months, with successive relapse 2 years later.

Treatment of chromomycosis with a CO_2 laser. Kuttner BJ, Siegle RJ. J Dermatol Surg Oncol 1986;12:965–8.

Description of the successful use of a CO_2 laser in the treatment of localized chromoblastomycosis.

Successful treatment of chromomycosis using carbon dioxide laser associated with topical heat applications. Hira K, Yamada H, Takahashi Y, Ogawa H. J Eur Acad Dermatol Venereol 2002;16:273–5.

Case report of a 59-year-old male patient with a 6-year history of chromoblastomycosis at presentation who was successfully treated with the application of topical heat followed by treatment with CO_2 laser to eradicate the unresponsive remnants of the lesion.

Ajoene and 5-fluorouracil in the topical treatment of *Cladophialophora carrionii* **chromoblastomycosis in humans: a comparative open study.** Perez-Blanco M, Valles RH, Zeppenfeldt GF, Apitz-Castro R. Med Mycol 2003;41:517–20.

An open comparative trial to assess the safety and effectiveness of topical ajoene (garlic-derived natural compound) and 5-fluorouracil in the treatment of localized chromoblastomycosis. Results of the trial appear to support the clinical use of ajoene in the control of this very difficult cutaneous mycosis.

Evidence levels A Double-blind study   B Clinical trial ≥ 20 subjects   C Clinical trial < 20 subjects   D Series ≥ 5 subjects   E Anecdotal case reports

Chronic actinic dermatitis

Sandra Albert, Roy A Palmer, John L M Hawk

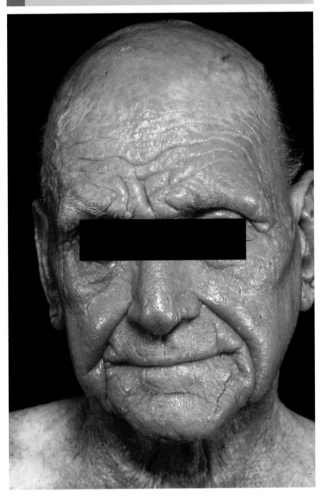

Chronic actinic dermatitis (CAD) is a UV and sometimes visible radiation-induced eczema affecting predominantly the face, upper chest, neck, and exposed areas of the limbs; rarely it may disseminate towards erythroderma. It is frequently associated with *contact sensitivity* to airborne allergens such as fragrances, colophony, and sesquiterpene lactone from plants of the Compositae family. Although it most often affects the elderly, recently it has been noted to present at an earlier age in occasional patients with atopic eczema.

MANAGEMENT STRATEGY

Once fully evolved, CAD is generally persistent, although it may gradually remit over years. Treatment involves the *restriction of exposure to UV* and in addition, in patients sensitive to it, visible radiation. Patients should be advised about behavioral measures (such as virtual avoidance of sunlight between about 10 a.m. and 4 p.m.), wearing of protective clothing such as long-sleeved shirts made of close weave materials, broad-brimmed hats, and the possible use of filtering window films. *Broad-spectrum high-factor sunscreens* of low allergenicity should be applied liberally every 2–3 h. *Avoidance of any relevant contact allergens* is also important.

Superpotent or potent *topical corticosteroids* and the regular use of emollients should essentially always be prescribed. Intermittent courses of *systemic corticosteroids* 30–60 mg daily, tapered over several weeks, may be used to bring acute flares under control, followed by maintenance with topical corticosteroids and other general measures described above. If control remains poor, *azathioprine* 100–200 mg (1–2.5 mg/kg) daily may be introduced, usually in lower doses initially, with increases as required; because azathioprine efficacy may develop only slowly over 4–6 weeks, oral corticosteroids may be needed initially in addition for several weeks. Thiopurine methyl transferase (TPMT) assay is a useful screening test before such therapy – patients with low levels are more prone to myelotoxicity. Possible adverse effects include gastrointestinal intolerance, bone marrow suppression, and liver toxicity, and appropriate blood tests should be undertaken at regular intervals. *Cyclosporine* in doses of 2.5–5 mg/kg daily is perhaps a more effective alternative, but possible side-effects include renal impairment and hypertension, which are initially reversible. *Psoralen and UVA (PUVA) therapy* under cover of reducing oral corticosteroids may then be tried if these measures are unsuccessful, one regimen being to start patients on 0.6 mg/kg 8-methoxypsoralen (8-MOP) followed by an initial UVA dose of 0.1–0.25 J/cm^2 with increments of 0.1–0.25 J/cm^2 at each session thereafter, provided the previous dose is tolerated. After, for example, a daily or alternate day regimen for 3–4 weeks, the frequency of therapy may then be reduced very gradually to once weekly, then once monthly maintenance doses according to clinical response. A potent topical corticosteroid should be applied to all exposed areas just after the irradiation. Narrowband 311 nm UVB (TL-01) therapy has been shown to be useful in other photodermatoses such as polymorphic light eruption and actinic prurigo, and might well be expected to be beneficial in CAD also, though confirmatory studies remain to be undertaken.

SPECIFIC INVESTIGATIONS

- Patch and photopatch tests
- Phototesting (UVA, UVB, visible light)

Contact and photocontact sensitization in chronic actinic dermatitis: sesquiterpene lactone mix is an important allergen. Menagé H du P, Ross JS, Norris PG, Hawk JLM, White IR. Br J Dermatol 1995;132:543–7.

In a study of 89 patients with CAD, cutaneous phototesting was done by recording the minimal erythema doses following exposure to graded irradiation doses at a series of wavelengths between 300 and 600 nm with a monochromator. All patients had abnormal responses: 83% to UVB and UVA, 9% to UVB alone, and 8% to UVB, UVA and visible light. On patch testing 72% had positive reactions, the most common allergens being sesquiterpene lactone mix (36%), fragrance mix (21%), and colophony (20%). Photopatch testing resulted in 11% having positive reactions, including 7% who had positive photopatch tests to sunscreen agents.

Contact allergy to sunscreen chemicals in photosensitivity dermatitis/actinic reticuloid syndrome (PD/AR) and polymorphic light eruption (PLE). Bilsland D, Ferguson J. Contact Derm 1993;29:70–3.

Ten of 45 patients with CAD reacted to a sunscreen agent, suggesting that this is occasionally an explanation for at least some of the eczema on exposed sites. Benzophenones (mexenone, oxybenzone) are the most frequent sensitizers.

FIRST LINE THERAPIES

■ Photoprotective measures	C
■ Avoidance of relevant contact allergens	C
■ Topical corticosteroids	C
■ Topical emollients	C

Chronic actinic dermatitis: a retrospective analysis of 44 cases referred to an Australian photobiology clinic. Yap LM, Foley P, Crouch R, Baker C. Australas J Dermatol 2003;44:256–62.

Avoidance of sunshine and allergens combined with the use of sunscreens and topical corticosteroids provided symptomatic relief in only 36% of patients: the remainder required systemic immunosuppressive agents or phototherapy.

Photosensitivity dermatitis/actinic reticuloid syndrome in an Irish population: a review and some unusual features. Healy E, Rogers S. Acta Derm Venereol 1995;75:72–4.

Nine patients were treated with sunscreens, emollients, topical corticosteroids, and antigen avoidance as the first line of therapy. Six responded, five also requiring intermittent courses of oral corticosteroids during the early phase; two achieved complete clinical remission while four remained well controlled with topical corticosteroids.

A double blind controlled study to assess the effect of pretreatment with a potent topical steroid on the phototest response of photosensitivity dermatitis and actinic reticuloid syndrome (PD/AR). (Abstract) Lowe JG, Ferguson J. Scot Med J 1989;34:509.

Phototesting in eight patients with CAD after 3 days of twice daily topical applications of 0.05% betamethasone dipropionate ointment increased the minimal erythema dose by a factor of 11 and moved it into the normal range in four patients; no change was noted in a control group of nine normal subjects, or on the side treated with the ointment base alone in the patients.

Protective effect of various types of clothes against UV radiation. Berne B, Fischer T. Acta Derm Venereol 1980;60: 459–60.

The light protective effects of 20 commonly used textiles were studied; tightly woven material was better than loose weave, and dark colors and double layering had additive effects. Blue denim gave the best results, with a protection factor of 1700 – far better than any sunscreen.

SECOND LINE THERAPIES

■ Azathioprine	A
■ Cyclosporine	D
Phototherapy	
■ PUVA	C
■ UVB	C
■ Topical tacrolimus	D

Azathioprine treatment in chronic actinic dermatitis: a double-blind controlled trial with monitoring of exposure to ultraviolet radiation. Murphy GM, Maurice PDL, Norris PG, et al. Br J Dermatol 1989;121:639–46.

In a study of 18 severely affected patients, with the complete subsidence of itch and eczematous change being considered as remission, five of eight patients on azathioprine 50 mg three times daily achieved remission, one other improved, one defaulted at 6 weeks due to gastrointestinal symptoms, and one did not improve over 8 weeks of therapy. None of the ten patients on placebo improved significantly.

Azathioprine in dermatology: a survey of current practice in the UK. Tan BB, Gawkrodger DJ, English JSC. Br J Dermatol 1997;136:351–5.

A questionnaire survey of 253 UK-based dermatologists demonstrated that 68% use azathioprine in CAD, 66% alone, and the others as a corticosteroid-sparing agent. Most used a dosage of 100 mg daily, only 13% prescribing it by body weight (1–2.5 mg/kg daily). CAD had the highest proportion of perceived efficacy (62%) among all the disorders treated with the drug.

Actinic reticuloid: response to cyclosporine. Norris PG, Camp RDR, Hawk JLM. J Am Acad Dermatol 1989;21:307–9.

Two patients who failed to respond adequately to oral and topical corticosteroids, PUVA or azathioprine responded favorably to cyclosporine 2.5–4 mg/kg daily. One patient relapsed on stopping therapy following an increase in serum creatinine levels; the other continued to do well on the medication.

Actinic reticuloid. A clinical photobiologic, histopathologic, and follow-up study of 16 patients. Toonstra J, Henquet CJ, van Weelden H, et al. J Am Acad Dermatol 1989;21:205–14.

Fifteen patients were treated with broadband UVB phototherapy five times a week at a starting dose of one-tenth of their minimal erythema dose, with gradual increments according to skin response. Thirteen patients showed good clinical improvement and increased sunlight tolerance. Discontinuation of maintenance therapy gradually resulted in relapse.

PUVA therapy of chronic actinic dermatitis. Hindson C, Spiro J, Downey A. Br J Dermatol 1985;113:157–60.

Four patients with severe CAD were treated with psoralen photochemotherapy (PUVA) twice weekly, with a starting UVA dose of 0.25 J/cm^2 and increments of 0.25 J/cm^2 to 1 J/cm^2 up to a maximum dose of 10 J/cm^2. Hydrocortisone 1% to the face and betamethasone valerate

Evidence levels A Double-blind study B Clinical trial ≥ 20 subjects C Clinical trial < 20 subjects D Series ≥ 5 subjects E Anecdotal case reports

ointment to the rest of the body were applied immediately after the first six exposures. All patients had a marked response and remained controlled thereafter on twice monthly treatments at 10 J/cm².

Treatment of chronic actinic dermatitis with tacrolimus ointment. Uetsu N, Okamoto H, Fujii K, et al. J Am Acad Dermatol 2002;47:881–4.

Six patients regularly applied tacrolimus ointment 0.1% to the face; symptoms were greatly improved by 4 weeks. The treatment remained effective during follow-up over 0.5–2.5 years.

Erythrodermic chronic actinic dermatitis responding only to topical tacrolimus. Evans AV, Palmer RA, Hawk JLM. Photodermatol Photoimmunol Photomed 2004;20:59–61.

An erythrodermic patient who had resisted or failed to tolerate standard oral immunosuppressive treatments and phototherapy responded well to topical tacrolimus 0.1%.

THIRD LINE THERAPIES

■ Hydroxychloroquine	D
■ Oral retinoids	E
■ Retinoids with PUVA	E
■ Danazol	E
■ Topical mechlorethamine	E
■ Mycophenolate	E

Chronic actinic dermatitis. An analysis of 51 patients evaluated in the United States and Japan. Lim HW, Morison WL, Kamide R, et al. Arch Dermatol 1994;130:1284–9.

General photoprotective measures, sunscreens, and topical corticosteroids were used in all patients. Azathioprine 50–200 mg was also commonly used. Hydroxychloroquine 200 mg once or twice daily was said (without further qualification) to give a partial to good response in nine patients and PUVA with oral corticosteroids to help seven patients, while four apparently responded well to cyclosporine, and two to etretinate.

Chronic actinic dermatitis responding to danazol. Humbert P, Drobacheff C, Vigan M, et al. Br J Dermatol 1991;124:195–7.

A patient with CAD having low α_1-antitrypsin levels treated with danazol 600 mg daily responded dramatically within 20 days, relapsed on stopping the medication, and again improved on reinstituting it; he remained well after 18 months on the drug. Danazol increases serum levels of α_1-antitrypsin/protease inhibitors in those with low levels, and an imbalance of proteases and antiproteases has been implicated as a cause of abnormal inflammatory responses in several dermatoses. There are no other reports of efficacy for danazol.

Aromatic retinoid–oral photochemotherapy (RePUVA) for actinic reticuloid. Hunziker T, Zala L, Krebs A. Dermatologica 1983;166:6311–3.

Etretinate 0.8–0.25 mg/kg followed by PUVA was more effective than oral PUVA alone in this patient.

Successful treatment of actinic reticuloid induced by whole-body topical application of mechlorethamine. Volden G, Falk ES, Wisløff-Nilssen J, et al. Acta Derm Venereol 1981;61:353–4.

Topical therapy with freshly prepared mechlorethamine (nitrogen mustard), 10 mg dissolved in 50 mL of water, was applied daily for 4 weeks, stopped due to skin irritation, and then reinstituted about 3 months later for a further 3 weeks. There was both clinical and histologic improvement and increased sunlight tolerance.

Mycophenolate in psoralen-UV-A desensitization therapy for chronic actinic dermatitis. Nousari HC, Anhalt GJ, Morison WL. Arch Dermatol 1999;135:1128–9.

Two patients better tolerated PUVA therapy by being immunosuppressed beforehand with prednisolone and mycophenolate.

Coccidioidomycosis

Wanda Sonia Robles

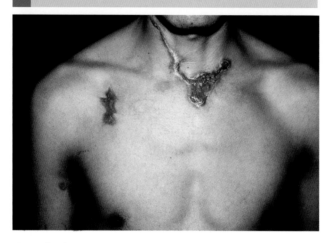

Coccidioidomycosis is a primary respiratory fungal infection caused by the soil-inhabiting fungus *Coccidioides immitis*. The disease may become progressive, in some instances with severe or fatal forms. The condition is endemic in the desert areas of the Southwest of the USA and also in parts of Central and South America. Cases have, however, been reported in Southern Europe and in Asia. Primary infection of the skin is rare. However, the majority of patients with disseminated coccidioidomycosis present with cutaneous manifestations. Clinical features vary from mild inapparent respiratory tract infection to acute disseminated fatal disease. Primary lung involvement is the commonest form of infection; it is sometimes asymptomatic but may simulate flu-like illness. This may be associated with erythema multiforme or erythema nodosum.

MANAGEMENT STRATEGY

In the primary pulmonary infection, no specific therapy is required. *Amphotericin B* has been the drug of choice for the disseminated forms of the disease. *Oral itraconazole, fluconazole,* and *ketoconazole* are advocated in the localized form of infection or lesions restricted to the skin.

As this is a potentially life-threatening disease, early diagnosis is of paramount importance. Dermatologists should be aware that the combination of atypical skin changes, pulmonary infiltrates, and a history of travel to endemic areas of the disease may represent infection. The treatment of choice for cutaneous coccidioidomycosis is currently *oral azole antifungal agents*, the most commonly used being *itraconazole* at a dose of 400 mg daily which is continued for 6 months after clinical response. Follow-ups are required for years in view of the frequent relapse rates after discontinuation of the treatment. Other oral azole antifungal agents, including *fluconazole* and *ketoconazole*, are advocated in a localized form of infection or in lesions restricted to the skin. More recently, case reports of treatment of disseminated nonmeningeal and coccidioidal meningitis with a new triazole antifungal agent, *voriconazole*, have documented success. Disseminated coccidioidomycosis in immunosuppressed or critically ill patients has also been successfully treated with *caspofungin*. This is the first of a new class of antifungal agents, the *echinocandins*, which

interfere with fungal cell wall synthesis by inhibition of glucan synthesis. The advent of highly active antiretroviral therapy (HAART) has seen a decrease in the incidence of fungal infections over the last 5 years in countries where this treatment is widely available, in comparison with countries that cannot afford this treatment. However, in endemic areas, coccidioidomycosis is still a risk in HIV-infected individuals, solid-organ transplant recipients, and patients with hematologic malignancies. For these patients, long-term prophylactic treatment with fluconazole may be considered.

SPECIFIC INVESTIGATIONS

- Direct microscopy
- Culture
- Serologic tests
- Serology for HIV/AIDS (where relevant)

The characteristic globular spherules may be seen in potassium hydroxide mounts of infected material: sputum, CSF, or pus. However, laboratory diagnosis depends on the isolation of the fungus in culture. In the mycelial form, the fungus is highly infectious, so cultures should be handled with care.

Coccidioidomycosis in the acquired immunodeficiency syndrome. Bronnimann DA, Adam RD, Galgiani JN, et al. Ann Intern Med 1987;106:372–9.

Report of 27 patients with AIDS in Arizona, seven of whom had concurrent coccidioidomycosis. A retrospective review of 300 patients with coccidioidal infection identified only 13 without AIDS.

FIRST LINE THERAPIES

■ Amphotericin B	D

Practice guidelines for the treatment of coccidioidomycosis. Infectious Diseases Society of America. Galgiani JN, Ampel NM, Catanzaro A, et al. Clin Infect Dis 2000;30: 658–61.

Management involves definition of the extent of infection. Relatively localized lung infection often requires only periodic follow-up. Patients with extensive infection or with immunosuppression need antifungal chemotherapy. Amphotericin B is the drug of choice in patients with respiratory failure or rapidly progressive infection. For more chronic manifestations of the disease, treatment with fluconazole, itraconazole, or ketoconazole is advocated. Duration of therapy varies from several months to years.

Chronic progressive coccidioidal pneumonitis. Report of six cases with clinical, roentgenographic, serologic, and therapeutic features. Bayer AS, Yoshikawa TT, Guze LB. Arch Intern Med 1979;139:536–40.

Report of six patients with pulmonary coccidioidomycosis who were previously healthy individuals. Serologic tests were very helpful in establishing the diagnosis, as the clinical presentation was indolent, resulting in long diagnostic delays. Five of these patients received treatment with intravenous amphotericin B greater than or equal to 30 mg/kg total.

Successful treatment of disseminated coccidioidomycosis with amphotericin B lipid complex. Koehler AP, Cheng AF, Chu KC, et al. J Infect 1998;36:113–5.

Case report of a Chinese patient in Hong Kong who had disseminated disease successfully treated with amphotericin B lipid complex (ABLC).

Use of newer antifungal therapies in clinical practice: what do the data tell us? Perfect JR. Oncology 2004;18: 15–23.

This review paper clearly states the importance of making an early diagnosis and also gives a good guide on the best use of the available antifungal drugs for both prophylaxis and treatment. ABLC and liposomal amphotericin B are advocated to be as effective as amphotericin B deoxycholate but less nephrotoxic.

A good review on new antifungal drugs.

Intrathecal amphotericin in the management of coccidioidal meningitis. Stevens DA, Shatsky SA. Semin Respir Infect 2001;16:263–9.

This review advocates the use of intrathecal amphotericin B as a way to avoid the toxicity of intra-CSF amphotericin treatment.

A good review.

Use of liposomal amphotericin B in the treatment of disseminated coccidioidomycosis. Antony S, Dominguez DC, Sotelo E. J Natl Med Assoc 2003;95:982–5.

Report of an immunosuppressed patient on long-term steroid therapy successfully treated with liposomal amphotericin B (AmBisome).

Coccidioidomycosis: case report and update on diagnosis and management. Kim A, Parker SS. J Am Acad Dermatol 2002;46:743–7.

This paper advocates the use of amphotericin B to treat coccidioidal meningitis or acute, aggressive pulmonary disease. Regarding the use of azoles, advice given by this paper is that clinical trials that have used ketoconazole, itraconazole, and fluconazole at doses of 400 mg daily have done so for a period of 3–6 months. Continuation of the medication is recommended for an additional 6 months after the disappearance of the clinical lesions.

SECOND LINE THERAPIES

■ Fluconazole	A
■ Itraconazole	A
■ Ketoconazole	B

Treatment of coccidioidal meningitis with fluconazole. Tucker RM, Galgiani JN, Denning DW, et al. Rev Infect Dis 1990;12(suppl 3):S380–9.

Eighteen patients with coccidioidal meningitis were treated with fluconazole at doses of 50–400 mg daily. Mean duration of treatment was 9.8 months. Among the 15 evaluable patients, success was observed in 10 (67%), one had a partial response, and four failed to respond. Two patients relapsed on discontinuation of treatment.

Fluconazole therapy for coccidioidal meningitis. The NIAID Mycoses Study Group. Galgiani JN, Catanzaro A, Cloud GA, et al. Ann Intern Med 1993;119:28–35.

Uncontrolled clinical trial including 50 consecutive patients with coccidioidal meningitis. Forty-seven were evaluated. Twenty-five had received no previous treatment and nine were HIV-positive. Thirty-seven of 47 responded to treatment with fluconazole. Response rates were similar in patients with or without previous therapy.

Fluconazole in the treatment of chronic pulmonary and nonmeningeal disseminated coccidioidomycosis. NIAID Mycoses Study Group. Catanzaro A, Galgiani JN, Levine BE, et al. Am J Med 1995;98:249–56.

A multicenter, open-label, single-arm study. Of 78 patients enrolled, 22 had soft tissue, 42 had chronic lung, and 14 had skeletal coccidioidomycosis. Forty-nine had at least one concomitant disease, seven of whom had HIV infection. Patents were given fluconazole 200 mg daily. Nonresponders were increased to 400 mg daily. Length of treatment was 4–8 months. Among 75 evaluable patients, a satisfactory response was observed in 12 (86%) of those with bone, 22 (55%) of those with lung, and 16 (76%) of those with soft tissue disease. It was concluded that fluconazole 200 or 400 mg/day is well tolerated and moderately effective for the treatment of nonmeningeal coccidioidomycosis, but the relapse rate is high.

Itraconazole treatment of coccidioidomycosis. NIAID Mycoses Study Group. Graybill JR, Stevens DA, Galgiani JN, et al. Am J Med 1990;89:282–90.

A multicenter study including 51 patients with nonmeningeal coccidioidomycosis. Patients were treated with itraconazole 100–400 mg daily for periods up to 39 months. Forty-seven patients entered evaluation. Forty-four completed therapy. Of these, 25 (57%) achieved remission. The authors concluded that itraconazole is effective and well tolerated in patients with coccidioidomycosis.

Comparison of oral fluconazole and itraconazole for progressive, nonmeningeal coccidioidomycosis. A randomized, double-blind trial. Galgiani JN, Catanzaro A, Cloud GA, et al. Ann Intern Med 2000;133:676–86.

In this randomized, double-blind, placebo-controlled trial, 198 patients were treated with either fluconazole 400 mg daily or itraconazole 200 mg twice daily. Success rates at 12 months were similar and both drugs were well tolerated. Neither drug was statistically superior in efficacy in nonmeningeal disease, although there was a trend toward greater efficacy with itraconazole.

Ketoconazole treatment of coccidioidomycosis: evaluation of 60 patients during three years of study. DeFelice R, Galgiani JN, Campbell SC, et al. Am J Med 1982;72:681–7.

Assessment of 60 patients with coccidioidal infection treated with ketoconazole. These included patients with chronic pulmonary disease, with soft tissue lesions, and with bone involvement. It was observed that soft tissue lesions improved rapidly (mean of 34 days) on treatment with 200 mg daily. Seven patients relapsed on discontinuation of therapy. Remission was observed in patients who had received ketoconazole for 6–17 months.

Ketoconazole therapy of progressive coccidioidomycosis. Comparison of 400- and 800-mg doses and observations at higher doses. Galgiani JN, Stevens DA, Graybill JR, et al. Am J Med 1988;84:603–10.

A randomized clinical trial involving 112 patients with progressive pulmonary, skeletal, or soft tissue infections. Success rate was similar for the two groups; however, relapse rates were higher in those requiring doses of >400 mg. It was concluded that higher doses of ketoconazole offer little or no benefit for patients with nonmeningeal forms of the disease.

Ketoconazole treatment of coccidioidal meningitis. Graybill JR, Stevens DA, Galgiani JN, et al. Ann N Y Acad Sci 1988;544:488–96.

Fifteen patients with coccidioidal meningitis were treated with high-dose ketoconazole for up to 4 years. Five patients were treated with ketoconazole alone; the others received combination therapy with intrathecal amphotericin B. The clinical responses appeared to be similar.

THIRD LINE THERAPIES

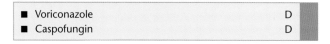

■ Voriconazole	D
■ Caspofungin	D

Successful treatment of coccidioidal meningitis with voriconazole. Cortez KJ, Walsh TJ, Bennett JE. Clin Infect Dis 2003;36:1619–22.

Case report of a 47-year-old male with coccidioidal meningitis successfully treated with voriconazole after failure to respond to fluconazole treatment. This patient developed a photosensitivity reaction after 10 weeks of treatment, which improved on lowering the dose.

Successful treatment of disseminated nonmeningeal coccidioidomycosis with voriconazole. Prabhu RM, Bonnell M, Currier BL, Orenstein R. Clin Infect Dis 2004; 39:e74–7.

Report of an adult male with disseminated nonmeningeal coccidioidomycosis, unsuccessfully treated with both amphotericin B deoxycholate and liposomal amphotericin B, who responded to voriconazole therapy.

Treatment of meningeal coccidioidomycosis with caspofungin. Hsue G, Napier JT, Prince RA, et al. Antimicrob Chemother 2004;54:292–4.

Use of the echinocandins (caspofungin) in the treatment of disseminated coccidioidomycosis in a renal transplant recipient. Antony S. Clin Infect Dis 2004;39:879–80.

Newer systemic antifungal agents: pharmacokinetics, safety and efficacy. Boucher HW, Groll AH, Chiou CC, Walsh TJ. Drugs 2004;64:1997–2020.

Caspofungin (the first available echinocandin) and voriconazole (the first available second-generation triazole) have greatly expanded the antifungal armamentarium available to physicians in the treatment of life-threatening systemic fungal infections.

A very good review.

Cryptococcosis

Wanda Sonia Robles

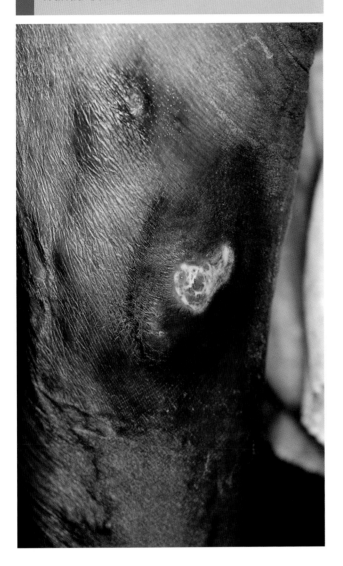

Cryptococcosis is an acute, subacute, or chronic infection caused by an encapsulated yeast known as *Cryptococcus neoformans* which is a significant human pathogen. There are two variants of this fungus: *C. neoformans* var. *neoformans* (seen in all patients including those with HIV) and *C. neoformans* var. *gattii* (rare in AIDS patients). Clinical presentation varies from localized to disseminated disease and the organism has a marked predisposition for the brain and meninges even when occasionally the skin and other organs may also be involved.

It is most commonly seen in patients with AIDS or other forms of immunodeficiency, including those receiving immunosuppressive treatment, renal or liver transplant recipients, and patients with hematologic malignancies, but it can occur in the immunocompetent host. Cutaneous manifestations are usually due to disseminated cryptococcosis. Primary cutaneous infections by inoculation are quite exceptional. Cutaneous lesions in the disseminated disease may precede or follow the signs of systemic involvement of the central nervous system (CNS) and lungs. Clinical features include mucous membrane lesions, cystic slow-growing subcutaneous or verrucous nodules, cellulitis,

molluscum-like lesions, acneiform papules or pustules, erythematous indurated plaques, or even punched-out ulcers with rolled edges.

MANAGEMENT STRATEGY

Cryptococcal infection, if left untreated, is a fatal disease. Optimal treatment very much depends on whether the patient has AIDS. In non-AIDS cryptococcal infection, the main treatment is *intravenous amphotericin B* at a dose of 0.3 mg/kg daily, combined with *oral flucytosine* at a dose of 150 mg/kg daily (depending on renal function) for a period of 6 weeks. This combination should be used in most cases, except in patients known to have cryptococcal infections especially localized to the skin with no evidence of systemic involvement after investigation. In the latter patients, *fluconazole* at a dose of 400–600 mg daily may be of benefit. Treatment of cryptococcal infection in AIDS is more complicated, as these patients are always at risk of recurrence and therefore maintenance therapy is necessary. In these patients, initial treatment is with amphotericin B, with or without flucytosine, for 7–14 days, with good initial remission. This is followed by long-term maintenance treatment with oral fluconazole 200–400 mg daily. There is now evidence that it may be possible to stop therapy in AIDS patients receiving highly active antiretroviral therapy (HAART), provided the CD4 cell count increases to in excess of 100 cells/μL while receiving HAART. *Itraconazole* has also been reported as an alternative for long-term treatment. In view of its rarity, prevention of cryptococcosis in the general population is not necessary. Suppressive treatment is also necessary in the case of immunocompromised non-AIDS patients. Be aware of the possibility of cryptococcosis in patients receiving treatment with infliximab.

Both fluconazole and itraconazole have been advocated for consolidation therapy in AIDS patients.

SPECIFIC INVESTIGATIONS

- Direct microscopy plus India ink or nigrosin stains to demonstrate cryptococcal capsules
- Culture and demonstration of pigmentation on Niger seed agar
- Cryptococcal antigen test (by latex agglutination or ELISA)
- Presence of mucopolysaccharide capsule staining with mucicarmine in histology
- Serology for HIV/AIDS

Cutaneous cryptococcosis in a patient with cutaneous T-cell lymphoma receiving therapy with photopheresis and methotrexate. Frieden TR, Bia FJ, Heald PW, et al. Clin Infect Dis 1993;17:776–8.

Report of a patient with advanced cutaneous T cell lymphoma who developed disseminated mainly pulmonary and cutaneous cryptococcosis after receiving therapy with photopheresis and methotrexate twice weekly.

Cellulitis as first clinical presentation of disseminated cryptococcosis in renal transplant recipients. Horrevorts AM, Huysmans FT, Koopman RJ, Meis JF. Scand J Infect Dis 1994;26:623–6.

Two renal transplant patients with cellulitis treated empirically for presumed bacterial erysipelas without response were described as having cellulitis due to *C. neoformans*. In both cases, the cellulitis was the presenting feature of disseminated cryptococcosis.

Cutaneous cryptococcosis in a diabetic renal transplant recipient. Gupta RK, Khan ZU, Nampoory MR, et al. J Med Microbiol 2004;53:445–9.

Case report of a diabetic renal transplant patient who developed cellulitis and was successfully treated with AmBisome followed by fluconazole. Diagnosis and correct treatment resulted in complete resolution of the condition.

Cutaneous cryptococcosis mimicking bacterial cellulitis in a liver transplant recipient: case report and review in solid organ transplant recipients. Singh N, Rihs JD, Gayowski T, Yu VL. Clin Transplant 1994;8:365–8.

Report of a liver transplant recipient presenting with pain and edema of the lower leg including his foot, with erythema and heat. Evidence of cryptococcal cellulitis was found, but the clinical presentation was indistinguishable from an acute bacterial cellulitis. The patient went on to develop concomitant cryptococcal septic arthritis, with evidence of cryptococcal antigen in the synovial fluids.

Cryptococcal necrotizing fasciitis with multiple sites of involvement in the lower extremities. Basaran O, Emiroglu R, Arikan U, et al. Dermatol Surg 2003;29:1158–60.

Case report of necrotizing fasciitis of the legs caused by *C. neoformans* in a renal transplant patient. Treatment was successfully carried out with AmBisome for 21 days, followed by oral itraconazole 200 mg daily. On discharge, the patient was continued on oral fluconazole for a total of 6 weeks.

Cryptococcal cellulitis in a patient on prednisone monotherapy for myasthenia gravis. Lafleur L, Beaty S, Colome-Grimmer MI, et al. Cutis 2004;74:165–70.

Cellulitis is a rare manifestation of cutaneous cryptococcosis, and certainly, this should be included in the differential diagnosis of cellulitis in patients on low-dose steroids who do not respond to antibiotic treatment.

Cutaneous manifestations of disseminated cryptococcosis. Dimino-Emme L, Gurevitch AW. J Am Acad Dermatol 1995;32:844–50.

Description of seven patients with disseminated cryptococcosis with a range of cutaneous manifestations. AIDS was confirmed as a predisposing factor in six of these patients. Response to treatment was recorded as variable with amphotericin B, flucytosine, and fluconazole.

Cutaneous cryptococcosis in corticosteroid-treated patients without AIDS. Vandersmissen G, Meuleman L, Tits G, et al. Acta Clin Belg 1996;51:111–7.

Two non-AIDS patients on immunosuppressive treatment with corticosteroids were described as having developed subcutaneous cryptococcal infection. Successful treatment was carried out with oral fluconazole for 6 weeks.

Cutaneous cryptococcosis mimicking basal cell carcinoma in a patient with AIDS. Ingleton R, Koestenblatt E, Don P, et al. J Cutan Med Surg 1998;3:43–5.

Report of a case of subcutaneous cryptococcosis with multiple lesions mimicking basal cell carcinoma in a patient with AIDS. There was no evidence of systemic involvement.

Cryptococcosis: an unusual opportunistic infection complicating B-cell lympho-proliferative disorders. Melzer M, Colbridge M, Keenan F, et al. J Infect 1998;36:220–2.

Report of two patients with Waldenstrom's macroglobulinemia and chronic lymphocytic leukemia who developed cryptococcosis and were successfully treated with systemic amphotericin B and flucytosine.

Large crusted ulceration of the scalp: first manifestation of cryptococcosis in an AIDS patient. Nicolas C, Truchetet F, Christian B, et al. Ann Dermatol Venereol 2000;127:188–90.

Report of a case of cutaneous cryptococcosis localized to the scalp, possibly as a first manifestation of AIDS. The patient was successfully treated with fluconazole.

Clinical presentation of primary cutaneous cryptococcosis may be misleading and it may also be the first sign in immunocompromised patients.

Cryptococcosis during systemic glucocorticosteroid treatment. Lauerma AI, Jeskanen L, Rantanen T, et al. Dermatology 1999;199:180–2.

Report of a patient on treatment with systemic steroids for 4 years for lung sarcoidosis. The patient developed a papular eruption, which became ulcerated. Histologic examination of a skin biopsy showed granulomatous inflammation and this was treated as sarcoidosis without success. After 1 year, a biopsy was repeated and skin fungal culture revealed the presence of *C. neoformans*. The patient was successfully treated with amphotericin B and flucytosine and this was then followed by treatment with fluconazole.

FIRST LINE THERAPIES

■ Amphotericin B	C
■ Flucytosine plus amphotericin B (flucytosine levels should be monitored)	B
■ Fluconazole	A

Combination antifungal therapies for HIV-associated cryptococcal meningitis: a randomised trial. Brouwer AE, Rajanuwong A, Chierakul W, et al. Lancet 2004;363:1764–7.

A randomized controlled trial to assess the fungicidal activity of combinations of amphotericin B, flucytosine, and fluconazole for the treatment of cryptococcosis. The study concluded that clearance of crytococci from the CSF was exponential and significantly faster with amphotericin B plus flucytosine than with amphotericin B alone, amphotericin B plus fluconazole, or triple therapy.

Cryptococcosis in human immunodeficiency virus-negative patients in the era of effective azole therapy. Pappas PG, Perfect JR, Cloud GA, et al. Clin Infect Dis 2001;33:690–9.

A multicenter case study of HIV-negative patients with cryptococcosis from 1990 to 1996. Patients with pulmonary disease were administered fluconazole and patients with CNS disease usually received amphotericin B. Two-thirds of these latter patients also received fluconazole for consolidation therapy. Therapy was reported as successful in 74% of patients. The overall mortality was 30% and mortality due to cryptococcosis was 12%.

Fluconazole therapy for cryptococcosis in non-AIDS patients. Yamaguchi H, Ikemoto H, Watanabe K, et al. Eur J Clin Microbiol Infect Dis 1996;15:787–92.

Multicenter study involving 44 patients with cryptococcal infection without AIDS. Treatment evaluated was fluconazole 200–400 mg daily. The overall clinical response rate was 89%: 48% clinical cure and 41% clinically improved.

A multicentre, randomized, double-blind, placebo-controlled trial of primary cryptococcal meningitis prophylaxis in HIV-infected patients with severe immune deficiency. Chetchotisakd P, Sungkanuparph S, Thinkhamrop B, et al. HIV Med 2004;5:140–3.

This multicenter, randomized, controlled trial was set up to assess the efficacy and survival benefit of low-dose fluconazole (400 mg weekly) for primary prophylaxis of cryptococcal meningitis in patients with advanced HIV infection. The study concluded that this regimen certainly suggested survival benefits. The study involved 90 patients and undoubtedly a larger study is recommended to confirm these findings.

Adverse effects of a higher dosage of amphotericin B therapy for cryptococcal meningitis in patients with HIV infection. Hsieh SM, Hung C, Chen MY, et al. J Microbiol Immunol Infect 1998;31:233–9.

This study involved 13 patients with advanced HIV infection. Amphotericin B was used at the dose of 0.8–1.0 mg/kg daily for 26 days. The success rate was 85%.

A higher dose of amphotericin B can be successful in treatment of cryptococcal infection, even in AIDS patients with poor prognostic factors.

A prospective study of AIDS-associated cryptococcal meningitis in Thailand treated with high-dose amphotericin B. Pitisuttithum P, Tansuphasawadikul S, Simpson AJ, et al. J Infect 2001;43:226–33.

A prospective study carried out in adults with cryptococcal meningitis associated with AIDS. High-dose amphotericin B (0.7 mg/kg daily) followed by oral azole treatment were used to determine the kinetics of cryptococci in CSF and prognostic factors affecting survival. The study concluded that high-dose amphotericin B is not as effective as previously thought, with cumulative mortality at 2 weeks, 4 weeks, and 1 year of 16%, 24%, and 76%, respectively.

SECOND LINE THERAPIES

■ Flucytosine (controversial)	B
■ Flucytosine plus fluconazole	C
■ Itraconazole	B
■ Voriconazole	B

Voriconazole treatment for less-common, emerging, or refractory fungal infections. Perfect JR, Marr KA, Walsh TJ, et al. Clin Infect Dis 2003;36:1122–31.

A multicenter, controlled, clinical trial to assess the efficacy, tolerability, and safety of voriconazole as salvage treatment for patients with refractory and intolerant-to-treatment fungal infections, as well as primary treatment for patients with infections for which there is no approved treatment. The efficacy rate for voriconazole in the treatment of cryptococcosis was 38.9%. Voriconazole was reported to be well tolerated, and discontinuation of treatment was observed only in less than 10% of patients.

Flucytosine therapy for cryptococcosis. Hospenthal ER, Bennet GH. Clin Infect Dis 1998;27:260–4.

A retrospective review of 27 patients treated with flucytosine monotherapy between 1968 and 1973. Flucytosine therapy was associated with an overall response rate of 43%; 57% failed to respond. Resistance was noted to have developed in isolates from six (50%) of 12 patients for whom therapy failed. This study showed that the treatment was well tolerated and that failure was not invariably associated with the development of resistance. However, this is a recognized risk.

Successful treatment of disseminated cryptococcosis in a liver transplant recipient with fluconazole and flucytosine, an all oral regimen. Singh N, Gayowski T, Marino IR. Transpl Int 1998;11:63–5.

Case report of the use of fluconazole 800 mg daily plus flucytosine also administered orally. Serology became negative at 6 weeks of treatment.

A controlled trial of itraconazole as primary prophylaxis for systemic fungal infections in patients with advanced human immunodeficiency virus infection in Thailand. Chariyalertsak S, Supparatpinyo K, Sirisanthana T, Nelson KE. Clin Infect Dis 2002;34:277–84.

In this prospective, double-blind trial, 129 patients with HIV infection and CD4+ lymphocyte counts of <200 cells/μL were randomized to receive either oral itraconazole 200 mg daily or a matched placebo. The study concluded that primary prophylaxis with oral itraconazole is well tolerated and prevents both cryptococcosis and *Penicillium marneffei* infection in patients with advanced HIV infection. However, it was not associated with a survival advantage in patients with advanced HIV disease.

The efficacy of fluconazole 600 mg/day versus itraconazole 600 mg/day as consolidation therapy of cryptococcal meningitis in AIDS patients. Mootsikapun P, Chetchotisakd P, Anunnatsiri S, Choksawadphinyo K. J Med Assoc Thai 2003;86:293–8.

In this trial, HIV-infected patients with primary cryptococcal meningitis who had been treated with amphotericin B for 2 weeks were randomized to receive either fluconazole 600 mg daily or itraconazole 600 mg daily for 10 weeks. The results indicated that treatment with either fluconazole or itraconazole at the dose of 600 mg daily has the same efficacy in AIDS patients suffering from cryptococcal meningitis. In addition, the results were suggestive that the higher-dose regimens may be superior to treatment regimens using lower doses of these medications.

Pulmonary cryptococcosis after initiation of anti-tumor necrosis factor-alpha therapy. Hage CA, Wood KL, Winer-Muram HT, et al. Chest 2003;124:2395–7.

Pneumonia due to *Cryptococcus neoformans* in a patient receiving infliximab: possible zoonotic transmission from

a pet cockatiel. Shrestha RK, Stoller JK, Honari G, et al. Respir Care 2004;49:606–8.

Cavitating pneumonia after treatment with infliximab and prednisone. Arend SM, Kujiper EJ, Allaart CF, et al. Eur J Clin Microbiol Infect Dis 2004;23:638–41.

These three papers highlight the increasing incidence of pulmonary disease in patients receiving infliximab.

Practice guidelines for cryptococcal disease. Infectious Diseases Society of America. Saag MS, Graybill RJ, Larsen RA, et al. Clin Infect Dis 2000;30:710–8.

A subcommittee of the National Institute of Allergy and Infectious Diseases (NIAID) Mycoses Study Group evaluated available data on the treatment of cryptococcal infection. The choice of treatment was based on both the anatomic site of involvement and the immune status of the host. For immunocompetent hosts with symptomatic infection, recommended treatment is fluconazole 200–400 mg daily for 36 months; this includes patients with non-CNS involvement, a positive serum cryptococcal antigen titer >1:8, or urinary tract or cutaneous disease. For patients unable to tolerate fluconazole, itraconazole 200–400 mg daily for 6–12 months is an alternative. For patients with more severe disease, amphotericin B 0.5–1 mg/kg daily for 6–10 weeks is recommended. For immunocompetent hosts with CNS disease, standard therapy comprises amphotericin B 0.7–1.0 mg/kg daily plus flucytosine 100 mg/kg daily for 6–10 weeks. An alternative regimen is amphotericin B 0.7–1.0 mg/kg daily plus flucytosine 100 mg/kg daily for 2 weeks, followed by fluconazole 400 mg daily for a minimum of 10 weeks. Fluconazole 'consolidation' therapy may be continued for as long as 6–12 months, depending on the clinical status of the patient. Non-HIV immunocompromised hosts should be treated in the same way as those with CNS disease, regardless of the site of involvement. For HIV patients with isolated pulmonary or urinary tract disease, fluconazole 200–400 mg daily is indicated. It is recommended that all HIV-infected individuals continue prophylactic treatment for life. In individuals unable to tolerate fluconazole, itraconazole 200–400 mg daily is an alternative. For patients with more severe disease, a combination of fluconazole 400 mg daily plus flucytosine 100–150 mg/kg daily may be used for 10 weeks, followed by fluconazole maintenance treatment.

Patients with HIV infection and cryptococcal meningitis, induction therapy with amphotericin B 0.7–1.0 mg/kg daily plus flucytosine 100 mg/kg daily for 2 weeks, followed by fluconazole 400 mg daily for a minimum of 10 weeks, is the treatment of choice. After 10 weeks of treatment, the dose of fluconazole may be reduced to 200 mg daily.

Amphotericin B in lipid formulations can be used for patients with renal impairment. An alternative to the use of amphotericin B is fluconazole 400–800 mg daily plus flucytosine 100–250 mg/kg daily for 6 weeks. It is worth noting that toxicity with this regimen is high.

Cutaneous larva migrans

Bridgette Cave, Anthony Abdullah

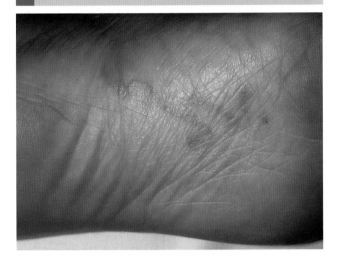

Cutaneous larva migrans (CLM) is a cutaneous lesion produced by percutaneous penetration and migration of larvae of various nematodes, mainly *Ancylostoma braziliense*, *A. caninum*, *Uncinaria stenocephala*, *Bunostonum phlebotomum*, *Ancylostoma duodenale* and *Necator americanus*. The clinical picture is that of characteristic erythema and serpiginous, sinuous, macular or papular linear lesions due to the presence of moving parasites. The common sites involved are the feet, hands and buttock, and people at risk include plumbers, pest controllers, farm workers, sea bathers, and children playing in sandpits.

MANAGEMENT STRATEGY

Cutaneous larva migrans is self-limiting: most lesions resolve after 1–3 months because the human is a 'dead-end host'. Usually, however, the lesions are extremely itchy, and can be extensive so treatment is often required. There are topical and systemic treatment options. Topical treatment usually takes the form of *thiabendazole* in a suitable lipophilic vehicle. The systemic treatments that are normally utilized by the authors include oral *albendazole* 400 mg daily for 3 days. Another option that may be considered as an alternative, second line therapy is *ivermectin*, given as a single dose of 12 mg orally. *Cryotherapy* using liquid nitrogen is rarely effective because larvae may not be killed by freezing.

SPECIFIC INVESTIGATIONS

- Clinical appearance is characteristic.

FIRST LINE THERAPIES

■ Topical thiabendazole in a lipophilic vehicle	D
■ Systemic albendazole	B

Efficacy and tolerability of thiabendazole in a lipophil vehicle for cutaneous larva migrans. Chatel G, Scolari C, Gulletta M, et al. Arch Dermatol 2000;136:1174–5.

A small series of patients treated with a lipophilic formulation of thiabendazole. The treatment consisted of topical applications (twice daily for 5 days) of 15% thiabendazole (prepared by crushing the tablets of thiabendazole in the lipophilic base ointment) in a lipophilic vehicle of base fat cream (24 g) and dimethyl sulfoxide gel (35 g). All patients experienced a clinical resolution within a median of 48 h after the beginning of treatment. No adverse effects and no recurrence had occurred in any patient at 3-month follow-up.

Treatment with topical thiabendazole ointment at 10–15% concentration in a hydrophilic vehicle has shown 98% efficacy within a median of 10 days of treatment and with no contraindications.

Cutaneous larva migrans: clinical features and management of 44 cases presenting in the returning traveller. Blackwell V, Vega-Lopez F. Br J Dermatol 2001;145:434–7.

Five patients received 10% thiabendazole cream topically for 10 days and four were cured. Thirty-one patients received oral albendazole 400 mg daily for 3–5 days and 24 were cured (77%). Four needed no treatment.

Treatment of larva migrans cutanea (creeping eruption): a comparison between albendazole and traditional therapy. Albanese G, Venturi C, Galbiati G. Int J Dermatol 2001;40: 67–71.

Experience of treating 56 patients of which 34 received oral albendazole. A prompt and definitive cure was achieved in all 56. The therapeutic effectiveness of the various methods was equivalent, but in the study's opinion albendazole should be considered the first choice because it was extremely well tolerated and patient compliance was good. Of the other patients 13 received cryotherapy, six oral thiabendazole, two cryotherapy and albendazole, and one cryotherapy and thiabendazole.

Effectiveness of a new therapeutic regimen with albendazole in cutaneous larva migrans. Veraldi S, Rizzitelli G. Eur J Dermatol 1999;9:352–3.

Twenty-four adult Caucasian patients were treated with oral albendazole according to a new therapeutic regimen (400 mg/day for 7 days). No other topical or systemic drug was used, nor any physical treatment. All patients were cured at the end of the therapy. No recurrence was observed. No side effects were reported, nor was any laboratory abnormality recorded.

Perianal cutaneous larva migrans in a child. Grassi A, Angelo C, Grossa MG, Paradisi M. Pediatr Dermatol 1998; 15:367–9.

The authors suggest that the oral administration of albendazole is safe and effective in children.

SECOND LINE THERAPIES

■ Systemic ivermectin	B

A randomized trial of ivermectin versus albendazole for the treatment of cutaneous larva migrans. Caumes E, Carriere J, Datry A, et al. Am J Trop Med Hyg 1993;49:641–4.

A comparison of efficacy between oral ivermectin (12 mg) and oral albendazole (400 mg). Twenty-one patients were randomly assigned to receive ivermectin (n = 10) or albendazole (n = 11). All patients who received ivermectin responded and none relapsed (cure rate 100%). All except one patient in the group receiving albendazole responded, but five relapsed after a mean of 11 days (cure rate 46%; p = 0.017). No major adverse effects were observed. The authors suggest that a single 12 mg dose of ivermectin is more effective than a single 400 mg dose of albendazole.

Cutaneous larva migrans in travellers: a prospective study, with assessment of therapy with ivermectin. Bouchaud O, Houze S, Schiemann R, et al. Clin Infect Dis 2000;31:493–8.

An update of epidemiologic data and evaluation of therapeutic efficacy of ivermectin (a single dose of 200 μg/kg was used). Sixty-four patients were studied. The initial diagnosis was wrong in 55% of patients. The cure rate after a single dose of ivermectin was 77%. For 14 patients, one or two supplementary doses were necessary, and the overall cure rate was 97%. The median times required for pruritus to disappear and lesions to resolve were 3 and 7 days, respectively. No systemic adverse effects were reported. Single-dose ivermectin therapy appears to be effective and well tolerated, although several treatments are sometimes necessary.

Treatment of 18 children with scabies or cutaneous larva migrans using ivermectin. Del Mar Saez-De-Ocariz M, McKinster CD, Orozco-Covarrubias L, et al. Clin Exp Dermatol 2002;27:264–7.

Eighteen children (aged 14 months to 17 years) of which seven had CLM. All seven were cured with a single dose of ivermectin with no significant adverse effects. In the authors' experience ivermectin is a safe and effective alternative treatment of cutaneous parasitosis in children.

THIRD LINE THERAPIES

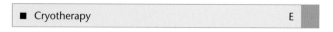
| ■ Cryotherapy | E |

Treatment of larva migrans cutanea (creeping eruption): a comparison between albendazole and traditional therapy. Albanese G, Venturi C, Galbiati G. Int J Dermatol 2001;40: 67–71.

As mentioned under albendazole, 13 patients in this study received cryotherapy treatment alone and all were cured.

Studies relating to creeping eruption. Hitch JM, Iralu V. South Med J 1960;53:447–53.

One method of treating CLM involves freezing with liquid nitrogen. This is rarely effective, however, because the larvae are ahead of the advancing track and can be missed, and because larvae may not be killed by freezing (larvae survived 5 min of exposure to −25°C in this study).

Evidence levels **A** Double-blind study **B** Clinical trial ≥ 20 subjects **C** Clinical trial < 20 subjects **D** Series ≥ 5 subjects **E** Anecdotal case reports

Darier's disease

Susan M Cooper, Susan M Burge

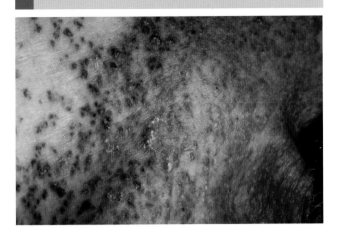

Darier's disease is an uncommon cutaneous disease characterized by persistent greasy, hyperkeratotic papules. It is inherited as an autosomal dominant trait. A mutation in a gene on chromosome 12q23–q24 that encodes for a sarco/endoplasmic reticulum calcium ATPase pump (SERCA 2) is causative in both generalized and localized disease.

MANAGEMENT STRATEGY

The warty, keratotic papules, which usually appear before the age of 20, can be malodorous, irritate, and look unsightly. The flexures can be a particular problem, as plaques here are frequently hypertrophic and may smell very unpleasant. Initial treatment is aimed at controlling irritation. *Simple emollients, soap substitutes,* and *topical corticosteroid* creams are helpful. Keeping the skin cool by wearing comfortable pure cotton clothing helps. Sunblock is recommended for those with a history of photoaggravation.

In mild disease or linear disease reflecting a genetic mosaicism, *topical retinoids* may be sufficient. These include topical isotretinoin (0.05% and 0.1%), tretinoin cream, and tazarotene gel. Treatment is applied on alternate days to begin with, increasing to once daily if possible, as irritation is common. The addition of a topical corticosteroid (alternating with the retinoid) may alleviate some of the side effects. Superinfection with viruses and bacteria is frequent, so combined corticosteroid/antibiotic preparations are logical.

In more extensive disease, an *oral retinoid* is required. Etretinate, acitretin, and isotretinoin are effective. Teratogenicity is a problem and pregnancy is contraindicated for 2 years after stopping treatment with etretinate or acitretin and 1 month with isotretinoin. For this reason, isotretinoin is the usual choice in women of childbearing age. Treatment may be given either long term or as intermittent short courses. The usual starting dose of acitretin is 10–25 mg daily but this can be increased gradually. Isotretinoin is usually started at 0.5–1.0 mg/kg daily. In the UK, etretinate is only available on a named patient basis but may work where other retinoids have failed.

The rare vesiculobullous form of the disease may respond to *prednisolone.* Hypertrophic flexural disease, unresponsive to retinoids, may require surgery. A variety of

surgical approaches have been tried, including *electrosurgery, debridement,* and *laser.* Recurrence is a problem.

SPECIFIC INVESTIGATIONS

- Skin biopsy. The characteristic finding is focal acantholytic dyskeratosis. The acantholysis is suprabasal.
- Skin swab for bacterial and viral culture if infection is suspected.

Darier-White disease: a review of the clinical features in 163 patients. Burge SM, Wilkinson JD. J Am Acad Dermatol 1992;27:40–50.

Fourteen percent of patients in this series had herpes simplex complicating their Darier's disease.

Painful blisters arising in the typical lesions of Darier's disease are usually due to secondary infection with Staphylococcus aureus *or herpes simplex.*

FIRST LINE THERAPIES

■ Cool cotton clothing	E
■ Emollients	D
■ Topical retinoids	D

Management of Darier's disease. Burge S. Clin Exp Dermatol 1999;24:53–6.

A review of current treatments. Simple measures such as emollients and cotton clothing are stressed. The importance of counseling is highlighted.

In most genetic diseases, genetic counseling is important. Written information is often appreciated. Patient support groups – for example, DARDIS in the UK – can provide useful information.

Darier's disease. Cooper SM, Burge SM. Am J Clin Dermatol 2003;4:97–105.

A detailed review of the current management of Darier's disease.

Tazarotene gel for Darier's disease. Burkhart CG, Burkhart CN. J Am Acad Dermatol 1998;38:1001–2.

A single case report of Darier's disease responding to topical 0.05% tazarotene gel within 3 months. Tazarotene was alternated with a weak topical corticosteroid to reduce irritation.

Tazarotene gel in childhood Darier's disease. Micali G, Nasca MR. Pediatr Dermatol 1000;16:603–4.

Two childhood cases were treated successfully. Lesions resolved after 2 weeks, but the duration of remission was not given.

Topical isotretinoin in Darier's disease. Burge SM, Buxton PK. Br J Dermatol 1995;133:924–8.

Six of 11 patients improved when a test patch was treated with 0.05% isotretinoin. Erythema, burning, and irritation were common.

Acral Darier's disease successfully treated with adapalene. Cianchini G, Colonna L, Camaioni D, et al. Acta Derm Venereol 2001;81:57–8.

A single case report of acral Darier's disease responding to a synthetic retinoid, adapalene 0.1% gel. Lesions cleared after 4 weeks of treatment on the hands and 6 weeks on the soles.

SECOND LINE THERAPIES

■ Oral retinoids	B
■ Topical 5-fluorouracil	E

The efficacy of an aromatic retinoid, Tigason (etretinate), in the treatment of Darier's disease. Burge SM, Wilkinson JD, Miller AJ, Ryan TJ. Br J Dermatol 1981;104:675.

Seventeen of 18 patients benefited from etretinate, using doses of between 0.5 and 1.0 mg/kg.

Clinical and ultrastructural effects of acitretin in Darier's disease. Lauharanta J, Kanerva L, Turjanmaa K, Geiger JM. Acta Derm Venereol 1988;68:492–8.

Thirteen patients were treated with acitretin starting at 30 mg daily. Duration of treatment was 16 weeks. All showed some improvement, but side effects included itching (five patients) and hair loss (two patients).

Isotretinoin treatment of Darier's disease. Dicken CH, Bauer EA, Hazen PG, et al. J Am Acad Dermatol 1982;6(4 Pt 2 Suppl):721–6.

This multicenter open study assessed the effect of short and longer courses of treatment. The starting dose was 0.5 mg/kg, but longer courses were adjusted according to symptoms. Isotretinoin was very effective, but did not give long-term remission. Some patients were maintained on alternate-day or alternate-week regimens.

A double-blind comparison of acitretin and etretinate in the treatment of Darier's disease. Christopherson J, Geiger JM, Danneskiold-Samsoe P. Acta Derm Venereol 1992;72:150–2.

This small study compared the efficacy of treatment with acitretin and etretinate. The initial dose of both drugs was 30 mg daily for the first month, but this was individually adjusted for the 12 further weeks of the study. No significant difference was seen between the two groups.

Etretinate may work where acitretin fails. Bleiker TO, Bourke JF, Graham-Brown RA, Hutchinson PE. Br J Dermatol 1997;136:368–70.

Two patients with Darier's disease unresponsive to acitretin responded to etretinate.

Skeletal hyperostosis and extraosseous calcification in patients receiving long-term etretinate. Wilson D, Kay V, Charig M, et al. Br J Dermatol 1988;119:597–607.

Retinoids can cause diffuse skeletal hyperostosis and extraosseous calcification.

It is not yet clear if radiologic screening is necessary for asymptomatic patients on long-term treatment, but it is prudent to inquire about musculoskeletal problems in these patients.

Retinoids have many side effects, including mucosal dryness and soreness, skin fragility, and itching. They may cause hepatic dysfunction and hyperlipidemia. Liver function, cholesterol, and triglycerides should be monitored during treatment.

Topical 5-fluorouracil in the treatment of Darier's disease. Knulst AC, Baart de la Faille H, Van Vloten WA. Br J Dermatol 1995;133:463–6.

Two cases with therapy-resistant Darier's disease responded to topical 5-fluorouracil. Both patients were also taking oral retinoids.

THIRD LINE THERAPIES

■ Cyclosporine (eczematization only)	E
■ Oral contraceptive pill	E
■ Supplementary dietary fatty acids	E
■ Oral prednisolone (vesiculobullous only)	E
■ Laser (CO_2 and erbium:YAG)	E
■ Dermabrasion	E
■ Debridement	E
■ Photodynamic therapy	E

Darier's disease: severe eczematization successfully treated with cyclosporin. Shahidullah H, Humphreys F, Beveridge GW. Br J Dermatol 1994;131:713–16.

Cyclosporine may be helpful in widespread eczematized Darier's disease; however, cyclosporine had no effect on the underlying disease.

Oral contraceptives in the treatment of Darier-White disease – a case report and review of the literature. Oostenbrink JH, Cohen EB, Steijlen PM, Van de Kerkhof PCM. Clin Exp Dermatol 1996;21:442–4.

Many women report premenstrual exacerbation of their symptoms and some, but not all, improve in pregnancy. This is a report of a female treated with the combined oral contraceptive pill (ethinyl estradiol 50 µg, levonorgestrel 125 µg) whose skin became less itchy and less fragile on treatment.

Essential fatty acids in the treatment of Darier's disease. du Plessis PJ, Jacyk WK. J Dermatol Treat 1998;9:97–101.

Thirteen out of 16 patients responded to fatty acid supplements. This interesting observation needs to be confirmed.

Vesiculobullous Darier's disease responsive to oral prednisolone. Speight EL. Br J Dermatol 1998;139:934–5.

A patient with the rare vesiculobullous form of the disease responded to a short course of oral prednisolone.

Oral steroids may also be useful in the eczematized form.

Carbon dioxide laser vaporization of recalcitrant symptomatic plaques of Hailey-Hailey disease and Darier's disease. McElroy JA, Mehregan DA, Roenigk RK. J Am Acad Dermatol 1990;23:893–7.

Two patients with chronic, localized plaques unresponsive to other treatments had a good response to laser vaporization.

Efficacy of erbium:YAG laser ablation in Darier disease and Hailey-Hailey disease. Beier C, Kaufmann R. Arch Dermatol 1999;135:423–7.

Complete resolution was achieved in two patients treated with this laser. Lesions treated were in the axillae, scapular, upper arm, extremities, and neck regions. Follow-up in both cases was under 2 years.

Evidence levels A Double-blind study **B** Clinical trial ≥ 20 subjects **C** Clinical trial < 20 subjects **D** Series ≥ 5 subjects **E** Anecdotal case reports

Electrosurgical treatment of etretinate-resistant Darier's disease. Toombs EL, Peck GL. J Dermatol Surg Oncol 1989;15:1277–80.

Electrosurgery was effective in two cases unresponsive to etretinate.

Dermabrasion in Darier's disease. Zachariae H. Acta Derm Venereol 1979;59:184–5.

Five patients with severe disease were treated by dermabrasion. The skin was dermabraded down to and including the papillary dermis. Three-quarters of the treated skin remained disease-free 6 months later. Facial treatment was less successful than treatment to the trunk area.

The surgical treatment of hypertrophic Darier's disease. Wheeland RG, Gilmore WA. J Dermatol Surg Oncol 1985;11:420–3.

Recalcitrant, hypertrophic lesions were debrided under local anesthesia. Symptomatic and cosmetic improvement was maintained for 2 years.

Treatment of Darier's disease with photodynamic therapy. Exadaktylou D, Kurwa HA, Calonje E, Barlow RJ. Br J Dermatol 2003;149:606–10.

Six patients received photodynamic therapy with topical 5-aminolaevulinic acid as a photosensitizer. One patient could not tolerate the treatment, but the remaining five experienced sustained improvement. All had an initial inflammatory response that lasted 2 to 3 weeks.

Darier disease: sustained improvement following reduction mammaplasty. Cohen PR. Cutis 2003;72:124–6.

A woman with large breasts and recalcitrant submammary disease experienced a dramatic and sustained improvement in her submammary disease after reduction mammaplasty.

Darier's disease, an unusual problem and solution. Sprowson AP, Jeffery SL, Black MJ. J Hand Surg 2004;29:293–5.

A woman with intolerable nail disease benefited from surgery to all 10 fingernails. An eponychial flap was raised and the nail complex excised. A full-thickness skin graft was obtained from the groin. This was sutured into place with the proximal border of the graft tucked under the eponychial fold.

Decubitus ulcers

Joseph A Witkowski, Lawrence Charles Parish, Jennifer L Parish

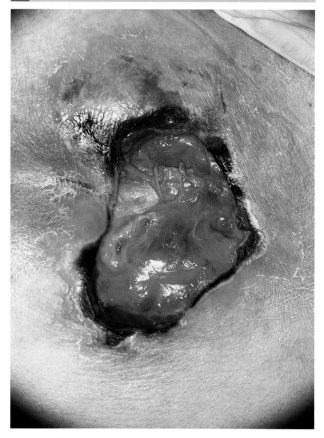

The decubitus ulcer represents a defect in the skin that can extend through the subcutaneous tissue and muscle layer to the underlying bone.

MANAGEMENT STRATEGY

Prevention

A patient in an ordinary bed who is at risk for developing a pressure sore should be repositioned at frequent intervals; however, the correct timing for turning has never been established. The regularity is determined by the level of risk for developing an ulcer and the duration of blanchable erythema. Pillows and foam wedges are used to maintain these positions and to keep bony prominences apart. Completely immobile patients should have their heels raised from the bed by a pillow or boot and not be placed on their trochanters, unless a specialized bed is utilized. To avoid the latter, use a 30° position from the horizontal lying on the side. The head of the bed should not be raised more than 30° from the horizontal for an extended period of time. Use lifting devices or draw sheets to reposition or to transfer patients, where possible. Finally, the patient should be placed on a pressure-reducing device such as foam, alternating air, gel or water mattress, when appropriate.

A patient sitting in a chair who is at risk for developing a decubitus ulcer should be repositioned frequently, perhaps every hour, and be taught to shift weight every 15 min. The wheelchair should be adjusted appropriately for each patient. A pressure-reducing device made of foam, gel, air, or a combination of each is indicated.

Despite these measures, many decubitus ulcers simply cannot be prevented.

Management

The management of skin lesions caused by pressure is based on four principles:

- elimination of relative pressure;
- removal of necrotic debris;
- maintenance of a moist wound environment;
- correction of the underlying contributing factors.

Elimination of sustained pressure

The patient should not lie on the ulcer. A patient who is at risk for developing additional ulcers and can assume a variety of positions without lying on the ulcer should be placed on a *static support surface (i.e. air, foam, or water)*. If the patient cannot assume various positions without laying on the ulcer or bottoms out while on a static surface, or if the ulcer does not heal after 2–4 weeks of optimal care, place the patient on *a dynamic support surface when possible (i.e. an alternating air overlay on the mattress, a low-air-loss bed, or an air-fluidized bed)*. If a patient has large deep ulcers (stage III or IV) on multiple sleep surfaces or has excess moisture on intact skin, use a low-air-loss bed or air-fluidized bed. A patient with an ulcer on the sitting surface should not sit, if possible.

Removal of necrotic debris

Surgical debridement is indicated for infected ulcers with necrotic debris and eschars other than those on the heel; however, the extent of tissue needed to be removed is highly variable. An eschar on the heel should be excised only if it is fluctuant, draining, or surrounded by cellulitis, and if the patient is septic.

Major debridement is performed in the operating room, but serial sharp debridement can be performed at the bedside. The use of *systemic antimicrobials* should be considered to prevent bacteremia during significant debridement. A *bone biopsy* is recommended while debriding ulcers when bone is exposed and for nonhealing deep ulcers (stage III or IV ulcers) after 2–4 weeks of optimal therapy.

Other ulcers can be *debrided by the use of saline wet to dry gauze* every 4–6 h or by the use of saline in a 35 mL syringe with an attached 19-gauge angiocatheter, or by whirlpool utilization. The use of enzymes should be reserved for ulcers that are not clinically infected. *Autolytic debridement* is indicated for noninfected ulcers that are not likely to become infected.

Debridement can also be indicated for staging of the ulcer. This assumes that staging is a requisite for treating the patient. While debridement is a useful therapeutic tool, complete elimination of necrotic tissue is unnecessary, as is daily surgical debridement.

Maintenance of a moist wound environment

The choice of a synthetic dressing depends on the presence of infection, amount of exudate, status of the periulcer skin and amount of pain experienced by the patient. *Saline dressings* and *alginates* are indicated for infected ulcers. *Synthetic*

Evidence levels A Double-blind study B Clinical trial ≥ 20 subjects C Clinical trial < 20 subjects D Series ≥ 5 subjects E Anecdotal case reports

dressings (i.e. films), are used on ulcers with minimal exudate, hydrocolloid wafers for moderate exudate, and foam wafers and alginates for ulcers with a large amount of exudate. Ulcers with fragile or dermatitic periulcer skin should be covered with hydrogel wafers or nonadherent foam wafers. All occlusive dressings relieve pain, but the hydrogel wafers are best for this purpose.

Correction of the underlying contributing factors

Patients may have associated illnesses that interfere with wound healing. Attention to the medical status is important. For example, diabetes mellitus, malnutrition, peripheral vascular disease, cardiac disease, malignancy, and even Alzheimer's disease may prevent any healing of an ulcer. Unfortunately, even the best of medical care may not permit healing. The clinician should keep in mind that the skin can fail just as any other organ in the body can fail.

General measures

Treatment of the decubitus ulcer can be simplified and made more effective, if the following recommendations are considered.

Saline should be used to clean most pressure lesions; soap and disinfectants are too irritating for more than occasional usage.

When ulcers are not infected, synthetic dressings should be changed only if they become dislodged or wound fluid escapes from under the dressing.

Periulcer skin must be kept dry not only to avoid maceration, but also to permit the dressing to adhere to the skin.

To obliterate dead space, loosely fill deep ulcers with a hydrocolloid, a hydrogel wound filler, or an alginate rope before applying a synthetic dressing. This same material should be placed under the edge of the ulcer when undermining is present. Bleeding after serial surgical debridement can often be controlled with an alginate dressing; the calcium alginate assists in the clotting pathway. Moistening with saline can loosen an alginate dressing that adheres to granulation tissue.

A clean ulcer that fails to show signs of healing or an ulcer with persistent excessive exudate, despite receiving optimal care, should be treated with an antibacterial agent (i.e. 1% silver sulfadiazine, cadexomer iodine, or triple antibiotic) for 2 weeks to decrease the bacterial burden. Increased bacterial burden may impede healing before clinical signs of infection become apparent. The odor of a malodorous ulcer can often be eliminated by application of metronidazole gel to the ulcer bed. Systemic antimicrobials are indicated for patients with bacteremia, sepsis, advancing cellulitis, or osteomyelitis.

Although most synthetic dressings relieve pain, treatment for moderate to severe pain can include topical anesthetics, nonsteroidal anti-inflammatory agents (NSAIDs), opiates, antidepressants and sedatives. Many patients with decubitus ulcers do not have pain.

Blanchable erythema and nonblanchable erythema

Blanchable erythema and nonblanchable erythema represent the initial development of the decubitus ulcer. The early lesions of nonblanchable erythema are bright red areas; later, they become dark red to purple. Both can be treated with adherent synthetic dressings, to protect the lesion from friction and shear, topical corticosteroids, or zinc oxide paste. The bright red lesion can also be treated with 2% nitroglycerin ointment – 0.5–1 cm of the ointment is applied over the lesion and covered with an impermeable plastic wrap (such as Saran®) for 12 h daily.

Decubitus dermatitis

Decubitus dermatitis is treated with topical corticosteroids, Vaseline® gauze, or a hydrogel wafer. Large bullae (when present) may be debrided before applying the dressing.

Superficial and deep ulcers

Superficial and deep ulcers without necrotic debris are treated with saline wet-to-wet gauze or an adherent synthetic dressing. Deep ulcers should be loosely filled with synthetic wound filler before applying a synthetic dressing. Ulcers that do not involve bone can also be treated with becaplermin gel and then packed with saline-moistened gauze once daily. The deep ulcer with necrotic debris requires debridement and then is treated as a clean ulcer.

Enzymatic debridement or the use of an antimetabolite can help manage the eschar. Covering the lesion with an adhesive occlusive dressing for several days will often soften the eschar before excision is undertaken. Faster softening can be accomplished by scarifying the lesion, applying an enzyme to the surface, and covering with an impermeable plastic wrap. The firmly adherent dry eschar that is not attached to underlying bone can often be separated from the surrounding skin with 5% 5-fluorouracil cream. After scarification and application of zinc oxide paste to protect the surrounding skin, 5-fluorouracil is applied to the eschar; including its margin, and then covered with an impermeable plastic wrap. Application is repeated every 8 h. When separation occurs, it can be excised.

Underlying contributing factors

Management of anemia, malnutrition, diabetes mellitus, and incontinence is essential. The patient should be ingesting approximately 30–35 calories/kg daily and 1.25–1.50 g protein/kg daily. Ascorbic acid 500 mg twice daily may enhance healing but this has not been proven. Keep in mind that the patient who is debilitated and has a multitude of other conditions may have no healing capabilities (skin failure).

SPECIFIC INVESTIGATIONS

- Categorize patient
- Stage decubitus ulcer
- Total protein, serum albumin
- Complete blood count

Clinical observation is the key to making the diagnosis. Cutaneous biopsies will not be helpful, although biopsies for aerobic and anaerobic bacteriological cultures could be useful if infection is suspected.

Categories of patients

Patients at risk need to be considered in terms of the underlying disease process:

- spinal cord injury in an otherwise healthy person;
- neurologic disease with no medical disease, but a devastating condition such as multiple sclerosis or a cerebral vascular accident compromising the body integrity;
- debilitation with a multitude of medical diseases affecting the patient (i.e. arteriosclerosis, diabetes mellitus, Parkinson's disease, Alzheimer's disease, malignancy, malnutrition and peripheral vascular disease);
- surgical procedures requiring lengthy positioning on the operating room table for cardiovascular or orthopedic procedures.

Grading or evaluation

Grading or evaluation can be accomplished by dermatologic observation and staging.

Dermatologic observation
Observe for:

- blanchable erythema;
- nonblanchable erythema;
- decubitus dermatitis;
- superficial ulcer;
- deep ulcer;
- eschar/gangrene.

Staging
Stages are as follows:

- stage I – nonblanchable erythema of intact skin;
- stage II – partial-thickness skin loss involving the epidermis and/or dermis;
- stage III – full-thickness skin loss with damage to the subcutaneous tissue that may extend down to, but not through, the underlying fascia;
- stage IV – full-thickness skin loss with extensive destruction, tissue necrosis or damage to muscle, bone or supporting structures.

Pressure sores among hospitalized patients. Allman RM, Laprade CA, Noel LB, et al. Ann Intern Med 1986;105:337–42.

Hypoalbuminemia, fecal incontinence, and fractures may identify bedridden patients at greatest risk for developing pressure ulcers.

Anaemia and serum protein alteration in patients with pressure ulcers. Fuoco U, Scivoletto G, Pace A, et al. Spinal Cord 1997;35:58–60.

All 40 patients with sacral pressure ulcers showed mild–moderate anemia with low serum iron and normal or increased ferritin and hypoproteinemia with albuminemia.

FIRST LINE THERAPIES

■ Eliminate pressure	C
■ Pressure reducing and relieving devices	C
■ Removal of necrotic debris	C
■ Maintenance of a moist wound environment	C
■ Synthetic dressings	B
■ Topical antibacterials	B
■ Nutrition	C
■ Dietary supplements	C

Eliminating pressure and relieving devices

An investigation of geriatric nursing problems in hospital. Norton D, McClaren R, Exton-Smith AN. London: Churchill Livingstone; 1975;238.

Patients who developed fewer pressure sores were those who were turned every 2–3 h.
This is based upon a book published in 1916.

Influence of 30 degrees laterally inclined position and the supersoft 3-piece mattress on areas of maximum pressure and implications for pressure sore prevention. Seiler WO, Allen S, Stahelin NB. Gerontology 1986;32:158–66.

When positioned directly on their trochanters, subjects had higher interface pressures and lower transcutaneous oxygen tension than when positioned off at an angle.

Shearing force as a factor in decubitus ulcers in paraplegics. Reichel SM. JAMA 1958;166:762–3.

As a result of shear, blood vessels in the sacral area become twisted and distorted, and the tissue may become ischemic and necrotic.

Drawsheets for prevention of decubitus ulcer. Witkowski JA, Parish LC. N Engl J Med 1981;305:1594.

Use of drawsheets decreased incidence of friction burns.

Decubitus prophylaxis: a prospective trial on the efficiency of alternating-pressure air mattresses and water mattresses. Andersen KE, Jensen O, Kvorning SA, Bach E. Acta Derm Venereol 1983;63:227–30.

The incidence of pressure ulcers in patients cared for on the hospital mattress was significantly greater than in patients on alternating-pressure air mattresses.

The effectiveness of preventive management in reducing the occurrence of pressure sores. Krouskop TA, Noble PC, Garber SL, Spencer WA. J Rehabil RD 1983;20:74–83.

Weight shifts are an effective means of reducing the risk of pressure ulcer formation.

Comparison of total body tissue interface pressure of specialized pressure-relieving mattresses. Hickerson WL, Slugocki GM, Thaker RL, et al. J Long Term Eff Med Implants 2004;14:81–94.

Pressure can be relieved by specialized mattresses and beds.

Mechanical loading and support surfaces. Agency for Health Care Policy and Research. Pressure ulcers in adults: prediction and prevention. Clinical Practice Guideline No. 3. May 1992. AHCPR Publ No. 92-0047.

An overview of pressure-relieving devices.

A clinical comparison of two pressure reducing surfaces in the management of pressure ulcers. Warner DJ. Decubitus 1992;5:52–5, 58–60, 62–4.

Pressure ulcers were shown to heal when a static support surface was used.

A randomized trial of low-air-loss beds for treatment of pressure ulcers. Ferrell BA, Osterweil D, Christenson PA. JAMA 1993;269:499–507.

Patients with pressure ulcers showed a significantly improved healing rate.

Evidence levels **A** Double-blind study **B** Clinical trial ≥ 20 subjects **C** Clinical trial < 20 subjects **D** Series ≥ 5 subjects **E** Anecdotal case reports

Air-fluidized beds or conventional therapy for pressure sores; a randomized trial. Allman RM, Walker JM, Hart MK, et al. Ann Intern Med 1987;107:641–8.

Patients with large pressure ulcers may benefit from the use of air-fluidized beds.

Lateral rotation mattresses for wound healing. Anderson C, Rappl L. Ostomy Wound Manage 2004;50:50–4,56,58.

Continuous lateral rotation therapy utilizes mattresses and beds that move the patient in a regular pattern around a longitudinal axis. In this study 10 patients with partial thickness ulcers healed in an average of 9.25 weeks and full-thickness ulcers healed in an average of 11.25 weeks.

Debridement

The care of decubitus ulcers, pressure ulcers. Michocki RJ, Lamy PP. J Geriatr Soc 1976;24;217–24.

The benefits of sharp debridement are based on expert opinion.

Debridement of cutaneous ulcer: medical and surgical aspects. Witkowski JA, Parish LC. Clin Dermatol 1991;9:585–93.

Debridement can be accomplished by cold steel cutting, by chemical application, or by autohemolytic destruction under an occlusive dressing.

Pressure ulcer treatment guide: quick reference guide for clinicians No. 15. Bergstrom N, Bennett MA, Carlson CE. Adv Wound Care 1995;6:22–44.

Histologic examination of bone biopsy specimens is the gold standard for diagnosing osteomyelitis.

Cleansing the traumatic wound by high pressure syringe irrigation. Stevenson TR, Thacker JG, Rodeheaver GT, et al. JACEP 1976;5:17–21.

Provides enough force to remove bacteria, other debris, and loosen eschar.

Conservation management of chronic wounds. Feedar JA, Kloth LC. In: Kloth LC, McCulloch JM, Feedar JA, eds. Wound healing; alternatives in management. Philadelphia: FA Davis; 1990.

More effective removal of debris can be accomplished by twice-daily wound treatment.

Collagenase in the treatment of dermal and decubitus ulcers. Rao DB, Sane PG, Georgiev EL. J Am Geriatr Soc 1975;23:22–30.

Enzymes can be used alone or in combination with other forms of debridement.

Dissolution of wound coagulum and promotion of granulation tissue under DuoDERM. Lydon MJ. Hutchinson JJ, Rippon M. Wounds 1989;1:95–106.

Enzymes normally present in wound fluid digest devitalized tissue when allowed to collect under a synthetic dressing for several days.

Antimicrobials

Relationship of quantitative wound bacterial counts to healing of decubiti: effect of topical gentamicin. Bendy RH Jr, Nuccio PA, Wolfe E, et al. Antimicrob Agents Chemother 1964;4:147–55.

Topical metronidazole gel: the bacteriology of decubitus ulcers. Witkowski JA, Parish LC. Int J Dermatol 1991;30:660–1.

Metronidazole gel eliminated the odor and anaerobic organisms.

Nutrition

The importance of dietary protein in healing pressure ulcers. Breslow RA, Hallfrisch J, Guy DG, et al. J Am Geriatr Soc 1993;4:357–62.

High protein with increased caloric contents may enhance pressure ulcer healing.

Ascorbic acid supplementation in the treatment of pressure sores. Taylor TV, Rimmer S, Day B, et al. Lancet 1974;11:544–6.

Healing was enhanced even in the absence of deficiency; however, in practice, this does not seem to be the case.

Old age, malnutrition, and pressure sores: an ill-fated alliance. Mathus-Vliegen EM. J Gerontol A Biol Sci Med Sci 2004;59:355–60.

Although vitamins A, B and C, proteins, and minerals such as zinc and copper promote healing in animal models, supplements of these offer disparate results in the clinic. The potential benefits of tube feeding may be lost due to diarrhea, bowel incontinence, and restricted mobility.

Nutritional interventions for preventing and treating pressure ulcers. Langer G, Schloemer G, Knerr A, et al. Cochrane Database Syst Rev 2003;4:CD003216.

There is no confirmation that enteral and/or parenteral nutrition prevents and/or promotes healing of decubitus ulcers.

SECOND LINE THERAPIES

■ Hydrocolloid wafer dressing	C

A comparison of the efficacy and cost-effectiveness of two methods of managing pressure ulcers. Colwell JC, Foreman MD, Trotter JP. Decubitus 1993;6:28–36.

A larger number of superficial and deep ulcers (stage II and III ulcers) healed with DuoDERM than with saline moist dressings.

THIRD LINE THERAPIES

■ Ketanserin ointment	B
■ Nitroglycerin ointment	D
■ Becaplermin gel	A
■ 5-Fluorouracil cream	D
■ Hyperbaric oxygen	E

Use of topical ketanserin in the treatment of skin ulcers: a double blind study. Janssen PA, Janssen H, Cauwenbergh G, et al. J Am Acad Dermatol 1989;21:85–90.

Ketanserin 2% was used topically in combination with routine measures in 25 patients with decubitus ulcers: there was a significant difference in healing rates in favor of ketanserin over placebo – 35% of ulcers were healed at 8 weeks compared to 15% in the placebo group.

Becaplermin gel in the treatment of pressure ulcers: a phase II randomized, double-blind, placebo-controlled study. Rees RS, Robson MC, Smiell JM, Perry BH. Wound Repair Regen 1999;7:141–7.

Recombinant human platelet-derived growth factor-BB (becaplermin, the active ingredient in Regranex®) gel in the treatment of chronic full-thickness pressure ulcers was compared with that of placebo gel. A total of 124 adults with pressure ulcers were assigned randomly to receive topical treatment with becaplermin gel 100 µg/g (n = 31) or 300 µg/g (n = 32) once daily alternated with placebo gel every 12 h, becaplermin gel 100 µg/g twice daily (n = 30), or placebo (n = 31) twice daily until complete healing was achieved or for 16 weeks. All treatment groups received a standardized regimen of good wound care throughout the study period. Once-daily treatment of chronic pressure ulcers with becaplermin gel 100 µg/g significantly reduced the median relative ulcer volume at endpoint compared with that of placebo gel (p < 0.025 for all comparisons). Becaplermin gel 300 µg/g did not result in a significantly greater incidence of healing than that observed with 100 µg/g.

Pressure ulcer accelerated healing with local injections of granulocyte macrophage-colony stimulating factor. El Saghir NS, Bizri AR, Shabb NS, et al. J Infect 1997; 35:179–82.

A single report of granulocyte macrophage-colony stimulating factor (GM-CSF) inducing accelerated healing of a sacral pressure ulcer in a bedridden patient with bilateral hemiplegia. GM-CSF was diluted and injected locally around and into the ulcer bed every 2–3 days for 2 weeks, then weekly for 4 weeks until complete healing occurred. New firm granulation tissue was noted within a few days. The ulcer showed 85% healing within 2 weeks and 100% by 2 months. The ulcer remained closed until the patient's sudden death 9 months later.

Hyperbaric oxygen therapy for chronic wounds. Kranke P, Bennett M, Roecki-Wiedmann I, Debus S. Cochrane Database Syst Rev 2004;2:CD004123.

There are no satisfactory studies available to prove that hyperbaric oxygen is useful in decubitus or arterial ulcers.

Evidence levels **A** Double-blind study   **B** Clinical trial ≥ 20 subjects   **C** Clinical trial < 20 subjects   **D** Series ≥ 5 subjects   **E** Anecdotal case reports

Delusions of parasitosis

Anjeli Krishnan, John Koo

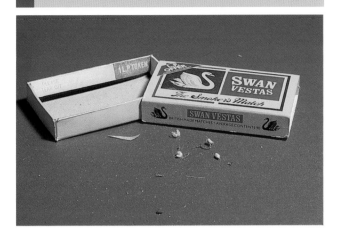

An uncommon primary psychiatric disorder, delusions of parasitosis is a form of monosymptomatic hypochondriacal psychosis, in which patients have a strong conviction that their skin is infested with parasites; this belief cannot be argued with reason, as is characteristic of most delusional disorders. No actual dermatologic disorder exists in these cases, or the patient grossly misinterprets an existing dermatologic condition, which is usually minor. Therefore, relatively normal skin can be altered by attempts to remove the perceived parasites. Many of these patients can have hallucinatory experiences as well that are compatible with their delusion. The common characteristic hallucinatory symptom these patients may experience is formication, which is manifested as sensations of cutaneous crawling, biting, or stinging. The condition has a bimodal age distribution, occurring in younger adults (both men and women) and the elderly (women more than men). The most common underlying psychopathologies in delusions of parasitosis are psychosis, depression, and anxiety; these can be severe enough to cause the patient to commit suicide.

MANAGEMENT STRATEGY

The physician should first establish *good patient rapport*. This begins with conducting a *thorough and complete skin examination*. A good skin examination sometimes entails deciding whether performing a biopsy may be worthwhile, if for no other reason than to maintain rapport with the patient. It is also important to rule out other conditions that may mimic delusions of parasitosis and cause symptoms of formication. For example, underlying neurologic disease such as multiple sclerosis, pernicious anemia (leading to vitamin B12 deficiency), and pellagra, other psychiatric illnesses such as schizophrenia, and substance abuse with cocaine or amphetamines should be excluded. In addition, delusions of parasitosis has been associated with certain endocrine diseases, especially hypothyroidism and diabetes mellitus, as well as with cardiovascular diseases, central nervous system dysfunctions, and hematologic disorders such as polycythemia vera. Finally, the presence of real skin disorders, such as

scabies and Grover's disease, should not be overlooked in the differential diagnosis of delusions of parasitosis. Also, the condition can develop after the patient, relative, or a pet has had a true parasitic infection, so ruling out the presence of a real infestation may be warranted. Importantly, when patients do not know the reason why they are itching, the clinician is wise to entertain a diagnosis other than delusions of parasitosis because patients with this condition are rigid in their mindset that 'parasites' are causing their symptoms.

Looking at various 'specimens' that the patient may bring to the dermatologist's office will demonstrate to the patient that his or her concerns are being taken seriously. Almost always, however, the specimens brought in by patients only show dry pieces of skin or other detritus. One should not make any comment that may reinforce the patient's delusional ideation, such as a statement that an organism responsible for the condition was found; an agreement such as this on the part of the clinician may ultimately render the patient more difficult to deal with, by making the patient even more firmly fixated on their erroneous belief systems. On the other hand, by definition, rational argument or trying to talk a patient out of a delusion is also generally counterproductive.

The most feasible way to reverse delusional ideation is to start the patient on an *antipsychotic medication*. If this medication is described as an antipsychotic agent, however, few, if any, patients will accept the treatment. On the other hand, if the option of treating with this medication is offered in a neutral way, emphasizing possible symptom reduction such as decreased crawling, biting, or stinging sensations, or a decrease in agitation or mental preoccupation, patients are often eager to start the medication.

The medication classically used to treat delusions of parasitosis is the traditional antipsychotic agent, *pimozide*, a neuroleptic and selective blocker of dopamine D2 receptors, which have been shown to contribute to psychosis. This medication can work well for patients, whether they have classic delusions of parasitosis or merely formications but are not delusional. The starting dose of pimozide is purposely kept low, and the dose is gradually increased until the optimal clinical response is attained, as evidenced by decreased mental preoccupation, formication, and agitation. The dosage of pimozide can be increased by as little as 1 mg increments, or as slowly as on a weekly basis until significant clinical response is noted, which is usually evident by the time the dosage is 4–6 mg daily. It is very rare that a patient will require a dose of more than 6 mg daily, and the use of greater than 10 mg daily is almost unheard of in the treatment of delusions of parasitosis. Once the patient reaches a stable, well-tolerated dose of the medication and agitation, mental preoccupation, and symptoms of formication have subsided, the dose can be maintained for a few months. During this time, if the patient continues to experience improvement, the dosage of pimozide can be decreased gradually by as slowly as 1 mg every 1–2 weeks until the minimum necessary dosage is determined or the patient is tapered off the pimozide altogether successfully.

If the clinical state deteriorates again in the future with a new episode of exacerbation of a delusional belief system and formication, the patient can be restarted on pimozide and again treated in a time-limited fashion to control the particular episode. Most patients with delusions of parasitosis can be treated on an episodic basis and can be tapered off pimozide after 2–3 months of usage, but some require long-term treatment with pimozide.

As pimozide blocks dopaminergic receptors, there is the possibility that extrapyramidal side effects such as stiffness in the muscles or joints or akathisia, an inner sensation of restlessness, may develop. Acute dystonic reaction and tardive dyskinesia are other potential adverse consequences associated with pimozide, although with the relatively low dosages of pimozide used to treat delusions of parasitosis, these side effects are rarely encountered. If these effects develop, however, they can be controlled with anticholinergic agents such as benztropine or diphenhydramine. Akathisia and pseudoparkinsonian side effects are not a reason for discontinuing treatment with pimozide provided that they are kept under control with one of these agents.

Because pimozide can theoretically prolong a QT interval or cause ventricular arrhythmias, it is advisable to consider checking pretreatment and post-treatment electrocardiograms (ECGs) periodically, especially in older patients or patients with a history of cardiac arrhythmia. It should be noted that in most cases, however, the risk of ECG abnormalities, including prolongation of the QT interval, is minimal with doses at or less than 10 mg daily. Caution must be exercised in prescribing pimozide for those with hepatic or renal dysfunction.

More recently, atypical antipsychotics, such as *risperidone* and *olanzapine*, have been used to treat patients with delusions of parasitosis. Atypical antipsychotics block more 5HT-2 receptors than D2 receptors. Serotonin has been shown to be a key player in some states of psychosis, most cases of obsessive–compulsive disorder, and self-mutilation, which can all potentially be manifest in patients with delusions of parasitosis. Thus, atypical antipsychotics, by blocking both serotonin and dopaminergic receptors, are thought theoretically to be an effective choice for treating this condition. Furthermore, the burden of side effects with atypical antipsychotics may be reduced compared with that of typical antipsychotics. Over the past several years, clinicians have reported several cases with good success using atypical antipsychotic agents. It is usually advisable to start at low doses of these agents and titrate upward as needed while avoiding side effects (between 0.5 mg once to twice daily and 2 mg twice daily). To date, however, there have been no randomized double-blind, placebo-controlled trials comparing the efficacy of pimozide to the atypical antipsychotics, and most of the medical literature on atypical antipsychotics is limited to case reports.

Once the delusional ideation is successfully treated, it may be beneficial to try to *refer the patient to a psychiatrist*. However, many successfully treated patients with delusions of parasitosis have not been treated by psychiatrists because of a continued refusal on the part of these patients to believe their condition is psychiatric in nature. Therefore, having dermatologists understand the use of pimozide may be the only way that most of these patients receive the treatment that they need. At the same time, the most difficult aspect of managing patients with delusions of parasitosis is trying to get their cooperation in taking pimozide. This difficulty arises as a result of the difference between the patient's belief system and the physician's understanding of how to treat the situation. Several sessions may be needed before the patient begins to trust the physician. In addition, these patients would be best served by *long-term follow-up*, even when their condition is under control, to ensure that the delusions have not recurred and that the patient has an ongoing, stable environment to return to when necessary. Also, monitoring for secondary problems such as cellulitis from excessive scratching of the skin will help prevent comorbidity.

SPECIFIC INVESTIGATIONS

These additional tests may be considered, depending on the patient's clinical presentation:

- Complete blood count
- Complete electrolyte panel, including serum potassium, blood urea nitrogen, and creatinine, and glucose
- Thyroid function tests
- Liver function tests
- Serum B12, ferritin
- ECG before initiation of pimozide
- Ask about recreational drug use
- Microscopy of specimens brought in by the patient

Delusions of parasitosis. A dermatologist's guide to diagnosis and treatment. Koo J, Lee CS. Am J Clin Dermatol 2001;2:285–90.

A good review of the diagnosis and treatment of delusions of parasitosis.

100 years of delusional parasitosis. Meta-analysis of 1,223 case reports. Trabert W. Psychopathology 1995;28:238–46.

A comprehensive review of delusions of parasitosis. The delusions were present on average 3 years prior to presentation to a healthcare provider. Social isolation seemed to be present in many patients as a premorbid condition. Full remission was observed in approximately half of the patients. Short preclinical courses may indicate better outcome. Comparing the patients of the prepsychopharmacological era (before 1960) with those after, the rate of full remissions increased from 34 to 52%.

Delusions of parasitosis. Lynch PJ. Semin Dermatol 1993; 12:39–45.

Another good review of the clinical features and treatment options for this condition.

FIRST LINE THERAPIES

■ Pimozide	B

The Michelson Lecture. Delusions of parasitosis. Lyell A. Br J Dermatol 1983;108:485–99.

A review of the condition with recommendations on the use of pimozide.

Delusional parasitosis: a dermatologic, psychiatric, and pharmacologic approach. Driscoll MS, Rothe MJ, Grant-Kels JM, Hale MS. J Am Acad Dermatol 1993;29:1023–33.

Pimozide is suggested as the first line of therapy for this psychodermatologic condition. Relapse often occurs on discontinuation of the drug.

Neurotropic and psychotropic drugs in dermatology. Tennyson H, Levine N. Dermatol Clin 2001;19:179–97.

This is a review article discussing the use of psychotropic drugs for psychodermatologic conditions such as delusions of parasitosis.

Evidence levels A Double-blind study **B** Clinical trial ≥ 20 subjects **C** Clinical trial < 20 subjects **D** Series ≥ 5 subjects **E** Anecdotal case reports

Delusions of parasitosis. A psychiatric disorder to be treated by dermatologists? An analysis of 33 patients. Zomer SF, DeWit RF, Von Cronswijk JE, et al. Br J Dermatol 1998;138:1030–2.

Of 33 patients with delusions of parasitosis, 24 were prescribed pimozide and only 18 patients took the medicine because it was difficult to convince them to take it. Of these 18 patients, five had full remission, four became less symptomatic, five were unchanged, and four died of unrelated causes.

Successful treatment of chronic delusional parasitosis. Mitchell C. Br J Psychiatry 1989;155:556–7.

This is a case report of successful treatment of delusions of parasitosis with pimozide.

Pimozide in delusions of parasitosis. Damiani JT, Flowers FP, Pierce DK. J Am Acad Dermatol 1990;22:312–13.

Another case report of the successful use of pimozide in treating delusions of parasitosis.

Delusions of infestation treated with pimozide: a follow-up study. Lindskov R, Baadsgaard O. Acta Derm Venereol 1985;65:267–70.

Fourteen patients were followed up for 19–48 months after pimozide therapy was completed – seven remained in remission, three had a relapse that required repeat treatment, and four responded poorly.

SECOND LINE THERAPIES

■ Risperidone	C
■ Olanzapine	C

Therapeutic update: use of risperidone for the treatment of monosymptomatic hypochondriacal psychosis. Elmer KB, George RM, Peterson K. J Am Acad Dermatol 2000;43:683–6.

The authors discuss risperidone as being highly effective for delusions of parasitosis while avoiding the negative long-term side effects of pimozide (as discussed above).

Risperidone in the treatment of delusions of infestation. DeLeon OA, Furmaga KM, Canterbury AL, Bailey LG. Int J Psychiatry Med 1997;27:403–9.

Risperidone was reported to be successful in three patients who had not responded to haloperidol or pimozide.

A case of monosymptomatic hypochondriacal psychosis treated with olanzapine. Weintraub E, Robinson C. Ann Clin Psychiatry 2000;12:247–9.

An elderly woman reported to have a good response with the atypical antipsychotic agent, olanzapine at lower doses than those needed to treat schizophrenia (2.5 mg as a starting dose titrated upward by 2.5 mg per week to a maximum of 10 mg daily).

Olanzapine is considered to offer considerable safety and side effect advantages over other agents in older patients.

Atypical antipsychotics in the treatment of delusional parasitosis. Wenning MT, Davy LE, Catalano G, Catalano MG. Ann Clin Psychiatry 2003;15:233–9.

Favorable results were observed utilizing atypical antipsychotics in five patients with delusions of parasitosis. The rationale for this treatment choice is discussed.

Dermatitis artefacta

John Koo, Anjeli Krishnan

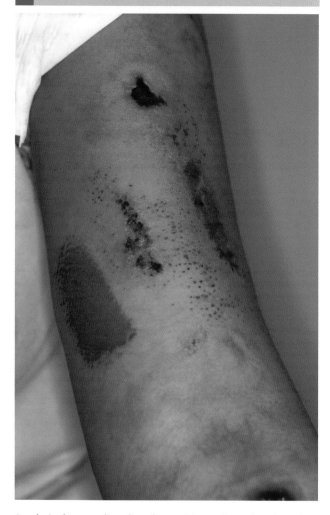

A relatively rare disorder, dermatitis artefacta is primarily a psychiatric condition in which a patient self-induces a variety of skin lesions to satisfy a conscious or unconscious psychological need. However, the patient will invariably deny responsibility for the injury. The method utilized to inflict the lesions is typically more elaborate than simple excoriations. In turn, the appearance of the lesions depends upon the manner in which they are created and can range from minor cuts to large areas of trauma, but is usually characterized by sharp geometric outlines surrounded by normal-looking skin on parts of the body easily contacted by the dominant hand. Chemical or thermal burns, injection of foreign materials, circulatory occlusion, and tampering with old lesions, such as existing scars or prior surgical incision sites, are some common methods of self-injury. More serious wounds can result in abscesses, gangrene, or other life-threatening infection. A large proportion of patients with dermatitis artefacta manifest borderline personality disorder. Interestingly, when the patient is asked about the manner in which the skin condition evolved, he or she is often vague, generally unmoved, and cannot provide sufficient detail, an unusual aspect of the illness termed the 'hollow history'.

MANAGEMENT STRATEGY

It is first important to rule out malingering as the etiology of the skin lesions. If the lesions were made deliberately for secondary gain such as disability or insurance benefits, the case is no longer considered psychiatrically based. These cases may eventually need to be dealt with legally.

Most of the treatment for dermatitis artefacta is symptomatic and supportive. *Protective dressings*, such as an Unna boot, can occlude the involved areas and protect against further self-injurious behavior.

Antidepressant medications, such as *selective serotonin reuptake inhibitors (SSRIs)*, may be helpful for patients with dermatitis artefacta who have primary or secondary depression. If there is clinical evidence of a psychotic process, *pimozide* could be considered empirically in resistant cases. There have also been recent case reports of patients responding to the atypical antipsychotic, *olanzapine*, when all other modes of therapies, including antidepressants and other antipsychotics, have failed.

Importantly, physicians should be aware that patients presenting with dermatitis artefacta have a psychiatric illness, and the skin lesions are often an appeal for help. However, presenting the illness to the patient as psychiatrically based may alienate him or her. Direct confrontation should be avoided if possible, and instead, *a supportive environment* and a *stable physician–patient relationship* should be fostered, often initially through short frequent office visits. The clinician should be nonjudgmental, empathize with the pain, discomfort, and restrictions imposed by the illness, and potentially explore life circumstances and possible stressors in the patient's life. In the case of an adolescent patient, the clinician should encourage the parents to become involved in identifying these psychosocial stressors and in helping to modify the patient's environment to meet his or her needs. However, most parents are resistant to this diagnosis and can be angry and critical toward the clinician, so using great tact is advisable. Once the patient establishes trust in the physician by means of a stable relationship, the physician may help the patient to recognize the psychosocial impact of the disorder and *recommend consultation with a psychiatrist* or psychotherapy. However, the patient may still not acknowledge psychogenic issues as the etiologic factors.

Most patients with dermatitis artefacta have a chronic, waxing and waning course. Thus, often when the patient's condition is under control, the physician should still follow him or her at regular intervals to ensure that the self-destructive behavior does not reinitiate. *Regular visits*, whether or not lesions are present, will help the patient feel cared for and diminish the need for self-mutilatory behavior as a call for help.

SPECIFIC INVESTIGATIONS

- Rule out malingering
- Rule out any organic dermatologic disease
- Assess for associated psychiatric disorders (i.e. depression)

Cutaneous manifestations of psychiatric disease that commonly present to the dermatologist – diagnosis and treatment. Koblenzer CS. Int J Psychiatry Med 1992;22:47–63.

This article describes common dermatological presentations of psychopathology, including dermatitis artefacta.

Self-mutilation and the borderline personality. Schaeffer CB, Carrol J, Abramowitz SI. J Nerv Ment Dis 1982;170: 468–73.

Patients with dermatitis artefacta usually have borderline personality disorder.

Psychiatric aspects of dermatitis artefacta. Fabisch W. Br J Dermatol 1980;102:29–34.

Some psychiatrists believe that the patient may have an underlying immature personality, with the dermatitis artefacta being 'an appeal for help'.

Self-inflicted injury: a follow-up study of 43 patients. Sneddon I, Sneddon J. Br Med J 1975;3:527–30.

Thirteen (39%) of 33 patients with dermatitis artefacta continued to have skin lesions or other disabling psychiatric disorders more than 12 years after diagnosis; 5% of patients with dermatitis artefacta developed anorexia nervosa.

Dermatitis artefacta in pediatric patients: experience at the National Institute of Pediatrics. Saez-de-Ocariz M, Orozco-Covarrubius L, Mora-Magaña I, et al. Pediatr Dermatol 2004;21:205–11.

In this study, the incidence of dermatitis artefacta is 1 in 23 000, and is considered a rarity in children; 12 of the 29 patients reported had an associated chronic illness, and seven patients displayed mild mental retardation.

FIRST LINE THERAPIES

■ Occlusive dressings	D
■ Psychotropic agents	D
■ Psychotherapy (even if only supportive)	D
■ Management of secondary cutaneous complications	D

Diagnostic clues to dermatitis artefacta. Joe EK, Li VW, Magro CM, Arndt KA, Bowers KE. Cutis 1999;63:209–14.

This is a case report of a 36-year-old man who had several of the classic features of dermatitis artefacta. The clinical and histopathologic features, diagnostic aids, approach to therapy, and prognosis for the condition are reviewed.

Training future dermatologists in psychodermatology. Van Moffaert M. Gen Hosp Psychiatry 1986;8:115–18.

Palliative dermatological measures such as occlusive bandages, ointments, or placebo drugs, as well as hospitalization that includes bathing and massaging by nurses, can have a therapeutic impact on the psychiatric problem by symbolizing the medical attention and care for which the patient with dermatitis artefacta is craving.

Psychodermatology: an overview. Van Moffaert M. Psychother Psychosom 1992;58:125–36.

Specific aspects of psychotherapy, behavioral treatment, and psychotropic agents are discussed.

Dermatitis artefacta. Van Moffaert M, Vermander F, Kint A. J Dermatol 1985;24:236–8.

Seven cases of patients with dermatitis artefacta illustrate the variety in psychiatric disorders and lead to a discussion of an appropriate approach to these difficult patients by the dermatologist and the dermatologic nursing staff.

Dermatitis artefacta. Clinical features and approach to treatment. Koblenzer CS. Am J Clin Dermatol 2000;1:47–55.

A good review article.

The self-inflicted dermatoses: a critical review. Gupta MA, Gupta AK, Haberman HF. Gen Hosp Psychiatry 1987;9: 45–52.

A good review article.

SECOND LINE THERAPIES

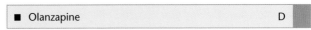

■ Olanzapine	D

Treatment of self-mutilation with olanzapine. Garnis-Jones S, Collins S, Rosenthal D. J Cutan Med Surg 2000;4:161–3.

Three patients successfully treated with low-dose olanzapine when multiple other therapies (including antidepressants and other antipsychotics) failed.

Olanzapine is effective in the management of some self-induced dermatoses: case reports. Gupta MA, Gupta AK. Cutis 2000;66:143–6.

Three patients with acne excoriee, factitious ulcers, and trichotillomania, respectively, responded to 2–4 weeks of olanzapine 2.5–5 mg daily.

Dermatitis herpetiformis

Ronald M Harris, John J Zone

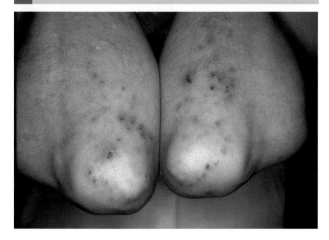

Dermatitis herpetiformis (DH) is a chronic, pruritic, papulovesicular eruption that primarily involves the extensor surfaces and scalp. The prevalence of DH is approximately 10–39 per 100 000 persons in the Caucasian population. DH is distinguished from other bullous diseases by characteristic histologic, immunologic, and associated gastrointestinal findings. Histologically, vesicle formation at the dermal–epidermal junction and infiltration of dermal papillary tips with neutrophils are seen. Immunofluorescence shows granular IgA localized in the dermal papillary tips of perilesional skin. All patients with DH have at least latent associated gluten-sensitive enteropathy, but only two-thirds have villous atrophy on intestinal biopsy.

MANAGEMENT STRATEGY

Although patients with DH can present with a spectrum of severity, the lesions of DH are invariably extremely pruritic and treatment is required for symptomatic relief. DH is a life-long disease; however, spontaneous remissions occur in 10–20% of cases.

Dapsone is the drug of choice for DH and is currently the only drug approved by the United States Food and Drug Administration for use in this disease. Initial treatment with dapsone 25 mg daily will usually improve pruritus within 24–48 h and the papulovesicular lesions within 1 week in adults. Correspondingly smaller doses should be used in children. Maintenance therapy is then adjusted on a weekly basis to maintain adequate suppression of symptoms. The average maintenance dose is 1 mg/kg daily. Despite adequate treatment, outbreaks of facial and scalp lesions are common.

Adherence to a gluten-free diet (GFD) often improves clinical symptoms in patients with DH. The advantages of gluten restriction include a reduction of dapsone dosage and its attendant complications, improvement of gastrointestinal symptoms (which range from crampy pain to overt diarrhea), and a therapy aimed at the cause rather than the symptoms of the disease. The increased risk of lymphoma incident to DH and celiac disease is also reduced with a GFD, but not with systemic agents like dapsone. Dapsone

improves the cutaneous lesions, but has no effect on intestinal disease. Strict adherence to a GFD is, however, challenging, and reintroduction of gluten can exacerbate symptoms of DH. A small percentage of patients may after a sustained remission on a GFD, successfully reintroduce gluten into their diet without deleterious effects on cutaneous or small intestinal disease. A small percentage of patients will not respond to gluten restriction. It is not possible to predict with certainty which patients will respond to a GFD. In the authors' opinion, a useful therapeutic strategy is the initial control of DH symptoms with dapsone, followed by gradual introduction of a GFD with subsequent tapering of suppressive medications. Oats have recently been found to be nontoxic in most patients with DH and may broaden the dietary options in an otherwise restrictive GFD.

Sulfapyridine is an alternative choice in patients who are intolerant to dapsone and has been shown to result in significant therapeutic efficacy. Sulfapyridine is started at 500 mg three times daily and is usually increased to a maximum maintenance dose of 1.5 g three times daily. Sulfapyridine, however, may not completely control symptoms at any dosage level and may be totally ineffective in some cases.

Other agents that have been reported to have a therapeutic benefit in DH include *nicotinamide, tetracycline* (or a combination of the two), *heparin, cyclosporine, colchicine*, and *systemic corticosteroids. Topical corticosteroid application* is generally inadequate when used alone to control DH symptoms. However, potent corticosteroids in gel form may provide relief for occasional lesions that develop on otherwise adequate dapsone or GFD therapy. This allows patients to treat lesions without increasing the dosage of dapsone.

SPECIFIC INVESTIGATIONS

- Biopsy for histology and immunofluorescence
- Complete blood count (CBC) and liver function tests (LFTs)
- Glucose-6-phosphate dehydrogenase levels
- IgA antiendomysial antibodies or tissue transglutaminase antibodies

Deposition of granular IgA relative to clinical lesions in dermatitis herpetiformis. Zone JJ, Meyer LJ, Petersen MJ. Arch Dermatol 1996;132:912–18.

It is now generally accepted that granular IgA deposition in perilesional clinically normal-appearing skin is the most reliable diagnostic criterion for DH. Although the combination of characteristic clinical and pathological features is highly suggestive of DH, the diagnosis of DH should not be made without the identification of granular IgA in dermal papillae.

Dermatitis herpetiformis and linear IgA bullous dermatosis. Smith EP, Zone JJ. Dermatol Clin 1993;3:511–26.

Hemolysis is the most common side effect of treatment with dapsone. Initial reduction of hemoglobin by 2–3 g is common, but subsequent partial compensation by reticulocytosis is the rule. Leukopenia and agranulocytosis may occur as well, usually within the first 2–12 weeks of therapy with dapsone. Recommendations for follow-up of patients on dapsone include baseline CBC and LFTs, weekly CBC for the first month, then monthly for 5 months. Chemistry profile and LFTs should be checked at 6 months and then annually to monitor for possible hepatotoxicity, changes in renal function, and hypoalbuminemia.

Anaemia in dermatitis herpetiformis. The role of dapsone-induced haemolysis and malabsorption. Cream J, Scott G. Br J Dermatol 1970;82:330.

Dapsone may produce severe hemolysis in patients with glucose-6-phosphate dehydrogenase deficiency (G6PD). Blacks and Caucasians of southern Mediterranean origin should be screened for G6PD deficiency before therapy is instituted. Methemoglobinemia is seldom a severe problem, but may be tolerated poorly in patients with G6PD deficiency.

Sensitivity and specificity of IgA-class antiendomysial antibodies for dermatitis herpetiformis and findings relevant to their pathogenic significance. Buetner EH, Chorzelski TP, Kumar V, et al. J Am Acad Dermatol 1986;15:467–73.

IgA class antiendomysial antibodies are highly specific for gluten-sensitive enteropathy and are found in approximately 70% of patients with DH who are not on a GFD. Antibody titers correlate with adherence to gluten restriction.

Dermatitis herpetiformis and coeliac disease are both primarily associated with HLA-DQ heterodimers. Spurkland A, Ingvarsson O, Falk ES, et al. Tissue Antigens 1997;49:29–34.

The same heterodimers of DQ2 and DQ8 associated with celiac disease have been found in a similar frequency in DH, suggesting a similar genetic basis for both entities, further suggesting the concept that DH is celiac disease of the skin.

FIRST LINE THERAPIES

■ Dapsone	C
■ GFD	C

Dermatitis herpetiformis and linear IgA bullous dermatosis. Smith EP, Zone JJ. Dermatol Clin 1993;3:511–26.

A good review article on treatment strategies for DH with dapsone. Dapsone is considered to be the drug of choice for the treatment of DH; however, there are no controlled clinical studies (i.e. double-blind studies or clinical trials on the efficacy of dapsone in the treatment of DH). The authors' personal observations corroborate the superior clinical efficacy of this agent.

25 years' experience of a gluten-free diet in the treatment of dermatitis herpetiformis. Garioch JJ, Lewis HM, Sargent SA, et al. Br J Dermatol 1994;131:541–5.

This is a retrospective study on a large series of patients with DH who were treated with a GFD – 60% of patients on the strict diet demonstrated a prolonged resolution of DH lesions. Patients on a partial GFD required substantially smaller doses of other medications such as dapsone. These authors consider a GFD to be the most appropriate therapy.

Gluten-free diet in dermatitis herpetiformis. I. Clinical response of skin lesions in 81 patients. Reunala T, Blomqvist K, Tarpila S, et al. Br J Dermatol 1977;97:473–80.

Patients with DH on a GFD substantially reduced their requirement for dapsone compared to patients on a normal diet. Almost 30% of patients were able to discontinue dapsone. Complete remission was seen only in patients on a GFD.

Absence of toxicity of oats in patients with dermatitis herpetiformis. Hardman CM, Garioch JJ, Leonard JN, et al. N Engl J Med 1997;337:1884–7.

Ten patients on a long-term GFD were given a mean of 62.5 g of oats for 12 weeks and showed no serologic or histologic evidence for recurrence of skin or intestinal disease. Avenin, the storage protein of oats is structurally different from gliadin and does not appear to induce an antibody response in these patients.

SECOND LINE THERAPIES

■ Sulfapyridine	E

Sulfonamides and sulfones in dermatologic therapy. Bernstein JE, Lorincs AL. Int J Dermatol 1981;20:81–8.

An extensive review of sulfonamides such as sulfapyridine. Sulfapyridine has been used extensively for the treatment of DH with variable clinical efficacy, but there are no controlled clinical studies of its use in the treatment of DH.

THIRD LINE THERAPIES

■ Tetracycline and nicotinamide	E
■ Heparin	E
■ Cyclosporine	E
■ Colchicine	D
■ Systemic corticosteroids	E

Dermatitis herpetiformis effectively treated with heparin, tetracycline and nicotinamide. Shah SAA, Ormerond AD. Clin Exp Dermatol 2000;25:204–5.

This is a case report of a patient with severe DH who was intolerant to dapsone and sulfapyridine. His DH lesions resolved with combination treatment consisting of subcutaneous low-dose heparin, nicotinamide 1.5 g daily in divided doses, and tetracycline 2 g daily. The patient was, however, on a GFD. The authors propose using this combination as a short-term measure in patients who are intolerant of dapsone.

Successful treatment of dermatitis herpetiformis with tetracycline and nicotinamide in a patient unable to tolerate dapsone. Zemtsov A, Nelder KH. J Am Acad Dermatol 1993;28:505–6.

This is a case report of a patient with DH who developed dapsone-induced agranulocytosis. She was treated with nicotinamide 500 mg three times daily and tetracycline 500 mg daily, with resolution of her skin lesions. She remained clear on nicotinamide and minocycline, 100 mg twice daily. She was not on a GFD.

A rare case of dermatitis herpetiformis requiring parenteral heparin for long-term control. Tan CC, Sale JE, Brammer C, Irons RP, Freeman JG. Dermatology 1996;192:185–6.

A patient with severe DH who was intolerant of dapsone and sulfapyridine was treated with parenteral heparin with complete resolution of her skin lesions within 1 week of therapy. This treatment is not practical for long-term management.

Efficacy of cyclosporine in two patients with dermatitis herpetiformis resistant to conventional therapy. Stenveld HJ, Starink TM, van Joost T, Stoof TJ. J Am Acad Dermatol 1993;28:1014–15.

Two patients with severe DH who were intolerant and/or unresponsive to conventional therapy were treated with cyclosporine (5–7 mg/kg daily) with resolution of skin lesions.

Dermatitis herpetiformis responsive to systemic corticosteroids. Lang PG. J Am Acad Dermatol 1985;13:513-15.

A patient with DH was treated successfully with a short course of prednisone and remained clear 4 months after discontinuation. He was successfully retreated with systemic corticosteroids for recurrence of the skin lesions.

Treatment of dermatitis herpetiformis with colchicine. Silver DN, Juhlin EA, Berczeller PH, McSorley J. Arch Dermatol 1980;116:1373–84.

Oral colchicine resulted in a significant improvement of skin lesions in three of four patients with DH. The authors suggest that colchicine may be used when dapsone or sulfapyridine is contraindicated.

Evidence levels **A** Double-blind study **B** Clinical trial ≥ 20 subjects **C** Clinical trial < 20 subjects **D** Series ≥ 5 subjects **E** Anecdotal case reports

Dermatologic non disease

Richard G Fried

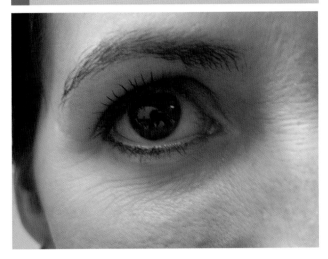

Dermatologic non disease (also known as body dysmorphic disorder [BDD]) is an alteration in perception of body image that causes preoccupation with a minimal or imagined defect in appearance. The preoccupation can be markedly excessive, causing clinically significant distress or impairment in social, occupational, or other important areas of functioning. Preoccupations commonly involve the face and head, with skin and hair being the most frequent areas of concern. Dermatologic preoccupations are distressing, time consuming, and difficult or impossible for patients to resist. Insight is typically poor and alterations in perception are often to delusional proportions. Most patients have ideas of reference, thinking that others take special notice or mock them for their perceived defect. Repetitive behaviors are present in almost all patients; excessive checking or grooming, constant need for reassurance, and skin picking are common. Risk of suicide is high, with approximately one-quarter of patients attempting suicide.

MANAGEMENT STRATEGY

Dermatologic non disease is common in dermatologic settings, with the prevalence estimated at 11.9%. Recognition of these patients is extremely important because they typically have a poor response to cosmetic dermatological treatments. Dissatisfaction, anger, and even aggression toward the treating dermatologist have been reported. Patients with dermatologic non disease often have associated psychiatric disorders including major depression, substance abuse and dependence, social phobia, and obsessive–compulsive disorder. Most of them also have a personality disorder. Appropriate psychiatric treatment can result in a generally favorable outcome

Typical body areas of preoccupation include the following.

■ The face – a preoccupation with facial itching and burning or obsessive preoccupation with imagined acne, scars, wrinkles, pigmentation, oiliness, redness, paleness, facial vessels, and facial hair is common. Preoccupation

with the nose, ears, and pore size is reported. Although others usually do not see these minimal or nonexistent flaws, patients can spend hours in front of mirrors, preventing them from working or socializing.

■ The scalp – dysesthesias (burning or itch) and obsession with imagined hair loss are common.

■ The genitals – scrotal, perineal, and perianal burning as well as vulvar redness and burning are common symptoms. Preoccupation with sexually transmitted disease or a neoplastic process is common. The symptoms can be incapacitating.

Patients presenting with extreme concern that appears out of proportion to their chief complaint accompanied by a paucity of objective physical findings should raise suspicion that dermatologic non disease may be present. Obsession, rumination, and extreme psychological distress are striking features. These patients usually report dissatisfaction with previous physicians and describe poor outcomes from past medical and surgical interventions. Skin picking and related behaviors, such as excessive tanning, excessive grooming, and a relentless need for reassurance are characteristic. Attempts at reassurance are inevitably futile because their perceptions and thinking are usually delusional, which by definition suggests that the distorted perceptions are unresponsive to logic and persuasion. The frequent presence of referential thinking further substantiates the delusional nature of the perceptions. Patients often wear heavy makeup and hats to hide their imperfections and perceived ugliness.

Patients with dermatologic non disease make unusual and excessive requests for cosmetic procedures with the belief that the procedure will transform or fix their lives. Almost always there is poor psychosocial functioning, with difficulties in relationships, school, and work. Depression is frequently evident, and previous suicide attempts are not infrequent.

Clinical interactions and consultations with these patients are typically long, difficult, and emotionally draining. Regardless of the actual length of time spent with them, patients often feel that they are not given adequate time and attention. It is inadvisable to perform procedures on these patients because less than 10% will be satisfied with the results of medical or surgical interventions.

Serotonin reuptake inhibitors (SRIs) and *cognitive–behavioral psychotherapy* are the treatments of choice. *Fluoxetine, fluvoxamine,* and *citalopram* are the best studied agents, but recent evidence suggests that all SRIs are probably effective. Higher dosing regimens than those used for depression are usually required. For example, fluoxetine and citalopram should be titrated to 60 mg daily while fluvoxamine should be increased to 300 mg daily at monthly intervals. Patients should receive a trial of 12–16 weeks before efficacy is assessed. If one agent fails, another should be substituted because some patients idiosyncratically respond more favorably to one agent over another. Interestingly, SRIs appear to be more effective than antipsychotic agents despite the fact that dermatologic non disease is frequently a delusional disorder. Only about 20% of patients will become free of their delusional thinking. However, the intrusiveness of the thoughts and distress will diminish sufficiently such that many patients will be able to resume some social and vocational functioning.

Cognitive–behavioral therapy (CBT) is a reality-based, in the present therapy that specifically focuses on the symptoms of dermatologic non disease. The key elements are known as exposure, response prevention, and cognitive restructuring. In exposure, patients expose the perceived defect in social situations. Response prevention consists of helping patients avoid their repetitive behaviors. Cognitive restructuring helps patients change their erroneous beliefs about their appearance and the importance attributed to their appearance. Ideally, treatment of dermatologic non disease should encompass both CBT and an SRI.

To initiate treatment or referral suggest to the patient in a gentle manner that they may have a body image disorder called body dysmorphic disorder (BDD). Convey your concern regarding the amount of their time being usurped by their preoccupation and their emotional distress. *Psychiatric referral* is preferable, but often not feasible. Dermatologists are encouraged to align themselves if possible with mental heath professionals who are experienced in treating this entity. Euphemisms such as 'skin-emotion specialist' reduce the stigma of psychiatric referral and may increase patient acceptance. If referral is not possible, treating with an SRI may be successful. If suicidal ideation and intent are present, *immediate hospitalization* is recommended.

SPECIFIC INVESTIGATIONS

■ Assess the quality of life, degree of distress, psychosocial impairment, and suicide risk

Depression, anxiety, anger, and somatic symptoms in patients with body dysmorphic disorder. Phillips KA, Siniscalchi JM, McElroy SL. Psychiatr Q 2004;75:309–20.

Seventy-five patients with BDD completed a symptom questionnaire assessing depression, anxiety, somatic/somatization, and anger–hostility. Compared to normal controls, BDD subjects had markedly elevated scores on all four scales, indicating severe distress and psychopathology. When treated with fluvoxamine, all symptoms significantly improved.

Quality of life for patients with body dysmorphic disorder. Phillips KA. J Nerv Ment Dis 2000;188:170–5.

This is the only published study looking at quality of life in patients with BDD. They were found to have a poorer mental health quality of life than reported for patients with other severe illnesses such type II diabetes mellitus, recent myocardial infarction, or depression.

These findings highlight the dramatic impact of a non disease.

33 cases of body dysmorphic disorder in children and adolescents. Albertini RS, Phillips KA. J Am Acad Child Adolesc Psychiatry 1999;38:453–9.

Thirty three cases were examined. Onset was usually during adolescence, but sometimes in childhood. Earlier identification and treatment may avert unnecessary cosmetic and medical interventions as well as suicide.

Gender differences in body dysmorphic disorder. Phillips KA, Diaz S. J Nerv Ment Dis 1997;185:570–7.

This study looked at a large series of patients with DSM-IV (Diagnostic and Statistical Manual of Mental Disorders, 4th edn) defined BDD and found that one-quarter of patients had attempted suicide. Female patients with severe symptoms are at greater risk.

Suicide in dermatological patients. Cotterill JA, Cunliffe WJ. Br J Dermatol 1997;137:246–50.

Sixteen patients who had committed suicide are described. Most of these patients had acne or BDD. Females with facial complaints and men with facial scarring appeared more at risk for suicide. The authors relate these findings to the possible preventive benefits of early isotretinoin to prevent scarring in patients predisposed to dermatologic non disease.

FIRST LINE THERAPIES

■ Serotonin reuptake inhibitors   A

A randomized placebo-controlled trial of fluoxetine in body dysmorphic disorder. Phillips KA, Albertini RS, Rasmussen SA. Arch Gen Psychiatry 2002;59:381–8.

This is the only placebo-controlled BDD pharmacotherapy study. In the 74 patients studied, fluoxetine was significantly more effective than placebo, with a response rate of 53% versus 18%.

Clomipramine versus desipramine crossover trial in body dysmorphic disorder: selective efficacy of a serotonin reuptake inhibitor in imagined ugliness. Hollander E, Allen A, Kwon J, et al. Arch Gen Psychiatry 1999;56:1033–9.

This double-blind crossover study of 29 randomized patients found clomipramine (an SRI) superior to desipramine (a non-SRI tricyclic antidepressant).

Efficacy and safety of fluvoxamine in body dysmorphic disorder. Phillips KA, Dwight MM, McElroy SL. J Clin Psychiatry 1998;59:165–71.

This open label study of fluvoxamine demonstrated that 19 (63%) of 30 patients with BDD responded to this SRI.

Delusionality and response to open-label fluvoxamine in body dysmorphic disorder. Phillips KA, McElroy SL, Dwight MM, et al. J Clin Psychiatry 2001;62:87–91.

Thirty patients with BDD were treated with fluvoxamine for 16 weeks in this open-label trial, and 63% of treated patients improved significantly. Both delusional and nondelusional patients responded similarly.

Change in psychosocial functioning and quality of life of patients with body dysmorphic disorder treated with fluoxetine: a placebo-controlled study. Phillips KA, Rasmussen SA. Psychosomatics 2004;45:438–44.

This was a 12-week placebo-controlled study of psychosocial functioning and mental health-related quality of life in 60 patients. At baseline, the patients had impaired psychosocial functioning and markedly poor mental health-related quality of life. Significant decrease in the severity of BDD was demonstrated along with improvement in functioning and quality of life.

An open label study of citalopram in body dysmorphic disorder. Phillips KA, Najar F. J Clin Psychiatry 2003;64: 715–20.

This open-label study found that 11 of 15 patients (73%) with DSM-IV documented BDD demonstrated a statistically significant improvement. Psychosocial functioning and quality of life also improved.

SECOND LINE THERAPIES

■ Cognitive–behavioral therapy	B

Cognitive–behavioral body image therapy for body dysmorphic disorder. Rosen JC, Reiter J, Orosan P. J Consult Clin Psychol 1995;63:263–9.

Exposure and response prevention was effective in 77% of 27 women treated with cognitive–behavioral group therapy for 8 weeks. Subjects in the treatment group improved more than those in the no-treatment waiting list control group.

Cognitive behavioral group therapy for body dysmorphic disorder: a case series. Wilhelm S, Otto MW, Lohr B, Deckersbach T. Behav Res Ther 1999;37:71–5.

Thirteen patients with BDD significantly improved after twelve group therapy sessions.

Body dysmorphic disorder: a cognitive behavioral model and pilot randomized controlled trial. Veale D, Gournay K, Dryden W, et al. Behav Res Ther 1996;34;717–29.

Nineteen patients were randomly assigned to cognitive–behavioral therapy or a waiting list control group. There was significantly greater improvement in BDD symptoms in the cognitive–behavioral therapy group.

THIRD LINE THERAPIES

■ Rational role play	E

Does rational role play enhance the outcome of exposure therapy in dysmorphophobia? A case study. Cromarty P, Marks I. Br J Psychiatry 1995;167:399–402.

Rational role play ('paradoxical discourse') was added to exposure plus cognitive restructuring for a dysmorphic delusion study comprised of 20-minute sessions 1 week apart. Previous exposure plus attempted cognitive restructuring had improved anxiety, phobias, work and social leisure, but not dysmorphic belief. Additional brief rational role play was followed by resolution of the dysmorphic belief. All measures remained much improved at 18-month follow-up.

Dermatomyositis

Jeffrey P Callen

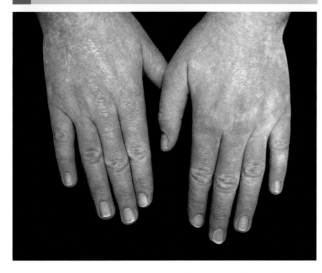

Dermatomyositis (DM) is one of the idiopathic inflammatory myopathies characterized by cutaneous disease, including a heliotrope rash, Gottron's papules, a violaceous erythema on extensor surfaces and in a photodistribution, and/or periungual changes. Patients with cutaneous lesions of DM most often have demonstrable muscle disease, muscle weakness of the proximal muscles, elevated enzymes such as creatine kinase or aldolase, or abnormal electromyograms or muscle biopsy findings. Some patients, however, have cutaneous disease that either precedes the onset of demonstrable muscle disease or occurs in its absence. DM in children and adolescents may be complicated by calcinosis. Adults with DM have a greater risk of having or developing a malignancy.

MANAGEMENT STRATEGY

Prior to treatment the patient should be thoroughly evaluated to assess the severity of the disease, the presence of systemic involvement such as pulmonary, cardiac, or gastrointestinal involvement, and the presence of malignancy.

The goal of management is to *reverse the weakness* and allow the patient to return to normal functional status. The *prevention of contractures* is also a consideration and the *prevention or treatment of calcinosis* is usually an issue in the management of children. Patients with cutaneous disease are troubled by extreme pruritus and the appearance of their skin and therefore request management even when the muscle disease has been effectively treated or is absent.

For the myopathy, *corticosteroid with or without an immunosuppressive agent* is the standard treatment. Most patients respond to these agents, but for those who do not, *high-dose intravenous immune globulin* may be of benefit. Patients with cutaneous disease are photosensitive and are treated with *sunscreens, topical corticosteroids, oral antimalarials,* or an *oral immunosuppressive*.

SPECIFIC INVESTIGATIONS

- A thorough evaluation to exclude other causes of myopathy
- Malignancy evaluation
- Serum aldolase or creatine kinase
- Electromyogram
- Muscle biopsy
- Magnetic resonance imaging (MRI) or ultrasound of muscle
- Assessment for the presence of systemic involvement (e.g. pulmonary disease, esophageal dysfunction, cardiac involvement)
- Assessment of myositis-specific antibodies

Scalp involvement in dermatomyositis. Often overlooked or misdiagnosed. Kasteler JS, Callen JP. JAMA 1994;272: 1939–41.

Skin lesions in patients with DM, particularly of the scalp, are often confused with psoriasis, seborrheic dermatitis, or lichen planus. Often the lesions simulate cutaneous lupus erythematosus.

Idiopathic inflammatory diseases of muscle. Wortmann RL. In: Weisman M, Weinblatt M, Louie J, eds. Treatment of the rheumatic diseases, 2nd edn. Philadelphia: WB Saunders; 2001:390–402.

This chapter details the evaluation and the types of muscle diseases that need to be excluded prior to classifying patients as having an idiopathic inflammatory myopathy.

Influence of age on characteristics of polymyositis and dermatomyositis in adults. Marie I, Hatron PY, Levesque H, et al. Medicine (Baltimore) 1999;78:139–47.

This group compared characteristics of younger versus older adults; it found that the incidence of malignancy was much higher in the older population, and therefore the prognosis for the older population was poorer.

Dermatomyositis as a presenting symptom of ovarian cancer. Nakanishi K, Cualing H, Husseinzadeh N. Obstet Gynecol 1999;94:836–8.

This is a case report of a 75-year-old woman with DM who was found to have an ovarian cancer. Other larger studies, including population-based studies from Scandinavia, have also demonstrated this association.

Women with DM should have a careful gynecologic evaluation.

MR imaging in amyopathic dermatomyositis. Lam WW, Chan H, Chan YL, et al. Acta Radiol 1999;40:69–72.

These authors conducted a prospective study to investigate the role of MRI in ten patients with amyopathic DM. Three patients demonstrated abnormal signal intensity in muscles on both T2 and fat suppression sequences. Thus, one-third of patients with DM and clinically normal muscles may have detectable muscle inflammation on MRI, indicating that MRI has a potential role for locating the relevant biopsy site and for longitudinal follow-up. MRI is useful for demonstrating subclinical muscle involvement in patients with the clinical diagnosis of amyopathic DM.

Dermatomyositis with normal muscle enzyme concentrations. A single-blind study of the diagnostic value of

magnetic resonance imaging and ultrasound. Stonecipher MR, Jorizzo JL, Monu J, et al. Arch Dermatol 1994;130:1294–9.

This single-blind study evaluated the use of MRI and ultrasound in five patients with classical DM but normal levels of serum muscle enzymes. Ultrasonography revealed hyperechogenicity, and MRI revealed high signals on T2-weighted images in several muscle groups of the patient with active myositis (positive control). Noninvasive examinations such as MRI and ultrasound are beneficial as adjunctive means of examination in the evaluation of patients with amyopathic DM or classical DM. Ultrasound appears to be the more cost-effective and simple test; MRI, although more expensive, may be more sensitive and specific.

The value of malignancy evaluation in patients with dermatomyositis. Callen JP. J Am Acad Dermatol 1982;6: 253–9.

DM has been linked to internal malignancy in adult patients, but the value of an extensive malignancy evaluation in patients with DM is controversial. Fifty seven patients who had DM with malignancies for whom data were available regarding the discovery of malignancy, have been analyzed: 53 of these were reported previously. There were 67 malignancies in the 57 patients. The malignancy preceded (26 cases), followed (23 cases), or occurred with the DM (18 cases). A 'blind' (nondirected) malignancy search was not of value in any of the cases analyzed. Rather, the tumors were discovered in 40 cases by history (preceding tumor or abnormal symptoms), in 14 cases by physical examination, and in 12 cases by abnormal laboratory findings (e.g. chest radiograph, urinalysis, stool guaiac). One case was not discovered until autopsy (adenocarcinoma of the broad ligament). Analysis of tumor sites further negates the value of a malignancy work-up because most tumors (>90%) occur in areas not amenable to a 'routine malignancy search'. In several instances patients had an extensive search without having complete physical examinations.

Malignancy evaluations should be directed by abnormalities found on history, physical findings, or routine laboratory testing.

A new approach to the classification of idiopathic inflammatory myopathy: myositis-specific autoantibodies define useful homogeneous patient groups. Love LA, Leff RL, Fraser DD, et al. Medicine (Baltimore) 1991;70:360–74.

This study compared the usefulness of myositis-specific autoantibodies (anti-aminoacyl-tRNA synthetases, anti-signal recognition particle [anti-SRP], anti-Mi-2 and anti-MAS) to the standard clinical categories (polymyositis, DM, overlap myositis, cancer-associated myositis, and inclusion body myositis) in predicting clinical signs and symptoms and prognosis in 212 adult patients. Patients with anti-amino-acyl-tRNA synthetase autoantibodies (n = 47), compared to those without these antibodies, had significantly more frequent arthritis, fever, interstitial lung disease, and 'mechanic's hands'; higher mean prednisone dose at survey; higher proportion of patients receiving cytotoxic drugs; and higher death rates. Those with anti-SRP antibodies (n = 7) had more frequent palpitations, myalgias, severe refractory disease, and higher death rates. Patients with anti-Mi-2 antibodies (n = 10) had increased 'V-sign' and 'shawl-sign' rashes and cuticular overgrowth and a good response to therapy. These findings suggest that myositis-specific autoantibody status is a more useful guide than clinical group in assessing patients with myositis. The authors pro-

posed that myositis-specific autoantibody status be incorporated into future studies of epidemiology, etiology, and therapy of myositis.

These antibodies are less common in patients with DM than in patients with polymyositis, and thus should remain investigational at the current time.

FIRST LINE THERAPIES

For cutaneous disease	
■ Sunscreens	E
■ Topical corticosteroids	E
■ Antimalarials – hydroxychloroquine or chloroquine	D
For muscle disease	
■ Systemic corticosteroids	B
■ Immunosuppressive agents – methotrexate, azathioprine	A

The use of pulse corticosteroid therapy for juvenile dermatomyositis. Paller AS. Pediatr Dermatol 1996;13:347–8.

This report details preliminary experience from the Children's Hospital in Chicago. It has been suggested that this method of administration might result in less toxicity from corticosteroids, and further that this therapy aids in the prevention of calcinosis.

Dermatomyositis: comparative studies of cutaneous photosensitivity in lupus erythematosus and normal subjects. Dourmishev L, Meffert H, Piazena H. Photodermatol Photoimmunol Photomed 2004;20:230–4.

About half of the patients with DM were found to have a reduced minimal erythema dose to UVB radiation. The action spectrum of DM remains unknown.

Cutaneous lesions of dermatomyositis are improved by hydroxychloroquine. Woo TY, Callen JP, Voorhees JJ, et al. J Am Acad Dermatol 1984;10:592–600.

DM is a collagen vascular disease with prominent cutaneous findings. Although the myositis often responds to therapy with corticosteroids and/or immunosuppressives, the cutaneous disease may not respond. Seven patients with cutaneous lesions of DM that had not responded to therapy were treated with hydroxychloroquine in an open study. Three patients had idiopathic DM, one had DM without myositis, one had DM with malignancy, one with an overlap syndrome and one had adolescent DM. The response to the addition of hydroxychloroquine was good in all patients, and three had total resolution of their skin lesions. In two patients the corticosteroid dosage could be tapered. Therapy with hydroxychloroquine did not appear to have any beneficial effect on the myositis. It was concluded that hydroxychloroquine may have a role as an adjuvant therapy for patients with cutaneous lesions of DM.

Prednisone and azathioprine for polymyositis: long-term follow up. Bunch TW. Arthritis Rheum 1981;24:45–8.

This follow-up study measured outcome after a double-blind, placebo-controlled trial of azathioprine had failed to demonstrate significant improvement. Unfortunately, this report dealt with the open-label experience following the previously reported 3-month controlled trial; however, there was significant improvement in the treated group and lower corticosteroid dosage.

SECOND LINE THERAPIES

For cutaneous disease	
■ Tacrolimus or pimecrolimus	D
■ Methotrexate	D
■ Mycophenolate mofetil	D
■ Intravenous immune globulin	A
For muscle disease	
■ Other immunosuppressive agents – cyclophosphamide, chlorambucil, mycophenolate mofetil, cyclosporine	D
■ Intravenous immune globulin	A

Topical tacrolimus 0.1% ointment for refractory skin disease in dermatomyositis: a pilot study. Hollar CB, Jorizzo JL. J Dermatol Treat 2004;15:35–9.

This is an open-label study of six patients with cutaneous lesions of DM who were treated with topical tacrolimus. A very good to excellent response was noted in two patients, a moderate response in one and essentially no response in three. This agent is worthy of a trial, but does not seem to be highly effective.

Low-dose methotrexate administered weekly is an effective corticosteroid-sparing agent for the treatment of the cutaneous manifestations of dermatomyositis. Kasteler JS, Callen JP. J Am Acad Dermatol 1997;36:67–71.

The records of 13 patients who received oral methotrexate in doses ranging from 2.5 to 30 mg weekly were reviewed. Their skin lesions had not been completely responsive to sunscreens, topical corticosteroids, oral prednisone, oral antimalarial therapy, and, in one patient each, chlorambucil and azathioprine. At the end of the study period, four of these 13 patients were free of all cutaneous manifestations of DM, and another four had almost complete clearing. In the remaining five patients, methotrexate induced moderate clearing of their cutaneous lesions. In all patients, the addition of methotrexate allowed a reduction in or discontinuation of other therapies including prednisone.

Mycophenolate mofetil in the treatment of severe skin manifestations of dermatomyositis: a series of 4 cases. Gelber AC, Nousari HC, Wigley FM. J Rheumatol 2000;27: 1542–5.

Four patients with classic skin manifestations and histologic evidence of DM who failed to respond to conventional therapy with corticosteroids, hydroxychloroquine and/or methotrexate were treated effectively with mycophenolate mofetil.

A controlled trial of high-dose intravenous immune globulin infusions as treatment for dermatomyositis. Dalakas MC, Illa I, Dambrosia JM, et al. N Engl J Med 1993;329:1993–2000.

These authors conducted a double-blind, placebo-controlled trial of intravenous immune globulin in 15 patients with biopsy-proved, treatment-resistant DM. The patients continued to receive prednisone (mean daily dose 25 mg) and were randomly assigned to receive one infusion of immune globulin (2 g/kg body weight) or placebo monthly

for 3 months, with the option of crossing over to the alternative therapy for three more months. The eight patients assigned to immune globulin showed a significant improvement in scores of muscle strength (p < 0.018) and neuromuscular symptoms (p < 0.035), whereas the seven patients assigned to placebo did not. With crossovers a total of 12 patients received immune globulin. Of these, nine with severe disabilities showed a major improvement to nearly normal function. Of 11 placebo-treated patients, none had a major improvement, three had a mild improvement, three had no change in their condition, and the condition of five worsened. Skin disease also responded in the treated patients.

Chlorambucil. An effective corticosteroid-sparing agent for patients with recalcitrant dermatomyositis. Sinoway PA, Callen JP. Arthritis Rheum 1993;36:319–24.

Five patients with recalcitrant DM were treated with oral chlorambucil, 4 mg daily, after discontinuation of the other immunosuppressive agent (azathioprine or methotrexate). Three patients were treated with a combination of prednisone and chlorambucil, and two with chlorambucil alone. Beneficial effects were noted within 4–6 weeks in all five patients, and corticosteroids were eventually discontinued in four. The chlorambucil was stopped after 13–30 months of treatment in four patients, and their disease remained in remission. Minimal chlorambucil toxicity was noted, consisting of leukopenia in two patients.

Although chlorambucil was effective, its potential for subsequent malignancy makes it a less desirable choice.

Cyclosporin A and intravenous immunoglobulin treatment in polymyositis/dermatomyositis. Danieli MG, Malcangi G, Plamieri C, et al. Ann Rheum Dis 2002;61:37–41.

This is a retrospective review of 20 patients, including 12 with DM. It suggests that combining prednisone, cyclosporine, and intravenous immune globulin was the most useful regimen.

Cyclosporin A versus methotrexate in the treatment of polymyositis and dermatomyositis. Vencovsky J, Jarosova K, Machacek S, et al. Scand J Rheumatol 2000;29:95–102.

Patients were randomly assigned to receive either methotrexate or cyclosporine in addition to prednisone. The methotrexate dosage was 7.5–15 mg/week and the dose of cyclosporine 3.0–3.5 mg/kg daily. Both groups improved. This is a small study of a heterogeneous group of patients treated with adequate doses of corticosteroid, but relatively low doses of the second agent.

THIRD LINE THERAPIES

■ Dapsone for cutaneous disease	E
■ Diltiazem for calcinosis	D
■ Etanercept	D
■ Infliximab	D
■ Total body irradiation	D

Regression of calcinosis during diltiazem treatment in juvenile dermatomyositis. Oliveri MB, Palermo R, Mautalen C, Hubscher O. J Rheumatol 1996;23:2152–5.

An 8-year-old girl with juvenile DM developed dystrophic calcifications 26 months after diagnosis. She also had severe corticosteroid-induced bone loss (osteoporosis). The calcifications turned into generalized heterotopic calcinosis with an exoskeleton-like pattern despite successful treatment of her myopathy with methylprednisolone and immunosuppressive drugs. She was subsequently treated with oral diltiazem (5 mg/kg daily) to control calcinosis and oral pamidronate (4 mg/kg daily) in addition to calcium and vitamin D supplementation, which she had been taking for 3 years. After 21 months of treatment, clinical and radiological examination revealed dramatic regression of the calcinosis. Bone mass reached normal levels, as determined by bone absorptiometry. Diltiazem, alone or in combination with other drugs, could be a useful therapy in patients with juvenile DM and pronounced calcifications.

Etanercept is effective in the treatment of polymyositis/dermatomyositis which is refractory to conventional therapy including steroids and other disease modifying agents. (Abstract) Saadeh CK. Arthritis Rheum 2000;43:S193.

This author reports her experience with four patients with DM/polymyositis that was refractory to corticosteroids and immunosuppressive agents. The focus of this abstract was on the muscle disease. It is not known whether this agent will be useful for the skin.

Anti-TNF-blockade with infliximab (Remicade) in polymyositis and dermatomyositis. Hengstman GJD, van den Hoogen FHJ, van Engelen BP, et al. Eur Neurol 2003;50:10–15.

One patient with DM and one with polymyositis were presented in this paper. Both the myopathy and the skin eruption responded in the patient with DM.

Response to total body irradiation in dermatomyositis. Kelly JJ, Madoc-Jones H, Adelman LS, Andres PL, Munsat TL. Muscle Nerve 1988;11:120–3.

Two patients with severe DM refractory to immunosuppressive therapy were treated with 150 rad of total body irradiation given over a period of 5 weeks. Both patients responded promptly with minimal side effects and remain in partial remission 42 and 18 months after completion of the treatment. Total body irradiation is effective in some patients with DM who are refractory to standard therapy.

Diaper dermatitis

Victoria M Yates

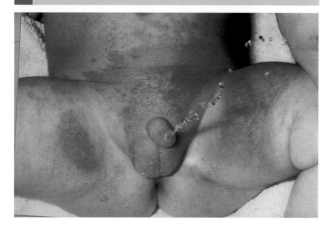

Diaper (napkin) dermatitis (DD) is a form of irritant contact dermatitis affecting the skin in closest contact with the diaper (buttocks, upper thighs, lower abdomen, and genitalia) and classically spares the inguinal creases. It may also be referred to as irritant diaper dermatitis (IDD). It can occur in any diapered individual regardless of age, but the peak incidence is in infants aged 8–12 months, and up to one in four infants are affected. Other dermatoses can affect the diaper area and may need to be excluded.

MANAGEMENT STRATEGY

Diapers cause occlusion, leading to an increase in skin wetness. Overhydration disrupts the stratum corneum ultrastructure leading to increased frictional damage between the skin and the diaper because the frictional coefficient of hydrated skin is substantially higher than that of dry skin. Alteration in skin barrier function and increased skin permeability increase susceptibility to irritation from the increased pH of the urine/feces mixture (fecal enzymes act on urine causing a rise in pH) and infection with microorganisms. *Candida albicans* is the only pathogen of importance, and when cultured has been shown to correlate with increased severity of DD. Management should therefore focus on *reducing overhydration and frictional damage in the napkin area*.

Frequent diaper change is one of the most important factors in treating and preventing DD. Good-quality diapers should be used such as superabsorbent disposable diapers, and changed a soon as possible after defecation. Newer 'breathable' disposable diapers may cause even less skin occlusion.

The *skin should be cleansed* to remove fecal material, avoiding soap, which strips the lipid layer from the stratum corneum. Water alone or water-dispersible cream, such as aqueous cream, or fragrance and alcohol-free baby wipes are suitable.

A *barrier ointment* should be applied at every diaper change to provide a lipid film over the surface of the skin and/or provide lipids that can penetrate into the stratum corneum, simulating the effects of normal intercellular lipids. This will reduce friction, skin wetting, and contact with urine and feces.

More severe DD may require treatment with a *low potency topical* corticosteroid, such as 1% hydrocortisone ointment.

This should be used with caution in the diaper area where there will be increased absorption. Proven or suspected *C. albicans* infection can be treated with a *topical antifungal preparation* or a *combined* corticosteroid *and antifungal preparation* such as hydrocortisone and miconazole or clotrimazole.

SPECIFIC INVESTIGATIONS

- ■ Skin swab for bacteriological and fungal culture
- ■ Skin biopsy
- ■ Patch testing
- ■ Zinc and biotin levels
- ■ HIV and syphilis serology

Diaper dermatitis: epidemiology. Kazaks EL, Lane AT. Pediatr Clin North Am 2000;47:909–14.

Recalcitrant or clinically atypical eruptions may signify rarer disorders, such as psoriasis, seborrheic dermatitis, Langerhans cell histiocytosis (Letterer-Siwe disease), acrodermatitis enteropathica (zinc deficiency), biotin deficiency, Netherton syndrome, perianal streptococcal disease, Kawasaki disease (mucocutaneous lymph node syndrome), pediatric HIV infection, congenital syphilis, and child abuse. Appropriate biochemical or bacteriological tests and a skin biopsy may be indicated.

Diaper dermatitis: a new clinical feature. Larralde M, Raspa ML, Silva H, et al. Pediatr Clin North Am 2000;47: 909–19

Among 53 infants seen with diaper dermatitis localized to the skin in contact with side band securing the diaper, the most common lesion was erythema in a triangular shape resembling a cowboy's holster. Positive patch tests in 70% of infants were thought to be due an irritant reaction to the glue component of the securing band of the diaper.

Microbiological aspects of diaper dermatitis. Ferrazzini G, Kaiser RR, Hirsig Cheung SK, et al. Microbiological aspects of diaper dermatitis. Dermatology 2003;206:136–41.

Forty eight children with healthy skin and 28 with diaper dermatitis were investigated for colonization of the skin with *Staphylococcus aureus* and *C. albicans*. Colonization by *C. albicans* was significantly more frequent in children with DD, whereas colonization with *S. aureus* was equally common in the two groups of children. There was a highly significant positive correlation between the severity of disease and extent of *C. albicans* colonization.

FIRST LINE THERAPIES

■ Increased frequency of diaper changes	B
■ Superabsorbent gel containing disposable diapers	A
■ Water repellent barrier creams	A

A review of the pathophysiology, prevention and treatment of irritant diaper dermatitis. Atherton DJ. Curr Med Res Opin 2004;20:645–9.

An excellent review article that discusses the pathophysiology of DD, the role of emollient formulations in the care of the diaper area, and selecting a barrier preparation for DD

Evidence levels A Double-blind study   B Clinical trial ≥ 20 subjects   C Clinical trial < 20 subjects   D Series ≥ 5 subjects   E Anecdotal case reports

management. Key points are the lack of controlled trials on traditionally used barrier preparations such as white soft paraffin, which is exceptionally occlusive and may not be suitable for long-term use, and zinc and titanium oxide hydrophilic pastes, which do not provide a very effective barrier. Two clinical trials have shown Bepanthen® ointment can help prevent and treat DD. All nonessential, potentially allergenic ingredients in barrier creams, such as perfumes, antiseptics and colorings, should be avoided.

Diaper dermatitis, frequency and severity among a general infant population. Jordan WE, Lawson KD, Berg RW, et al. Pediatr Dermatol 1986;3:198–207.

The frequency of diaper dermatitis in 1089 infants was significantly lower when the mean number of reported napkin changes was above average (over eight in 24 h) regardless of the type of napkin used.

Clinical studies with disposable diapers containing absorbent gelling materials: evaluation of effects on infant skin condition. Campbell RL, Seymour JL, Stone LC, Milligan MBA. J Am Acad Dermatol 1987;17:978–87.

Disposable infant diapers with absorbent gelling material (cross-linked sodium polyacrylate) can absorb many times their weight in fluid and when hydrated form a gel that keeps the urine stored away from the skin in the diaper core. In a double-blind comparative study of 1614 infants, absorbent gel-containing disposable diapers were closer to normal pH and were associated with reduced skin wetness and lower degrees of diaper dermatitis than conventional cellulose-core disposable or home-laundered cloth diapers.

Effects of breathable disposable diapers: reduced prevalence of *Candida* and common diaper dermatitis. Akin F, Spraker M, Aly R, et al. Pediatr Dermatol 2001;4:282–90.
The development of microporous membranes, which are permeable to air and vapor, but impervious to liquids, has provided a means of reducing occlusion in diapers. Infants wearing breathable gel-containing superabsorbent diapers experienced significantly less DD and confirmed *C. albicans* infection than infants wearing similar, but nonbreathable, diapers in a series of double-blind clinical trials. The inhibitory effect of breathable diapers on the survival of *Candida* was further confirmed in a controlled experiment with adult volunteers.

Effect of Bepanthen® ointment in the prevention and treatment of diaper rash on premature and full-term babies. Putet G, Guy B, Andres P, et al. Réal Pédiatr 2001;63:33–8.

It has been demonstrated in two controlled clinical trials that an ointment containing dexpanthenol, Betapathen® ointment, can help prevent and treat DD. This formulation also contains lanolin, which contains many of the lipid groups present in the human stratum corneum. It has been used extensively in Europe for many years and has recently become available in the UK.

SECOND LINE THERAPIES

■ 1% hydrocortisone ointment	D
■ Topical antibiotic/antifungal agent	B
■ Combined topical corticosteroid/antibiotic/ antifungal agent	B

Diaper dermatitis: a therapeutic dilemma. Results of a double-blind placebo controlled trial of miconazole nitrate 0.25%. Concannon P, Gisoldi E, Phillips S, et al. Pediatr Dermatol 2001;18:149–55

This placebo-controlled, randomized, double-blind, parallel-group trial compared the efficacy and safety of miconazole nitrate 0.25% in a zinc oxide/petrolatum base with that of the ointment base alone in treating over 200 infants with DD. Although an improvement was seen in the rash from baseline in both treatment groups, the results among patients receiving miconazole nitrate 0.25% were superior with respect to all outcome parameters after 5 days of treatment, with the improvement being most marked in the patients with the most severe DD and where *C. albicans* was cultured at baseline.

The treatment of napkin dermatitis: a double blind comparison of two steroid–antibiotic combinations. Bowring AR, Mackay D, Taylor FR. Pharmatherapeutica 1984;3:613–7.

Double-blind trial of 62 infants with moderate to severe napkin dermatitis comparing a miconazole/hydrocortisone preparation with a nystatin/benzalkonium chloride/ dimethicone/hydrocortisone preparation. Both treatments were equally effective with an 80% cure rate at 7 days, but miconazole/hydrocortisone was preferred because the nystatin preparation stained the napkins.

THIRD LINE THERAPIES

■ Continuous administration of petrolatum by disposable diaper	A
■ 2% eosin solution	C

Continuous topical administration of a petrolatum formulation by a novel disposable diaper. Odio MR, O'Connor RJ, Sarbaugh F, Baldwin S. Dermatology 2000;200:238–43.

Use of the formulation-treated diaper was associated with a significant reduction in diaper rash.

Efficacy of topical application of eosin compared with zinc oxide paste and corticosteroid cream for diaper dermatitis. Arad A, Mimouni D, Ben-Amitai D, et al. Dermatology 1999;199:319–22.

A 2% eosin solution was found to be superior to zinc oxide paste and clobetasone butyrate when complete healing of diaper dermatitis was the endpoint. However, in cases in which the corticosteroid cream was effective, it acted more rapidly. The red color of eosin made a double-blind study impossible and assessment of diaper dermatitis difficult, therefore weakening the conclusions of the study.

Discoid eczema

Neil H Cox

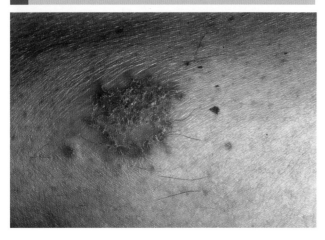

Discoid eczema comprises relatively well-defined, usually multiple, coin-sized plaques with itch and weeping from acute lesions. It primarily affects limbs (especially the legs), sometimes the trunk, and rarely the face or flexures.

MANAGEMENT STRATEGY

The discoid morphology of eczema has many etiologies. Discoid eczema is usually idiopathic in older patients, but similar lesions may occur due to contact allergic reactions, drug eruptions, as a pattern of hand and foot eczema, in atopic dermatitis (AD), as an 'id' eruption related to venous eczema, or locally (e.g. insect bite reactions, 'halo eczema' around melanocytic nevi).

There are few publications on the pathophysiology of discoid eczema to inform treatment. An association with dry skin (xerosis) is documented, and discoid lesions may appear during treatment with isotretinoin (which reduces sebum secretion). However, dry skin is not consistently present, and the morphology of discoid eczema differs from xerosis and asteatotic eczema.

One study suggested that patients with discoid eczema have a degree of xerosis similar to age-matched controls, but have stronger delayed hypersensitivity to allergens that permeate the skin due to scratching. A link with atopy has been proposed, but serum IgE levels are generally normal, and discoid variant AD is generally a persistent childhood pattern rather than a disease of older subjects. T lymphocyte subsets and increased mast cells in lesions are similar to those of AD.

Occult infections (e.g. dental abscess) and infections causing dry skin (e.g. leprosy) have rarely been linked with discoid eczema. *Helicobacter pylori* has been implicated, but the evidence is weak.

It is difficult to provide specific therapeutic strategies because of the various different causes and the paucity of pertinent publications; most reports are retrospective from individual departments or are anecdotal, rather than formal trials. The main therapeutic issues are:

- *other disorders may need to be excluded*, especially mycoses, psoriasis, Bowen's disease, mycosis fungoides, sarcoidosis;
- a *medication and alcohol history* should be taken;
- *patch testing* may be useful;
- the management of discoid eczema is generally similar to that of other eczemas – *emollients* appear to be helpful due to the link with dry skin;
- the mainstay of treatment is *topical corticosteroids* – severe itch in discoid eczema usually dictates that strong agents are applied; this is safe because the individual lesions are small, rarely affect thin skin sites such as the face or flexures, and usually respond to this approach;
- if weeping is present, *topical antiseptics* or *oral or topical antibiotics* may be combined with a corticosteroid;
- *tar-based treatments* and *impregnated bandages* may help;
- *systemic therapies* are rarely required.

Nummular eczema: an addition of senile xerosis and unique cutaneous reactivities to environmental aeroallergens. Aoyama H, Tanaka M, Hara M, et al. Dermatology 1999;199:135–9.

Mast cells, nerves and neuropeptides in atopic dermatitis and nummular eczema. Järvikallio A, Harvima IT, Naukkarinen A. Arch Dermatol Res 2003;295:2–7.

Nummular eczema of stasis origin. The backbone of a morphologic pattern of diverse etiology. Bendl BJ. Int J Dermatol 1979;18:129–35.

Eighty two of 113 patients with nummular eczema of uncertain etiology had varicose veins or lower leg edema, possibly causing autosensitization.

Therapeutic effects of antibacterial treatment for intractable skin diseases in *Helicobacter pylori*-positive Japanese patients. Sakurane M, Shiotani A, Furukawa FJ. Dermatology 2002;29:23–7.

Eleven of 15 cases of nummular dermatitis had a positive *H. pylori* (HP) test (a similar proportion as in the general population); skin lesions cleared in two and partially responded in four after HP eradication therapy.

SPECIFIC INVESTIGATIONS

- None usually required except to exclude differential diagnoses
- Consider medications as a cause
- Consider patch testing
- Bacteriology if secondary infection likely
- Consider occult infections in resistant cases

Medications and alcohol

Drugs that may cause discoid eczema include gold, methyldopa, and interferon-α/ribavirin. A high alcohol intake is associated with discoid eczema.

Pityriasis rosea and discoid eczema: dose related reactions to treatment with gold. Wilkinson SM, Smith AG, Davis MJ, et al. Ann Rheum Dis 1992;51:881–4.

Discoid eczematous lesions occur in up to 30% of patients on gold therapy, and this is possibly dose-related rather than allergic.

Cutaneous disease and alcohol misuse. Higgins EM, du Vivier AW. Br Med Bull 1994;50:85–98.

Documents a strong link between discoid eczema and alcohol consumption.

Patch testing

Patch testing can be helpful. Larger series suggest a 50% positive test rate, with clinical relevance in many. However, these are based on testing patients with chronic or therapy-resistant discoid eczema (i.e. a selected, potentially unrepresentative, group); most reports are anecdotal. Implicated agents include chromate, nickel, mercury, thimerosal, rubber chemicals, formaldehyde, neomycin, fragrances, aloe, ethylene diamine, cyanoacrylate glue and epoxy resin. Oral metal challenge tests rarely induce flares of discoid eczema. Irritants may also cause discoid eczema.

Patch testing in discoid eczema. Fleming C, Parry E, Forsyth A, Kemmett D. Contact Derm 1997;36:261–4.

Retrospective study of persistent and severe discoid eczema – 24 of 48 cases were positive and 16 were relevant, to rubber chemicals, formaldehyde, neomycin, chromate and nickel.

Patch testing in discoid eczema. Khurana S, Jain VK, Aggarwal K, Gupta S. J Dermatol 2002;29:763–7.

Positive tests in 28 of 50 patients with relatively chronic discoid eczema, mainly to dichromate, nickel, cobalt and fragrance.

Challenge with metal salts. (II). Various types of eczema. Veien NK, Hattel T, Justesen O, Nørholm A. Contact Derm 1983;9:407–10.

FIRST-LINE THERAPIES

■ Topical corticosteroids ± antibacterial agents	C
■ Emollients	C
■ Tar-based preparations	C
■ Oral antibiotics	C
■ Oral antihistamines	C
■ Topical doxepin	A

Most of these are standard treatments for discoid eczema; however, in terms of evidence grading, most studies include a variety of different eczemas, but few specifically identify results for discoid eczema, and comparative trials do not appear to be available.

Topical corticosteroids ± antibacterial agents

Topical corticosteroids are the usual first-line therapy. Trial evidence is limited to pharmaceutically-sponsored studies that are not specific to discoid eczema.

Use of antibacterial agents (e.g. clioquinol) or antibiotics is based on the fact that lesions are often moist and crusted. Secondary staphylococcal infection, as in AD, may aggravate the eczematous process. In AD, evidence for a long-term benefit from antibiotic therapy is mixed, although there may be benefit from short-term use of antiseptic/antibiotic agents in conjunction with topical corticosteroids.

Occlusion over a topical corticosteroid has been reported to lead to lesion clearance in previously therapy-resistant patients with discoid lesions due to AD.

As with other itchy dermatoses, sedating antihistamines may help symptoms – the increase in mast cells in lesions discussed above provides the rationale for this approach. However, histamine itself has not been shown to be important.

Successful treatment of therapy-resistant atopic dermatitis with clobetasol propionate and a hydrocolloid occlusive dressing. Volden G. Acta Derm Venereol Suppl (Stockh)1992;176:126–8.

Nummular AD lesions cleared rapidly.

Tar preparations

Tar preparations, historically used in the treatment of discoid eczema, have been superseded by potent topical corticosteroids as first line therapy. Also tar impregnated bandages.

Nummular eczema. A review, follow-up and analysis of a series of 325 cases. Cowan MA. Acta Derm Venereol 1961; 41:453–60.

Tar preparations were the main treatment. Recurrent crops of lesions occurred in 25%, and relapse when treatment was discontinued in 53%, presumably representing the natural history of the disease, but possibly reflecting the limitations of therapy available at the time (other options were hydrocortisone or superficial X-ray therapy).

Doxepin

Studies suggest that doxepin has a short-term effect on itch only.

The antipruritic effect of 5% doxepin cream in patients with eczematous dermatitis. Drake LA, Millikan LE. Arch Dermatol 1995;131:1403–8.

Significant improvement in itch at 1 day, not at 7 days.

SECOND-LINE THERAPIES

■ Phototherapy (broadband or narrowband UVB [311 nm])	E
■ Photochemotherapy (psoralen plus UVA [PUVA])	E
■ Topical immune modulators	E
■ Cyclosporine	E
■ Intralesional corticosteroid injection	E
■ Oral corticosteroids	E

Formal trials of these treatments in discoid eczema are lacking and therefore the evidence gradings are weak; however, all are useful in AD or other dermatitis (see gradings in Atopic Dermatitis, page 62), and are therefore likely to be effective in discoid eczema. Personal experience is that narrowband UVB or cyclosporine are useful if required.

UVB and PUVA

PUVA is beneficial in AD and in hand dermatitis (controlled trials), and in nodular prurigo and allergic contact dermatitis (open studies).

Photochemotherapy beyond psoriasis. Honig B, Morison WL, Karp D. J Am Acad Dermatol 1994;31:775–90.

Review article. Nothing specific to discoid eczema, but several eczemas respond to PUVA.

Half-side comparison study on the efficacy of 8-methoxypsoralen bath-PUVA versus narrow-band ultraviolet B phototherapy in patients with severe chronic atopic dermatitis. Der-Petrossian M, Seeber A, Honigsmann H, Tanew A. Br J Dermatol 2000;142:39–43.

Both were equivalent (at equi-erythemogenic doses) in AD.

Phototherapies also reduce staphylococci and superantigens, and therefore may improve eczema with weeping and infection.

Antimicrobial effects of phototherapy and photochemotherapy in vivo and in vitro. Yoshimura M, Namura S, Akamatsu H, Horio T. Br J Dermatol 1996;135:528–32.

Antimicrobial effects are apparent after a single exposure.

Suppressive effect of ultraviolet (UVB and PUVA) radiation on superantigen production by *Staphylococcus aureus*. Yoshimura-Mishima M, Namura S, Akamatsu H, Horio T. J Dermatol Sci 1999;19:31–6.

Topical immune modulators

Hand dermatitis: a review of clinical features, therapeutic options, and long-term outcomes. Warshaw E, Lee G, Storrs FJ. Am J Contact Derm 2003;14:119–37.

One review recommends topical tacrolimus or pimecrolimus for nummular hand dermatitis. No evaluable evidence presented.

Cyclosporine

Side effects (drug interactions, hypertension, nephrotoxicity) limit cyclosporine therapy in older patients with discoid eczema, compared with AD. It is possibly useful for intermittent short-term treatment.

Long-term efficacy and safety of cyclosporin in severe adult atopic dermatitis. Berth-Jones J, Graham-Brown RA, Marks R, et al. Br J Dermatol 1997;136:76–81.

Open study of 100 patients with AD, with mostly good responses.

Oral corticosteroids

Oral corticosteroids are generally unnecessary. Intralesional corticosteroid injection is impractical, except in patients who have a small number of persistent thickened lesions.

THIRD LINE THERAPIES

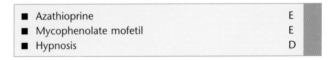

■ Azathioprine	E
■ Mycophenolate mofetil	E
■ Hypnosis	D

As for second line therapies formal trials of these treatments in discoid eczema are lacking and therefore the evidence gradings are weak; however, all are useful in AD or other dermatitis (see gradings in Atopic Dermatitis, page 62), and are therefore likely to be effective in discoid eczema.

Azathioprine is used in the treatment of several dermatoses, including various eczemas. It is likely to be beneficial in discoid eczema, although a study of azathioprine prescribing by UK dermatologists did not identify this as a current indication.

Mycophenolate mofetil is a 'recommended treatment' for nummular hand dermatitis (in Warshaw E, *et al.*, cited above), but there is no evidence.

Azathioprine in dermatological practice. An overview with special emphasis on its use in non-bullous inflammatory dermatoses. Scerri L. Adv Exp Med Biol 1999;445:343–8.

Documents efficacy of azathioprine in AD and pompholyx.

Azathioprine in dermatology: a survey of current practice in the UK. Tan BB, Lear JT, Gawkrodger DJ, English JSC. Br J Dermatol 1997;136:351–5.

Questionnaire of 248 dermatologists showed that none was using azathioprine for discoid eczema.

Hypnosis in dermatology. Shenefelt PD. Arch Dermatol 2000;136:393–9.

Hypnosis as a complementary therapy may improve lesions or itch in discoid eczema.

Discoid lupus erythematosus

Maryanna C Ter Poorten, Bruce H Thiers

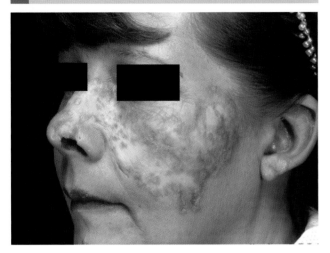

Discoid lupus erythematosus (DLE) is the most common form of chronic cutaneous lupus erythematosus. Lesions predominate in sun-exposed areas, especially the face, upper chest, and upper back. Early lesions consist of sharply demarcated, erythematous, often hyperpigmented, hyperkeratotic papules and small plaques with adherent scale; the individual lesions spread peripherally, leaving atrophic central scarring with alopecia, telangiectasia, and depigmentation.

MANAGEMENT STRATEGY

The lesions of DLE are quite characteristic, especially in their later stages. When the diagnosis is in doubt, a skin biopsy should be performed. The histologic findings are usually diagnostic, although direct immunofluorescence examination can be obtained in questionable cases. A complete history and physical examination should be performed, looking for signs of systemic disease. Laboratory examinations to be obtained include a complete blood count with differential, erythrocyte sedimentation rate, serum chemistry profile, and urinalysis. Serum should be screened for antinuclear antibodies (ANA) and Ro(SSA)/La(SSB) antibodies. It should be emphasized that although, as mentioned above, DLE is the most common form of chronic cutaneous lupus erythematosus, most patients do not have systemic involvement. Risk factors for systemic disease include widespread skin lesions, anemia or leukopenia, and a positive ANA, especially when the titer is high. Despite the relative infrequency of internal involvement, aggressive treatment of DLE is warranted because the scarring from the disease can be devastating. The characteristic 'carpet tack' scale associated with lesions indicates follicular involvement, and the disease leads to permanent scarring alopecia. Moreover, the depigmentation in fully evolved lesions can be disfiguring, especially in dark-skinned individuals. The goal of therapy is to halt the inflammatory process quickly and effectively to prevent these changes. The predominance of lesions in exposed areas emphasizes the urgency for prompt effective therapy.

Patients should be counseled on the role of UV light in the provocation of skin lesions, and a program of *sun avoidance* and *sunscreen use* should be instituted. *Corticosteroids,* either topical or intralesional, are the cornerstone of initial therapy for patients with limited involvement. *Hydroxychloroquine* and *other antimalarial drugs* appear to afford a measure of photoprotection and are often quite effective, although their onset of action is relatively slow. *Systemic retinoids* are useful, especially for hyperkeratotic lesions. *Dapsone,* which is more commonly used for lesions of bullous lupus erythematosus, is occasionally effective for patients with DLE. Treatments reserved for refractory cases include *cytotoxic agents, gold,* and *interferon-α.* The role of *thalidomide* in the treatment of DLE is evolving. Other drugs or modalities anecdotally reported to be effective in the treatment of DLE include *clofazimine, sulfasalazine, monoclonal antibodies,* and *laser ablation* of lesions.

SPECIFIC INVESTIGATIONS

- ■ Autoantibody studies
- ■ Indicators of systemic disease

Guidelines of care for cutaneous lupus erythematosus. American Academy of Dermatology. Drake LA, Dinehart SM, Farmer ER, et al. J Am Acad Dermatol 1996;34:830–6.

This article summarizes the latest recommendations for the diagnosis, management, and evaluation of patients with cutaneous lupus erythematosus. The most important points are discussed above in 'Management strategy'. It is emphasized that less than 10% of patients with DLE as their only initial disease manifestation will ever have significant clinical evidence of systemic lupus erythematosus (SLE).

FIRST LINE THERAPIES

■ Sunscreens	B
■ Topical or intralesional corticosteroids	B
■ Topical immunosuppressive agents	C

Phototesting and photoprotection in LE. Walchner M, Messer G, Kind P. Lupus 1997;6:167–74.

Cutaneous lupus erythematosus is a disease that is precipitated and aggravated by exposure to UV light; therefore, sun protection and sun avoidance are vital in its management. A broad-spectrum sunscreen that includes protection against both UVB (sun protection factor 15) and UVA (e.g. containing Parsol® 1789) should be used. Opaque physical sunscreens such as titanium dioxide, red veterinary petrolatum, and zinc oxide can provide broad-spectrum protection, and may be particularly helpful. UV blocking filters should be considered for home and automobile windows, and diffusion shields may provide benefit on fluorescent lights. Conversely, the patient (and the referring internist) should be reminded to limit the use of potentially photosensitizing drugs.

Successful treatment of chronic skin diseases with clobetasol propionate and a hydrocolloid occlusive dressing. Volden G. Acta Derm Venereol 1992;72:69–72.

Topical and intralesional corticosteroids play an important role in the management of DLE; however, their use involves a delicate balancing act because the disease ultimately causes cutaneous atrophy, which is also a side effect of long-term local corticosteroid use. Potent topical corticosteroid preparations are more effective than weaker preparations, but are also more likely to cause atrophy. Only active lesions should be treated. Likewise, larger lesions, which may show residual scarring and central atrophy, and erythema, scaling and hyperkeratosis at the periphery, should only be treated in the areas of disease activity. Occlusive dressings may provide additional therapeutic benefit, but increase the risk of atrophy and other topical corticosteroid-related side effects. Less potent preparations are preferred for facial lesions. If these are ineffective, stronger compounds can be used, provided their application is restricted only to areas of active inflammation.

Topical tacrolimus therapy of resistant cutaneous lesions in lupus erythematosus: a possible alternative. Lampropoulos CE, Sangle S, Harrison P, Hughes GR, D'Cruz DP. Rheumatology (Oxford) 2004;43:1383–5.

Pimecrolimus 1% cream for cutaneous lupus erythematosus. Kreuter A, Gambichler T, Breuckmann F, et al. J Am Acad Dermatol 2004;51:407–10.

The macrolactam immunosuppressive agents, tacrolimus and pimecrolimus, have been reported anecdotally to be effective in the treatment of lesions of DLE. Although probably not as effective as superpotent topical corticosteroid preparations, they may have a role when cutaneous atrophy, either disease or treatment-related, is a concern.

SECOND LINE THERAPIES

■ Antimalarial drugs	B
■ Systemic retinoids	B
■ Dapsone	D

Management of skin disease in lupus. Callen JP. Bull Rheum Dis 1997;46:4–7.

Antimalarial drugs are the favored long-term treatment for DLE and are effective in many patients in whom topical therapy alone is unsuccessful. In most patients, 6 weeks of treatment is needed before they begin to exert their effect, and therefore concomitant treatment is indicated, at least initially, in most patients. Hydroxychloroquine is most often used, chloroquine being reserved for unresponsive patients. Both drugs can cause a characteristic antimalarial retinopathy and thus periodic (every 6 months) ophthalmological examinations are necessary. Quinacrine, which is not a significant cause of retinopathy, has become increasingly difficult to obtain. It may be used alone or in combination with other antimalarial agents.

Isotretinoin for refractory lupus erythematosus. Shornick JK, Formica N, Parke AL. J Am Acad Dermatol 1991;24:49–52.

Oral retinoids, either isotretinoin or acitretin, are useful in the treatment of DLE, particularly the hypertrophic variety. Their teratogenic effects must be respected, especially because patients with DLE are often women of childbearing age. The long-term adverse effects of retinoids, including hypertriglyceridemia and possible bony abnormalities, must also be considered in constructing a treatment plan. As with other treatments for DLE, the disease occasionally flares, even with continued treatment.

A case of SLE with acute, subacute and chronic lesions successfully treated with dapsone. Neri R, Mosca M, Bernacchi E, Bombardieri S. Lupus 1999;8:240–3.

Dapsone is most often used in the treatment of bullous cutaneous lupus erythematosus. Occasionally, however, it has been reported to be effective in patients with DLE.

THIRD LINE THERAPIES

■ Cytotoxic agents	D
■ Thalidomide	D
■ Gold	D
■ Interferon-α	D
■ Clofazimine	D
■ Sulfasalazine	D
■ Monoclonal antibodies	D
■ Laser therapy	D

Management of antimalarial-refractory cutaneous lupus erythematosus. Callen JP. Lupus 1997;6:203–8.

Cytotoxic agents, including azathioprine, cyclophosphamide, and methotrexate, have been used in patients with DLE resistant to conservative management. However, although the scarring from the disease can be quite disfiguring, the use of cytotoxic drugs for this indication is limited by their significant toxicities.

Low-dose thalidomide therapy for refractory cutaneous lesions of lupus erythematosus. Housman TS, Jorizzo JL, McCarty MA, et al. Arch Dermatol 2003;139:50–4.

Thalidomide in cutaneous lupus erythematosus. Pelle MT, Werth VP. Am J Clin Dermatol 2003;4:379–87.

Thalidomide has been used in the treatment of patients with cutaneous lupus erythematosus refractory to other modalities. The response is variable. Again, it must be emphasized that the disease typically affects young women of childbearing age, and the teratogenic potential of the drug should not be ignored. Sensory neuropathy is another potential complication of thalidomide administration.

Treatment of chronic discoid lupus erythematosus with an oral gold compound (auranofin). Dalzial K, Going G, Cartwright PH, et al. Br J Dermatol 1986;115:211–6.

Gold has been used in the treatment of patients with DLE, but its use has been limited to small series. Physicians prescribing gold should be familiar with its unique toxicities.

Response of discoid and subacute cutaneous lupus erythematosus to recombinant interferon alpha-2a. Nicolas JF, Thivolet J, Kanitakis J, Lyonnet S. J Invest Dermatol 1990;95:142S–154S.

Interferon-α-2a has been administered both systemically and intralesionally for the treatment of DLE. Although it has in some cases been successful, the response is variable. The use of interferon may be somewhat counterintuitive because more recent data suggest a role for interferon-α in the pathogenesis of SLE.

Evidence levels **A** Double-blind study **B** Clinical trial ≥ 20 subjects **C** Clinical trial < 20 subjects **D** Series ≥ 5 subjects **E** Anecdotal case reports

Clofazimine: a review of its medical uses and mechanisms of action. Arbiser JL, Moschella SL. J Am Acad Dermatol 1995;32:241–7.

Clofazimine has been used successfully to treat some patients with DLE.

Treatment of discoid lupus erythematosus with sulfasalazine: 11 cases. Delaporte E, Catteau B, Sabbagh N, et al. Ann Dermatol Venereol 1997;124:151–6.

A few patients with DLE have been treated with sulfasalazine. This series of 11 patients included seven complete responders, one partial responder, and three patients who failed to respond. Sulfasalazine is a potentially photosensitizing drug, and its use should be limited to patients with resistant disease that has not responded to more conventional therapy.

Treatment of severe cutaneous lupus erythematosus with a chimeric CD4 monoclonal antibody, cM-T412. Prinz JC, Meurer M, Reiter C, et al. J Am Acad Dermatol 1996;34:244–52.

A chimeric CD4 monoclonal antibody was used to treat five patients with severe cutaneous lupus erythematosus. Many experienced a longlasting decrease in disease activity, healing of skin lesions, and a reconstituted responsiveness to conventional treatment. Although there was a substantial depletion of circulating CD4[+] T lymphocytes, no clinical signs of immunosuppression were noted.

Successful treatment of discoid lupus erythematosus with argon laser. Kuhn A, Becker-Wegerich PM, Ruzicka T, Lehmann P. Dermatology 2000;201:175–7.

A few patients with treatment-resistant DLE have undergone laser therapy. The treated skin lesions improve after a few sessions while disease activity continues in untreated lesions. Induction of DLE lesions by a Koebner-type reaction has been reported. Further investigation is needed before any conclusions can be drawn about the usefulness of this modality in the long-term management of patients with DLE.

Dissecting cellulitis of the scalp and folliculitis decalvans

Andrew JG McDonagh

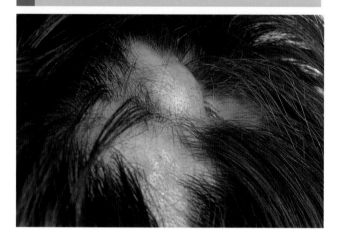

Dissecting cellulitis of the scalp

Dissecting cellulitis is a rare, chronic progressive inflammatory disease of the scalp and affects predominantly the vertex and occipital scalp of males, mainly from the second to the fourth decade. Dissecting cellulitis may occur in association with hidradenitis suppurativa and acne conglobata to form the 'follicular occlusion or retention triad'. The suggested common pathogenic mechanism includes follicular retention, intense folliculitis, and granulomatous changes, leading to interconnecting sinuses along with abscess formation. Patchy alopecia is associated with extensive fibrosis and scarring, which may become keloidal.

MANAGEMENT STRATEGY

Dissecting cellulitis is characterized by a chronic, progressive course with temporary improvement on treatment followed by relapses when treatment is discontinued. There are no large therapeutic clinical trials and recommendations for therapy are based on case reports or small series. Inflammatory tinea capitis (kerion) and the very rare case of occult squamous carcinoma should be excluded. Although no specific pathogenetic organisms have been isolated, bacteriology swabs should be obtained and the antibiotic sensitivity of organisms reviewed.

In mild cases or when disease is limited, *improved scalp hygiene* and the use of *antiseptics, topical antibiotics* (based on bacterial culture results), *intralesional corticosteroid injections* and periodic *aspiration of fluctuant lesions* may be adequate. At an early stage, *systemic antibiotics* such as *tetracycline* and *clindamycin* reduce inflammation and can control disease. In more severe cases a *combination of systemic antibiotics and*

corticosteroids may be effective. *Isotretinoin* has been shown to provide sustained remission if continued for at least 4 months after clinical control is achieved, at a dose of 0.75–1.0 mg/kg daily. Oral *zinc sulfate* has received anecdotal reports of success when used long term.

X-ray epilation of affected areas has been superseded by *laser epilation* before the stage of massive inflammation occurs. Resistant cases may require *surgical excision and skin grafting*.

SPECIFIC INVESTIGATIONS

- Swabs for bacteriology
- Scrapings and plucked hair roots for mycology
- Scalp biopsy for histology and fungal culture

Inflammatory tinea capitis (kerion) mimicking dissecting cellulitis. Sperling LC, Major MC. Int J Dermatol 1991;30: 190–2.

Two cases of highly inflammatory tinea capitis eventuating in scarring alopecia. In any inflammatory alopecia in adults, tinea capitis should be excluded. If scalp scrapings and plucked hair roots do not show spores, and superficial fungal culture gives negative results, a biopsy for histology and fungal culture should be performed.

Dissecting cellulitis of the scalp in 2 girls. Ramesh V. Dermatologica 1990;180:48–50.

Two girls with dissecting cellulitis, and in one of these *Pseudomonas aeruginosa* was isolated from sinus discharge. The role of infection in perpetuating the condition is highlighted.

Squamous cell carcinoma arising in dissecting perifolliculitis of the scalp. Curry SS, Gaither DH, King LE. J Am Acad Dermatol 1981;4:673–8.

A case of squamous cell carcinoma arising in dissecting folliculitis of the scalp that was fatally aggressive. Early diagnosis and treatment are essential.

Folliculotropic mycosis fungoides with large cell transformation presenting as dissecting cellulitis of the scalp. Gillam AC, Lessin SR, Wilson DM, Salhany KE. J Cutan Pathol 1997;24:169–75.

A patient with follicular mycosis fungoides presenting in a manner similar to dissecting cellulitis of the scalp with nonhealing, draining nodular lesions.

FIRST LINE THERAPIES

Scalp hygiene	D
Topical antibiotics	D
Systemic antibiotics	D
Intralesional corticosteroid injection	D
Incision and drainage	D

Acquired scalp alopecia. Part II. A review. Sullivan JR, Kossard S. Australas J Dermatol 1999;40:61–72.

A good review article on the treatment of pustular scarring alopecia, including dissecting folliculitis.

Perifolliculitis capitis abscedens et suffodiens. Moyer DG, Williams RM. Arch Dermatol 1962;85:118–24.

A report of six cases treated with systemic antibiotics.

Evidence levels **A** Double-blind study **B** Clinical trial ≥ 20 subjects **C** Clinical trial < 20 subjects **D** Series ≥ 5 subjects **E** Anecdotal case reports

Perifolliculitis capitis abscedens et suffodiens (dissecting cellulitis of the scalp). Jolliffe DS, Sarkany I. Clin Exp Dermatol 1977;2:291.

A discussion of the therapeutic difficulties inherent in this disorder and report of a mild case of dissecting folliculitis responding well to oral oxytetracycline 1 g daily for 2 months.

SECOND LINE THERAPIES

■ Systemic corticosteroids	E
■ Isotretinoin (oral)	D
■ Isotretinoin (topical)	E

Perifolliculitis capitis: successful control with alternate day corticosteroids. Adrian RM, Arndt KA. Ann Plast Surg 1980;4:166–9.

The authors used initially high-dose oral prednisolone after intravenous antibiotics had failed to control dissecting cellulitis. Maintenance with 5 mg prednisolone on alternate days for 2 years is reported.

Dissecting cellulitis of the scalp: response to isotretinoin. Scerri L, Williams HC, Allen BR. Br J Dermatol 1996;134: 1105–8.

Three patients with dissecting cellulitis of the scalp showed a sustained therapeutic response to isotretinoin. The authors recommend that isotretinoin should be given initially at 1 mg/kg daily and maintained at a dose not less than 0.75 mg/kg daily for at least 4 months after clinical remission is achieved. Long-term post-treatment follow-up of two of the patients showed sustained benefit.

Perifolliculitis capitis abscedens et suffodiens. Herman A, David M, Pitlik S, Tiqva P. Int J Dermatol 1992;31:746.

A case of dissecting cellulitis responding to isotretinoin at 0.8 mg/kg daily.

Perifolliculitis capitis abscedens et suffodiens successfully controlled with topical isotretinoin. Karpouzis A, Giatromanolaki A, Sivridis E, Kouskoukis C. Eur J Dermatol 2003;13:192–5.

Dissecting cellulitis in an 18-year-old white patient was controlled with topical isotretinoin.

If this therapy could be shown to be effective in larger clinical trials, this would represent a major advance in the treatment of this difficult disease.

THIRD LINE THERAPIES

■ Excision and grafting	E
■ Laser epilation	E
■ X-ray epilation	E
■ Systemic zinc sulfate	E

Dissecting cellulitis of the scalp. Williams CN, Cohen M, Ronan SG, Lewandowski CA. Plast Reconstr Surg 1986;77: 378–82.

Four patients with extensive scalp disease showing a favorable response to wide excision and split-thickness skin graft.

Perifolliculitis capitis abscedens et suffodiens. Moyer DG, Williams RM. Arch Dermatol 1962;85:378.

Scalping and grafting recommended for intractable dissecting cellulitis of the scalp.

Use of an 800-nm pulsed-diode laser in the treatment of recalcitrant dissecting cellulitis of the scalp. Boyd AS, Binhlam JQ. Arch Dermatol 2002;138:1291–3.

Complete clearance of disease poorly responsive to multiple drugs after four treatments at monthly intervals with remission maintained 6 months after laser epilation.

Treatment of perifolliculitis capitis abscedens et suffodiens with carbon dioxide laser. Glass LF, Berman B, Laub D. J Dermatol Surg Oncol 1989;15:673–6.

Perifolliculitis capitis abscedens et suffodiens. McMullen FH, Zeligman I. Arch Dermatol 1956;73:256–63.

With recurrence of dissecting cellulitis following topical and systemic treatment, some benefit is obtained from X-ray epilation.

Successful treatment of dissecting cellulitis and acne conglobata with oral zinc. Kobayashi H, Aiba S, Tagami H. Br J Dermatol 1999;141:1136–8.

A case report of a patient with dissecting cellulitis and acne conglobata responding to oral zinc sulfate 135 mg three times daily for 12 weeks. The dose was reduced to 260 mg daily for 7 weeks with no recurrence, but 1 week after stopping zinc therapy, scalp nodules recurred. Oral zinc was resumed and scalp lesions diminished within 8 weeks. Afterwards, disease was well controlled for 1 year on zinc sulfate 135 mg daily.

Perifolliculitis capitis abscedens et suffodiens (Hoffman): complete healing associated with oral zinc therapy. Berne B, Venge P, Ohman S. Arch Dermatol 1985;121:1028–30.

The patient was treated with an initial dose of 90 mg of Zn^{2+} (corresponding to 400 mg of zinc sulfate three times daily). Complete healing was seen after 3 months, when the dose was halved, and after an additional $2^1/_2$ months, therapy was stopped. No relapse occurred during a 5-year follow-up.

Folliculitis decalvans

Folliculitis decalvans is a rare progressive purulent folliculitis of the scalp resulting in follicular atrophy and subsequent scarring alopecia. 'Tufted folliculitis' is a characteristic of the disorder in evolution, with multiple hair tufts emerging from inflamed and crusted follicular orifices.

The etiology is unknown. Impaired immune responses, *Staphylococcus aureus* infection, nevoid lesions, and seborrheic states have been suggested as playing a role in its pathogenesis, though much controversy surrounds the role of each factor. Gram-positive organisms are usually present during active disease phases.

Folliculitis decalvans may affect any hairbearing region – scalp, face, axillae, pubes, and inner thighs. Scalp disease affects both sexes. In other sites it is confined to adult males. It occurs predominantly in men from adolescence onwards and in women between the third and sixth decades.

MANAGEMENT STRATEGY

Treatment of this chronic and progressive disease is notoriously difficult. *Underlying diseases such as immune deficiency or fungal infection* should be sought. *Staphylococcus aureus* or other Gram-positive organisms are present in follicular pustules and sometimes also in the anterior nares. *Bacteriology swabs* should be taken for culture and to determine sensitivity.

Topical and systemic antibiotics are the mainstay of treatment. Systemic antibiotics such as *tetracycline, minocycline, flucloxacillin, vancomycin* and *third generation cephalosporins* may inhibit the extension of disease, but only for as long as they are administered. *Rifampin* has been proposed as the most beneficial therapeutic option in recalcitrant cases, but should not be used as monotherapy because of the rapid emergence of resistance. A regimen of systemic *rifampin* 300 mg twice daily and *clindamycin* 300 mg twice daily for 10 weeks has produced marked improvement with infrequent relapse after one or more treatment courses. Prolonged courses of *dapsone* can also be beneficial.

Systemic corticosteroids suppress the inflammatory response and may provide moderate temporary improvement. There have been anecdotal reports of success using oral *zinc sulfate (in combination with fusidic acid).* Treatments that destroy hair follicles and prevent hair regrowth may be considered – these include *superficial X-ray irradiation, laser epilation, cryosurgery,* and *surgical excision.* Improvement has also been reported with shaving the scalp. *Keratolytics* and *tar shampoos* may reduce the scaling and erythema that herald extension of the disease.

SPECIFIC INVESTIGATIONS

- Swabs for bacteriology of follicular pustules and carrier sites
- Fungal microscopy and culture
- Scalp biopsy
- Immune deficiency screen

Acquired scalp alopecia. Part II: A review. Sullivan JR, Kossard S. Australas J Dermatol 1999;40:61–72.

A case of an individual with HIV infection who developed severe folliculitis decalvans after commencing triple antiviral therapy.

Folliculitis decalvans with hypocomplementaemia. (Abstract) Fraser NG, Grant PW. Br J Dermatol 1982; 107(suppl 22):88.

A case of a 12-year-old girl with folliculitis decalvans, recurrent nasal sores, bronchitis and secondarily infected chilblain reactions on her feet. She also had low C3 and C4 levels.

Folliculitis decalvans and cellular immunity – 2 brothers with oral candidiasis. Shitara A, Igareshi R, Morohashi M. Jpn J Dermatol 1974;28:133.

Severe folliculitis decalvans in two siblings who also had chronic oral candidiasis; defective cell-mediated immunity was demonstrated.

Tufted folliculitis of the scalp; a distinctive clinicohistological variant of folliculitis decalvans. Amnessi G. Br J Dermatol 1998;138:799–805.

Purulent material from dilated follicules was sampled in ten patients. *Staph. aureus* was isolated in all cases, whereas fungal cultures were negative.

Folliculitis decalvans. Bogg A. Acta Derm Venereol 1963;43: 14–24.

In most cases, culture revealed the presence of *Staph. aureus* in the affected follicles. The presence of organisms is likely to contribute to the pathogenesis.

FIRST LINE THERAPIES

Topical antibiotics	
■ Fusidic acid	E
Systemic antibiotics	
■ Rifampin and clindamycin	D
■ Tetracycline, minocycline, flucloxacillin, vancomycin, and third generation cephalosporins	E

Folliculitis decalvans including tufted folliculitis: clinical, histological and therapeutic findings. Powell JJ, Dawber RPR, Gatter K. Br J Dermatol 1999;140:328–33.

Eighteen patients with folliculitis decalvans treated with a combination of oral rifampin 300 mg twice daily and clindamycin 300 mg twice daily for 10 weeks. Ten of the 18 patients responded well with no evidence of recurrence 2–22 months after one course of treatment, and 15 of the 18 responded after two to three courses.

Tufted folliculitis of the scalp: a distinctive clinicohistological variant of folliculitis decalvans. Annessi G. Br J Dermatol 1998;138:799–805.

A useful review of the strengths and limitations of topical and oral antibiotics for folliculitis decalvans.

Folliculitis decalvans – response to rifampicin. Brozena SJ, Cohen LE, Fenske NA. Cutis 1988;42:512–5.

A recalcitrant case of folliculitis decalvans with excellent response to rifampin 600 mg daily for 10 weeks. There was no response with zinc, even in supraphysiological doses.

Folliculitis decalvans. Bogg A. Acta Derm Venereol 1963; 43:14–24.

A case of folliculitis decalvans responding to treatment with fusidic acid.

No information about treatment protocol was given.

A case of lupoid sycosis or ulerythema sycosiforme beginning in infancy. Lowenthal LJ. Br J Dermatol 1957;69:443–9.

A case of progressive follicular scarring alopecia beginning in infancy was treated with oxytetracycline 250 mg four times daily for 2 weeks. At the end of this course all redness, scaling, and infiltration had disappeared. Two months later, without any further treatment, the improvement was maintained.

SECOND LINE THERAPIES

■ Fusidic acid and oral zinc sulfate	E
■ Dapsone	E
■ Prednisolone and isotretinoin	E

Evidence levels A Double-blind study **B** Clinical trial ≥ 20 subjects **C** Clinical trial < 20 subjects **D** Series ≥ 5 subjects **E** Anecdotal case reports

Dapsone treatment of folliculitis decalvans. Paquet P, Pierard GE. Ann Dermatol Venereol 2004;131:195–7.

Two cases of folliculitis decalvans treated with dapsone 75–100 mg daily with clearance of pustular folliculitis after 1–2 months. Moderate relapse occurred within a few weeks of stopping dapsone; remission was sustained for 1–3 years on a maintenance dose of dapsone 25 mg daily.

Folliculitis decalvans. Abeck D, Korting HC, Braun-Falco O. Acta Derm Venereol 1992;72:143–5.

Three patients with folliculitis decalvans, followed up for more than a year responded to a combination of oral and topical fusidic acid and oral zinc sulfate. Each patient received a 3-week oral course of fusidic acid 500 mg 3 three times daily and a 6-month course of zinc sulfate 200 mg twice daily, after which the dose was reduced to 200 mg daily. Treatment with fusidic acid and zinc sulfate was started simultaneously. In addition, 1.5% fusidic acid in a cream base was applied topically for the first 2 weeks.

Simultaneous occurrence of folliculitis decalvans capillitii in identical twins. Douwes KE, Landthaler M, Szeimies R-M. Br J Dermatol 2000;143:195–7.

The use of oral prednisolone with low-dose isotretinoin to control folliculitis decalvans is described.

THIRD LINE THERAPIES

■ Surgical excision	E
■ Keratolytics and tar shampoo	E
■ Superficial X-ray therapy	E
■ Nd:YAG laser	E

Tufted hair folliculitis. Tong AK, Baden HP. J Am Acad Dermatol 1989;21:1096–9.

Successful treatment of tufted folliculitis by surgical excision.

Tufted hair folliculitis. A study of 4 cases. Leulmo-Aguilar J, Gonzalez-Castro U, Castells-Rodelas A. Br J Dermatol 1993;128:454–7.

The authors consider that erythema and scaling herald extension of the disease process and that treatment with keratolytics and tar shampoo is important.

Nd:YAG laser treatment of recalcitrant folliculitis decalvans. Parlette EC, Kroeger N, Ross EV. Dermatol Surg 2004;30:1152–4.

Remission achieved by laser epilation in an African-American patient.

Based on the optical properties of light in skin, the Nd:YAG laser is the best for laser depilation in dark individuals.

Drug eruptions

Neil H Shear

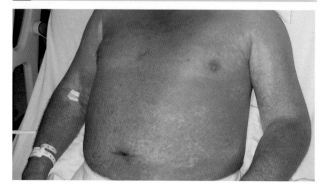

Drug eruptions are drug-induced diseases, often with a known etiology, but a poorly understood pathogenesis. Drug eruptions are common adverse events. Mild eruptions may be as common as one in ten exposures with some marketed drugs. Severe eruptions with systemic involvement occur in one in 3000 exposures, but life-threatening eruptions such as toxic epidermal necrolysis (TEN) are much less common.

The image above shows widespread exanthematous eruption. This can be localized to skin or, in the presence of fever, may be a systemic reaction.

MANAGEMENT STRATEGY

There are two steps in diagnosing drug eruptions. First, determine the morphology, most commonly among exanthematous ('maculopapular eruption'), urticarial, blistering, or pustular. Second, look for signs of systemic involvement, such as fever, lymphadenopathy, or malaise. Examples of simple eruptions, without systemic disease, are maculopapular eruption (unfortunately the most common drug eruption has no official name), urticaria, fixed drug eruption, and drug-induced acne. Examples of complex eruptions with systemic disease are hypersensitivity drug reaction, serum sickness-like reaction, Stevens–Johnson syndrome and TEN, and acute generalized exanthematous pustulosis.

After a diagnosis is considered, it is important to identify the relevant drug exposure, consider a differential diagnosis, and remember that each drug exposure has a possible etiologic role. Some are more likely than others, but it is rare that a single drug is the only culprit.

Treatment involves *stopping drugs that have a high probability of being the cause, while providing supportive therapy of symptoms*. Laboratory investigations may identify internal organ toxicity and systemic therapy may be considered. The patient should be *advised of the interpretation of the adverse event*, what drugs were likely causes, whether tests will help confirm the cause, and what drugs should be avoided in the future. For severe reactions relatives may need to be notified by the patient because some systemic reactions have a genetic susceptibility.

SPECIFIC INVESTIGATIONS

- Skin biopsy
- Vital signs
- Physical exam
- Hemogram
- Liver enzymes
- Urinalysis

FIRST LINE THERAPIES

■ Topical corticosteroids	E
■ Oral antihistamines	E
■ Nonsteroidal anti-inflammatory drugs	E

Most exanthems and urticarial eruptions are pruritic. Topical corticosteroids and oral antihistamines are usually soothing. If Benadryl® (diphenhydramine) is used, it is important to recognize that it may cross-react with some drugs, and could make the eruption worse. Febrile symptoms may be helped by ibuprofen. Acetaminophen (paracetamol) could compromise hepatic toxicity, but is often used. Clinical trials of therapy for most simple drug eruptions have not been conducted.

Guidelines of care for cutaneous adverse drug reactions. Drake LA, Dinehart SM, Farmer ER, et al. J Am Acad Derm 1996;35:458–61.

Treatment for cutaneous eruptions includes topical corticosteroids, antihistamines, topical antipruritic agents, baths (with or without additives), and emollients.

SECOND LINE THERAPIES

■ Systemic corticosteroids	E
■ Cyclosporine	D
■ Intravenous immunoglobulin G (IVIG)	C
■ Ocular care	E
■ Debridement and artificial skin membrane	E
■ Pain control	E

In complex reactions, severe discomfort or pending organ failure may require the use of oral corticosteroids. The optimal dose is unknown, but we use 1 mg/kg daily of prednisone to bring the reaction under control and prevent progression. If prednisone is used for complex, systemic reactions, it may take months to withdraw the corticosteroid due to flares of symptoms. Without prednisone, the reaction may take weeks to settle.

Systemic corticosteroids in the phenytoin hypersensitivity syndrome. Chopra S, Levell NJ, Cowley G, Gilkes JJ. Br J Derm 1996;134:1109–12.

Anticonvulsant hypersensitivity syndrome: treatment with corticosteroids and intravenous immunoglobulin. Mostella J, Pieroni R, Jones R, Finch CK. South Med J 2004;97:319–21.

A patient is described who developed hypersensitivity syndrome reaction and was treated with the combination of corticosteroids and immunoglobulin therapy. The clinical manifestations improved during corticosteroid and immunoglobulin therapy and then recurred after withdrawal of corticosteroids. After the reinstitution of corticosteroids with a prolonged taper, the signs and symptoms resolved completely.

Treatment of toxic epidermal necrolysis with cyclosporin A. Arevalo JM, Lorente JA, Gonzalez-Herrada C, Jimenez-Reyes J. J Trauma 2000;48:473–8.

A retrospective case series of eleven patients with TEN treated with cyclosporin A (3 mg/kg daily enterally every 12 h) is reported. Treatment with cyclosporin A was associated with a rapid re-epithelialization rate and a low mortality rate compared to patients treated with cyclophosphamide and corticosteroids (0 vs 50%, respectively).

Relief is often rapid and the drug can be stopped in under 1 week of therapy.

Analysis of intravenous immunoglobulin for the treatment of toxic epidermal necrolysis using SCORTEN: the University of Miami experience. Trent JT, Kirsner RS, Romanelli P, Kerdel FA. Arch Dermatol 2003;139:39–43.

A retrospective analysis of 16 consecutive patients with TEN who were treated with IVIG (1 g/kg daily for 15 patients) was completed. Treatment with IVIG significantly decreased the mortality rate (one patient died) compared to the SCORTEN-predicted mortality rate.

The use of IVIG is controversial. Some studies suggest that it is very helpful in reducing the mortality rate from TEN. It has never been shown to reduce the risk of permanent eye damage. Recommended dosages are 1 g/kg daily for 4 days.

Intravenous immunoglobulin does not improve outcome in toxic epidermal necrolysis. Shortt R, Gomez M, Mittman N, Cartotto R. J Burn Care Rehabil 2004;25:246–55.

A retrospective cohort review was used to compare outcomes in TEN patients who received IVIG (n = 16) compared to those who did not receive IVIG (n = 16). There was no significant difference in the mortality rate between the IVIG group (25%) and the control group (38%), though there was a trend towards less severe wound progression in patients who received IVIG.

Up to 25% of TEN patients can die so it is important to institute therapy early. An intensive care or burn unit is superior to a medical ward. Oxygenation, eye care, skin care, and pain control are critical.

Analysis of the acute ophthalmic manifestations of the erythema multiforme/Stevens–Johnson syndrome/toxic epidermal necrolysis disease spectrum. Power WJ, Ghoraishi M, Merayo-Lloves J, et al. Ophthalmology 1995;102:1669–76.

Topical antibiotic and corticosteroid usage, frequent lubrication, and the occasional use of therapeutic soft common lenses are common modalities of treatment used; however, the efficacy of such local treatments has never been evaluated in a prospective manner.

In TEN it is important to be mindful of ocular scarring. Topical cleansing and use of a glass rod daily to prevent adhesions is very important.

OTHER THERAPIES

■ Counseling	E
■ Drug testing	C
■ Inform patient of support groups	E

Anticonvulsant hypersensitivity syndrome: incidence, prevention and management. Knowles SR, Shapiro LE, Shear NH. Drug Saf 1999;21:489–501.

Patients with a history of anticonvulsant hypersensitivity syndrome should be counseled about potentially cross-reacting medications. Family counseling is a critical part of patient management in serious idiosyncratic reactions. The patient should carry a notification of the sensitivity (e.g. a MedicAlert® bracelet).

Patients need to have a clear understanding that they have had a drug eruption and the risk of sequelae, the drugs that they need to avoid in future, and the risks of future exposure.

Clinical experience with penicillin skin testing in a large inner-city STD clinic. Gadde J, Spence M, Wheeler B, et al. JAMA 1993;270:2456–63.

Skin testing with both major and minor penicillin determinants is safe using current recommendations, and both reagents are necessary for maximizing the identification of sensitized subjects. Routine penicillin skin testing can facilitate the safe use of penicillin in 90% of individuals with a previous history of penicillin allergy.

Guidelines for performing skin tests with drugs in the investigation of cutaneous adverse drug reactions. Barbaud A, Goncalo M, Bruynzeel D, Bircher A. Contact Derm 2001;45:321–8.

Guidelines suggest that drug skin tests should be performed 6 weeks to 6 months after complete healing of the cutaneous adverse drug reaction. Drug patch tests are performed using the commercialized form of the drug diluted at 30% with petrolatum and/or water. Drug prick and intradermal tests are performed with sequential dilutions of the commercialized form of the drug.

Drug testing is not widely available. Skin testing for penicillin allergy is very useful, but patch testing and intradermal testing may be required. Penicillin metabolites are also needed in the testing regimen (major and minor determinants). Allergists with an interest in drug reactions may have the proper reagents. Patch testing has been used and is investigational.

Disease management of drug hypersensitivity: a practice parameter. Bernstein I, Gruchalla R, Lee R, et al. Ann Allergy Asthma Immunol 1999;83:665–700.

This document provides guidelines for the management and diagnosis of patients with histories of adverse drug reactions, including cutaneous eruptions. The principle of a graded challenge is based on the administration of small doses of the drug with incremental progression at regular intervals until a therapeutic dose is achieved.

Drug provocation tests in patients with a history suggesting an immediate drug hypersensitivity reaction. Messaad J, Sahla H, Benahmed S, et al. Ann Intern Med 2004;140:1001–6.

Single-blinded administration of increasing doses of the suspected drug, up to the usual daily dose, were administered to 898 patients with suspected immediate drug allergy. There were 17.6% positive drug provocation test results.

Oral re-challenge with the drug in question has been used, but this cannot be recommended in most cases. The clinical question should be 'What drug can the patient use in future?' not 'What drug caused the reaction?'

Eosinophilic fasciitis

Brian S Fuchs, Marsha L Gordon

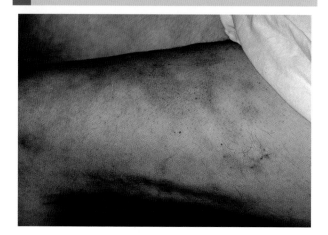

Eosinophilic fasciitis (EF) is a rare fibrosing disorder characterized by the rapid onset of symmetric woody induration of the extremities. Clinically, the progression of EF is marked by edema followed by dimpling of the skin and a peau d'orange appearance evolving into symmetric induration of the extremities and, less frequently, the trunk. Typically, the hands, feet, and face are spared. Although the etiology is unknown, vigorous exercise has been reported before the onset of EF in many cases.

MANAGEMENT STRATEGY

EF must be distinguished from scleroderma, from which it is differentiated by its lack of sclerodactyly, Raynaud's phenomenon, and serologic markers. EF has a more rapid onset than scleroderma, is associated with a peripheral eosinophilia, and usually responds to corticosteroid therapy. EF must also be differentiated from eosinophilia myalgia syndrome, which is caused by the ingestion of contaminated tryptophan.

Underlying hematologic disorders such as significant cytopenias, myeloproliferative disorders, leukemias, and aplastic anemia may be associated with EF and must be checked for. Additionally, simvastatin and trichloroethylene have been associated with this disorder, and a history of their ingestion must be ruled out.

EF *may resolve spontaneously*, but treatment helps prevent the progression to flexion contractures and impaired mobility. The response may be defined by clinical improvement resulting in a softening and loosening of fibrosed skin with improvement of contractures and better mobility. Serum aldolase levels may be a useful indicator of disease activity. Magnetic resonance imaging (MRI) has been employed in diagnosing EF and in monitoring the effectiveness of treatment.

The first line agent for EF is *prednisone*, initially at a dosage of 40–60 mg daily. A clinical response usually is noted within the first few weeks, and then the dose is slowly tapered over several months to an alternate-day regimen.

Patients who have an incomplete response or fail to respond to prednisone may benefit from the addition of *hydroxychloroquine* at a dose of 200–400 mg daily. Hydroxychloroquine alone has also been used successfully.

Clinical improvement with no recurrence after 1 year has been reported with *cyclosporine* 3.7 mg/kg daily tapered to 2.5 mg/kg. There has also been success with an aggressive course of *pulse methylprednisolone*, 1 g daily for 5 days, in conjunction with cyclosporine 150 mg twice daily.

Cimetidine 400 mg every 6–12 h, has been helpful in some cases. *Methotrexate, azathioprine, chloroquine, D-penicillamine, ketotifen, sulfasalazine, griseofulvin*, and *psoralen and UVA (PUVA)* have all been reported to have beneficial effects.

SPECIFIC INVESTIGATIONS

- Complete blood count
- Serum aldolase
- MRI
- History to exclude tryptophan, simvastatin, or trichloroethylene ingestion

Eosinophilic fasciitis. Sibrack LA, Mazur EM, Hoffman R, Bollet AJ. Clin Rheum Dis 1982;8:443–54.

Peripheral eosinophilia is typically present during active disease except in those patients who have an associated aplastic marrow. The eosinophilia is often transient, and may precede the clinical diagnosis.

Patients with eosinophilic fasciitis should have a bone marrow examination to identify myelodysplasia. Brito-Babapulee F. Br J Dermatol 1997;137:316–7.

EF may be associated with significant cytopenias and myeloproliferative disorders. Therefore, those patients who have abnormal complete blood counts should have a bone marrow examination.

Serum aldolase level is a useful indicator of disease activity in eosinophilic fasciitis. Fujimoto M, Sato S, Ihn H, et al. J Rheumatol 1995;22:563–5.

Three patients with EF are reported to have increased aldolase levels, which normalize with corticosteroid treatment and rise with recurrence of skin sclerosis.

Use of magnetic resonance imaging in diagnosing eosinophilic fasciitis. Report of two cases. Al-Shaikh A, Freeman C, Avruch L, McKendry RJR. Arthritis Rheum 1994;37:1602–8.

MRI is a useful noninvasive tool for diagnosing EF and for monitoring the effectiveness of therapy.

Eosinophilic fasciitis associated with tryptophan ingestion: a manifestation of eosinophilia myalgia syndrome. Gordon ML, Lebwohl MG, Phelps RG, et al. Arch Dermatol 1991;127:217–20.

Ingestion of contaminated tryptophan is associated with a very similar clinical entity called eosinophilia myalgia syndrome.

Eosinophilic fasciitis. A pathologic study of twenty cases. Barnes L, Rodnan GP, Medsger TA, Short D. Am J Pathol 1979;96:493–517.

Deep fascia and subcutaneous tissue are infiltrated with lymphocytes, plasma cells, histiocytes and eosinophils early in the course of the disease. Sclerosis of the dermis with increased collagen occurs later in the course of the disease.

FIRST LINE THERAPIES

■ Systemic corticosteroids	B
■ Pulsed methylprednisolone	E

Eosinophilic fasciitis: clinical spectrum and therapeutic response in 52 cases. Lakhanpal S, Ginsburg WW, Michet CJ, et al. Semin Arthritis Rheum 1988;17:221–31.

Of the 52 cases, 34 patients were treated with prednisone dosages ranging from 40 to 60 mg daily. The remaining 18 patients were treated with either hydroxychloroquine, colchicine, D-penicillamine, or no medication. Twenty of the 34 patients treated with prednisone had a partial response (>25% improvement) and five had complete resolution, detected after 3–6 months. Eight of the nine patients who had a poor response were treated with the addition of hydroxychloroquine at a dose of 200–400 mg daily. Two responded completely, two had an improvement of over 50%, and three were lost to follow-up. Eight patients also responded to treatment with hydroxychloroquine alone – two had complete resolution, four had a partial response, and the others were lost to follow-up. Relapses occurred in some patients and responses were not predictive of future recovery with the same therapy.

Diffuse fasciitis with eosinophilia: a steroid-responsive variant of scleroderma. Britt WJ, Duray PH, Dahl MV, Goltz RW. J Pediatr 1980;97:432–4.

A patient with EF responded completely to prednisone 40 mg/m^2 daily for 1 month, tapered to decreasing dosages every other day over 6 months.

Eosinophilic fasciitis. Helfman T, Falanga V. Clin Dermatol 1994;12:449–55.

Approximately 60% of patients with EF respond to prednisone at a dose of 40–60 mg daily within weeks of treatment.

A good review article.

Eosinophilic fasciitis associated with autoimmune thyroid disease and myelodysplasia treated with pulsed methylprednisolone and antihistamines. Farrell AM, Ross JS, Bunker CB. Br J Dermatol 1999;140:1169–99.

A 74-year-old man with EF associated with autoimmune thyroid disease and myelodysplasia responded to a combination of prednisolone, pulsed methylprednisolone, and antihistamines.

SECOND LINE THERAPIES

■ Hydroxychloroquine	C
■ Cyclosporine	D
■ Methotrexate	E
■ Cimetidine	C

Eosinophilic rheumatic disorders. Claw DJ, Crofford LJ. Rheum Clin North Am 1995;21:231–46.

Hydroxychloroquine at a dose of 200–400 mg daily can be used either alone or in combination with corticosteroids.

In the series by Lakhanpal et al. (see above) hydroxychloroquine was also shown to be highly effective.

Eosinophilic fasciitis following exposure to trichloro-ethylene: successful treatment with cyclosporin. Hayashi N, Igarashi A, Matsuyama T, Harada S. Br J Dermatol 2000;142:830–2.

This case report demonstrated clinical improvement within 1 month of treatment with cyclosporine 3.7 mg/kg daily tapered to 2.5 mg/kg daily with no recurrence after 1 year.

Eosinophilic fasciitis responsive to treatment with pulsed steroids and cyclosporine. Valencia IC, Chang A, Kirsner RS, Kerdel FA. Int J Dermatol 1999;38:369–72.

A significant clinical response within 3 weeks was shown with pulsed methylprednisolone 1 g daily for 5 days, in conjunction with cyclosporine 150 mg twice daily.

Treatment of eosinophilic fasciitis with methotrexate. Pouplin S, Daragon A, Le Loet X. J Rheumatol 1998;25:606–7.

In an effort to eliminate unwanted side effects of corticosteroids, methotrexate 15 mg intramuscularly given once a week, can be added to corticosteroid therapy as it is tapered.

The fasciitis-panniculitis syndromes. Clinical and pathologic features. Naschitz JE, Boss JH, Misselevich I, et al. Medicine 1996;75:6–16.

Complete and partial remission on cimetidine, at 400 mg twice daily, occurred in nine and five patients, respectively. Only three did not respond to cimetidine monotherapy.

The fasciitis-panniculitis syndrome: clinical spectrum and response to cimetidine. Naschitz JE, Yeshurun D, Zuckerman E, et al. Semin Arthritis Rheum 1992;21:211–20.

Six of eight patients treated with cimetidine improved significantly within 6 months. One patient's lesions remitted after 1 year, and the other patient's lesions did not respond. After 4 years, therapy was discontinued and no relapses were seen.

Eosinophilic fasciitis responsive to cimetidine. Solomon G, Barland P, Rifkin H. Ann Intern Med 1982;97:547–9.

Cimetidine's effectiveness in treating EF may be due to its role in blocking histamine-2 receptors on suppressor T lymphocytes and other cells. In 1982, cimetidine was first described as a therapeutic option when a patient's EF lesions resolved after initiating cimetidine, 400 mg every 6 h, as treatment of a presumptive ulcer.

THIRD LINE THERAPIES

■ PUVA	E
■ Extracorporeal photochemotherapy	D
■ Ketotifen	E
■ D-penicillamine	E
■ Azathioprine	E
■ Chloroquine	E
■ Griseofulvin	E
■ Sulfasalazine	E
■ Surgery	E

Eosinophilic fasciitis treated with psoralen-ultraviolet A bath photochemotherapy. Schiener R, Behrens-Williams SC, Gottlober P, et al. Br J Dermatol 2000;142:804–7.

PUVA had promising results within 6 months without side effects in a 56-year-old patient.

Extracorporeal photochemotherapy in the treatment of eosinophilic fasciitis. Romano C, Rubegni P, De Aloe G, et al. J Eur Acad Dermatol Venereol 2003;17:10–3.

Three patients were treated with extracorporeal photochemotherapy with a UVAR XTS apparatus on two consecutive days at 2-week intervals for the first 3 months, followed by treatment every 4 weeks dependent on response. After 1 year of therapy two patients showed a considerable improvement in clinical parameters.

Ketotifen – a therapeutic agent of eosinophilic fasciitis? Ching DWT, Leibowitz MR. J Intern Med 1992;231:555–9.

Ketotifen (a mast cell stabilizer) at 2 mg dosage twice daily was effective in remitting a patient's EF lesions. There were no relapses after 4 months of no further treatment.

Eosinophilic fasciitis: review and report of six cases. Nassonova VA, Ivanova MW, Akhnazarova VD, et al. Scand J Rheumatol 1979;8:225–33.

Some patients may respond to D-penicillamine at 125–375 mg daily to a maximal dose of 750 mg daily, azathioprine 50 mg once or twice daily, or chloroquine.

Griseofulvin for eosinophilic fasciitis. Giordano M, Ara M, Cicala C, et al. Arthritis Rheum 1980;23:1331–2.

In the light of its use in progressive systemic sclerosis, griseofulvin may be useful for patients with EF through its influence on collagen metabolism.

Eosinophilic fasciitis with late onset arthritis responsive to sulfasalazine. Jones AC, Doherty M. J Rheumatol 1993; 20:750–1.

In this patient, there was a complete response to 2 g daily of sulfasalazine within 3 months.

Surgical management of eosinophilic fasciitis of the upper extremity. Suzuki G, Itoh Y, Horiuchi Y. J Hand Surg 1997; 22:405–7.

Although one patient required a second operation for recurrence, all four patients experienced improved mobility a few weeks after fasciectomy with follow-up oral prednisolone. The recovery after surgery occurred sooner than with conservative management.

Epidermal nevi

Warren R Heymann, Robert Burd

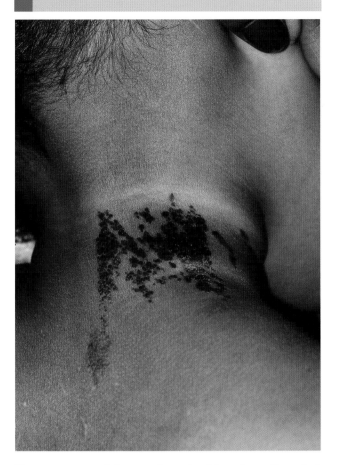

There are several forms of nevi arising from the pluri-potential stem cells of the embryonic ectoderm. The most common are verrucous epidermal nevi, which are best treated with an ablative procedure using either surgical or laser technology. Other inflammatory nevi may respond to topical or systemic therapy.

MANAGEMENT STRATEGY

The pluripotential stem cell in the embryonic ectoderm can develop into any of the cell types found within the epidermis and skin adnexa. Therefore there are many potential nevi that may develop from these cell types. Epidermal nevi may be classified according to the predominant cell type. However, there may be different cell populations or overlap between different areas within the same nevus.

This chapter will concentrate on nevi derived from keratinocytes. Of these, the verrucous epidermal nevus is the most common. Other forms include an inflammatory linear verrucous epidermal nevus (ILVEN), an acantholytic or Darier-like nevus, an epidermolytic form, and linear porokeratosis. Very rarely an epidermal nevus may be associated with other birth defects and a number of epidermal nevus syndromes have been described.

Verrucous epidermal nevi may be localized, segmental, and rarely systematized. There is evidence to support the theory that these nevi may develop as a result of mosaicism and hence may be transmitted to future offspring.

There are very few case reports of malignant change within epidermal nevi and the most troublesome feature is their appearance. It has been postulated that there are dermal influences that drive the differentiation and growth of the epidermis. Thus *surgical management* of these nevi is difficult for the following reasons. Superficial treatments, which only remove the epidermis, have a high recurrence rate, whereas excision or more aggressive ablative procedures may produce unacceptable scarring. *Laser* technology provides the surgeon with more precise tools to maximize efficacy while minimizing scarring. Alternatively for very widespread lesions a variety of *topical regimens*, as well as *systemic retinoids* have been reported to produce some benefit. ILVEN shares many features with psoriasis and certain cases respond to antipsoriatic therapies such as *topical vitamin D analogues*, *corticosteroids*, and *dithranol*. This has led some authors to suggest that this condition is a nevoid form of psoriasis.

Epidermolytic and acantholytic nevi are more likely to respond to treatment with retinoids.

SPECIFIC INVESTIGATION

- Skin biopsy
- X-ray, imaging studies (MRI, CT scans), and ophthalmologic examinations

The diagnosis can usually be made on the clinical appearance and distribution of the lesion alone. However, a skin biopsy will not only confirm the diagnosis, but may also determine the predominant cell type and the presence of inflammatory changes, acantholysis, or dysplasia. This can be helpful in determining which therapeutic modality is most likely to succeed. More importantly in the case of epidermolytic nevi, patients should be informed that there is a possibility that the mutation could be transmitted to their offspring with the risk that they may have generalized cutaneous involvement. Biopsy can also indicate the rare occurrence of squamous cell carcinoma, which can develop in epidermal nevi.

Epidermal nevus syndromes refer to the association of epidermal nevi with extracutaneous manifestations involving the central nervous system, eyes, or bones. The evaluation for extracutaneous disease is based on the clinical extent of the epidermal nevi in conjunction with related organ signs and symptoms.

Epidermolytic hyperkeratosis: generalized form in children from parents with systematized linear form. Nazzaro V, Ermacora E, Santucci B, Caputo R. Br Dermatol 1990;122:417–22.

A report of the inheritance of a generalized epidermolytic hyperkeratosis from parents with a nevoid form of the condition. There is the possibility of making a prenatal diagnosis.

Squamous cell carcinoma arising in a verrucous epidermal naevus. Ichikawa T, Saiki M, Kaneko M, Saida T. Dermatology 1996;193:135–8.

A case report of a squamous cell carcinoma arising in a 74-year-old man with an epidermal nevus, plus a review of the literature, which revealed 18 previous reports of malignant change in epidermal nevi.

Epidermal nevus syndromes. Sugarman JL. Semin Cutan Med Surg 2004;23:145–57.

Several subsets of the epidermal nevus syndrome have been delineated including the nevus sebaceus syndrome, Proteus syndrome, child syndrome, Becker nevus syndrome, nevus comedonicus syndrome, and phakomatosis pigmentokeratotica.

Epidermal nevus syndromes: clinical findings in 35 patients. Vidaurri-de la Cruz H, Tamayo-Sanchez L, Duran-McKinster C, et al. Pediatr Dermatol 2004;21:432–9.

Of patients with epidermal nevi, 10–18% may have disorders of the eye, skeletal, and nervous systems.

Verrucous epidermal nevi

FIRST LINE THERAPIES

■ Excision under local anesthetic	D
■ Shave or curettage under local anesthetic	D
■ Cryotherapy	E

Very small nevi can be excised to leave an acceptable scar, and this is therefore the treatment of choice. However, for larger lesions or for those in cosmetically sensitive sites this may not be possible. For larger lesions shave excision will restore the normal contour of the skin, but invariably there is a color mismatch. Cryotherapy can also ablate the nevus and produce a softer, though often hypopigmented, scar. All these procedures have the benefit of being cost-effective and easily performed.

Comparison of treatment modalities for epidermal nevus: a case report and review. Fox BJ, Lapins NA. J Dermatol Surg Oncol 1983;9:879–85.

A case report of treatment for a verrucous epidermal nevus. Review of the treatment modalities then available indicated that surgical excision was only suitable for small lesions, superficial dermabrasion often led to recurrence, and if performed more deeply could result in hypertrophic scarring. Similar considerations applied to cryosurgery.

Epidermal nevus: surgical treatment by partial-thickness skin excision. Dellon AL, Luethke R, Wong L, Barnett N. Ann Plast Surg 1992;28:292–6.

A case report of treatment of a systematized epidermal nevus by partial-thickness skin excision. This cleared the nevus, but led to extensive hypertrophic scarring.

SECOND LINE THERAPIES

■ Laser ablation	B
■ Dermabrasion	E
■ Ruby laser	E
■ Erbium:YAG laser	C

A resurfacing procedure either mechanically by dermabrading or with laser technology using either the erbium-YAG or CO_2 laser can produce very acceptable results. However, both these techniques are operator dependent, and in the case of laser therapy, access to expensive equip-ment is necessary. Darkly pigmented nevi may be treated using pigmented lesion lasers such as the ruby laser.

Laser therapy of verrucous epidermal naevi. Hohenleutner U, Landthaler M. Clin Exp Dermatol 1993;18:124–7.

A series of 43 patients (41 with verrucous epidermal nevi and two with ILVEN) treated with either the argon laser or the CO_2 laser. Soft, papillomatous lesions responded well to the argon laser, whereas hard keratotic nevi did not respond. A better response was seen to the CO_2 laser, but there was a tendency to hypertrophic scarring with this laser.

CO_2 laser treatment of epidermal nevi: long-term success. Boyce S, Alster TS. Dermatol Surg 2002;28:611–4.

Three females, aged between 15 and 19 years, presented with extensive grouped verrucous papules and plaques on the face, trunk, and extremities. A pulsed CO_2 laser was used to vaporize the lesions using 500 mJ pulse energy, 3 mm spot size, and 7 W of power. All lesions healed without incident. No lesional recurrence was observed 10–13 months after treatment except in one small area of the ankle in one patient.

It is debatable whether one should consider follow-up of 10–13 months 'long-term'.

Pulsed erbium:YAG laser ablation in cutaneous surgery. Kaufmann R, Hibst R. Lasers Surg Med 1996;19:324–30.

A small series of six epidermal nevi treated with the erbium:YAG laser by superficial precise etching of lesional skin only. Good results with no scarring or pigmentary change were seen up to 6 months after the procedure.

Er:YAG laser treatment of verrucous epidermal nevi. Park JH, Hwang ES, Kim SN, Kye YC. Dermatol Surg 2004;30:378–81.

Twenty patients with verrucous epidermal nevi were treated with the erbium:YAG laser. After a single treatment, successful elimination of the verrucous epidermal nevi was observed in 15 patients. Five patients (25%) showed a relapse within the first year following treatment.

Successful treatment of dark-coloured epidermal nevus with ruby laser. Baba T, Narumi H, Hanada K, Hashimoto I. J Dermatol 1995;22:567–70.

Five darkly pigmented epidermal nevi were successfully cleared following one to four treatments with a ruby laser in the normal mode. Two patients subsequently had hypo-pigmentation of the treated site.

THIRD LINE THERAPIES

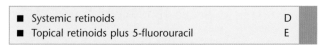

■ Systemic retinoids	D
■ Topical retinoids plus 5-fluorouracil	E

For very extensive and cosmetically troublesome lesions systemic retinoids can reduce the hyperkeratosis, but they need to be continued long term if the benefit is to be maintained. The topical combination of retinoic acid and 5-fluorouracil has also been reported to achieve a desirable cosmetic improvement, but it demands good patient compliance.

Systemic retinoid therapy of systematised verrucous epidermal naevus. Happle R, Kastrup W, Macher E. Dermatologica 1977;155:200–5.

Evidence levels A Double-blind study **B** Clinical trial ≥ 20 subjects **C** Clinical trial < 20 subjects **D** Series ≥ 5 subjects **E** Anecdotal case reports

Report of the use of etretinate in the treatment of a widespread verrucous epidermal nevus.

A case of verrucous epidermal naevus successfully treated with acitretin. Taskapan O, Dogan B, Baloglu H, Harmanyeri Y. Acta Derm Venereol 1998;78:475–6.

Report of a case of verrucous epidermal nevus on a 20-year-old patient that responded to acitretin 75 mg daily. The nevus started to recur 6 weeks after cessation of therapy.

Management of linear verrucous epidermal naevus with topical 5-fluorouracil and tretinoin. Nelson BR, Kolansky G, Gillard M, et al. J Am Acad Dermatol 1994;30:287–8.

A case report of the use of a combination of tretinoin 0.1% cream and 5% 5-fluorouracil applied twice daily under occlusion. The lesion responded well, but was seen to recur 3–4 weeks after therapy was stopped

Topical tretinoin and 5-fluorouracil in the treatment of linear verrucous epidermal nevus. Kim JJ, Chang MW, Shwayder T. J Am Acad Dermatol 2000;43:129–32.

There was significant improvement in this 7-year-old boy with an extensive, facial epidermal nevus using the concept of combination therapy for these lesions.

Inflammatory/dysplastic epidermal nevi

Nevi that have inflammatory, epidermolytic, acantholytic, or dysplastic features may respond to medical therapy more effectively than surgical treatment.

FIRST LINE THERAPIES

■ Topical corticosteroids	D

Topical corticosteroids are often used as first line therapy, but the response is often variable. There are few clinical data on the use of topical corticosteroids and their use appears to be empirical rather than evidence based; nevertheless they are relatively cheap and safe.

SECOND LINE THERAPIES

■ Topical calcipotriol/tacalcitol	D
■ Topical retinoids	E
■ Topical dithranol	E

ILVEN have been shown to respond to a variety of antipsoriatic modalities, leading some authors to believe that it is a nevoid form of psoriasis.

Topical calcipotriol for the treatment of inflammatory linear verrucous epidermal nevus. Zvulunov A, Grunwald MH, Halvy S. Arch Dermatol 1997;133:567–8.

A report of the use of calcipotriol in the treatment of an ILVEN.

Successful therapy of an ILVEN in a 7-year-old girl with calcipotriol. Bohm I, Bieber T, Bauer R. Hautarzt 1999; 50:812–4.

A report on the successful use of calcipotriol in the treatment of an ILVEN. After 8 weeks of use the ILVEN had cleared and remained clear for 25 weeks after treatment was stopped.

Dithranol in the treatment of inflammatory linear verrucous epidermal nevus. De Mare S, van de Kerkhof PC, Happle R. Acta Dermatol Venereol 1989;69:77–80.

A letter reports the use of topical dithranol in the treatment of ILVEN.

THIRD LINE THERAPIES

■ Pulsed dye laser	E
■ CO_2 laser	E
■ Surgical excision	D

Inflammatory linear verrucous epidermal nevus: successful treatment with the 585 nm flashlamp-pumped pulsed dye laser. Alster TS. J Am Acad Dermatol 1994;31:513–4.

The pulsed dye laser has been reported to be successful in the treatment of ILVEN; this may be related to its effects on psoriatic lesions.

Pulsed dye laser for inflammatory linear verrucous epidermal nevus. Sidwell RU, Syed S, Harper JI. Br J Dermatol 2001;144:1267–9.

Three cases of ILVEN in children ranging in age from 2 to 8 years were treated successfully with the pulsed dye laser. The authors surmise that the destruction of capillaries by the laser decreases the release of inflammatory mediators.

Carbon dioxide laser therapy for an inflammatory linear verrucous epidermal nevus: a case report. Ulkur E, Celikoz B, Yuksel F, Karagoz H. Aesthetic Plast Surg 2004;28:428–30.

A case of ILVEN was treated with the CO_2 laser. All symptoms, including erythema, excoriation, granulation, and pruritus, disappeared, leaving a pale pigmentation.

Full-thickness surgical excision for the treatment of inflammatory linear verrucous epidermal nevus. Lee BJ, Mancini AJ, Renucci J, et al. Ann Plast Surg 2001;47:285–92.

The authors report four patients with extensive ILVEN treated successfully with full-thickness surgical excision.

Epidermodysplasia verruciformis

Slawomir Majewski, Stefania Jablonska

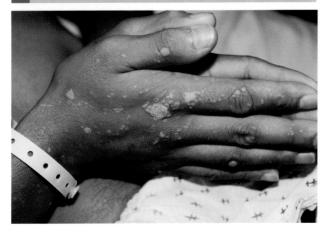

Epidermodysplasia verruciformis (EV) is a life-long genetic disease associated with specific, potentially oncogenic human papillomavirus types (HPV5 and HPV8) and various nononcogenic EV HPVs. Benign warty-type lesions appear in early childhood (usually by the age of 6–8 years), and are disseminated all over the body. Cutaneous cancers, which start to develop in the fourth to fifth decades of life, occur in over half of those with EV. UV radiation acts as a co-carcinogen, so cancers and precancerous lesions are present mostly on uncovered skin. An EV-like eruption has been reported in some individuals with HIV infection.

MANAGEMENT STRATEGY

No compound acts directly on HPV, so no therapy produces a complete and sustained clearance of lesions associated with oncogenic EV HPVs. The management of EV associated with oncogenic HPVs is in essence limited to prophylaxis – first of all *protection from UV radiation*, which is the most harmful cancer cofactor for EV. Light avoiding behavior, high sun protection factor sunscreens, and light protecting clothing and window blinds are suggested. Other cancer cofactors, such as arsenic (possibly relevant in countries where high water arsenic concentrations are found), immunosuppressants, and skin radiotherapy must be avoided. Premalignant and troublesome benign lesions that characterize the disease can be treated by a variety of *destructive surgical techniques* (cryotherapy, shave excision, curettage, excision, laser), or chemical agents (*trichloroacetic acid* or *5-fluorouracil*). Agents that modify keratinization such *as topical and oral retinoids* and *vitamin D analogs* may help. Agents that have specific antiviral activity such as *interferons (IFNs)*, and immune response enhancing agents like *imiquimod* have been utilized. Finally, large areas of involved facial skin can be *excised and grafted* in those severely affected by pre and frank malignancy. The graft should be taken from unexposed areas.

SPECIFIC INVESTIGATIONS

- Careful clinical inspection of cutaneous lesions
- Family history and examination of other family members
- Skin biopsy.
- Tissue HPV typing
- Consider HIV testing

Epidermodysplasia verruciformis. Jablonska S. In: Friedman RJ, ed. Cancer of the skin. Philadelphia; WB Saunders Co; 1991:101–13.

The histology of EV-specific lesions is highly characteristic with pronounced cytopathic effect.

Epidermodysplasia verruciformis-like eruption complicating human immunodeficiency virus infection. Barzegar C, Paul C, Saiag P, et al. Br J Dermatol 1998;139:122–7.

Three patients with HIV infection presented with disseminated pityriasis versicolor-like skin lesions. Histological examination showed features characteristic of EV. Hybridization studies demonstrated the presence of HPV5 DNA in two patients and HPV20 in one.

FIRST LINE THERAPIES

■ UV avoidance	E
■ Surgical destruction of premalignant and malignant lesions	E
■ Topical 5-fluorouracil	E
■ Topical retinoids	E

Epidermodysplasia verruciformis. Majewski S, Jablonska S. In: Sterling JC, Tyring SK, eds. Human papillomaviruses. Clinical and scientific advances. New York: Arnold; 2001: 90–101.

Epidermodysplasia verruciformis. Immunological and non-immunological surveillance mechanisms: role in tumor progression. Majewski S, Jablonska S, Orth G. Clin Dermatol 1997;15:321–34.

Benign widespread lesions can be treated locally with 0.05–0.1% retinoic acid. This is more effective if combined with 5% 5-fluorouracil ointment. Actinic keratoses and keratotic changes in EV, due to frequent progression into malignancy, should be prophylactically removed.

SECOND LINE THERAPIES

■ Topical IFN	E
■ Systemic IFN	E
■ Oral retinoids	E
■ Vitamin D3 analogs	E
■ Imiquimod	E
■ Photodynamic therapy (PDT)	E

Response of warts in epidermodysplasia verruciformis to treatment with systemic and intralesional alpha interferon. Androphy EF, Dvoretzky I, Maluish AE. J Am Acad Dermatol 1984;11:197–202).

Evidence levels A Double-blind study **B** Clinical trial > 20 subjects **C** Clinical trial < 20 subjects **D** Series ≤ 5 subjects **E** Anecdotal case reports

The systemic and intralesional IFNs α, β, and γ were unsuccessful, although some lesions cleared during the therapy, reappearing after the treatment was stopped.

Some authors reported the results of systemic IFN therapy as satisfactory because of the decrease of skin lesions. However, the improvement was transient with relapse after the application was stopped.

Epidermodysplasia verruciformis with multiple mucosal carcinomas treated with pegylated interferon alfa and acitretin. Gubinelli E, Posterato P, Cocuroccia B, Girolomoni G. J Dermatolog Treat 2003;14:184–8.

Marked improvement, but not clearance, of disseminated wart-like lesions of EV was reported after combined therapy with oral acitretin and pegylated IFN.

Calcitriol and isotretinoin combination therapy for precancerous and cancerous skin lesions. Skopinska M, Majewski S, Bollag W, Jablonska S. J Dermatolog Treat 1996;9:418–22

Therapy with oral retinoids and vitamin D3 (calcitriol) was found to be partially effective in premalignant skin lesions in the general population, therefore it could be tried in EV.

Ro 10-9359 in epidermodysplasia verruciformis. Preliminary report. Jablonska S, Obalek S, Wolska H, Jarzabek-Chorzelska M. In: Orfanos CE, ed. Retinoids. Berlin: Springer-Verlag; 1981:401–5.

Marked improvement, especially in patients with EV and disseminated plane wart-like lesions.

Epidermodysplasia verruciformis: association with isolated IgM deficiency and response to treatment with acitretin. Iraji F, Faghihi G. Clin Exp Dermatol 1999;25:41–3.

Slight improvement during therapy with 0.5 mg/kg acitretin, but relapse on discontinuation.

Treatment of epidermodysplasia verruciformis with a combination of acitretin and interferon alfa-2a. Anadolu R, Oskay T, Erdem C. J Am Acad Dermatol 2001;45:296–9.

Slight improvement with combination therapy.

Treatment of localized epidermodysplasia verruciformis with tacalcitol ointment. Hayashi J, Matsui C, Matsui T. Int J Dermatol 2002;41:817–20.

Minimal improvement only.

Imiquimod 5% cream in the treatment of Bowen's disease. MacKenzie-Wood A, Kossard S, Launey J, et al. J Am Acad Dermatol 2001;44:462–70.

Imiquimod has proved to be effective in actinic keratosis, Bowen's disease and superficial basal cell carcinomas; however, imiquimod may be useful only in decreasing viral load and inducing regression of single premalignancies and basaliomas in patients with EV. There is only one anecdotal report on an improvement of EV lesions with imiquimod (personal communication, Stockfleth E. World Congress of Dermatology, Paris, 2002).

Epidermodysplasia verruciformis treated using topical 5-aminolaevulinic acid photodynamic therapy. Karrer S, Szeimies RM, Abels C, et al. Br J Dermatol 1999;140:935–8.

A 65-year-old woman had had wart-like lesions on her hands, lower arms and forehead for about 45 years. In-situ hybridization (HPV types 5, 8, 12, 14, 19–23, 25, 36) of skin biopsies confirmed a diagnosis of EV. 20% 5-aminolaevulinic acid PDT was utilized, and at 3 weeks the cosmetic result was excellent. At 12 months a few lesions had recurred on the hands.

THIRD LINE THERAPIES

■ Skin grafts	D

Skin autografts in epidermodysplasia verruciformis: human papillomavirus-associated cutaneous changes need over 20 years for malignant conversion. Majewski S, Jablonska S. Cancer Res 1997;57:4214–6.

The only beneficial treatment for advanced cases of EV with steadily appearing numerous, premalignant and malignant lesions is removal of the entire skin of the forehead and replacement with skin taken from nonexposed parts. In 22 years of follow-up there has not been any malignancy within the grafted skin, although premalignant and early malignant changes developed around it.

Epidermolysis bullosa

Ysabel M Bello, Anna F Falabella, Lawrence A Schachner

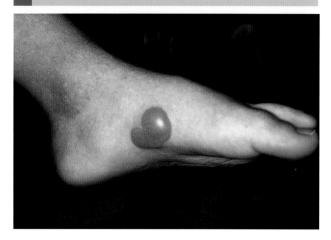

Epidermolysis bullosa is a complex group of mechanobullous disorders characterized by painful blister formation as a result of minor trauma to the skin. With the exception of the acquisita type, epidermolysis bullosa is an inherited disorder. Hereditary epidermolysis bullosa can be grouped into three major types according to the level of blister formation: epidermolytic or simplex, junctional, and dermolytic or dystrophic. The disease can involve the skin, mucosae, and internal organs. The severity of epidermolysis bullosa ranges from mild to severe, and skin involvement can be localized or generalized. Epidermolysis bullosa acquisita is discussed on page 191.

MANAGEMENT STRATEGY

The management of inherited epidermolysis bullosa has classically been *supportive: avoidance of trauma, treatment of infections, and nutritional support.* More recent efforts have been directed at trying to improve the ability to heal wounds and prevent new wound formation by treating the underlying disease.

Trauma avoidance to intact skin is important but difficult. Sewing foam pads into the lining of clothing is helpful, especially over the elbows, knees, and other pressure points. Minimizing trauma to wounds is also vital. Mepilex® is a nonadherent, absorbent polyurethane foam pad that can be applied, removed and reapplied to wounds with little discomfort, no trauma to the wound bed, and no disruption of wound healing. Other nonadherent dressings, such as white petrolatum-impregnated gauzes, hydrogels, and foams can be used and held in place with soft, roller gauze bandages or elastic tube dressings.

Avoidance of wound infection is also critical to promote more rapid wound healing and avoid overwhelming infections and sepsis, which are associated with an increased mortality rate. *Topical antibiotics* are routinely used, but should be rotated monthly to avoid the development of resistant organisms. Cutaneous infections unresponsive to topical measures need to be treated with *systemic antibiotics,*

but the chronic use of systemic antibiotics is not recommended as a preventive measure.

Some common nutritional problems include chewing and swallowing difficulties, malnutrition, constipation, and vitamin and mineral deficiencies. Avoidance of malnutrition depends on *active and continuous nutritional support.* Early nutritional supplementation can promote better childhood growth rates and encourage healing of skin lesions. In patients who develop esophageal strictures, intensive nutritional support has been reported as necessary to achieve good results even associated with balloon dilatation. Daily multivitamin and zinc supplementation has been recommended. Anemia may be profound in epidermolysis bullosa, and oral iron replacement is mandatory for patients with iron deficiency, and erythropoietin has been recommended if the level is below 500 mU/mL. Some have recommended intravenous iron therapy for patients resistant to oral replacement.

A variety of *skin grafts* have been used to treat the wounds of epidermolysis bullosa, including split-thickness skin grafts, allogeneic and autogeneic cultured keratinocytes, and cryopreserved acellular human dermis. Several trials have reported impressive results with Apligraf®, a bilayered, tissue-engineered skin derived from neonatal foreskin that contains living keratinocytes and fibroblasts. Another allogeneic composite cultured skin (OrCel®) has been approved by the United States Food and Drug Administration to treat hands and donor sites in patients with recessive dystrophic epidermolysis bullosa.

Many systemic therapies such as *psoralens in combination with UVA irradiation, corticosteroids, vitamin E, cyclosporine, antimalarials, retinoids, phenytoin, tetracycline* and *cyproheptadine* have been used, but their efficacy is unproven.

Most believe that future efforts to treat the underlying causes of epidermolysis bullosa will incorporate cutaneous gene transfer.

SPECIFIC INVESTIGATIONS

- Skin biopsy for electron microscopy
- Immunohistochemical techniques
- Genetic studies

Update on inherited bullous dermatoses. Marinkovich MP. Dermatol Clin 1999;17:473–85.

Electron microscopy is the gold standard for determination of the level of the blistering and can provide additional information on the morphology of intermediate filaments, hemidesmosomes, and anchoring fibrils.

Vesiculobullous diseases. Tidman MJ, Garzon MC. In: Schachner LA, Hansen RC, eds. Pediatric dermatology, 3rd edn. New York: Churchill Livingstone; 2003.

Immunohistochemistry techniques, such as immunofluorescence antigen mapping can reveal the level of the split by defining its location relative to proteins expressed at various levels of the basement membrane zone.

Molecular pathology of the cutaneous basement membrane zone. Mellerio JE. Clin Exp Dermatol 1999;24:25–32.

The major forms of epidermolysis bullosa are caused by mutations in ten different genes encoding skin structural proteins. Determination of the candidate gene has implications for establishing the prognosis in affected individuals,

Evidence levels **A** Double-blind study **B** Clinical trial ≥ 20 subjects **C** Clinical trial < 20 subjects **D** Series ≥ 5 subjects **E** Anecdotal case reports

DNA-based prenatal diagnosis, clinical management, and the development of newer forms of treatments.

FIRST LINE THERAPIES

■ Sterile dressing and topical antibiotics	B
■ Nutritional support	C

Management of epidermolysis bullosa in infants and children. Bello YM, Falabella AF, Schachner LA. Clin Dermatol 2003;21:278–82.

Open or only partially healed erosions are best covered with polymyxin, bacitracin, or silver sulfadiazine and then covered with either petrolatum-impregnated gauze or non-adherent synthetic dressing. Such dressings are usually changed daily. Mupirocin may be substituted for those infected sites unresponsive to milder antibiotics, but is best avoided for routine use because of the potential for development of resistance.

Mupirocin-resistant *Staphylococcus aureus* after long-term treatment of patients with epidermolysis bullosa. Moy JA, Caldwell-Brown D, Lin An, et al. J Am Acad Dermatol 1990;22:893–5.

A long-term, open study in 47 patients with epidermolysis bullosa who were treated with topical 2% mupirocin (Bactroban®) ointment to decrease bacterial infection and promote wound healing reported evidence of appearance of bacterial strains with decreased sensitivity to mupirocin. Clinical improvement and culture negativity were observed in four patients after treatment with oral antibiotic sensitive to *Staphylococcus aureus*.

Resistance of S. aureus to mupirocin is a growing problem worldwide and argues against the routine use of this antibiotic for prophylaxis against cutaneous infections.

Nutrition management of patients with epidermolysis bullosa. Birge K. J Am Diet Assoc 1995;95:575–9.

This report provides information based on 80 patients with epidermolysis bullosa. Estimation of protein and energy requirements should consider catch-up growth, percentage of body surface blistered, and presence of infection. Impaired nutrient intake because of chewing and swallowing problems requires more aggressive therapy, such as restorative dental therapy, dilatation of esophageal strictures, or placement of a gastrostomy tube for feeding. A high-fiber diet and adequate fluid intake may help alleviate constipation. Vitamin and mineral supplementation is recommended.

Scarring of the gastrointestinal tract may contribute to malabsorption of nutrients as well as medications.

Esophageal strictures in children with recessive dystrophic epidermolysis bullosa: experience of balloon dilatation in nine cases. Fujimoto T, Lane GJ, Miyano T, et al. J Pediatr Gastroenterol Nutr 1998;27:524–9.

Intensive nutritional support followed by balloon dilatation is a treatment of choice for esophageal strictures complicating recessive epidermolysis bullosa.

Gastrostomy and growth in dystrophic epidermolysis bullosa. Haynes L, Atherton DJ, Ade-Ajayi N, et al. Br J Dermatol 1996;134:872–9.

A significantly improved growth rate and improved quality of life for both child and family followed the establishment of supplementary gastrostomy feeding in 13 patients.

Correction of the anemia of epidermolysis bullosa with intravenous iron and erythropoietin. Fridge JL, Vichinsky EP. J Pediatr 1998;132:871–3.

A transfusion-dependent chronic anemia is seen in some types of epidermolysis bullosa. Four children, whose anemia failed to respond to oral iron became transfusion independent after treatment with intravenous iron and human recombinant erythropoietin.

SECOND LINE THERAPIES

■ Skin grafts	C

Cultured keratinocyte allografts and wound healing in severe recessive dystrophic epidermolysis bullosa. McGrath JA, Schofield OM, Ishida-Yamamoto A, et al. J Am Acad Dermatol 1993;29:407–19.

In ten patients with recessive dystrophic epidermolysis bullosa, cultured keratinocytes were applied to part of the wound, with another part left ungrafted. The only distinguishing findings were a moderate analgesic effect induced by the graft.

Tissue-engineered skin (Apligraf) in the healing of patients with epidermolysis bullosa wounds. Falabella AF, Valencia IC, Eaglstein WH, Schachner LA. Arch Dermatol 2000;135:1219–22.

Open-label uncontrolled study of 15 patients with 69 acute wounds and nine chronic wounds who were treated with tissue-engineered skin; 79% of the wounds were healed a week later. The patients and their families considered that healing with the tissue-engineered skin was faster and less painful, and that quality of life was improved, compared to healing with conventional dressings.

Graftskin therapy in epidermolysis bullosa. Fivenson DP, Scherschun L, Choucair M, et al. J Am Acad Dermatol 2003;48:886–92.

Second series of 96 sites treated with Apligraf in nine patients reported rapid healing with over 90% closure of 94 treated sites.

Surgical management of hands in children with recessive dystrophic epidermolysis bullosa: use of allogeneic composite cultured skin grafts. Eisenberg M, Llewelyn D. Br J Plast Surg 1998;51:608–13.

Composite cultured skin allografts were used as a partial substitute for autografts on digits and were used over donor sites in the course of 16 operations performed on seven children with recessive dystrophic epidermolysis bullosa and syndactyly and flexor contracture of the fingers.

THIRD LINE THERAPIES

■ Phenytoin	A
■ Tetracycline	C
■ Cyproheptadine	C
■ Gene therapy	E

Lack of efficacy of phenytoin in recessive dystrophic epidermolysis bullosa. Epidermolysis Bullosa Study Group. Caldwell-Brown D, Stern RS, Lin AN, Carter DM. N Engl J Med 1992;327:163–7.

This article reports the results of a randomized, double-blind, placebo-controlled, crossover trial in 36 patients that compared phenytoin versus placebo in the treatment of dystrophic epidermolysis bullosa. The authors reported no significant differences in disease activity (number of blisters and erosions) between the two groups.

Two familial cases of epidermolysis bullosa simplex successfully treated with tetracycline. Malkinson FD. Arch Dermatol 1999;135:997–8.

Suppression of the formation of new bullae was observed in two patients with epidermolysis bullosa simplex after treatment with tetracycline. Tetracycline may modulate the enzyme activity that controls matrix degradation, thereby reducing the formation of bullae.

Treatment of epidermolysis bullosa simplex with tetracycline. Veien NK, Buus SK. Arch Dermatol 2000;136:424–5.

A number of patients using tetracycline were observed over a 7-year period. The article reports an increase in bulla formation during the summer months, but healing was more rapid and less painful while patients took the tetracycline.

Tetracycline and epidermolysis bullosa simplex: a double-blind, placebo-controlled, crossover randomized clinical trial. Weiner M, Stein A, Cash S, et al. Br J Dermatol 2004;150:613–4.

A limited number of patients – six of 12 patients completed at least the first arm, four experienced a reduction in the total number of EB lesions; in contrast two experienced an increased number of lesions after 4 months of active therapy (oral tetracycline administered 1000 mg every morning and 500 mg every evening). The risk of tetracycline-induced dental discoloration in children needs to be balanced against the severity and chronicity of the symptoms.

Is cyproheptadine effective in the treatment of subjects with epidermolysis bullosa simplex? Neufeld-Kaiser W, Sybert VP. Arch Dermatol 1997;133:251–2.

An unblinded, non-placebo-controlled study in a small cohort of patients receiving systemic cyproheptadine for 6 weeks reported a marked patient dropout (nine of 13). This dropout rate prevented the authors from determining whether the reduction in blister formation and symptoms seen during the study was related to the medication.

Cutaneous gene therapy. Khavari PA, Krueger GG. Advances in clinical research. Dermatol Clin 1997;15:27–35.

Some types of epidermolysis bullosa may require that only the corrective gene be expressed in the appropriate location in skin. Other forms of epidermolysis bullosa may pose an additional challenge by requiring the elimination of the *trans* dominant effects of expressed mutant proteins.

Evidence levels A Double-blind study **B** Clinical trial ≥ 20 subjects **C** Clinical trial < 20 subjects **D** Series ≥ 5 subjects **E** Anecdotal case reports

Epidermolysis bullosa acquisita

Lawrence S Chan

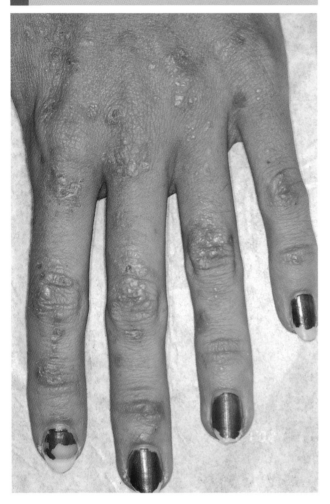

Epidermolysis bullosa acquisita is a rare, acquired, chronic, autoimmune, blistering disease of skin and mucous membranes, affecting primarily elderly individuals and occurring predominantly at trauma-prone skin areas (the non-inflammatory mechanobullous scarring subset) or widespread skin areas (the generalized inflammatory non-scarring subset). IgG or IgA autoantibodies targeting the skin basement membrane component type VII collagen (anchoring fibrils) and trauma are apparently the major contributing factors for the blistering process. The subset of patients with predominantly mucous membrane involvement is addressed on page 405 (Mucous membrane pemphigoid).

MANAGEMENT STRATEGY

Epidermolysis bullosa acquisita is known to be resistant to medical therapies, especially the non-inflammatory mechanobullous subset. For an immune-mediated blistering disease associated with autoantibodies that target skin component, the logical approach is to modify the immune response to reduce the production and effect of the autoantibodies to their target antigen type VII collagen.

However, no target-specific treatment is available. Thus the currently available non-target-specific immunosuppressives not only reduce the immune responses against autoantigen, but also suppress the patient's response against pathogens, resulting in a general immunodeficiency state. Therefore, in treating patients with this disease, every effort should be made to use anti-inflammatories rather than immunosuppressives, use lowest possible doses of immunosuppressives for the shortest duration, and replace immunosuppressives with other anti-inflammatory medications whenever suitable. A commonly used initial regimen is *systemic corticosteroid with either or both azathioprine and dapsone* as a corticosteroid-sparing agent. For adult patients without significant medical problems, a combination of oral prednisone (1 mg/kg daily), azathioprine (1–2 mg/kg daily), and dapsone (100–200 mg daily) can be started. Because of its rarity, no well-controlled clinical trial has been performed for epidermolysis bullosa acquisita. The following therapeutic guidelines are derived primarily from case reports of small groups or single patients.

Other therapeutic agents have been reported to be beneficial for this disease. *Colchicine* (1–2 mg daily) has been reported to significantly improve the disease. *Cyclosporine* (5–9 mg/kg daily) has been shown to be beneficial in reducing blister formation and speeding up healing. *Intravenous immunoglobulin G* treatment (400 mg/kg daily) has also been demonstrated to reduce new blister formation and facilitate healing. In addition, *extracorporeal photochemotherapy*, *mycophenolate mofetil*, and *humanized anti-Tac monoclonal antibodies* have been used successfully in treating this disease in some patients.

In addition to medical treatments, patients with this disease should be instructed to *avoid physical trauma* as much as possible. Vigorous rubbing of their skin and the use of harsh soaps and hot water should also be avoided. The patients should be instructed to *care for open wounds promptly* and to recognize local skin infection and *seek medical attention when infection occurs.*

SPECIFIC INVESTIGATIONS

- Skin biopsy and serum for direct and indirect immunofluorescence, respectively, to detect IgG or IgA class skin basement membrane-specific autoantibodies
- Serum for enzyme-linked immunosorbent assay (ELISA) to detect IgG or IgA class type VII collagen-specific autoantibodies
- Gastrointestinal (GI) work-up for inflammatory bowel disease

Epidermolysis bullosa acquisita: ultrastructural and immunological studies. Yaoita H, Briggaman RA, Lawley TJ, et al. J Invest Dermatol 1981;76:288–92.

Identification of the skin basement-membrane autoantigen in epidermolysis bullosa acquisita. Woodley DT, Briggaman RA, O'Keefe EJ, et al. N Engl J Med 1984;310: 1007–13.

Direct immunofluorescence detects IgG deposits linearly at the dermal–epidermal junction in all patients. Indirect immunofluorescence detects IgG circulating autoantibodies bound to the dermal side of salt-separated normal skin substrate in about 50% patients with this disease.

Development of an ELISA for rapid detection of anti-type VII collagen autoantibodies in epidermolysis bullosa acquisita. Chen M, Chan LS, Cai X, et al. J Invest Dermatol 1997;108:68–72.

ELISA assay using eukaryotically expressed recombinant protein of the non-collagenous (NC1) domain of type VII collagen is the most sensitive and specific method for detecting IgG class autoantibodies in patients with this disease.

IgA-mediated epidermolysis bullosa acquisita: two cases and review of the literature. Vodegel RM, de Jong MC, Pas HH, Jonkman MF. J Am Acad Dermatol 2002;47:919–25.

In rare cases IgA class rather than IgG class autoantibodies were found to target the type VII collagen, resulting in a clinical phenotype indistinguishable from the classic IgG-mediated disease. However, IgA-mediated disease tends to have less tendency to form scar and is more responsive to dapsone treatment.

Epidermolysis bullosa acquisita and inflammatory bowel disease. Raab B, Fretzin DF, Bronson DM, et al. JAMA 1983; 250:1746–8.

Inflammatory bowel disease, particularly Crohn's disease, is strongly associated with this disease. All patients should be questioned for symptoms of inflammatory bowel disease. If symptoms are present, a comprehensive GI work-up is indicated.

The epidermolysis bullosa acquisita antigen (type VII collagen) is present in human colon and patients with Crohn's disease have autoantibodies to type VII collagen. Chen M, O'Toole EA, Sanghavi J, et al. J Invest Dermatol 2002;118:1059–64.

The presence of type VII collagen in the gut and autoantibodies to type VII collagen in patients with inflammatory bowel disease without skin manifestations supports a link between the gut and the skin.

FIRST LINE THERAPIES

■ Systemic corticosteroids	D
■ Azathioprine	D
■ Dapsone	D

Epidermolysis bullosa acquisita – a pemphigoid-like disease. Gammon WR, Briggaman RA, Woodley DT, et al. J Am Acad Dermatol 1984;11:820–32.

Five patients with the generalized inflammatory subset of disease responded, at least partially, to prednisone (40–120 mg daily), with or without the addition of azathioprine (100 mg daily).

Bullous pemphigoid and epidermolysis bullosa acquisita: presentation, prognosis, and immunotherapy in 11 children. Edwards S, Wakelin SH, Wojnarowska F, et al. Pediatr Dermatol 1998;15:184–90.

A survey of five childhood-onset cases showed good clinical responses to combined corticosteroids and dapsone, as well as a good long-term prognosis.

Epidermolysis bullosa acquisita responsive to dapsone therapy. Hughes AP, Callen JP. J Cutan Med Surg 2001;5: 397–9.

One patient who failed to respond to prednisone (40 mg daily) plus tetracycline and niacinamide achieved complete control of blistering activities after 2 months on dapsone (150 mg daily).

SECOND LINE THERAPIES

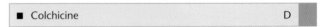

■ Colchicine	D

Colchicine for epidermolysis bullosa acquisita. Cunningham BB, Kirchmann TT, Woodley DT. J Am Acad Dermatol 1996;34:781–4.

Four patients with the non-inflammatory mechanobullous subset of disease, some refractory to prednisone treatment, were treated with oral colchicine (1–2 mg daily), with or without the addition of cyclophosphamide (50 mg daily). In all patients, there was substantial clinical improvement in the decrease of skin fragility and spontaneous blister formation. An initial dose of 0.4–0.6 mg daily is recommended with an increase by 0.6 mg daily each week until diarrhea develops. The patients are instructed to take the highest tolerable doses. Other than diarrhea, the long-term administration of colchicine (up to 4 years) was well tolerated. The side effect of diarrhea, however, makes it questionably suitable for those patients who have associated inflammatory bowel disease.

THIRD LINE THERAPIES

■ Intravenous immunoglobulin G	D
■ Cyclosporine	D
■ Extracorporeal photochemotherapy	D
■ Anti-Tac monoclonal antibody	E
■ Mycophenolate mofetil	E

Severe, refractory epidermolysis bullosa acquisita complicated by an oesophageal stricture responding to intravenous immune globulin. Harman KE, Whittam LR, Wakelin SH, Black MM. Br J Dermatol 1998;139:1126–7.

The patient had the non-inflammatory mechanobullous subset of disease and esophageal stricture, and was refractory to prednisone (up to 80 mg daily), dapsone (100 mg daily), cyclophosphamide (150 mg daily), and azathioprine (3 mg/kg daily). The patient was treated with courses of intravenous immunoglobulin G (0.4 g/kg daily) on five consecutive days at 4–6-week intervals as a monotherapy, resulting in a dramatic fall in the circulating titers of anti-basement membrane IgG autoantibodies, reduction of new blister formation, and disappearance of dysphagia. However, not all patients reported in the literature responded to this treatment. The major disadvantage of this regimen is the extremely high cost.

Oral cyclosporine in the treatment of inflammatory and noninflammatory cases. A clinical and immunopathologic analysis. Gupta AK, Ellis CN, Nickoloff BJ, et al. Arch Dermatol 1990;126:339–50.

Two patients with epidermolysis bullosa acquisita (subset not defined) were treated with oral cyclosporine (6 mg/kg daily) for a total of 8 weeks. These patients experienced gradual decrease in the frequency of new blister and erosion formation. The known renal toxicity of cyclosporine makes it questionable as a suitable long-term regimen and warranted only as a last-resort measure.

Treatment of refractory epidermolysis bullosa acquisita with extracorporeal photochemotherapy. Gordon KB, Chan LS, Woodley DT. Br J Dermatol 1997;136:415–20.

Three patients with non-inflammatory mechanobullous subset of disease, refractory to conventional therapy (prednisone, azathioprine) and colchicine were treated with this immunomodulatory regimen. The patients were given oral dose of 1–1.5 mg/kg of crystalline 8-methoxypsoralen 90 min prior to photopheresis treatment and underwent a discontinuous leukophoresis. The leukocyte-enriched portion of blood was passed through a photo cassette, exposing it to 2 J/cm^2 of UVA over 3 h. The patients underwent a total of six to seven cycles of treatment at 3-week intervals, with each cycle consisting of treatments on two consecutive days. All three patients had improvement by objective measurement of their disease activity (increased suction blister time – an indication of increased dermal–epidermal adhesion strength, and decreased titers of anti-basement membrane autoantibodies by indirect immunofluorescence). Two of these patients had significant improvement by subjective measurement (decreased frequency of new blister formation and elimination of oral mucosal lesions) during the course of treatment and continued to improve over the 6 months following the treatment period. All patients tolerated the procedure well and none stopped the treatment due to side effects. One patient required antiemetics for nausea due to oral 8-methoxypsoralen. One patient required inhaled bronchodilator therapy for worsening of chronic obstructive pulmonary disease immediately after therapy.

The practical use of this regimen is somewhat limited by the availability of photopheresis and the high cost.

Treatment of epidermolysis bullosa acquisita with the humanized anti-Tac mAb daclizumab. Egan CA, Brown M, White JD, Yancey KB. Clin Immunol 2001;101:146–51.

Humanized monoclonal antibody to Tac, a fragment of IL-2 receptor (CD25) of activated T cells, at a dose of 1 mg/kg (6–12 intravenous treatments at 2–4-week intervals), has shown effectiveness as a corticosteroid-sparing agent in one of three patients, without complication. Two other patients treated with the same medication did not have observable clinical improvement, though there was a substantial reduction of CD25$^+$ T cells.

Mycophenolate mofetil in epidermolysis bullosa acquisita. Kowalzick L, Suckow S, Zuiegler H, et al. Dermatology 2003;207:332–4.

Mycophenolate mofetil (1 g twice daily) was used successfully, in conjunction with plasmapheresis as a corticosteroid-sparing agent in one patient with epidermolysis bullosa acquisita not controlled by azathioprine (150 mg daily) and prednisolone (60 mg daily). The clinical improvement was associated with a reduction in autoantibody titers.

Erythema annulare centrifugum

Linda Y Hwang, Julia E Haimowitz

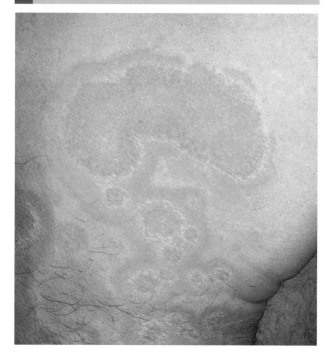

Erythema annulare centrifugum (EAC) is a gyrate erythema characterized by minimally pruritic, polycyclic, erythematous patches or plaques that expand up to 2–3 mm/day and clear centrally. There are two forms: the more common superficial form has trailing scale at the inner borders of the erythema, whereas the deep form has erythematous induration without scale. EAC may persist for decades, with a mean duration of 2.8 years, and treatment is often difficult.

MANAGEMENT STRATEGY

EAC represents a hypersensitivity reaction to any of a myriad of conditions; therefore a *search for and treatment of an underlying disease* is the primary management strategy.

Concurrent infection is the most common underlying association. Fungal, bacterial, viral, mycobacterial, and parasitic pathogens have been reported. Typically, the infection is cutaneous and separate from the EAC eruption. Dermatophytosis is implicated in up to 48% of EAC patients. Thus, the skin, especially the feet, groin, and nails, should be carefully examined for tinea. Other anecdotal reports of associated skin infections include molluscum contagiosum, herpes virus infection, and *Phthirus pubis* infestation. Less commonly, the infection is internal, and intestinal *Giardia* or *Candida* spp. infection, latent Epstein-Barr virus infection, chronic viral hepatitis, appendicitis, urinary tract *Escherichia coli*, and nematode infestations have been reported.

EAC may be associated with either benign or malignant hematologic and solid neoplasms. This paraneoplastic phenomenon is thought to result from hypersensitivity to tumor proteins released by these neoplasms. However, in the absence of strong clinical suspicion, an extensive search for malignancy is not recommended. Should neoplasia be identified, EAC activity correlates with tumor response to treatment.

Ingested agents, especially medications, may be associated with EAC. Anecdotal reports of associated medications include acetazolamide, amitriptyline, ampicillin, cimetidine, cyclopenthiazide, cotrimoxazole, etizolam, gold, hydrochlorothiazide, ibuprofen, iron, neutradonna (aluminum silicate and belladonna), oxprenolol, piroxicam, salicylates, spironolactone, thiacetazone, chloroquine, and hydroxychloroquine. Early reports of antimalarials as a cause of EAC may be debated; what was considered EAC in these reports may actually have been unrecognized forms of subacute cutaneous lupus erythematosus. EAC may also be caused by hypersensitivity to other ingested agents, such as blue cheese *Penicillium* sp.

Other conditions associated with EAC include thyroid disease, liver disease, hypereosinophilic syndrome, sarcoidosis, surgical trauma, linear IgA dermatosis, and autoimmune diseases such as relapsing polychondritis, rheumatoid arthritis, and polyglandular autoimmune disease. EAC may also be seen with pregnancy and hormonal fluctuations due to menstruation. One form of EAC, described as autoimmune progesterone dermatitis, can be reproduced by intradermal and patch testing to progesterone and may involve helper TH1-type cytokines. EAC may even be familial; there has been one report involving identical twins.

Once the underlying condition is treated, EAC usually resolves. Frequently, however, the cause is elusive, and treatment becomes empiric and temporizing. *Topical corticosteroids* may provide symptomatic relief and may improve its appearance. In one report of EAC with unknown etiology, all lesions cleared after *topical calcipotriene (calcipotriol)* use. A trial of *empiric antimicrobials* may be helpful to eradicate an underlying, clinically undetected infection. If these more conservative treatments fail, the patient's perceived need for treatment should be reassessed because stronger treatments may be more harmful than the condition itself. *Systemic glucocorticoids* can usually suppress EAC, but EAC commonly recurs after the course is completed. If EAC is very disabling to the patient, other *systemic immunomodulators* may need to be considered.

EAC should be distinguished from the following clinical mimickers: tinea corporis, granuloma annulare, sarcoidosis, mycosis fungoides, psoriasis, pityriasis rosea, tinea versicolor, cutaneous lupus erythematosus, especially the subacute variant, annular erythema of Sjögren's syndrome, granuloma faciale, necrolytic migratory erythema, bullous pemphigoid, secondary syphilis, Hansen's disease, annular urticarial and fixed drug reactions, annular erythema of infancy, and other reactive erythemas such as erythema multiforme, erythema gyratum repens, erythema migrans, and erythema marginatum. Such clinical possibilities are ruled out by history, examination and routine histologic examination.

Evidence levels A Double-blind study B Clinical trial ≥ 20 subjects C Clinical trial < 20 subjects D Series ≥ 5 subjects E Anecdotal case reports

SPECIFIC INVESTIGATIONS

- Punch biopsy for histologic examination
  superficial type: focal spongiosis, superficial perivascular lymphocytic infiltrate
  deep type: superficial and deep perivascular lymphohistiocytic infiltrate
- Perilesional direct immunofluorescence
- Full skin exam for potential skin infections
- Direct mycology and culture of suspected EAC lesion and site of potential dermatophyte infection
- Intradermal trichophyton or candidal skin injection and tuberculin test to test for underlying infection
- Systemic work-up, if indicated: complete blood count, liver function tests, urinalysis, chest radiography initial screen; if warranted, antinuclear antibody, Ro and La antibodies, thyroid stimulating hormone, malignancy work-up including serum protein electrophoresis

Linear IgA dermatosis presenting with erythema annulare centrifugum lesions: report of three cases in adults. Dippel E, Orfanos CE, Zouboulis C. J Eur Acad Dermatol Venereol 2000;15:167–70.

Linear IgA bullous dermatosis initially presenting as an annular erythema in three cases.

Bullous pemphigoid occasionally presents in a similar way.

Gyrate erythema. White JW Jr. Dermatol Clin 1985;3:129–39.

Allergic confirmation that some cases of erythema annulare centrifugum are dermatophytids. Jillson OF. AMA Arch Dermatol Syphilol 1954;70:54–8.

Erythema annulare centrifugum and intestinal *Candida albicans* infection – coincidence or connection? (Letter) Schmid MH, Wollenber A, Sander CA, Beiber T. Acta Derm Venereol 1997;77:93–4.

Intradermal trichophyton and candidal skin injection tests may demonstrate a local cutaneous hypersensitivity. These tests may help confirm this reaction pattern and support a trial of empiric antifungals despite an inability to locate the site of a pathogen.

Erythema annulare centrifugum: a review of 24 cases with special reference to its association with underlying disease. Mahood JM. Clin Exp Dermatol 1983;8: 383–7.

A basic work-up for internal disease may include a complete blood cell count, liver function tests, urinalysis, and chest radiograph.

Erythema annulare centrifugum: results of a clinicopathologic study of 73 patients. Weyers W, Diaz-Cascajo C, Weyers I. Am J Dermatopathol 2003;25:451–62.

Clinicopathologic analysis of 66 cases of erythema annulare centrifugum. Kim KJ, Chang SE, Choi JH, et al. J Dermatol 2002;29:61–7.

Erythema annulare centrifugum induced by molluscum contagiosum. Furue M, Akasu R, Ohtake N, Tamaki K. Br J Dermatol 1993;129:646–7.

Erythema annulare centrifugum induced by generalized *Phthirus pubis* infestation. Bessis D, Chraibi H, Guillot B, Guilhou JJ. Br J Dermatol 2003;149:1291.

Erythema annulare centrifugum. A case due to tuberculosis. Burkhart CG. Int J Dermatol 1982;21:538–9.

Recurrent acute appendicitis with erythema annulare centrifugum. Sack DM, Carle G, Shama SK. Arch Intern Med 1984;144:2090–2.

Erythema annulare centrifugum and *Escherichia coli* urinary infection. Borbujo J, de Miguel C, Lopez A, et al. Lancet 1996;347:897–8.

Erythema annulare centrifugum associated with ascariasis. Hendricks AA, Lu C, Elfenbein GJ, Hussain R. Arch Dermatol 1981;117:582–5.

Erythema annulare centrifugum associated with liver disease. Tsuji T, Kadoya A. Arch Dermatol 1986;122:1239–40.

Erythema annulare centrifugum and Graves' disease. Braunstein BL. Arch Dermatol 1982;118:623.

Erythema annulare centrifugum with autoimmune hepatitis. Gulati S, Mathur P, Saini D, et al. Indian J Pediatr 2004;71:541–2.

Erythema annulare centrifugum as the presenting sign of the hypereosinophilic syndrome: observations on therapy. Shelley WB, Shelley ED. Cutis 1985;35:53–5.

Sarcoidosis presenting as erythema annulare centrifugum. Altomare GF, Capella GL, Frigerio E. Clin Exp Dermatol 1995;20:502–3.

Erythema annulare centrifugum following pancreaticobiliary surgery. Thami GP, Sachdeva A, Kaur S, et al. J Dermatol 2002;29:347–9.

Linear IgA dermatosis presenting with erythema annulare centrifugum lesions: report of three cases in adults. Dippel E, Orfanos CE, Zouboulis C. J Eur Acad Dermatol Venereol 2001;15:167–70.

Erythema annulare centrifugum and relapsing polychondritis. Ingen-Housz S, Venutolo E, Pinquier L, et al. Ann Dermatol Venereol 2000;127:735–9.

Erythema annulare centrifugum in a patient with polyglandular autoimmune disease type 1. Garty B. Cutis 1998;62:231–2.

Erythema annulare centrifugum associated with pregnancy. Choonhakam C, Seramethakun P. Acta Derm Venereol 1998;78:237–8.

Autoimmune progesterone dermatitis manifested as erythema annulare centrifugum: confirmation of progesterone sensitivity by in vitro interferon-gamma release. Halevy S, Cohen AD, Lunenfeld E, Grossman N. J Am Acad Dermatol 2002;47:311–3.

Annular erythema in identical twins. Watsky KL, Hansen T. Cutis 1989;44:139–40.

Annular erythema in childhood – a new eosinophilic dermatosis. Kunz M, Hamm K, Brocker EB, Hamm H. Hautarzt 1998;49:131–4.

FIRST LINE THERAPIES

■ Treatment of underlying condition	E
■ Discontinue potential causative medications	E
■ Topical corticosteroids	E

Erythema annulare centrifugum as the presenting sign of Hodgkin's disease. Yaniv R, Shpielberg O, Shpiro D, et al. Int J Dermatol 1993;32:59–60.

Erythema annulare centrifugum and Hodgkin's disease: association with disease activity. Leimert JT, Corder MP, Skibba CA, Gingrich RD. Arch Intern Med 1979; 139:486–7.

Erythema annulare centrifugum associated with piroxicam. Hogan DJ, Blocka KLN. J Am Acad Dermatol 1985; 13:840–1.

Erythema annulare centrifugum caused by aldactone. Carsuzaa F, Pierre C, Dubegny M. (French) Ann Dermatol Venereol 1987;114:375–6.

Ampicillin induced erythema annulare centrifugum. Gupta HL, Sapra SM. J Indian Med Assoc 1975;65:307–8.

Etizolam-induced superficial erythema annulare centrifugum. Kuroda K, Yabunami H, Hisanaga Y. Clin Exp Dermatol 2002;27:34–6.

Amitriptyline-induced erythema annulare centrifugum. Garcia-Doval I, Peteiro C, Toribio J. Cutis 1999;63:35–6.

Erythema annulare centrifugum associated with gold sodium thiomalate therapy. Tsuji T, Nishimura M, Kimura S. J Am Acad Dermatol 1992;27:284–7.

Erythema annulare centrifugum: an unusual case due to hydroxychloroquine sulfate. Hudson LD. Cutis 1985;36: 129–30.

Erythema annulare centrifugum due to hydroxychloroquine sulfate and chloroquine sulfate. Ashurst PJ. Arch Dermatol 1967;95:37–9.

Erythema annulare centrifugum associated with piroxicam. Hogan DJ, Blocka KL. J Am Acad Dermatol 1985; 13:840–1.

Erythema annulare centrifugum. A case due to hypersensitivity to blue cheese penicillium. Shelley WB. Arch Dermatol 1964;90:54–8.

All the above reports confirm resolution of EAC with treatment of or withdrawal of the trigger.

SECOND LINE THERAPIES

■ Empiric antimicrobials	E
■ Topical or systemic antipruritics	E

Empiric broad-spectrum antibiotics or antifungal agents have been advocated, but the evidence base regarding efficacy is slim.

THIRD LINE THERAPIES

■ Systemic corticosteroids	E
■ Immunomodulatory agents	E
■ Topical calcipotriene (calcipotriol)	E

Erythema annulare centrifugum. Seidel DR, Burgdorf WHC. In: Demis DJ, et al., eds. Clinical dermatology. Philadelphia: Lippincott Williams & Wilkins; 1999:1–4.

Calcipotriol for erythema annulare centrifugum. Gnaiadecki R. Br J Dermatol;2002;146:317–9.

A single anecdote of a woman with a 3-year history of EAC that was resistant to topical and systemic glucocorticoids, antifungals, and psoralen plus ultraviolet A treatment. After 3 months of treatment with topical calcipotriol the lesions cleared completely and did not recur during a 6-month follow-up period.

As yet, there are no reports of the use of topical tacrolimus or pimecrolimus in EAC, but they would seem a reasonable option to try.

Evidence levels **A** Double-blind study **B** Clinical trial ≥ 20 subjects **C** Clinical trial < 20 subjects **D** Series ≥ 5 subjects **E** Anecdotal case reports

Erythema dyschromicum perstans

Christine Soon, Sanjay Agarwal, John Berth-Jones

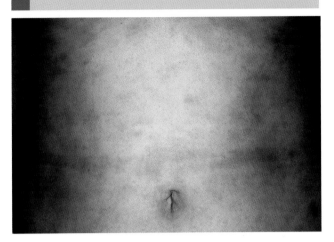

Erythema dyschromicum perstans (EDP) is an acquired, generalized cutaneous hypermelanosis of unknown etiology. It has been linked in the past to lichen planus, but its exact relationship to this disease remains uncertain. Clinically it presents as asymptomatic ashen–gray–blue macules of varying sizes, most commonly on the trunk and proximal extremity. It has been reported most frequently in dark-skinned Latin-American people although all racial groups can be affected.

MANAGEMENT STRATEGY

No controlled trial of any treatment modality has been reported. Treatment regimens including sun protection, peeling lotions, antibiotics, topical hydroquinone, topical corticosteroid therapy, antimalarials, and griseofulvin have proven ineffective. Although EDP may persist for many years, there have been reports of *spontaneous resolution*. *Camouflage creams* can be prescribed for cosmetic purposes. The treatments discussed below have also been tried with varying success.

SPECIFIC INVESTIGATIONS

■ Biopsy	

There is vacuolar degeneration of the basal layer associated with pigmentary incontinence. Dermal vessels are surrounded by an infiltrate of lymphocytes and histiocytes and there are many melanophages.

EDP may need to be differentiated from the late stage of pinta. Dark-field examination and serological tests for syphilis should be done to exclude this treponematosis in suspected cases.

FIRST LINE THERAPIES

■ No therapy	D

Erythema dyschromicum perstans. A follow-up study from Northern Finland. Palatsi R. Dermatologica 1977; 155:40–4.

A series of four patients were followed up for 2 years. Three of the four showed spontaneous resolution.

SECOND LINE THERAPIES

■ Clofazimine 100 mg daily for 3 months	D
■ Vitamin A	D

Involvement of cell adhesion and activation molecules in the pathogenesis of erythema dyschromicum perstans (ashy dermatitis). The effect of clofazimine therapy. Baranda L, Torres-Alvarez B, Cortes-Franco R, et al. Arch Dermatol 1997;133:325–9.

This was a prospective clinical and immunohistochemical study indicating that clofazimine reduces the inflammatory response in EDP. Four of six patients treated with clofazimine 100 mg daily showed marked improvement after 3 months of treatment.

Clinical trial with clofazimine for treating erythema dyschromicum perstans. Evaluation of cell-mediated immunity. Piquero-Martin J, Perez-Alfonzo R, Abrusci V, et al. Int J Dermatol 1989;28:198–200.

Eight patients were studied to determine the possible use of clofazimine in EDP. Seven had excellent to good responses and one had a marginal response.

The results suggest that clofazimine 100 mg daily for 3 months is useful in the treatment of EDP.

Vitamin A in the treatment of lichen planus pigmentosus. Bhutani LK. Br J Dermatol 1979;100:473–4.

Lichen planus pigmentosus is considered by some to be the same entity as EDP. Vitamin A was prescribed in pulses of 100 000 units daily for 15 days. Up to ten such pulses were given. Of 140 patients, 28 showed a 'good' to 'excellent' response (50–100% clearance).

THIRD LINE THERAPIES

■ Dapsone 100 mg daily for 3 months	E
■ Oral corticosteroid therapy	E

Erythema dyschromicum perstans: response to dapsone therapy. Kontochristopoulos G, Stavropoulos P, Panteleos D, Aroni K. Int J Dermatol 1998;37:796–8.

Two cases of EDP responded to dapsone 100 mg daily. The duration of therapy ranged from 8 to 12 weeks.

Erythema dyschromicum perstans: a case report and review. Osswald SS, Proffer LH, Sartori CR. Cutis 2001; 68:25–8.

One case of EDP with active inflammatory areas responded to 3 weeks of oral corticosteroid therapy. The authors do not state the dose.

Erythema elevatum diutinum

Helen S Young, Ian Coulson

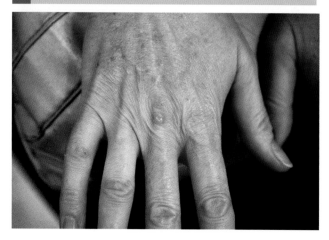

Erythema elevatum diutinum (EED) is a rare neutrophilic dermatosis consisting of violaceous, brown, or red papules, plaques and nodules over the extensor surfaces of the joints and buttocks. Cases have a female preponderance and there is a peak onset in the sixth decade, with a smaller peak in childhood. EED is thought to be a form of immune complex-mediated vasculitis although its etiology remains unclear. Infections (including HIV and streptococcal), hematologic abnormalities, autoimmune diseases and other conditions have been associated.

MANAGEMENT STRATEGY

EED is a chronic disease; there are only a few well-documented instances of spontaneous long-term resolution.

Dapsone 100 mg daily remains the initial treatment of choice. The response may be partial and dose dependent.

Corticosteroids have also been effective in patients with EED. Topical betamethasone and topical fluocinolone have been used under occlusion with good effect. In other patients both intralesional and systemic corticosteroids (prednisolone 30–40 mg daily) have produced favorable responses.

Sulfonamides (sulfamethoxypyridazine 500 mg once daily and sulfapyridine 0.5–1 mg three times daily), *nicotinamide* 100 mg three times daily, *colchicine* 0.5 mg twice daily with 0.5 mg three times daily for 3–4 days to abate minor disease flares, and *chloroquine* 300 mg daily have produced resolution of lesions.

EED has been reported in association with diseases such as HIV infection, hematological disorders, inflammatory bowel disease, celiac disease and ophthalmic disorders (peripheral keratitis), and evidence of these should be sought. In these patients treatment of the associated condition has been reported as beneficial to EED resolution. There are case reports suggesting that EED may be associated with the following drug treatments – interferon-β, erythropoietin, antituberculosis chemotherapy, and cisplatin.

SPECIFIC INVESTIGATIONS

- Full blood count
- Immunoglobulins and serum electrophoresis/immunofixation electrophoresis
- Antineutrophil cytoplasmic antibodies (ANCAs)
- HIV risk factors enquiry
- Histology

Erythema elevatum diutinum: a clinical and histopathologic study of 13 patients. Yiannias JA, El-Azhary RA, Gibson LE. J Am Acad Dermatol 1992;26:38–44.

Of 13 patients with EED, six had associated hematologic abnormalities, with IgA monoclonal gammopathy occurring most frequently.

Erythema elevatum diutinum and IgA paraproteinaemia: 'a preclinical iceberg'. Chowdhury M, Inaloz HS, Motley RJ, Knight AG. Int J Dermatol 2002;41:368–70.

The technique of immunofixation electrophoresis is more sensitive than immunoelectrophoresis and uses a combination of zone electrophoresis and immunoprecipitation with specific antisera to detect monoclonal immunoglobulins or light chains at very low concentrations in serum and urine. This is useful in EED because patients may have associated paraproteinemias, which in some cases, may undergo malignant transformation.

The authors note that in monoclonal disorders there is extensive asymptomatic tumor proliferation and possible malignant transformation in 20% of patients during long-term follow-up. It was recommended that there should be lengthy follow-up and monitoring for patients with both EED and IgA paraproteinemia due to the risk of progression to IgA myeloma.

Antineutrophil cytoplasmic antibodies of IgA class in neutrophilic dermatoses with emphasis on erythema elevatum diutinum. Ayoub N, Charuel JL, Diemert MC, et al. Arch Dermatol 2004;140:931–6.

In a study to evaluate the prevalence of ANCAs in EED, IgA ANCAs were present in all patients with EED (n = 10). It was therefore suggested that ANCAs (particularly IgA class) may be useful paraclinical markers in EED.

Erythema elevatum diutinum and HIV infection: a report of five cases. Muratori S, Carrera C, Gorani A, Alessi E. Br J Dermatol 1999;141:335–8.

The largest case series of patients with EED and HIV infection, bringing the total number of reported cases of EED in people with HIV infection to 16. Streptococcal infection seemed to trigger exacerbations in four of five patients. EED can simulate Kaposi's sarcoma and bacillary angiomatosis, which may be particularly confusing in the context of an HIV-seropositive patient. Histopathological confirmation of the diagnosis is therefore advocated.

Erythema elevatum diutinum: an ultrastructural case study. Lee AY, Nakagawa H, Nogita T, Ishibashi Y. J Cutan Pathol 1989;16:211–7.

An electron microscopic study of a patient with EED demonstrating that the characteristic histopathologic changes in early lesions include leukocytoclastic vasculitis and a massive dermal infiltrate of neutrophils, histiocytes/macrophages, and Langerhans cells. In late lesions the inflammatory infiltrate is replaced by fibrosis, with a dermal infiltrate of lymphocytes, histiocytes/macrophages, and Langerhans cells.

FIRST LINE THERAPIES

■ Dapsone	D
■ Dapsone plus antiretroviral in HIV-associated disease	E
■ Corticosteroids	D

Erythema elevatum diutinum: a clinicopathological study. Wilkinson SM, English JSC, Smith NP, et al. Clin Exp Dermatol 1992;17:87–93.

Dapsone 100 mg daily was the most effective therapy in this series of 13 patients with EED. Responses were often partial and dose dependent. Other effective treatments included sulfa drugs, corticosteroids, and chloroquine.

Dapsone may be ineffective once nodules appear; treatment of associated concomitant conditions is often beneficial to EED outcome.

Nodular erythema elevatum diutinum in an HIV-1 infected woman: response to dapsone and antiretroviral therapy. (Letter). Suarez J, Miguelez M, Villalba R. Br J Dermatol 1998;138:706–7.

Report of a 37-year-old woman with HIV-1 infection and EED whose lesions completely resolved over 3 weeks after treatment with oral antiretroviral therapy and oral dapsone 100 mg once daily. Over 2 months her CD4 count increased and her serum P24 antigen levels diminished. The authors concluded that the therapeutic approach to patients with EED associated with HIV infection should focus on reducing circulating P24 antigen with adequate antiretroviral therapy in addition to conventional dapsone treatment.

Nodular lesions of erythema elevatum diutinum in patients infected with the human immunodeficiency virus. LeBoit PE, Cockerell CJ. J Am Acad Dermatol 1993;28:919–22.

A clinicopathologic study of four patients with HIV infection who had unusual nodular lesions of EED. None of the patients responded to treatment with oral dapsone and the authors commented that the observed lack of response to dapsone may reflect the preponderance of fibrosis rather than neutrophils in these advanced lesions.

Peripheral keratitis associated with erythema elevatum diutinum. Aldave AJ, Shih JL, Jovkar S, McLeod SD. Am J Ophthalmol 2003;135:389–90.

Report of a 25-year-old with EED who was diagnosed 15 months later with an inflammatory peripheral keratitis of the left eye. The sclerokeratitis was thought to represent an ocular extension of the patient's cutaneous vasculitis. Dapsone therapy was initiated and resulted in rapid resolution of both the cutaneous and ocular inflammation.

Although dapsone is recommended as first line treatment for EED its use has been based solely on multiple anecdotal reports and small case series rather than on blinded controlled clinical trials.

SECOND LINE THERAPIES

■ Other sulfonamides	D
■ Chloroquine	D
■ Nicotinamide and tetracycline	E
■ Colchicine	E

Erythema elevatum diutinum treated with niacinamide and tetracycline. Kohler IK, Lorinez AL. Arch Dermatol 1980;116:693–5.

Case report of a 60-year-old woman with EED, which completely cleared following 4 weeks of treatment with oral nicotinamide 100 mg three times daily and oral tetracycline hydrochloride 250 mg four times daily. Following this, oral nicotinamide alone was sufficient for disease suppression, although recurrent lesions were apparent on cessation of therapy.

Erythema elevatum diutinum – a case successfully treated with colchicine. Henriksson R, Hofer PA, Hornqvist R. Clin Exp Dermatol 1989;14:451–3.

A case report of a 68-year-old man with EED refractory to treatment with oral dapsone who responded well to treatment with colchicine 0.5 mg twice daily over 6 weeks. Disease flares were noted on stopping colchicine, which was maintained at a dose of 0.5 mg twice daily. Minor flares were abated by temporarily increasing colchicine to 0.5 mg three times daily for 3–4 days without provoking diarrhea.

THIRD LINE THERAPIES

■ Gluten-free diet	E
■ Cyclophosphamide	E
■ Plasma exchange	E
■ Reduction in cyclosporine dose	E
■ Colectomy	E

Erythema elevatum diutinum in association with coeliac disease. Tasanen K, Raudasoja R, Kallioinen M, Ranki A. Br J Dermatol 1997;136:624–7.

This case report describes a 47-year-old woman who presented with clinically and histologically typical EED in whom previously undiagnosed celiac disease was found. Treatment with dapsone was partially effective, but complete healing of the EED lesions was achieved only after the introduction of a strict gluten-free diet. Maintenance treatment with a gluten-free diet only was required.

Erythema elevatum diutinum in a patient with relapsing polychondritis. Bernard P, Bedane C, Delrous JL, et al. J Am Acad Dermatol 1992;26:312–5.

A 69-year-old man with a history of relapsing polychondritis developed EED, which responded to treatment with oral cyclophosphamide 100 mg daily and prednisolone 20 mg daily. Cyclophosphamide was discontinued after 2 months and subsequently the prednisolone was tapered to 15 mg daily. This association suggests that EED may represent a cutaneous manifestation of a systemic vasculitis.

Erythema elevatum diutinum associated with IgA paraproteinemia successfully controlled with intermittent plasma exchange. Chow RKP, Benny WB, Coupe RL, et al. Arch Dermatol 1996;132:1360–4.

Intermittent plasma exchange has been reported to control EED associated with IgA paraproteinemia successfully.

Erythema elevatum diutinum after liver transplantation: disappearance of the lesions associated with a reduction

in cyclosporin dosage. Hernandez-Cano N, De Lucas R, Lazaro TE, et al. Pediatr Dermatol 1998;15:411–2.

Lesions of EED resolved following a reduction in cyclosporine dosage in a 10-year-old patient who had previously received a cadaveric hepatic allograft because of Alagille disease.

Erythema elevatum diutinum – an unusual association with ulcerative colitis. Buahene K, Hudson M, Mowat A, et al. Clin Exp Dermatol 1991;16:204–6.

A 58-year-old woman developed EED during a severe acute exacerbation of ulcerative colitis, which resolved following colectomy.

Evidence levels **A** Double-blind study **B** Clinical trial ≥ 20 subjects **C** Clinical trial < 20 subjects **D** Series ≥ 5 subjects **E** Anecdotal case reports

Erythema multiforme

Nicholas M Craven, Jean Revuz

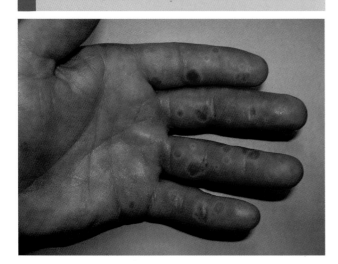

Erythema multiforme (EM) is a distinct cutaneous reaction pattern to a variety of stimuli. It usually runs a self-limiting course and has a tendency to recur. It is defined by the presence of 'typical' three-zone target lesions, with a predominantly acral distribution. The presence of mucosal involvement at more than one site distinguishes EM major from EM minor. EM major can be distinguished from Stevens-Johnson syndrome (see page 657).

MANAGEMENT STRATEGY

The etiology of EM is unknown in 30–50% of cases. The most commonly recognized precipitant is herpes simplex virus (HSV) infection, both types I and II. HSV-specific DNA has been isolated from lesional tissue in 60–70% of cases (even in patients with no recorded association with HSV). Orf, histoplasmosis, and a variety of other infections have been implicated in some cases. An extensive list of drugs has been reported to trigger EM. Rare cases are attributed to contact hypersensitivity, lupus erythematosus, carcinomas (kidney, ovary, and stomach) and sarcoidosis. The luteal phase of the menstrual cycle and exogenous administration of progesterone have been associated with worsening of EM.

Most cases, particularly EM minor, run a self-limiting course. Symptomatic measures include *oral antihistamines* and *mild to moderate potency topical corticosteroids* to reduce pruritus. If there is proven secondary infection *oral antibiotics* (e.g. erythromycin) may be indicated. Any treatable underlying condition identified should be addressed. Recurrent EM (> 6 attacks per year) may respond to long-term *acyclovir (aciclovir)*. In acyclovir-resistant cases of EM a variety of other therapies can be helpful (see below).

Mucosal manifestations of EM are a source of morbidity and occur in up to 70% of cases. The commonest sites affected are the buccal mucosa and lips. Symptomatic measures include *mouthwashes* (e.g. tetracycline with or without nystatin or 0.2% chlorhexidine gluconate), a *soft diet, topical anesthetics* (lidocaine gel, benzocaine lozenges or 0.15% benzydamine hydrochloride) and *topical corticosteroids* (e.g.

0.1% triamcinolone acetonide paste). Budesonide or beclomethasone inhalers (1 puff three to four times daily) provide an alternative method of delivering local corticosteroid to the inflamed mucosal surfaces. Short courses of high-dose *oral prednisolone* may be needed for severe oral disease. Strict eye care to reduce secondary infection and scarring includes *saline washes* for removal of crusts, *local antibiotics* (e.g. chloramphenicol with or without corticosteroids), and frequent *debridement of tarsal and bulbar conjunctival adherences.*

SPECIFIC INVESTIGATIONS

■ Histology/immunofluorescence

EM is a clinical diagnosis. Histology may be useful in atypical cases. It may be necessary to exclude other bullous diseases that present with oral manifestations, such as pemphigus vulgaris or cicatricial pemphigoid, with direct immunofluorescence.

Investigations directed at determining the underlying trigger factors include culture or serological testing for HSV or other infections, especially Mycoplasma pneumoniae, *as indicated by clinical findings.*

Clinical characteristics of childhood erythema multiforme, Stevens-Johnson syndrome and toxic epidermal necrolysis in Taiwanese children. Lam NS, Yang YH, Wang LC, et al. J Microbiol Immunol Infect 2004;37:3667–70.

This study included 19 cases of EM, eight cases of Stevens-Johnson syndrome, and one case of toxic epidermal necrolysis. The most common etiology in EM was infection, and the most common implicated organism was *M. pneumoniae* (42.1%).

FIRST LINE THERAPIES

■ Acyclovir   A

Recurrent erythema multiforme: clinical features and treatment in a large series of patients. Schofield JK, Tatnall FM, Leigh IM. Br J Dermatol 1993;128:542–5.

Review of 65 patients with recurrent EM – 71% had episodes triggered by HSV infection. In one patient, EM was related to the menstrual cycle and could be precipitated by intramuscular progesterone injection. Treatment with standard doses of acyclovir for HSV was relatively disappointing; continuous acyclovir 400 mg twice daily for 6 months was more effective, with disease remission in some responders. Some patients responded to dapsone, antimalarials, azathioprine, and human immunoglobulin.

A double-blind, placebo-controlled trial of continuous aciclovir therapy in recurrent erythema multiforme. Tatnall FM, Schofield JK, Leigh IM. Br J Dermatol 1995;132:267–70.

Acyclovir 400 mg twice daily for 6 months suppressed EM in seven of 11 patients (including one with apparently idiopathic EM). Two patients went into complete remission.

A therapeutic trial of acyclovir is justified even when clinical evidence of HSV is lacking. Acyclovir 400 mg twice daily can be administered for 6 months to 2 years because it has a good long-term safety profile. It is probably of little use for an acute episode once the herpetic lesion or EM eruption has developed.

Very low dose acyclovir can be effective as prophylaxis for post-herpetic erythema multiforme. Williams RE, Lever R. Br J Dermatol 1991;124:111.

Acyclovir 200 mg daily was effective prophylaxis for recurrent EM in one patient.

Recurrent erythema multiforme unresponsive to acyclovir prophylaxis and responsive to valacyclovir continuous therapy. Kerob D, Assier-Bonnet H, Esnault-Gelly P, et al. Arch Dermatol 1998;134:876–7.

A reduced response to acyclovir may be due to the low oral bioavailability of the drug, and one of the second generation antivirals such as valacyclovir (500 mg daily) or famciclovir (250 mg twice daily) may need to be substituted.

SECOND LINE THERAPIES

■ Dapsone	C
■ Azathioprine	C
■ Thalidomide	B
■ Potassium iodide	C
Oral EM	
■ Topical corticosteroid	B
■ Antifungal therapy	B
■ Levamisole	A
■ Prednisolone	D

Recurrent erythema multiforme: clinical features and treatment in a large series of patients. Schofield JK, Tatnall FM, Leigh IM. Br J Dermatol 1993;128:542–5.

Dapsone in a dose of 100–150 mg daily induced partial or complete suppression of EM in eight of nine patients. Azathioprine 100–150 mg daily was effective in 11 patients resistant to other treatments. Relapse of EM occurred on discontinuation of treatment.

Dapsone-responsive persistent erythema multiforme. Mahendran R, Grant JW, Norris PG. Dermatology 2000;200:281–2.

Dapsone 100 mg daily was effective in controlling EM in a patient with ovarian malignancy.

Characteristics of the oral lesions in patients with cutaneous recurrent erythema multiforme. Farthing PM, Maragou P, Coates M, et al. J Oral Pathol Med 1995;24:9–13.

In this series of 82 patients with typical cutaneous EM, 70% had oral mucosal involvement. Five patients with resistant disease were controlled with azathioprine 100–150 mg daily.

Azathioprine therapy in the management of persistent erythema multiforme. Jones RR. Br J Dermatol 1981;105:465–7.

Azathioprine 100–150 mg daily was effective in two patients and permitted reduction of corticosteroid dosage.

Thalidomide for recurrent erythema multiforme. Moisson YF, Janier M, Civatte J. Br J Dermatol 1992;126:92–3.

Recurrent EM responded to thalidomide 100–200 mg daily in two patients.

Treatment by thalidomide of chronic multiforme erythema: its recurrent and continuous variants. A retrospec-

tive study of 26 patients. (French) Cherouati K, Claudy A, Souteyrand P, et al. Ann Dermatol Venereol 1996;123:375–7.

Thalidomide reduces the duration of episodes of EM by 11 days on average. Remission can be maintained with low-dose (25–50 mg daily) thalidomide.

Potassium iodide in erythema nodosum and other erythematous dermatoses. Horio T, Danno K, Okamoto H, et al. J Am Acad Dermatol 1983;9:77–81.

Fourteen of 16 subjects with EM (six related to HSV infection) responded within 1 week to 300 mg three times daily of potassium iodide. Gastrointestinal and cutaneous side effects can occur with this treatment.

Erythema multiforme – response to corticosteroid. Ting HC, Adam BA. Dermatologica 1984;169:175–8.

Thirteen patients with EM minor treated with systemic corticosteroids were compared with twelve treated without. Apart from a shorter duration of fever, the corticosteroid-treated group did not respond better than the non-corticosteroid-treated group.

Oral EM

Open preliminary clinical trial of clobetasol propionate ointment in adhesive paste for treatment of chronic oral vesiculoerosive diseases. Lozada-Nur F, Huang MZ, Zhou GA. Oral Surg Oral Med Oral Pathol 1991;71:283–7.

Clobetasol propionate 0.05% ointment mixed 1:1 with Orabase® paste twice to three times daily was helpful in four patients with chronic oral EM.

Topically applied fluocinonide in an adhesive base in the treatment of oral vesiculoerosive diseases. Lozada F, Silverman S Jr. Arch Dermatol 1980;116:898–901.

Topical application of 0.05% fluocinonide in an adhesive base was used in 16 patients with oral EM. All responded to therapy, and remission was induced in some cases.

Oral erythema multiforme: clinical observations and treatment of 95 patients. Lozada-Nur F, Corsky M, Silverman S Jr. Oral Surg Oral Med Oral Pathol 1989;67:36–40.

As 19 of 29 patients with oral EM and oral candidiasis responded to antifungal therapy, a possible etiological role for these organisms in EM was suggested in this paper.

Only two of these 29 patients had skin lesions. The nature of the skin lesions was not described.

Levamisole in the treatment of erythema multiforme: a double-blind trial in fourteen patients. Lozada F. Oral Surg Oral Med Oral Pathol 1982;53:28–31.

Fourteen patients with severe oral EM were treated in this crossover trial with levamisole 150 mg daily or placebo, 3 days a week for 4–8 weeks. Nine of 12 experienced a decrease in severity and duration of attacks, and seven reported a reduction in disease frequency for up to 2 years after the trial.

The presence or absence of skin involvement is not mentioned in this study.

Clinical response to levamisole in thirty-nine patients with erythema multiforme. An open prospective study. Lozada-Nur F, Cram D, Gorsky M. Oral Surg Oral Med Oral Pathol 1992;74:294–8.

Evidence levels **A** Double-blind study **B** Clinical trial ≥ 20 subjects **C** Clinical trial < 20 subjects **D** Series ≥ 5 subjects **E** Anecdotal case reports

Levamisole 150 mg daily 3 days a week was effective in 31 of 39 patients with oral EM. Prednisolone 5–30 mg daily was required for 18 patients in addition to levamisole. The most common side effects from levamisole were rash, tiredness, weakness, myalgia, taste change, and insomnia. The white cell count needs to be monitored in patients on levamisole because there is a risk of drug-induced granulocytopenia.

Nineteen patients are recorded as having skin disease, but the lesions are not described.

Prednisone and azathioprine in the treatment of patients with vesiculoerosive oral diseases. Lozada F. Oral Surg Oral Med Oral Pathol 1981;52:257–63.

In this open trial, two patients with oral EM required lower doses of prednisolone (15–20 mg alternate days) when treated simultaneously with azathioprine (50 mg daily).

Recurrent oral erythema multiforme. Clinical experience with 11 patients. Bean SF, Quezada RK. JAMA 1983;249: 2810–2.

In this retrospective study, patients with severe recurrent oral EM involvement were treated with prednisolone 40–60 mg daily, subsequently tapered over 2–3 weeks. This decreased the time taken for oral erosions to heal, but did not influence recurrences.

Some authorities, however, believe that use of corticosteroids in EM increases the frequency and chronicity of attacks.

THIRD LINE THERAPIES

■ Antimalarials	D
■ Human immunoglobulin	D
■ Interferon-α (IFN-α)	E
■ Tamoxifen	E
■ Zinc sulfate	E
■ Cimetidine	E
■ Cyclosporine	E
■ Pulsed methylprednisolone	E

Recurrent erythema multiforme: clinical features and treatment in a large series of patients. Schofield JK, Tatnall FM, Leigh IM. Br J Dermatol 1993;128:542–5.

The use of normal human immunoglobulins and antimalarials was reported in a few patients in this study. Intramuscular human immunoglobulin 750 mg once a month caused suppression of EM in 11 of 13 patients. One respon-

der remained in remission after therapy was discontinued. There was a 50% success rate with antimalarials (both hydroxychloroquine and mepacrine) used in four patients.

Recurrent erythema multiforme and chronic hepatitis C: efficacy of interferon alpha. Dumas V, Thieulent N, Souillet AL, et al. Br J Dermatol 2000;142:1248–9.

One patient with recurrent EM and hepatitis C virus infection responded to two courses of IFN-α (9 MU weekly for 6 and 8 months).

Progesterone-induced erythema multiforme. Wojnarowska F, Greaves MW, Peachey RD, et al. J R Soc Med 1985;78: 407–8.

EM linked to the luteal phase of the menstrual cycle was controlled with tamoxifen.

Topical treatment of recurrent herpes simplex and postherpetic erythema multiforme with low concentrations of zinc sulphate solution. Brody I. Br J Dermatol 1981;104: 191–4.

Treatment of the skin at the site of the herpetic infection with zinc sulfate solution prevented relapse of post-herpetic EM over a 2-year period of observation in one patient. For the skin, 0.025–0.05%, and for the oral mucous membrane, 0.01–0.025% zinc sulfate solution was used.

Cimetidine prevents recurrent erythema multiforme major resulting from herpes simplex virus infection. Kurkcuoglu N, Alli N. J Am Acad Dermatol 1989;21:814–5.

EM resistant to acyclovir responded to cimetidine 400 mg three times daily in one patient.

Cyclosporine therapy for bullous erythema multiforme. Wilkel CS, McDonald CJ. Arch Dermatol 1990;126:397–8.

High-dose cyclosporine (5–10 mg/kg daily) suppressed an atypical bullous eruption with histologic features of EM. The use of cyclosporine permitted tapering of the corticosteroid dosage.

High-dose systemic corticosteroids can arrest recurrences of severe mucocutaneous erythema multiforme. Martinez AE, Atherton DJ. Pediatr Dermatol 2000;17:87–90.

A child with recurrent EM major (associated with severe ulcerative stomatitis, conjunctival inflammation, and urethritis) responded to pulsed intravenous methylprednisolone 20 mg/kg daily for three consecutive days, but not to oral prednisolone 3 mg/kg daily. Intravenous methylprednisolone stopped progression of the acute attack and repeated treatments induced remission.

Erythema nodosum

Robert A Allen, Richard L Spielvogel

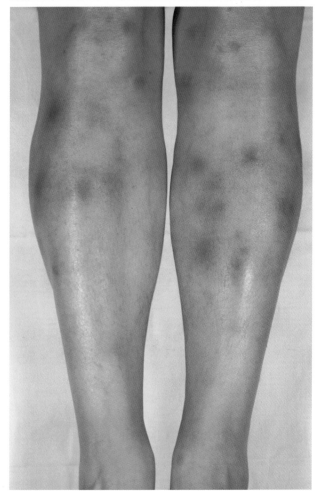

Erythema nodosum (EN) is a septal panniculitis that manifests as tender, erythematous nodules and plaques located primarily on the extensor surfaces of the lower extremities. Numerous causes have been implicated, including reactions to medications, infections, chronic inflammatory states, and rarely, malignancies. There is a tendency towards spontaneous regression, which usually takes place in 6 months or less.

MANAGEMENT STRATEGIES

Treatment of EN should be aimed at the suspected or documented etiology. The most common etiologies are a variety of infections and drugs. Unfortunately, even after extensive evaluation many cases are classified as idiopathic. Infectious agents include, but are not limited to:

- *Yersinia enterocolitica, Salmonella enteritidis, Giardia lamblia, Streptococcus, Shigella*, and *Klebsiella* spp., and HIV, and
- the infectious agents causing tuberculosis, brucellosis, psittacosis, cat scratch disease, chancroid, tularemia, campylobacter septicemia, blastomycosis, sporotrichosis, coccidioidomycosis, histoplasmosis, and fungal kerions.

Sarcoidosis, inflammatory bowel disease (Crohn's disease and ulcerative colitis), Behçet's syndrome, Sweet's syndrome, and malignancies such as lymphomas have also been implicated.

Drugs are also common inciting agents. The most common cause is oral contraceptive use, but medicines such as iodides, bromides, and sulfonamides have been implicated. Echinacea supplements are a recently reported cause.

Skin biopsy is generally not necessary if the history and physical signs are suggestive of EN. Inflammation is characteristically seen mainly in the subcutis in the septa between fat lobules. Fibrosis and increased thickness of the intralobular septa are usually seen, and radial arrays of macrophages around blood vessels are characteristic. A biopsy is usually helpful in ruling out other forms of panniculitis, and if an infectious cause is in the differential diagnosis, some tissue may be sent for culture.

Treatment consists primarily of *bed rest, activity reduction, nonsteroidal anti-inflammatory agents (NSAIDs),* and *potassium iodide.* Various NSAIDs have been used successfully, including naproxen and indomethacin. Treatment with potassium iodide has recently regained popularity. We recommend a supersaturated solution of potassium iodide of five drops three times daily in orange juice. This dose is increased by one drop per dose per day until clinical effectiveness is achieved. Hypothyroidism can result from long-term use.

Hydroxychloroquine 200 mg twice a day has been used with limited success. *Dapsone* was successful in a patient who developed EN after starting isotretinoin for acne fulminans. *Systemic corticosteroids* may also be helpful in refractory cases or to 'jump start' therapy.

SPECIFIC INVESTIGATIONS

- Anti-streptolysin O (ASO) titer, throat culture
- Chest radiograph
- Purified protein derivative standard (PPD) tuberculosis skin test
- Skin biopsy

Erythema nodosum: a review. Soderstrom RM, Krull EA. Cutis 1978;21:806–10.

Streptococcal infection is the most common etiologic agent and sarcoidosis is the most common disease associated with EN.

All patients should have a chest radiograph, ASO titer, throat culture, and PPD.

Erythema nodosum and associated diseases – a study of 129 cases. Cribier B, Caille A, Heid E, Grosshans E. Int J Dermatol 1998;37:667–72.

Streptococcal infection was the most common cause of EN and sarcoidosis the second most common cause.

Erythema nodosum: a study of 160 cases. Atanes A, Gomez N, de Toro J, et al. Med Clin (Barc) 1996;9:169–72.

Of 160 cases reviewed, the majority were due to sarcoidosis, followed by drugs, streptococcal infection, and tuberculosis, respectively.

FIRST LINE THERAPIES

■ NSAIDs	E
■ Potassium iodide	B

Evidence levels A Double-blind study B Clinical trial ≥ 20 subjects C Clinical trial < 20 subjects D Series ≥ 5 subjects E Anecdotal case reports

Suppression of erythema nodosum by indomethacin. Ubogy Z, Persellin RH. Acta Derm Venereol 1982;62:265–7.

Three patients with EN secondary to streptococcal pharyngitis were treated with indomethacin 100–150 mg orally for 2 weeks with excellent results, after having failed to respond to treatment with erythromycin, penicillin, and aspirin.

Chronic erythema nodosum treated with indomethacin. Barr WG, Robinson JA. Ann Intern Medicine 1981;95:659.

Idiopathic EN in a 32-year-old woman that had been unsuccessfully treated with aspirin, resolved with indomethacin 25 mg three times daily for 1 month.

Control of chronic erythema nodosum with naproxen. Lehman CW. Cutis 1980;26:66–7.

A 28-year-old woman with recurrent EN refractory to phenylbutazone and aspirin was treated with naproxen 250 mg orally twice daily for 1 month, with cessation of symptoms within 96 h and clearing in 14 days. Relapses occurred after stopping therapy, but cleared promptly with reinstitution of naproxen.

Potassium iodide in erythema nodosum and other erythematous dermatoses. Horio T, Danno K, Okamoto H, et al. J Am Acad Dermatol 1983;9:77–81.

Twelve of 16 patients treated with potassium iodide experienced improvement in a few days, with complete resolution in 10–14 days. Six had recurrent attacks over 1–12 months with resolution upon repeat dosing with potassium iodide. Of those who did not respond well, most received treatment 2–14 months after the onset of symptoms, indicating that earlier treatment is better. All patients with positive C-reactive protein responded well, and those with high fevers and arthralgias also responded well.

Potassium iodide may be a reasonable choice for those patients who cannot tolerate NSAIDs or corticosteroids. A saturated solution of potassium iodide (SSKI) may be made more palatable by adding the solution to orange juice.

Treatment of erythema nodosum and nodular vasculitis with potassium iodide. Schultz EJ, Whiting DA. Br J Dermatol 1976;94:75–8.

Twenty four of 28 patients with EN experienced improvement in 48 h and resolution in 2 weeks with 300–900 mg daily of potassium iodide.

Potassium iodide in dermatology. A 19th century drug for the 21st century – uses, pharmacology, adverse effects, and contraindications. Sterling JB, Heymann WR. J Am Acad Dermatol 2000;43:691–7.

An excellent review article.

SECOND LINE THERAPIES

■ Colchicine	E
■ Hydroxychloroquine	E
■ Prednisone	E

Traitement de l'eretheme noueux par la colchicine. De Coninck P, Baclet JL, Di Bernardo C, et al. Presse Med 1984;13:680.

Five women were treated with colchicine (2 mg daily for 3 days, then 1 mg daily for 2–4 weeks). Improvement was seen within 72 h, with no recurrences once colchicine was stopped.

Erythema nodosum treated with colchicine. Wallace S. JAMA 1967;202:144.

One patient with EN was successfully treated with colchicine.

Hydroxychloroquine in the treatment of chronic erythema nodosum. Alloway JA, Franks LK. Br J Dermatol 1995; 132:661–70.

A 38-year-old woman with a 24-year history of EN with almost monthly flares was treated with hydroxychloroquine 200 mg orally twice daily. Within 3 months she had a dramatic reduction in lesions and remained stable for at least 6 months. Previously she had occasionally responded to acetaminophen (paracetamol), but not aspirin or indomethacin. One previous flare had responded to prednisone.

Hydroxychloroquine and chronic erythema nodosum. Jarrett P, Goodfield MJD. Br J Dermatol 1996;134:373.

A 52-year-old with idiopathic EN was treated with hydroxychloroquine 200 mg orally twice daily and prednisone 15 mg four times daily for 8 weeks with improvement. Prednisone was stopped and 8 weeks later the hydroxychloroquine dose was cut by half, but the patient experienced a flare and the original dose was restarted. After three more months the hydroxychloroquine was stopped, though intermittent dosing was required. The patient had previously been unresponsive to NSAIDs and prednisone.

THIRD LINE THERAPIES

■ Dapsone	E
■ Extracorporeal monocyte granulocytapheresis	E
■ Erythromycin	E
■ Mycophenolate mofetil	E
■ Infliximab	E

Acne fulminans and erythema nodosum during isotretinoin therapy responding to dapsone. Tan B, Lear J, Smith A. Clin Exp Dermatol 1997;22:26–7.

Acne fulminans and EN that occurred in a patient 3 weeks after starting isotretinoin responded to dapsone without oral prednisone.

Prior to the use of isotretinoin for acne fulminans, dapsone was frequently utilized because it may help control both the acne and the EN. The improvement of EN may be secondary to the improvement of acne fulminans.

Extracorporeal monocyte granulocytapheresis was effective for a patient of erythema nodosum concomitant with ulcerative colitis. Fukunaga K, Sawada K, Fukuda Y, et al. Ther Apher Dial 2003;7:122–6.

A patient with ulcerative colitis and EN that failed to respond to high-dose corticosteroids recovered from both conditions after monocyte granulocytapheresis once a week for 5 weeks. He was also on 2250 mg of 5-aminosalicylic acid daily.

Severe erythema nodosum due to Behçet's disease responsive to erythromycin. Kaya TI, Tursen U, Baz K, et al. J Dermatolog Treat 2003;14:124–7.

A patient with refractory Behçet's disease and EN responded to coincidental treatment with erythromycin for erythrasma.

Use of mycophenolate mofetil in erythema nodosum. Boyd AS. J Am Acad Dermatol 2002;47:968–9.

A patient taking estrogen replacement developed EN that was unresponsive to many treatments, including discontinuing hormone therapy and azathioprine. The EN cleared with an increasing dose of mycophenolate mofetil to 750 mg twice a day and remained clear after a slow taper.

Dermatologic manifestations of Crohn disease in children: response to infliximab. Kugathasan S, Miranda A, Nocton J, et al. J Pediatr Gastroenterol Nutr 2003;37:150–4.

One child in a series of four patients with Crohn's disease had resistant concurrent EN. The patient cleared with infliximab 5 mg/kg (anti-tumor necrosis factor [TNF]-α antibody) and was maintained on 6 mercaptopurine. The conditions associated with Crohn's disease in the other children (pyoderma gangrenosum, orofacial Crohn's, and lymphedema) also cleared.

Erythrasma

Melissa C Barkham, Andrew G Smith

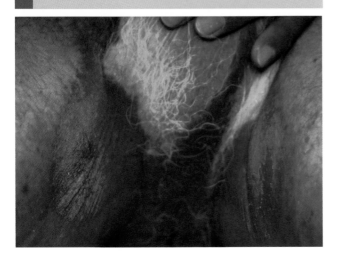

In its most typical form, erythrasma is characterized by well-defined reddish-brown flexural plaques, which show minimal fine scaling and no tendency to central clearing. In type VI skin there is often significant hyperpigmentation. It may also present with maceration, and rarely vesiculation of the toe clefts and nonflexural discoid plaques.

Erythrasma is usually associated with infection of the skin with *Corynebacterium minutissimum*, a bacterium which is frequently found on normal skin. Examination of infected skin under Wood's (long wave UV) light (illustrated above) shows characteristic coral red fluorescence due to the organism's production of coproporphyrin III. Erythrasma is more common in people with diabetes mellitus, obesity, or atopy, in old age, and in warm, humid climates.

MANAGEMENT STRATEGY

Erythrasma is frequently a trivial infection, but therapy may be requested because of the cosmetic appearance of the rash or because of pruritus. Toe web infection may lead to fissuring of the skin and secondary infection with streptococci, thus justifying therapy of the primary erythrasma infection.

Topical imidazoles such as miconazole, clotrimazole and econazole (but not ketoconazole) are effective treatments that have the advantage of being effective against concomitant fungal infection and, to some extent, against complicating Gram-positive bacterial infection. These preparations neither stain nor irritate.

The *topical antibiotics* fusidic acid and framycetin sulfate are probably equally effective. Whitfield's (benzoic acid compound) ointment is effective, but may be too irritant to use in the flexures.

For widespread infection *oral erythromycin or clarithromycin* may be considered. A combination of oral and topical treatment is sometimes required for stubborn interdigital infections.

Prophylaxis with antibacterial soap may help prevent recurrence.

SPECIFIC INVESTIGATIONS

- Examination under Wood's light
- Potassium hydroxide (KOH) preparation of skin scrapings

Chains of rods may be seen microscopically in KOH-mounted preparations of the skin scrapings. Their identification may be facilitated by methylene blue staining. Coinfection with dermatophytes or *Candida albicans* is common, particularly in interdigital erythrasma, so the presence of fungal hyphae or yeasts should be sought. Culture is difficult because the organisms do not always grow satisfactorily.

Skin biopsy is generally not indicated. If done, it provides an example of an 'invisible dermatosis' (i.e. no more than a sparse superficial perivascular infiltrate of lymphocytes). Gram staining may demonstrate the organism as basophilic rods and filaments in the stratum corneum.

FIRST LINE THERAPIES

■ Miconazole cream	A
■ Clotrimazole cream	C
■ Econazole cream	D

Treatment of erythrasma with miconazole. Pitcher DG, Noble WC, Seville RH. Clin Exp Dermatol 1979;4:453–6.

Twenty three patients were treated with miconazole cream and 25 with Whitfield's ointment twice daily for 2 weeks. In both groups a clearance rate of 88% was obtained, but irritation was a problem with Whitfield's ointment.

A clinical double-blind trial of topical miconazole and clotrimazole against superficial fungal infections and erythrasma. Clayton YM, Knight AG. Clin Exp Dermatol 1976;1:225–32.

This trial was primarily a comparison of the two preparations in dermatophyte infection, but 11 patients with erythrasma were also studied – six treated with miconazole, five with clotrimoxazole, both twice daily. All patients in both groups were free of infection at 4 weeks.

The vesiculobullous form of interdigitoplantar erythrasma. Grigoriu D, Delacretaz J. Dermatologica 1976;152: 1–7.

Seven cases of this unusual variant of erythrasma are described, with a variety of treatments, which include the effective use of econazole cream.

SECOND LINE THERAPIES

■ Fusidic acid cream	D
■ Whitfield's ointment	D
■ Framycetin ointment	D
■ Clindamycin lotion or solution	E

Specific topical treatment for erythrasma. Macmillan AL, Sarkany I. Br J Dermatol 1970;82:507–9.

All eight patients treated with 2% fusidic acid ointment twice daily for 2 weeks were cured. The cream is preferable for flexural lesions.

The treatment of erythrasma in a hospital for the mentally subnormal. Seville RH, Sommerville DA. Br J Dermatol 1970;82:502–6.

Eight of nine patients were cured with framycetin ointment twice daily for 2 weeks. Whitfield's ointment was effective in 23 of 24 patients. Both proved superior to tolnaftate cream, which benefited only six of 19 treated patients.

THIRD LINE THERAPIES

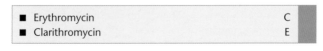

■ Erythromycin	C
■ Clarithromycin	E

The treatment of erythrasma in a hospital for the mentally subnormal. Seville RH, Sommerville A. Br J Dermatol 1970; 82:502–6.

Twenty patients were treated with erythromycin 250 mg four times daily for 7 days. Nearly all cases with involvement of the axillae and groins, but only about two-thirds of toe web infections were cured.

Erythrasma owing to an unusual pathogen. Dellion S, Morcel P, Vignon-Pennamen D, Felton A. Arch Dermatol 1996;132:716–7.

A case of widespread plaques of erythrasma, caused unusually by *Corynebacterium afermentans*, cured by 15 days of treatment with erythromycin 1.5 g daily. Usually 1 g daily for 5 days will be effective.

Erythrasma treated with single-dose clarithromycin. Wharton JR, Wilson PL, Kincannon JM. Arch Dermatol 1998; 134:671–2.

Three patients treated with a single 1 g dose of clarithromycin showed no sign of residual disease at 2 weeks.

Evidence levels A Double-blind study   B Clinical trial ≥ 20 subjects   C Clinical trial < 20 subjects   D Series ≥ 5 subjects   E Anecdotal case reports

Erythroderma

Michelle A Thomson, John Berth-Jones

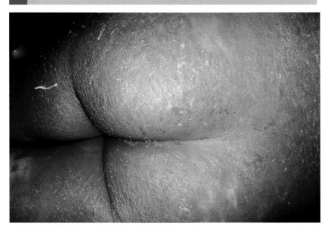

Table 1 Cutaneous diseases that may present with or develop into erythroderma

Atopic dermatitis	Lupus erythematosus
Bullous pemphigoid	Pemphigus foliaceous
Contact allergic dermatitis	Pityriasis rubra pilaris
Cutaneous T-cell lymphoma	Psoriasis
Dermatomyositis	Reiter's syndrome
Dermatophytosis	Sarcoid
Graft vs host disease	Seborrheic dermatitis
Hailey-Hailey disease	Scabies
Ichthyoses	Stasis dermatitis
Lichen planus	

Table 2 Drugs that may induce erythroderma

Allopurinol	Isoniazid
Amiodarone	Lithium
Antimalarials	Omeprazole
Aspirin	Para-aminosalicylic acid
Captopril	Penicillins
Carbamazepine	Phenothiazines
Cephalosporins	Quinidine
Cimetidine	Ranitidine
Codeine phosphate	Sulfonamides
Diaminodiphenyl sulfone (dapsone)	Sulfonylureas
Diltiazem	Thiazides
Diphenylhydantoin (phenytoin)	Trimethoprim
Epoprostenol	Vancomycin
Gold	

Erythroderma (exfoliative dermatitis) is persistent, severe, generalized inflammation of the skin. By convention the term tends to be reserved for cases where at least 90% of the skin is involved. Although the erythema is a constant feature, the scaling or exfoliation is highly variable. The condition arises as a 'reaction pattern' in a diverse range of circumstances (see Tables 1 and 2) including genodermatoses and congenital disorders such as severe ichthyoses and ichthyosiform erythrodermas; severe cases of dermatoses such as psoriasis, atopic or seborrheic or contact allergic dermatitis; cutaneous T-cell lymphoma; allergic reactions to drugs; and reactions to internal malignancies (especially lymphoma and other lymphoreticular malignancies). In addition to this multitude of known causes, a proportion of cases develop without any apparent trigger and remain 'idiopathic'.

MANAGEMENT STRATEGY

Erythroderma, especially when fulminant, is a life-threatening state of skin failure, which demonstrates vividly that the skin is as vital to life as any internal organ. The dangers arise from the loss of an effective barrier to entry of bacteria, from the loss of thermoregulation, from increased fluid loss through evaporation or exudation, from loss of protein due to the increased proliferative and metabolic activity, which accompany uncontrolled desquamation, and from the risk of high-output cardiac failure. All these hazards are greatest in the very young and the elderly. Many patients who are otherwise healthy can tolerate a chronic or permanently erythrodermic state. By contrast, elderly patients with fulminant disease may develop septicemia and die within a matter of hours.

Many aspects of the management of a patient with erythroderma are similar regardless of the etiology, and it is often necessary to treat a case without knowing the cause. However, for optimal management in the longer term it is vital to establish a more precise diagnosis when possible. In many cases there has been pre-existing skin disease and the diagnosis may be quite clear from the history, but when erythroderma arises de novo establishing the cause can be difficult or impossible. A careful drug history should always be obtained and this should include all over-the-counter and herbal remedies. Erythroderma has been associated with the use of St John's wort. Severe pruritus may suggest underlying lymphoma. Although findings on examination may be entirely nonspecific, there may be clues such as bullae indicating the presence of bullous pemphigoid or pemphigus foliaceous. Severe scaling is suggestive of psoriasis. Sparing of the flexures may suggest papuloerythroderma of Ofuji. Lymphadenopathy is often present, but is more often reactive than malignant.

Histology of the skin often proves as nonspecific as the clinical features and merely shows features of dermatitis. Occasionally, however, the presence of atypical large lymphocytes will point to a diagnosis of cutaneous T-cell lymphoma, or there may be features suggestive of psoriasis, a lichenoid reaction, or pityriasis rubra pilaris. Repeated or multiple biopsies are sometimes helpful.

Patients with acute onset of erythroderma are *usually best managed in a hospital bed because frequent observations and intensive supportive care are required and bed rest may be highly therapeutic.* All nonessential drugs should be withdrawn. Frequent applications of abundant quantities of *bland emollients* such as petrolatum are required to soothe the skin and these help to partially restore the barrier. Careful attention must be paid to *hydration and nutrition.*

The use of more active pharmaceutical intervention requires careful consideration. Some patients with erythroderma have multiple drug allergies. Immunosuppressive drugs may be considered to be contraindicated if malignancy is suspected (particularly cutaneous lymphoma).

Topical treatments may be far more irritant than expected, and systemic absorption will be greater than usual. *Prophylactic antibiotics* such as *erythromycin* are often given orally. *Corticosteroids* are often applied topically. *Antihistamines* are often prescribed, but act largely as sedatives.

If a diagnosis can be established, withdrawal of a causal drug or specific treatment for an underlying dermatosis, combined with the supportive measures described above, will usually produce rapid improvement in the erythroderma. When a firm diagnosis cannot be made, treatment may have to be directed at the most likely cause, based on the clinical and histologic features.

SPECIFIC INVESTIGATIONS

- Hematology
- Skin biopsy
- Monitoring of temperature and vital signs
- Monitoring of renal function
- Blood cultures
- T-cell receptor analysis
- Lymph node biopsy
- Screening for connective tissue disease
- Immunodeficiency screen
- Potassium hydroxide (KOH) preparation and fungal culture

T-cell receptor gene analysis in the diagnosis of Sézary syndrome. Russell-Jones R, Whittaker S. J Am Acad Dermatol 1999;41:254–9.

A discussion of the criteria used for diagnosis of Sézary syndrome. The demonstration of large atypical lymphocytes in peripheral blood (so-called 'Sézary cells') is not specific for this condition because these are often observed in benign reactive erythrodermas. Only when they comprise 20% or more of the circulating peripheral blood mononuclear cells do they reliably distinguish Sézary syndrome from other erythrodermas.

Diagnostic and prognostic importance of T-cell receptor gene analysis in patients with Sézary syndrome. Fraser-Andrews EA, Russell-Jones R, Woolford AJ, et al. Cancer 2001;92:1745–52.

The definitive diagnostic criteria for patients with Sézary syndrome should include the presence of a clonal T cell receptor gene rearrangement. Clonal patients have a poor prognosis and are likely to die from leukemia/lymphoma, whereas nonclonal patients may have a reactive, inflammatory T-cell disorder.

Mycosis fungoides and the Sézary syndrome. Kim YH, Hoppe RT. Semin Oncol 1999;26:276–89.

The prognosis of patients with mycosis fungoides is considered highly dependent on the initial presentation. Patients who present with limited patch/plaque disease have an overall long-term survival similar to a matched control population. Patients who have tumorous or erythrodermic skin involvement have a less favorable prognosis.

Bullous pemphigoid presenting as exfoliative erythroderma. Alonso-Llamazares J, Dietrich SM, Gibson LE. J Am Acad Dermatol 1998;39:827–30.

A patient with bullous pemphigoid presented with exfoliative erythroderma without any blistering. The diagnosis was based on the demonstration of circulating antibodies to the basement membrane zone, with an epidermal pattern on salt-split skin, and the presence of eosinophilic spongiosis in the skin biopsy.

Paraneoplastic dermatomyositis presenting as erythroderma. Nousari HC, Kimyai-Asadi A, Spegman DJ. J Am Acad Dermatol 1998;39:653–4.

A patient with gastric adenocarcinoma presented with erythrodermic dermatomyositis. Histology showed an interface dermatitis.

Idiopathic erythroderma: a follow-up study of 28 patients. Sigurdsson V, Toonstra J, van Vloten WA. Dermatology 1997;194:98–101.

During the median follow-up of 33 months, 35% of the patients went into remission and 52% improved. Three patients, all females, had persistent erythroderma. Two of these progressed to cutaneous T-cell lymphoma (one to Sézary syndrome and one to mycosis fungoides).

Inherited ichthyoses: a review of the histology of the skin. Scheimberg I, Harper JI, Malone M, Lake BD. Pediatr Pathol Lab Med 1996;16:359–78.

A review of the histologic features in 46 cases of congenital ichthyosis. Features of bullous ichthyosiform erythroderma, Netherton's syndrome, and neutral lipid storage disease can be recognized on routine hematoxylin and eosin staining. Electron microscopy, frozen sections, and other diagnostic techniques may also be required.

Congenital erythrodermic psoriasis: case report and literature review. Salleras M, Sanchez-Regana M, Umbert P. Pediatr Dermatol 1995;12:231–4.

A girl who suffered from erythroderma, palmoplantar hyperkeratosis, and scalp desquamation since birth. A skin biopsy at 1 year of age showed features of psoriasis. She was successfully treated with acitretin at the age of four. Plaque psoriasis developed at the age of seven.

Erythroderma due to dermatophyte. Gupta R, Khera V. Acta Derm Venereol 2001;81:70.

Dermatophytosis rarely presents as erythroderma. In this case, the presence of multiple mycelia without spores in KOH preparation confirmed the clinical suspicion of dermatophytosis. The scaling and erythema completely cleared with oral fluconazole 150 mg daily and miconazole nitrate cream 2% topically.

Severe subacute cutaneous lupus erythematosus presenting with generalized erythroderma and bullae. Mutasim DF. J Am Acad Dermatol 2003;48:947–9.

A patient presented with an erythrodermic and bullous form of subacute cutaneous lupus erythematosus. Serologic evaluation revealed a markedly elevated titer of antinuclear antibody (ANA) and La/SS-B antibodies. She later developed classic discrete lesions of subacute cutaneous lupus erythematosus. This case highlights the need to perform an autoimmune screen in cases where the etiology remains uncertain.

Neonatal and infantile erythrodermas. Pruszkowski A, Bodemer C, Fraitag S, et al. Arch Dermatol 2000;136:875–80.

The underlying cause of neonatal erythroderma is often difficult to ascertain. An immunodeficiency must be suspected in cases of severe erythroderma. The prognosis is poor in immunodeficiency disorders and severe cases of Netherton's syndrome and psoriasis.

FIRST LINE THERAPIES

■ Bed rest in hospital	C
■ Emollients	C

SECOND LINE THERAPIES

■ Topical corticosteroids	C
■ Psoralen and UVA (PUVA)	C
■ Systemic corticosteroids	C
■ PUVA with retinoid	E

Cushing's syndrome induced by topical steroids used for the treatment of non-bullous ichthyosiform erythroderma. Borzyskowski M, Grant DB, Wells RS. Clin Exp Dermatol 1976;1:337–42.

Salicylism from topical salicylates: review of the literature. Brubacher JR, Hoffman RS. J Toxicol Clin Toxicol 1996; 34:431–6.

Calcipotriol and hypercalcaemia. Dwyer C, Chapman RS. Lancet 1991;338:764–5.

Significant absorption of topical tacrolimus in 3 patients with Netherton syndrome. Allen A, Siegfried E, Silverman R, et al. Arch Dermatol 2001;137:747–50.

Patients with Netherton's syndrome have a skin barrier dysfunction that puts them at risk for increased percutaneous absorption. Tacrolimus levels should be carefully monitored to prevent systemic absorption and associated side effects.

Reports illustrating the potential for unexpected toxicity due to systemic absorption of topical medications through erythrodermic skin.

Treatment of papuloerythroderma of Ofuji with Re-PUVA: a case report and review of the therapy. Mutluer S, Yerebakan O, Alpsoy E, et al. J Eur Acad Dermatol Venereol 2004;18:480–3.

Papuloerythroderma of Ofuji is a disease of elderly men characterized by intensely pruritic and widespread red, flat-topped papules with sparing of the folds and creases. A case of PEO in a 60-year-old man who responded to retinoid plus PUVA (Re-PUVA) is discussed.

Treatment of severe erythrodermic acute graft-versus-host disease with photochemotherapy. Kunz M, Wilhelm S, Freund M, et al. Br J Dermatol 2001;144:901–22.

A 34-year-old male patient with grade IV graft-versus-host disease (GVHD) who did not respond to a combination of three different high-dose immunosuppressive agents.

The benefit of PUVA treatment for acute GVHD is well known, but successful treatment of severe GVHD is less common.

Ofuji papuloerythroderma: report of a European case. Bettoli V, Mantovani L, Altieri E, Strumia R. Dermatology 1993;186:187–9.

A patient in whom the disease improved after systemic corticosteroids and PUVA.

A dermatitis-eosinophilia syndrome. Treatment with methylprednisolone pulse therapy. Dahl MV, Swanson DL, Jacob HS. Arch Dermatol 1984;120:1595–7.

A case in which erythroderma developed after a wasp sting and persisted for 4 months despite intensive topical therapy and oral corticosteroids. Pulsed methylprednisolone, 2 g intravenously, repeated after a week, cleared the erythroderma.

THIRD LINE THERAPIES

■ Cyclosporine	D
■ Cytotoxic drugs/antimetabolites	C
■ Systemic retinoids	C
■ Extracorporeal photochemotherapy	C
■ UVA1 phototherapy	C
■ Topical calcipotriol	E
■ Photopheresis and infliximab	E
■ Infliximab	E
■ Alemtuzumab	E
■ Daclizumab	E
■ Bexarotene	E
■ Carbamazepine	E

Treatment of resistant severe psoriasis with systemic cyclosporine. Picascia DD, Garden JM, Freinkel RK, Roenigk HH. J Am Acad Dermatol 1987;17:408–14.

One of several reports of erythrodermic psoriasis responding to cyclosporine.

Psoriatic erythroderma and bullous pemphigoid treated successfully with acitretin and azathioprine. Roeder C, Driesch PV. Eur J Dermatol 1999;9:537–9.

A 59-year-old man with severe psoriasis who developed bullous pemphigoid was successfully treated with a combination of acitretin and azathioprine, avoiding the use of systemic corticosteroids.

Methotrexate for psoriasis. Boffa MJ, Chalmers RJ. Clin Exp Dermatol 1996;21:399–408.

Methotrexate is considered especially useful in acute generalized pustular psoriasis and psoriatic erythroderma.

A useful review article.

An appraisal of acitretin therapy in children with inherited disorders of keratinization. Lacour M, Mehta-Nikhar B, Atherton DJ, Harper JI. Br J Dermatol 1996;134:1023–9.

A review of the authors' experience of using acitretin and etretinate in 46 children with severe ichthyoses and erythrodermas. Acitretin therapy is considered safe and effective provided that the minimal effective dose is maintained and that side effects are carefully monitored.

Treatment of classic pityriasis rubra pilaris. Dicken CH. J Am Acad Dermatol 1994;31:997–9.

Classical pityriasis rubra pilaris almost always progresses to erythroderma. This is a retrospective review of 75 cases.

Retinoids are considered to offer the best chance of complete clearing. Methotrexate should be considered if retinoids fail or cannot be used.

Extracorporeal photopheresis in Sézary syndrome: hematologic parameters as predictors of response. Evans AV, Wood BP, Scarisbrick JJ, et al. Blood 2001;98:1298–1301.

Data analyzed from 23 patients with Sézary syndrome undergoing monthly extracorporeal photopheresis as the sole therapy for up to 1 year showed that 57% achieved a reduction in erythema greater than 25% from baseline.

Complete remission of lichen-planus-like graft-versus-host disease (GVHD) with extracorporeal photochemotherapy (ECP). Gerber M, Gmeinhart B, Volc Platzer B, et al. Bone Marrow Transplant 1997;19:517–19.

A report of a 45-year-old female patient who underwent marrow transplantation for chronic myeloid leukemia and developed two episodes of acute GVHD. The first responded well to cyclosporine and corticosteroids. The second episode, which was erythrodermic, proved resistant to this regimen. Twelve cycles of extracorporeal photochemotherapy produced a lasting complete remission.

Photopheresis therapy for cutaneous T-cell lymphoma. Duvic M, Hester JP, Lemak NA. J Am Acad Dermatol 1996; 35:573–9.

A report on 34 evaluable patients. Complete or partial remission was achieved in 50% of the patients. All responders except one had erythroderma.

"High-dose" UVA1 therapy of widespread plaque-type, nodular, and erythrodermic mycosis fungoides. Zane C, Leali C, Airò P, et al. J Am Acad Dermatol 2001;44:629–33.

In this series of 13 patients, 11 patients showed complete clinical and histological responses to 100 J/cm^2 UVA1 daily until remission. Unirradiated control lesions did not improve. Serious short-term side effects were not recorded. "High-dose" UVA1 seems at least as effective as PUVA in the treatment of cutaneous mycosis fungoides.

Bullous congenital ichthyosiform erythroderma: safe and effective topical treatment with calcipotriol ointment in a child. Bogenrieder T, Landthaler M, Stolz W. Acta Derm Venereol 2002;83:52–5.

A report of the safe and long-term (>3 years) use of topical calcipotriol ointment in a nine-year-old boy with a keratinization disorder.

Successful treatment of Netherton's syndrome with topical calcipotriol. Godic A, Dragos V. Eur J Dermatol 2004;14:115–17.

Monitoring the decrease of circulating malignant T cells in cutaneous T-cell lymphoma during photopheresis and interferon therapy. Ferenczi K, Yawalkar N, Jones D, Kupper TS. Arch Dermatol 2003;139:909–13.

A patient with stage IV cutaneous T cell lymphoma (CTCL) who was treated with photopheresis and low-dose interferon showed a dramatic reduction in the percentage of the malignant T-cell population paralleled by clinical skin improvement from initial generalized erythroderma to undetectable skin disease.

Erythrodermic, recalcitrant psoriasis: clinical resolution with infliximab. Rongioletti F, Borenstein M, Kirsner R, Kerdel F. J Dermatolog Treat 2003;14:222–5.

The report describes a patient with erythrodermic psoriasis that failed all previous therapies over a 12-year period and responded to treatment with infliximab. The potential utility of infliximab as a therapeutic alternative for erythrodermic psoriasis is discussed.

Case number 29: hitting three with one strike: rapid improvement of psoriatic arthritis, psoriatic erythroderma, and secondary renal amyloidosis by treatment with infliximab (Remicade). Fiehn C, Andrassy K. Ann Rheum Dis 2004;63:232.

A 64-year-old woman with a 30-year history of psoriasis, polyarticular psoriatic arthritis, and newly diagnosed renal insufficiency failed to respond to low-dose prednisolone. Treatment with 200 mg infliximab intravenously (3.3 mg/kg) relieved joint pain and reduced joint swelling and the erythroderma disappeared.

Successful treatment of chemotherapy-refractory Sézary syndrome with alemtuzumab (Campath-1H). Gautschi O, Blumenthal N, Streit M, et al. Eur J Haemotol 2004;72:61–3.

A 32-year-old male patient with advanced stage, extensively pretreated Sézary syndrome with very pruritic erythroderma that had not responded to PUVA or interferon-α and progressed on chemotherapy. Following treatment with alemtuzumab (30 mg intravenously three times weekly for 10 weeks), itching resolved rapidly and almost complete remission was achieved within 3 months of starting this treatment.

Phase 2 study of alemtuzumab (anti-CD52 monoclonal antibody) in patients with advanced mycosis fungoides/Sézary syndrome. Lundin J, Hagberg H, Repp R, et al. Blood 2003;101:4267–71.

This study evaluated the efficacy and safety of alemtuzumab in 22 patients. Clinical responses were recorded in more than 50% of patients with advanced mycosis fungoides/Sézary syndrome with a preference for erythrodermic versus plaque/tumor stage of disease.

Humanized monoclonal anti-CD25 antibody as a novel therapeutic option in HIV-associated psoriatic erythroderma. Dichmann S, Mrowietz, Schopf E, Norgauer J. J Am Acad Dermatol;47:635–6.

The successful use of daclizumab in a patient with HIV-associated psoriatic erythroderma. The monoclonal anti-CD25 antibody therapy did not influence the controlled HIV parameters during continuous antiretroviral therapy.

The treatment of cutaneous T-cell lymphoma with a novel retinoid. Heald P. Clin Lymphoma 2000;1:S45–9.

Four patients with erythrodermic CTCL were treated with high-dose oral bexarotene and all patients showed rapid (within 2 weeks) improvement of erythroderma.

Optimizing bexarotene therapy for cutaneous T-cell lymphoma. Talpur R, Ward S, Apisarnthanarax N, Breuer-Mcham J, Duvic M. J Am Acad Dermatol 2002;47:672–84.

Evidence levels A Double-blind study **B** Clinical trial ≥ 20 subjects **C** Clinical trial < 20 subjects **D** Series ≥ 5 subjects **E** Anecdotal case reports

Therapeutic efficacy of carbamazepine in a HIV-1-positive patient with psoriatic erythroderma. Smith KJ, Decker C, Yeager J, et al. J Am Acad Dermatol 1997;37:851–4.

This is a case report of a patient with HIV infection and erythrodermic psoriasis who was inadvertently treated with carbamazepine 200–400 mg daily. His erythroderma cleared, but then recurred when the carbamazepine was discontinued. Upon retreatment, the erythroderma cleared again.

Erythrokerato-dermas

Gabriele Richard

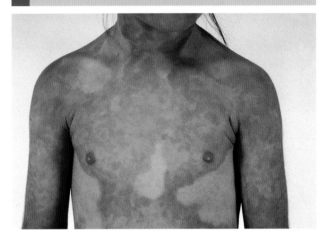

Erythrokeratodermas are a clinically and genetically heterogeneous group of rare inherited disorders of cornification characterized by two distinct morphologic features: localized hyperkeratosis and erythema. The hallmark of erythrokeratodermia variabilis (EKV) is the seemingly independent occurrence of transient, figurate erythema and hyperkeratosis, which can be localized or generalized. Progressive symmetric erythrokeratoderma (PSEK) is characterized by fixed, slowly progressive, symmetric and well-defined hyperkeratotic plaques with underlying erythema predominantly on the extensor surface of the extremities, on the trunk, and on the face.

MANAGEMENT STRATEGY

Erythrokeratodermas are heritable, chronic disorders that often require life-long treatment. Management depends on the severity and extent of hyperkeratosis, which may vary over time, and from patient to patient. The spectrum may range from fixed hyperkeratotic plaques over the knees and elbows to generalized hyperkeratosis with accentuated skin markings and peeling or thickened plates with a spiny, hystrix-like appearance.

The *topical management* of erythrokeratodermas is often disappointing but it remains a therapeutic cornerstone. Topical treatment of patients with mild, localized hyperkeratosis is symptomatic and focuses on hydration, lubrication, and keratolysis. While in some patients *emollients* such as petrolatum, lanolin, stearyl alcohol, cetyl alcohol, or isopropyl palmitate twice daily may suffice, most patients require topical treatment with *keratolytic agents*. Lactic acid (6–12%) and urea (5–20%) applied once or twice daily in combination with emollients are effective, although their use may be limited, especially in children, because of irritation. Other α-hydroxy acids, salicylic acid (3–6%), propylene glycol, glycolic acid (11%), topical vitamin D analogs, or combinations of these are alternative treatment options. Topical treatment with *retinoids* and derivatives has been successful in some patients but ineffective in others. In addition, avoidance of trauma to the skin, such as sudden temperature changes, friction, and mechanical irritation, may be beneficial.

Systemic retinoids are the treatment of choice in erythrokeratodermas with extensive or generalized skin involvement. While they are highly effective in EKV, the therapeutic response in PSEK is less satisfactory. As is the case for other disorders of cornification, the effect of acitretin or etretinate is superior to that of systemic isotretinoin. It seems advantageous to start at low doses of acitretin for 3–6 weeks, and then to gradually increase the dosage until the desired therapeutic effect is achieved. The minimal effective maintenance dose for patients with EKV is usually lower than for patients with PSEK. Both morphologic components respond well to retinoid treatment, resulting in rapid and dramatic improvement or clearing of the hyperkeratosis and significant moderation of the erythema, although the latter cannot be completely suppressed. Nevertheless, the use of retinoids should always be considered carefully since chronic therapy is required to attain continuing results, and long-term side effects, especially in children, may ensue. Anecdotally, *PUVA therapy* has been beneficial in the treatment of PSEK.

The variable erythema in EKV often results in cosmetic concerns, which can be limited by masking uncovered skin with makeup and camouflage. Serious discomfort due to burning and pruritus, which may accompany the variable erythema in some patients, remains a therapeutic challenge.

SPECIFIC INVESTIGATIONS

- Family history
- Histopathology

Family study of erythrokeratodermia figurata variabilis. Itin P, Levy CA, Sommacal-Schopf D, Schnyder UW. Hautarzt 1992;43:500–4.

Thorough studies in a large five-generational EKV family with 29 affected individuals revealed valuable clinical data on age of onset, relationship between erythema and hyperkeratosis, precipitating factors, frequency of palmoplantar involvement, and natural history of EKV.

Erythrokeratoderma progressiva symmetrica: report of 10 cases. Ruiz-Maldonado R, Tamayo L, del Castillo V, Lozoya I. Dermatologica 1982;164:133–41.

Clinical investigation of 10 patients with PSEK, six of whom belonged to three families with autosomal dominant inheritance, two were sporadic cases, and two cases were the product of consanguineous unions suggestive of autosomal recessive inheritance. While eight patients were treated conventionally with topical keratolytics with moderate results, two patients achieved complete remission under treatment with systemic retinoids.

Is erythrokeratoderma one disorder? A clinical and ultrastructural study of two siblings. MacFarlane AW, Chapman SJ, Verbov JL. Br J Dermatol 1991;124:487–91.

Clinical presentations of EKV and PSEK with identical electron microscopic features were observed in the same family, and raised the question as to whether these two disorders are indeed separate entities.

Mutations in the human connexin gene *GJB3* cause erythrokeratodermia variabilis. Richard G, Smith LE, Bailey RA, et al. Nat Genet 1998;20:366–9.

Evidence levels **A** Double-blind study **B** Clinical trial ≥ 20 subjects **C** Clinical trial < 20 subjects **D** Series ≥ 5 subjects **E** Anecdotal case reports

Disease-causing missense mutations in the connexin gene *GJB3*, which is localized on chromosome 1p35.1 and encodes the gap junction protein β-3 (connexin-31, Cx31), were identified in four families with EKV. The study provided evidence that intercellular communication mediated by gap junctions is crucial for epidermal differentiation and response to external factors.

Mutation in the gene for connexin 30.3 in a family with erythrokeratodermia variabilis. Macari F, Landau M, Cousin P, et al. Am J Hum Genet 2000;67:1296–301.

Report of a pathogenic mutation in the connexin gene *GJB4*, encoding Cx30.3, in an extended EKV family. The data suggest that EKV is genetically heterogeneous and may be caused by mutations in at least two structurally and functionally related connexin genes.

Genetic heterogeneity in erythrokeratodermia variabilis: novel mutations in the connexin gene *GJB4* (Cx30.3) and genotype-phenotype correlations. Richard G, Brown N, Rouan F, et al. J Invest Dermatol 2003;120:601–9.

In a large cohort of patients, these authors identified six different missense mutations of *GJB4* (Cx30.3) in five families and a sporadic case of EKV. In two families, these mutations were associated with the occurrence of rapidly changing erythematous patches with prominent, circinate, or gyrate borders, suggesting that this feature is specific to Cx30.3 defects.

FIRST LINE THERAPIES

■ Emollients	E
■ Topical keratolytics	E
■ Topical retinoids	E

Erythrokeratodermia variabilis. Report of 3 clinical cases and evaluation of the topical retinoic acid treatment. Lacerda e Costa MH, de Brito Caldeira J. Med Cutan Ibero Lat Am 1975;3:281–7.

Topical retinoic acid (0.1% cream) treatment of three patients with EKV substantially reduced hyperkeratosis. Discontinuation resulted in prompt relapse.

Erythrokeratoderma variabilis: case report and review of the literature. Knipe RC, Flowers FP, Johnson FR Jr, et al. Pediatr Dermatol 1995;12:21–3.

Topical therapy with retinoic acid proved ineffective in an infant with EKV.

The pharmacology of topical therapy. Arndt KA, Mendenhall PV, Sloan KB, Perrin JH. In: Fitzpatrick TB, ed. Dermatology in General Medicine. 4ᵗʰ edn. New York: McGraw-Hill; 1993:2837–46.

In-depth summary of topical formulations, vehicle ingredients, and applications.

SECOND LINE THERAPIES

■ Acitretin, etretinate	C
■ Isotretinoin	E

Acitretin in the treatment of erythrokeratodermia variabilis. van de Kerkhof PC, Steijlen PM, van Dooren-Greebe RJ, Happle R. Dermatologica 1990;181:330–3.

A patient with EKV had been successfully treated for 3 years with etretinate (on average 25 mg daily), while subsequent therapy with isotretinoin (20 mg daily) for 2 years was less efficient. Systemic therapy with acitretin at an initial dose of 35 mg daily for 8 weeks, reduced to a maintenance dose of 25–35 mg daily, resulted in a striking and sustained clinical improvement and decreased hyperkeratosis and dermal inflammation on histologic skin evaluation.

Compared to the other retinoids, acitretin was found to elicit similar effects as etretinate at lower initial doses, and thus was regarded as the first choice in treatment of EKV.

Acitretin for erythrokeratodermia variabilis in a 9-year-old girl. Graham-Brown RAC, Chave TA. Pediatr Dermatol 2002;19:510–2.

Oral treatment with acitretin 1 mg/kg daily resulted in complete clearing of the skin within 3 weeks. This positive therapeutic effect could be maintained with a reduced dose of 0.66 mg/kg daily.

[Erythrokeratodermia progressiva symmetrica Darier-Gottron with generalized expression]. Emmert S, Küster W, Schauder S, et al. Hautarzt 1998;49:666–71. In German.

Two patients of a family with PSEK responded very well to oral treatment with acitretin. One patient was treated with 0.4 mg/kg daily for 3 months and showed improvement of hyperkeratosis even 3 months after discontinuation. The other patient required only intermittent therapy, twice a year, with 10 mg daily acitretin for 2 weeks.

Treatment of erythrokeratodermia variabilis with oral retinoid (Ro 10-9359). van der Schroeff JG, Suurmond D. In: Orfanos CE, et al., eds. Retinoids: Advances in Basic Research and Therapy. Berlin: Springer; 1981:295–301.

Ten patients from two different families with EKV were treated with etretinate for between 6 and 36 months. An initial dose of 0.5–0.9 mg/kg daily produced desquamation and clearing of hyperkeratotic plaques already after 2 weeks, while the erythematous patches remained. Two to three months of therapy with a reduced maintenance dose of between 0.1 mg/kg and 0.5 mg/kg daily resulted in complete clearance of the hyperkeratotic component and the erythema was significantly diminished. The clinical improvement was accompanied by a normalization of the histologic findings, in particular hyperkeratosis and hypergranulosis.

Retinoids. Peck GL, DiGiovanna JJ. In: Fitzpatrick TB, ed. Dermatology in General Medicine. 5ᵗʰ edn. New York: McGraw-Hill; 1999:2810–20.

Extensive review on pharmacology, use, and toxicity of retinoids.

Oral retinoid (Ro 10-9359) in children with lamellar ichthyosis, epidermolytic hyperkeratosis and symmetrical progressive erythrokeratoderma. Tamayo L, Ruiz-Maldonado R. Dermatologica 1980;161:305–14.

Five children with PSEK demonstrated dramatic improvement under systemic therapy with etretinate. Treatment was considered efficient and tolerable, with manageable side effects.

Progressive symmetric erythrokeratodermia. Histological and ultrastructural study of patient before and after

treatment with etretinate. Nazzaro V, Blanchet-Bardon C. Arch Dermatol 1986;122:434–40.

Treatment of a PSEK patient with etretinate diminished hyperkeratotic plaques and reduced mitochondrial swelling in granulocytes as well as the number of lipid-like vacuoles in corneocytes observed by electron microscopy.

Is the use of Ro 10-9359 (Tigason) in children justified? Van der Rhee HJ, van Gelderen HH, Polano MK. Acta Derm Venereol 1980;60:274–5.

Excellent therapeutic results were noted in three children with EKV treated with an initial dose of 0.6–1 mg/kg etretinate, and were maintained with half the dose over 1 year.

Oral synthetic retinoid treatment in children. DiGiovanna JJ, Peck GL. Pediatr Dermatol 1983;1:77–88.

In one patient with EKV, marked improvement was achieved with oral isotretinoin therapy. Side effects, toxicity, and therapeutic guidelines of retinoid therapy are discussed.

Erythrokeratodermia variabilis treated with isotretinoin. A clinical, histologic, and ultrastructural study. Rappaport IP, Goldes JA, Goltz RW. Arch Dermatol 1986;122:441–5.

Isotretinoin therapy (80 mg daily) in an adult patient with EKV resulted in almost complete clinical clearing of hyperkeratotic plaques and substantial reduction of erythema after 4 months. A skin biopsy under treatment revealed diminished hyperkeratosis and papillomatosis on light microscopy as well as normalization of the number of lamellar bodies observed by electron microscopy.

THIRD LINE THERAPIES

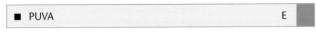

■ PUVA   E

[Gottron's erythroderma congenitalis progressiva symmetrical]. Levi L, Beneggi M, Crippa D, Sala GP. Hautarzt 1982;33:605–8. In German.

In one family with PSEK, an adult patient was treated with aromatic retinoid for 8 weeks, while her child received PUVA therapy for a total of 63 J/cm² UVA. Both treatments were effective and reduced hyperkeratosis, but PUVA attained superior results.

Evidence levels   **A** Double-blind study   **B** Clinical trial ≥ 20 subjects   **C** Clinical trial < 20 subjects   **D** Series ≥ 5 subjects   **E** Anecdotal case reports

Erythromelalgia

Cato Mørk, Knut Kvernebo

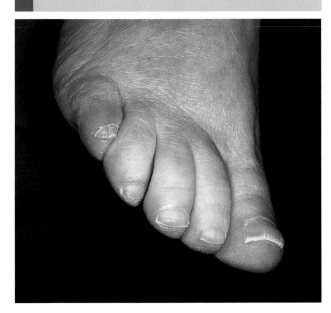

Erythromelalgia is a symptom complex characterized by burning extremity pain, pain aggravated by warming, pain relieved by cooling, erythema of affected skin, and increased temperature of affected skin. The symptoms and findings are usually intermittent and not present during physical examination. Our hypothesis of pathogenesis is that symptoms are caused by maldistribution of skin perfusion, with increased thermoregulatory flow through anatomical and functional arteriovenous anastomoses and a relative deficit in nutritional flow.

MANAGEMENT STRATEGY

The severity of symptoms varies from mild discomfort (most common) to completely disabling pain and gangrene. In daily clinical work the terms mild, moderate, and severe may be useful. The treatment strategy is dependent on the patient's medical history. Acute disease has a tendency to get better, whereas chronic disease tends to have a stable course. Spontaneous remissions have occurred without treatment. *Underlying diseases (secondary erythromelalgia), such as myeloproliferative, connective tissue, cardiovascular, infectious and neurological diseases, diabetes mellitus, vasculitis, and neoplasia should be sought and optimally treated.* Drug-induced erythromelalgia has been reported secondary to calcium channel blockers, bromocriptine, norepinephrine (noradrenaline), pergolide, ticlopidine, cyclosporine, iodine contrast, mushroom, and mercury poisoning.

All patients benefit from *local skin cooling* (applying cold objects or surfaces such as cold floors, wet sand, and towels, air-conditioned rooms, or immersion in buckets of cool or ice water) and from *elevation of the affected limb.* Comfortable shoes to relieve pressure over the soles of the feet can help. *Aggravating factors such as warmth, exercise, dependency of the extremity, and tight shoes and gloves, and even alcohol intake in some cases, should be avoided.*

Contact with The Erythromelalgia Association (www.erythromelalgia.org) may be of help for doctors and patients in the management of erythromelalgia.

The wide spectrum of published approaches in the management of erythromelalgia reflects the heterogeneity in the etiology of erythromelalgia and the lack of documented effects of treatment. Only two controlled clinical trials have been published. The main reason may be the low prevalence of erythromelalgia, the heterogeneity of patients, and the lack of laboratory diagnostic methods. No single medication or treatment modality has been universally helpful, maybe because erythromelalgia, in our minds, is not a specific disease, but a condition with one common pathogenetic mechanism, arteriovenous shunting. This view is analogous to the recognized fact that inflammation is not a specific disease, but a physiological response to stimuli such as infection, trauma, and tumor. Before designing a treatment regimen, the patient's condition should be classified according to whether it is primary or secondary, the etiology (for secondary cases), and its severity. Analgesics, including opiate analgesics, have limited effect. A few patients become free of symptoms with small doses of *acetylsalicylic acid.* Numerous drugs have been used with varying success. Case reports or series of patients have shown beneficial effect with *vasodilators* (prostaglandin E1/prostacyclin or analogues, sodium nitroprusside, naftidrofuryl, calcium channel blockers). Other drugs that may be of benefit are *antidepressants* and *gabapentin.* Calcium channel blockers may help some, but exacerbate others.

We suggest that most patients start with low dosages and then increase gradually depending on effect and side effects. Sometimes combinations have proven more helpful than a single drug. If partial improvement is achieved with one drug, antidepressants and gabapentin could be added. Vasoconstrictor therapy (norepinephrine [noradrenaline], epinephrine [adrenaline], β-blockers) and sympathectomy may exacerbate erythromelalgia and are probably contraindicated.

Numerous treatment alternatives based on single case reports are presented in the literature. Anecdotally, nitroglycerin ointment, capsaicin cream, ketanserin, methysergide, pizotifene, β-blockers, cyproheptadine or other antihistamines, carbamazepine, clonazepam, corticosteroids or other immunosuppressants, hyperbaric O_2-treatment, pentoxifylline, phenoxybenzamine, opiates, spinal cord stimulation, biofeedback, epidural blocks, transcutaneous electrical nerve stimulation, sympathectomy, phenoxybenzamine, prazosin, and hypnotherapy have been presented as effective. From our personal experience with 160 patients with erythromelalgia and based on extensive studies of pathophysiology, we believe that vasoconstrictor therapy and sympathectomy should not be given, though there are some positive reports in the literature. The Erythromelalgia Association survey of 2003 reports more than 50 therapies for erythromelalgia based on 222 respondents.

Erythromelalgia – a condition caused by microvascular arteriovenous shunting. Kvernebo K. VASA 1998;27 (suppl 51):3–39.

Erythromelalgia: studies on pathogenesis and therapy. (Doctoral thesis) Mørk C. Faculty of Medicine, University of Oslo (ISBN 82-8072-146-0 No 173); June 2004. Available on www.erythromelalgia.org.

SPECIFIC INVESTIGATIONS

- Exclude erythromelalgia secondary to hematologic, metabolic, connective tissue, cardiovascular, infectious, neurological, musculoskeletal, or neoplastic diseases
- Drug history of exposure to calcium channel blockers, bromocriptine, vasoconstrictors, norepinephrine (noradrenaline), pergolide, ticlopidine, cyclosporine, iodine contrast, mushroom, mercury
- Full blood count with white cell differential count
- Serum chemistry including blood sugar
- Antinuclear antibody, RA latex
- HIV testing

Natural history of erythromelalgia: presentation and outcome in 168 patients. Davis MDP, O'Fallon WM, Rogers RS III, Rooke TW. Arch Dermatol 2000;136:330–6.

The largest retrospective study presented on erythromelalgia. An increase in mortality and morbidity is demonstrated, and the comorbidities and causes of death are reported.

Erythromelalgia: a clinical study of 87 cases. Kalgaard OM, Seem E, Kvernebo K. J Int Med 1997;242:191–7.

Classification, etiology, and prognosis of erythromelalgia are presented. The findings in this material are the main basis for the proposed investigations.

Erythromelalgia: a pathognomonic microvascular thrombotic complication in essential thrombocythemia and polycythemia vera. Van Genderen PJJ, Michiels JJ. Semin Thromb Hemost 1997;23:357–63.

Erythromelalgia is seen secondary to platelet aggregation and peripheral microvascular occlusion in myeloproliferative disorders and may, untreated, progress to peripheral gangrene. Remission is observed after treatment of the myeloproliferative disorder.

Erythromelalgia as a paraneoplastic syndrome in a patient with abdominal cancer. Mørk C, Kalgaard OM, Kvernebo K. Acta Derm Venereol 1999;79:394.

Erythromelalgia in a patient with AIDS. Mørk C, Kalgaard OM, Myrvang B, Kvernebo K. J Eur Acad Dermatol Venereol 2000;14:498–500.

FIRST LINE THERAPIES

■ Treatment of underlying disease	C
■ Cooling	C
■ Aspirin	D
■ Prostaglandins/prostacyclin or oral analogues	A

Several accompanying diseases, conditions, and pharmacological substances have been described as associated with erythromelalgia. A beneficial effect on the symptoms of erythromelalgia after successful treatment or elimination of the primary condition indicates a causal relationship.

Immersion of an affected limb in cold water or exposure to cold air temperature will make patients feel better for a limited time, but can create problems such as tissue breakdown of the skin, infection, reactive flaring, and ulcers that heal slowly. Cooling of

the skin may, through microvascular stasis, increase the arteriovenous shunting.

Aspirin and platelet-lowering agents for the prevention of vascular complications in essential thrombocythemia. Michiels JJ. Clin Appl Thromb Hemost 1999;5:247–51.

Aspirin 250–500 mg daily or less may abolish the symptoms completely in erythromelalgia secondary to myeloproliferative conditions. The response is probably due to the antiplatelet effect. A reduction of platelet numbers by cytostatic treatment may also lead to relief.

The Erythromelalgia Association Survey 2003. *www.erythromelalgia.org.*

In a survey 128 respondents had used aspirin (80–250 mg daily) – four reported complete, 17 moderate, and 22 minimal relief; 78 had no improvement and six reported worsening of their symptoms.

Aspirin should be tried in all EM patients without contraindications.

Erythromelalgia – a condition caused by microvascular arteriovenous shunting. Kvernebo K. VASA 1998;27(suppl 51):3–39.

Based on the hypothesis of arteriovenous shunting prostaglandin E1 (PGE1) and prostacyclin was tried as an intravenous infusion to enhance nutritive skin perfusion in severe erythromelalgia. Nine of ten patients benefited from PGE1 given as a continuous infusion for 3 days, starting with 6, then 10, and finally 12 ng/kg per min.

Erythromelalgia: a personal perspective. Belch JJF. J Dermatol Treat 1992;3:153–8.

Case reports of the use of prostacyclin.

Prostacyclin reduces symptoms and sympathetic dysfunction in erythromelalgia in a double-blind randomized pilot study. Kalgaard OM, Mørk C, Kvernebo K. Acta Derm Venereol 2003;83:442–4.

For the first time in a double-blind, randomized study, reduced symptoms and sympathetic dysfunction were demonstrated. Eight patents were treated with prostacyclin infusion and four with placebo infusion.

The prostaglandin E1 analog misoprostol reduces symptoms and microvascular arteriovenous shunting in erythromelalgia – a double-blind, crossover, placebo-compared study. Mørk C, Salerud EG, Asker CL, Kvernebo K. 2004;122:587–93.

This first properly designed placebo-controlled clinical trial for the treatment of erythromelalgia demonstrated that misoprostol (0.4–0.8 mg daily) reduced symptoms significantly more than placebo, as determined by pain and cooling scores, and global assessment. Furthermore, misoprostol reduced pain and hyperemia, induced by central body heating when compared with baseline recordings at baseline and after placebo treatment. Misoprostol is recommended as first line treatment.

SECOND LINE THERAPIES

■ Gabapentin	C
■ Antidepressants	C
■ Sodium nitroprusside	D

Evidence levels **A** Double-blind study **B** Clinical trial ≥ 20 subjects **C** Clinical trial < 20 subjects **D** Series ≥ 5 subjects **E** Anecdotal case reports

Erythromelalgia pain managed with gabapentin.
McGraw T, Kosek P. Anesthesiology 1997;86:988–90.

Two patients with beneficial effect are reported. This effect is compatible with a report of thin-fiber neuropathy in erythromelalgia.

The Erythromelalgia Association Survey 2003. *www. erythromelalgia.org.*

In a survey 129 members of The Erythromelalgia Association reported use of gabapentin with complete (n = 7), moderate (n = 48) or minimal (n = 22) relief. Fifty sufferers reported no improvement or worsening.

The treatment is safe and generally well tolerated and could easily be combined with other drugs.

Erythromelalgia: response to serotonin reuptake inhibitors. Rudikoff D, Jaffe IA. J Am Acad Dermatol 1997;37:281–3.

Two patients responded to venlafaxine, and one patient to sertraline.

Serotonin is a vasoactive substance that may cause vasodilatation.

Association of erythromelalgia and Raynaud's disease responding to a serotonin reuptake inhibitor. Maldonado NR, Acaso MCA, Castano AH, Izquierdo RM. J Dermatol Treat 1999;10:141–4.

Report of one single case.

The Erythromelalgia Association Survey 2003. *www. erythromelalgia.org.*

190 reports of the use of antidepressants are given in The Erythromelalgia Association survey, mostly with minimal or no improvement. The use of venlafaxine was reported to give the most beneficial effect.

Erythromelalgia – a condition caused by microvascular arteriovenous shunting. Kvernebo K. VASA 1998;27 (suppl 51):3–39.

Sodium nitroprusside given parenterally for 7 days in increasing doses (1, 3, and 5 µg/kg per min) was successful in two patients with severe erythromelalgia. Microvascular perfusion measurements documented the effect.

Sodium nitroprusside treatment in erythromelalgia. Özsoylu S, Coskun T. Eur J Paediatrics 1984;141:185–7.

Report of one single case.

THIRD LINE THERAPIES

■ Magnesium	C
■ Calcium channel blockers	C
■ Naftidrofuryl	E
■ Nonsteroidal anti-inflammatory drugs (NSAIDs)	D
■ Mexiletine	E

High-dose oral magnesium treatment of chronic, intractable erythromelalgia. Cohen JS. Ann Pharmacother 2002;36:255–60.

Magnesium is a naturally occurring calcium channel blocker. Eight of 13 patients reported improvement, four no

response, and one deterioration using magnesium sulphate, up to 1166 mg daily.

The Erythromelalgia Association Survey 2003. *www. erythromelalgia.org.*

Forty six of 75 respondents using magnesium reported no effect or worsening following magnesium treatment.

Erythromelalgia: new theories and new therapies. Cohen JS. J Am Acad Dermatol 2000;43: 841–7.

Recommendations for the use of calcium channel blockers (diltiazem) are given.

The Erythromelalgia Association Survey 2003. *www. erythromelalgia.org.*

Sixty nine respondents had used calcium channel blockers with complete (n = 2), moderate (n = 8), and minimal (n = 7) relief of symptoms; 26 reported no improvement and 26 reported worsening of the condition.

Possible erythromelalgia-like syndrome associated with nifedipine in a patient with Raynaud's phenomenon. Sunahara JF, Gora-Harper ML, Nash KS. Ann Pharmacother 1996;30:484–6.

Calcium channel blockers may be helpful for patients with erythromelalgia, but can also cause or exacerbate symptoms.

Erythromelalgia. Belch JJF. In: Tooke JE, Lowe GDO, eds. A Textbook of Vascular Medicine. London: E. Arnold Publishers Ltd; 1996:342–52.

This group from Scotland proposed the combination of naftidrofuryl oxalate (a vasodilator) and amitriptyline (an antidepressant).

Natural history of erythromelalgia: presentation and outcome in 168 patients. Davis MDP, O'Fallon WM, Rogers RS III, Rooke TW. Arch Dermatol 2000;136:330–6.

Twenty five of 49 patients reported a response to NSAIDs.

Erythromelalgia relieved by piroxicam in a patient with allergy to aspirin. Levesque H, Cailleux N, Vuillermet P, et al. Therapie 1991;46:499–500.

Lidocaine and mexiletine therapy for erythromelalgia. Kuhnert SM, Phillips WJ, Davis MD. Arch Dermatol 1999;135:1447–9.

A single case.

A case of primary erythromelalgia improved by mexiletine. Jang HS, Jung D, Kim S, et al. Br J Dermatol 2004;151: 708–10.

A single case.

Natural history of erythromelalgia: presentation and outcome in 168 patients. Davis MDP, O'Fallon WM, Rogers RS III, Rooke TW. Arch Dermatol 2000;136:330–6.

Reports responses to 20 different treatment regimens based on a survey questionnaire from 99 patients.

Erythropoietic protoporphyria

Maureen B Poh-Fitzpatrick

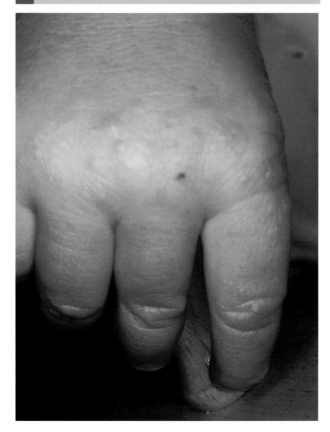

Erythropoietic protoporphyria is caused by ferrochelatase gene mutations resulting in abnormally high levels of protoporphyrin, a photoactive intermediary of heme synthesis, in erythrocytes, plasma, bile, and feces. Oxygen-dependent acute cutaneous phototoxicity is elicited by long UV and visible light radiation; cholelithiasis and progressive liver failure may supervene. Hypochromic microcytic anemia, when present, is typically mild and rarely requires treatment.

MANAGEMENT STRATEGY

Protoporphyric photosensitivity is rarely managed adequately by *sun avoidance* alone (i.e. lifestyle changes, protective clothing, physical barriers). *Topical sunscreens* containing *titanium dioxide, zinc oxide, iron oxide,* or *dihydroxyacetone* block or filter long UV and visible light spectra, offering additional relief. Epidermal melanization and hyperplasia achieved with *UVB* or *psoralen plus UVA (PUVA) phototherapy* also increase sunlight tolerance. Oral agents believed to photoprotect by quenching excited oxygen species include *beta-carotene, cysteine, vitamin E, vitamin C, flavonoids,* and possibly *pyridoxine. Antihistamines* may attenuate phototoxic flaring. Gallstones are managed *surgically.* Exacerbators of protoporphyrin-induced hepatotoxicity (alcohol, cholestatic drugs, dietary carbohydrate restriction) are best avoided.

Deteriorating liver function is only sporadically reversible by *enteric sorbents (cholestyramine, activated charcoal;* which interrupt enterohepatic porphyrin recirculation), *bile acids* (which stimulate biliary protoporphyrin secretion), *blood transfusion or exchange, hematin infusion,* or *glucose loading* (which retard endogenous porphyrinogenesis), *iron* (to increase protoporphyrin conversion to heme), or various combinations thereof. It is postulated that *cimetidine* inhibits porphyrinogenesis. When indicated, *liver transplantation* is aided by measures to reduce peri- and intraoperative porphyrin levels (*exchange transfusion, hematin infusion, plasmapheresis*). Operating room lamps should be filtered to exclude wavelengths that can severely damage porphyrin-photosensitized skin and internal organs. *Bone marrow transplantation* would be curative but is not warranted in uncomplicated cases.

SPECIFIC INVESTIGATIONS

- Porphyrin analyses in erythrocytes, serum or plasma, urine, feces
- Hematological profile, iron studies if anemic
- Liver function profile, liver imaging and biopsy if clinically indicated

Erythropoietic protoporphyria. Todd DJ. Br J Dermatol 1994;131:751–66.

An excellent review of clinical, laboratory, genetic, and therapeutic aspects of the disease.

Hepatobiliary implications and complications in protoporphyria. A 20-year study. Doss MO, Frank M. Clin Biochem 1989;22:223–9.

Among 55 patients with protoporphyria impaired liver function was observed in 19, cirrhosis in seven, and fatal liver failure in two. Coproporphyrinuria appeared early in the course of progressive protoporphyric hepatotoxicity.

Symptomatic liver failure probably occurs in approximately 5% of all cases. Because urine in uncomplicated protoporphyria is typically free of excess porphyrins, surveillance for mild excess coproporphyrinuria might identify patients with asymptomatic hepatic dysfunction in whom early medical intervention might be more successful.

FIRST LINE THERAPIES

■ Topical sunscreens, physical barriers	C
■ Beta-carotene	B

Efficiency of opaque photoprotective agents in the visible light range. Kaye ET, Levin JA, Blank IH, et al. Arch Dermatol 1991;127:351–5.

Iron oxide increases the light-blocking efficacy and cosmetic acceptability of 'white paste' sunscreens containing zinc oxide or titanium dioxide.

Erythropoietic protoporphyria: IV. Protection from sunlight. Fusaro RM, Runge WJ. Br Med J 1970;1:730–1.

Seven patients had prolonged sunlight tolerance after applying a 3% dihydroxyacetone and 0.13% lawsone skin cream causing brown coloration of stratum corneum.

Most 'sunless tanning' formulations contain dihydroxyacetone and can be used to augment other photoprotectors.

Evidence levels   **A** Double-blind study   **B** Clinical trial ≥ 20 subjects   **C** Clinical trial < 20 subjects   **D** Series ≥ 5 subjects   **E** Anecdotal case reports

Beta-carotene therapy for erythropoietic protoporphyria and other photosensitivity diseases. Mathews-Roth MM, Pathak MA, Fitzpatrick TB, et al. Arch Dermatol 1977;113: 1229–32.

Of 133 patients with protoporphyria, 84% had approximately threefold increased sunlight tolerance after ingesting pharmaceutical grade beta-carotene.

The same efficiently absorbed beta-carotene is available without prescription (Lumitene™, Tischcon). Doses producing serum levels of approximately 800 µg/dL (30–120 mg a day in children, 120–300 mg a day in adults, in two to three doses with meals), should be started 4–6 weeks before seasonal symptoms are anticipated. Efficacy varies, and is nil in some patients. Increased lung cancer among heavy smokers treated with beta-carotene in two cancer prevention clinical trials raises concern about its use in smokers.

SECOND LINE THERAPIES

■ Phototherapy (UVB, PUVA)	D

Narrow-band (TL-01) UVB phototherapy: an effective preventative treatment for the photodermatoses. Collins P, Ferguson J. Br J Dermatol 1995;132:956–63.

Six patients with protoporphyria had increased sunlight tolerance after serial narrowband UVB treatments.

Photo(chemo)therapy and general management of erythropoietic protoporphyria. Roelandts R. Dermatology 1995;190:330–1.

PUVA can increase sun tolerance in protoporphyria; other treatments are reviewed.

THIRD LINE THERAPIES

■ Cysteine	A
■ Antihistamines	D
■ Vitamin E	D
■ Vitamin C	B
■ Pyridoxine	E
■ Flavonoids	E
■ Iron	D
■ Cholestyramine, activated charcoal	D
■ Blood transfusion or exchange	D
■ Hematin infusion	D
■ Plasmapheresis	E
■ Bile acids	D
■ Liver transplantation	C
■ Bone marrow transplantation	E

A double-blind study of cysteine photoprotection in erythropoietic protoporphyria. Mathews-Roth MM, Rosner B, Benfell K, Roberts JE. Photodermatol Photoimmunol Photomed 1994;10:244–8.

This placebo-controlled crossover trial in 16 subjects found that cysteine 500 mg orally twice daily for 8 weeks significantly prolonged time to erythema in UVA and visible light phototesting. Subjective assessment of sunlight tolerance also favored cysteine. Mild to moderate gastrointestinal disturbances occurred in six subjects taking cysteine.

Inhibition of photosensitivity in erythropoietic protoporphyria with terfenadine. Farr PM, Diffey BL, Matthews JNS. Br J Dermatol 1990;122:809–15.

Ingestion of this H1 receptor antagonist 60–120 mg twice daily for 48 h, followed by blue light phototesting, significantly reduced the flare surrounding, but not erythema within, phototest sites of seven subjects, compared with pretreatment reactions.

Antihistamines have not provided much relief in clinical practice.

Cimetidine reduces erythrocyte protoporphyrin in erythropoietic protoporphyria. Yamamoto S, Hirano Y, Horie Y. Am J Gastroenterol 1993;88:1465–6.

This H2 receptor antagonist (800 mg four times daily orally) was given to a patient with protoporphyric liver disease. Erythrocyte protoporphyrin fell from approximately 16 000 to approximately 11 000 µg/dL during treatment. Cimetidine inhibition of heme synthesis was postulated.

Only three porphyrin measurements were obtained: before and immediately after 2 weeks of cimetidine, and approximately 2 weeks after discontinuation. More data are required to establish reproducibility and mechanism.

Possible use of vitamins E and/or C in erythropoietic protoporphyria. Johnson JA, Fusaro RM. JAMA 1973;224: 901–2.

These antioxidants are postulated to quench porphyrin-generated oxyradicals in vivo. Vitamin E has been used sporadically in protoporphyria, usually as an adjunctive therapy, but robust data supporting efficacy are lacking.

A double-blind, placebo-controlled, crossover trial of oral vitamin C in erythropoietic protoporphyria. Boffa MJ, Ead RD, Reed P, Weinkove C. Photodermatol Photoimmunol Photomed 1996;12:27–30.

Vitamin C 1 g daily orally for 4 weeks was subjectively assessed by nine of 12 patients to be associated with less photosensitivity compared to placebo.

Relief of the photosensitivity of erythropoietic protoporphyria by pyridoxine. Ross JB, Moss MA. J Am Acad Dermatol 1990;22:340–2.

Two patients given oral pyridoxine dosages varying from 100 mg a day to 100 mg three times daily to 1 g each morning reported increased sunlight tolerance.

Treatment of erythropoietic protoporphyria with hydroxyethylrutosides. Schoemaker JH, Bousema MT, Zijlstra H, van der Horst FA. Dermatology 1995;191:36–8.

A flavonoid mixture was ingested by a patient for 3 months, during which time phototesting and subjective assessment indicated decreased photosensitivity.

Iron therapy for hepatic dysfunction in erythropoietic protoporphyria. Gordeuk VR, Brittenham GM, Hawkins CW, et al. Ann Intern Med 1986;105:27–31.

Carbonyl iron 400–4000 mg daily by mouth was given for 15 weeks to a patient with protoporphyria, iron deficiency anemia, and early liver dysfunction. Erythrocyte porphyrin fell, photosensitivity improved, and liver function normalized.

In a subsequent report on the same case, ferrous sulfate 300 mg daily by mouth was started when liver function and porphyrin levels worsened again. Liver function again normalized and remained stable for several years (Mercurio MG, Prince G, Weber FL Jr, et al. J Am Acad Dermatol 1993;29:829–33).

Erythropoietic protoporphyria and iron therapy. McClements BM, Bingham A, Callendar ME, Trimble ER. Br J Dermatol 1990;122:423–4.

Oral ferrous fumarate 580 mg a day was followed by florid photosensitivity in a patient previously tolerant of iron supplements. Abnormal liver enzymes improved and erythrocyte protoporphyrin diminished after iron discontinuation.

Iron supplementation in protoporphyria is contentious. Patients have been both better and worse after iron.

Fecal protoporphyrin excretion in erythropoietic protoporphyria: effect of cholestyramine and bile acid feeding. McCullough AJ, Barron D, Mullen KD, et al. Gastroenterology 1988;94:177–81.

Ingesting cholestyramine 12 g a day, but not bile acids 300–900 mg a day, increased fecal protoporphyrin excretion threefold in one patient with hepatic dysfunction. Liver function and photosensitivity improved after 1 year of cholestyramine.

Bile acid ingestion was associated with improved liver function and erythrocyte porphyrin levels in another patient who eventually succumbed to liver failure (Doss MO, Frank M. Clin Biochem 1989;22:223–9). Efficacy remains uncertain, but bile acids in conjunction with an enteric sorbent in selected cases is rational therapy.

Liver failure in protoporphyria: long-term treatment with oral charcoal. Gorchein A, Foster GR. Hepatology 1999;29:995–6.

A patient with rapidly deteriorating hepatic function given activated charcoal 10–12.5 g orally four times a day for 2 years exhibited improved liver function, and blood porphyrin and photosensitivity diminished.

Other treatments included blood transfusions, vitamin supplements, amiloride, ranitidine and lactulose, so it is difficult to assess their relative merits.

Perioperative measures during liver transplantation for erythropoietic protoporphyria. Meerman L, Verwer R, Sloof MJH, et al. Transplantation 1994;57:155–8.

Protocols for exchange transfusion and shielding of operating room lamps during liver transplantation are detailed for two patients.

The value of intravenous heme–albumin and plasmapheresis in reducing postoperative complications of orthotopic liver transplantation for erythropoietic protoporphyria. Reichheld JH, Katz E, Banner BF, et al. Transplantation 1999;67:922–8.

A 3-month course of heme infusions (4 mg daily-to-weekly), a high carbohydrate diet (300 g daily) plus intravenous glucose, ursodeoxycholic acid (900 mg a day orally), and cholestyramine (10 g three times a day orally) initially appeared to improve severe liver dysfunction in a patient with protoporphyria, who then suddenly deteriorated and required urgent transplantation. Intensive heme infusions (daily for 18 days), plasmaphereses (twelve 1–1.5 volume exchanges over 19 days) and blood transfusions (14 units packed cells over 19 days) reduced blood porphyrins prior to successful liver transplantation performed in illumination filtered to exclude 300–480 nm wavelengths.

A barrage of medical therapy is typical in protoporphyric crises, when it is rational to consider any treatments that might reverse deterioration or contribute to successful transplantation, even on chiefly theoretical grounds.

Treatment of recurrent allograft dysfunction with intravenous hematin after liver transplantation for erythropoietic protoporphyria. Dellon ES, Szczepiorkowski ZM, Dzik WH, et al. Transplantation 2002;73:911–5.

Hematin given intermittently for 2 years after protoporphyric hepatopathy recurred 700 days post-transplantation was well-tolerated and aided achievement and maintenance of disease remission in the allograft.

Erythropoietic protoporphyria: altered phenotype after bone marrow transplantation for myelogenous leukemia in a patient heteroallelic for ferrochelatase gene mutations. Poh-Fitzpatrick MB, Wang X, Anderson K, et al. J Am Acad Dermatol 2002;46:861–6.

A symptomatic woman with protoporphyria harboring two ferrochelatase gene mutations developed leukemia. Bone marrow transplantation from a mildly affected sibling with only one mutation and minimally elevated blood porphyrin resulted in a marked reduction of the recipient's protoporphyrin levels and cutaneous photosensitivity, as well as leukemia remission.

Extramammary Paget's disease

Erine A Kupetsky, Robin M Levin

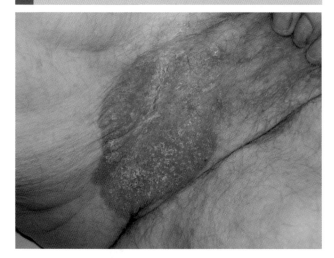

Extramammary Paget's disease (EMPD) is an infiltration of the epidermis with Paget's cells. It occurs in apocrine-bearing areas of the body such as the vulvar, scrotal, penile, perianal, anal, axillary, and umbilical areas and less commonly on the cheek, eyelids, and external auditory canal. EMPD can present as a primary neoplasm or as epidermotropic metastases from an underlying contiguous gastrointestinal or genitourinary malignancy or other internal malignancy (25% of the time). Typically, EMPD presents in Caucasian postmenopausal women and Caucasian middle-aged men with a non-healing erythematous, eczematous, and/or ulcerative macule or patch. Clinically, EMPD may be confused with and treated as eczema, contact dermatitis, or even a fungal or bacterial infection. A lesion on a sun-exposed area can be misdiagnosed as an actinic keratosis or squamous cell carcinoma. Erythema in the involved area in an underpants pattern usually suggests dermal metastases.

MANAGEMENT STRATEGY

Clinical suspicion of EMPD should warrant a biopsy for staining with hematoxylin and eosin (H&E), which will demonstrate the presence of Paget's cells. Immunohistochemical stains are helpful in ruling out other diseases in the histologic differential. Cytokeratin 7 immunostain is a good marker for EMPD, but staining for *ras* oncogene P21 or finding other immunophenotypes such as cytokeratin 7+ or cytokeratin 20 in Paget's cells suggests an underlying regional internal malignancy and can warrant sentinel node biopsy. Paget's cells will also stain positive for carcinoembryonic antigen (CEA), gross cystic disease fluid, epithelial membrane antibody, and with periodic acid–Schiff stain, alcian blue (at pH 2.5), and other mucin stains, such as colloidal iron and mucicarmine.

Typically, EMPD is treated with surgical excision – specifically wide local excision or Mohs micrographic surgery. Extensive disease may warrant more radical treatment such as hemi or total vulvectomy or scrotectomy.

It may be because of the delay in diagnosis of EMPD that extensive areas of epidermis are involved, and often, with wide local excision, margins are positive. Therefore, Mohs surgery is preferred because irregular or clinically unapparent margins can be examined intraoperatively, which reduces the likelihood of positive margins and preserves tissue. Topical 5-fluorouracil (5-FU) preoperatively and topical δ-aminolevulinic acid and Wood's light used 16–18 h preoperatively are useful because they delineate the extent of the margins for Mohs surgery.

Surgical excision can be preceded or followed by radiation or chemotherapy with some success. These adjuvant therapies are rarely successful when used alone.

SPECIFIC INVESTIGATIONS

- Full body skin examination and palpation of all lymph nodes
- Skin biopsy for H&E and immunostains
- Cancer screening – fecal occult blood, urinalysis, Papanicolaou (Pap) smear, prostate-specific antigen (PSA), CEA, colonoscopy, gastroendoscopy
- Radioimaging and/or ultrasound of involved region if needed
- Colposcopy if needed
- Urethrocystoscopy if needed

Extramammary Paget's disease. Wilde JL. *www. emedicine.com* 2002.

An overview of the pathophysiology, morbidity, mortality, and epidemiology of the disease.

FIRST LINE THERAPIES

Wide local excision–lymph node dissection	B
Mohs micrographic surgery	C
Aminolevulinic acid–photodynamic therapy (ALA–PDT)	D

Indications for lymph node dissection in the treatment of EMPD. Tsutsumida A, Yamamoto Y, Minakawa H, et al. Dermatol Surgery 2003;29:21–4.

Prospective study in which 34 patients with genital or perineal EMPD were treated with wide local excision with 2–5 cm normal skin margin, including superficial and deep fascia. Histopathologic or clinical presentations of metastasis led to biopsy and subsequent dissection of lymph nodes. An invasion of EMPD into subcutaneous tissues was correlated with 100% lymph node metastasis and death. The rate of survival for those with invasion to the reticular dermis was 33%. None of those with carcinoma in situ or microinvasion to the papillary dermis had lymph node metastasis and they had a 100% 5-year survival rate.

Penoscrotal EMPD: A review of 33 cases in a 20-year experience. Lai YL, Yang WG, Tsay PK, et al. Plast Reconstr Surg 2003;112:1017–23.

Retrospective review of 33 patients with penoscrotal involvement, of whom 31 were treated with wide local excision. Wide local excision with reconstruction by split-thickness graft was preferred because of its esthetic and functional benefits. Table comparing local recurrence, distant metastasis, and mortality after this surgery.

Prognosis and management of EMPD and the association with secondary malignancies. Pierie JP, Choudry U, Muzikansky A, et al. J Am Coll Surg 2003;196:45–50.

Retrospective study of 33 patients with EMPD treated with different modalities from 1971 to 1998 found that complete local excision and re-excisions, if required, were preferred because of the lower rates of recurrence when compared to hemivulvectomy and radiation therapy.

Comparison of Mohs micrographic surgery and wide local excision for EMPD. O'Connor WJ, Lim KK, Zalla MJ, et al. Dermatol Surg 2003;29:723–7.

Retrospective review of 95 patients treated at the Rochester and Scottsdale Mayo Clinics between 1976 and 2001. Compared to wide local excision, patients treated with Mohs surgery had a lower recurrence rate than patients treated with wide local excision.

Photodynamic therapy for the treatment of extramammary Paget's disease. Shieh S, Dee AS, Cheney RT, et al. Br J Dermatol 2002;146:1000–5.

A retrospective review of five patients at the Roswell Park Cancer Institute between 4/20/95 and 2/1/01 with a total of 16 EMPD lesions treated with 20% topical ALA and then PDT; 11 of 16 lesions had failed Mohs excision or laser prior to PDT. No patient had internal malignancy. This therapy achieved good cosmetic results and after 6 months 50% of the lesions had clinically responded, 19% had partially responded, and 31% had minimally responded.

SECOND LINE THERAPIES

■ Low-dose mitomycin C, etoposide, and cisplatin	D
■ Systemic 5-FU and cisplatin	E
■ Radiation	D

Low-dose mitomycin C, etoposide, and cisplatin for invasive vulvar Paget's disease. Watanabe Y, Hoshiai H, Ueda H, et al. Int J Gynecol Cancer 2002;12:304–7.

A report of three patients with invasive EMPD without underlying carcinoma who declined surgery and were all treated with low-dose mitomycin C, etoposide, and cisplatin. One patient achieved a full clinical response, two partially responded (and underwent surgery); all patients were without recurrence at 10-month follow-up.

Chemotherapy was a good prepartial vulvectomy adjunct that resulted in smaller resection, avoidance of skin grafting, and therefore, better cosmesis.

Trial of low-dose 5-fluorouracil/cisplatin therapy for advanced extramammary Paget's disease. Kariya K, Tsuji T, Schwartz RA. Dermatol Surg 2004;30:341–4.

One patient with EMPD and bone and visceral metastases was treated intravenously for 6 weeks. He had no local recurrences aside from the bone metastases.

Extramammary Paget's disease: outcome of radiotherapy with curative intent. Luk NM, Yu KH, Yeung WK, et al. Clin Dermatol 2003;28:360–3.

In this case series, six patients were studied, two of whom were primarily treated with radiotherapy. The patients were followed for from 1.2 to 14.8 years. Of the two patients treated with radiotherapy, one patient, who had underlying adenocarcinoma, died of metastasis. The other patient, however, was alive with no evidence of disease after 2 years of radiation therapy.

THIRD LINE THERAPIES

■ Androgen receptor antagonist	E
■ Liposomal doxorubicin	E
■ Imiquimod 5% cream	E
■ Topical 5-FU	E
■ Fluorescein preoperatively (with UV light)	E
■ Topical bleomycin	E
■ CO_2 laser, Nd:YAG laser	E

Expression of structurally unaltered androgen receptor in extramammary Paget's disease. Fujimoto A, Takata M, Hatta N, Takehara K. Lab Invest 2000;80:1465–71.

A review of 30 cases of EMPD revealing that 80% of the cases, and four of six lymph node metastases showed unchanged nuclear androgen receptor expression. Because of this, the authors postulated that hormone therapy may be useful or effective, at least in advanced cases of EMPD. For males, use maximum antiandrogen therapy; for females, medroxyprogesterone acetate is suggested.

Liposomal doxorubicin for treatment of metastatic chemorefractory vulvar adenocarcinoma. Huang GS, Juretzka M, Ciaravino G, et al. Gynecol Oncol 2002;87:313–18.

A case report of a 65-year-old patient with metastatic adenocarcinoma and associated EMPD refractory to multiple chemotherapeutic agents, radiation, and radical vulvectomy with lymph node dissection who developed multiple-site metastases and was partially responsive to doxorubicin.

Successful treatment of extramammary Paget's disease of the scrotum with 5% imiquimod cream. Berman B, Spencer J, Villa A, et al. Clin Exp Dermatol 2003;28(suppl 1):36–8.

A case report of a 68-year-old white man whose EMPD lesion was refractory to Mohs surgery 4 years earlier and who was treated with imiquimod 5% cream for 6 weeks. Clearance was achieved by week 4, and at 6 months he remained clinically free of disease.

Extramammary Paget's disease of the scrotum: treatment with topical 5-fluorouracil and plastic surgery. Bewley AP, Bracka A, Staughton RC, Bunker CB. Br J Dermatol 1994;131:445–6.

Topical 5-FU may be used preoperatively to better delineate the lesion, to achieve lesion reduction before surgery, for residual tumor, or for recurrence.

Vulvar Paget disease: fluorescein-aided visualization of margins. Misas JE, Cold CJ, Hall FW. Obstet Gynecol 1991;77:156–9.

Used prior to modified radical vulvectomy, fluorescein showed 99.8% sensitivity and 98% specificity for EMPD cells and guided the successful excision of all neoplastic tissue.

Treatment of recurrent Paget's disease of the vulva with topical bleomycin. Watring WG, Roberts JA, Lagase LD, et al. Cancer 1978;41:10–11.

Four patients with recurrent noninvasive disease had a complete response to bleomycin.

Paget's disease of the vulva treated by combined surgery and laser. Ewing TL. Gynecol Oncol 1991;43:137–40.

There are significant limitations with this technique due to an inability to show histologic clearing and the lack of depth necessary for destruction of adnexal structures. It is therefore only potentially useful for those patients with superficial lesions.

Flushing

Jonathan K Wilkin

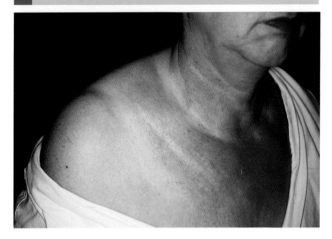

Flushing is a transient reddening of the face and frequently other areas, including the neck, upper chest, pinnae, and epigastric area. Flushing is the visible sign of a generalized increase in cutaneous blood flow despite the limited distribution of the erythema.

MANAGEMENT STRATEGY

The first step in the management of a patient with a flushing disorder is a specific diagnosis because therapy is individualized according to the specific factors causing the flushing, and there is no broad-spectrum antiflushing treatment. The first algorithmic step is to distinguish between autonomic neural-mediated flushing in which eccrine sweating occurs at the time of the flushing ('wet flushing') and direct vasodilator-mediated flushing in which there is no accompanying eccrine sweating ('dry flushing'). The 'dry flushing' reactions are further divided into those with prominent dysesthesia and those without.

Patients with dry flushing and no dysesthesia have circulating vasodilator substances that are either exogenous or endogenous. Exogenous vasodilator agents are almost always elicited from the patient's history. Patient diaries listing all foods, beverages, medications, activities, etc., can not only pinpoint the inciting agent, but also the temporal relationship can be convincing, for both patient and physician. The usual strategy for most vasodilator agents is *simple avoidance of the agent*, although *niacin (nicotinic acid) therapy for hyperlipidemia* and *tamoxifen for breast cancer* are important exceptions for which antiflushing therapies can permit continued treatment with the offending agent.

Finally, endogenous circulating vasodilator agents, typically from underlying neoplasias, are suggested by both multiple stimuli that provoke flushing (rather than one or a few provocative agents) and prominent features associated with the flushing attack. The differential diagnosis is usually generated from the prominent associated feature. Itching or urticaria with flushing suggests circulating mast cell mediators – examples include systemic mastocytosis and mast cell leukemia. Flushing following an attack of hypertension, pallor, tachycardia, palpitations, and sweating suggests pheochromocytoma. Flushing with diarrhea can occur with cholinergic urticaria, cholinergic erythema, anxiety reactions, intolerance to foods, menopausal flushing, the dumping syndrome (a common complication of gastric surgery), diabetes mellitus, pancreatic cholera (watery diarrhea syndrome, Verner-Morrison syndrome), medullary carcinoma of the thyroid, pheochromocytoma, multiple endocrine neoplasia syndromes II and III, mastocytosis, and carcinoid syndrome.

SPECIFIC INVESTIGATIONS

- 5-Hydroxyindoleacetic acid (5-HIAA) urine test
- Histamine urine test
- Serotonin blood/platelet test
- Histamine plasma test

The red face: flushing disorders. Wilkin JK. Clin Dermatol 1993;11:211–23.

The first step in diagnosing a flushing reaction is to determine the mechanism: autonomic neural-mediated flushing, which includes eccrine sweating ('wet flush'), versus flushing from agents that act directly on vascular smooth muscle ('dry flush'). This review describes the three types of blushing, including the type that responds to a low-dose, long-acting nonselective β-blocker, such as nadolol 40 mg every morning. The use of aspirin to block niacin-induced flushing, and amitriptyline to treat facial dysesthesia, is described.

Flushing reactions in the chemotherapy patient. Wilkin JK. Arch Dermatol 1992;128:1387–9.

Chemotherapy causes of flushing are reviewed, along with other drugs that cause flushing.

Flushing reactions. Wilkin JK. In: Rook AJ, Maibach H, eds. Recent advances in dermatology. New York: Churchill Livingstone; 1983:157–87.

This reviews categories of flushing reactions with catalogs of specific causes.

Influence of a serotonin- and dopamine-rich diet on platelet serotonin content and urinary excretion of biogenic amines and their metabolites. Kema IP, Schellings AM, Meiborg G, et al. Clin Chem 1992;38:1730–6.

Serotonin, catecholamines, histamine, and their metabolites in urine, platelets, and tumor tissue of patients with carcinoid tumors. Kema IP, de Vries EG, Slooff MJ, et al. Clin Chem 1994;40:86–95.

The platelet serotonin level by high performance liquid chromatography (HPLC) and gas chromatography/mass spectrometry (GC/MS) has a higher sensitivity for the detection of carcinoid tumors and is more consistently elevated than urinary 5-HIAA. Carcinoid flushing may occur with foregut carcinoids, which can have a low rate of serotonin production. Also, in contrast to urinary 5-HIAA, platelet serotonin is not influenced by the consumption of a serotonin-rich diet.

The quantitative 24-h urinary 5-HIAA level is useful in the follow-up of carcinoid tumors with a high serotonin production rate. It is also useful initially for diagnosis, but only when it is positive during a low-serotonin diet. If the urinary 5-HIAA level is not elevated in a patient with flushing and other features characteristic of carcinoidosis, the platelet or blood serotonin level should be obtained.

Evidence levels A Double-blind study **B** Clinical trial ≥ 20 subjects **C** Clinical trial < 20 subjects **D** Series ≥ 5 subjects **E** Anecdotal case reports

FIRST LINE THERAPIES

■ Ice chips	B
■ Aspirin	B
■ Hormone replacement	A

Oral thermal-induced flushing in erythematotelangiectatic rosacea. Wilkin J. J Invest Dermatol 1981;76:15–8.

It is heat, not caffeine, that causes the flushing from drinking hot coffee.

Sucking on ice chips can abort mild menopausal, thermal, or spicy food-induced flushing.

Aspirin blocks nicotinic acid-induced flushing. Wilkin JK, Wilkin O, Kapp R, et al. Clin Pharmacol Ther 1982;31:478–82.

Not only does aspirin block niacin flushing, but other cyclooxygenase inhibitors (nonsteroidals) also block this prostaglandin-mediated flushing reaction. Importantly, the inhibition of cyclooxygenase does not reduce the lipid-lowering effect of niacin.

Although 1 g of aspirin 1 h before taking the niacin will greatly suppress the flushing reaction, a substantial number of the patients taking niacin are already taking nonsteroidals, mostly for rheumatologic conditions. Generally, all that is needed is to change the time of dosing to 1 h before the niacin, rather than adding a second nonsteroidal drug and risking toxicity.

Aspirin attenuation of alcohol-induced flushing and intoxication in Oriental and Occidental subjects. Truitt EB, Gaynor CR, Mehl DL. Alcohol 1987;1(suppl):595–9.

Eight Oriental and three Occidental subjects sensitive to alcohol manifested as facial flushing were given 0.64 g of aspirin 1 h before vodka in orange juice at levels known to cause flushing. Facial flushing was markedly reduced after aspirin pretreatment.

Combined versus sequential hormonal replacement therapy: a double-blind, placebo-controlled study on quality of life-related outcome measures. Bech P, Munk-Jensen N, Obel EB, et al. Psychother Psychosom 1998;67:259–65.

In a double-blind, placebo-controlled study of 105 early postmenopausal women, hormone replacement therapy was superior to placebo for many symptoms including hot flushing.

SECOND LINE THERAPIES

■ H1 and H2 antihistamines	C
■ Clonidine	A

Scombroid Fish Poisoning – Pennsylvania, 1998. Centers for Disease Control and Prevention. MMWR Morb Mortal Wkly Rep (CDC) 2000;49:398–400.

Four adults in Pennsylvania had facial flushing, nausea, diarrhea, sweating, headache, metallic taste, and burning sensations in the mouth occurring within 5 min to 2 h after eating tuna. Scombroid fish poisoning has been associated primarily with the consumption of tuna, mahi-mahi, and bluefish. Certain bacteria on such fish can grow in warm temperatures and produce enzymes that liberate histamine and other products from precursors in fish flesh.

The association of features of histamine toxicity (flushing, itching, hives, nausea, diarrhea, etc.) and the ingestion of fish should alert the physician to the possibility of scombroid fish poisoning. Both H1 and H2 antihistamines may be sufficient symptomatic therapy, and epinephrine (adrenaline) and systemic corticosteroids considered for more severe cases.

Histamine receptor antagonism of intolerance to alcohol in the Oriental population. Miller NS, Goodwin DW, Jones FC, et al. J Nerv Mental Dis 1987;175:661–7.

Each of 17 subjects received placebo, diphenhydramine 50 mg, and cimetidine 300 mg, singly and in combination, 1 h before ethanol in a soft drink at a level sufficient to produce flushing. Cimetidine given alone blocked the flushing significantly more than diphenhydramine alone or placebo, but less than the combined antihistamines.

The obvious disadvantages are that nonsteroidals can worsen an alcohol-provoked gastritis, and sedating antihistamines can enhance the alcohol-induced drowsiness. Patients should be screened for alcohol abuse using CAGE or a similar instrument and warned about gastritis and sedation before prescribing combination pretreatment consisting of cimetidine, a non-sedating H1 antihistamine, and a nonsteroidal. The author has found that such a combination pretreatment greatly reduces the flushing and headache from red wine in sensitive subjects.

Primary care for survivors of breast cancer. Burstein HJ, Winer EP. N Engl J Med 2000;343:1086–94.

Table 4 on p. 1089 summarizes a variety of nonestrogenic agents used to ameliorate hot flashes. Selective serotonin reuptake inhibitors received the most favorable comments.

Although the focus of this article is on breast cancer survivors, the list of nonestrogenic agents is useful for all women for whom estrogenic agents are contraindicated or not desirable. Clonidine patches are frequently associated with a contact dermatitis, so the author favors oral clonidine.

Menopausal flushing: double-blind trial of a non-hormonal medication. Clayden JR, Bell JW, Pollard P. Br Med J 1974;1:409–12.

Clonidine (Dixarit) for menopausal flushing. Edington RF, Chagon J-P, Steinberg WM. Can Med Assoc J 1980;123:23–6.

A pronounced placebo effect was seen in both trials, with clonidine contributing an additional significant measure of control.

Clonidine reduces the intensity and frequency of menopausal hot flushes, including the sometimes drenching sweat, but it seldom eliminates either the flushing or the eccrine sweating. The author prescribes the 0.1 mg tablet size and asks the patient to crush one tablet each day, taking half the powder in the morning and the other half in the evening. Many patients experience dry mouth or sedation during the first week of therapy, but after a week or two these side effects are no longer a problem for most patients. Patients who do not respond to this 0.05 mg twice-daily regimen only rarely in the author's experience respond to higher doses.

THIRD LINE THERAPIES

■ Somatostatin analogues	E
■ Excision for carcinoid tumors	D

Treatment of type II gastric carcinoid tumors with somatostatin analogues. Tomassetti P, Migliori M, Caletti GC, et al. N Engl J Med 2000;343:551–4.

This is a report of three patients with multiple type II gastric carcinoids treated with lanreotide or octreotide acetate. In all three patients there was a reduction in size and number of the carcinoid tumors after 6 months of somatostatin analogue treatment and complete disappearance of tumors after 1 year. A report of regression of a type III gastric carcinoid with octreotide is also cited.

Although all three types of gastric carcinoid tumors are usually removed surgically, somatostatin analogues, especially the longer-acting octreotide acetate (20 mg intramuscularly every 28 days), provide a successful medical option.

Evidence levels A Double-blind study B Clinical trial ≥ 20 subjects C Clinical trial < 20 subjects D Series ≥ 5 subjects E Anecdotal case reports

Follicular mucinosis

Bav Shergill, Malcolm Rustin

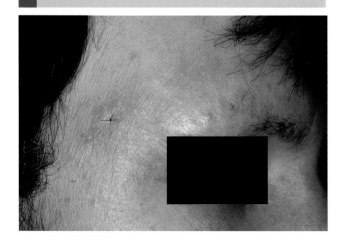

Follicular mucinosis is characterized histologically by mucinous degeneration of the follicular outer root sheaths and sebaceous glands with an inflammatory infiltrate composed of lymphocytes, histiocytes, and eosinophils. Lesions consist of erythematous, scaly and infiltrated plaques with follicular papules or prominent follicular orifices, and may demonstrate alopecia (alopecia mucinosa). Benign follicular mucinosis tends to affect younger patients (under 40 years of age), with a small number of lesions, usually situated on the head and neck. Although lesions may resolve spontaneously within 2 years, a more generalized benign form, with lesions on the trunk and extremities, may run a chronic relapsing course over many years. Follicular mucinosis is associated with lymphoma, particularly mycosis fungoides, in 15–30% of cases. It is still unclear whether follicular mucinosis is a transitional state evolving into mycosis fungoides in these cases. No single clinical or histological feature predicts which patients will have a benign course, although patients found to have mycosis fungoides rarely had initial lesions on the head and neck. Associated lymphoma tends (although not invariably) to be associated with age over 30 years, a wider distribution of lesions, and possibly systemic features such as night sweats, weight loss or lymphadenopathy.

MANAGEMENT STRATEGY

There is no standard therapy for follicular mucinosis. Because spontaneous resolution occurs in the benign forms, *observation* alone is certainly justified, particularly in the younger patient with limited disease. However, the need for *follow-up and evaluation to exclude lymphoma* must be emphasized. Follicular mucinosis associated with mycosis fungoides or other neoplastic or inflammatory disorders is managed by treating the underlying associated condition.

SPECIFIC INVESTIGATIONS

- Skin biopsy
- Immunohistochemistry and T cell gene receptor analysis may be helpful adjuncts to skin biopsy
- Consider investigations to rule out lymphoma or other underlying disorders dependent on the presenting clinical features (general examination, plain radiology, and CT scans)

The cutaneous mucinoses. Truhan AP, Roenigk HH. J Am Acad Dermatol 1986;14:1–18.

Follicular mucinosis: a critical reappraisal of clinico-pathologic features and association with mycosis fungoides and Sézary syndrome. Cerroni L, Fink-Puches R, Bäck B, Helmut K. Arch Dermatol 2002;138:182–9.

Two excellent reviews of the follicular mucinosis literature, including histopathology and investigation.

FIRST LINE THERAPIES

■ Topical and intralesional corticosteroids	D
■ Dapsone	E
■ Mepacrine	E
■ Tetracycline	E

Follicular mucinosis: a study of 47 patients. Emmerson RW. Br J Dermatol 1969;81:395–413.

Topical or intralesional corticosteroids improved surface eczematous change in eight of 22 patients with benign disease whose lesions resolved spontaneously within 2 years. Deeper follicular and dermal changes were not affected. Resolution was considered to have occurred independently of treatment. Six of ten patients with benign chronic disease of more than 2 years' duration showed slight improvement with topical or intralesional corticosteroids.

Alopecia mucinosa: a follow-up study. Coskey RJ, Mehregan AH. Arch Dermatol 1970;102:193–4.

Topical or intralesional corticosteroids were applied to seven patients with one or two facial lesions. All lesions resolved, as did lesions in two untreated patients. In patients with more than two lesions, including extremity lesions, nine of 15 patients given topical corticosteroids had complete clearance of their lesions.

Urticaria-like follicular mucinosis responding to dapsone. Al Harthi F, Kudwah, A, Ajlan A, Nuaim A, Shehri F. Acta Derm Venereol 2003;83:389–90.

Itchy urticaria-like papules on the face, chest, and back of a 25-year-old man for 2 years responded to dapsone 100 mg daily long term after previously failing to respond to oral prednisolone. Attempts to drop the dosage resulted in recurrence.

Follicular mucinosis presenting as acute dermatitis and response to dapsone. Rustin MHA, Bunker C, Levene GM. Clin Exp Dermatol 1989;14:382–4.

Facial follicular mucinosis clinically resembling acute extensive dermatitis in a 34-year-old man rapidly responded to dapsone 100 mg daily and topical clobetasol propionate; 6 months of maintenance therapy was required.

Atypical follicular mucinosis controlled with mepacrine. Sonnex TS, Ryan T, Dawber RPR. Br J Dermatol 1981;105 (suppl 19):83–4.

Facial lesions in a 39-year-old man responded to mepacrine 100 mg twice daily. Lesions redeveloped on cessation of therapy.

A case of follicular mucinosis treated successfully with minocycline. Yotsumoto S, Uchimiya H, Kanzaki T. Br J Dermatol 2000;142:841–2.

A 36-year-old man presented with itchy papular lesions on his head, nape, and chest. After histological confirmation of the diagnosis, indomethacin was tried (no time specified), but was not effective. Minocycline 100 mg daily for 6 weeks induced complete remission.

Follicular mucinosis presenting as an acneiform eruption: report of four cases. Wittenberg GP, Gibson LE, Pittelkow MR, el-Azhary RA. J Am Acad Dermatol 1988;38:849–51.

Facial acneiform lesions in a 21-year-old woman responded well to tetracycline (dose not recorded) and benzoyl peroxide gel. There was a minor improvement in the facial papules of a 31-year-old man with minocycline 100 mg daily for 4 months.

SECOND LINE THERAPIES

■ Isotretinoin	E
■ Psoralen and UVA (PUVA)	E
■ UVA1	E
■ Indomethacin	E
■ Interferon (IFN)	E
■ Superficial radiotherapy	D
■ Systemic corticosteroids	E

Follicular mucinosis successfully treated with isotretinoin. Guerriero C, De Simone C, Guidi B, et al. Eur J Dermatol 1999;9:22–4.

A 33-year-old man with facial lesions and no systemic disease was treated with isotretinoin 0.5 mg/kg daily. After 2 months remission was achieved, with tapering of the dose of isotretinoin after a further 3 weeks.

Follicular mucinosis presenting as an acneiform eruption: report of four cases. Wittenberg GP, Gibson LE, Pittelkow MR, el-Azhary RA. J Am Acad Dermatol 1998;38:849–51.

Two women under 40 years of age had acneiform facial lesions. One had decreased numbers and size of lesions following tretinoin gel 0.01% daily and oral pentoxifylline 400 mg three times daily, followed 2 years later by isotretinoin 40 mg daily. The second significantly improved following isotretinoin 40 mg daily and intermittent clobetasol cream.

Follicular mucinosis treated with PUVA. Kenicer KJA, Lakshmipathi T. Br J Dermatol 1982;107 Suppl 22:48–9.

A 79-year-old woman with facial, truncal, and limb papules with no evidence of systemic disease failed to respond to topical corticosteroids and localized radiother-

apy (1000 rad over 5 days). After a total of 98 treatments of PUVA over five months, with total exposure dose 454 J/cm^2, she remained disease free.

Treatment of idiopathic mucinosis follicularis with UVA1 cold light phototherapy. Von Kobyletzki G, Kreuter JA, Nordmeier R, et al. Dermatology 2000;201:76–7

A 26-year-old Caucasian woman with itchy follicular papules on the trunk for 7 months was diagnosed histologically and started on potent corticosteroids with no success. A UVA1 cold light source (340–530 nm) was used five times a week for 3 weeks and induced remission that had been sustained at 3 months.

Follicular mucinosis: response to indomethacin. Kodama H, Umemura S, Nohara N. J Dermatol 1988; 15:72–5.

Plaques and papules on the face and back of a 48-year-old man with no signs of cutaneous lymphoma were unresponsive to topical corticosteroids, UVA or dapsone. Indomethacin 1% in white petrolatum was applied topically until the lesions disappeared. Oral indomethacin 75 mg daily reduced untreated lesions, but was not tolerated. The patient was lesion-free at 5-year follow-up.

Successful treatment of primary progressive follicular mucinosis with interferons. Meissner K, Weyer U, Kowalzick L, Altenhoff J. J Am Acad Dermatol 1991;24:848–50.

A 37-year-old man had a 5-year history of facial, truncal, and upper extremity lesions with alopecia, and no evidence of systemic disease. Isotretinoin, dapsone, and systemic corticosteroids were unhelpful. Increasing doses of recombinant IFN-α-2b up to 9 million IU/m^2 were administered subcutaneously three times weekly, with recombinant IFN-γ 100 μg subcutaneously daily each fourth week. For 4 months, 5 million IU of IFN-α-2b was injected intralesionally into the chin lesion three times weekly. Slight relapse led to increasing the dosage of IFN-α to 10 million IU/m^2. Complete remission was achieved by week 46. The treatment was well tolerated.

Follicular mucinosis: a study of 47 patients. Emmerson RW. Br J Dermatol 1969;81:395–413.

Two patients with benign disease lasting more than 2 years were treated with X-rays 400 rad and had complete resolution. Two patients with benign chronic disease treated with X-rays (dose not recorded) had no benefit.

Acneiform follicular mucinosis. Passaro EMC, Silveira MT, Valente NYS. Clin Exp Derm 2004;29:396–8.

A 36-year-old man presented with a 1 year history of acneiform follicular mucinosis was commenced on 40 mg of prednisolone for 20 days. His symptoms improved quickly and the prednisolone was weaned off by day 48. He was clear for 7 months at time of writing.

Alopecia mucinosa: a follow-up study. Coskey RJ, Mehregan AH. Arch Dermatol 1970;102:193–4.

Patients with one or two facial lesions were given superficial X-ray therapy in a weekly dose of 75 rad for four weeks (three cases) or a combination of X-ray therapy and topical corticosteroid cream (six cases). In all cases lesions resolved.

Evidence levels A Double-blind study B Clinical trial ≥ 20 subjects C Clinical trial < 20 subjects D Series ≥ 5 subjects E Anecdotal case reports

Folliculitis

Beverley Adriaans

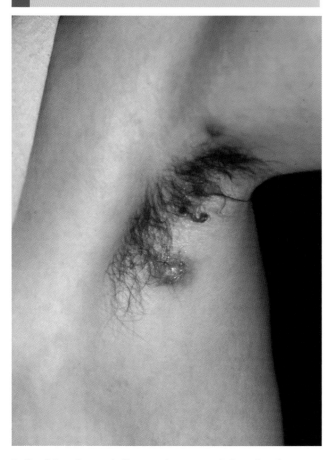

Folliculitis refers to inflammation around the pilosebaceous unit. Inflammation may result from infections with Gram-positive bacteria (usually *Staphylococcus aureus*), Gram-negative bacteria, yeasts (*Pityrosporum* and *Candida* spp.), viruses, parasites (*Demodex* spp.) and fungi. Immuno-compromised patients, particularly those with HIV infection, develop a variety of follicular inflammatory lesions caused by bacteria and viruses, and a characteristic sterile eosinophilic folliculitis. Pregnancy and drugs (e.g. corticos-teroids) may also be associated with folliculitis. Patients taking retinoids are susceptible to staphylococcal folliculitis. Patients with atopic eczema frequently develop infective follicular lesions from which *S. aureus* is isolated. Gram-negative folliculitis follows long-term antibiotic therapy for acne. The superficial follicular lesions on the face are usually associated with coliforms, which may also be isolated from the nose. Cultures from deeper cysts often grow *Escherichia coli* or *Proteus*, *Klebsiella* or *Enterobacter* spp. Jacuzzi bathers may develop a widespread folliculitis due to *Pseudomonas aeruginosa*. Folliculitis barbae, though usually staphylococcal, may also be caused by *Candida albicans*. Pityrosporum folliculitis, a widespread follicular eruption on the trunk and back, is caused by *Pityrosporum* yeasts. Although the disease is more common in hot, humid countries, it may occur worldwide and is found in normal and immunocompromised patients. Viral folliculitis may occur with molluscum contagiosum and herpes simplex viruses, even in immuno-competent individuals, although extensive folliculitis caused by these viruses is more common in the immunosuppressed host.

The noninfectious forms of folliculitis may be associated with sun exposure (superficial actinic folliculitis), occupational contact with oils or tars, epilation (traumatic folliculitis), or systemic diseases. The latter include Behçet's disease, renal disease (perforating folliculitis/Kyrle's disease), Reiter's syndrome, inflammatory bowel disease, connective tissue disease including mixed connective tissue disease and rheumatoid arthritis, and blood dyscrasias.

Folliculitis decalvans is a chronic progressive scalp folli-culitis from which staphylococci are frequently isolated. It causes scarring and subsequent hair loss (see Folliculitis decalvans, page 174).

MANAGEMENT STRATEGY

Folliculitis associated with trauma or occupation (e.g. epilation, tar, or oils) may improve if the precipitants are removed.

For the infective forms of folliculitis, treatment should aim at eradicating the infection, preventing recurrent disease, particularly by eradicating nasal carriage if colo-nized by staphylococci, and modifying any of the underly-ing predisposing factors if possible. The treatments include *topical antibiotics or antiseptics*, *systemic antibiotics* or a com-bination of these. Although little evidence-based informa-tion is available on these treatments, clinical evidence supports the use of topical antibiotics and antiseptics for localized infections. Widespread or extensive infections should be treated with oral antibiotics.

Corticosteroid-induced folliculitis usually settles when these agents are stopped, although this may take several weeks.

SPECIFIC INVESTIGATIONS

- Lesional swabs for culture and sensitivity (moistened in agar or sterile water) from pustules
- Nasal swabs from those with recurrent infections
- Skin scrapings from pustules for Gram stain and mycology
- In those suspected of being immunocompromised – complete blood count, glucose, renal function, immunoglobulin levels, HIV status
- Patients with follicular lesions associated with underlying systemic disease – complete blood count, autoimmune profile

Staphylococci. Aly R. In: Lesher JL, ed. An Atlas of Micro-biology of the Skin. New York: Parthenon Publishing Group; 2000:15–9.

FIRST LINE THERAPIES

Topical therapy	
■ Povidone-iodine, acetic acid or gentamicin for *Pseudomonas aeruginosa*	A
■ Fusidic acid or mupirocin for *Staphylococcus aureus*	A
■ Topical corticosteroid for eosinophilic pustular folliculitis	C
■ Permethrin cream for *Demodex* spp.	D
Oral therapy	
■ Flucloxacillin or fusidic acid for *Staphylococcus* spp.	A
■ Itraconazole for *Pityrosporum* spp.	C
■ Dapsone for eosinophilic pustular folliculitis	C
■ Phototherapy for eosinophilic pustular folliculitis	C

Topical therapy

Optimum outpatient therapy of skin and skin structure infections. Failla DM, Pankey GA. Drugs 1994;49:172–8.

Most cases of pseudomonal folliculitis require no treatment. If the infection is widespread, however, topical povidone-iodine, 1% acetic acid soaks, or gentamicin cream are useful.

A comparison of sodium fusidate ointment and mupirocin ointment in superficial skin sepsis. Morley PAR, Munot LD. Curr Med Res Opin 1988;11:142–8.

These antibiotics were equally effective in 354 patients.

Eosinophilic pustular folliculitis. A comprehensive review of treatment options. Ellis E, Scheinfield N. Am J Clin Dermatol 2004;5:189–97.

There are no controlled trials for any of the treatment options for this condition. This review covers all the treatments reported recently.

The clinical importance of demodex folliculorum presenting with non specific facial signs and symptoms. Karincaoglu Y, Bayram N, Aycan O, Esrefoglu M. J Dermatol 2004;31:518–26.

5% permethrin cream was helpful.

Systemic therapy

A comparison of fusidic acid and flucloxacillin in the treatment of skin and soft-tissue infections. Eur J Clin Res 1994;5:97–106.

Flucloxacillin 500 mg three times daily and 500 mg fusidic acid over 5–10 days resulted in an equal improvement in these infections.

Fusidic acid tablets in patients with skin and soft-tissue infection: a dose-finding study. Carr WD, Wall AR, Georgala-Zervogiani S, et al. Eur J Clin Res 1994;5:87–95.

Fusidic acid 500 mg daily was approximately as effective as 1.5 g daily.

Skin diseases associated with *Malassezia* species. Gupta AK, Batra R, Bluhm R et al. J Am Acad Dermatol 2004;51:785–98.

Oral itraconazole is effective for extensive pityrosporum folliculitis.

SECOND LINE THERAPIES

Oral antibiotics	
■ Clindamycin or azithromycin for *Staphylococcus* spp.	A
■ Systemic ketoconazole for *Pityrosporum* spp.	D

Comparison of two regimens of oral clindamycin versus dicloxacillin in the treatment of mild to moderate skin and soft tissue infections. Blaszczyk-Kostanecka M, Dobozy A, Dominguez-Soto L, et al. Curr Ther Res Clin Exp 1998;59: 341–53.

In this prospective, randomized study, clindamycin 150 mg four times a day, clindamycin 300 mg twice daily, and dicloxacillin 250 mg four times a day for 7–14 days were compared in patients with skin infections including folliculitis. There was no difference in the healing or the relapse rates. Patients were followed for up to 3 weeks after completing treatment.

A comparative study of the efficacy, safety and tolerance of azithromycin, dicloxacillin and flucloxacillin in the treatment of children with acute skin and skin structure infections. Rodrigues-Solares A, Pérez-Gutiérrez F, Prosperi J, et al. J Antimicrob Chemother 1993;31(suppl E): 103–9.

This was an open, randomized study to compare a 3-day regimen of azithromycin with a 7-day course of dicloxacillin and flucloxacillin in the treatment of acute skin infections in children. Bacteriological cure was similar with all treatment regimens.

Evidence levels A Double-blind study **B** Clinical trial ≥ 20 subjects **C** Clinical trial < 20 subjects **D** Series ≥ 5 subjects **E** Anecdotal case reports

Fox–Fordyce disease

Ian Coulson

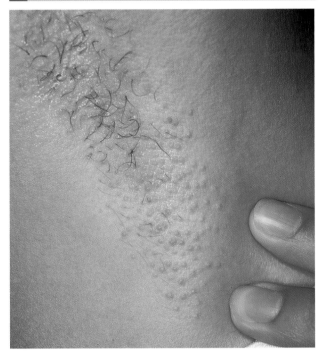

Obliteration of the follicular infundibulum with keratin in the apocrine gland bearing skin is the cause of this rare, paroxysmally intensely itchy condition. Apocrine sweat retention and rupture of the gland duct under periods of apocrine sudomotor stimulation, particularly emotional stress, results in the development of an itchy spongiotic intraepidermal vesicle. Itchy, domed, flesh-colored or keratotic papules developing peripubertally in the apocrine areas of the axillae and pubic and periareolar skin characterize this condition, which predominates in women. Sparsity of axillary hair is usual. Improvement in pregnancy and during the administration of the oral contraceptive pill has led to speculation of an endocrine etiology, but this has been unsubstantiated by blood sex hormone investigations. It has been reported in Turner's syndrome.

MANAGEMENT STRATEGY

There are no controlled trials of any agents in Fox–Fordyce disease.

Topical and intralesional corticosteroids are frequently tried and may be of limited benefit, but atrophy in the axillary area will limit the potency and duration of use. Topical *tretinoin* has been reported to reduce itch, but its alternation with a mild corticosteroid may be needed to reduce retinoid irritancy. *Clindamycin* lotion may be of help. The *oral contraceptive pill (OCP)* may bring relief to some women. Oral *isotretinoin* may give temporary help. *Electrocautery* and *excision* of the periareolar skin may offer permanent solutions. A recent report advocates an ingenious method of removal of the apocrine glands using a microliposuction cannula.

SPECIFIC INVESTIGATIONS

> ■ Biopsy

Fox–Fordyce disease: diagnosis by transverse histologic sections. Stashower ME, Krivda SJ, Turiansky GW. J Am Acad Dermatol 2000;42:89–91.

Transverse sectioning demonstrates the follicular plugging and infundibular spongiosis more readily than conventional sections.

Axillary perifollicular xanthomatosis resembling Fox–Fordyce disease. Kossard S, Dwyer P. Australas J Dermatol 2004;45:146–8.

There are occasional conditions to consider in the differential diagnosis!

FIRST LINE THERAPIES

■ Topical and intralesional corticosteroids	D
■ Topical clindamycin	E
■ Oral contraceptive pill	D
■ Topical retinoids	D
■ UVB	D

The treatment of Fox–Fordyce disease. Shelley WB. JAMA 1972;222:1069.

A concise review of the therapies available to that date. The author admits that sometimes all fails and relief may only come at the menopause.

A new treatment of Fox–Fordyce disease. Helfamn RJ. South Med J 1962;55:681–4.

A single report of successful symptom relief of axillary lesions with 10 mg/mL triamcinolone diluted with an equal volume of 1% lidocaine to four sites on nine occasions over 3 months.

Fox-Fordyce disease. Control with tretinoin cream. Giacobetti R, Caro WA, Roenigk HH Jr. Arch Dermatol 1979;115:1365–6.

A single report of 0.1% tretinoin cream applied to the axillae on alternate nights resulting in reduction of itch and regrowth of hair. Local retinoid irritation was controlled with 1% hydrocortisone cream.

Fox-Fordyce disease – successful treatment with topical clindamycin in alcoholic propylene glycol solution. Feldmann R, Masouye I, Chavaz P, Saurat JH. Dermatology 1992;184:310–3.

A single report of axillary, pubic, and inguinal area Fox–Fordyce disease responding to 1% clindamycin in an alcoholic propylene glycol solution within 1 month (clindamycin 10 mg/mL; propylene glycol 50 mg/mL; isopropyl alcohol 0.5 mg/mL; water). Nine months later, the treatment was stopped and no recurrence was observed. The authors speculate that the keratolytic effect of propylene glycol may have been responsible for the therapeutic effect.

Fox–Fordyce disease. Treatment with an oral contraceptive. Kronthal HI, Pomeranz JR, Sitomer G. Arch Dermatol 1965;91:243–5.

Two female patients responded to a high estrogen dose combined OCP, norethynodrel and mestranol.

Treatment of Fox–Fordyce disease. Pinkus H. JAMA 1973;223:924.

Erythemogenic doses of UVB (once weekly for 4–6 weeks) produced longlasting relief to several patients.

SECOND LINE THERAPIES

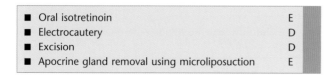

■ Oral isotretinoin	E
■ Electrocautery	D
■ Excision	D
■ Apocrine gland removal using microliposuction	E

Fox-Fordyce disease in a male patient – response to oral retinoid treatment. Effendy I, Ossowski B, Happle R. Clin Exp Dermatol 1994;19:67–9.

Oral treatment with isotretinoin (30 mg daily for 8 weeks then 15 mg daily for 2 months) resulted in temporary relief. Relapse occurred 3 months after discontinuation.

Fox–Fordyce disease in the post-menopausal period treated successfully with electrocoagulation. Pasricha JS, Nayyar KC. Dermatologica 1973;147:271–3.

Electrocoagulation to a level of 3–4 mm under local anesthetic produced a permanent resolution of symptoms in the axillae of two patients.

Surgical treatment of areolar hidradenitis suppurativa and Fox–Fordyce disease. Chavoin J-P, Charasson T, Barnard J-D. Ann Chir Plast Esthet 1994;39:233–8.

A simple technique involving dermal detachment of the areola, excision of the underlying apocrine glands, and reattachment of the areola with good cosmetic results.

This treatment has not proven beneficial long term.

Axillary Fox–Fordyce disease treated with liposuction-assisted curettage. Chae KM, Marschall MA, Marschall SF. Arch Dermatol 2002;138:452–4.

A novel technique of curettage removal of the apocrine glands using a small liposuction cannula with symptom relief, great cosmesis, and a follow-up at publication of 8 months. A liposuction cannula was introduced through a stab incision in the axilla and, with the aperture of the cannula turned up toward the underside of the dermis, the deeper dermis was curetted to create inflammation and subsequent fibrosis. The same technique can be used to treat axillary hyperhidrosis.

Evidence levels A Double-blind study   **B** Clinical trial ≥ 20 subjects   **C** Clinical trial < 20 subjects   **D** Series ≥ 5 subjects   **E** Anecdotal case reports

Furunculosis

Beverley Adriaans

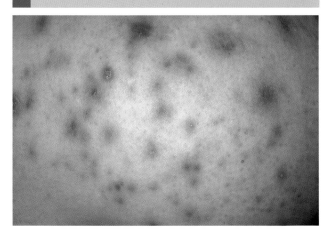

Furunculosis, the term used to describe what are commonly known as 'boils', is a deep infection of the hair follicle apparatus. Lesions can occur on any hairbearing area, including the nares. The infection, caused by *Staphylococcus aureus*, usually involves the subcutaneous tissues as well as the dermis. Multiple hair follicles may be involved, resulting in a carbuncle. These large suppurative lesions may be very painful and have multiple draining sites. The head and neck area are commonly involved. Although patients may have recurrent disease the majority show no immunological defects. Most are nasal carriers of *Staph. aureus*. The organism may also be carried in other hairbearing areas. Increasingly, community acquired methicillin-resistant *Staph. aureus* (MRSA) infections have been reported. Rarely myiasis may present with furunculosis.

MANAGEMENT STRATEGY

Isolated lesions should be *incised and drained*, and oral *antistaphylococcal* antibiotics should be reserved for those with numerous lesions, substantial surrounding cellulitis, or fever. Nasal carriage of staphylococci should be sought in those with recurrent disease and eradicated with either *nasal fusidic acid* or *mupirocin*. Unresponsive recurrent disease may be controlled by either *low-dose clindamycin* or a *fluoroquinolone* antibiotic such as *ciprofloxacin*.

Predisposing factors should be eliminated if possible.

Common bacterial skin infections. Stulberg DL, Penrod MA, Blatny RA. Am Fam Physician 2002;67:254.

An overview of skin infections including furunculosis.

Community-onset methicillin-resistant *Staphylococcus aureus* associated with antibiotic use and the cytotoxin Panton-Valentine leukocidin during a furunculosis outbreak in rural Alaska. Baggett HC, Hennessy TW, Rudolph K, et al. J Infect Dis 2004;189:1565–73.

Community-onset MRSA reports are increasing, and infections often involve soft tissue. This article considers that selective antibiotic pressure for drug-resistant strains may be at play.

SPECIFIC INVESTIGATIONS

- Culture and sensitivity of pus
- Nasal swab (moistened)
- Neutrophil count

Skin and skin structure infections in the patient at risk: carrier state of *Staphylococcus aureus*. Tauzon CU. Am J Med 1984;76:166–71.

Carriage of staphylococci in the nares may predispose to outbreaks of infection in nurseries and in postoperative patients, and may lead to more severe infections in the immunocompromised host. Factors predisposing to carriage are varied and carriage rates are greater in patients with renal failure, diabetes mellitus, and drug abusers. *Staphylococcus aureus* may be carried in the nose, throat, umbilicus, groin, rectum, and other body sites.

Recurrent staphylococcal furunculosis: bacteriology and epidemiology in 100 cases. Hedstrom SA. Scand J Infect Dis 1981;13:115–9.

Occasionally patients with Job's syndrome and cyclic neutropenia develop recurrent furunculosis. A white cell count should be estimated. Alcoholics, diabetics, and drug abusers may be predisposed to recurrent furunculosis.

Furunculosis and IgG subclass deficiency. Mahe E, Girszin N, Descamps V, Crickx B. Dermatology 2004; 209:189–197.

Immunodeficiency may present with furunculosis. Immunoglobulin levels may be helpful.

FIRST LINE THERAPIES

■ Surgery – incision and drainage	C
■ Eradication of nasal carriage of staphylococci	B
■ Topical antibiotics – fusidic acid	A
■ Systemic antibiotics	
■ Flucloxacillin	C
■ Low-dose clindamycin	B

Treatment and prevention of recurrent staphylococcal furunculosis: clinical and bacteriological follow-up. Hedstrom SA. Scan J Infect Dis 1985;17:55–8.

Sodium fusidate ointment was used as a prophylactic agent to prevent nasal furunculosis. Patients used the ointment twice daily for a month, with cessation of furuncles in ten of 20 patients. Controls took antibiotics systemically, and three of 20 had no furuncles. After a year, those who used topical therapy had fewer recurrent lesions than those who had taken systemic therapy.

Comparison of two regimens of oral clindamycin versus dicloxacillin in the treatment of mild to moderate skin and soft tissue infections. Blaszcyk-Kostanecka M, Dobozy A, Dominguez-Soto L, et al. Curr Ther Res Clin Exp 1998;59: 341–53.

A prospective, double-blind, randomized study carried out in 14 countries throughout Asia. The study included a number of infections including furuncles (which were not incised and drained). Treatment varied between 7 and 14 days, with no difference found between the three regimens (clindamycin 150 mg four times daily, clindamycin 300 mg twice daily, or dicloxacillin 250 mg four times daily). Flucloxacillin will be the dicloxacillin equivalent in the UK.

SECOND LINE THERAPIES

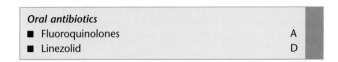

Oral antibiotics
■ Fluoroquinolones — A
■ Linezolid — D

A multicenter, double blind, double placebo comparative study of grepafloxacin versus ofloxacin in the treatment of skin and skin structure infections. Arata J, Matsuura Y, Umemura S, et al. Japanese J of Chemother 1997;45:506–24.

Two fluoroquinolones were compared for efficacy. There were no significant differences in the improvement rates or in the side effect profiles of the drugs. Patients were treated for 7 days and evaluated by day 7. Relapse rates (not mentioned) would have been helpful.

Treatment of bacterial skin and skin structure infections. Guay DR. Expert Opin Pharmacother 2003;4:1259–75.

Although most skin infections are still treated with β-lactams, macrolides, and lincosamides (clindamycin), antimicrobial resistance may lead to treatment failures. Some of the newer agents such as linezolid, quinupristin/dalfopristin and moxifloxacin are discussed. At present these are not used often.

THIRD LINE THERAPIES

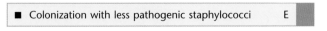

■ Colonization with less pathogenic staphylococci — E

Recurrent staphylococcal infection in families. Steele R. Arch Dermatol 1980;116:189–90.

A different, less pathogenic strain of *Staph. aureus* was inoculated into the nose of family members to try to prevent spread of staphylococci among the family in an attempt to minimize recurrent infections. Patients and their family members also took oral antibiotics prior to inoculation.

Geographic tongue

Alison J Bruce, Roy S Rogers III

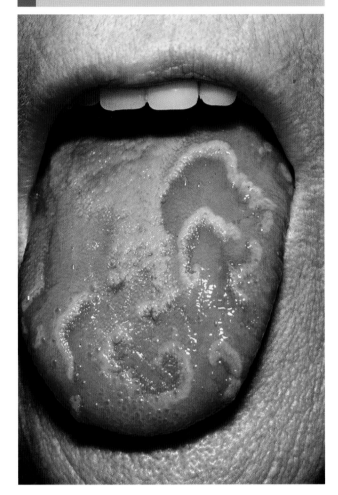

Geographic tongue is a reactive mucosal inflammatory condition characterized by arcuate or annular alternating hypertrophic or atrophic filiform papillae producing a geographic pattern. It may be an asymptomatic incidental finding. Some patients complain of a sore, burning sensation, particularly in atrophic areas of the tongue. Similar changes may occur in oral sites other than the tongue (geographic stomatitis).

MANAGEMENT STRATEGY

Geographic tongue is a common glossitis affecting 2% of the population. There is no racial predilection, and the condition may be seen in patients of all ages, but more often in children than adults. Because geographic tongue is usually asymptomatic, no treatment is necessary other than reassurance that the nature of the condition is benign, reactive, and self-limiting, and that it is not a sign of systemic illness. Geographic tongue often will remit spontaneously, but may persist for years. Occasional patients may be symptomatic, complaining of a burning discomfort. Effective therapy can be challenging.

The changes of geographic tongue may occur in patients with psoriasis vulgaris, pustular psoriasis, Reiter's disease,

pityriasis rubra pilaris, or the atopic diathesis. The clinician should also consider acute or chronic atrophic candidiasis.

For those patients whose geographic tongue is symptomatic, measures that may be considered include *avoidance of hot, spicy, or acidic foods; gentle brushing of the tongue; avoidance of harsh antibacterial mouthwashes, chewing gum, and breath mints; and soothing rinses with saline solutions.* Occasionally, the topical application of *fluorinated corticosteroid* or *elixir of diphenhydramine* 12.5–25.0 mg/5 mL after meals and at bedtime may be recommended. *Topical anesthetic rinses or gels* provide temporary relief. *Anti-yeast treatments* may be palliative.

SPECIFIC INVESTIGATIONS

- Culture for candidiasis
- Medical evaluation as for burning mouth syndrome

Geographic stomatitis: a critical review. Hume WJ. J Dent 1975;3:25–43.

The topic and the differential diagnosis are reviewed carefully.

Culture of the tongue for yeast organisms may help direct therapy. Some patients require reassurance that they do not have a systemic illness. A laboratory evaluation along the lines discussed for burning mouth syndrome would be reasonable to exclude systemic causes.

FIRST LINE THERAPIES

■ Avoidance of spicy food, mouthwashes, chewing gum, and breath mints	D
■ Topical fluorinated corticosteroids such as 0.05% fluocinonide gel	C
■ Topical antihistamines	C
■ Anti-yeast therapy	E

Symptomatic benign migratory glossitis: report of two cases and literature review. Sigal MJ, Mock D. Pediatr Dent 1992;14:392–6.

Management with topical corticosteroids and topical antihistamines is discussed.

Glossitis and other tongue disorders. Byrd JA, Bruce AJ, Rogers RS III. Dermatol Clin 2003;21:123–34.

Review of geographic and other tongue disorders.

Oral psoriasis. Bruce AJ, Rogers RS III. Dermatol Clin 2003;21:99–104.

The concept of the geographic tongue as the mucosal equivalent of psoriasis is discussed.

Painful geographic tongue (benign migratory glossitis) in a child. (Letter) Menni S, Boccardi D, Crosti C. J Eur Acad Dermatol Venereol 2004;18:737–8.

SECOND LINE THERAPIES

■ Topical anesthetics	C
■ Topical tretinoin	E
■ Discontinue dentifrices and other oral flavoring agents	D
■ Topical tacrolimus	E

Glossodynia and other disorders of the tongue. Powell FC. Dermatol Clin 1987;5:687–93.

Despite concerns, tretinoin may be used on mucosal surfaces in a judicious manner.

The treatment of geographic tongue with topical Retin-A solution. Helfman RJ. Cutis 1979;24:179–80.

The use of topical Retin-A solution is described in three cases.

Anecdotally we have used tacrolimus 0.1% ointment for symptomatic geographic tongue with occasional improvement.

THIRD LINE THERAPIES

■ 5% carbol fuchsin paint	E
■ 0.5% gentian violet paint	E

Disorders of the oral cavity and lips. Pindborg JJ. In: Rook A, Wilkinson DS, Elbing FJG, eds. Textbook of Dermatology, 3rd edn, vol 2. Oxford: Blackwell Scientific Publications; 1979:1900.

Compliance, because of the color, is a challenge.

Gianotti–Crosti syndrome

Carlo Gelmetti

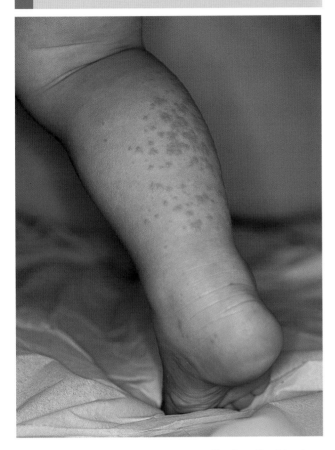

Gianotti–Crosti syndrome was originally described in three children in 1955 by Ferdinando Gianotti as a disease characterized by an erythematous papular eruption symmetrically distributed on the face, buttocks, and extremities of children. Besides the typical topography of the dermatosis, Gianotti also pointed out that the disease had mild, if any, constitutional symptoms, was not preceded by fever or by severe prodromes, the lesions had a simultaneous evolution, and the course of the disease was quite long (3–6 weeks). The term 'Gianotti–Crosti syndrome' is now used to include all eruptive acrolocated dermatoses clinically characterized by papular or papulovesicular lesions that are caused by a range of viruses. These almost always run a benign and self-healing course over a few weeks. The first virus associated with this eruption was hepatitis B virus (HBV), but many others have since been documented.

MANAGEMENT STRATEGY

The diagnosis of Gianotti–Crosti syndrome is clinical. Like many other viral exanthems it mainly affects children of pre-school age, though occasional adult cases have occurred. The typical eruption consists of monomorphic, flat, lentil-sized lesions symmetrically distributed on the face, buttocks, and limbs. The lesions are papular or papulovesicular, sometimes edematous, and rarely purpuric. They may coalesce over the elbows and knees. The trunk, antecubital and popliteal surfaces are usually spared, though a transient rash may be noted on the trunk in the early stage of the eruption. Mucous membranes are not affected. In the early eruptive phase the Koebner phenomenon may be elicited. In children less than 1 year of age the lesions may be edematous, while in adolescents and young adults they tend to be consistently papular. The eruption develops within a week, typically beginning on the thighs and buttocks, then involving the extensor aspects of the arms, and finally involving the face. Individual lesions look hemispherical, are a few millimeters in diameter (lesions of 8–10 mm in diameter are uncommon), and vary in color from rose to red-brown. The pruritus is usually mild and excoriation is never seen. The lesions fade in 3–4 weeks with mild desquamation, and relapse is rare. A longer course of up to 6–8 weeks is occasionally seen. Inguinal and axillary lymphadenopathy is common, but not invariable. Nodes are moderately enlarged, of elastic consistency, and mobile.

In cases associated with hepatitis B the hepatitis begins at the same time as, or 1–2 weeks after, the onset of the dermatitis. The liver is usually enlarged, but not tender; jaundice is exceptional. There are high serum levels of liver enzymes and the various viral markers become detectable in the serum of all patients depending on the duration of infection. Serious complications are very rare, though some patients have developed chronic periportal hepatitis. Abnormalities in the peripheral blood are inconsistent: there may be a leukopenia or a slight leukocytosis with 2–15% of monocytes; the erythrocyte sedimentation rate is not raised.

In hepatitis B-negative cases, hepatomegaly and liver function abnormalities, if present, are slight: serum transaminases rarely are higher than 100 U/mL. In these cases, the liver involvement can be explained by the fact that some viruses that can provoke Gianotti–Crosti syndrome are considered among the minor hepatitic viruses (e.g. Epstein–Barr virus [EBV]).

There is no specific treatment for the rash. We do not recommend any topical or systemic drug; however, when itching is present *oral antihistamines* or *topical antipruritics* can be prescribed for their symptomatic effect. Although mild topical corticosteroids are sometimes used, the benefit is not firmly established. Systemic absorption of superpotent topical corticosteroids could prolong or delay recovery from the disease.

In cases associated with hepatitis B, the *hepatitis must be treated*. It is also important to investigate and treat other members of the family who may be carriers of the HBV or may benefit from vaccination. Prophylactic vaccination against HBV, which has been introduced in the past two decades, will potentially eradicate all cases of Gianotti–Crosti syndrome due to this virus, as has happened in Italy where such vaccination was instituted in 1983 and is routinely administered to all newborns. The present vaccine is not only effective against hepatitis, but also seems to decrease the incidence of hepatocellular carcinoma. *Other infective causes may require treatment* if identified.

SPECIFIC INVESTIGATIONS

- Liver enzymes
- Viral serology for hepatitis A, HBV, hepatitis delta virus, EBV, cytomegalovirus
- Total IgE – paper radioimmunosorbent test (PRIST); and specific IgE – radioallergosorbent test (RAST)

Other possible causes include coxsackievirus, adenovirus, enterovirus, human herpesvirus-6, reovirus, varicella, roseola, rotavirus, respiratory syncytial virus, Lyme borreliosis, *Mycoplasma pneumoniae*, and immunization.

Gianotti–Crosti syndrome caused by acute hepatitis B virus genotype D infection. Michitaka K, Horiike N, Chen Y, et al. Intern Med 2004;43:696–9.

A 12-year-old girl with Gianotti–Crosti syndrome caused by HBV infection revealed elevation of transaminase, positivity for HBsAg, and an IgM type anti-HB core. The eruption and level of transaminase improved, and HBsAg became negative within 2 months of onset. Analysis of the virus revealed a rare serotype of HBsAg.

Gianotti–Crosti syndrome associated with endogenous reactivation of Epstein–Barr virus. Terasaki K, Koura S, Tachikura T, Kanzaki T. Dermatology 2003;207:68–71.

A 6-year-old girl with Gianotti–Crosti syndrome had infectious mononucleosis at the age of 3 years. Because the titer of anti-EBV capsid antigen antibody was high at 1280 and the titer of early antigen DR IgG, which increases during the early stage of reactivation, was high at 80 during the recovery stage, the patient was diagnosed as having Gianotti–Crosti syndrome associated with reactivation of EBV.

A prospective case control study of the association of Gianotti–Crosti syndrome with human herpesvirus 6 and human herpesvirus 7 infections. Chuh AA, Chan HH, Chiu SS, et al. Pediatr Dermatol 2002;19:492–7.

In two infants with Gianotti–Crosti syndrome, active HHV-6 infection was demonstrated by detection of viral DNA in the absence of antibody in the acute plasma specimens and HHV-6 DNA viral loads of more than 5.3 log10 genome copies/5 μL in the whole blood specimens, a profile previously shown to be diagnostic of recent primary HHV-6 infection.

Gianotti–Crosti-Syndrom nach Impfung. Haug S, Schnopp C, Ring J, et al. Hautarzt 2002;53:683–5.

Four infants developed Gianotti–Crosti syndrome 6–8 days after immunization (hepatitis A, hepatitis B, diphtheria, tetanus, pertussis, *Haemophilus influenzae*, measles, mumps, rubella).

Vaccination may be a relevant etiologic factor and should be considered in infants presenting with Gianotti–Crosti syndrome.

Gianotti–Crosti syndrome and allergic background. Ricci G, Patrizi A, Neri I, et al. Acta Derm Venereol 2003; 83:202–5.

In twenty-nine children with Gianotti–Crosti syndrome and 59 age- and sex-matched controls, the presence of atopic dermatitis (24.1%) was significantly higher (p < 0.005) than in the control group (6.8%). In addition, the percentage of patients with total IgE greater than +2 SD for age was higher than in controls (27.6 vs 13.7%), as was the percentage of specific IgE present (31 vs 17.2%).

FIRST LINE THERAPIES

■ Systemic antihistamines	E
■ Topical corticosteroids	E
■ Topical antiseptics	E
■ Topical antipruritics	E
■ Systemic corticosteroids	E
■ Systemic antibiotics	E
■ Emollients	E
■ Vitamin C	E
■ Interferon-α	B
■ Hepatitis B vaccine	B

Gianotti–Crosti syndrome: clinical, serologic and therapeutic data from nine children. Boeck K, Mempel M, Schmidt T, Abeck D. Cutis 1998;62:271–4.

In nine children with Gianotti–Crosti syndrome therapeutic interventions included systemic antihistamines, topical clioquinol lotion 1%, topical corticosteroids, and systemic methylprednisolone. Skin lesions resolved after 2–4 weeks in treated as well as in nontreated children. Whole-body involvement seemed to correlate with severe pruritus and additional general symptoms, requiring more intensive therapy.

Infection aiguë à *Mycoplasma pneumoniae*: nouvelle cause de syndrome de Gianotti–Crosti. Angoulvant N, Grezard P, Wolf F, et al. Presse Med 2000;29:1287.

A bacterial origin of Gianotti–Crosti syndrome could justify treatment with antibiotics.

Infantile acrodermatitis of Gianotti–Crosti and Lyme borreliosis. Baldari U, Cattonar P, Nobile C, et al. Acta Derm Venereol 1996;76:242–3.

One patient was treated with ceftriaxone (500 mg intramuscularly daily for 30 days) and the second with josamycin (250 mg daily for 14 days).

Truncal lesions do not exclude a diagnosis of Gianotti–Crosti syndrome. Chuh AA. Australas J Dermatol 2003;44:215–6.

Although most patients with Gianotti–Crosti syndrome only have the typical acrally distributed eruption, additional truncal lesions, if few in number, do not exclude the diagnosis. Topical calamine lotion and a sedating oral antihistamine were prescribed. The truncal lesions subsided in 3 weeks, and there was remission of all lesions after 6 weeks.

Hepatitis B: virus, pathogenesis and treatment. Grob PJ. Vaccine 1998;16(suppl):S11–6.

Treatment of hepatitis B with interferon has become accepted, resulting in the elimination of the virus in up to 30–40% of cases, though the mechanism of action is still poorly understood.

Evidence levels A Double-blind study **B** Clinical trial ≥ 20 subjects **C** Clinical trial < 20 subjects **D** Series ≥ 5 subjects **E** Anecdotal case reports

Glossodynia/ burning mouth syndrome

Lisa A Drage, Alison J Bruce, Roy S Rogers III

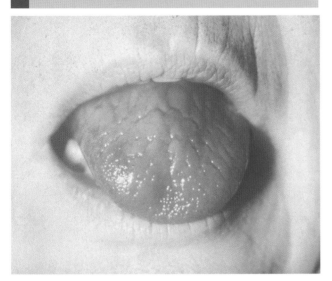

Burning mouth syndrome refers to those patients with mouth pain who have normal oral physical findings. The burning sensation may localize to specific sites such as the tongue, palate, or lip or it may be a generalized oral pain. As many oral mucosal diseases (e.g. lichen planus, herpes simplex, recurrent aphthous stomatitis, aphthous ulcers) also cause mouth pain, a thorough oral examination to exclude other primary mucosal alterations must be done before considering burning mouth syndrome (BMS).

MANAGEMENT STRATEGIES

Identification and *treatment of all correctable causes of mouth pain* should be emphasized. Conditions most commonly associated with mouth pain include psychiatric illness (depression, anxiety, and cancer phobia), xerostomia (drug-related, secondary to connective tissue diseases, or aging), nutritional deficiency (iron, vitamin B6, vitamin B12, folate, zinc), and allergic contact stomatitis (particularly to flavorings and food additives). Multiple associated factors are commonly present and demand concurrent treatment.

Geographic tongue is also associated with burning mouth pain. Other less common etiologies include candidiasis, denture-related oral pain, denture sore mouth, menopause, and use of angiotensin-converting enzyme (ACE) inhibitors.

A directed history and physical examination with emphasis on a thorough oral exam must be completed. All medications must be assessed for xerostomic potential. Direct questions about depression, anxiety, and fear of cancer should be asked. Exacerbations with food or other oral preparations (e.g. toothpaste, mouthwash, gum) should be elicited. A history of pain starting with dental work or

dentures as well as parafunctional behaviors (tongue thrusting, clenching, and bruxism) should be documented.

Treatment should be based on the results of a directed history, thorough oral exam, and laboratory investigation. It should be tailored to the individual patient. Initially, treatment should be based on the suspected cause of the mouth pain rather than used in an algorithmic manner. If there are no identifiable causes of the mouth symptoms, then a *trial of a chronic pain protocol*, similar to the medical management of other neuropathic pain conditions, would be appropriate.

SPECIFIC INVESTIGATIONS

- A thorough history emphasizing:
  - medications that can cause xerostomia
  - dental work and denture history
  - oral care and habits
  - history or symptoms of depression, anxiety, or fear of cancer
- Oral examination specifically checking for any sign of erythema, candidiasis, xerostomia, or abnormal mucosal changes
- Laboratory tests:
  - complete blood count
  - iron, total iron binding capacity, iron saturation, ferritin
  - vitamin B6, vitamin B12, folate, zinc
  - fasting plasma glucose, glycosylated hemoglobin
- Biopsy (only if indicated on the basis of an abnormal oral examination)
- Culture for candidiasis
- Patch testing (including oral flavors and preservatives)
- Psychiatric evaluation if indicated by history and review of systems
- Further consultation if indicated by dentistry, neurology, or otorhinolaryngology

Clinical assessment and outcome in 70 patients with complaints of burning or sore mouth. Drage LA, Rogers RS. Mayo Clin Proc 1998;74:223–8.

Seventy patients with a burning or sore mouth were retrospectively reviewed. The report lists etiologic agents of burning or sore mouth symptoms. Multiple etiologic factors were present in 37% of patients. The most frequently associated conditions were psychiatric disease (30%), xerostomia (24%), geographic tongue (24%), nutritional deficiency (21%), and allergic contact stomatitis to food additives (13%). Tables on appropriate management and evaluation are included, and 70% of patients improved with tailored therapy.

Psychiatric comorbidity in patients with burning mouth syndrome. Bogetto F, Malina G, Ferro G, et al. Psychosom Med 1998;60:378–85.

In a case-controlled study, 102 patients with BMS were evaluated according to the diagnostic criteria of Diagnostic and Statistical Manual of Mental Disorders (DSM)-IV. High rates (71.6%) of comorbid psychiatric diagnoses were found, most commonly depressive disorders and generalized anxiety disorder. BMS also occurred in the absence of psychiatric diagnoses (28.4%).

FIRST LINE THERAPIES

Tailor treatment to suspected cause of mouth pain	
■ Avoidance of irritants, especially alcohol-based mouthwashes and highly flavored dentifrices	E
■ Avoidance of allergens documented on patch testing, especially flavorings and food additives such as propylene glycol, sorbic acid, cinnamon, mint	E
■ Discontinuation of ACE inhibitors	D
■ Sialogogues or artificial saliva for xerostomia	E
■ Discontinuation of medications that cause xerostomia	E
■ Assessment for parafunctional habits: clenching, tongue thrusting	E
■ Reassurance that cancer is not present	E
■ Denture evaluation and adaptation	C
■ Replacement of vitamin B6, vitamin B12, iron, zinc, or folate	B
■ Anti-yeast agents	C
■ Appropriate evaluation and treatment of underlying psychiatric disease	C

The burning mouth syndrome. Huang U, Rothe MJ, Grant-Kels JM. J Am Acad Dermatol 1996;34:91–8.

Review of BMS with emphasis on contact allergy association. Evaluation and management strategies.

Type III burning mouth syndrome: psychological and allergic aspects. Lamey PJ, Lamb AB, Hughes A, et al. J Oral Pathol Med 1994;23:216–9.

Of 33 patients with intermittent BMS (type III), 65% had positive patch tests to food additives or flavorings, and 80% of this group improved with avoidance of the documented allergen.

Stomatodynia (burning mouth) as a complication of enalapril therapy. Triantos D, Kanakis P. Oral Dis 2004; 10:244–5.

A case report of BMS that improved after discontinuing enalapril. Summary of ten additional cases of ACE inhibitors associated with burning mouth in the literature.

Patients complaining of a burning mouth. Main DMG, Basker RM. Br Dent J 1983;154:206–11.

In this study, 50% of cases of burning mouth were attributed to errors in denture design. With replacement of dentures, the patients improved. Onset of symptoms coincident with denture implementation or at the site of a denture should prompt patient referral for a formal dental consultation.

Candidiasis may induce glossodynia without objective manifestation. Osaki T, Yoneda K, Yamamoto T, et al. Am J Med Sci 2000;319:100–5.

Of 98 patients, 26 had no objective signs of candidiasis, but had hyposalivation and overgrowth of *Candida* spp. on laboratory examination. Glossal pain subsided with treatment (3% amphotericin mouthwash solution).

SECOND LINE THERAPIES

After evaluation, if no cause of mouth pain is identified consider one of the following:	
■ Low dose of tricyclic antidepressant	C
■ Low dose benzodiazepine or doxepin	C
■ Topical capsaicin	E
■ Topical clonazepam	B
■ Gabapentin	E

Topical clonazepam in stomatodynia: a randomized placebo-controlled study. Gremeau-Richard C, Woda A, Navez ML, et al. Pain 2004;108:51–7.

Forty-eight patients with BMS 'sucked and spat' a 1 mg tablet of clonazepam or placebo three times daily for 14 days. The decrease in pain scores was significantly more pronounced in the clonazepam than in the placebo group. The authors hypothesize that clonazepam acts locally to disrupt the mechanism(s) causing burning.

An open-label dose escalation pilot study of the effect of clonazepam in burning mouth syndrome. Grushka M, Epstein J, Mott A. Oral Surg Oral Med Oral Pathol Oral Radiol Endod 1998;86:557–61.

Clonazepam (a benzodiazepine) was used in increasing doses (starting at 0.25 mg and increased by 0.25 mg weekly if continued); 70% of patients noted some improvement. The authors propose that the action may be separate from the anxiolytic effect of benzodiazepines.

Oral medicine in practice: burning mouth syndrome. Lamey PJ, Lewis MAO. Br Dent J 1989;167:197–200.

These authors recommend doxepin (75–150 mg at night) for patients with depression, anxiety, or parafunctional habits.

Clinical characteristics and management outcome in burning mouth syndrome: an open study of 130 patients. Gorsky M, Silverman S, Chinn H. Oral Surg Oral Med Oral Pathol 1991;72:192–5.

Treatment with chlordiazepoxide (a benzodiazepine) was associated with remission in 15% of patients.

Effectiveness of gabapentin for treatment of burning mouth syndrome. White TL, Kent PF, Kurtz DB, Emko P. Arch Otolaryngol Head Neck Surg 2004;130:786–8.

Report of a case of BMS responsive to gabapentin, gradually increasing to the dose to 300 mg three times a day.

Capsaicin in burning mouth syndrome: titration strategies. Spice R, Hagen NA. J Otolaryngol 2004;33:53–4.

A commercial hot pepper product is used to combat burning mouth. Clear guidelines on use are included.

Burning mouth syndrome. Grushka M, Epstein JB, Gorsky M. Am Fam Physician 2002;65:615–20.

A practical review on the multiple etiologies and management of BMS.

THIRD LINE THERAPIES

■ Cognitive behavioral therapy	B
■ Alpha lipoic acid	C

Cognitive therapy in the treatment of patients with resistant burning mouth syndrome: a controlled study. Bergdahl J, Anneroth G, Perris H. J Oral Pathol Med 1995;24:213–5.

A randomized control study examining the effects of cognitive therapy on resistant BMS in comparison to a 'placebo' attention program. There was a statistically significant reduction in pain intensity for those receiving cognitive therapy.

Burning mouth syndrome (BMS): double blind controlled study of alpha-lipoic acid (thioctic acid) therapy. Femiano F, Scully C. J Oral Pathol Med 2002;31:267–9.

Sixty patients with BMS received 200 mg alpha-lipoic acid (an over-the-counter supplement) or placebo three times daily for 2 months: 74% of treated patients showed 'decided improvement' compared with 0% on placebo. Alpha-lipoic acid (thioctic acid) is an antioxidant and the authors speculate that BMS is a neuropathy related to free radical production.

Gonorrhea

Patrice Morel

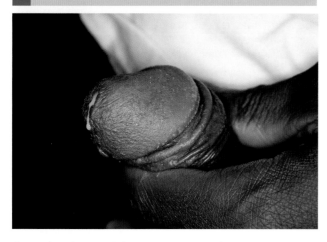

Gonorrhea is one of the commonest and most severe sexually transmitted diseases. It is caused by the Gram-negative aerobic diplococcus *Neisseria gonorrhoeae*, which primarily infects the mucous membranes of the urethra, endocervix, rectum, and pharynx. The infection may be asymptomatic.

MANAGEMENT STRATEGY

Individuals with gonorrhea should be treated as promptly as possible:

- to prevent regional infection such as epididymitis or pelvic inflammatory disease leading to infertility or ectopic pregnancy;
- to prevent disseminated gonococcal infection, which occurs in about 1–3% cases;
- to stop transmission to sexual partners.

Urethritis is typically characterized by a discharge of mucopurulent or purulent material and by burning during urination. Dysuria may be the only symptom.

Gonococcal cervicitis is characterized by a mucopurulent or purulent endocervical exudate. However, a cervical discharge is not specific for a gonococcal infection, and gonococcal infection of the cervix is often asymptomatic.

Pharyngeal infection is asymptomatic in more than 90% of cases.

Rectal infection is prevalent in homosexual men. It causes anal discharge and pain. In females, rectal infection results from spread through vaginal secretions and does not necessarily imply anal intercourse.

Patients in whom gonorrhea is suspected should be investigated for *N. gonorrhoeae* using the most sensitive and specific tests, though empiric treatment of the symptoms may be recommended for patients at high risk for infection who are unlikely to return for a follow-up evaluation. In this circumstance, the recommended *antibiotic treatment must be effective against all strains of N. gonorrhoeae*, including the penicillinase producing and the high-level tetracycline-resistant *N. gonorrhoeae* strains.

Patients infected with *N. gonorrhoeae* are often co-infected with *Chlamydia trachomatis*. A co-treatment effective against *C. trachomatis* should be considered.

Patients should be instructed:

- to return for evaluation if symptoms persist or recur after completion of therapy, and
- to abstain from sexual intercourse until they and their sex partners are cured.

SPECIFIC INVESTIGATIONS

> **Men**
> - Microscopy of Gram-stained urethral secretion
> - Culture on Thayer-Martin medium
>
> **Women**
> - Culture on Thayer-Martin medium

Male urethritis with and without discharge. A clinical and microbiological study. Janier M, Lassau F, Casin I, et al. Sex Transm Dis 1995;22:244–52.

Neisseria gonorrhoeae was found in 21% of patients with urethral discharge and in no patient without discharge. A systemic treatment for *N. gonorrhoeae* in patients without discharge in the absence of proven contact with an infected patient is not recommended.

Gonorrhoea in men: clinical and diagnostic aspects. Sherrard J, Barlow D. Genitourin Med 1996;72:422–6.

Urethral gonorrhea was diagnosed by microscopy in 94.4% of symptomatic men and in 81.1% of asymptomatic men; so, culture should be considered essentially for asymptomatic patients.

Gonorrhoea in women. Diagnostic, clinical and therapeutic aspects. Barlow D, Phillips I. Lancet 1978;1:761–4.

In women, culture is necessary (endocervical, urethral and rectal swabs) because of the low sensitivity of microscopy of Gram-stained endocervical (37–50%) and urethral (20%) smears.

Microbiological diagnosis of gonorrhoea. Jephcott AE. Genitourin Med 1997;73:245–52.

Many antigen detection tests are available. The choice of a particular system will be based on weighing up its relative advantages and disadvantages.

Epidemiology and treatment of oropharyngeal gonorrhoea. Hutt DM, Judson FN. Ann Intern Med 1986;104:655–8.

Gonococci were grown from expectorated saliva in 34 of 51 cultures from patients with oropharyngeal gonorrhea, suggesting transmissibility and providing another reason for ensuring effective treatment.

Disseminated gonococcal infection (DGI)

DGI results from gonococcal bacteremia with the possibility of petechial or pustular acral skin lesions, arthralgia, tenosynovitis, or septic arthritis. The infection may be complicated by perihepatitis and rarely by endocarditis and meningitis.

FIRST LINE THERAPIES

■ Cefixime 400 mg orally in a single dose	B
■ Ceftriaxone 125 mg intramuscularly in a single dose	B

Oral cefixime versus intramuscular ceftriaxone in patients with uncomplicated gonococcal infections. Portilla I, Lutz B, Montalvo M, Mogabgab J. Sex Transm Dis 1992; 19:94–8.

The 400 mg dose of cefixime cured 97% of uncomplicated urogenital and anorectal gonococcal infections. The advantage of cefixime is that it can be administered orally.

Drugs of choice for the treatment of uncomplicated gonococcal infections. Moran JS, Levine WC. Clin Infect Dis 1995;20(suppl 1):s47–s65.

Ceftriaxone in a single injection of 125 mg provides sustained, high bactericidal levels in the blood. Extensive clinical experience indicates that ceftriaxone cures 99% of uncomplicated urogenital and anorectal infections and 94% of pharyngeal infections. Up to now no case of gonorrhea caused by *N. gonorrhoeae* resistant to ceftriaxone has been reported.

SECOND LINE THERAPIES

■ Ciprofloxacin 500 mg orally in a single dose	B
■ Ofloxacin 400 mg orally in a single dose	B

Sexually transmitted diseases. Treatment guidelines 2002. Centers for Disease Control and Prevention. MMWR Recomm Rep 2002;51(RR-6):1–78.

In published clinical trials, ciprofloxacin has cured 99.8% of uncomplicated urogenital and anorectal infections. Ofloxacin is also effective, curing 98.6% of uncomplicated infections. Levofloxacin can be used in place of ofloxacin as a single dose of 250 mg.

Fluoroquinolone resistance in *Neisseria gonorrhoeae*, Hawaii, 1999, and decreased susceptibility to azithromycin in *N. gonorrhoeae*, Missouri, 1999. Centers for Disease Control and Prevention. MMWR 2000;49:833–7.

Fluoroquinolone therapy has been recommended by the CDC since 1993 because it is an inexpensive, oral and single-dose therapy. However, because of increased prevalence of fluoroquinolone-resistant *N. gonorrhoeae* in Asia, the Pacific Islands, other places in the United States or United Kingdom, fluoroquinolones are no longer recommended for treating gonorrhoea acquired in those locations. Instead, ceftriaxone or cefixime should be used.

Increases in fluoroquinolone-resistant *Neisseria gonorrhoeae* among men who have sex with men. United States, 2003 and revised recommendations for gonorrhea treatment, 2004. Centers for Disease Control and Prevention. MMWR Morb Mortal Wkly Rep 2004;53:335–8.

Local and national data suggest that the prevalence of quinolone-resistant *N. gonorrheoae* among men who have sex with men infected with gonorrhea is close to or exceeds 5%. In this situation fluoroquinolones should no longer be used.

THIRD LINE THERAPIES

■ Spectinomycin 2 g intramuscularly in a single dose	B

Spectinomycin resistance in *Neisseria* spp. due to mutations in IGSrRNA. Galimand M, Gerbaud G, Courvalin P. Antimicrob Agents Chemother 2000;44:1365–6.

It is possible, though rare, for a patient to be infected with a spectinomycin-resistant *N. gonorrhoeae* strain; spectinomycin is expensive and must be injected. Therefore, spectinomycin is useful for treatment of patients who cannot tolerate cephalosporins and quinolones.

Efficacy of azithromycin 1 g single dose in the management of uncomplicated gonorrhoeae. Habib AR, Fernando R. Int J STD AIDS 2004;15:240–2.

Azithromycin cured 98.8% of uncomplicated gonorrhea. *However the emergence of* N. gonorrhoeae *with decreased susceptibility to azithromycin has been described and azithromycin is not recommended (CDC, 2002). Azithromycin one dose of 1 g orally or doxycycline 100 mg twice daily for 7 days must be added to the treatment of gonorrhea if chlamydia is not ruled out.*

SPECIAL CONSIDERATIONS

■ Pharyngeal infection
■ DGI
■ Pregnancy
■ Ophthalmia neonatorum

Pharyngeal infection

Treating uncomplicated *Neisseria gonorrhoeae* infections: is the anatomic site of infection important? Moran JS. Sex Transm Dis 1995;22:39–47.

A systematic review of published therapeutic trials of various antimicrobial regimens for the biological cure of uncomplicated gonorrhea has shown that pharyngeal infection is more difficult to cure. Cephalosporin and quinolone regimens are the best choice. They are likely to cure at least 80% of pharyngeal infections. Spectinomycin is unreliable (i.e. only 52% effective) against pharyngeal infections.

Disseminated gonococcal infection

Sexually transmitted diseases. Treatment guidelines 2002. Centers for Disease Control and Prevention. MMWR Recomm Rep 2002;51(RR-6):1–78.

Hospitalization is recommended for initial therapy. The experts recommend ceftriaxone 1 g intramuscularly or intravenously every 24 h as the initial regimen.

Pregnancy

Treatment of gonorrhoea in pregnancy. Cavenee MR, Farris JR, Spalding TR, et al. Obstet Gynecol 1993;81:33–8.

Two hundred and fifty two pregnant women with gonorrhea were randomly assigned to receive ceftriaxone 250 mg intramuscularly, spectinomycin 2 g intramuscularly, or amoxicillin 3 g orally with probenecid 1 g orally. The overall efficacy was 95, 95, and 89%, respectively. There was no increased incidence of congenital malformations. Ceftriaxone and spectinomycin are the best choice. Pregnant women should not be treated with quinolones or tetracyclines.

Ophthalmia neonatorum

1998 guidelines for treatment of sexually transmitted diseases. Centers for Disease Control and Prevention. MMWR Recomm Rep 1998;47(RR-1):1–111.

Gonococcal ophthalmia is strongly suggested when typical Gram-negative diplococci are identified in conjunctival exudate, justifying presumptive treatment for gonorrhea after appropriate cultures for *N. gonorrhoeae* are obtained. The recommended regimen is ceftriaxone 25–50 mg/kg intravenously or intramuscularly in a single dose, not to exceed 125 mg. Local treatment, with or without systemic antibiotic, is inappropriate.

Evidence levels **A** Double-blind study **B** Clinical trial ≥ 20 subjects **C** Clinical trial < 20 subjects **D** Series ≥ 5 subjects **E** Anecdotal case reports

Graft versus host disease

*Dwayne Montie, Carmen E Kannee,
Carlos H Nousari*

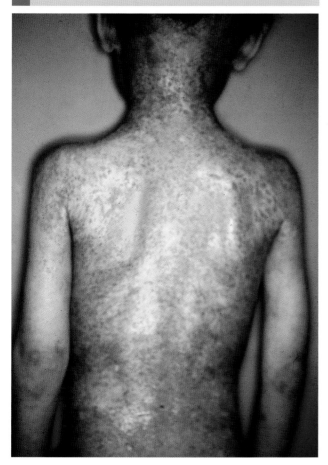

Graft versus host disease (GvHD) classically affects the skin, liver, and gastrointestinal tract and almost always occurs in the setting of allogenic bone marrow transplants. Acute GvHD (aGvHD) occurs within 1–3 weeks after transplantation and typically presents as a maculopapular eruption, which may progress to erythroderma and less commonly to a toxic epidermal necrolysis-like eruption. Chronic GvHD (cGvHD) is characteristically seen later than 3 months after transplantation as mucocutaneous lichenoid and/or sclerodermatous disease.

MANAGEMENT STRATEGY

Cyclosporine and methotrexate as sole or combined therapy are the most common drugs used for prophylaxis of aGvHD. Although the combination of cyclosporine with methotrexate has become the standard, other combinations using *sirolimus, mycophenolate mofetil,* and *systemic corticosteroids* are currently being evaluated.

Several randomized studies in myeloablative and non-myeloablative allogenic bone marrow transplantation have shown that the combination of cyclosporine with mycophenolate mofetil had similar incidences of aGvHD and comparable survival rates when compared with the combination of cyclosporine and methotrexate. However, the combination with mycophenolate mofetil was associated with faster hematopoietic engraftment and thus less morbidity.

Recent prospective studies have shown that *tacrolimus* as monotherapy or in combination with methotrexate may be associated with less morbidity than methotrexate as sole therapy or in combination with cyclosporine.

The role of prednisone remains unclear and is not part of the standard regimen for prophylaxis of aGVHD. In spite of showing similar survival rates, studies have shown that the addition of prednisone to any of current standard therapies is associated with increased morbidity.

The first line therapy for aGvHD is *systemic corticosteroids.* A typical regimen includes the addition of prednisone at 1–2 mg/kg daily to an optimized dose of *cyclosporine.*

The response to first line therapy was found to be the single most important factor predicting improved long-term survival. If there is no response to corticosteroids, second line therapy should be initiated, this includes *mycophenolate mofetil, tacrolimus, antithymocyte globulin,* and *sirolimus.*

In cases of refractory aGvHD, third line therapy includes *biologic agents. Supportive care* is also critical in the management and incudes cessation of oral intake, total parenteral nutrition with hyperalimentation, antibiotic and antiviral prophylaxis, and pain control. In patients with mild aGvHD with only cutaneous involvement, topical corticosteroids and *antipruritic agents* may help to control the symptoms.

Treatment of cGvHD depends on the extent of the organ involvement. Patients with localized skin disease require only topical therapy, while those with extensive disease (generalized skin disease per se, or localized cutaneous with internal organ involvement) require systemic therapy. The standard systemic treatment is the combination of *systemic corticosteroids with calcineurin inhibitor,* for example prednisone 1–2 mg/kg daily with cyclosporine 5–10 mg/kg daily or tacrolimus 0.03 mg/kg daily. *Thalidomide and tacrolimus as sole therapies or combined with mycophenolate mofetil* have been found to be effective and safe in corticosteroid-refractory disease, though standard regimens are still lacking for these patients. Unlike the lichenoid variant, which shows a high response rate to *phototherapy,* the sclerodermatous form seems to respond better to *etretinate* or *extracorporeal photopheresis.*

Successful use of *mycophenolate mofetil, sirolimus, hydroxychloroquine, cyclophosphamide, pentostatin and monoclonal antibodies against cytokines, specially anti-TNF-α,* have also been reported as salvage therapy.

Supportive therapy with good nutrition, physical therapy, dental hygiene, and skin lubrication is also important.

SPECIFIC INVESTIGATIONS

Acute GvHD
■ Skin biopsy
■ Liver function tests

Histopathology of graft-vs.-host reaction (GvHD) in human recipients of marrow from HL-A-matched sibling donors. Lerner KG, Kao GF, Storb R, et al. Transplant Proc 1974;6:367–71.

Skin biopsy is useful for confirming the diagnosis of aGvHD and for grading the severity of acute cutaneous GvHD.

Bone marrow transplantation. Thomas ED, Storb R, Clift RA, et al. N Engl J Med 1975;292:895–902.

Bilirubin levels in association with extent of skin involvement and volume of diarrhea are used in the grading of aGvHD, which reflects prognosis.

> *Chronic GvHD*
> - Skin biopsy
> - Liver function tests
> - Schirmer's test
> - Pulmonary function tests
> - Complete blood count
> - Serum immunoglobulins

Clinical importance of confirming or excluding the diagnosis of chronic graft-versus host disease. Jacobsohn D, Montross S, Anders V, Vogelsang G. Bone Marrow Transplant 2001;28:1047–51.

Retrospective analysis of 123 patients referred to the GvHD clinic at the Johns Hopkins Oncology Center from 1994 to 1998 with a diagnosis of active cGvHD. Of these, nine patients (7%) had no evidence of cGVHD, and 25 patients (20%) had inactive cGVHD. Many of these patients were found to have other processes accounting for their ongoing symptoms.

Acute GvHD

FIRST LINE THERAPIES

■ Corticosteroids (with optimization of cyclosporine for prophylaxis)	A
■ Cyclosporine with mycophenolate mofetil	A
■ Sirolimus with tacrolimus	B

Treatment of acute graft-versus-host disease after allogeneic marrow transplantation. Randomized study comparing corticosteroids and cyclosporine. Kennedy MS, Deeg HJ, Storb R, et al. Am J Med 1985;78:978–83.

This trial comparing corticosteroids and cyclosporine, showing response rates of 41 and 60%, respectively, was done in the early days when GvHD prophylaxis consisted only of methotrexate. In the cyclosporine era, corticosteroids are now the drug choice.

A prospective randomized trial comparing cyclosporine and short course methotrexate with cyclosporine and mycophenolae mofetil for GVHD prophylaxis in myeloablative allogenic bone marrow transplantation. Bolweel B, Sobecks R, PohlmanB, et al. Bone Marrow Transplant 2004; 34:621–5.

GvHD prophylaxis with cyclosporine and mycophenolate mofetil is associated with faster hematopoietic engraftment, decreased incidence of mucositis, and similar incidence of aGvHD and comparable survival when compared to cyclosporine and methotrexate.

Sirolimus and tacrolimus without methotrexate as graft-versus-host disease prophylaxis after matched related donor peripheral blood stem cell transplantation. Cutler C, Kim HT, Hochberg E, et al. Biol Blood Marrow Transplant 2004;10:328–36.

This trial showed that sirolimus and tacrolimus without methotrexate resulted in an overall survival rate of 93 and 97%, respectively, at 100 days post transplantation. The incidence of mucositis and other transplant-related toxicity was modest while engraftment was prompt.

SECOND LINE THERAPIES

■ Antithymocyte globulins (ATG)	C
■ Biologics (such as anti-IL2R and anti-CD52)	B

Treatment of established human graft-versus-host disease by anti-thymocyte globulin. Storb R, Gluckman E, Thomas ED, et al. Blood 1974;44:56–75.

Twelve of 19 patients showed resolution of aGvHD.

Low dose alemtuzumab (Campath) in myeloablative allogeneic stem cell transplantation for CD52-positive malignancies: decreased incidence of acute graft-versus-host-disease with unique pharmacokinetics. Khouri IF, Albitar M, Saliba RM, et al. Bone Marrow Transplant 2004; 33:833–7

At 3 months post-transplantation, 11 of 12 patients had achieved 100% donor chimerism.

THIRD LINE THERAPIES

■ Extracorporeal photopheresis	B
■ PUVA	B
■ Biologics (infliximab, etanercept)	B

Extracorporeal photochemotherapy in the treatment of severe steroid-refractory acute graft-versus host disease: A pilot study. Greinix HT, Volc-Platzer B, Kalhs P, et al. Blood 2000;96:2426–31.

Three months after initiation of extracorporeal photochemotherapy in 21 patients with corticosteroid-refractory aGvHD, 60% achieved complete resolution of GvHD manifestations. Responses were achieved in 60% of patients with either cutaneous or liver involvement, but in none with gut involvement.

Treatment of acute graft-versus-host disease with PUVA (psoralen and ultraviolet irradiation): results of a pilot study. Wiesmann A, Weller A, Lischka G, et al. Bone Marrow Transplant 1999;23:151–5.

The vast majority of 20 patients treated with PUVA for aGvHD had a good response in terms of skin improvement and reduction of corticosteroid dosage.

Tumor necrosis factor-alpha blockade for the treatment of acute GVHD. Couriel D, Saliba R, Hicks K et al. Blood 2004;104:649–54.

In this study including 134 corticosteroid-refractory aGVHD patients, infliximab was well tolerated and effective with an overall response rate of 67%.

Evidence levels   **A** Double-blind study   **B** Clinical trial ≥ 20 subjects   **C** Clinical trial < 20 subjects   **D** Series ≥ 5 subjects   **E** Anecdotal case reports

Chronic GvHD

FIRST LINE THERAPIES

Systemic	
■ Systemic corticosteroid and calcineurin inhibitor	A
■ Corticosteroid alone	A

Therapy for chronic graft-versus-host disease: a randomized trial comparing cyclosporine plus prednisone vs prednisone alone. Koc S, Leisenring W, Flowers ME, et al. Blood 2002;100:48–51.

The use of cyclosporine in combination with prednisone was associated with higher mortality rates related to transplant or relapse when compared with prednisone alone, but with less corticosteroid-related morbidity, and with the same overall survival.

SECOND LINE THERAPIES

Systemic	
■ Thalidomide	B
■ Tacrolimus and mycophenolate mofetil	B
■ Tacrolimus	B
Lichenoid cutaneous cGvHD	
■ PUVA	B
Sclerodermatous cutaneous cGvHD	
■ Etretinate	B
■ Extracorporeal photochemotherapy	C

Thalidomide for the treatment of chronic GvHD. Vogelsang GB, Farmer ER, Hess AD, et al. N Engl J Med 1992; 325:1055–8.

Complete and partial responses were seen in 32 and 27% of the 44 refractory and high-risk patients treated with thalidomide.

Thalidomide after allogeneic haematopoietic stem cell transplantation: activity in chronic but not in acute graft-versus-host disease. Kulkarni S, Powles R, Sirohi B, et al. Bone Marrow Transplant 2003;32:165–70.

Thalidomide was used after failure to respond to the combination of cyclosporine and corticosteroids with or without other agents. None of the 21 patients responded and all died of aGvHD. Of 59 patients with cGvHD, 13 had a complete and eight had a partial response.

Salvage therapy for refractory chronic graft-versus-host disease with mycophenolate mofetil and tacrolimus. Mookerjee B, Altomonte V, Vogelsang G. Bone Marrow Transplant 1999;24:517–20.

Of 26 patients with refractory disease, 46% improved.

FK506 treatment of graft-versus-host disease developing or exacerbating during prophylaxis and therapy with cyclosporin and/or immunosuppressants. Japanese FK506 BMT Study Group. Kanamaru A, Takemoto Y, Kakishita E, et al. Bone Marrow Transplant 1995;15:885–9.

Good to marked responses were observed in 12 of 26 patients with cGvHD who had failed to respond to cyclosporine and other immunosuppressive therapy.

Amelioration of steroid resistant chronic graft versus host mediated liver disease via tacrolimus treatment. Nagler A, Menachem Y, Ilan Y. J Hematother Stem Cell Res 2001;10: 411–7.

Retrospective study of 15 patients with chronic graft versus host-mediated liver disease treated with tacrolimus – five had a complete response and four had a partial response.

Treatment of chronic graft-versus-host disease with ultraviolet irradiation and psoralen (PUVA). Vogelsang GB, Wolff D, Altomonte V, et al. Bone Marrow Transplant 1996; 17:1061–7.

Of 40 patients treated with PUVA, 31 improved, with 16 achieving a complete response when PUVA was added to their GvHD regimen. However, no extracutaneous improvement was noted.

Etretinate therapy for refractory sclerodermatous chronic graft-versus-host disease. Marcellus DC, Altomonte VL, Farmer ER, et al. Blood 1999;93:66–70.

Twenty of 27 patients who had sclerodermatous GvHD showed improvement in terms of skin softening and increased range of movement.

THIRD LINE THERAPIES

Systemic	
■ Extracorporeal photochemotherapy	C
■ Mycophenolate mofetil	C
■ Hydroxychloroquine	B
■ Pulse cyclophosphamide	C
■ Pentostatin	C
■ Infliximab	C
■ Etanercept	C
■ Rituximab	D
■ Daclizumab	E
Lichenoid cutaneous cGvHD	
■ UVB	E
■ Clofazimine	B
■ UVA1 and mycophenolate mofetil	E
Sclerodermatous cutaneous cGvHD	
■ Etretinate	B
■ Extracorporeal photochemotherapy	C
Oral GvHD	
■ Topical corticosteroids	C
■ Topical cyclosporine	D
■ Intraoral PUVA	E
■ Oral UVB	E

Pulse cyclophosphamide for corticosteroid-refractory graft-versus-host disease. Mayer J, Krejci M, Doubek M, et al. Bone Marrow Transplant 2005;35:699–705.

In a retrospective study of 15 patients who had not responded to corticosteroids (nine with aGvHD, three with GvHD after donor leukocyte infusion, and three with progressive cGvHD, pulse cyclophosphamide at a median dose of 1 g/m² was very effective in the treatment of skin (100% response), liver (70% response), and oral cavity (100% response). Severe intestinal GvHD responded poorly. The toxicity profile was acceptable.

Influence of extracorporeal photopheresis on clinical and laboratory parameters in chronic graft versus host disease and anaysis of predictors of response. Seaton ED, Szydlo RM, Kanfer E, et al. Blood 2003;102:1217–23.

Of 21 patients with cutaneous cGvHD treated with extracorporeal photopheresis, one had a complete response and nine had partial responses. Of 25 patients with liver cGvHD, eight had a partial response, and of six patients with oral cGvHD three had a partial response.

Mycophenolate mofetil (MMF) for the treatment of acute and chronic GVHD is effective and well tolerated but induces a high risk of infectious complications: a series of 21 BM or PBSC transplant patients. Baudard M, Vincent A, Moreau P, et al. Bone Marrow Transplant 2002;30:287–95.

Retrospective study with mycophenolate mofetil used as first line in four patients. The best responses were gastrointestinal tract (60%), oral (33%), and nonsclerodermatous skin (43%) GvHD. There was a high incidence of opportunistic infections.

Hydroxychloroquine for the treatment of chronic graft-versus-host disease. Gilman AL, Chan KW, Mogul A, et al. Biol Blood Marrow Transplant 2000;6:327–34.

Three complete responses and 14 partial responses were seen in 32 patients with corticosteroid-resistant or corticosteroid-dependent cGvHD treated with hydroxychloroquine 12 mg/kg. All responders tolerated a reduction in their corticosteroid dose of over 50% while receiving hydroxychloroquine.

Chronic sclerodermic graft-versus-host disease refractory to immunosuppressive treatment responds to UVA1 phototherapy. Grundmann-Kollmann M, Behrens S, Gruss C, et al. J Am Acad Dermatol 2000;42:134–6.

A patient with chronic sclerodermatous GvHD who did not respond to cyclosporine–prednisone and mycophenolate mofetil–prednisone combinations improved with low-dose UVA1 therapy in combination with mycophenolate mofetil.

Chronic graft-versus-host disease treated with UVB phototherapy. Enk CD, Elad S, Vexler A, et al. Bone Marrow Transplant 1998;22:1179–83.

One patient with lichenoid lesions had complete clearing.

Treatment of chronic graft-versus-host disease with ultraviolet irradiation and psoralen (PUVA). Vogelsang GB, Wolff D, Altomonte V, et al. Bone Marrow Transplant 1996;17:1061–7.

PUVA with a glass fiber extension was used to treat intraoral GvHD.

Topical cyclosporine in a bioadhesive for treatment of oral lichenoid mucosal reactions: an open label clinical trail. Epstein JB, Truelove EL. Oral Surg Oral Med Oral Pathol Oral Radiol Endod 1996;82:532–6.

Three of four patients with oral GvHD improved.

TNF-α inhibition for the treatment of cGvHD. Couriel D, Saliba R, Hicks K, et al. Blood 2002;100:847a.

Twenty six patients were treated with infliximab 10 mg/kg weekly for 3 weeks. Response was complete in 16 cases with partial responses in another two. Higher response rates were observed in disease affecting the upper (100%) and lower (73%) gastrointestinal tract, and skin (50%).

Recombinant human tumor necrosis factor receptor fusion protein as complementary treatment for cGvHD. Chiang KY, Abhyankar S, Bridges K, et al. Transplantation 2002;73:665–7.

Ten patients were treated with etanercept – only eight were evaluable and seven had partial responses.

Treatment of chronic graft-versus-host disease with anti-CD20 chimeric monoclonal antibody. Ratanatharathorn V, Ayash L, Reynolds C, et al. Biol Blood Marrow Transplant 2003;9:505–11.

Eight patients with corticosteroid-refractory chronic GvHD were treated with an anti-CD20 chimeric monoclonal antibody (rituximab) by intravenous infusion at a weekly dose of 375 mg/m^2 for 4 weeks. Four patients responded to treatment with ongoing resolution or improvement ranging from 265 to 846 days after therapy.

Treatment of steroid refractory acute and chronic graft-versus-host disease with daclizumab. Willenbacher W, Basara N, Blau IW, et al. Br J Haematol 2001;112:820–3.

Sixteen patients (12 with aGvHD and four with cGvHD) received daclizumab (1 mg/kg) on five occasions over 3 weeks post-transplantation. Responses were observed in nine patients (six aGvHD, three cGvHD). Fourteen patients acquired infections during daclizumab treatment and three deaths were infection related.

Evidence levels **A** Double-blind study **B** Clinical trial ≥ 20 subjects **C** Clinical trial < 20 subjects **D** Series ≥ 5 subjects **E** Anecdotal case reports

Granuloma annulare

Andrew Ilchyshyn

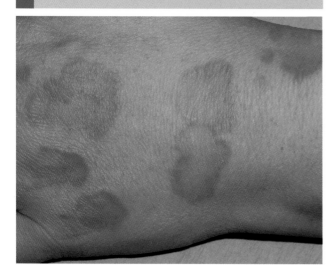

Granuloma annulare is a skin disease of unknown etiology which may present a number of different clinical pictures. It is characterized histologically by necrobiosis of collagen surrounded by a lymphohistiocytic infiltrate. The disease usually resolves spontaneously, with no long-term sequelae.

MANAGEMENT STRATEGY

The diagnosis can often be made clinically in the annular, localized form of granuloma annulare, but a skin biopsy may be required to confirm the diagnosis of the more unusual varieties (generalized, papular umbilicated, perforating, and subcutaneous). Once the diagnosis is established, it is prudent to check the urine for sugar and thus exclude diabetes mellitus.

Since the majority of cases of granuloma annulare do not give rise to any symptoms, the need for any active treatment should be considered carefully; in many cases, reassurance that the disease is benign and will resolve spontaneously is sufficient. Lesions that are painful or unsightly may justify more active treatment, though the level of evidence to support the efficacy of many of the treatments used is poor.

In the localized variety of granuloma annulare, treatment with either *cryotherapy* or *topical corticosteroids* could be tried. Cryotherapy using liquid nitrogen or nitrous oxide may be effective. If required, this treatment can be repeated at intervals of 3–4 weeks. Clobetasol propionate (Dermovate®) lotion, occluded with a hydrocolloid dressing and changed at weekly intervals, can be used for a period of 4–6 weeks. Alternatively, 0.1 mL injections of triamcinolone acetonide (5 mg/mL) may be used to produce even infiltration of lesions, this treatment being repeated, if necessary, at intervals of 6–8 weeks. Treatment of refractory lesions has included *scarification* and the use of *intralesional interferon*. Large, tumid lesions may require excision.

Generalized granuloma annulare may be persistent and its unsightly appearance causes patients to seek active treatment, though the results of therapy are often disappointing. *PUVA*, using oral or topical psoralens, may be used, but relapses occur and a period of maintenance photochemotherapy may be required. UVA alone has been used with reported beneficial results. Both *etretinate* and *isotretinoin* have been associated with improvement or clearance of generalized granuloma annulare. *Topical tacrolimus* has been used in this disease, with greater success in generalized granuloma annulare than in the localized variety. Other reported treatments for this condition include *dapsone, cyclosporine, systemic corticosteroids, chlorambucil, antimalarials, potassium iodide, pentoxifylline, nicotinamide* (niacinamide), *topical vitamin E, fumaric acid esters, defibrotide,* and *efalizumab.*

SPECIFIC INVESTIGATIONS

- ■ Check urine for glucose

Unlike necrobiosis lipoidica, in which there is a strong association with diabetes mellitus, the relationship between granuloma annulare and diabetes is not clear. Nevertheless, it would seem sensible to use the diagnosis of granuloma annulare as a cue to exclude undiagnosed diabetes, and at least check the urine for sugar.

Carbohydrate tolerance in patients with granuloma annulare. Study of fifty-two cases. Haim S, Freidman-Birnbaum R, Haim N, et al. Br J Dermatol 1973;88:447–51.

The incidence of abnormal carbohydrate tolerance in 39 patients with localized granuloma annulare was 23.1% and similar to a control population, compared with an incidence of 76.9% in 13 patients with generalized disease.

Absence of carbohydrate intolerance in patients with granuloma annulare. Gannon TF, Lynch PJ. J Am Acad Dermatol 1994;30:662–3.

Glycosylated hemoglobin levels were found to be normal in the study population of 23 patients with granuloma annulare, 13 of whom had localized lesions and 10 with the generalized form of the disease.

Localised granuloma annulare is associated with insulin-dependent diabetes mellitus. Muhlemann MF, Williams DDR. Br J Dermatol 1984;111:325–9.

This retrospective study looked at 557 insulin-dependent diabetics and found that 16 of them had granuloma annulare, a significantly greater figure than the 0.9 cases that might have been expected.

Localized granuloma annulare

FIRST LINE THERAPIES

■ Cryotherapy	B
■ Intralesional corticosteroids	C
■ Topical corticosteroids	E

Successful outcome of cryosurgery in patients with granuloma annulare. Blume-Peytavi U, Zouboulis CC, Jacobi H, et al. Br J Dermatol 1994;130:494–7.

Of 31 patients with granuloma annulare, 22 were treated with liquid nitrogen and 9 with nitrous oxide. All treated lesions responded, with 80.6% clearing after a single freeze thaw cycle. In the patients treated with liquid nitrogen, there were four cases of persistent atrophic scars where large lesions had been treated.

It should be possible to prevent cryoatrophy by avoiding freeze thaw cycles of greater than 10 s, and taking care not to overlap treatment areas.

Granuloma annulare and necrobiosis lipoidica treated by jet injector. Sparrow G, Abell E. Br J Dermatol 1975;93:85–9.

Injections of 0.1 mL of triamcinolone (5 mg/mL) into lesions of granuloma annulare produced a complete response in 68% of patients, after a mean of 2.9 treatments carried out at 6–8-week intervals. About half the patients suffered recurrences, which are reported to have responded to retreatment.

Successful treatment of chronic skin diseases with clobetasol propionate and a hydrocolloid occlusive dressing. Volden G. Acta Derm Venereol 1992;72:69–71.

In this trial, clobetasol propionate under hydrocolloid occlusion was used in a variety of chronic skin diseases. One of three cases of granuloma annulare showed a complete response after 4 weeks' treatment.

This treatment modality has the advantage of being painless, but the evidence for its efficacy is not at all strong.

A contact dermatitis reaction to clobetasol propionate cream associated with resolution of recalcitrant, generalised granuloma annulare. Agarwal S, Berth-Jones J. J Dermatol Treat 2000;11:279–82.

A single patient was cleared of disseminated lesions of granuloma annulare by topical clobetasol propionate; however, the patient developed contact sensitization to the medication, raising the possibility that this reaction may also have played a therapeutic role.

SECOND LINE THERAPIES

■ Intralesional interferon	C
■ Scarification	E
■ Surgery	E

Treatment of granuloma annulare by local injections with low-dose recombinant human interferon gamma. Weiss JM, Muchenberger S, Schöpf E, Simon JC. J Am Acad Dermatol 1998;39:117–9.

This paper describes a small trial in which three patients with localized granuloma annulare were treated with intralesional injections of recombinant human interferon-γ (2.5×10^5 IU/lesion) on 7 consecutive days and thereafter three times weekly for a further 2 weeks. All lesions had cleared at the end of the treatment period.

Scarification treatment of granuloma annulare. Wilkin JK, DuComb D, Castrow FF. Arch Dermatol 1982;118:68–9.

Two patients are described in whom lesions of granuloma annulare were treated successfully by scarification, using the point of a 19-gauge injection needle drawn across lesions to produce capillary bleeding. Treatment was carried out weekly for 8 weeks, and every 2–3 weeks thereafter.

Surgical pearl: surgical treatment of tumor-sized granuloma annulare of the fingers. Shelley WB, Shelley ED. J Am Acad Dermatol 1997;37:473–4.

The report is of a case of nodular granuloma annulare treated with shave excision, allowing the wound to heal by second intention.

Generalized granuloma annulare

FIRST LINE THERAPIES

■ Photochemotherapy	C
■ Systemic isotretinoin	C
■ Dapsone	C
■ Topical tacrolimus	E

Photochemotherapy of generalised granuloma annulare. Kerker BJ, Huang CP, Morison WL. Arch Dermatol 1990;126:359–61.

In this study, five patients with diffuse granuloma annulare were treated with PUVA, using oral methoxsalen, two to three times weekly. All patients cleared after a period of 3–4 months, but four relapsed after PUVA was stopped. These patients responded to further treatments.

PUVA therapy of diffuse granuloma annulare. Hindson TC, Spiro JG, Cochrane H. Clin Exp Dermatol 1988;13:26–7.

This report is of three patients who were treated with oral PUVA. Two cleared after 6 months of therapy and the third was almost clear at the end of 12 months. Only one patient achieved a longstanding remission.

There have been similar reports with oral PUVA using 5-methoxypsoralen, and also with bath PUVA and polythene sheet bath PUVA.

Resolution of disseminated granuloma annulare with isotretinoin. Schleicher SM, Milstein HJ, Lim SJ. Int J Dermatol 1992;31:371–2.

Six women treated with isotretinoin showed complete or almost complete resolution of diffuse granuloma annulare.

In the reported cases, the dose of isotretinoin used has not always been clear. After looking at a number of reports, doses tend to be about 40 mg daily, with improvement occurring after about 3 months. There is a report in which etretinate was used successfully in this condition, but none that mention acitretin.

The response of generalised granuloma annulare to dapsone. Czarnecki DB, Gin D. Acta Derm Venereol 1986;66:82–4.

Six patients with generalized granuloma annulare were treated with dapsone at a dose of 100 mg daily. All showed a complete response, with five subjects clearing within 8 weeks, and four were documented to have remained clear for 4–20 months after stopping dapsone therapy.

Sulphone treatment of granuloma annulare. Steiner A, Pehamberger H, Wolff K. J Am Acad Dermatol 1985;13:1004–8.

This study of dapsone in granuloma annulare found that while 7 of 10 patients with generalized granuloma annulare

Evidence levels A Double-blind study   B Clinical trial ≥ 20 subjects   C Clinical trial < 20 subjects   D Series ≥ 5 subjects   E Anecdotal case reports

showed a complete or partial response, all patients relapsed within 3 months of stopping dapsone.

Successful treatment of disseminated granuloma annulare with topical tacrolimus. Jain S, Stephens CJM. Br J Dermatol 2004;150:1042–3.

This report is of four patients who were treated with tacrolimus for a period of 6 weeks, during which time two showed complete clearance, maintained for at least 6 weeks, and two had marked improvement.

SECOND LINE THERAPIES

■ Cyclosporine	E
■ Systemic corticosteroids	E
■ Chlorambucil	D
■ Antimalarials	D
■ Pentoxifylline	E
■ Topical vitamin E	E
■ Nicotinamide	E
■ Fumaric acid esters	E
■ Defibrotide	E
■ Efalizumab	E

Cyclosporine in the treatment of generalised granuloma annulare (letter). Ho VC. J Am Acad Dermatol 1995;32:298.

This letter describes two patients, both of whom were treated with cyclosporine, initially at a dose of 4 mg/kg, for a period of 3 months. The first case showed complete resolution but relapsed within a month of stopping treatment; the second did not respond despite an increase in the dose of cyclosporine.

Cyclosporin for the treatment of granuloma annulare. Fiallo P. Br J Dermatol 1998;138:369–70.

Two women were treated with cyclosporine 3 mg/kg, and their granuloma annulare cleared within a month. No recurrence was noted during a follow-up period of a year.

Low-dose chlorambucil in the treatment of generalised granuloma annulare. Kossard S, Winkelmann RK. Dermatologica 1979;158:443–50.

Chlorambucil 2 mg twice daily was used to treat six patients, five of whom showed a marked improvement by 12 weeks. The authors state that chlorambucil should only be considered in refractory cases of granuloma annulare in which there is a compelling requirement for therapy, and then only used for a maximum period of 12 weeks.

Antimalarials for control of disseminated granuloma annulare in children. Simon M, von den Driesch P. J Am Acad Dermatol 1994;31:1064–5.

Six children achieved complete clearance within 4–6 weeks of starting hydroxychloroquine, and remained clear for a mean period of $2\frac{1}{2}$ years. The dose of hydroxychloroquine was 3 mg/kg daily in four subjects and 6 mg/kg daily in the other two.

Potassium iodide in the treatment of disseminated granuloma annulare. Smith JB, Hansen CD, Zone JJ. J Am Acad Dermatol 1994;30:791–2.

A double-blind, placebo-controlled, crossover trial of 10 patients concluded that oral potassium iodide does not show an advantage over placebo in the treatment of disseminated granuloma annulare.

Additional reports of responses in single cases include the following.

Generalised granuloma annulare successfully treated with pentoxifylline. Rubel DM, Wood G, Rosen R, Jopp-McKay A. Australas J Dermatol 1993;34:103–8.

Disseminated granuloma annulare: therapy with vitamin E topically. Burg G. Dermatology 1992;184:308–9.

Response of generalised granuloma annulare to high-dose niacinamide. Ma M, Medenica M. Arch Dermatol 1983; 119:836–9.

Granuloma annulare, generalised. Larralde J. Arch Dermatol 1963;87:777–8.

A case report describing the use of systemic steroids in generalized granuloma annulare.

Treatment of disseminated granuloma annulare with fumaric acid esters. Kreuter A, Gambichler T, Altmeyer A, Brockmeyer NH. BMC Dermatol 2002;2:5.

A case of disseminated granuloma annulare treated with defibrotide: complete clinical remission and progressive hair darkening. Rubegni P, Sbano P, Fimiani M. Br J Dermatol 2003;149:437–8.

Disseminated granuloma annulare resolved with the T-cell modulator efalizumab. Goffe BS. Arch Dermatol 2004; 140:1287–8.

Disseminated granuloma annulare cleared during the treatment of psoriasis with efalizumab.

Granuloma faciale

Susan E Handfield-Jones

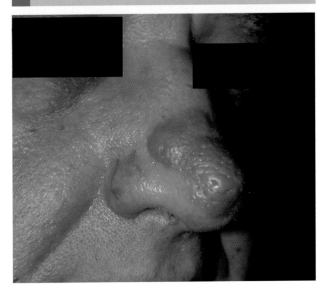

Granuloma faciale is a rare form of localized, fibrosing vasculitis, usually confined to the face. Lesions are purplish-red, but can be skin-colored or brown. With time lesions become raised plaques and nodules with accentuation of follicular openings. There are isolated reports of lesions of similar histology in the eye and upper airways.

MANAGEMENT STRATEGY

The lesions can be disfiguring, but are not usually painful, itchy, or the cause of functional problems. They grow slowly and are persistent, with documented cases of lesions remaining unchanged for 8 years. Spontaneous resolution is reported, but is very uncommon. The condition is more common in white men in middle age.

The clinical differential diagnosis includes lupus pernio, lymphocytoma cutis, persistent insect bite reactions, and lymphoma. The clinical diagnosis should be confirmed by biopsy. Histology shows a dense infiltrate in the upper dermis, sometimes extending more deeply. The epidermis is spared and there is a Grenz zone. The infiltrate is mixed, but eosinophils and neutrophils predominate. Vasculitis with leukocytoclasis is a feature, and in older lesions fibrosis is seen. Peripheral blood eosinophilia is sometimes found. The histological differential diagnosis includes erythema elevatum diutinum and angiolymphoid hyperplasia with eosinophilia.

Reports of treatment success and failure are anecdotal because of the rarity of the condition. There are no formal trials of therapy. *Intralesional corticosteroid* is often the initial treatment of choice. In patients with localized disease destructive methods such as *cryotherapy, surgery* and *laser treatment* are used. *Dapsone* and other systemic agents have been used with variable effect.

SPECIFIC INVESTIGATIONS

- Skin biopsy
- Hematology (complete blood count)

FIRST LINE THERAPIES

■ Intralesional, topical, or occluded corticosteroids	E
■ Laser therapy	E
■ Cryotherapy	E
■ Cryotherapy and intralesional corticosteroids	D
■ Surgery	E

The choice of therapy depends on the size, site, and thickness of the lesions. For patients with multiple, widespread lesions not responding to topical corticosteroids, systemic treatment, such as dapsone could be considered. A single small nodular lesion might be better treated with intralesional corticosteroid or surgical excision.

Granuloma faciale treated with intradermal dexamethasone. Arundell FD, Burdick KH. Arch Dermatol 1960;82: 437–8.

Intralesional corticosteroids are commonly referred to in texts, but there is a paucity of written data. Triamcinolone acetonide, triamcinolone hexacetonide, and dexamethasone have all been used. Patients should be warned of the risk of skin atrophy and pigment change.

Laser treatment

The majority of reports of laser treatment use the tunable dye laser. There are reports of response to argon and CO_2 laser treatment in the literature and more recently to potassium-titanyl-phosphate laser.

Granuloma faciale successfully treated with long-pulsed tuneable dye laser. Chatrath V, Rohrer TE. Dermatol Surg 2002;28:527–9.

Scar-free clearing after three treatments with no recurrence after 9 months

Treatment of granuloma faciale with pulsed dye laser. Elston DM. Cutis 2000;65:97–8.

Response to treatment in a patient refractory to topical corticosteroid and dapsone.

Treatment of granuloma faciale with the 585-nm pulsed dye laser. Ammirati CT, Hruza GJ. Arch Dermatol 1999; 135:903–5.

Two treatments with 585 nm laser resulted in complete scar-free resolution with no recurrence at 6 years.

New treatment modalities for granuloma faciale. Ludwig E, Allam J-P, Bieber T, Novak N. Br J Dermatol 2003;149:634–7.

Report of two cases of sizeable faciale lesions responding rapidly to Laserscope potassium-titanyl-phosphate 532 nm laser.

Granuloma faciale: treatment with the argon laser. Apfelberg DB, Druker D, Maser MR, et al. Arch Dermatol 1983;119:573–6.

Evidence levels A Double-blind study **B** Clinical trial ≥ 20 subjects **C** Clinical trial < 20 subjects **D** Series ≥ 5 subjects **E** Anecdotal case reports

A report of three cases, resistant to intralesional corticosteroids, responding to argon laser with no recurrence from 5 to 23 months. A 'white, collagenous scar' resulted.

Carbon dioxide laser treatment of granuloma faciale. Wheeland RG, Ashley JR, Smith DA, et al. J Dermatol Surg Oncol 1984;10:730–3.

A single treatment resulted in healing with no discernible scar. There was no recurrence at 1 year.

Cryosurgery effective for granuloma faciale. Zacarian SA. J Dermatol Surg Oncol 1985;11:11–3.

The lesion resolved in 4 weeks after open spray cryosurgery using a single freeze–thaw cycle, 1 min freeze, and did not recur for 10 years. The lesion was biopsy proven and had not responded to several intralesional injections of triamcinolone.

Granuloma faciale: successful treatment of nine cases with a combination of cryotherapy and intralesional corticosteroid injection. Dowlati B, Firooz A, Dowlati Y. Int J Dermatol 1997;36:548–51.

Cryotherapy for 20–30 s was followed immediately with triamcinolone acetonide 5 mg/mL intralesionally. Treatment was repeated every 3 weeks. The total number of treatments given varied from patient to patient.

Recurrent facial plaques following full-thickness grafting. Phillips DK, Hymes SR. Arch Dermatol 1994;130:1436–7.

Surgery is mentioned in many papers, but recurrence can occur, even following full-thickness excision and grafting.

Granuloma faciale: comparison of different treatment modalities. Dinehart SM, Gross DJ, Davis CM, Herzberg AJ. Arch Otolaryngol Head Neck Surg 1990;116:849–51.

Combined electrosurgery and dermabrasion was compared with CO_2 laser treatment in a patient with two similar lesions. Skin texture at 6 weeks was better in the laser treated side, but laser treatment was more time consuming.

SECOND LINE THERAPIES

■ Dapsone	E
■ Topical tacrolimus 0.1%	E

On the efficacy of dapsone in granuloma faciale. Van de Kerkhof PCM. Acta Derm Venereol 1994;74:61–2.

A 4 cm plaque showed 'impressive improvement' with dapsone 200 mg daily. Dapsone needs care with monitoring and many patients would not tolerate 200 mg daily.

Many authors mention dapsone as a treatment that has been tried but failed.

New treatment modalities for granuloma faciale. Ludwig E, Allam J-P, Bieber T, Novak N. Br J Dermatol 2003;149:634–7.

A single case of extensive lesions on the forehead showing partial response to treatment with topical tacrolimus.

THIRD LINE THERAPIES

■ Clofazimine	E
■ Topical psoralen with UVA (PUVA)	E

Granuloma faciale mimicking rhinophyma: response to clofazimine. Gomez-de la Fuente E, del Rio R, Guerra A, et al. Acta Derm Venereol 2000;80:144.

A patient with a 10-year history of a plaque on the nose with histological diagnosis of granuloma faciale was treated with 300 mg clofazimine once daily for 5 months with 'remarkable improvement'. Two similar reports are cited.

Granuloma faciale: treatment with topical psoralen and UVA. Hudson LD. J Am Acad Dermatol 1983;8:559.

Marked improvement resulted from 24 J/cm² UVA given over 10 weeks, with no evidence of residual lesion at 6 months.

OTHER THERAPIES

There are reports of treatment with intralesional gold and bismuth, radiotherapy, oral colchicine, isoniazid, potassium arsenite, testosterone, and antimalarials, but within the past 25 years there are no reports of successful response to these agents.

Granuloma inguinale

Patrice Morel

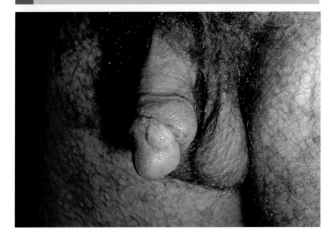

Granuloma inguinale (donovanosis), is an infection causing progressive granulomatous ulceration of the genital, inguinal, and perineal skin. It is extremely rare in Western Europe and in the USA, but is still endemic or epidemic in India, South Africa, and Brazil, and among aborigines in Australia. The causative organism is *Calymmatobacterium granulomatis* (an intracellular Gram-negative bacillus). Transmission of this infection is frequently, but not exclusively, sexual.

MANAGEMENT STRATEGY

Patients with donovanosis should be treated

- to prevent the gradual development of the disease that may lead to genital deformity or a life-threatening disseminated infection;
- to prevent transmission to sexual partners;
- to prevent the risk of concomitant transmission of HIV.

In the absence of randomized controlled trials, antibiotic treatment of donovanosis is based on the results of clinical experience and individual reports, usually involving relatively small numbers of patients.

Trimethoprim–sulfamethoxazole or *doxycycline* is recommended by the Centers for Disease Control and Prevention (CDC) (2002). *Azithromycin* is recommended in the Australian Antibiotic Guidelines (1996–7). Many other antibiotics are also effective (e.g. *ciprofloxacin, ceftriaxone, erythromycin*). The addition of an *aminoglycoside (gentamicin)* is recommended by the CDC if lesions do not respond within the first few days of therapy.

The therapy should be continued until all lesions have healed completely (except for the 4-week azithromycin regimen). A relapse may occur 6–18 months later despite effective initial therapy. Surgical excision may be necessary for extensive disease unresponsive to medical treatment.

Sexual partners of patients who have granuloma inguinale should be examined and treated if they:

- had sexual contact with the patient during the 60 days preceding the onset of symptoms in the patient, and

- have clinical signs and symptoms of the disease (CDC, 1998).

SPECIFIC INVESTIGATIONS

- Microscopic evaluation of either tissue smears or biopsy specimen stained with Wright's or Giemsa stain
- Culture in human peripheral blood monocytes and in Hep-2 cells
- Polymerase chain reaction (PCR) test

Genital ulcer disease: accuracy of clinical diagnosis and strategies to improve control in Durban, South Africa. O'Farrell N, Hoosen AA, Coetzee KD, Van den Ende J. Genitourin Med 1994;70:7–11.

One hundred men and 100 women with genital ulcers were recruited to investigate the accuracy of clinical diagnosis in genital ulcer disease (GUD). The clinical diagnostic accuracy for donovanosis was relatively high (63% in men, 83% in women). When compared with other causes of GUD, donovanosis ulcers bled to the touch, were larger, and were not usually associated with inguinal lymphadenopathy.

Donovanosis. Hart G. Clin Infect Dis 1997;25:24–32.

For laboratory confirmation of donovanosis, the preferred method involves demonstration of typical intracellular Donovan bodies within large mononuclear cells that are visualized in smears prepared from lesions or biopsy specimens. The large mononuclear cells are 25–90 μm in diameter, with a vesicular or pyknotic nucleus. There are around 20 intracytoplasmic vacuoles containing pleomorphic Donovan bodies in either young noncapsulated or mature capsulated forms.

Culture of the causative organism of donovanosis (*Calymmatobacterium granulomatis*) in Hep-2 cells. Carter J, Hutton S, Sriprakash KS, et al. J Clin Microbiol 1997;35: 2915–17.

With the positive culture of *C. granulomatis* in Hep-2 cells, it is now possible to test in-vitro susceptibility of *C. granulomatis* to antibiotics and to provide a ready source of DNA and antigenic material to enable the development of serological tests and possibly, in the future, a vaccine.

A colorimetric detection system for *Calymmatobacterium granulomatis*. Carter JS, Kemp DJ. Sex Transm Infect 2000; 76:134–6.

A colorimetric PCR test was developed that could be used by well-equipped diagnostic laboratories. Molecular techniques should help to answer some remaining questions about donovanosis (e.g. nonsexual contamination, autoinoculation).

Granuloma inguinale. Rosen T, Tschen JA, Ramsdell W, et al. J Am Acad Dermatol 1984;11:433–7.

A report of 20 cases of granuloma inguinale in Houston, Texas. Evidence supports the venereal transmission of the infection. Three heterosexual patients had intercourse with the same prostitute during a single evening and all developed lesions 2 weeks later. The occurrence of donovanosis in young children and the low prevalence of the disease among sexual partners are cited as evidence against sexual transmission in some cases.

Evidence levels A Double-blind study   **B** Clinical trial ≥ 20 subjects   **C** Clinical trial < 20 subjects   **D** Series ≥ 5 subjects   **E** Anecdotal case reports

Infants born to infected mothers may acquire infection at birth and develop lesions of the umbilicus and sexual organs as well as disseminated infection.

Donovanosis. Seghal VN, Sharma HK. J Dermatol 1992;19: 32–46.

Although genitalia are the sites of primary lesions most frequently encountered, many cases report extragenital lesions due to autoinoculation, direct contiguous spread, or spread via the blood stream to the bones, joints, lung, liver, and spleen.

Donovanosis. O'Farell N. Sex Transm Infect 2002;78:452–7.

The donovanosis elimination programme among Aboriginals in Australia appears successful and is a model that could be adopted in other donovanosis endemic areas.

FIRST LINE THERAPIES

■ Azithromycin 500 mg orally daily for 7 days or 1 g orally weekly for 4 weeks	B
■ Erythromycin 500 mg orally four times daily for at least 3 weeks	B
■ Trimethoprim–sulfamethoxazole one double-strength tablet orally twice daily for at least 3 weeks	B

Donovanosis: treatment with azithromycin. Bowden FJ, Savage J. Int J STD AIDS 1998;9:61.

Australian authors say that they have treated over 100 patients with donovanosis with azithromycin with no primary treatment failures. They recommend two treatment regimens: 500 mg orally daily for 7 days or 1 g orally weekly for 4 weeks. The 1996–7 edition of the Australian Antibiotic Guidelines lists azithromycin as the first-line agent for donovanosis. The drug is listed as a B1 agent in pregnancy, meaning that it can be used for the treatment of antenatal patients with the disease.

Clinico-epidemiologic features of granuloma inguinale in the era of acquired immune deficiency syndrome. Jamkhedkar PP, Hira SK, Shroff HJ, Lanjewar DN. Sex Transm Dis 1998;25:196–200.

Indian authors treated 50 patients with granuloma inguinale (21 HIV positive and 29 HIV negative) with their 'standard treatment regimen' of erythromycin 2 g orally daily. The ulcers took longer to heal in the seropositive group (mean 25.7 vs 16.8 days).

Erythromycin is less convenient to administer than azithromycin.

Granuloma inguinale. Rosen T, Tschen JA, Ramsdell W, Moore J, Markham B. J Am Acad Dermatol 1984;11:433–7.

Twenty patients with granuloma inguinale were treated with trimethoprim–sulfamethoxazole. The drug proved to be a safe and effective therapy. It is currently recommended for a minimum of 3 weeks by the CDC.

Trimethoprim–sulfamethoxazole has been used extensively in India, with consistently good results.

SECOND LINE THERAPIES

■ Doxycycline 100 mg orally twice daily for at least 3 weeks	C
■ Ciprofloxacin 750 mg orally twice daily	C

National guidelines for the management of donovanosis (granuloma inguinale). Clinical Effectiveness Group. Sex Transm Infect 1999;75(suppl 1):S38–9.

Doxycycline has not been individually assessed prospectively and recommendations are based on trials carried out with older tetracyclines, which are assumed to be equivalent to doxycycline, which is chosen for more convenient twice daily dosing. Doxycycline is also recommended by the CDC (2002).

Treatment of donovanosis with norfloxacin. Ramanan CR, Sarma PSA, Ghorpade A, Das M. Int J Dermatol 1990;29: 298–9.

Ten patients with donovanosis were treated with norfloxacin in an oral dose of 400 mg twice daily. The time taken for complete healing was 2–11 days. The CDC recommends ciprofloxacin rather than norfloxacin as an alternative regimen.

THIRD LINE THERAPIES

■ Ceftriaxone 1 g intramuscularly daily	C
■ Gentamicin 1 mg/kg intravenously every 8 h	C
■ Surgical treatment	E

Ceftriaxone in the treatment of chronic donovanosis in Central Australia. Merianos A, Gilles M, Chuah J. Genitourin Med 1994;70:84–9.

Eight women and four men with chronic (mean duration 3 years) donovanosis were treated with a single daily injection of 1 g ceftriaxone diluted in 2 mL of 1% lidocaine. Clinical improvement was dramatic in most lesions and four patients healed completely without recurrence after a total 7–10 g of ceftriaxone. The drug is safe in pregnancy.

1998 Guidelines for treatment of sexually transmitted diseases. Centers for Disease Control and Prevention. MMWR Recomm Rep 1998;47(RR-1):1–116.

The CDC recommends the addition of an aminoglycoside (gentamicin) if lesions do not respond within the first few days of therapy.

Surgical treatment of granuloma inguinale. Bozbora A, Erbil Y, Berber E, Ozarmagan S. Br J Dermatol 1998;138: 1079–81.

Longstanding and complicated disease (multiple fistulas and abscesses unresponsive to antibiotics) may require surgical treatment.

SPECIAL CONSIDERATIONS

- ■ Pregnancy
- ■ HIV infection

Pregnant and lactating women should be treated with the erythromycin or azithromycin regimens.

People with HIV infection should be treated following the regimens cited above. The addition of gentamicin should be considered.

Granulomatous cheilitis

Julia E Haimowitz, Linda Y Hwang

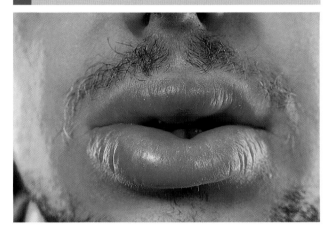

Orofacial granulomatosis describes a clinical entity of recurrent, persistent orofacial swelling with histologic evidence of noncaseating granulomatous inflammation. Orofacial swelling most commonly involves the lips and is known as granulomatous cheilitis (CG) or Miescher's cheilitis granulomatosa. Melkersson–Rosenthal syndrome (MRS) describes the triad of recurrent orofacial edema, recurrent facial nerve palsy, and lingua plicata (fissured tongue). Monosymptomatic CG or oligosymptomatic forms of MRS are recognized.

MANAGEMENT STRATEGY

The dermatologic treatment of MRS predominantly involves therapy for CG. Because the etiology of MRS/CG is unknown, a variety of therapeutic strategies have been attempted. No randomized clinical trial comparisons have been performed. Rarely, spontaneous remissions of CG have been reported.

Treatment of CG is directed at preventing permanent labial deformity. Conservative measures for acute CG include *cold compresses* and *oral antihistamines* for reducing edema and *ointments* to protect against fissuring of the lips. Most therapeutic regimens include *corticosteroid therapy*, either topical, intralesional, or systemic, as an initial empiric therapy. Responses are generally favorable, but temporary.

Mild cases of CG may improve with *triamcinolone* or *clobetaso*l in Orabase®. Triamcinolone acetonide 10 mg/mL injections at doses ranging from 0.5–1.5 mL per lip at weekly or biweekly intervals are helpful. In resistant cases, the concentration of triamcinolone can be increased to 20 mg/mL. Nerve blocks may be used to limit discomfort from infiltration of corticosteroids, thus allowing higher-volume injections. Systemic corticosteroids are rarely indicated. However, in those patients with severe edema or those who fail to respond to intralesional therapy, short courses of prednisone 40–60 mg daily for 3–6 weeks can be beneficial. The addition of *minocycline* 100 mg twice daily or *tetracycline* 500 mg daily to prednisone therapy may prevent disease rebound after corticosteroid therapy is discontinued.

Clofazamine may be tried when a patient becomes dependent upon or fails to respond to corticosteroids. The patient should be informed about side effects such as transient orange-pink skin discoloration, nausea, and vomiting. Fatal enteropathy, the most severe side effect, usually occurs at much higher doses than those recommended for CG. Monotherapy with *metronidazole*, *hydroxychloroquine*, or *thalidomide*, although less well substantiated, can be attempted.

The chronic and recurrent nature of CG may lead to permanent lip swelling. Patients with permanent esthetic deformity or functional impairment may benefit from *cheiloplasty*, but should be advised that surgery may not be curative. Surgery should only be performed when more conservative approaches have failed and when the disease is quiescent. Many authors recommend *postoperative intralesional corticosteroids* to minimize recurrence.

There is an extensive differential diagnosis for CG (see below). The clinician must be aware that CG may be an initial manifestation of Crohn's disease or sarcoidosis and a systemic evaluation should be performed when indicated. A search for underlying odontogenic infections or allergenic sensitizers should be undertaken.

SPECIFIC INVESTIGATIONS

- Biopsy for histopathologic examination, polarization, and stains/cultures for fungi and acid-fast bacilli
- Complete blood count, and chemistry profile, including serum calcium
- Angiotensin-converting enzyme level
- Chest radiograph
- C1-esterase inhibitor, C1-esterase inhibitor functional assay, C1, C2, and C4 levels
- Consultation with dental professional, if odontogenic infection suspected
- Consultation with gastroenterologist, if malabsorption or enteritis suspected
- Patch testing and food allergy testing

Cheilitis granulomatosa. van der Waal RIF, Schulten EAJM, van de Scheur MR, et al. Eur Acad Dermatol Venereol 2001; 15:519–23.

Melkersson–Rosenthal syndrome: a review of 36 patients. Greene RM, Rogers RS III. J Am Acad Dermatol 1989;21: 1263–70.

Orofacial granulomatosis. Armstrong DKB, Burrows D. Int J Dermatol 1995;34:830–3.

These articles review MRS and discuss possible etiologies and differential diagnoses. The differential diagnosis of facial edema includes sarcoidosis, Crohn's disease, hereditary angioedema, anaphylaxis, infectious granulomas, erysipelas, chronic herpes simplex labialis, dentoalveolar abscess, contact dermatitis, lymphatic/venous obstruction, double lip, Ascher's syndrome, eosinophilic fasciitis, facial edema with eosinophilia, mucocele, hemangioma, lymphangioma, and neoplastic infiltrates. A careful history and physical examination, in addition to the specific investigations listed, may disclose an etiologic factor. If intestinal symptoms or biochemical evidence of malabsorption exist, a gastrointestinal work-up for Crohn's disease is recommended.

Melkersson–Rosenthal syndrome and cheilitis granulomatosa. A clinicopathologic study of thirty-three patients with special reference to their oral lesions. Worsaae N, Christensen KC, Schiødt M, Reibel J. Oral Surg Oral Med Oral Pathol 1982;54:404–13.

The elimination of odontogenic infectious foci led to inactivity of orofacial edema over a 3-month period in 11 of 16 patients.

Contact hypersensitivity in patients with orofacial granulomatosis. Armstrong DKB, Biagonia P, Lamey, Burrows D. Am J Contact Dermat 1997;1:35–8.

In this study, 48 patients were investigated and ten showed positive reactions to an oral battery on standard patch testing. Of these ten, seven showed an improvement on an elimination diet. In most cases, this was not a complete result. Improvement was noted from 2 weeks to 4 months after commencing the elimination diet.

A subgroup of patients with CG may have a sensitivity to an identifiable agent. Implicated allergens include cinnamon, cinnamaldehyde, benzoic acid, sodium benzoate, tartrazine, piperitone, carvone, carmoisine, sunset yellow, monosodium glutamate, cobalt, and others. In selected patients, patch testing (including an oral series) and an elimination diet may be beneficial.

FIRST LINE THERAPIES

■ Intralesional corticosteroids	C
■ Oral corticosteroids	C

Management of cheilitis granulomatosa. Williams PM, Greenberg MS. Oral Surg Oral Med Oral Pathol 1991;72: 436–9.

CG of the lower lip was successfully managed with intralesional triamcinolone hexacetonide 20 mg/mL. Doses of 2–3 mL were injected into 10 to 15 sites on the lower lip weekly for 4 weeks, biweekly for 1 month, monthly for 2 months, and bimonthly for 4 months.

Triamcinolone acetonide 0.05–10 mg/mL injections at weekly to monthly intervals can be effective.

Intralesional steroid injection after nerve block anesthesia in the treatment of orofacial granulomatosis. Sakuntabhai A, MacLeod RI, Lawrence CM. Arch Dermatol 1993;129:477–80.

Mental and infraorbital nerve blocks permitted the painless introduction of high-volume intralesional triamcinolone acetonide 10 mg/mL (3.0–3.5 mL for one lip, 5–10 mL for both lips) in five patients with orofacial granulomatosis. Of the three patients available for follow-up, all experienced return to near normal lip size within 6 weeks of therapy, though one patient required four treatments over a 2-year period.

No studies comparing high-dose to low-dose intralesional corticosteroids exist. Increasing the concentration of triamcinolone used is an alternative to high-volume injections.

Melkersson–Rosenthal syndrome and orofacial granulomatosis. Rogers RS III. Dermatol Clin 1996;14:371–9.

Occasional short courses of systemic corticosteroids may be used for more severe and symptomatic episodes of CG. Oral prednisone 1–1.5 mg/kg daily tapered over 3–6 weeks may be effective.

SECOND LINE THERAPIES

■ Clofazamine	C
■ Oral corticosteroids and minocycline/tetracyline	E

Cheilitis granulomatosa Miescher: treatment with clofazamine and review of the literature. Ridder GJ, Fradis M, Löhle E. Ann Otol Rhinol Laryngol 2001;110:964–7.

The authors present the case of a 15-year-old girl whose lip swelling was treated with clofazamine 100 mg daily. Regression of swelling was noted after 30 days of treatment. Thereafter, 100 mg of clofazimine three times a week was given for 3 months. Her lip eventually returned to normal size. The patient was followed up for 6 years with no recurrence of the disease.

This article reviews multiple case reports and small case series of clofazamine therapy. There was great variability in the response to clofazamine therapy.

Melkersson–Rosenthal syndrome: clinical, pathologic, and therapeutic considerations. Sussman GL, Yang WH, Steinberg S. Ann Allergy 1992;69:187–94.

Clofazimine 100 mg four times weekly for 3–11 months was used to treat ten patients with chronic lip edema associated with MRS. Complete remissions occurred in five of ten patients, partial clinical responses occurred in three of ten patients, and two patients had no clinical response.

Other studies have reported efficacy with a regimen consisting of clofazimine 100 mg daily for 10 days, followed by 200–400 mg weekly for 3–6 months.

Melkersson–Rosenthal syndrome in childhood: successful management with combination steroid and minocycline therapy. Stein SL, Mancini AJ. J Am Acad Dermatol 1999; 41:746–8.

A 12-year-old girl with orofacial granulomatosis and a fissured tongue, and a 10-year-old boy with orofacial granulomatosis were successfully treated with the combination of prednisone 0.6–1.0 mg/kg daily and minocycline 100 mg twice daily. Prednisone was tapered over 2–4 months during continuous minocycline therapy.

The authors' experience with monotherapy in MRS included treatment failures with minocycline and rapid rebound with prednisone discontinuation.

Chronic lip edema with particular reference to the Melkersson–Rosenthal syndrome (MRS). Fisher AA. Cutis 1990;45:144–6.

Prednisone 10 mg on alternate days and tetracycline 500 mg daily, given for 2.5 years, led to a 60% reduction in lip edema in a 29-year-old patient with MRS.

THIRD LINE THERAPIES

■ Cheiloplasty with postoperative intralesional corticosteroids	C
■ Thalidomide	E
■ Metronidazole	E
■ Hydroxychloroquine	E
■ Tranilast	E
■ Danazol	E

Evidence levels **A** Double-blind study **B** Clinical trial ≥ 20 subjects **C** Clinical trial < 20 subjects **D** Series ≥ 5 subjects **E** Anecdotal case reports

Cheilitis granulomatosa: successful treatment with combined local triamcinolone injections and surgery. Krutchkoff D, James R. Arch Dermatol 1978;114:1203–6.

A man with CG for 15 years was treated with triamcinolone acetonide injections 10 mg/mL over 6 months, followed by upper and lower cheiloplasty; 4 months later, repeat cheiloplasty of the upper lip revealed granulomas that were more numerous and larger than those observed on initial biopsy. Postoperative corticosteroid injections at biweekly and then monthly intervals maintained remission. The authors recommend that corticosteroid injections be continued postoperatively to prevent exaggerated recurrences.

Once clinical stability is reached, corticosteroid injections at 4–6-month intervals may be appropriate.

Long-term results after surgical reduction cheiloplasty in patients with Melkersson–Rosenthal syndrome and cheilitis granulomatosa. Ellitsgaard N, Andersson AP, Worsaae N, Medgyesi S. Ann Plast Surg 1993;31:413–20.

A reduction cheiloplasty was performed on 13 patients (seven with MRS, six with CG) due to permanent labial swelling, and a follow-up study was done 16 years later (median). All 13 patients were satisfied with their results, despite postoperative disease activity in six patients.

Lip reduction cheiloplasty for Miescher's granulomatous macrocheilitis (cheilitis granulomatosa) in childhood. Oliver DW, Scott MJL. Clin Exp Dermatol 2002;27:129–31.

Lip reduction cheiloplasty provided successful treatment of CG in an 11-year-old boy. The child had physical improvement after surgery, as well as a considerable gain in his self-confidence. The authors describe the development of lip tissue, suggesting that surgery can be safely undertaken in young children, if necessary.

The surgical management of Melkersson–Rosenthal syndrome. Glickman LT, Gruss JS, Birt BD, Kohli-Dang N. Plast Reconstr Surg 1992;89:815–21.

Treatment of Miescher's cheilitis granulomatosa in Melkersson–Rosenthal syndrome. Camacho F, Garcia-Bravo, Carrizosa A. Eur Acad Derm Venereol 2001;15:546–9.

The authors conclude that the best treatment for resistant CG is surgery with immediate injection of triamcinolone, followed by a course of oral tetracycline.

Melkersson–Rosenthal syndrome: reduction cheiloplasty utilizing a transmodiolar labial suspension suture. Cederna PS, Fiala TGS, Smith DJ, Newman MH. Aesth Plast Surg 1998;22:102–5.

Successful treatment of granulomatous cheilitis with thalidomide. Thomas P, Walchner M, Ghoreschi K, Rocken M. Arch Dermatol 2003;139:136–8.

A 39-year-old woman with CG was initially treated with clofazimine at 200 mg daily, but developed a morbilliform eruption 2 weeks into therapy. Her condition failed to respond to other conventional therapies, necessitating another therapeutic option. As tumor necrosis factor (TNF)-α is a key chemokine found in most types of acute and chronic inflammation, thalidomide was considered as a treatment. The patient was treated with thalidomide 100 mg daily orally for 6 months and the lip swelling almost completely resolved. Thalidomide treatment was then reduced to 100 mg every other day for 2 months, with no recurrence observed. Therapy was stopped and the patient remained without signs of relapse for 1 year.

The potential for serious adverse effects on thalidomide therapy, including teratogenicity and peripheral neuropathy, necessitates close patient observation.

Cheilitis granulomatosa treated with metronidazole. Miralles J, Barnadas MA, de Moragas JM. Dermatology 1995;191:252–3.

A 30-year-old woman with monosymptomatic MRS and a negative gastrointestinal work-up was successfully treated with metronidazole 750–1000 mg daily for an 8-month tapering course.

Metronidazole has also been useful in two patients with CG associated with Crohn's disease. Treatment failures are also reported.

Cheilitis granulomatosa: report of six cases and review of the literature. Allen CM, Camisa C, Hamzeh S, Stephens L. J Am Acad Dermatol 1990;23:444–50.

Decreased swelling was observed in both lips of a patient with CG after treatment with hydroxychloroquine 200 mg daily for 3 months, followed by 400 mg daily for 3 months. Complete reduction of the lip size to normal did not occur and other forms of treatment were necessary.

Hydroxychloroquine has been reported to be efficacious in CG associated with Crohn's disease. Chloroquine therapy has not been successful in MRS.

Successful treatment of cheilitis granulomatosa with tranilast. Kato T, Tagami H. J Dermatol 1986;13:402–3.

Tranilast, an anti-allergic agent, was administered orally at a dose of 240 mg daily to a 46-year-old woman with CG. Three weeks after initiation of therapy, improvement was noted. Lip swelling was dramatically suppressed and no recurrence was noted during the following 12 months.

This case report is from Japan. Tranilast is not widely available.

Danazol. Madanes AE, Farber M. Ann Intern Med 1982;96:625–30.

In one case, danazol was reported to improve MRS (personal communication).

While danazol is useful in hereditary angioedema by increasing hepatic synthesis of C1 esterase inhibitor, it is unclear how it would affect a granulomatous disease. Anecdotal accounts of treatment failures with danazol are also reported.

Hailey–Hailey disease

Robin AC Graham-Brown, Susan M Burge

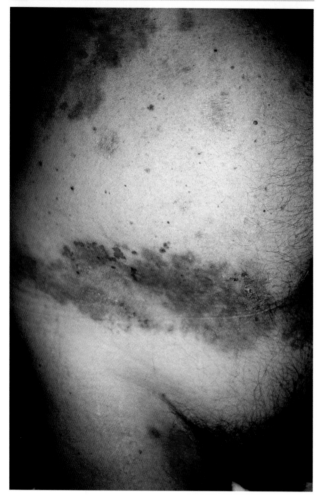

Hailey–Hailey disease is a rare blistering disorder first described by two medical brothers in 1939 and characterized by recurrent vesicles and erosions, particularly involving flexural areas. Signs may appear for the first time from the late teens to the third or fourth decades. The disease is generally of relatively limited extent, though widespread and severe involvement can occur. The most commonly affected sites are the axillae, groins, intertriginous areas such as the inframammary folds, and the neck. Lesions may also occur on the trunk and in the antecubital and popliteal fossae. A seborrheic dermatitis-like involvement of the scalp has also been described.

Hailey–Hailey disease is a dominantly inherited condition caused by a primary defect in a Ca^{2+} pump mechanism. There are clinical and histopathologic similarities with Darier's disease (see page 143) and Grover's disease (see page 661).

MANAGEMENT STRATEGY

The lesions of Hailey–Hailey disease are frequently precipitated by friction. Infection with various bacteria, yeasts, and viruses also appears to be an aggravating factor in some patients. Thus, avoidance of precipitating trauma and skin infections can help to reduce the frequency and severity of outbreaks.

Simple anti-infective agents, topical or systemic, reduce the severity of exacerbations and remain the mainstay of treatment. Topical *tetracyclines, fusidic acid,* and *imidazoles* have all been recommended. *Tetracyclines* are probably the best systemic agents. If secondary infection with herpes simplex is suspected, *appropriate antiviral therapy* should be instituted.

Combining anti-infective therapy with *topical corticosteroids* seems to be particularly helpful, but corticosteroids alone may reduce the severity of lesions. Generally, moderate to potent agents are required, though some patients gain benefit from milder preparations. Caution should be exercised with long-term use because the axillae and groins are prone to atrophy. The use of the topical calcineurin inhibitor *tacrolimus,* either alone or in combination with topical corticosteroids, has recently been reported to be effective and is certainly worth trying. Some success has also been recorded with *calcitriol.*

Patients with Hailey–Hailey disease are at high risk of developing contact allergic dermatitis, and patch testing should be performed if there is a poor response to therapy.

At one time, *superficial (Grenz) rays* were in vogue, but access is now difficult.

Patients with major exacerbations may benefit from a *short course of systemic corticosteroids,* but control seldom lasts, and there may be a rebound of the disease on withdrawal.

Systemic alternatives that have been tried in severe disease include *dapsone, cyclosporine, methotrexate,* and *retinoids,* but there is little evidence for their effectiveness beyond anecdotal case reports.

There may be a place for surgical approaches to disease of limited extent, including *excision and grafting, dermabrasion, CO_2 laser vaporization,* and the use of *botulinum toxin* to reduce sweating.

SPECIFIC INVESTIGATIONS

- Biopsy
- Microbiologic cultures for bacteria, yeast, and herpes virus
- Consider patch testing to topical medicaments

FIRST LINE THERAPIES

■ Anti-infectives and antibiotics	C
■ Topical corticosteroids	C

Hailey–Hailey disease: the clinical features, response to treatment and prognosis. Burge SM. Br J Dermatol 1992; 126:275–82.

In this series 86% of patients found combinations of topical corticosteroids and anti-infective agents helpful, especially if they were started as soon as the patient noticed the onset of discomfort.

This is an excellent article and remains a key review of clinical and therapeutic aspects of Hailey–Hailey disease.

SECOND LINE THERAPIES

■ Tacrolimus	E
■ Calcitriol	E
■ Systemic corticosteroids	E
■ Dapsone	E
■ Cyclosporine	E

Topical tacrolimus ointment is an effective therapy for Hailey–Hailey disease. Sand C, Thomsen HK. Arch Dermatol 2003;139:1401–2.

Treatment of Hailey–Hailey disease with tacrolimus ointment and clobetasol propionate foam. Umar SA, Bhattacharjee P, Brodell RT. J Drugs Dermatol 2004;3:200–3.

The authors recommend alternating clobetasol and tacrolimus.

Treatment of Hailey–Hailey disease with topical calcitriol. Bianchi L, Chimenti M, Giunta A. J Am Acad Dermatol 2004;51:475–6.

Generalized Hailey–Hailey disease. Marsch WC, Stüttgen G. Br J Dermatol 1978;99:553.

The use of systemic corticosteroids was successful in controlling particularly extensive Hailey–Hailey disease, but cessation of therapy resulted in significant rebound of the disease.

Benign familial chronic pemphigus treated with dapsone. Sire DJ, Johnson BL. Arch Dermatol 1971;103:262.

Topical cyclosporine in chronic benign familial pemphigus (Hailey–Hailey disease). Jitsukawa K, Ring J, Weyer U, et al. J Am Acad Dermatol 1992;27:625–6.

Benign familial pemphigus responsive to cyclosporin, a possible role for cellular immunity in pathogenesis. Ormerod AD, Duncan J, Stankler L. Br J Dermatol 1991;124:299–300.

Benign familial chronic pemphigus (Hailey–Hailey disease) responds to cyclosporin. Berth-Jones J, Smith SG, Graham-Brown RA. Clin Exp Dermatol 1995;20:70–2.

These papers report small numbers or individual case reports of apparent success. Tacrolimus and calcitriol are at least safe. Dapsone is generally safe and may be worth a try. Cyclosporine has a long, daunting list of side effects, but can be used safely if doses do not exceed 5 mg/kg and patients are properly monitored.

THIRD LINE THERAPIES

■ Surgical excision	E
■ Dermabrasion	E
■ CO$_2$ laser therapy	E
■ Botulinum toxin A	E
■ Grenz rays	D
■ Methotrexate	E
■ Oral retinoids	E

Surgical eradication of familial benign chronic pemphigus from the axillae. Shelley WB, Randall P. Arch Dermatol 1969;100:275.

Dermabrasion of Hailey–Hailey disease. Zachariae H. J Am Acad Dermatol 1992;27:136.

Familial benign chronic pemphigus (Hailey–Hailey disease): treatment with carbon dioxide laser vaporization. Kartamaa M, Reitamo S. Arch Dermatol 1992;128:646.

Surgery must remain a last resort in this condition, especially as the authors themselves report some recurrences, either around the edges of the treated areas or on further friction or trauma.

Intracutaneous botulinum toxin A versus ablative therapy of Hailey–Hailey disease – a case report. Konrad H, Karamfilov T, Wollina U. J Cosmet Laser Ther 2001;3:181–4.

A single report using intracutaneous botulinum toxin A in a standard fashion as used to treat hyperhidrosis. Remission occurred.

Botulinum toxin type A for the treatment of axillary Hailey–Hailey disease. Lapiere JC, Hirsh A, Gordon KB, et al. Dermatol Surg 2000;26:371–4.

After one treatment with a low dose of botulinum toxin type A, partial improvement of the treated axilla was observed. With subsequent treatment of both axillae with the recommended dose for axillary hyperhidrosis, a sustained complete remission of the disease in the treated axillae was seen.

Grenz-ray treatment of familial benign chronic pemphigus. Sarkany I. Br J Dermatol 1959;71:247.

Methotrexate for intractable benign familial chronic pemphigus. Fairris GM, White JE, Leppard BJ, Goodwin PG. Br J Dermatol 1986;115:640.

A single report of a patient with extensive disease resistant to topical corticosteroids and antibiotics, responding to methotrexate at a dose of 15 mg a week.

Vesiculobullous Hailey–Hailey disease: successful treatment with oral retinoids. Hunt MJ, Salisbury EL, Painter DM, Lee S. Australas J Dermatol 1996;37:196–8.

A single case of generalized vesiculobullous Hailey–Hailey eruption. His past history revealed classical symptoms of limited Hailey–Hailey disease for 34 years. Various therapeutic modalities including topical and oral antibiotics, oral prednisone, and dapsone failed to achieve sustained remission. Treatment with low-dose oral etretinate (25 mg daily) produced marked clinical improvement with complete suppression of new vesicle formation after 6 weeks.

Hemangiomas

Adelaide A Hebert, Yuchi C Chang

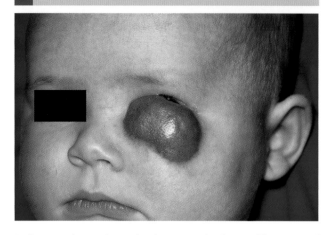

A hemangioma is a benign neoplastic proliferation of endothelial cells and is the most common soft tissue tumor of infancy. The incidence of hemangiomas in a general newborn nursery is between 1 and 2.6%, but may be as high as 10% in the Caucasian population. Hemangiomas occur four times more frequently in female infants and also demonstrate a predilection for premature infants.

MANAGEMENT STRATEGY

Approximately 55% of hemangiomas present at birth, with the remainder arising in the first weeks of life. Initially, mature cutaneous hemangiomas grow rapidly for the first 3–9 months. After this characteristic proliferative phase, the lesions typically cease growing at 18 months of age, and subsequent spontaneous involution is the rule. Most will involute slowly over a period of 2–6 years, usually completing the process by age 7–10 years. About half of the children with hemangiomas will have normal skin after involution, but the rest may have residual changes, including telangiectasias, atrophy, fibrofatty residuum, and scarring. Therefore, for the majority of uncomplicated hemangiomas, treatment typically consists of *active nonintervention*. This involves a thorough explanation of the pathogenesis and natural history of the hemangioma to the patient and parents with close follow-up visits.

It is important to differentiate benign, common hemangiomas from other vascular anomalies because the pathophysiology, treatment modalities, and prognoses are significantly different. Vascular malformations and tumors such as the kaposiform hemangioendothelioma (KE), and tufted angioma (TA) differ from hemangioma in clinical and histological appearance as well as growth rate and involutional tendencies. In particular, KE and TA are associated with the Kasabach–Merritt syndrome and its accompanying coagulopathy, whereas common hemangiomas are not. Recent studies in immunoreactivity have shown that hemangiomas express high endothelial immunoreactivity for GLUT1, a glucose transporter protein present in the brain, retina, and placenta, but absent from vascular malformations. In addition, hemangiomas are highly immunoreactive for FcγRII, merosin, and Lewis Y antigens, markers present in placental chorionic villi, but absent from

normal skin, granulation tissue, pyogenic granulomas, or vascular malformations. The majority of common hemangiomas occur as solitary lesions, but organ system involvement or, rarely, syndromes such as diffuse neonatal hemangiomatosis and PHACES (posterior fossa malformation, hemangiomas, cardiac anomalies, eye abnormalities, and sternal cleft/supraumbilical raphe) can also occur.

Although the natural course of hemangiomas is self-limited, treatment is probably indicated for approximately 25%, including the 5% that ulcerate and the 20% that may compress, obstruct, or distort vital structures, such as the larynx, eyes, ears, and nose. Local treatment of ulcerative lesions includes gentle cleansing, application of *topical antibiotics*, and occasional *wet-to-dry dressings*. *Occlusive dressings with zinc oxide paste, hydrocolloid gels, or topical antibiotics* may be particularly useful in areas prone to trauma or superinfection, such as the anogenital region.

Medical management of low-risk hemangiomas has traditionally centered around the administration of *corticosteroids, either topically or intralesionally.* Intralesional triamcinolone acetonide, 10–40 mg/mL, in doses of 3–5 mg/kg, may be injected for small lesions (1–2 cm in diameter) on the lip, nasal tip, cheek, or ear, but must be used with caution for periocular hemangiomas. Though rare, serious side effects, such as central retinal artery occlusion, have been reported with intralesional injections of periocular lesions. The response rate for intralesional administration may be similar to that for systemic therapy. *Class I topical corticosteroids* may also be used, though there is a paucity of data in the medical literature regarding this modality. One group of investigators used *clobetasol propionate* cream, 0.05%, in treating periocular hemangiomas. Other less frequently used management options include *cryosurgery, surgical excision* (especially for pedunculated lesions), and *laser therapy*.

Systemic corticosteroids are the mainstay of therapy for larger, deforming, endangering, or life-threatening lesions, and are usually indicated during their growth phase. *Prednisone or prednisolone* can be given at doses from 2 to 4 mg/kg daily from 2–3 months and then gradually tapered over several months. Stopping treatment before adequate therapeutic response may result in rebound growth. Approximately one-third of patients will show an accelerated rate of involution, but another one-third may have no response to this treatment modality. Therapy should be discontinued if no response is noted within 3–6 weeks. The most important side effect to consider with systemic corticosteroids is immune suppression, and the patient's pediatrician should be aware of this treatment before administering live attenuated viral vaccines. Other reported risks include hypothalamic–pituitary–adrenal axis suppression, growth delays, pseudotumor cerebri, and avascular bone necrosis. *Surgical excision, laser treatment* (especially flashlamp-pumped pulsed dye laser), and *cryosurgery*, either alone or in combination with corticosteroids, may also be employed in certain cases.

For endangering or life-threatening lesions refractory to systemic corticosteroids, *interferon alfa-2a* or *2b* may be used. The typical delivery route is subcutaneously at a dose of 3 million units/m² daily for 6–12 months. Side effects include transient neutropenia, fever, elevated liver enzymes, and flu-like symptoms. In addition, there are rare reports in the literature of neurotoxicity, specifically spastic diplegia, which may develop in 5–10% of patients. For the exceptional recalcitrant hemangioma, other treatments include *cyclophosphamide, vincristine,* and *embolization.* Another currently evolving treatment is the use of *angiogenesis inhibitors.*

SPECIFIC INVESTIGATIONS

- ■ Ultrasound with Doppler
- ■ MRI

The diagnosis of hemangioma is usually made clinically, and the above investigations may only be needed in atypical cases, to monitor progress of treatment, establish the extent of the vascular lesion, or screen for other complications.

Soft-tissue vascular anomalies: utility of US for diagnosis. Paltiel HJ, Burrows PE, Kozakewich HPW, et al. Radiology 2000;214:747–54.

Doppler ultrasonography is an available, low-cost, non-invasive method to confirm the diagnosis of a vascular anomaly, monitor therapeutic response, or preclude the involvement of visceral organs. Hemangiomas can be differentiated from vascular malformations on ultrasonography by distinguishing features such as the presence of a solid tissue mass.

Hemangioma from head to toe: MR imaging with pathologic correlation. Vilanova JC, Barcelo J, Smirniotopoulos JG, et al. Radiographics 2004;24:367–85.

MRI is a useful noninvasive imaging technique to diagnose, characterize, and determine the extent of vascular lesions. On MRI T2-weighted images, hemangiomas have the characteristic appearance of multiple lobules, similar to a bunch of grapes.

Although not specifically mentioned in this article, infants with large, segmental, plaque-like facial hemangiomas should have MRI head evaluation for possible posterior fossa brain abnormalities as a component of the PHACES syndrome.

FIRST LINE THERAPIES

■ Topical corticosteroids	D
■ Intralesional corticosteroids	B
■ Systemic corticosteroids	B

Systemic corticosteroids are the mainstay of therapy for life-threatening or endangering hemangiomas. In contrast, topical and intralesional administration remain first line therapies for relatively uncomplicated cases.

Topical treatment of periocular capillary hemangioma. Elsas F, Lewis A. J Pediatr Ophthalmol Strabismus 1994;31: 153–6.

Five patients with sight-threatening periocular hemangiomas were treated with the ultrapotent topical corticosteroid clobetasol propionate 0.05% cream. Therapy was well tolerated, with involution proceeding at a slower rate than with intralesional therapy, but eliminating the risk of central retinal artery occlusion (Shorr N, Seiff SR. Central retinal artery occlusion associated with periocular corticosteroid injection for juvenile hemangioma. Ophthalmic Surg 1986; 17:229–31).

This may be a useful initial treatment for lesions that are not amenable to injection.

Intralesional corticosteroid therapy in proliferating head and neck hemangiomas: a review of 155 cases. Chen MT, Yeong EK, Horng SY. J Pediatr Surg 2000;35:420–3.

In this retrospective study, 155 hemangiomas of the head and neck region treated with intralesional corticosteroid injections (three to six injections of triamcinolone acetonide 10 mg/mL in monthly intervals with four mean injections per lesion) were analyzed. At the 1 month visit, 85% of hemangiomas showed greater than 50% reduction, with superficial hemangiomas showing the most improvement. Perioral hemangiomas appeared the most recalcitrant to intralesional corticosteroid treatment.

Oral corticosteroid use is effective for cutaneous hemangiomas. Bennett ML, Fleischer AB, Chamlin SL, et al. Arch Dermatol 2001;137:1208–13.

This meta-analysis of ten case series with 184 patients analyzed the efficacy of systemic corticosteroids in the treatment of cutaneous hemangiomas. The mean age of infants at initiation of therapy was 4.5 months at an average prednisone dose equivalent to 2.9 mg/kg. The mean response rate was 84%, and the mean rate of rebound growth after treatment cessation was 36%. Treatment with higher doses of corticosteroids resulted in a higher response rate, but greater adverse effects. The average incidence of side effects was 35% (behavior changes, irritability, cushingoid appearance, and transient growth delay).

Treatment of hemangiomas of infants with high doses of prednisone. Sadan N, Wolach B. J Pediatr 1996;128:141–6.

In this prospective 24-year study, 60 patients with hemangiomas were treated with oral prednisone at an initial dose of either 3 or 5 mg/kg daily for a period of 6–12 weeks. Treatment failure occurred in only 7% of patients while 68% experienced excellent and rapid results.

SECOND LINE THERAPIES

■ Interferon alfa-2a or 2b	B
■ Laser therapy	B
■ Surgical excision	D
■ Becaplermin gel for ulcerated lesions	D

Interferon alfa-2a therapy for life-threatening hemangiomas of infancy. Ezekowitz RA, Mulliken JB, Folkman J. N Engl J Med 1992;326:1456–63.

Twenty infants with life-threatening or vision-threatening hemangiomas who failed corticosteroid therapy were treated with up to 3 million units/m^2 daily of interferon alfa-2a; 90% of the infants experienced a 50% or greater regression in their lesions by 7.8 months of treatment. Side effects were transient, including fever, neutropenia, and skin necrosis. No long-term effects were documented after a mean follow-up period of 16 months.

Regression of infancy hemangiomas with recombinant IFN-alpha 2b. Garmendia G, Miranada N, Borroso S, et al. J Interferon Cytokine Res 2002;21:31–8.

In this prospective study of 39 children with complicated hemangiomas, interferon-alfa-2b was injected (3 million IU/m^2 daily) for 6 months. Of the 38 patients that completed

6 months of treatment, 71.1% experienced regression and 28.9% had stable disease. Adverse effects included a flu-like syndrome (79%), increased alanine aminotransferase (28%), anorexia (19%), and local site reaction at the injection site (19%).

Although not observed in this study, spastic diplegia is a documented and potentially irreversible complication of this treatment and should be considered prior to initiation of therapy.

Flashlamp-pumped pulsed dye laser for hemangiomas in infancy: treatment of superficial vs. mixed hemangiomas. Poetke M, Philipp C, Berlien HP. Arch Dermatol 2000;136: 628–32.

A prospective study of 165 children with 225 separate hemangiomas treated with flashlamp-pumped pulsed dye laser demonstrated that this therapy produced excellent results in treating superficial hemangiomas. However, this method was less successful in treating deeper lesions because the efficacy of the laser was limited by the depth of the vascular proliferation.

Pulsed dye laser therapy promotes epithelialization and is also a safe and effective means of treating ulcerated hemangiomas.

Treatment of facial hemangiomas: the present status of surgery. Demiri EC, Pelissier P, Genin-Etcheberry T, et al. Br J Plast Surg 2001;54:665–74.

In this retrospective study, 35 patients (2.5 months to 35 years of age) underwent surgical treatment for complicated facial hemangiomas with good postoperative outcomes. Tumors on the forehead and glabellar areas were elliptically excised and closed primarily. Nasal tip hemangiomas were removed and nasal tip remodeling done for cartilaginous damage. Periocular hemangiomas were excised and secondary operative procedures such as skin flaps and grafts were used for reconstruction. The authors note that early surgical excision of periocular, nasal tip, and labial tumors gives superior results to delayed treatment.

Response of ulcerated perineal hemangiomas of infancy to becaplermin gel, a recombinant human platelet-derived growth factor. Metz BJ, Rubenstein MC, Levy ML, Metry DW. Arch Dermatol 2004;140:867–70.

Eight infants were treated with becaplermin gel 0.01% for ulcerated perineal hemangiomas of infancy. Rapid ulcer healing occurred in all patients within 3–21 days (average, 10.25 days).

The rapid healing achieved with 0.01% becaplermin gel allows a reduction in the risk of secondary infection, pain, and the need for hospitalization, as well as in the costs that often accumulate from multiple follow-up visits and long-term therapy.

THIRD LINE THERAPIES

■ Vincristine	E
■ Embolization	D
■ Cyclophosphamide	E
■ Angiogenesis inhibitors	E

Vincristine as a treatment for a large haemangioma threatening vital functions. Fawcett SL, Grant I, Hall PN, et al. Br J Plast Surg 2004;57:168–71.

A 21-month-old infant with a large, deep hemangioma in the beard distribution, necessitating multiple hospital admissions for respiratory and feeding difficulties, was treated with vincristine after failing to respond to systemic corticosteroid therapy. Vincristine (1.5 mg/m²) was administered in weekly doses for 1 month with improvement in feeding, speech, and external appearance of the lesion with no adverse effects.

Although reports of success achieved with vincristine exist in the literature, data are anecdotal at best.

Embolization of hepatic hemangiomas in infants. Kullendorff CM, Cwikiel W, Sandstrom S. Eur J Pediatr Surg 2002;12:348–52.

Two infants with hepatic cavernous hemangiomas complicated by congestive heart failure were treated successfully by coil and glue embolizations. One patient, however, continued to suffer gastrointestinal complications due to growth of the hemangioma into the intestine and needed partial resection of the hemangioma even after embolization.

Aggressive interventions, such as embolization and resection, are viable options when there are life-threatening symptoms and medical management fails.

Infantile hemangioma: clinical resolution with 5% imiquimod cream. Martinez MI, Sanchez-Carpintero I, North PE, et al. Arch Dermatol 2002;138:881–4.

Two infants with frontal scalp hemangiomas were successfully treated with imiquimod within 3–5 months of therapy. Imiquimod was initially applied three times per week and then increased to every other day. Erythema and crusting occurred, necessitating frequent rest periods. Virtually complete clinical regression was achieved with no recurrence and no hair loss at the 4-month follow-up visit. Imiquimod induces antiangiogenic cytokines such as interferon-α, interleukin-12, and tissue inhibitor of metalloproteinase-1 (TIMP-1), all of which may play active roles in the response of hemangiomas to imiquimod.

Responses to anti-angiogenic therapies. Paller, AS. J Investig Dermatol Symp Proc 2000;5:83–6.

This review article discusses the role of angiogenesis in the proliferation of vascular tumors and potential antiangiogenic agents. Treatment options currently under investigation include batimastat, thrombospondin, angiostatin, and interleukin-12. Such agents have a direct antiangiogenic effect or target a specific step in the migration, adhesion, and proliferation of endothelial cells during angiogenic recruitment. Obstacles in the use of antiangiogenic therapies include the cost of production and limited methods of medication administration. Further animal studies and safety studies in humans need to be conducted prior to routine use of these agents.

Evidence levels **A** Double-blind study **B** Clinical trial ≥ 20 subjects **C** Clinical trial < 20 subjects **D** Series ≥ 5 subjects **E** Anecdotal case reports

Hereditary angioedema

Malcolm W Greaves

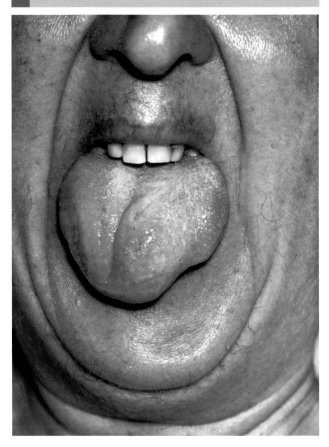

Classical hereditary angioedema (HAE), is an autosomal dominantly inherited disease due to mutations in the C1-esterase inhibitor (C1-INH) gene on chromosome 11 (11q12–q13.1), and is manifested by painless, nonpruritic swellings of subcutaneous and submucosal tissues, including abdominal organs and the upper airway. It is characterized by a quantitative (type 1, 85%) or functional (type 2, 15%) defect of the inhibitor of the first component of complement (C1-INH). Recently hereditary angioedema type 3 has been reported exclusively in women, with no detectable abnormality of complement components (Bork K, Barnstedt S-E, Koch P, Traupe H. Hereditary angioedema with normal C1-inhibitor activity in women. Lancet 2000;356:213–17).

MANAGEMENT STRATEGY

Therapy for HAE is dependent upon three considerations:

- relief of acute angioedema, especially preservation of the airway;
- long-term prophylaxis,
- prevention of relapse due to dental and surgical interventions.

Acute angioedema

Acute presentations of HAE are treated optimally with intravenous, vapor-sterilized, *C1-INH concentrate*. This treatment is safe and no proven cases of viral transmission have been reported (Safety and efficacy of pasteurised C1 inhibitor concentrate (Berinert P) in hereditary angioedema: a review. De Serres J, Groner A, Lindner J. Transfus Apheresis Sci 2003;29:247–54). Reduction in swelling is usually significant in minutes, and substantial within 2–3 hours. *Fresh frozen plasma (FFP)*, which contains C1-INH, can be used if concentrate is unavailable; however, FFP carries a higher risk of inadvertent viral transmission (HIV, hepatitis) and could exacerbate angioedema due to presence of C1 esterase substrate. Although *subcutaneous epinephrine (adrenaline)* (0.3 mg every 3 min) may be helpful, parenterally administered corticosteroids, and antihistamines are not effective for HAE. Laryngeal edema may require *tracheostomy, intubation, and/or other life-support measures.*

Long term prophylaxis

Generally long-term prophylaxis is appropriate in those patients with at least one or more attacks of angioedema per month, and in those with severe symptoms. However, patients could have infrequent attacks and still present with laryngeal edema. Even first-episode angioedema can be fatal. The 17-α-alkylated androgens *danazol* and *stanozolol* are first line prophylactic medications that are extremely efficacious in preventing asphyxia in type 1 and type 2 HAE. The dose of androgen should be adjusted to obtain clinical remission at the lowest possible dose, regardless of C1-INH or C4 levels. Side effects include hirsuties, deepening of voice, and menorrhagia. In some patients, alternate-day therapy can be achieved. Hepatocellular adenoma and hepatocellular carcinoma have been reported in patients on long-term danazol. Other prophylactic therapies include *antifibrinolytics (e.g. tranexamic acid, ε-aminocaproic acid [EACA])*, but these are of less certain value. In patients with mild infrequent attacks: *avoidance of provoking factors including estrogens and angiotensin converting enzyme (ACE) inhibitors* may be sufficient. In general angiotensin receptor II antagonists are deemed well tolerated in patients with reactions to ACE inhibitors.

Prevention of relapse due to dental and surgical interventions

In all patients, prior to elective surgical, dental or other invasive procedures, *higher-dose androgens can be used for 5–10 days*. If an emergency procedure is necessary, C1-INH concentrate or FFP can be administered.

Patients with HAE should all wear a *MedicAlert® disc* stating the diagnosis and emergency treatment.

SPECIFIC INVESTIGATIONS

- Complement levels (C4, C2, C1q)
- C1-INH immunoreactive level
- Functional assay for C1-INH

Angioedema. (CME article) Kaplan AP, Greaves MW. J Am Acad Dermatol 2005;In press.

Type I HAE is characterized by low antigenic and functional plasma levels of normal C1-INH. Type II HAE is characterized by normal or elevated antigenic levels of a dysfunctional mutant C1-INH together with functional C1-INH. In those patients with a low C4, but with normal C1-INH levels, a functional assay should be obtained to identify type II disease. A depressed C1q level in addition to low C4 and C1-INH levels is characteristic of acquired C1-INH-deficient angioedema (AAE). Causes include B cell lymphoma, cryoglobulinemia, and presence of autoantibodies against C1-INH itself.

Hereditary and acquired C1 inhibitor deficiency: biological and clinical characteristics in 235 patients. Agostini A, Cicardi M. Medicine 1992;71:206–15.

C4 level is the best screening test. A decreased value is typical between attacks and it is almost undetectable during an attack.

A multicentre evaluation of the diagnostic efficiency of serological investigations for C1 inhibitor deficiency. Gompels MM, Lock RJ, Morgan JE, et al. J Clin Path 2002; 55:145–7.

All patients with suspected C1-INH deficiency should have serum C4 measured. If C4 is normal, it is unnecessary to proceed to C1-INH analysis. If C4 is low, then C1-INH function should be analyzed. A combination of low C4 and low C1-INH function has a 98% specificity and 96% predictive value for C1-INH deficiency and is a very effective screening procedure.

Acute angioedema

FIRST LINE THERAPIES

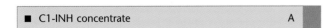

■ C1-INH concentrate   A

Treatment of 193 episodes of laryngeal edema with C1 inhibitor concentrate in patients with hereditary angioedema. Bork K, Barnstedt S-E. Arch Intern Med 2001; 161:714–18.

A series of 193 episodes of laryngeal edema treated with 500–1000 units (500 units initially, then repeated in 30–60 min if necessary) of concentrate were compared to cases that did not receive concentrate. The relief of symptoms occurred, on average, at 42 minutes after injection.

C1-INH concentrate has also been effective as short-term prophylaxis in labor induction, tonsillectomy, and maxillofacial surgery. Long-term prophylaxis has not generally been advocated due to lack of availability, cost, and potential for infectious transmission. However, this may be considered in children, pregnant women, and patients who do not respond to or tolerate androgens or antifibrinolytics, or if these drugs are contraindicated.

Treatment of hereditary angioedema with a vapor-heated C1 inhibitor concentrate. Waytes AT, Rosen FS, Frank MM. N Engl J Med 1996;334:1630–4.

Two randomized, placebo-controlled, double-blind studies evaluated the safety and efficacy of vapor-heated infusions of C1-INH concentrate in acute attacks (22 patients) and as prophylaxis (six patients). In the pro-

phylaxis arm, concentrate was administered every third day; in the treatment arm, concentrate was begun within 5 h of symptoms. A dose of 25 units/kg was used in both groups. Compared to placebo, significantly lower daily symptom scores were found in the prophylaxis group, and a shorter duration of symptoms was found in the treatment group (55 vs 563 min). No toxicity was demonstrated and after 4 years of observation there was no evidence of seroconversion to HIV or hepatitis B or C.

A randomized, controlled trial to study the efficacy and safety of C1 inhibitor concentrate in treating hereditary angioedema. Kunschak M, Engl W, Maritsch F, et al. Transfusion 1998;38:540–9.

A study that clearly demonstrates that the administration of C1-INH concentrate is far more effective than placebo (7.62 h vs 15.35 h) in relieving attacks. The C4 levels are increased within 12–24 h.

C1-INH is not readily accessible in the USA, but can be obtained in Europe from Berinert HS, Aventis Behring (Liederbach, Germany), or Immuno (Vienna, Austria).

C1-esterase inhibitor transfusions in patients with hereditary angioedema. Visnetin DE, Yang WH, Karsh J. Ann Allergy Asthma Immunol 1998;80:457–61.

C1-INH concentrate was very effective in abating attacks of HAE in seven of 13 patients. The mean duration of an attack in treated patients was 50 ± 8 min, compared to 1–4 days in the untreated group.

SECOND LINE THERAPIES

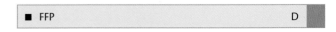

■ FFP   D

This is effective and can be used if C1-INH concentrate is unavailable. It is not virally inactivated and, being larger in volume, requires a longer infusion time.

Replacement therapy in hereditary angioedema: successful treatment of two patients with fresh frozen plasma. Pickering RJ, Kelley JR, Good RA, Gewurz H. Lancet 1969;1:326–30.

Apart from the risk of virus infection, using FFP carries the potential for exacerbation of attacks due to its content of complement substrates.

Long-term prophylaxis of hereditary angioedema

FIRST LINE THERAPIES

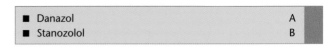

■ Danazol   A
■ Stanozolol   B

How do we treat patients with hereditary angioedema? Cicardi M, Zingale L. Transfus Apheresis Sci 2003;29:221–7.

In a study of 141 patients, danazol and stanozolol proved equally effective; less than 10% of patients failed to obtain significant remission. Normalization of C1-INH is not required. These authors start with a run-in period of

Evidence levels A Double-blind study B Clinical trial ≥ 20 subjects C Clinical trial < 20 subjects D Series ≥ 5 subjects E Anecdotal case reports

400–600 mg daily of danazol for 1 month, slowly tapering to 100–200 mg daily to determine the minimum dose that will cause remission (C1-INH level around 50% of normal; C4 within normal range; complete remission of angioedema).

Treatment of hereditary angioedema with danazol. Gelfand JA, Sherins RJ, Alling DW, Frank MM. N Engl J Med 1976;295:1444–8.

A randomized, placebo-controlled, double-blind trial demonstrated the effectiveness of danazol 200 mg three times daily as prophylaxis. Nine patients participated in 93 courses of therapy. The patients were crossed over after 28 days of therapy, unless an attack occurred sooner.

Long-term treatment of hereditary angioedema with attenuated androgens: a survey of a 13-year experience. Cicardi M, Bergamaschini L, Cugno M, et al. J Allergy Clin Immunol 1991;87:768–73.

The authors report their experience with attenuated androgens used for long-term prophylaxis. In 54 of 56 patients resolution of symptoms was achieved. The lowest effective daily dose usually did not exceed 2 mg for stanozolol and 200 mg for danazol. Twenty four patients were observed for more than 5 years. Hepatic cell necrosis occurred in one patient treated with stanozolol 4 mg daily for 1 year.

Side effects of long-term prophylaxis with attenuated androgens in hereditary angioedema: comparison of treated and untreated patients. Cicardi M, Castelli R, Zingale LC, Agostoni A. J Allergy Clin Immunol 1997;99: 194–6.

Thirty six patients with HAE were treated with attenuated androgens for a median of 125.5 months and compared to 34 patients with HAE who never received prophylaxis. The main side effects were menstrual irregularities (15 of 36) and weight gain (14 of 36). A statistically significant increase in arterial hypertension occurred in 25% of treated patients. Significant changes in hepatic enzymes and ultrasounds were not found. Stanozolol seemed to have fewer side effects than danazol.

Side effects in female patients may be troublesome, including menstrual disturbance, deepening of voice, and hirsuties. In males, monitoring of prostate changes should be carried out. All patients should have regular liver function tests. Attenuated androgens are contraindicated in pregnancy.

SECOND LINE THERAPIES

■ EACA	A
■ Tranexamic acid	A

Hereditary and acquired C1-inhibitor deficiency: biological and clinical characteristics in 235 patients. Agostoni A, Cicardi M. Medicine (Baltimore) 1992;71:206–15.

Twelve of 15 patients had initially effective prophylaxis with tranexamic acid, but this agent was only effective long term in 28% whereas danazol was effective long term in 97%.

Epsilon aminocaproic acid therapy of hereditary angioneurotic edema: a double blind study. Frank MM, Sergent JS, Kane MA, Alling DW. N Engl J Med 1972;286: 808–12.

EACA (16 g daily) in a double-blind crossover trial prevented attacks of angioedema in four of five patients over a 2-year period. Common side effects consisted of weakness and increased fatigability. A follow-up open trial led to control of symptoms on 7–10 g daily of EACA.

Higher dose therapy (24–30 g) has led to elevation of creatine phosphokinase and aldolase levels and muscle necrosis.

Long-term treatment of C1 inhibitor deficiency with ε-aminocaproic acid in two patients. Van Dellen RG. Mayo Clin Proc 1996;71:1175–8.

Two patients were successfully treated with EACA (8–10 g daily) over a period of 12–23 years. No adverse effects were found.

EACA therapy can also be used as short-term prophylaxis for minor procedures, but due to its potential thrombotic effects, it should be discontinued before major surgery.

Tranexamic acid therapy in hereditary angioneurotic edema. Sheffer AL, Austen KF, Rosen FS. N Engl J Med 1972;287:452–4.

Patients participated in a randomized, placebo-controlled, double-blind crossover trial over a 4–13-month period. Seven of 12 patients receiving tranexamic acid 1 g three times daily achieved a complete or near-complete cessation of attacks. Four additional patients experienced a moderate response.

Tranexamic acid is more potent than EACA and has been reported to cause fewer side effects.

Treatment of hereditary angioneurotic oedema with tranexamic acid. A random double-blind cross-over study. Blohme G. Acta Med Scand 1972;192:293–8.

High-dose antifibrinolytics (e.g. tranexamic acid 1 g every 3–4 h) have been administered early in acute attacks with efficacy. Compared to androgens, antifibrinolytics are less effective. In one study they effectively controlled attacks 28% of the time, compared to 97% effectiveness for androgens. However, antifibrinolytics may have a more favorable side effect profile, especially in children.

THIRD LINE THERAPIES

■ C1-INH concentrate	C

Long-term prophylaxis with C1 inhibitor (C1 INH) concentrate in patients with recurrent angioedema caused by hereditary and acquired C1 INH deficiency. Bork K, Witzke GL. J Allergy Clin Immunol 1989;83:677–82.

C1-INH concentrate 500 units once or twice weekly for 1 year or more was reported.

Pharmacokinetic parameters of C1 inhibitor concentrate in 40 patients with hereditary angioedema (HAE) – a prospective study. Martinez-Saguer I, Muller W, Aygoren Pursun E, et al. Haemophilia 2002;8:574–80.

C1-INH concentrate can be used in long-term prophylaxis of HAE.

Prevention of relapse due to dental and surgical interventions

■ FFP	B
■ Danazol	B
■ C1-INH concentrate	C

Hereditary angioedema: the use of fresh frozen plasma for prophylaxis in patients undergoing oral surgery. Jaffe CJ, Atkinson JP, Gelfand JA, et al. J Allergy Clin Immunol 1975;55:386–93.

FFP (2 units) was found to be effective in six patients undergoing seven episodes of dental surgery. Two units of FFP were given 1 day prior to the surgery.

Others have effectively used danazol (600 mg daily) or stanozolol (6–8 mg daily) 5–10 days preoperatively to 3 days postoperatively.

The efficacy of short-term danazol prophylaxis in hereditary angioedema patients undergoing maxillofacial and dental procedures. Farkas H, Gyeney L, Gidofalvy E, et al. J Oral Maxillofac Surg 1999;57:404–8.

Twelve patients with a history of angioedema after dental procedures received danazol 600 mg 4 days preoperatively and 4 days postoperatively for dental or maxillofacial procedures. None experienced angioedema.

Other preoperative options include 500–1000 units of C1-INH concentrate or antifibrinolytic agents.

Hereditary angioedema: uncomplicated faciomaxillary surgery using short term C1 inhibitor replacement therapy. Leimgruber A, Jacques WA, Spaeth PJ. Int Arch Allergy Immunol 1993;101:107–12.

Tranexamic acid: preoperative prophylactic therapy for patients with hereditary angioneurotic edema. Sheffer AL, Fearon DT, Austen KF, Rosen FS. J Allergy Clin Immunol 1977;60:38–40.

Hereditary angioedema: treatment in children

Clinical management of hereditary angio-edema in children. Farkas H, Harmat G, Fust G, et al. Pediatr Allergy Immunol 2002;13:153–61.

Based on data from 26 patients, these authors advise use of C1-INH concentrate for emergency treatment of acute attacks. Tranexamic acid or danazol should be used for short or long-term prophylaxis. Apart from one instance of delayed menarche, no adverse events were experienced.

Treatment of hereditary angioedema type 3

Hereditary angioedema type 3, angioedema associated with angiotensin II receptor antagonists and female sex. Bork K. Am J Med 2004;116:644.

Bork describes two unrelated female patients who had normal C1-INH and C4 levels and who experienced severe exacerbations of hereditary angioedema following administration of losartan and valsartan, respectively.

Acute attacks do not respond to C1-INH concentrate, and antihistamines or corticosteroids are ineffective. The value of antifibrinolytics is unproven. For prevention danazol is worth trying, but substantiation of its value is awaited. All patients should avoid angiotensin-2-receptor antagonists (sartans) and estrogens because these are known to provoke attacks in affected women. Possibly bradykinin antagonists or kallikrein inhibitors, currently under development, may offer some future benefit to these patients.

Hereditary hemorrhagic telangiectasia

Mitchell S Cappell, Oscar Lebwohl

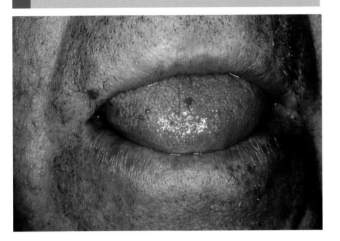

Hereditary hemorrhagic telangiectasia (HHT), an autosomal dominant disease, produces a syndrome of multiple orocutaneous telangiectasias, especially on the face, lips, tongue, oral mucosa, and hands, together with multiple internal telangiectasias, especially in the nose and gastrointestinal tract. Cutaneous lesions typically are 3–10 mm wide, macular, bright red, nonpulsatile, and spidery in shape, with a fine reticular internal structure. They tend to blanch under pressure (with diascopy). They slowly increase in size and number with age. Although the dermatologic lesions are usually a minor cosmetic problem, the nasal and gastrointestinal lesions frequently bleed significantly and repeatedly. Chronic blood loss may result in iron deficiency anemia, while acute blood loss may cause hypovolemia and systemic hypotension. Infrequent syndromic manifestations include hypoxia from pulmonary arteriovenous shunts; cerebral ischemia or abscess from systemic shunts; and portal hypertension, biliary tract disease, or high-output cardiac failure from intrahepatic shunts. The basic lesion is probably a defect in the wall of small vessels that leads to direct arteriovenous communications without intervening capillaries. Various mutations in the gene encoding endoglin (ENG) or in the gene encoding activin receptor-like kinase 1 (ALK-1) usually underlie this defect.

MANAGEMENT STRATEGY

The diagnosis of HHT is straightforward in patients with the triad of mucocutaneous telangiectasia, recurrent epistaxis, and a compatible family history. Patients may have telangiectasia solely on the face with rosacea or with lupus erythematosus, but lack the other manifestations of HHT. Patients with sporadic gastrointestinal angiodysplasia are differentiated from patients with HHT by clinical presentation in old age, a paucity of the characteristic lesions, a negative family history, and exclusive gastrointestinal involvement without epistaxis.

For epistaxis, the bleeding severity is determined by inspection, vital signs, and laboratory tests. The bleeding site is precisely localized by nasal examination using bright shadow-free illumination, with a headlight or head mirror, and spot suction, with a fine caliber rigid tube. For gastrointestinal bleeding, the bleeding severity is indicated by patient history, vital signs, physical findings, rectal examination, nasogastric aspiration, and transfusion requirements. The bleeding site and source are conclusively diagnosed by gastrointestinal endoscopy.

Choice of therapy depends upon bleeding site, severity, and chronicity as well as individual physician expertise. Significant acute blood loss is treated with *intravenous fluid resuscitation*, with *transfusion of packed erythrocytes as needed*. Chronic blood loss is treated with *iron* and, if needed, *folate supplementation*.

Epistaxis is initially treated by nonspecific local therapy such as *nasal packing* to tamponade the bleeding and *topical vasoconstrictors* to decrease local blood flow. *Estrogen with progesterone* is used to prevent or arrest chronic epistaxis by promoting vascular integrity. Significant, refractory, chronic epistaxis is definitively treated by *septal dermoplasty*.

Actively bleeding gastrointestinal telangiectasias are treated at endoscopy by *thermocoagulation, electrocoagulation, photocoagulation, or argon plasma coagulation*. Chronically bleeding gastrointestinal telangiectasias may be treated with *estrogen and progesterone. Surgical resection* is reserved for well localized, active bleeding from gastrointestinal telangiectasias refractory to other therapy because these patients tend to subsequently re-bleed from telangiectasias at other sites. Where available, *angiographic embolization* can obviate the need for gastrointestinal surgery.

SPECIFIC INVESTIGATIONS

- Serial hematocrit determinations
- Serum iron, total iron binding capacity (TIBC), and ferritin level
- Esophagogastroduodenoscopy
- Colonoscopy
- Capsule endoscopy
- Angiography

Clinical spectrum of hereditary hemorrhagic telangiectasia (Osler–Weber–Rendu disease). Peery WH. Am J Med 1987;82:989–97.

Review of clinical manifestations and management of HHT.

Evidence of small-bowel involvement in hereditary hemorrhagic telangiectasia: a capsule-endoscopic study. Ingrosso M, Sabba C, Pisani A, et al. Endoscopy 2004;36: 1074–9.

Recent study demonstrating a high frequency of small bowel telangiectasias in elderly patients with HHT as detected by capsule endoscopy. Chronic blood loss from these intestinal lesions may contribute to iron deficiency anemia from HHT.

Liver disease in patients with hereditary hemorrhagic telangiectasia. Garcia-Tsao G, Korzenik JR, Young L, et al. N Engl J Med 2000;343:931–6.

Review of the clinical findings in eight patients with high-output cardiac failure, six with portal hypertension, and five with biliary tract disease caused by intrahepatic shunts with HHT.

Serial hematocrit determinations are important, particularly for acute bleeding, to determine the need for transfusions of packed erythrocytes. Serum levels of iron, TIBC, and ferritin are important, particularly for chronic bleeding, to determine the need for iron replacement therapy. Upper gastrointestinal bleeding, usually manifested by hematemesis or melena, should be investigated by esophagogastroduodenoscopy. Lower gastrointestinal bleeding, usually manifested by hematochezia, melena, or fecal occult blood, should be investigated by colonoscopy. Barium contrast radiography or virtual colonoscopy should not be performed to evaluate lower gastrointestinal bleeding in patients with HHT because the telangiectasias are mucosal and macular and not visualized with barium contrast. Small intestinal bleeding, usually manifested by hematochezia, melena, or fecal occult blood, can be investigated by capsule endoscopy, after exclusion of upper and lower gastrointestinal bleeding by the aforementioned endoscopic tests. At endoscopy telangiectasias appear as intensely red maculae due to the high oxygen content in erythrocytes within vessels supplied by arteries without intervening capillaries. Telangiectasias are distinguished from the very common lesions caused by endoscopic trauma by lesion identification during endoscopic intubation as opposed to identification during endoscopic extubation with trauma, by a finely reticular (fern-like) internal structure due to a vascular tuft, by an irregular (fern-like) border as opposed to a round border with trauma, by an abrupt lesion margin as opposed to an indistinct margin with trauma, and by lesions lying flush (coplanar) with mucosa. Additionally, colonic lesions from endoscopic trauma usually occur at sharp colonic turns, during endoscopic looping, or after endoscopic suctioning.

Angiography is indicated for active gastrointestinal bleeding when esophagogastroduodenoscopy and colonoscopy have failed to diagnose the source of bleeding. The angiographic hallmarks of telangiectasias are a vascular tuft or tangle resulting from the local mass of irregular vessels, an early and intensely filling vein resulting from a direct arteriovenous connection without intervening capillaries, and persistent opacification beyond the normal venous phase (slowly emptying vein), attributed to vascular tortuosity. Telangiectasias bleed only intermittently, and extravasation of contrast material from telangiectasias is infrequently detected at angiography.

FIRST LINE THERAPIES

For epistaxis	
■ Nasal packing	A
■ Septal dermoplasty	A
For gastrointestinal bleeding	
■ Endoscopic thermocoagulation, electrocoagulation, argon plasma coagulation, or photocoagulation	B
■ Angiographic embolization	B
■ Segmental bowel resection	A
For epistaxis or gastrointestinal bleeding	
■ Oral estrogen with progesterone	B

Septal dermoplasty – ten years experience. Saunders WH. Trans Am Acad Ophthalmol Otolaryngol 1968;72:153–60.

Classic report describing a marked reduction in the frequency and severity of epistaxis in 125 patients undergoing septal dermoplasty, mostly for HHT, during a 10-year period. No significant surgical complications occurred.

Nasal packing often temporarily stems epistaxis by vascular tamponade. Septal dermoplasty is indicated for severe and recurrent epistaxis, especially from anterior nasal mucosa. In this procedure, skin, removed from the upper thigh, is grafted onto the anterior nasal septum and floor to cover and protect the fragile mucosal telangiectasias from local trauma. The procedure is well-tolerated using only local anesthesia, and complications, other than recurrent epistaxis, are rare. Septal dermoplasty is effective in more than 75% of cases. Failure results from inadequate graft coverage with bleeding from lesions at the border or beyond the grafted area.

Mucosal vascular malformations of the gastrointestinal tract: clinical observations and results of neodymium: yttrium-aluminum-garnet laser therapy. Gostout CJ, Bowyer BA, Ahlquist DA, et al. Mayo Clin Proc 1988;63: 993–1003.

Gastrointestinal bleeding from telangiectasias was successfully controlled in nine of ten patients with HHT and in 72 of 83 patients with sporadic telangiectasias by endoscopic photocoagulation with the YAG laser. Three gastrointestinal perforations occurred in 243 laser treatment sessions.

Long-term results of treatment of vascular malformations of the gastrointestinal tract by neodymium YAG laser photocoagulation. Naveau S, Aubert A, Poynard T, Chaput JC. Dig Dis Sci 1990;35:821–6.

Thirteen patients with HHT had a decrease in transfusion requirements for 2–3 years after endoscopic photocoagulation of bleeding gastrointestinal telangiectasias. This decrease, however, was not statistically significant and successful treatment required multiple endoscopic sessions (median of seven) due to the large number of telangiectasias in HHT.

At endoscopy, isolated actively bleeding telangiectasias are treated with endoscopic thermocoagulation, electrocoagulation, argon plasma coagulation, or photocoagulation. Most endoscopists prefer thermocoagulation, electrocoagulation, or argon plasma coagulation over photocoagulation due to lower equipment costs and simpler therapeutic techniques. These endoscopic therapies are relatively safe and highly successful at achieving hemostasis when performed by an experienced endoscopist. However, patients with HHT often subsequently re-bleed from other, untreated, gastrointestinal telangiectasias and therefore require multiple sessions of endoscopic therapy to treat other lesions to prevent re-bleeding. Angiographic embolization or segmental bowel resection is reserved for active severe bleeding localized to a single region, and refractory to medical and endoscopic therapy.

Diagnosis and management of gastrointestinal bleeding in patients with hereditary hemorrhagic telangiectasia. Longacre AV, Gross CP, Gallitelli M, et al. Am J Gastroenterol 2003;98:59–65.

In a nonrandomized, long-term observational study, the mean hemoglobin level increased and the chronic transfusion requirements decreased in about three-fourths of 17 patients after instituting chronic estrogen hormonal therapy, either alone or with other therapies, for gastrointestinal bleeding from HHT.

Treatment of bleeding gastrointestinal vascular malformations with oestrogen–progesterone. Van Custen E, Rutgeerts P, Vantrappen G. Lancet 1990;335:953–5.

In a double-blind, placebo-controlled, crossover trial of ten patients with frequent and severe gastrointestinal bleeding from HHT, the number of transfusions significantly decreased from 10.9 units of packed erythrocytes in controls

Evidence levels   A Double-blind study   B Clinical trial ≥ 20 subjects   C Clinical trial < 20 subjects   D Series ≥ 5 subjects   E Anecdotal case reports

receiving placebo to 1.1 units in patients treated with estrogen–progesterone during a 6-month period.

Estrogen–progesterone therapy for bleeding gastrointestinal telangiectasias in chronic renal failure: an uncontrolled trial. Bronner MH, Pate MB, Cunningham JT, Marsh WH. Ann Intern Med 1986;105:371–4.

Blood transfusion requirements decreased from 1.2 units/month to 0.21 units/month of packed erythrocytes after instituting estrogen and progesterone therapy in seven patients with gastrointestinal bleeding from telangiectasias associated with renal failure.

Use of estrogen in treatment of familial hemorrhagic telangiectasia. Harrison DFN. Laryngoscope 1982;92:314–20.

A report of successful control of epistaxis with estrogen therapy in 67 patients with HHT, with few complications.

Several studies have reported a markedly decreased incidence in chronic gastrointestinal or nasal bleeding from telangiectasias after instituting estrogen therapy, either alone or with progesterone. Estrogen therapy can be combined with other therapies, such as local endoscopic therapy, for greater efficacy. Despite controversy concerning efficacy, this therapy should be considered before performing gastrointestinal or nasal surgery for chronic bleeding because of the low risk of this therapy and the risk of recurrent bleeding after surgery. Estrogen therapy is less desirable in males than females because it can cause feminization.

SECOND LINE THERAPIES

For epistaxis	
■ Arterial ligation	B
■ Topical vasoconstrictors	B
■ Cryosurgery, electrical cautery, argon plasma coagulation	B
■ Arterial embolization	B
■ Submucosal resection	C
■ Topical aminocaproic acid	D
For gastrointestinal bleeding	
■ Oral aminocaproic acid therapy	D

Brief report: treatment of bleeding in hereditary hemorrhagic telangiectasia with aminocaproic acid. Saba HI, Morelli GA, Logrono LA. N Engl J Med 1994;330:1789–90.

Case report of rapid and sustained decrease in the frequency and severity of bleeding from the nose and gastrointestinal tract in two patients with HHT treated with aminocaproic acid.

Local nonspecific therapy of arterial ligation, cryosurgery, electrical cautery, argon plasma coagulation, or submucosal resection provide temporary but impermanent relief of epistaxis from HHT. Moreover, these treatments can cause mucosal scarring, which diminishes the efficacy of subsequent septal dermoplasty. Local nonspecific topical therapy, with either vasoconstrictors or aminocaproic acid, is unlikely to produce scarring. Nonspecific therapies are indicated only for temporary relief of acute bleeding.

Aminocaproic acid therapy aims to promote thrombosis and retard bleeding by inhibiting proteolysis of fibrin by plasmin. Oral aminocaproic acid therapy has had mixed success and should be viewed as a temporary and second line therapy. Aminocaproic acid rarely causes hypotension or rhabdomyolysis.

Herpes simplex

Jane C Sterling

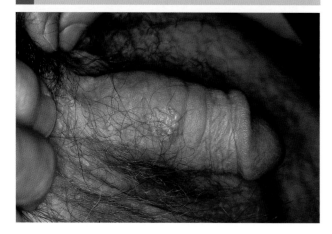

Herpes simplex virus (HSV) infects skin and mucous membranes causing inflammation and damage to keratinocytes, seen as small blisters on a background of erythema. The primary infection may be obvious or subclinical; once latency is established in sensory ganglia, the virus may reactivate to produce visible lesions. In immunosuppression, disease can be chronic and antiviral resistance can develop.

MANAGEMENT STRATEGY

Both primary and reactivation episodes are usually self-limiting and may require no treatment. Antiviral therapy, in the form of *acyclovir* and related drugs, is available for topical and systemic use and is usually the most effective form of treatment. Anogenital herpes, either primary infection or a reactivation episode, will frequently respond to *topical acyclovir* applied five times daily for 5 days. *Oral acyclovir*, 200 mg five times daily for 5 days, will usually reduce the time to healing and duration of virus shedding in both cutaneous and anogenital herpes. Topical or systemic treatment for an acute episode should be started early in the episode to have most benefit. In addition, pain relief may be necessary.

In severe or frequently recurrent disease, or in immunosuppressed individuals, antiviral treatment is recommended and measures may be taken to avoid any precipitating factors. *UV protection* may help to reduce viral reactivation in herpes labialis. Oral acyclovir has been used extensively as prophylaxis, but needs to be taken for several weeks or months. The dose of 400 mg twice daily for acyclovir is most likely to produce a decrease in the frequency of reactivation episodes. There is a potential risk of selection of resistant strains of virus with long-term therapy, but this is rare even in immunosuppressed patients. The risk of herpetic reactivation at bone marrow transplantation or mother-to-baby transmission in women with HSV infection can be reduced by prophylactic therapy.

A failure of response to acyclovir may be due to the poor absorption and rapid clearance following ingestion or to the emergence of acyclovir resistance. *Valacyclovir,* a prodrug of acyclovir, and *famciclovir,* a prodrug of penciclovir, have improved bioavailability and are alternatives to acyclovir. Efficacy of oral valacyclovir can be as good as intravenous

acyclovir. *Topical idoxuridine* and the related *trifluorothymidine (TFT)* have also been used. In immunosuppressed individuals, intravenous therapy with acyclovir, or the more toxic *foscarnet* or *cidofovir,* may be necessary. *Vidarabine, interferons,* and *interleukin-2* and other agents have also been used, but without reliable effect. Herpes simplex is a common precipitating cause of episodes of recurrent erythema multiforme, which can be reduced in frequency by prophylactic antiviral therapy.

SPECIFIC INVESTIGATIONS

- Electron microscopy of blister fluid
- Viral culture from swab of lesion
- Immunocytology of blister floor cells
- Skin biopsy of atypical lesion
- Herpes simplex serology
- Assessment of immune function

The diagnosis may be obvious clinically. In atypical disease, laboratory confirmation is essential. In unexplained persistent or severe disease, immunodeficiency should be excluded.

FIRST LINE THERAPIES

■ Topical acyclovir	A
■ Oral acyclovir	A
■ Topical idoxuridine	A
■ Valacyclovir (for prophylaxis)	B
■ Sunscreen	A

Primary cutaneous or genital infection
A trial of topical acyclovir in genital herpes simplex infections. Corey L, Nahmias AJ, Guinan ME, et al. N Engl J Med 1982;306:1313–19.

Oral acyclovir, 200–400 mg five times daily for 5 days, reduced the time of pain and viral shedding in both primary and recurrent infection. Topical acyclovir also significantly reduced the duration of active disease.

Acute reactivation episodes – cutaneous
Successful treatment of herpes labialis with topical acyclovir. Fiddian AP, Yeo JM, Stubbings R, Dean D. Br Med J 1983;286:1699–701.

In a double blind, placebo-controlled trial on 89 patients, acyclovir 5% cream applied five times daily for 5 days for acute recurrent herpes labialis produced a reduction in symptoms and a shortening of the duration of the episode.

Failure of aciclovir cream in treatment of recurrent herpes labialis. Shaw M, King M, Best JM, et al. Br Med J 1985; 291:7–9.

No significant benefit was obtained from topical 5% acyclovir applied five times daily in a double blind, placebo-controlled, crossover trial on 45 patients who suffered 72 episodes of recurrent herpes labialis.

Treatment of herpes labialis with acyclovir. Review of three clinical trials. Raborn GW, McGaw WT, Grace M, Percy J. Am J Med 1988;85:39–42.

Oral acyclovir, five times daily for 5 days, was helpful. Two topical formulations were evaluated: 5% acyclovir in a modified aqueous cream base exhibited favorable trends, but 5% acyclovir in a polyethylene base was ineffective.

Treatment of recurrent herpes simplex labialis with oral acyclovir. Spruance SL, Stewart JCB, Rowe NH, et al. J Infect Dis 1990;161:185–90.

Herpes labialis was less painful and quicker to heal in 114 patients treated before the development of blistering with 400 mg acyclovir, five times daily for 5 days, compared to 60 given placebo treatment. The development of blisters and the size of the lesion were not affected by treatment.

Early application of topical 15% idoxuridine in dimethylsulfoxide shortens the course of herpes simplex labialis: a multicenter placebo-controlled trial. Spruance SL, Stewart CB, Freeman DJ, et al. J Infect Dis 1990;161:191–7.

Idoxuridine 15% solution, applied six times daily for 4 days starting within 1 h of the onset of symptoms of a recurrence, significantly reduced pain and time to healing compared to 2% idoxuridine or dimethylsulfoxide alone.

Acute reactivation episodes – genital

Treatment of recurrent genital herpes simplex infections with oral acyclovir. Reichman RC, Badger GJ, Mertz GJ, et al. JAMA 1984;251:2103–7.

In a study of 250 patients with recurrent genital herpes, acyclovir, 200 mg five times daily for 5 days, reduced the time to healing and the duration of viral shedding compared to placebo, especially when treatment was started very early in the course of an episode.

Prophylactic treatment – for frequent reactivation, recurrent severe attacks, at bone marrow transplantation, or before delivery

Prevention of ultraviolet-light-induced herpes labialis by sunscreen. Rooney JF, Bryson Y, Mannix ML, et al. Lancet 1991;338:1419–22.

Using an experimental system of UV exposure to induce reactivation of herpes, 71% of 38 patients using a placebo developed lesions, whereas none developed in 35 patients using sunscreen.

Long-term acyclovir suppression of frequently recurring genital herpes simplex virus infection. Mertz GJ, Jones CC, Mills J, et al. JAMA 1988;260:201–6.

Of 519 patients who had had at least six episodes of reactivation of genital herpes in the preceding year 44% remained symptom free during a year of treatment with acyclovir 400 mg twice daily, whereas only 2% of 431 placebo-treated patients were episode free.

Acyclovir prophylaxis to prevent herpes simplex virus recurrence at delivery: a systematic review. Sheffield JS, Hollier LM, Hill JB, et al. Obstet Gynecol 2003;102:1396.

A review of evidence for potential reduction of transmission from mother to baby by acyclovir suggests 200 mg four times daily or 400 mg twice daily from 36 weeks gestation until after delivery.

Valacyclovir prophylaxis for the prevention of Herpes simplex virus reactivation in recipients of progenitor cell transplantation. Dignani MC, Mykietiuk A, Michelet M, et al. Bone Marrow Transplant 2002;29:263–7.

Comparison of intravenous acyclovir, oral valacyclovir, or no prophylaxis following bone barrow transplantation in over 100 patients showed equal efficacy of the two antivirals.

SECOND LINE THERAPIES

■ Valacyclovir	A
■ Famciclovir	A

Valaciclovir versus aciclovir in patient initiated treatment of recurrent genital herpes: a randomised, double blind clinical trial. Bodsworth NJ, Crooks RJ, Borelli S, et al. Genitourin Med 1997;73:110–16.

Valacyclovir 500 mg twice daily and acyclovir 200 mg five times daily for 5 days were equally effective in reducing the duration of signs, symptoms, and viral shedding in recurrent genital herpes episodes.

Valaciclovir for the suppression of recurrent genital herpes simplex virus infection: a large-scale dose range-finding study. Reitano M, Tyring S, Lang W, et al. J Infect Dis 1998;178:603–10.

Valacyclovir, 1 g daily, 250 mg twice daily, or acyclovir 400 mg twice daily were the most effective dose regimens for reducing the frequency of recurrences of HSV infection in a trial of 1479 patients.

Oral famciclovir for the suppression of recurrent genital herpes: a randomized controlled trial. Diaz-Mitoma F, Sibbald RG, Shafran SD, Saltzman RL. JAMA 1998;280:887–92.

Four hundred and forty five patients received either famciclovir or placebo for 1 year. Approximately 80% of famciclovir treated patients were recurrence free at 6 months compared to 27% of those treated with placebo.

THIRD LINE THERAPIES

■ Vidarabine	C
■ Foscarnet	C
■ Cidofovir	C

Foscarnet treatment of acyclovir-resistant herpes simplex virus infection in patients with acquired immunodeficiency syndrome: preliminary results of a controlled, randomized, regimen-controlled trial. Hardy WD. Am J Med 1992;92(suppl 2A):30s–5s.

Twenty five patients with AIDS and acyclovir-resistant HSV infection were treated with foscarnet infusions for 2 weeks and then either for a further 8 weeks with 40 mg/kg daily or without further maintenance therapy. Healing of lesions was quickest in those treated for a total of 10 weeks.

A controlled trial comparing foscarnet with vidarabine for acyclovir-resistant mucocutaneous herpes simplex in the acquired immunodeficiency syndrome. Safrin S, Crumpacker C, Chatis P, et al. N Engl J Med 1991;325:551–5.

Foscarnet 40 mg/kg every 8 hours produced healing of acyclovir-resistant herpetic lesions within 4 weeks in eight patients with AIDS, while no improvement occurred in six similar patients treated with vidarabine 15 mg/kg daily.

Treatment with intravenous (S)-1-[hydroxy-2-(phosphonylmethoxy)propyl]-cytosine of acyclovir-resistant mucocutaneous infection with herpes simplex virus in a patient with AIDS. Lalezari JP, Drew WL, Glutzer E, et al. J Infect Dis 1994;170:570–2.

Treatment with four intravenous infusions of 5 mg/kg/week of HPMPC (cidofovir) produced 95% healing in a patient with severe resistant herpetic lesions.

A randomized, double-blind, placebo-controlled trial of cidofovir gel for the treatment of acyclovir-unresponsive mucocutaneous herpes simplex virus infection in patients with AIDS. Lalezari J, Schacker T, Feinberg J, et al. J Infect Dis 1997;176:892–8.

Twenty patients with AIDS applied 0.3% or 1% cidofovir gel once daily for 5 days; 50% healed or improved compared to 0% of the ten placebo-treated patients. Cidofovir produced local inflammation in a quarter of patients.

OTHER THERAPIES

Trifluorothymidine 0.5% ointment in the treatment of aciclovir-resistant mucocutaneous herpes simplex in AIDS. Amin AR, Robinson MR, Smith DD, Luque AE. AIDS 1996;10:1051–3.

Three patients responded to topical TFT applied five times daily for 14 days and then maintenance twice daily. Healing of previously acyclovir-resistant lesions occurred within 3 weeks.

Leukocyte interferon for treating first episodes of genital herpes in women. Pazin GJ, Harger JH, Armstrong JA, et al. J Infect Dis 1987;156:891–8.

Interferon given over 14 days reduced the time to healing of primary genital herpes, but did not alter risk of subsequent recurrence.

Herpes zoster

Richard Ashton

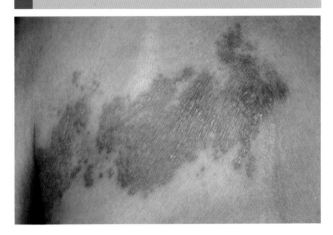

Herpes zoster is an acute vesicular eruption, usually located within a single dermatome, resulting from reactivation of the varicella zoster virus. The rash is self limiting and heals spontaneously after 2 weeks, but may leave scarring, especially if it becomes secondarily infected. Before, during, and after the eruption, pain within the affected dermatome is usual, but persisting pain lasting longer than 3 months (post-herpetic neuralgia, PHN) is debilitating and is the complication that the physician hopes to prevent with prompt treatment.

MANAGEMENT STRATEGY

Treatment of herpes zoster is aimed at promoting rapid healing of the skin lesions, reducing acute pain, and preventing any scarring. Most importantly, effective treatment seeks to prevent the occurrence of PHN. This chronic pain syndrome may be particularly debilitating and is most likely to occur in the elderly, with prodromal pain in the affected dermatome, greater severity of the acute pain, and a severe rash.

Herpes zoster is seven times more common in immuno-compromised patients, especially those who are HIV positive. Indeed any patient under the age of 40 years who develops zoster should be suspected of being HIV positive.

The antiviral drugs *acyclovir, valacyclovir* (prodrug of acyclovir), *famciclovir* (converted to penciclovir) and *brivudin* are the treatments of choice. Acyclovir and penciclovir are analogues of guanosine. They are converted to the triphosphate (firstly by viral thymidine kinase and then by cellular kinases), which inhibits viral DNA polymerase by competitive inhibition of guanosine triphosphate. These drugs are only activated in the presence of virus, and are effective only if the virus is actively replicating. Thus they are of no use as a preventative treatment or after the active replicating phase of zoster. Oral acyclovir is poorly absorbed (15–20%), so a high dose (800 mg) given five times daily for 7 days is needed. Famciclovir (250 mg) and valacyclovir (1 g) are both much better absorbed and can be given three times daily for 7 days. Brivudin has greater antiviral potency than the others, but is not available in the United States or UK at present. It is given once daily (125 mg). All have been shown to reduce the acute pain, accelerate healing, prevent scar-

ring, and possibly reduce the incidence of PHN. They have an excellent safety profile. Headache, nausea, diarrhea, and CNS, renal, and hepatic dysfunction can occur. Due to better absorption, famciclovir and valacyclovir may be slightly more effective. These antiviral drugs are expensive and only effective in the acute phase of zoster.

Indications for antiviral treatment are:

1. within 48 h of the onset of the rash;
2. up to 72 h of onset in the following: age over 50; affecting the ophthalmic branch of the fifth cranial nerve; immunocompromised; if new vesicle formation is still occurring.

The evidence for antivirals preventing true PHN (as opposed to pain associated with the acute episode) is still debatable, but logically it seems right to treat the above groups.

Foscarnet (given intravenously 40 mg/kg body weight three times daily) is effective against acyclovir-resistant strains of the virus because it does not rely on viral kinases for phosphorylation.

Corticosteroids have been used in conjunction with antivirals with the aim of reducing PHN. They may help to reduce acute pain and aid rash resolution, but no improvement in the incidence or severity of PHN has been seen. The tricyclic antidepressants *amitriptyline, desipramine* and *nortriptyline* (the latter is better tolerated and is recommended) and *gabapentin* (a new anticonvulsant) have been shown to be helpful. It is possible that prophylactic treatment with low doses of nortriptyline (10–20 mg at night) as soon as zoster is diagnosed may be helpful in the high-risk group (over age 60 years).

Topical measures do not help except for *lidocaine patches* and *capsaicin cream*. The latter can cause an intense burning sensation after application, which reduces many patients' compliance.

Patients with established PHN may benefit from 45 mg of controlled-release *oxycodone* with improved pain relief and reduction of allodynia. Beneficial effects of *tramadol* have also been demonstrated.

Asymptomatic reactivation of the varicella-zoster virus and contact with patients with chickenpox may enhance cell-mediated immunity. Frequent contact with children (even without chickenpox) seems to reduce the incidence of zoster. Vaccination of children against varicella may result in an increased incidence of zoster because there will be fewer opportunities for those with latent varicella-zoster infection to boost their immunity. However, the vaccine virus may be less likely to become dormant and reactive, so vaccination would be beneficial in those who have been vaccinated. Vaccination of adults may be helpful.

SPECIFIC INVESTIGATIONS

- Tzanck smear
- Viral culture
- Serology
- Electron microscopy
- Check HIV status in appropriate cases

In most cases investigation is not required to establish the diagnosis.

FIRST LINE THERAPIES

Antiviral agents	
■ Acyclovir	A
■ Famciclovir	A
■ Valacyclovir	A

Effect of oral acyclovir on pain resolution in herpes zoster: a reanalysis. Huff JC, Drucker JL, Clemmer A, et al. J Med Virol 1993;41(suppl 1):93–6.

Acyclovir reduced chronic zoster-associated pain (median duration of pain 20 days vs placebo 62 days) in 187 immunocompetent patients.

Famciclovir for the treatment of acute herpes zoster: effects on acute disease and postherpetic neuralgia. A randomized, double-blind, placebo controlled trial. Tyring S, Barbarash RA, Nahlik JE, et al. Ann Intern Med 1995;123: 89–96.

Famciclovir recipients had faster resolution of pain following an acute episode than those receiving placebo.

Antiviral therapy for herpes zoster: randomized, controlled clinical trial of valacyclovir and famciclovir therapy in immunocompetent patients 50 years and older. Tyring SK, Beutner KR, Tucker BA, et al. Arch Fam Med 2000;9:863–9.

Valacyclovir is comparable to famciclovir in the resolution of zoster-associated pain and PHN.

SECOND LINE THERAPIES

Agents to reduce post-herpetic neuralgia	
■ Lidocaine patch	A
■ Tricyclic antidepressants (e.g. nortriptyline)	A
■ Gabapentin	A
■ Oxycodone	A

Topical lidocaine patch relieves post-herpetic neuralgia more effectively than a vehicle topical patch: results of an enriched enrollment study. Galer BS, Rowbotham MC, Perander J, et al. Pain 1999; 80:533–8.

A lidocaine patch is an effective form of pain relief. There is no systemic uptake nor does the dose need to be increased over time to maintain effectiveness.

Amitriptyline versus placebo in postherpetic neuralgia. Watson CP, Evans RJ, Reed K, et al. Neurology 1982;32: 671–3.

Amitriptyline is effective in the treatment of PHN, and this benefit is independent of its antidepressant action.

The effects of pre-emptive treatment of postherpetic neuralgia with amitriptyline: a randomized, double-blind, placebo-controlled trial. Bowsher D. J Pain Symptom Manage 1997;13:327–31.

Low-dose amitriptyline given at the time of the acute zoster rash may reduce the incidence of PHN in 'at-risk patients' (i.e. those over 60 years of age).

Nortriptyline versus amitriptyline in post-herpetic neuralgia: a randomized trial. Watson CPN, Vernich L, Chipman M, et al. Neurology 1998; 51:1166–71.

Nortriptyline is equally efficacious as amitriptyline but is better tolerated, so it is the anti-depressant of choice in preventing and treating PHN. Nortriptyline is given as 10–20 mg daily and gradually increased until effective up to a maximum of 150 mg daily.

Gabapentin for the treatment of post-herpetic neuralgia: a randomized controlled trial. Rowbotham M, Harden N, Stacey B, et al. JAMA 1998;280:1837–42.

Gabapentin is effective in the treatment of pain and sleep interference associated with PHN. Mood and quality of life also improve. It is given as 300 mg three times daily.

Efficacy of oxycodone in neuropathic pain: a randomized trial in post-herpetic neuralgia. Watson CPN, Babul N. Neurology 1998;50:1837–41.

Patients on slow-release oxycodone (dose range 20–60 mg) had significantly greater pain relief and reduction in allodynia and disability.

THIRD LINE THERAPIES

■ Contact with varicella or with children	C
■ Vaccination of children or adults	E
■ Corticosteroids	E
■ Topical capsaicin	A
■ Topical nonsteroidal anti-inflammatory cream	C
■ Tramadol	B
■ Sympathetic nerve block	C
■ Transcutaneous electrical stimulation	C

Contacts with varicella or with children and protection against herpes zoster in adults: a case controlled study. Thomas SL, Wheeler JG, Hall AJ. Lancet 2002;360:678–82.

Social contact with many children outside the household or occupational contacts with children ill with chickenpox results in a graded protection against zoster.

Acyclovir with and without prednisone for the treatment of herpes zoster. A randomized placebo-controlled trial. Whitley RJ, Weiss H, Gnann JW Jr, et al. Ann Intern Med 1996;125:376–83.

There was no statistical difference between acyclovir plus prednisone and acyclovir alone in the resolution of pain during the 6 months after the acute episode.

Postherpetic neuralgia and topical capsaicin. Watson CP, Evans RJ, Watt VR. Post-herpetic neuralgia and topical capsaicin. Pain 1988;33:333–40.

Topical capsaicin (0.025%) was used to treat 33 patients, of whom 39% had a good result.

A randomized vehicle-controlled trial of topical capsaicin in the treatment of postherpetic neuralgia. Watson CPN, Tyler KL, Bickers DR, et al. Clin Ther 1993;15:510–26.

A double-blind study with 143 patients comparing capsaicin 0.075% cream with vehicle. Capsaicin was effective. The response was maintained in 86% of 77 patients who entered a subsequent open-label follow-up phase of 2 years' duration. The only side effect was the burning or stinging at sites of application.

Benzydamine cream for the treatment of post-herpetic neuralgia: minimum duration of treatment periods in a

Evidence levels A Double-blind study B Clinical trial ≥ 20 subjects C Clinical trial < 20 subjects D Series ≥ 5 subjects E Anecdotal case reports

cross-over trial. McQuay HJ, Carroll D, Moxon A, et al. Pain 1990;40:131–5.

Some patients benefit.

Treatment of pain due to post-herpetic neuralgia with tramadol: results of an open, parallel pilot study vs clomipramine with and without levomepromazine. Gobel H, Stadler T. Clin Drug Invest 1995;10:208–14.

A weak opioid μ-receptor agonist and monoamine-reuptake inhibitor resulted in effective pain relief for nine of ten patients.

Treatment of herpes zoster with sympathetic blocks. Tenicela R, Lovasik D, Eaglstein W. Clin J Pain 1985;1:63–7.

Twenty patients enrolled with acute herpetic pain (< 6 weeks). Nine of ten treated with bupivacaine 0.25% were pain free after 1–4 daily treatments, whereas two of ten treated with electrolyte placebo were pain free.

Transcutaneous electrical nerve stimulation for chronic pain. Bates JA, Nathan PW. Anaesthesia 1980;35:817–22.

One-third of patients treated were continuing to use treatment after 1 year, and one-quarter after 2 years. The rest stopped treatment because it was ineffective, made the pain worse, or the pain became worse after stopping treatment.

Hidradenitis suppurativa

Gregor BE Jemec

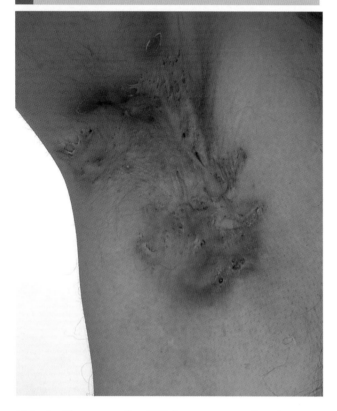

Hidradenitis suppurativa (HS) is a common chronic recurrent multifocal disease of skin and subcutaneous tissues affecting inverse (flexural) areas where it causes inflammation, scarring, and sinus formation. It is a follicular disease, distinct from acne vulgaris, staphylococcosis, and furunculosis. Pain and suppuration cause considerable morbidity and significantly impair quality of life.

MANAGEMENT STRATEGY

No pathognomonic test exists. Early diagnosis relies on recognition of recurrent, multifocal, painful inflammatory lesions, often bilaterally, in the axillae and anogenital regions. Age of onset is usually after the teenage period.

According to Hurley, stage I lesions are often 'blind' boils (i.e. deep and rounded). Gradually scarring and sinus formation occur in separate areas of the affected regions (stage II), and ultimately scarring and sinuses coalesce to form stage III lesions. Early lesions may remit with treatment. Once sinus tracts are established the treatment options are more limited and the disease is more chronic. Patients can often be managed by a structured approach, though many will ultimately require surgery.

Clinically HS can often be distinguished from furunculosis (often large boils and not limited to inverse areas) and epidermal cysts (usually solitary lesions). Microbiology is most useful in the later stages of disease when superinfection with organisms such as anaerobic streptococci or *Streptococcus milleri* may occur. Early lesions are frequently sterile

on routine culture of swabs. Suspicion of mycobacterial infection, metastasis, or Crohn's disease requires specific investigations.

Current medical practice is mainly empirical. A three-stage approach gives structure to patient management. The first stage consists of topical treatment. *Topical clindamycin* has been shown to have an effect on early lesions in a double blind, placebo-controlled study. *Systemic tetracycline* may be used as an alternative (500 mg orally twice daily). This treatment can be supplemented with regional prophylactic treatment with *azelaic acid cream* once daily.

Specific treatment should be directed at superinfections, and can involve *oral clindamycin* 300 mg twice daily or *dicloxacillin* 500 mg three times daily. Hormonal therapy with *cyproterone acetate* may be helpful for some females, but requires high and continued use, which raises safety concerns.

The second stage of treatment involves *intralesional corticosteroids* or *minor surgery* (i.e. localized excisions or exteriorization of sinus tracts).

The third stage of treatment involves *major surgery* or *palliative medication*. Surgical intervention should involve excision of the affected tissue or careful laying open of all sinus tracts, but not lancing. The recurrence rate is inversely proportional to the extent of surgery: wide extensive surgery may offer a better chance of remission. Palliative medication includes systemic anti-inflammatory drugs such as *oral corticosteroids, cyclosporine, or infliximab*. An initial anti-inflammatory response may be followed by relapse, and superinfection may intervene as a further complication. HS shows little sign of improvement with isotretinoin.

General measures that reduce smoking and pressure and shearing forces at affected sites are advisable, as is weight loss in the obese.

SPECIFIC INVESTIGATIONS

- Histopathology
- Microbiology

Hidradenitis suppurativa: disease of follicular epithelium rather than disease of apocrine glands. Yu CC, Cook MG. Br J Dermatol 1990;122:763–9.

Squamous epithelium-lined structures (probably abnormal dilated hair follicles) are a more constant diagnostic feature than inflammation of apocrine glands.

The microbiology of hidradenitis suppurativa. Jemec GBE, Faber M, Gutschick E, Wendelboe P. Dermatology 1996;193: 203–6.

Bacteria are found in 50% of lesions.

FIRST LINE THERAPIES

■ Antibiotics – clindamycin and tetracycline	B
■ Surgery	B

Topical treatment of hidradenitis suppurativa with clindamycin. Clemmensen OJ. Int J Dermatol 1983;22:325–8.

Topical clindamycin for 3 months was significantly more effective than placebo in early lesions.

A randomized trial of topical clindamycin vs. systemic tetracycline in hidradenitis suppurativa with special reference to disease assessment. Jemec GBE, Wendelboe P. J Am Acad Dermatol 1998;39:971–4.

Clinical equivalence of efficacy between topical clindamycin and oral tetracycline in 46 patients.

Axillary hyperhidrosis, apocrine bromhidrosis, hidradenitis suppurativa, and familial benign pemphigus: surgical approach. Hurley HJ. In: Roenigk RK, Roenigk HHJ, eds. Dermatologic surgery: principles and practice. New York: Marcel Dekker; 1989;717–43.

A good synthesis of long clinical experience.

Extent of surgery and recurrence rate of hidradenitis suppurativa. Ritz P, Runkel N, Haier J, Buhr HJ. Int J Colorectal Dis 1998;13:164–8.

Drainage alone carries a recurrence rate of up to 100%; radical excision has a recurrence rate of 25% at a median interval of 20 months.

SECOND LINE THERAPIES

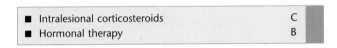

■ Intralesional corticosteroids	C
■ Hormonal therapy	B

A double-blind controlled cross-over trial of cyproterone acetate in females with hidradenitis suppurativa. Mortimer PS, Dawber RP, Gales MA, Moore RA. Br J Dermatol 1986;115:263–8.

Equal clinical effect from cyproterone acetate (plus ethinyl estradiol) and a 50 μg ethinyl estradiol contraceptive pill.

Hidradenitis suppurativa: pathogenesis and management. Slade DEM, Powell BW, Mortimer PS. Br J Plast Surg 2003;56:45–61.

Although the use of intralesional corticosteroids is mentioned anecdotally, this article offers an excellent approach to the therapeutic options available to patients with HS.

THIRD LINE THERAPIES

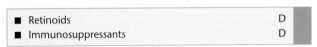

■ Retinoids	D
■ Immunosuppressants	D

Failure of treatment of familial widespread hidradenitis suppurativa with isotretinoin. Norris JF, Cunliffe WJ. Clin Exp Dermatol 1986;11:579–83.

Pure HS without acne vulgaris or conglobata does not respond to isotretinoin.

Long-term results of isotretinoin in the treatment of 68 patients with hidradenitis suppurativa. Boer J, van Gemert JP. J Am Acad Dermatol 1999;40:73–6.

Isotretinoin had generally poor effect; any effect was mainly in mild disease. The condition cleared in 11 of 68 patients. Doses ranged between 0.5 and 0.8 mg/kg daily for 4–6 months.

Infliximab for hidradenitis suppurativa. Sullivan TP, Welsh E, Kerdel FA, et al. Br J Dermatol 2003;149:1046–9.

Objective and subjective improvement in five treated cases.

Cyclosporin-responsive hidradenitis suppurativa. Buckley DA, Rogers S. J R Soc Med 1995;88:289–90.

Immunosuppressant therapy can be helpful, but care is required in the presence of infection.

Histoplasmosis

Wanda Sonia Robles

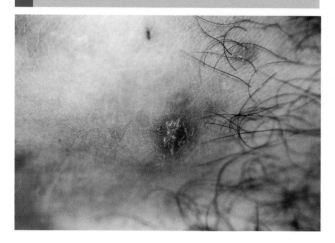

Histoplasmosis is an acute or chronic, highly infectious disease caused by the fungus *Histoplasma capsulatum* or the closely related *H. duboisii*. This is an intracellular organism which primarily infects the lungs, where it is usually asymptomatic. The infection is usually contracted through inhalation of spores in dry soil or bird or bat droppings. Most infections are self-limiting but the disease occasionally becomes disseminated, especially in immunosuppressed individuals, including those with AIDS. Other sites then involved include the liver, spleen, kidneys, central nervous system, and skin. Cutaneous lesions are usually multiple small nodules which may ulcerate. The infection caused by *H. capsulatum* is widely distributed throughout the world. It is highly endemic in the USA, particularly in the Mississippi and the Ohio valleys. Infections with *H. duboisii* have been reported only from Africa.

In addition to the skin lesions of disseminated disease, which are likely to be seen only in a patient who is clearly ill, histoplasmosis may present to the dermatologist as a cause of erythema multiforme, erythema nodosum, or toxic erythema.

MANAGEMENT STRATEGY

Pulmonary forms of histoplasmosis in the acute phase may resolve spontaneously but should be treated. The treatment of choice for many cases of both histoplasmosis and African histoplasmosis is *itraconazole*, which is very effective. However, *amphotericin B* should be used for extensive infections, where the patient is acutely sick, or as initial therapy in AIDS patients. The majority of patients requiring initial treatment with amphotericin B respond quickly and can then continue treatment with itraconazole to finish their course of therapy. Other alternatives are *fluconazole, ketoconazole*, and *sulfonamides*.

SPECIFIC INVESTIGATIONS

- Microscopy and culture of sputum, blood, bone marrow, or biopsy material
- Histology
- Serology
- Serology for HIV/AIDS (where relevant)

Disseminated histoplasmosis in persons infected with human immunodeficiency virus. Hajjeh RA. Clin Infect Dis 1995;21(suppl 1):S108–10.

Disseminated histoplasmosis is an AIDS-defining illness that occurs in approximately 5% of AIDS patients who are resident in endemic areas of the USA. This paper reviews current treatment of histoplasmosis with consideration of the role of chemoprophylaxis using itraconazole in endemic areas.

Disseminated histoplasmosis presenting with cutaneous lesions in a patient with acquired immunodeficiency syndrome. Angius AG, Viviani MA, Muratori S, et al. J Eur Acad Dermatol Venereol 1998;10:182–5.

Case report of a 54-year-old homosexual male with AIDS-related Kaposi sarcoma who developed cutaneous lesions and fever due to disseminated histoplasmosis. The patient was successfully treated with itraconazole 200 mg daily. Attention is drawn to the fact that patients with HIV/AIDS may develop histoplasmosis even in nonendemic areas.

Diffuse ulcerations due to disseminated histoplasmosis in a patient with HIV. Scheinfeld N. J Drugs Dermatol 2003;2: 189–91.

Case report of a patient who developed disseminated histoplasmosis while on antiretroviral therapy and with a CD4 count of 525 mm^3.

FIRST LINE THERAPIES

■ Itraconazole	B
■ Amphotericin B	B

Practice guidelines for the management of patients with histoplasmosis. Infectious Diseases Society of America. Wheat J, Sarosi G, McKinsey D, et al. Clin Infect Dis 2000;30: 688–95.

This paper includes treatment of patients with the more common form of histoplasmosis. Treatment options include itraconazole, fluconazole, ketoconazole, amphotericin B, liposomal amphotericin B, amphotericin B colloidal suspension, and amphotericin B lipid complex.

Itraconazole treatment of disseminated histoplasmosis in patients with the acquired immunodeficiency syndrome. AIDS Clinical Trial Group. Wheat J, Hafner R, Korzun AH, et al. Am J Med 1995;98:336–42.

A multicenter, nonrandomized, prospective trial. All patients involved in this study had AIDS and were treated with itraconazole 300 mg twice daily for 3 days and then 200 mg twice daily for 12 weeks. Evaluation of 59 patients showed that 50 (85%) responded well to therapy. Five withdrew from the study because of progressive infection, one died within the first week of therapy without improvement, two withdrew because of toxicity of the medication, and one

Evidence levels **A** Double-blind study **B** Clinical trial ≥ 20 subjects **C** Clinical trial < 20 subjects **D** Series ≥ 5 subjects **E** Anecdotal case reports

was lost to follow-up. Resolution of systemic symptoms occurred after a median of 3 weeks in the less severely affected and 6 weeks in the moderately severe cases. Fungemia cleared after a median of 1 week.

Itraconazole is safe and effective in the treatment of mild disseminated histoplasmosis in patients with AIDS. For patients with moderately severe or severe histoplasmosis, amphotericin B is the drug of first choice and this can be switched to itraconazole after clinical improvement.

Management of histoplasmosis. Kauffman CA. Expert Opin Pharmacother 2002;3:1067–72.

This paper highlights the importance of the infection in endemic areas of histoplasmosis where millions of people are exposed. However, it also highlights the fact that most people may have a self-limiting infection which does not require treatment. The ones that require treatment are those with disseminated infection, pulmonary infection, or focal organ involvement. The treatment of choice for severe infection is amphotericin B, and itraconazole is given to patients with mild to moderate infection.

A good review.

Disseminated histoplasmosis in children: the role of itraconazole therapy. Tobon AM, Franco L, Espinal D, et al. Pediatr Infect Dis J 1996;15:1002–8.

A study involving seven children, five girls and two boys, aged 1–14 years. All had confirmed diagnosis of disseminated histoplasmosis and malnourishment, but no underlying disease. All patients were treated with itraconazole at a dose of 7.2 mg/kg daily for a period varying from 3 to 12 months, depending on individual responses. The study concludes that itraconazole is effective in the treatment of disseminated histoplasmosis in children.

Itraconazole maintenance treatment for histoplasmosis in AIDS: a prospective, multicenter trial. Hecht FM, Wheat J, Korzun AH, et al. J Acquir Immune Defic Syndr Hum Retrovirol 1997;16:100–7.

A prospective, multicenter, open-label study involving 46 patients with AIDS and mild to moderate disseminated histoplasmosis. All patients had successfully completed 12 weeks of induction treatment with itraconazole and were then treated with itraconazole 200 mg once daily (n = 42) or 400 mg once daily (n = 4) as maintenance. From the start of the maintenance therapy, the estimated 1-year survival rate was 73%. The authors concluded that itraconazole 200 mg daily is effective in preventing relapse of disseminated histoplasmosis in patients with AIDS. The medication was generally well tolerated but attention is drawn to possible drug interactions and liver damage.

African histoplasmosis: therapeutic efficacy of itraconazole. Velho GC, Cabral JM, Massa A. J Eur Acad Dermatol Venereol 1998;10:77–80.

A report of a patient with African histoplasmosis who was unsuccessfully treated for 7 years with ketoconazole. Treatment with itraconazole 100 mg daily for 9 months was successful. No evidence of relapse was observed during the 3-year follow-up period.

Itraconazole prophylaxis for fungal infections in patients with advanced human immunodeficiency virus infection: randomized, placebo-controlled, double-blind study. National Institute of Allergy and Infectious Diseases Mycoses Study Group. McKinsey DS, Wheat LJ, Cloud GA, et al. Clin Infect Dis 199;28:1049–56.

A prospective, randomized, double-blind trial involving 295 patients with advanced HIV infection randomized to receive itraconazole capsules at a dose of 200 mg daily or placebo. Itraconazole significantly delayed time to onset of histoplasmosis and cryptococcosis. No benefit was observed in survival. The medication was generally well tolerated. Itraconazole is therefore recommended for primary prophylaxis against histoplasmosis and cryptococcosis in patients with HIV infection.

Disseminated histoplasmosis successfully treated with liposomal amphotericin B following azathioprine therapy in a patient from a nonendemic area. Poveda F, Carcia-Alergria J, de las Nieves MA, et al. Eur J Clin Microbiol Infect Dis 1998;17:357–9.

Case report of a 22-year-old Spanish male who developed disseminated histoplasmosis in a nonendemic area. The patient had been treated with azathioprine and prednisolone for 4 weeks before presentation. Acute presentation may have represented reactivation of a latent infection as a complication of the immunosuppressive treatment.

Safety and efficacy of liposomal amphotericin B compared with conventional amphotericin B for induction therapy of histoplasmosis in patients with AIDS. Johnson PC, Wheat LT, Cloud GA, et al. US National Institute of Allergy and Infectious Diseases Mycoses Study Group. Ann Intern Med 2002;137:105–9.

A multicenter, randomized, controlled trial to compare liposomal amphotericin B with conventional amphotericin B for induction therapy of moderate to severe disseminated histoplasmosis in patients with AIDS. Results reported a clinical success in 64% of patients treated with conventional amphotericin B compared with 88% of patients receiving liposomal amphotericin B. Culture conversion rates were similar. This study concludes that liposomal amphotericin B is a less toxic alternative to conventional amphotericin B and is associated with improved survival.

Case report. Successful therapy of disseminated histoplasmosis in AIDS with liposomal amphotericin B. Rieg GK, Shah PM, Helm EB, Just-Nubling G. Mycoses 1999;42:117–20.

Case report of a 36-year-old HIV-positive patient who developed disseminated infection with *H. capsulatum*. Treatment was initiated with amphotericin B for 24 days. Symptoms recurred 14 days after therapy was discontinued. Liposomal amphotericin B was subsequently started, with rapid improvement of clinical signs. Maintenance therapy with itraconazole 600 mg daily was initiated and reduced to 400 mg daily after 2 weeks. This was continued for 2 years, until the patient died of other complications of HIV infection.

Clearance of fungal burden during treatment of disseminated histoplasmosis with liposomal amphotericin B versus itraconazole. Wheat LJ, Cloud G, Johnson PC, et al. AIDS Clinical Trials Group; Mycoses Study Group of NIAID. Antimicrob Agents Chemother 2001;45:2354–7.

The evaluation of the efficacy of liposomal amphotericin B and itraconazole treatment of disseminated histoplasmosis in patients with AIDS was made in two separate closed clinical trials. The clinical response rates were similar: 86%

with liposomal amphotericin B versus 85% with itraconazole. However, the authors observed a more rapid clearance of fungemia with the use of liposomal amphotericin B than with itraconazole.

SECOND LINE THERAPIES

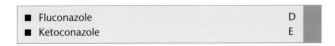

■ Fluconazole	D
■ Ketoconazole	E

Fluconazole therapy for histoplasmosis. The National Institute of Allergy and Infectious Diseases Mycoses Study Group. McKinsey DS, Kauffman FA, Pappas PG, et al. Clin Infect Dis 1996;23:996–1001.

A randomized controlled trial. Of 27 evaluable patients, two had progressive acute pulmonary histoplasmosis, 11 had chronic pulmonary histoplasmosis, and 14 had disseminated histoplasmosis. Nineteen patients were treated with fluconazole 400 mg daily (two of these received 800 mg daily for a period of their treatment), seven were treated with fluconazole 200 mg daily, and one was treated with 800 mg daily. Successful treatment is reported in 17 (63%) of 27 cases; no substantial toxicity was reported. The authors conclude that fluconazole is only moderately effective and should be reserved for patients intolerant to itraconazole.

Treatment of histoplasmosis with fluconazole in patients with acquired immunodeficiency syndrome. National Institute of Allergy and Infectious Diseases Acquired Immunodeficiency Syndrome Clinical Trials Group and Mycoses Study Group. Wheat J, MaWhinney S, Hafner R, et al. Am J Med 1997;103:223–32.

A multicenter, open-label, nonrandomized, prospective trial. All patients had AIDS and mild to moderately severe disseminated histoplasmosis. They were treated with fluconazole 1600 mg once on the first day, then 800 mg once daily for 12 weeks (induction therapy), and patients who improved clinically were then given maintenance fluconazole 400 mg daily for 1 year. Thirty-six of 49 patients responded to induction therapy. Of the seven patients who failed induction therapy because of progression of histoplasmosis, one died from the infection. Two of the 49 withdrew due to liver toxicity. Of the 36 patients who entered into the maintenance phase of the study, 11 (35%) relapsed,

including one who died. The relapse-free rate at 1 year was 53%. Fluconazole 800 mg daily was considered a safe and moderately effective induction therapy for mild or moderately severe disseminated histoplasmosis in patients with AIDS. Fluconazole 400 mg daily is less effective than itraconazole 200–400 mg daily or amphotericin B 50 mg weekly as maintenance therapy to prevent relapse. This is based on historic comparison.

African histoplasmosis: report of two patients treated with amphotericin B and ketoconazole. Akpuaka FC, Gugnani HC, Iregbulam LM. Mycoses 1998;41:363–4.

Report of two patients with African histoplasmosis successfully treated with combined therapy.

Life-threatening histoplasmosis complicating immunotherapy with tumor necrosis factor alpha antagonists infliximab and etanercept. Lee JH, Slifman NR, Gershon SK, et al. Arthritis Rheum 2002;46:2565–70.

This paper reviewed the US Food and Drug Administration's passive surveillance database for monitoring postlicensure adverse events in patients treated with infliximab and etanercept. Infliximab was licensed in 1998 for treatment of Crohn's disease and etanercept was licensed in 1998 for treatment of rheumatoid arthritis. The authors were able to identify all reports received through July 2001 and 10 cases of *H. capsulatum* infection were reported. Of the 10 patients with histoplasmosis, nine required treatment in an intensive care unit and one died. This suggests that acute life-threatening histoplasmosis may be a complication of immunotherapy with tumor necrosis factor-α antagonists.

Safety of discontinuation of maintenance therapy for disseminated histoplasmosis after immunologic response to antiretroviral therapy. Goldman M, Zackin R, Fichtenbaum CJ, et al. AIDS Clinical Trials Group A5038 Study Group. Clin Infect Dis 2004;38:1485–9.

This was a prospective observational study to assess the safety of stopping maintenance therapy for disseminated histoplasmosis in patients with HIV infection after treatment with antiretroviral therapy. The study concluded that discontinuation of antifungal therapy appears to be safe in patients with previously treated disseminated histoplasmosis who have sustained immunologic improvement with antiretroviral therapy.

Hydroa vacciniforme

Herbert Hönigsmann

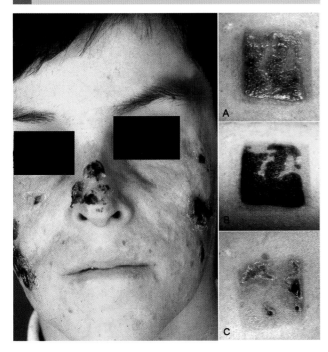

Hydroa vacciniforme is a very rare, idiopathic photo-dermatosis that principally starts in childhood, frequently resolving by adolescence or young adulthood. It is charac-terized by recurrent crops of papulovesicles or vesicles, most commonly on the face and the dorsa of the hands, but other sun-exposed areas of the skin may also be involved. The vesicles resolve with pock-like scarring. The disease was first described by Bazin in 1862 and it is possible that before the clear definition of erythropoietic protoporphyria by Magnus et al. in 1961, some cases may have been protoporphyria rather than hydroa because of the similarity of symptoms. Some recent reports of an association with Epstein–Barr virus (EBV) infection are interesting, but not all these cases are typical – they are associated with lymphoma and may not represent the usual form of hydroa vacciniforme.

MANAGEMENT STRATEGY

Hydroa vacciniforme usually presents in childhood, with sometimes spontaneous improvement during adolescence. Parents generally seek specialist advice because their children are unable to tolerate sunshine (play outdoors or travel abroad) and because the eruption can result in considerable scarring, both causing significant morbidity.

Hydroa vacciniforme is almost always refractory to any treatment, but *restriction of sun exposure, appropriate clothing, and regular use of broad-spectrum sunscreens with an effective UVA filter* can help in mild to moderate disease. Windows in the car and home can be covered with certain films that filter UV wavelengths less than 380 nm.

In patients with more severe disease, however, courses of *narrowband UVB phototherapy* or *psoralen with UVA (PUVA)* administered as for polymorphic light eruption may help

occasionally. Both phototherapy regimens usually consist of thrice weekly treatments for an average of 3–4 weeks. It is important to administer these therapies carefully to avoid provoking disease exacerbations.

Antimicrobial therapy has also been tried as have antimalarials and systemic immunosuppressive therapy, including intermittent oral corticosteroids, but although occasionally helpful, none of these appear to be reliably effective. Beta-carotene used in several studies, however, was mostly shown to be ineffective.

For severe and refractory hydroa vacciniforme unre-sponsive to other therapies, immunosuppressive agents including *azathioprine* and *cyclosporine* may be effective, but thalidomide does not seem to be. However, the use of immunosuppressive drugs for an admittedly unpleasant, but otherwise benign disease should be considered carefully.

In two reports, *dietary fish oil* rich in omega-3 polyunsat-urated fatty acids, was associated with clinical improvement in three of four patients. The mechanism may be through inhibition of prostanoid production and by their proposed buffering effect against free radical-induced damage.

The rare nature of this condition means that there are no large or randomized trials. Evidence for treatment is based on case series or single reports.

SPECIFIC INVESTIGATIONS

- Erythrocyte and plasma protoporphyrin levels, red cell photohemolysis, and stool analysis
- Photoprovocation testing with UVA
- Serology for antinuclear antibody and extractable nuclear antigens
- Urinary amino acids
- Screening for EBV infection and detection of EBV-infected cells by T cell receptor gamma gene rearrangement with polymerase chain reaction

A porphyrin screen will exclude erythropoietic proto-porphyria.

Photoprovocation testing induces typical blisters. Light tests are abnormal in the UVA range. Photographs to the right of the figure show the result of photoprovocation with UVA (three times 30 J/cm² on three consecutive days): A. After 24 h; B. After 48 h; C. After 2 weeks.

Serology for antinuclear antibody and extractable nuclear antigens (anti-Ro, La and Sm), will exclude bullous lupus erythematosus, which quite commonly can be ruled out by its clinical symptoms.

Rare cases have been associated with metabolic disor-ders, such as Hartnup disease, so aminoaciduria should be ruled out.

Screening for EBV is required only if lymphoma is suspected.

Hydroa vacciniforme – Aktionsspektrum. Jaschke E, Hönigsmann H. Hautarzt 1981;32:350–3.
Successful photoprovocation with UVA in one case.

Hydroa vacciniforme: induction of lesions with ultraviolet A. Halasz CL, Leach EE, Walther RR, Poh-Fitzpatrick MB. J Am Acad Dermatol 1983;8:171–6.
Successful photoprovocation with UVA in one case.

Hydroa vacciniforme: a review of ten cases. Sonnex TS, Hawk JLM. Br J Dermatol 1988;118:101–8.

Successful photoprovocation with UVA in several cases.

Hydroa vacciniforme: a clinical and follow-up study of 17 cases. Gupta G, Man I, Kemmett D. J Am Acad Dermatol 2000;42:208–13.

Eight of 14 patients were sensitive in the UVA spectrum. UVA provocation tests showed a papulovesicular response in six of 14 patients.

There is now strong evidence that UVA radiation is the causal factor. In addition to reduced UVA minimal erythema dose values, repetitive broad-spectrum UVA has been shown to reproduce lesions that are clinically and histologically identical to those produced by natural sunlight and that heal with scarring. All cases seen so far by the present author (HH) had their action spectrum in the UVA range.

Hydroa vacciniforme occurring in association with Hartnup disease. Ashurst PJ. Br J Dermatol 1969;81:486–92.

This was a case report of a single patient.

Urinary amino acids should be checked to exclude aminoacidurias.

Epstein–Barr virus-associated lymphoproliferative lesions presenting as a hydroa vacciniforme-like eruption: an analysis of six cases. Cho KH, Lee SH, Kim CW, et al. Br J Dermatol 2004;151:372–80.

A report of six patients and review of the literature.

This type of sunlight-induced rash may well be a different entity, but this requires further investigations.

FIRST LINE THERAPIES

■ High-factor broad-spectrum sunscreens and behavioral sunlight avoidance	C

Hydroa vacciniforme: a clinical and follow-up study of 17 cases. Gupta G, Man I, Kemmett D. J Am Acad Dermatol 2000;42:208–13.

Disease in nine of 15 patients was controlled satisfactorily with high-factor, broad-spectrum sunscreens and behavioral sunlight avoidance.

Hydroa vacciniforme: a review of ten cases. Sonnex TS, Hawk JLM. Br J Dermatol 1988;118:101–8.

Disease severity was reduced in eight of ten patients using either Coppertone Supershade 15® or ROC Factor 10®.

Most sunscreens offer good UVB but not UVA protection. The new Dundee sunscreen Reflectant Sun Screen, which is available from Tayside Pharmaceuticals, Ninewells Hospital, and Medical School, Dundee DD1 9SY, UK, offers better protection in the UVA and visible spectrum.

Borrowing from museums and industry: two photo-protective devices. Dawe R, Russell S, Ferguson J. Br J Dermatol 1996;135:1016–7.

The Museum 200 Film (manufactured by Sun Guard, Florida, USA) prevents transmission of all wavelengths less than 380 nm.

This is a clear, lightweight film that can stick onto any glass surface without causing visual impairment. It may be a useful adjunct in the treatment of most photodermatoses but in some

patients with hydroa vacciniforme, particularly those who are sensitive in the 380–400 nm wavelengths, it may not be beneficial.

SECOND LINE THERAPIES

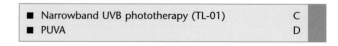

■ Narrowband UVB phototherapy (TL-01)	C
■ PUVA	D

Narrow-band UVB (TL-01) phototherapy: an effective preventative treatment for the photodermatoses. Collins P, Ferguson J. Br J Dermatol 1995;132:956–63.

This was an open clinical trial in which four patients were treated on average ten times on a daily basis. Two of these patients reported an increase in tolerance to sunshine from 1 h to 3–6 h.

Hydroa vacciniforme: a clinical and follow-up study of 17 cases. Gupta G, Man I, Kemmett D. J Am Acad Dermatol 2000;42:208–13.

Five of 15 patients who had not responded to conservative measures were treated with narrowband UVB phototherapy. In three patients there was good or moderate disease control. In the other two patients, narrowband UVB phototherapy was not helpful.

Hydroa vacciniforme: a review of ten cases. Sonnex TS, Hawk JLM. Br J Dermatol 1988;118:101–8.

Two of ten patients were treated with UVB with improvement in their disease.

It is likely that broadband UVB was used in this report but the methodology is unclear.

Hydroa vacciniforme – Aktionsspektrum. Jaschke E, Hönigsmann H. Hautarzt 1981;32:350–3.

One patient received PUVA therapy with good control of his disease.

Hydroa vacciniforme: a review of ten cases. Sonnex TS, Hawk JLM. Br J Dermatol 1988;118:101–8.

There was a flare of hydroa vacciniforme in the one patient treated with PUVA.

Photosensitivity disorders: cause, effect and management. Millard TP, Hawk JL. Am J Clin Dermatol 2002;3:239–46.

A review of the management of various photodermatosis with reference to the use of UVB and PUVA.

THIRD LINE THERAPIES

■ Antimalarials	D
■ Beta-carotene	E
■ Azathioprine	E
■ Cyclosporine	E
■ Dietary fish oil	E
■ Thalidomide	E

Hydroa vacciniforme: a review of ten cases. Sonnex TS, Hawk JLM. Br J Dermatol 1988;118:101–8.

Four of ten patients were treated with either hydroxychloroquine (two patients) or chloroquine (two patients). Hydroxychloroquine 100 mg daily was ineffective, but the

Evidence levels   **A** Double-blind study   **B** Clinical trial ≥ 20 subjects   **C** Clinical trial < 20 subjects   **D** Series ≥ 5 subjects   **E** Anecdotal case reports

two patients on chloroquine (100–125 mg daily) had a reduction in the severity of their disease.

Hydroa vacciniforme. Bickers DR, Demar LK, DeLeo V, et al. Arch Dermatol 1978;114:1193–6.

One patient treated with hydroxychloroquine 200 mg twice daily reported an improvement in his disease.

Hydroa vacciniforme: an unusual clinical manifestation. Leenutaphong V. J Am Acad Dermatol 1991;25:892–5.

One patient treated with chloroquine phosphate 500 mg daily did not find it beneficial.

Hydroa vacciniforme. Ketterer R, Morier P, Frenk E. Dermatology 1994;189:428–9.

One patient treated with chloroquine 100 mg daily and broad-spectrum sunscreens showed good disease control.

It is unclear whether the response was due to chloroquine or the sunscreen.

Hydroa vacciniforme. Bickers DR, Demar LK, DeLeo V, et al. Arch Dermatol 1978;114:1193–6.

Two patients reported an improvement of their disease with beta-carotene 180 mg daily.

Hydroa vacciniforme: induction of lesions with ultraviolet A. Halasz CLG, Leach EE, Walther RR, Poh-Fitzpatrick MB. J Am Acad Dermatol 1983;8:171–6.

The one patient treated with beta-carotene 180 mg daily reported some subjective improvement.

Hydroa vacciniforme: diagnosis and therapy. Goldgeier MH, Nordlund JJ, Lucky AW, et al. Arch Dermatol 1982;118:588–91.

Beta-carotene 120 mg daily for 2 months in the one patient was ineffective.

Hydroa vacciniforme presenting in an adult successfully treated with cyclosporin A. Blackwell V, McGregor JM, Hawk JLM. Clin Exp Dermatol 1998;23:73–6.

Azathioprine 2.5–3.5 mg/kg daily was ineffective in the one patient studied.

See additional report on use of azathioprine below.

Hydroa vacciniforme presenting in an adult successfully treated with cyclosporin A. Blackwell V, McGregor JM, Hawk JLM. Clin Exp Dermatol 1998;23:73–6.

There was good control of disease with cyclosporin A 3 mg/kg daily over a 2-month period.

The report does not provide details of follow-up.

Hydroa vacciniforme: traitement par huiles de poisson (Maxepa®). Modeste AB, Cordel N, Balguerie X, et al. Ann Dermatol Venereol 2001;128:247–9.

One patient was treated successfully after unsuccessful treatment with antimalarials.

Dietary fish oil as a photoprotective agent in hydroa vacciniforme. Rhodes LE, White SI. Br J Dermatol 1998;138: 173–8.

Three patients were treated with dietary fish oil, five capsules daily for 3 months. Mild to good improvement was noted in two patients and no improvement in the third.

The latter patient responded to azathioprine. The action of fish oils may be through inhibition of prostanoid production and by their proposed buffering effect against free radical-induced damage.

Hydroa vacciniforme: major and minor forms. Cruces MJ, de la Torre C. Photodermatol 1986;3:109–10.

In the one patient treated with thalidomide there was initial improvement.

Hydroa vacciniforme presenting in an adult successfully treated with cyclosporin A. Blackwell V, McGregor JM, Hawk JLM. Clin Exp Dermatol 1998;23:73–6.

In the one patient, thalidomide 100 mg daily was ineffective.

Hyperhidrosis

James AA Langtry

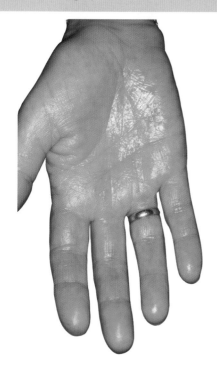

Hyperhidrosis is the result of increased secretion of eccrine sweat. This can be annoying, disabling (at work or socially), or indicative of an underlying systemic disease. The eccrine gland is unusual in that the sympathetic sudomotor fibers are cholinergic rather than adrenergic.

Disease associations

The classification of hyperhidrosis is variously described. Two approaches to classification are *idiopathic/pathologic* and *neural/non-neural*.

Idiopathic hyperhidrosis is defined as excessive sweating that is symmetrical, localized to the palms, soles, or axillae (singly or in combination), and independent of thermoregulation. Craniofacial hyperhidrosis is a similar but rarer condition. The other characteristics include its episodic nature, occurrence in response to stimuli, and onset on or after puberty; there is commonly a family history. There is an absence of bromhidrosis and little or no seasonal variation. *Pathologic* hyperhidrosis may be localized or generalized. Localized hyperhidrosis may result from injury to the central or peripheral nervous systems, syringomyelia, neuritis, myelitis, tabes dorsalis, or localized vascular diseases, including cold injury, arteriovenous malformation (AVM), and erythrocyanosis. Localized hyperhidrosis can occur as a functional nevus in which a normal number of eccrine glands are oversensitive to acetylcholine. Localized areas of hyperhidrosis can develop as a compensatory phenomenon when extensive anhidrosis develops in Ross' syndrome (bilateral Holmes Adie pupils, tendon areflexia, generalized anhidrosis, and compensatory islands of hyperhidrosis). Hyperhidrosis may occur in hereditary conditions, including blue rubber bleb nevus syndrome. The causes of generalized hyperhidrosis include: febrile illnesses; metabolic and endocrine diseases (diabetes, hyperthyroidism, gout, acromegaly, pregnancy, porphyria, pheochromocytoma, carcinoid syndrome, alcohol intoxication); congestive cardiac failure and shock; internal malignancy; CNS diseases (tumors and injury); and hereditary syndromes (Chediak–Higashi syndrome and phenylketonuria).

The *neural/non-neural* classification is based on the efferent sudomotor pathway, which consists of the cerebral cortex (emotional – the equivalent of idiopathic hyperhidrosis), hypothalamus (thermoregulatory, exercise, drugs, infection, metabolic, cardiovascular, vasomotor, neurologic), medulla (syringomyelia, auriculotemporal syndrome), spinal cord (syringomyelia, injury, tabes dorsalis), sympathetic ganglia, and postganglionic fibers. Facial surgery (particularly of the parotid) and trauma may result in localized gustatory sweating (Frey's syndrome). Hyperhidrosis of *non-neural* causes include local heat, local changes in blood flow (arteriovenous malformation), and drugs (cholinergic).

MANAGEMENT STRATEGY

The management of idiopathic hyperhidrosis is discussed.

Oral anticholinergic drugs and *minor tranquilizers* produce a dose-related inhibition of sweating and are therefore limited by side effects. Anticholinergic effects, including dry mouth, pupillary dilatation and photophobia, glaucoma, urinary retention, constipation, vomiting, and tachycardia, may occur at a dose that produces satisfactory sweat inhibition. Some, however, advocate the use of *glycopyrronium bromide* (Robinul®), 2 mg up to three times daily. *Propantheline*, 15 mg three times daily, is an alternative. Other systemic drugs which have been used include the calcium channel blocker *diltiazem*, the CNS inhibitor *clonidine*, and *tricyclic antidepressants*, although these are the subject of few anecdotal reports. Local treatments, including medical, electrical, or surgical modalities, aim to stop or reduce sweating sufficiently to control symptoms. Treatments with the lowest risk should be considered first, as dictated by the severity of the condition and in discussion with the patient to assess the balance of risk and benefit.

Topical aluminum chloride hexahydrate (ACH) 20–25% solution in ethanol is the first line treatment. The mechanism of action appears to result from occlusion of the intraepidermal eccrine duct below the level of the stratum corneum. Correct application technique is critical to compliance; in the axillae, the solution should be applied nightly to the unshaven skin, with or without occlusion, and washed off the following morning before daytime sweating is established. The presence of moisture results in the formation of hydrochloric acid and resultant skin irritation. Mild potency topical corticosteroids may be used to reduce the common problem of skin irritation, which is the usual reason for treatment failure. ACH solution should not be applied again in the morning. An oral anticholinergic (e.g. 1 mg of sodium glycopyrrolate) 45 min before application of ACH may increase the efficacy of ACH by reducing sweating at the time of application, allowing the ACH to be retained on the skin and exert its effect on the sweat pores. The oral anticholinergic may be discontinued after several treatments have initiated a reduction in sweating.

Hyperhidrosis may take 2–3 weeks to be controlled, at which time application can be reduced to once each week, or at an interval that maintains control. Other topical

Evidence levels   **A** Double-blind study   **B** Clinical trial ≥ 20 subjects   **C** Clinical trial < 20 subjects   **D** Series ≥ 5 subjects   **E** Anecdotal case reports

therapies include formaldehyde, which is a common contact sensitizer, and glutaraldehyde, which stains the skin. *Methenamine gel* releases formaldehyde but does not appear to produce contact allergy frequently, and has been used in the past.

Iontophoresis is the process of introducing salt ions in solution through the skin into the tissues and may be effective in treating palmoplantar and axillary hyperhidrosis. Several iontophoretic devices are commercially available. Current is transmitted to electrodes in two trays filled with tap water, and the hands or feet are placed flat in the bottom of the trays. The current is increased until the patient experiences slight discomfort (average 15 mA on the palms and 20 mA on the soles). A special electrode for axillary use is available for some of the iontophoretic devices. The mechanism of reduction in sweating is not known. Current densities below the threshold of damage to the acrosyringium are employed and mechanical obstruction does not occur. Iontophoresis is contraindicated in pregnancy and in patients with cardiac pacemakers and metal implants. Twenty-minute sessions three times a week are continued until sweating is sufficiently reduced: thereafter, once- or twice-monthly maintenance therapies are instituted. Anticholinergic drugs such as glycopyrridium bromide may also be introduced by electrophoresis. A recent report suggests that botulinum toxin delivered by iontophoresis to the palms may be effective in the treatment of palmar hyperhidrosis.

Oral anticholinergic drugs, topical treatments, and iontophoresis may produce effective palliation of hyperhidrosis. More aggressive treatments may be sought, however, as a result of treatment failure, inconvenience of the treatments, or side effects.

Botulinum toxin injected intradermally produces sustained anhidrosis and has been used recently to treat axillary, palmar, facial, and other sites of focal hyperhidrosis. There are eight known serotypes of botulinum toxin, type A exotoxin (BTX-A) being the one that is commercially available as BOTOX® and Dysport®. These different commercially available BTX-A products differ in their potency and are not equivalent unit for unit. Botulinum toxin type B (BTX-B; Neurobloc®) has been shown to be effective in the treatment of axillary hyperhidrosis. This may be used as an alternative to BTX-A products, especially where antibody formation has resulted in a loss of clinical benefit to BTX-A. It is recommended that experience be gained with one of the products. It produces its effect by irreversibly blocking release of acetylcholine from cholinergic junctions. Treatment of the axilla is simple and well tolerated. Multiple injections, 2 cm apart, are performed in the axillary vault corresponding to the area of maximum sweating (an area of approximately 200 cm²). Palmar skin is painful to inject (may require a regional wrist block), injection is less well tolerated, and there is a potential for producing weakness of the intrinsic hand musculature. It is not a practical treatment for plantar hyperhidrosis. Inactivation of affected cholinergic junctions is permanent, but through the normal process of turnover and repair, new cholinergic junctions are produced, so the effect is temporary. Onset of anhidrosis after injection occurs at 24–72 h and lasts 3–6 months.

A number of surgical techniques have been employed in the management of axillary hyperhidrosis. These include:

- Cryotherapy (very painful and poorly tolerated).
- Methods that remove subcutaneous tissue alone. A number of skin flap/incisions are described to gain access to the subcutaneous axillary tissues, and the deep dermis and adjacent subcutis are trimmed away. Subcutaneous curettage and axillary liposuction are other methods described for achieving this objective.
- Methods that excise skin and subcutaneous tissue.
- Methods that combine cutaneous excision and resection of subcutaneous tissue.

Selective ablation of the sympathetic innervation of the palms, axillae, and soles reduces sweating effectively. A number of side effects are associated with sympathectomy, including compensatory hyperhidrosis, Horner's syndrome, pneumothorax, and intraoperative cardiac arrest. Satisfactory long-term results are generally achieved, although recurrence of sweating may occur. It is best reserved for severe palmar hyperhidrosis (upper thoracic sympathectomy T2–T3 ganglia), avoiding denervation of the axillary sweat glands and thereby minimizing side effects. This is performed as an open surgical technique or endoscopically (by a transthoracic route) using electrocautery or laser. Percutaneous chemical sympathectomy with ethanol has also been used, a technique that can be employed for lumbar sympathectomy to treat plantar hyperhidrosis. Ejaculatory failure, impotence, and anorgasmia are likely sequelae, however, and it is not generally recommended.

SPECIFIC INVESTIGATIONS

Tests are not necessary for diagnosis of idiopathic hyperhidrosis, although colorimetric sweating patterns (starch iodine) can be useful to define areas of maximum sweating, and gravimetric tests can be used for quantification.

Investigation appropriate to the clinical history and physical signs is necessary when hyperhidrosis is not idiopathic (thyroid function, urinary metanephrines and 5-hydroxyindoleacetic acid [5-HIAA], blood glucose).

FIRST LINE THERAPIES

■ Topical ACH solution in ethanol	B

Aluminium chloride hexahydrate versus palmar hyperhidrosis. Evaporimeter study. Goh CL. Int J Dermatol 1990; 29:368–70.

A single-blind study of unilateral palmar treatment with 20% ACH daily for 4 weeks in 12 patients. Efficacy was reported for all patients; however, four experienced skin irritancy, three patients clearing after 1 week of stopping treatment, and one patient withdrew from the study.

Axillary hyperhidrosis. Local treatment with aluminium-chloride hexahydrate 25% in absolute ethanol with and without supplementary treatment with triethanolamine. Glent-Madsen L, Dahl JC. Acta Derm Venereol 1988;68: 87–9.

A randomized, double-blind, half-sided experiment in 30 volunteers. Triethanolamine in 50% ethanol was applied after treatment to one axilla, to neutralize the pH and reduce skin irritation. The combined treatment was found to be less irritant but also less effective in reducing sweating, although the reduction in efficacy was not noted by the volunteers.

SECOND LINE THERAPIES

■ Topical anticholinergics	D
■ Oral anticholinergics	D
■ Iontophoresis	B
■ Botulinum A neurotoxin	A
– Botulinum A neurotoxin delivered by Dermojet®	C
– Botulinum A neurotoxin delivered by iontophoresis	D
■ Botulinum B neurotoxin	C
■ Liposuction and surgical excision (axillae only)	C
■ Sympathectomy	B

The use of topical glycopyrrolate in the treatment of hyperhidrosis. Seukeran DC, Highet AS. Clin Exp Dermatol 1998;23:204–5.

Topical glycopyrrolate 0.5% in aqueous solution was effective in the treatment of hyperhidrosis of the scalp and forehead after other treatments had proved ineffective.

Topical anticholinergics have been used successfully in gustatory hyperhidrosis in diabetics and in Frey's syndrome.

Propantheline bromide in the management of hyperhidrosis associated with spinal cord injury. Canaday BR, Stanford RH. Ann Pharmacother 1995;29:489–92.

Generalized hyperhidrosis after spinal injury was suppressed with careful titration of propantheline, starting at 15 mg daily and increasing to 15 mg three times daily.

Treating hyperhidrosis [Letter]. Klaber M, Catterall M. BMJ 2000;321:703.

The authors advocate the use of oral glycopyrrolate as a safe and convenient therapy in the doses outlined in the text above.

Iontophoresis with alternating current and direct current offset (AC/DC iontophoresis): a new approach for the treatment of hyperhidrosis. Reinauer S, Neusser A, Schauf G, Holzle E. Br J Dermatol 1993;129:166–9.

Palmar hyperhidrosis was controlled after an average of 11 treatments, with both the conventional DC and the AC/DC iontophoresis units studied. The AC/DC method, however, eliminated skin irritation and discomfort.

Treatment of hyperhidrosis by a battery operated iontopheretic device. Holzle E, Ruzicka T. Dermatologica 1986; 172:41–7.

The average duration of treatment with the Hidrex® device used was 14 months, without relapse (four patients were treated for more than 3 years).

Treatment of hyperhidrosis. Heymann WR. J Am Acad Dermatol 2005;52(3 Pt 1):509–10.

An editorial review of the treatment options available for hyperhidrosis, focusing on the current status of botulinum toxin.

Botulinum toxin A for axillary hyperhidrosis (excessive sweating). Heckmann M, Ceballos-Baumann AO, Plewig G. N Engl J Med 2001;344:488–93.

A multicenter trial in 145 patients with axillary hyperhidrosis, comparing 200 U and 100 U of BTX-A (Dysport®) per axilla. Changes in the rates of sweat production were measured gravimetrically. Two weeks after the injections, the mean rate of sweat production was slightly less in the 200 U injected axilla, and sweat reduction in both was significantly more than with placebo. After 24 weeks, sweat rates after 100 and 200 U were almost identical and less than half the baseline rate. Ninety-eight percent of the patients said they would recommend this therapy to others.

Botulinum toxin therapy for palmar hyperhidrosis. Shelley WB, Talanin NY, Shelley ED. J Am Acad Dermatol 1998;38:227–9.

Four patients with severe palmar hyperhidrosis were treated under regional nerve blocks of the median and ulnar nerve. Anhidrosis lasted for 12, 7, 7, and 4 months, respectively, and one patient experienced mild weakness of a thumb lasting 3 weeks.

Double-blind trial of botulinum A toxin for the treatment of focal hyperhidrosis of the palms. Schnider P, Binder M, Auff E, et al. Br J Dermatol 1997;136:548–52.

Significant reduction in sweating for 13 weeks is reported in this randomized, placebo-controlled, double-blind, within-group study of 11 patients with palmar hyperhidrosis. Two patients reported reversible minor weakness of powerful handgrip at BTX-A injected sites.

A double-blind, randomized, comparative study of Dysport® vs. Botox® in primary palmar hyperhidrosis. Simonetta Moreau M, Cauhepe C, Magues JP, Senard JM. Br J Dermatol 2003;149:1041–5.

Eight patients were treated with intradermal injections of BOTOX® in one palm and Dysport® in the other (using a conversion factor of 1 : 4) after regional nerve blocks. Similar efficacy was reported for the two BTX-A products.

Botulinum toxin type B: a new therapy for axillary hyperhidrosis. Nelson L, Bachoo P, Holmes J. Br J Plast Surg 2005;58:228–32.

Efficacy of BTX-B (Neurobloc®) was demonstrated in the treatment of 13 patients with axillary hyperhidrosis.

Treatment of plantar hyperhidrosis with botulinum toxin type A. Vadoud-Seyedi J. Int J Dermatol 2004;43:969–71.

Plantar hyperhidrosis in 10 patients, treated with BTX-A delivered via needleless injector (Dermojet®), is reported. Seven patients were symptom-free for 5 months following treatment.

BOTOX® delivery by iontophoresis. Kavanagh GM, Oh C, Shams K. Br J Dermatol 2004;151:1093–5.

Two patients with palmar hyperhidrosis had treatment with BTX-A (BOTOX®) delivered by iontophoresis. Control of approximately 70% was achieved for 3 months, without side effects.

Liposuction for the treatment of axillary hyperhidrosis. Lillis PJ, Coleman WP. Dermatol Clin 1990;8:479–82.

The authors suggest that this technique shows promise as the surgical treatment of choice for axillary hyperhidrosis resistant to other modalities.

Surgical treatment of axillary hyperhidrosis in 123 patients. Bretteville-Jensen G, Mossing N, Albrechsten R. Acta Derm Venereol 1975;55:73–8.

Excision of the axillary vault and reconstruction with a modified 'Z'-plasty is described. Of the 123 patients studied, 57% achieved a 75–100% reduction of axillary sweating and 36% achieved a 50–75% reduction. Complications included hematomas in six patients, limited flap necrosis in five, and minor complications in 10. There were no cases of keloid formation or restricted arm movement from wound contracture.

Endoscopic thoracic sympathectomy for primary hyperhidrosis of the upper limbs: a critical analysis and longterm results of 480 operations. Herbst F, Plas EG, Fuggo R, Fritsch A. Ann Surg 1994;220:86–90.

Complete satisfaction was reported by 67% and partial satisfaction by 27% of patients. Patients treated for axillary hyperhidrosis alone were less satisfied. The side effects reported included compensatory hyperhidrosis in 67%, gustatory sweating in 51%, and Horner's syndrome in 2.5%.

Transthoracic endoscopic sympathectomy for palmar hyperhidrosis in children and adolescents: analysis of 350 cases. Lin TS. J Laparoendosc Adv Surg Tech A 1999;9:331–4.

A total of 699 sympathectomies were performed in 350 patients aged 5–17 years (mean 12.9 years). There were no surgical deaths. The mean follow-up was 25 months (range 5–44 months), with highly satisfactory results reported in 95% of patients, although compensatory hyperhidrosis (86%) affected the axillae (12%), back (86%), abdomen (48%), or lower limbs (78%). The recurrence rates of palmar hyperhidrosis were 0.6% in the first year, 1.1% in the second, and 1.7% in the third.

THIRD LINE THERAPIES

■ Biofeedback and behavioral modification	D
■ Diltiazem	E
■ Clonazepam	E
■ Clonidine	E

Use of biofeedback in treating chronic hyperhidrosis. Duller P, Gentry WD. Br J Dermatol 1980;103:143–8.

Biofeedback and behavioral modification can be tried, but is helpful in only a small number of patients.

Emotional eccrine sweating. A heritable disorder. James WD, Schoomaker EB, Rodman OG. Arch Dermatol 1987;123:925–9.

Two members of a family with palmar hyperhidrosis showed decreased palmar sweat secretion during administration of diltiazem.

Unilateral localized hyperhidrosis responding to treatment with clonazepam. Takase Y, Tsushimi K, Yamamoto K, et al. Br J Dermatol 1992;126:416.

A single case of unilateral hyperhidrosis responding to this benzodiazepine antiepileptic agent.

Clonidine treatment in paroxysmal localized hyperhidrosis. Kuritzky A, Hering R, Goldhammer G, Bechar M. Arch Neurol 1984;41:1210–1.

Improvement of paroxysmal localized hyperhidrosis is described in two patients with oral clonidine hydrochloride 0.25 mg three times a day. Control of sweating was maintained with continuous treatment at 12-month follow-up.

Hypertrichosis and hirsutism

John B O'Driscoll

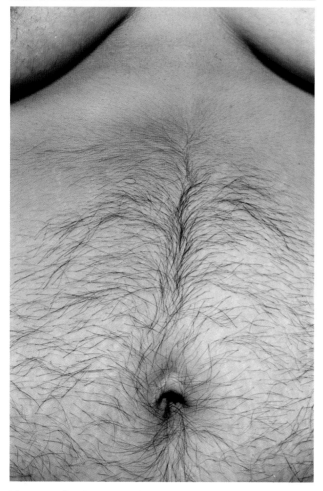

The growth of excessive hair is a common complaint. Hirsutism is the presence of excessive terminal hair in women at sites in which it is usually considered to be a male secondary sexual characteristic. Hypertrichosis is increased hair growth not confined to such sites.

Hypertrichosis may be congenital or acquired. Causes of acquired hypertrichosis include drugs (e.g. cyclosporine, diphenylhydantoin, minoxidil, penicillamine, cortisol), thyroid dysfunction, porphyria, and anorexia nervosa.

Hirsutism may result from either adrenal and/or ovarian overproduction of androgens and/or enhanced sensitivity of the hair follicles.

Racial and genetic factors play a role in hair growth and the perception of what is abnormal hair growth is very subjective and dependent on cultural and social factors in the community where the woman lives.

MANAGEMENT STRATEGY

Any specific underlying cause for hypertrichosis or hirsutism should be treated. Treatment of drug-induced hypertrichosis is straightforward; administration of the drugs should be stopped. Similarly in neoplastic disease of the ovary or adrenals the tumor should be removed. Congenital adrenal hyperplasia due to congenital enzyme deficiencies is treated with glucocorticoids to suppress excess adrenocorticotropic hormone (ACTH) and inhibit adrenal androgen secretion.

Most women complaining of hirsutism do not have a specific underlying medical disorder. A majority do, however, have polycystic ovaries. Patients with polycystic ovaries may be insulin resistant, and if obese, weight loss should be advised. This may help the hirsutism, but is also important from the cardiovascular and general health viewpoint.

Cosmetic measures including *physical hair removal* are of great value regardless of the severity of the excess hair growth and should be the first line therapy.

Dark hair can be *bleached with hydrogen peroxide preparations.*

Depilatory methods, such as *shaving and chemical depilatories*, remove hair from the surface of the skin. Shaving is a reasonable technique to use and does not lead to an increased rate of hair growth, though the blunt tip of shaved hair may appear coarser than unshaven hair. Shaving of areas other than axillae or legs is, however, unacceptable to many women. Chemical depilatories are simple and painless to use, but often lead to irritation.

Epilatory methods involve the removal of the intact hair with the root. Temporary epilation can be achieved by *plucking*, *wax treatment*, or the *use of epilatory devices*. Side effects of plucking may include postinflammatory hyperpigmentation, folliculitis, pseudofolliculitis, and scarring. Permanent epilation can only be achieved by *electrolysis*. Side effects of electrolysis can include pain, scarring, and postinflammatory hypopigmentation or hyperpigmentation. Success depends to a large extent on the skill of the electrologist.

Several different *lasers* have been introduced for hair removal and *intense pulsed light devices* (using broad-spectrum multi-wavelength light sources) have also been used. The lack of comparative data makes it difficult for both physicians and patients to choose the most effective laser or pulsed light treatment for hair removal. None of the devices used at present have been proven to destroy hair permanently.

Eflornithine cream has recently been introduced as a topical hair growth retardant and may benefit some patients.

In trials of systemic therapy the parameters used to assess hirsutism are diverse and often subjective. There is no standardization of methods of measurement and this limits comparison of treatments.

If systemic therapy is required then the first choice is generally an *oral contraceptive and/or spironolactone*. Estrogens in oral contraceptives reduce androgen synthesis and decrease the free androgen levels by increasing sex hormone binding globulin levels. The progestogen in the contraceptive should either be *cyproterone acetate* (not licensed in the USA) or of low androgenicity such as *desogestrel*. The benefits of high dose reversed sequential cyproterone acetate treatment over the contraceptive pill alone are arguable and may entail more side effects.

Spironolactone is an aldosterone antagonist that reduces androgen synthesis, binds androgen receptors, and reduces 5-α-reductase activity in tissue. Spironolactone has been shown to be tumorigenic in chronic toxicity studies in animals, though this is of doubtful relevance in humans. In published studies of women with hirsutism, effective doses of spironolactone have been mostly in the range 100–200 mg daily. In some women doses as low as 25 mg daily may be of benefit. It is not specifically licensed for the treatment of hirsutism in the UK.

SPECIFIC INVESTIGATIONS

- Testosterone level
- Ultrasound scan of pelvis for polycystic ovaries
- Consider need for urinary free cortisol, dexamethasone suppression test, and 17-hydroxyprogesterone

The main object of investigation is the exclusion of organic disease requiring specific treatment. History and examination will identify those patients who need other investigations such as urinary free cortisol excretion or overnight dexamethasone suppression test for suspected Cushing's syndrome, and a short ACTH stimulation test and measurement of plasma 17-hydroxyprogesterone for congenital adrenal hyperplasia. A single measurement of serum testosterone should be part of the routine assessment of women with hirsutism and if the level is greater than 4 nmol/L a full endocrine work-up is indicated.

A prospective study of the prevalence of clear-cut endocrine disorders and polycystic ovaries in 350 patients presenting with hirsutism or androgenic alopecia. O'Driscoll JB, Momtora H, Higginson J, et al. Clin Endocrinol 1994;41:231–6.

Eight of 350 patients presenting with hirsutism and/or androgenic alopecia had clear-cut endocrine disorders; 60% of the patients had polycystic ovaries identifiable on ultrasound scan. The authors of this study concluded that for the exclusion of enzyme deficiencies and virilizing tumors, clinical assessment and a single serum testosterone measurement will suffice.

FIRST LINE THERAPIES

■ Treat specific underlying conditions if appropriate	A
■ Weight loss if obese with polycystic ovaries	A
■ Temporary hair removal/disguise	B
■ Electrolysis	B
■ Laser therapy	B
■ Eflornithine	A

Electrosurgery using insulated needles: epilation. Kobayashi T. J Dermatol Surg Oncol 1985;11:993–1000.

The results for 39 patients, compiled 6 months to 1 year after the final epilations, showed almost no or extremely reduced hair regrowth with almost no scarring.

Permanent hair removal by normal-mode ruby laser. Dierickx CC, Grossman MC, Farinelli WA, Anderson RR. Arch Dermatol 1998;134:837–42.

Nonscarring alopecia can be induced by a single treatment with high-fluence ruby laser pulses. Miniaturization of the terminal hair follicles seems to account for this response.

Two years after laser exposure, four of 13 participants still had significant hair loss at laser treated sites.

Methods of hair removal. Olsen EA. J Am Acad Dermatol 1999;40:143–55.

A good review article on methods of hair removal.

Topical eflornithine. Barman JA, McClellan K. Am J Clin Dermatol 2001;2:1–5.

A summary of the effects of this new topical agent; 32% of patients with facial hirsutism were judged as successful responders after 24 weeks of treatment twice daily with a 15% eflornithine cream, and 70% of patients were regarded as having some response. Benefit was seen in some patients as soon as 2 weeks. White women responded better than black women. Within 8 weeks of stopping therapy all benefits were lost. Mild burning sensations were noted in 30% of users.

Eflornithine inhibits ornithine decarboxylase and thus reduces the rate of hair growth.

SECOND LINE THERAPIES

■ Oral contraceptives	B
■ Spironolactone	B

The treatment of hirsutism with a combination of desogestrel and ethinyl oestradiol. Dewis P, Petsos P, Newman M, Anderson DC. Clin Endocrinol 1985;22:29–36.

Androgen-dependent hair growth fell significantly in a group of 15 patients after 1 year of treatment with this oral contraceptive and ten of the 15 patients reported definite subjective improvement.

Spironolactone is an effective and well tolerated systemic antiandrogen therapy for hirsute women. Barth JH, Cherry CA, Wojnarowska F, Dawber RP. J Clin Endocrinol Metab 1989;68:966–70.

Twenty two hirsute women were treated with spironolactone in an open trial to determine whether it caused objective changes in hair growth. Among them, 18 women completed 12 months of therapy with 200 mg spironolactone daily. Daily hair volume production was reduced to 60% on the face, 52% on the arm, 34% on the abdomen, and 48% on the thigh.

THIRD LINE THERAPIES

■ Oral contraceptives plus high-dose cyproterone acetate	B
■ Flutamide	B
■ Gonadotropin releasing hormone (GnRH) agonist analogues	B
■ Finasteride	B
■ Cimetidine	D

Cyproterone acetate for severe hirsutism: results of a double-blind dose-ranging study. Barth JH, Cherry CA, Wojnarowska F, Dawber RP. Clin Endocrinol 1991;35:5–10.

Twenty one hirsute women received a contraceptive pill containing 35 µg ethinyl estradiol plus 2 mg cyproterone acetate. Twenty received this contraceptive pill plus 20 mg cyproterone acetate on days 1–10 and 19 received the contraceptive pill plus 100 mg cyproterone acetate on days 1–10. All three dose schedules produced significant reductions in clinical hair growth scores. There were no significant differences between the effect of different doses.

It was concluded that cyproterone acetate 2 mg daily appears to be as effective as higher doses in the therapy of hirsute women.

Treatment of hirsutism with the pure antiandrogen flutamide. Cusan L, Dupont A, Belanger A, et al. J Am Acad Dermatol 1990;23:462–9.

The effectiveness of the antiandrogen flutamide in combination with an oral contraceptive was studied in 22 patients with moderate to severe hirsutism.

A marked decrease in hirsutism, which reached the normal range at 7 months, was reported.

Flutamide therapy carries a significant risk of serious hepatotoxicity.

Gonadotrophin-releasing hormone analogues for hirsutism (protocol for a Cochrane review). Van der Spuy ZM, Tregoning SK. Cochrane Library 2001(2).

A number of researchers have reviewed the effects of GnRH agonist analogues on serum androgen levels in women who are hirsute and the preliminary results appear to be promising. The effectiveness of GnRH agonist analogue therapy with or without additional medical therapy has not been confirmed by systematic reviews.

GnRH analogues result in castrate levels of circulating plasma estrogens and androgens causing menopausal symptoms, including osteoporosis.

Finasteride treatment for one year in 35 hirsute patients. Bayram F, Muderris I, Sahin Y, Kelestimur F. Exp Clin Endocrinol Diabetes 1999;107:195–7.

Clinical improvement in the degree of hirsutism was observed in 26 of 35 patients receiving finasteride 5 mg daily over 12 months.

Finasteride is not licensed for use in women because of the risks of feminization of a male fetus.

Treatment of hirsutism with cimetidine. Golditch IM, Price VH. Obstet Gynecol 1990;75:911–13.

Twenty women with moderate to severe facial hirsutism were treated with cimetidine, 300 mg four times daily and nine were followed for 48 weeks or longer. Of these nine subjects who completed 48–72 weeks of treatment, only two showed a decrease in hirsutism. None of the 11 subjects treated for less than 48 weeks had any decrease in hirsutism.

The conclusion was that cimetidine, a weak antiandrogen, is not sufficiently effective to use in the treatment of hirsutism.

Evidence levels **A** Double-blind study **B** Clinical trial ≥ 20 subjects **C** Clinical trial < 20 subjects **D** Series ≥ 5 subjects **E** Anecdotal case reports

Ichthyoses

John J DiGiovanna

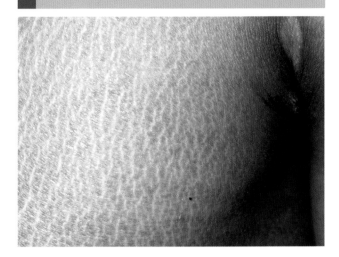

The ichthyoses are a heterogeneous group of scaly skin disorders including inherited and acquired forms. Presentation may be at birth or later in life, and severity spans a broad spectrum from mild ichthyosis vulgaris to the severe harlequin baby with a high mortality. Some patients have hypohidrosis with heat intolerance. In general, scaly skin retains moisture poorly, may be easily irritated, and is prone to enhanced penetration of topical drugs.

MANAGEMENT STRATEGY

The symptoms and severity of ichthyosis vary between patients and even within the same individual over time; therefore, it is important to tailor therapy to the individual patient. While diagnosis may be elusive in some patients, the approach to treatment is largely symptomatic, and dictated by clinical signs and symptoms. There are three key goals of agents used to treat ichthyosis: hydration, lubrication, and keratolysis.

In mild cases, *hydration and lubrication* may lead to satisfactory improvement. In cold, winter months, humidification of home, school, and work environments is important. *Bathing* can be one of the most effective methods for symptomatic improvement. Soaking softens stratum corneum, facilitating removal of thickened hyperkeratosis. During bathing, many patients will use mechanical debridement with roughly textured sponges (e.g. loofah) and abrasives (e.g. Buf-Puf®), or other creative tools to mechanically remove thick calloused areas that have been softened by soaking. Lubricating bath oils can be added to the water to help 'seal in' moisture. Lubricating creams and ointments should be applied generously while the skin is still moist. If the skin is allowed to dry and the humidified environment is lost, much of the absorbed moisture evaporates and will be lost.

As scaling becomes more severe, it becomes substantially more difficult to restore ichthyotic skin towards normal. In more severe cases, this can lead to cracking and fissuring. With increasing thickening of the stratum corneum, there can be a decrease in the range of motion around joints. *Keratolytic agents* are used to decrease keratinocyte adhesion, promoting desquamation of the stratum corneum, and to increase water binding, thereby enhancing hydration of the skin. Keratolytics, often formulated in lubricating vehicles, are widely available and range from very mild to potent. Commercially available formulations may include α-hydroxy acids (lactic acid, glycolic acid, etc.), salicylic acid, urea, or propylene glycol. Where available, many patients consider prescription brands such as LacHydrin®, with specifically developed vehicles, to be more effective than generic or compounded preparations of lactic acid. While a variety of *topical retinoid preparations* are available, their efficacy in the treatment of ichthyosis has been, in general, disappointing. More recently developed compounds such as *tazarotene* may be more useful in some patients.

The impaired barrier function of the skin in ichthyosis should be considered when using topicals over large areas of body surface. Transcutaneous salicylate intoxication can occur after application to large body surface areas, particularly in children because of their greater body surface area per unit weight.

The most severe forms of ichthyosis, including lamellar ichthyosis, congenital ichthyosiform erythroderma, epidermolytic hyperkeratosis, and erythrokeratodermia variabilis, usually respond well to *systemic retinoid therapy* with isotretinoin or acitretin, leading to significant physical and psychosocial benefits. There can be substantial improvement in skin function, including a decrease in scale, and improved heat tolerance and sweating. In some patients, there may be improvement in existing ectropion and a decrease in the tendency toward future ectropion development. Patients with epidermolytic hyperkeratosis can experience a decrease in hyperkeratosis, lesion extent, and frequency of secondary infection. Many forms of severe ichthyosis may respond more completely to acitretin compared with isotretinoin. However, because of slow elimination of acitretin from the body in conjunction with risk of teratogenicity, isotretinoin is preferable for women who may consider pregnancy in the future. When using isotretinoin, dosing can begin at 0.25–0.5 mg/kg daily and be increased as needed. In some patients, doses as high as 2 mg/kg daily may be needed. Acitretin is usually given at lower doses and may be started at 10–25 mg daily. Desquamation usually begins about 1–2 weeks after initiating systemic retinoid therapy.

Patients with epidermolytic hyperkeratosis should be started at a low dose of systemic retinoid, progressing slowly with increases, to avoid exacerbation of blistering. Blistering is common in epidermolytic hyperkeratosis and may be a sign of bacterial infection, requiring treatment with antibiotics.

Prior to initiation of systemic retinoid therapy, a baseline laboratory assessment including complete blood count, liver function tests, fasting cholesterol and triglycerides, and pregnancy testing for women of childbearing potential is performed. Strict contraceptive counseling is essential for women at risk for pregnancy. It is important that pregnancy be avoided not only during treatment with systemic retinoids but also until the drug is effectively eliminated from the body. Acitretin can persist in the body after discontinuation of the drug, which has led to the recommendation by the US Food and Drug Administration that pregnancy should not occur for at least 3 years after stopping the drug.

In the treatment of ichthyosis, improvement does not persist very long after discontinuation of therapy, which often leads to the retinoid therapy being continued long term. Long-term treatment involves a higher risk of chronic skeletal toxicity such as calcification of tendons and ligaments, hyperostoses, and osteoporosis, which may require periodic monitoring. Children on long-term therapy should have their growth monitored with a standardized growth chart. A periodic radiographic skeletal survey can monitor for skeletal toxicity and can include a lateral view of the cervical and thoracic spine, lateral view of the calcaneus (heel), and posteroanterior view of the pelvis. Chronic toxicity may be minimized by keeping the total retinoid dose as low as practicable. The dose of retinoid may be lowered with the use of combination therapy with keratolytic, hydrating, and lubricating topicals. Treatment of younger patients who are still growing entails the risk of the additional toxicity of premature epiphyseal closure.

SPECIFIC INVESTIGATIONS

- Dictated by clinical presentation (history, family history, physical examination) to determine which tests may be indicated to identify underlying etiology and/or associated abnormalities
- Hereditary ichthyosis
  - Steroid sulfatase activity
  - Fatty alcohol:NAD + oxidoreductase activity
  - Mutational analysis
- Acquired ichthyosis
  - Malignancy work-up
  - Infection (HIV, *Mycobacterium leprae*)
  - Skin biopsy (sarcoidosis)

Some forms of ichthyosis are associated with abnormalities in other organ systems. The clinical presentation, delineated by a complete history and physical examination, is the basis to determine which, if any, specific investigations are indicated.

Ichthyosiform dermatoses. Classification based on anatomic and biometric observations. Frost P, Van Scott EJ. Arch Dermatol 1966;94:113–26.

A classic article on the classification of the ichthyoses.

Ichthyosiform sarcoidosis. Cather JC, Cohen PR. J Am Acad Dermatol 1999;40:862–5.

In epidermolytic hyperkeratosis and in acquired ichthyosis secondary to sarcoidosis, skin biopsy examined under light microscopy can confirm the diagnosis.

X-linked ichthyosis: increased blood cholesterol sulfate and electrophoretic mobility of low-density lipoprotein. Epstein EH Jr, Krauss RM, Shackleton CH. Science 1981;214:659–60.

With a clinical presentation and family pedigree suggestive of X-linked recessive ichthyosis, steroid sulfate levels in serum can be measured to establish the diagnosis.

Mutations in the gene for transglutaminase 1 in autosomal recessive lamellar ichthyosis. Russell LJ, DiGiovanna JJ, Rogers GR, et al. Nat Genet 1995;9:279–83.

Mutations of keratinocyte transglutaminase in lamellar ichthyosis. Huber M, Rettler I, Bernasconi K, et al. Science 1995;267:525–8.

Mutations in the gene encoding transglutaminase 1 have been found in several families with lamellar ichthyosis. This finding allows for patient and prenatal diagnosis by mutational analysis.

Sjogren-Larsson syndrome. Deficient activity of the fatty aldehyde dehydrogenase component of fatty alcohol:NAD + oxidoreductase in cultured fibroblasts. Rizzo WB, Craft DA. J Clin Invest 1991;88:1643–8.

In Sjögren–Larsson syndrome (SLS) there is abnormal oxidation of fatty alcohol to fatty acid. If SLS is in the differential diagnosis because of neurologic manifestations (mental retardation, spasticity) and ophthalmologic findings (glistening white dots in retina), the diagnosis can be established by measuring the activity of the enzyme fatty alcohol:NAD + oxidoreductase (FAO) in cultured fibroblasts. Activity is deficient in SLS cells, and partially decreased in obligate SLS heterozygotes.

Prenatal diagnosis of Sjogren-Larsson syndrome using enzymatic methods. Rizzo WB, Craft DA, Kelson TL, et al. Prenat Diagn 1994;14:577–81.

Prenatal diagnosis can be achieved by measuring enzyme activity in cultured amniocytes or cultured chorionic villus cells.

Sjogren-Larsson syndrome is caused by mutations in the fatty aldehyde dehydrogenase gene. De Laurenzi V, Rogers GR, Hamrock DJ, et al. Nat Genet 1996;12:52–7.

The fatty aldehyde dehydrogenase (FALDH) enzyme is part of the FAO enzyme responsible for oxidation of fatty alcohol to fatty acid. Mutations have been identified in the FALDH gene, enabling prenatal diagnosis, in addition to diagnosis of affected patients and carriers, by mutational analysis.

Ichthyosiform dermatoses. DiGiovanna JJ. In: Freedberg IM, Eisen AZ, Wolff K, et al, eds. Fitzpatrick's Dermatology in General Medicine, 6th edn. New York: McGraw-Hill; 2003:481–505.

A work-up for malignancy may be indicated in certain patients with acquired ichthyosis.

Ichthyosiform conditions occurring in leprosy. Schulz EJ. Br J Dermatol 1965;77:151–7.

Acquired ichthyosis in concomitant HIV-1 and HTLV-II infection: a new association with intravenous drug abuse. Kaplan MH, Sadick NS, McNutt NS, et al. J Am Acad Dermatol 1993;29:701–8.

Acquired ichthyosis in association with leprosy or HIV can be identified by appropriate testing.

FIRST LINE THERAPIES

■ Hydration	E
– Humidification of environment	
– Bathing/soaking	
■ Lubrication	B
– Lotions	
– Creams	
– Ointments	

Ichthyosis: etiology, diagnosis, and management. DiGiovanna JJ, Robinson-Bostom L. Am J Clin Dermatol 2003;4:81–95.

Review of the ichthyoses, including etiologies, approach to diagnosis, and management.

Efficacy of urea therapy in children with ichthyosis. A multicenter randomized, placebo-controlled, double-blind, semilateral study. Kuster W, Bohnsack K, Rippke F, et al. Dermatology 1998;196:217–22.

Sixty children aged between 1 and 16 years were treated with Laceran® 10% urea lotion on one side, and Laceran® base on the other, for 8 weeks. On each side, a control area was left untreated. Improvement was 78% after 8 weeks for Laceran® 10% urea lotion and 72% for urea-free Laceran® lotion base. While urea was somewhat superior to base, the lotion base alone was effective.

SECOND LINE THERAPIES

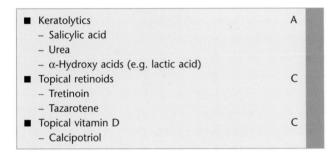

■ Keratolytics	A
– Salicylic acid	
– Urea	
– α-Hydroxy acids (e.g. lactic acid)	
■ Topical retinoids	C
– Tretinoin	
– Tazarotene	
■ Topical vitamin D	C
– Calcipotriol	

[Life threatening salicylate poisoning caused by percutaneous absorption in severe ichthyosis vulgaris]. Germann R, Schindera I, Kuch M, et al. Hautarzt 1996;47:624–7. In German.

Salicylate intoxication using a skin ointment. Chiaretti A, Schembri Wismayer D, Tortorolo L, et al. Acta Paediatr 1997;86:330–1.

Application of salicylic acid over large body surface areas has been associated with toxicity, especially in children. Signs and symptoms of salicylate intoxication include fever, dyspnea with respiratory alkalosis, oculogyric crisis, coma, and even death; and has been reported with concentrations as low as 10% salicylate and urea ointment.

Improved topical treatment of lamellar ichthyosis: a double-blind study of four different cream formulations. Ganemo A, Virtanen M, Vahlquist A. Br J Dermatol 1999;141: 1027–32.

Preparations including lactic acid can also be very effective for ichthyosis. This double-blind study compared Locobase® fatty cream containing a mixture of 5% lactic acid and 20% propylene glycol (LPL) to the same mixture in Essex® (Diprobase®) cream, and to Locobase® containing either lactic acid or propylene glycol. LPL had a superior therapeutic effect and was preferred by most patients.

Propylene glycol with occlusion for treatment of ichthyosis. Goldsmith LA, Baden HP. JAMA 1972;220: 579–80.

Aqueous propylene glycol in concentrations of 40–60% under occlusion may also be effective in softening hyperkeratotic skin of patients with ichthyosis.

Keratolytics: Salicylic acid is the oldest keratolytic and is used in concentrations ranging from 0.5% to 60%. Urea (5–20%), lactic acid, and propylene glycol in a variety of bases are also widely used.

Effect of topical tazarotene in the treatment of congenital ichthyoses. Hofmann B, Stege H, Ruzicka T, Lehmann P. Br J Dermatol 1999;141:642–6.

The topical receptor-selective retinoid tazarotene 0.05% gel was evaluated, relative to 10% urea ointment, in a heterogeneous group of 12 adult patients with congenital ichthyosis. Seventy-five percent of patients responded favorably, resulting in remission lasting up to 2 months. The only side effect was local irritation.

Efficacy, tolerability, and safety of calcipotriol ointment in disorders of keratinization. Results of a randomized, double-blind, vehicle-controlled, right/left comparative study. Kragballe K, Steijlen PM, Ibsen HH, et al. Arch Dermatol 1995;131:556–60.

Sixty-seven patients with disorders of keratinization were treated with calcipotriol ointment (50 μg/g) and placebo twice daily for up to 12 weeks (up to 120 g of calcipotriol ointment per week). Improvement was variable. No benefit was seen in palmoplantar keratoderma nor keratosis pilaris; 8 of 12 patients with Darier's disease withdrew.

Topical treatment of Sjogren-Larsson syndrome with calcipotriol. Lucker GP, van de Kerkhof PC, Cruysberg JR, et al. Dermatology 1995;190:292–4.

Two patients with SLS were treated with calcipotriol ointment versus ointment base for 12 weeks using a double-blind bilaterally paired comparison. Both patients had unilateral improvement on the calcipotriol treated side.

THIRD LINE THERAPIES

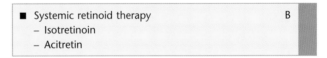

■ Systemic retinoid therapy	B
– Isotretinoin	
– Acitretin	

Treatment of lamellar ichthyosis and other keratinising dermatoses with an oral synthetic retinoid. Peck GL, Yoder FW. Lancet 1976;2:1172–4.

In a group of 13 patients treated with oral isotretinoin, there was near-complete clearing of the skin in five patients with lamellar ichthyosis, in two with Darier's disease, and in one with pityriasis rubra pilaris.

Oral synthetic retinoid treatment in children. DiGiovanna JJ, Peck GL. Pediatr Dermatol 1983;1:77–88.

Fifteen children with chronic disorders of keratinization and one with severe cystic acne were treated with oral isotretinoin for a mean of 20 months with an average dose of 2 mg/kg daily. Excellent response was seen in cystic acne, Darier's disease, lamellar ichthyosis, and congenital ichthyosiform erythroderma. Marked improvement was seen in keratosis palmaris et plantaris and erythrokeratodermia variabilis. Therapy was well tolerated.

Acitretin in the treatment of severe disorders of keratinization. Results of an open study. Blanchet-Bardon C,

Nazzaro V, Rognin C, et al. J Am Acad Dermatol 1991;24: 982–6.

Thirty-three patients with ichthyoses, palmoplantar hyperkeratosis, or Darier's disease were treated for a period of 4 months. Most patients showed marked improvement or remission.

An appraisal of acitretin therapy in children with inherited disorders of keratinization. Lacour M, Mehta-

Nikhar B, Atherton DJ, Harper JI. Br J Dermatol 1996;134: 1023–9.

Retrospective review of 29 children with ichthyosis who received acitretin since 1992. Overall improvement was considerable, with only three patients responding poorly. The starting dose was 0.5 mg/kg daily; irreversible side effects were not observed.

Impetigo

Robert Burd, Michael Sladden

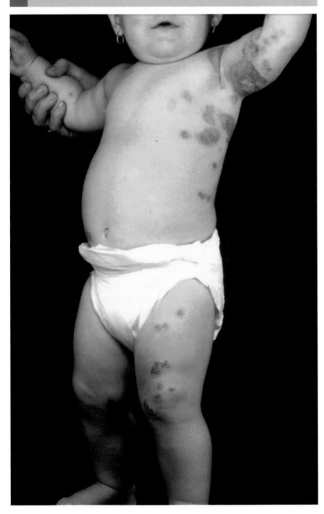

Impetigo is a superficial bacterial infection of the skin. The most common pathogen is *Staphylococcus aureus*, although β-hemolytic streptococci may also be implicated. The infection is highly contagious and can easily spread to other body sites or close contacts.

MANAGEMENT STRATEGY

The main aim of treatment is to eradicate the infecting bacteria. This allows rapid healing of skin lesions and controls the spread of infection. This requires the use of an appropriate antimicrobial delivered in an effective way. Antibiotics may be administered either orally or topically. The choice between topical or oral therapy depends on:

- the experience of the practitioner;
- the preference of the patient;
- the local bacterial resistance patterns;
- the cost and availability of local resources.

Staphylococcus aureus has been recognized as the major pathogen in both bullous and nonbullous impetigo in Europe. Traditionally, in the United States, nonbullous impetigo was considered to be caused primarily by streptococci, but recent evidence indicates that *S. aureus* is now the most common pathogen in both forms of impetigo in the United States as well.

Globally, the majority of isolates of *S. aureus* are resistant to penicillin. Erythromycin resistance is also becoming more prevalent.

In developing countries, where impetigo causes a significant burden of disease, streptococcus is often the predominant pathogen. In these countries, topical agents are expensive and may be unavailable. Treatment strategies have to be sufficiently flexible to meet local needs.

Historically, topical treatment of impetigo was ineffective due to the emergence of bacterial resistance to tetracyclines and gentamicin, and problematic because of contact sensitivity to topical antimicrobials. More recently introduced *topical antibiotics* are as effective as traditional *oral antibiotics*. When used in courses of less than 2 weeks, bacterial resistance does not appear to be a major problem.

Strains of bacteria causing impetigo are often extremely virulent. Patients therefore need to be educated on personal hygiene methods to avoid the spread of infection. The use of topical antiseptics and soaks to remove dried exudate and crusts has not been shown to be of benefit in the treatment of impetigo. However, commonsense would indicate that cleaning lesional skin with soap and water or a mild nonirritant antiseptic will aid the application of topical antibiotics and reduce the spread of infection.

Nasal carriage of *S. aureus* occurs in a high proportion of patients, and asymptomatic family members. Therefore in recurrent cases or multiple familial cases, *treatment of nasal and pharyngeal carriage* may be necessary.

SPECIFIC INVESTIGATIONS

- Gram stain
- Bacterial culture and sensitivity

A Gram stain of a swab from the lesion or exudate will reveal Gram-positive cocci, confirming the clinical diagnosis. Bacterial culture and sensitivity from a pretreatment swab is useful to assess suitable alternative antibiotics in cases that do not respond to conventional treatment.

Impetigo: a reassessment of etiology and therapy. Barton LL, Friedman AD. Pediatr Dermatol 1987;4:185–8.

S. aureus was the most common isolate in 71 patients with impetigo; only two patients had a pure isolate of group A β-hemolytic streptococci.

DNA heterogeneity of *Staphylococcus aureus* strains evaluated by Sma1 and SgrA1 pulsed field gel electrophoresis in patients with impetigo. Capoluongo E, Giglio A, Leonetti F, et al. Res Microbiol 2000;151:53–61.

Samples from lesional skin, nose, and pharynx were taken from 26 patients and their families and the strain of *S. aureus* was typed; 54% of the patients had the same strain in both the nose and the lesion. In over half the families at least one other family member was found to be carrying the same strain as the patient's lesion.

FIRST LINE THERAPIES

■ Topical mupirocin or fusidic acid	A
■ Oral flucloxacillin, cloxacillin, erythromycin, fusidic acid	A
■ Topical antiseptics	B

Oral or topical antibiotics with proven efficacy against *S. aureus* are the first choice in therapy.

Interventions for impetigo (Cochrane Review). Koning S, Verhagen AP, van Suijlekom-Smit LWA, et al. In: The Cochrane Library, Issue 2. Chichester, UK: John Wiley & Sons; 2004.

Systematic review of 57 trials including 3533 participants. There is good evidence that topical mupirocin and topical fusidic acid are equally, or more effective than oral antibiotics for people with limited impetigo. Topical antibiotics may be more effective, for example, than erythromycin because erythromycin resistance is becoming more common.

A systematic review and meta-analysis of treatments for impetigo. George A, Rubin G. Br J Gen Pract 2003;53:480–7.

Review of 16 trials concluding that both topical and oral antibiotics are effective treatments for impetigo.

Topical mupirocin treatment of impetigo is equal to oral erythromycin therapy. Mertz PM, Marshall DA, Eaglstein WH, et al. Arch Dermatol 1989;125:1069–73.

Seventy five patients were treated in an investigator-blinded study comparing topical mupirocin applied three times daily with oral erythromycin 30–50 mg/kg daily. The mupirocin-treated patients experienced similar clinical results as those treated with oral erythromycin, although mupirocin was superior in the microbiological eradication of *S. aureus*.

Common skin infections in children. Sladden MJ, Johnston GA. Br Med J 2004;329:95–9.

In this evidence-based review, the authors suggest using topical mupirocin or fusidic acid for 7 days in mild impetigo. They advise that oral antibiotics are reserved for recalcitrant, extensive, systemic disease.

Fusidic acid tablets in patients with skin and soft-tissue infection: a dose-finding study. Carr WD, Wall AR, Georgala-Zervogiani S, et al. Eur J Clin Res 1994;5:87–95.

Fusidic acid tablets, 250 mg twice daily, 500 mg twice daily, and the standard regimen of 500 mg three times daily, were compared in a randomized, double blind study in 617 patients with skin and soft tissue infections. Each treatment was given for 5–10 days. Cure rates after 5 days of treatment were 34.7, 37.8, and 37.2%, respectively. End of treatment cure rates were 75.5, 81.1, and 74.0%, respectively.

Impetigo. Current etiology and comparison of penicillin, erythromycin and cephalexin therapies. Demidovich CW, Wittler RR, Ruff ME, et al. Am J Dis Child 1990;144:1313–5.

A randomized trial of 73 children with impetigo treated with either penicillin V, erythromycin, or cefalexin. *S. aureus* was the most common pathogen and cefalexin the most

effective treatment, though erythromycin may be preferred on grounds of cost-effectiveness.

Topical 2% mupirocin versus 2% fusidic acid ointment in the treatment of primary and secondary skin infections. Gilbert M. J Am Acad Dermatol 1989;20:1083–7.

A double blind randomized trial of 70 patients with primary or secondary skin infections. In the patients with impetigo the degree of effectiveness favored mupirocin, though both treatments were very efficacious.

Cost-effectiveness of erythromycin versus mupirocin for the treatment of impetigo in children. Rice TD, Duggan AK, DeAngelis C. Pediatrics 1992;89:210–4.

Controlled clinical trial of topical mupirocin or oral erythromycin in 93 children with impetigo. Both treatments were highly effective. Mupirocin was more expensive, but caused significantly fewer side effects than erythromycin.

The frequency of erythromycin-resistant *Staphylococcus aureus* in impetiginized dermatoses. Misko ML, Terracina JR, Diven DG. Pediatr Dermatol 1995;12:12–5.

Despite significant in-vitro erythromycin resistance in a series of 98 outpatients, there was still a low frequency of treatment failure in this group. This suggested that erythromycin may still be a reasonable agent in the treatment of uncomplicated superficial skin infections in that community at that time.

The emergence of penicillin resistance, and erythromycin resistance is so common in isolates of S. aureus, *that alternative antibiotics should be considered.*

Hydrogen peroxide cream: an alternative to topical antibiotics in the treatment of impetigo contagiosa. Christensen OB, Anehus S. Acta Derm Venereol 1994; 74:460–2.

A prospective comparison of hydrogen peroxide cream with fusidic acid cream in 256 patients with impetigo. Over a 3-week treatment period, 92 patients of 128 (72%) in the hydrogen peroxide group were classified as healed, compared to 105 of 128 (82%) in the fusidic acid group. This difference was not statistically significant.

SECOND LINE THERAPIES

■ Intravenous antibiotics plus topical antibiotic	C
■ Rifampin (rifampicin)	D

Failure of first line therapy may indicate the presence of a resistant organism or poor patient compliance. The choice of antibiotic should be based on the sensitivities of organisms cultured from the pretreatment swab.

Addition of rifampin to cephalexin therapy for recalcitrant staphylococcal skin infections – an observation. Feder Jr HM, Pond KE. Clin Pediatr 1996;35:205–8.

Two children with staphylococcal infections failing to respond to standard antibiotics responded when rifampin was added.

Evidence levels **A** Double-blind study **B** Clinical trial ≥ 20 subjects **C** Clinical trial < 20 subjects **D** Series ≥ 5 subjects **E** Anecdotal case reports

THIRD LINE THERAPIES

■ Systemic antibiotic, topical antibiotic plus a formal antistaphylococcal regimen to reduce nasal and pharyngeal carriage	E

In recurrent cases, consider the possibility of nasal or pharyngeal colonization with the pathogenic S. aureus *in either the patient or a close family member. This may require eradication by the use of a systemic antibiotic in conjunction with the nasal application of a topical antibiotic and an antiseptic skin cleanser. Topical antiseptics have also proved useful in nosocomial outbreaks.*

Use of 0.3% triclosan (Bacti-Stat) to eradicate an outbreak of methicillin-resistant *Staphylococcus aureus* in a neonatal nursery. Zafar AB, Butler RC, Reese DJ, et al. Am J Infect Control 1995;23:200–8.

A nosocomial outbreak of infection with methicillin-resistant *S. aureus* (MRSA) in a neonatal nursery proved difficult to control even with aggressive conventional measures. The additional use of a handwashing and bathing soap containing 0.3% triclosan immediately ended the outbreak.

Prevention and control of nosocomial infection caused by methicillin-resistant *Staphylococcus aureus* in a premature infant ward: preventive effect of a povidone-iodine wipe of neonatal skin. Aihara M, Sakai M, Iwasaki M, et al. Postgrad Med J 1993;69(suppl 3):S117–21.

An outbreak of MRSA causing impetigo was halted by wiping the body surface of the infants with a diluted povidone-iodine solution (10% povidone-iodine; 1 : 100 dilution) to prevent colonization.

Irritant contact dermatitis

Nathaniel K Wilkin

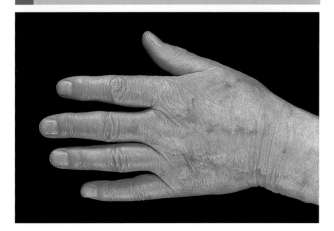

Irritant contact dermatitis (ICD) is a reaction to an irritant (i.e. an exogenous substance that damages the epidermis through physical or chemical mechanisms without triggering an immunological response). Acute ICD is usually attributable to a single irritant. Cumulative ICD usually results from chronic exposure to multiple irritants, often in association with endogenous factors such as atopy or stress. Chronic cumulative ICD usually involves the hands. ICD is common, often has a poor prognosis, has a significant economic impact for society, and seriously degrades the quality of life of affected individuals beyond the ability to work.

MANAGEMENT STRATEGY

The first step in any management strategy is *prevention*. Patients should be educated about proper skin care and protection including handwashing, the use of moisturizers, avoidance of common irritants, and the use of protective clothing like gloves and aprons when handling potentially irritating substances. Dermatologists can encourage primary prevention by counseling patients at higher risk because of endogenous factors (e.g. atopy) or exogenous factors (e.g. frequent occupational exposures in hairdressers). Secondary prevention includes measures to enable patients to remain employed without interfering with the resolution of the ICD. Chronic hand dermatitis is a common presentation, and patient education can be facilitated with a handout on lifestyle management principles directed at handwashing and moisturizing, occlusive moisturizing therapy at night, special protective modalities (such as type of glove to exclude specific irritants), and specific agents to avoid.

Azathioprine, cyclosporine, psoralen and UVA (PUVA), Grenz ray therapy, and *superficial radiotherapy* may be justified for short-term control for patients who are compliant with moisturization, use of protective modalities (gloves), and application of topical corticosteroids, and still have a severe disruption of their quality of life. Because the goal of such second-line therapies is to reduce the severity such that first-line therapies may become sufficient, patient selection is critical.

SPECIFIC INVESTIGATIONS

- Patch testing to environmentally relevant allergens
- Detailed case history of patient's work, habits, and hobbies

Thoughts on irritant contact dermatitis. Malten KE. Contact Dermatitis 1981;7:238–47.

Treatment should be directed at lessening the influence of every factor thought to be deleterious.

Clues to an accurate diagnosis of contact dermatitis. Rietschel RL. Dermatolog Ther 2004;17:224–30.

Patch testing, with known environmentally relevant allergens that is negative and sufficiently comprehensive would point to ICD, especially in the patients without atopy or psoriasis. A careful history and documentation of specific morphological changes on physical exam are essential when pursuing the presumptive diagnosis of ICD after negative patch testing.

Patch testing, a detailed history, and assessment of specific morphological changes provide for an accurate diagnosis and identify specific environmental factors the patient should avoid as completely as possible. Such documentation is also useful should medicolegal questions arise regarding impairment and job placement.

FIRST LINE THERAPIES

■ Physical skin protection	C
■ Emollients	C
■ Barrier creams	C
■ Topical corticosteroids	C
■ Topical calcineurin inhibitors	C

Therapeutic options for chronic hand dermatitis. Warshaw EM. Dermatol Ther 2004;17:240–50.

A review of the therapeutic alternatives for patients with recalcitrant hand dermatitis.

Effect of glove-occlusion on human skin (II). Ramsing DW, Agner T. Contact Dermatitis 1996;34:258–62.

Occlusive gloves worn for prolonged periods of time may impair skin barrier function. Wearing cotton gloves under the occlusive gloves can prevent this negative effect.

Protective gloves should be used for as short a time as possible and with cotton gloves under the occlusive gloves.

A randomized comparison of an emollient containing skin-related lipids with a petrolatum-based emollient as adjunct in the treatment of chronic hand dermatitis. Kucharekova M, Van de Kerkhof PCM, Van der Valk PGM. Contact Dermatitis 2003;48:293–9.

The frequent use of emollients is associated with significant improvement in hand dermatitis. No significant difference in the improvement was demonstrated for the emollient containing skin-related lipids.

The frequent use of emollients is an essential component of therapy. Traditional petrolatum-based emollients are accessible, inexpensive, and just as effective as an emollient containing skin-related lipids.

Double-blind, randomized trial of scheduled use of a novel barrier cream and an oil-containing lotion for

Evidence levels A Double-blind study B Clinical trial ≥ 20 subjects C Clinical trial < 20 subjects D Series ≥ 5 subjects E Anecdotal case reports

protecting the hands of health care workers. McCormick RD, Buchman TL, Maki DG. Am J Infect Control 2000;28: 302–10.

The scheduled use of petrolatum-oil-containing lotion or a barrier cream was associated with marked improvement (69% and 52%, respectively) in chronic hand irritant dermatitis.

It is debatable whether the distinction between 'skin care' and 'skin protection' is real. Side effects in using emollients and barrier creams are irritation and sensitization to their ingredients. A useful procedure is to include patch tests of those emollients and barrier creams anticipated to be used by the patient in the initial comprehensive patch testing evaluation of the chronic contact dermatitis.

Do topical corticosteroids modulate skin irritation in human beings? Assessment by transepidermal water loss and visual scoring. Van der Valk PGM, Maibach HI. J Am Acad Dermatol 1989;21:519–22.

Neither the corticosteroid products nor vehicle significantly influenced barrier function during repeated application of an irritant, sodium lauryl sulfate, in low concentration.

The first step must be the elimination, to the extent possible, of exposure to irritants. Until proven otherwise, no therapy should be considered sufficiently potent as to overcome the effects of continuing exposure to irritants.

An open-label pilot study to evaluate the safety and efficacy of topically applied tacrolimus ointment for the treatment of hand and/or foot eczema. Thelmo MC, Lang W, Brooke E, et al. J Dermatol Treatment 2003;14:136–40.

Pimecrolimus cream 1%: a potential new treatment for chronic hand dermatitis. Belsito DV, Fowler JF, Marks JG, et al. Cutis 2004;73:31–8.

The topical calcineurin inhibitor led to improvements over baseline in the open-label study and there was a trend toward greater clearance than vehicle in the pimecrolimus study.

Topical calcineurin inhibitors may have a role as an alternative to low-potency topical corticosteroids, in chronic irritant dermatitis in the patient with mild inflammatory changes who does not experience a burning sensation when the product is applied.

SECOND LINE THERAPIES

■ Cyclosporine	C
■ UVB therapy	C
■ PUVA therapy	C

Comparison of cyclosporine and topical betamethasone 17,21-dipropionate in the treatment of severe chronic hand eczema. Granlund H, Erkko P, Eriksson E, Reitamo S. Acta Derm Venereol 1996;76:371–6.

Low-dose oral cyclosporine at 3 mg/kg daily was compared with topical 0.05% betamethasone dipropionate in a randomized, double blind study of 41 patients with chronic hand dermatitis and an inadequate response to treatment with topical halogenated corticosteroids for at least 3–4 weeks and/or PUVA and avoidance of relevant contact allergens. Both treatment groups had similar improvement and similar relapse rates after successful treatment. Adverse events were slightly more common in patients treated with cyclosporine.

Low-dose cyclosporine may be a useful alternative treatment, though very high-potency topical corticosteroids can be effective in patients who do not have an adequate response to other mid- to high-potency topical corticosteroids.

PUVA-bath photochemotherapy (PUVA-soak therapy) of recalcitrant dermatoses of the palms and soles. Behrens S, von Kobyletzki G, Gruss C, et al. Photodermatol Photoimmunol Photomed 1999;15:47–51.

Almost two-thirds of patients showed complete remission at 8 weeks. Palmoplantar psoriasis responded best, followed by atopic dermatitis. Hyperkeratotic dermatitis displayed the poorest response rates.

A left–right comparison of UVB phototherapy and topical photochemotherapy in bilateral chronic hand dermatitis after 6 weeks' treatment. Simons JR, Bohnen IJWE, Van Der Valk PGM. Clin Exp Dermatol 1997;22:7–10.

Both UVB phototherapy and PUVA-soak therapy moderately improved the chronic hand dermatitis without a significant difference in efficacy between the two therapies. Side effects occurred more often on the PUVA-soak-treated side.

Given the similar improvement in chronic hand dermatitis and the increased side effects with PUVA-soak therapy, it would be prudent to begin treatment with UVB therapy and only use PUVA-soak therapy if the response is inadequate.

THIRD LINE THERAPIES

■ Superficial radiotherapy	A

Comparison of Grenz rays versus placebo in the treatment of chronic hand eczema. Cartwright PH, Rowell NR. Br J Dermatol 1987;117:73–6.

There was no difference in efficacy between Grenz rays (total dose 900 rad) and placebo.

A double-blind study of Grenz ray therapy in chronic eczema of the hands. Lindelöf B, Wrangsjö K, Liden S. Br J Dermatol 1987;117:77–80.

There was a statistically significant improvement in the scores of some signs and itching with Grenz rays (total dose 300 rad) compared with the untreated control.

Grenz ray or superficial radiotherapy is not an obvious 'go to' treatment when one second line treatment does not provide a sufficient response, but it may be tried for some additional advantage as an adjunct to intensive first line treatment with or without low-dose cyclosporine.

Juvenile plantar dermatosis

Stephen K Jones

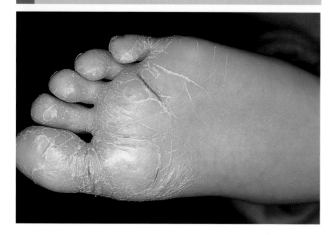

Juvenile plantar dermatosis is a specific condition comprising symmetrical erythema (sometimes with a polished 'billiard ball' appearance), scaling, and fissuring, primarily of the pressure areas of the foot. Vesiculation is never found. The commonest sites involved are the plantar aspects of the great toe, forefoot, heel, and very occasionally the fingertips and palms. The instep and the interdigital skin are rarely affected. The condition occurs almost exclusively in children, clearing around puberty.

MANAGEMENT STRATEGY

Juvenile plantar dermatosis usually presents in children between 4 and 7 years of age, though occasionally it presents before this. Most series suggest that it is a disease of the 'school years', with clearing in most patients by puberty. It is uncommon in adults. Spontaneous resolution can be expected in the majority of patients.

The main etiological factor is thought to be the occlusive effect of 'trainer' sports shoes and manmade fibers in hosiery, resulting in hyperhidrosis. This, some suggest, washes away surface lipids, which are already decreased because of the relative lack of sebaceous glands on the plantar surface of the foot. This hyperhidrosis is, therefore, followed by rapid dehydration of the skin on footwear removal. It is proposed that this maceration/dehydration renders the skin susceptible to trauma from, for example, sport. Avoidance of vigorous exercise may therefore be helpful in these patients.

The role of atopy is debated. Some series have found an increased incidence of atopy in patients and their families and, indeed, this condition was first referred to as 'atopic winter feet'. It has been argued that the atopic diathesis predisposes the skin of the foot to the traumatic effects of sport and vigorous activity and the effects of alternating hyperhidrosis and dehydration (see below). Other series, however, have found no increased incidence of atopy.

Investigations are unlikely to be helpful. Although some series have found positive patch tests in about 10% of cases, these are often irrelevant. Indeed, even when these are to footwear-related allergens, allergen avoidance rarely affects the clinical outcome.

Changing to nonocclusive footwear along with cotton socks or 'open' footwear has, therefore, been proposed as a therapeutic maneuver. *Emollients*, both to reduce fissuring and to reduce the dehydration that is said to occur on removing occlusive footwear, are reported as being helpful. *Topical corticosteroids* may be beneficial if there is an inflammatory component. *Occlusive bandages* containing zinc ointment, ichthammol or tar may help if hyperkeratosis and fissuring is a prominent feature. All the above often only help temporarily, and regular rotation of emollients may be required.

It is the impression of the author that this condition has become less common in recent years, possibly related to further changes in teenage 'fashion' and footwear materials.

SPECIFIC INVESTIGATIONS

■ Patch tests

Juvenile plantar dermatosis; a new entity. Mackie RM, Hussain SL. Clin Exp Dermatol 1976;1:253–60.

Thirteen of 102 patients showed a positive patch test. Eight were considered relevant, with reactions to footwear constituents. In none did subsequent changes in footwear affect the clinical outcome.

Common pediatric foot dermatoses. Guenst BJ. J Pediatr Health Care 1999;13:68–71.

A practical review differentiating the various forms of tinea pedis and shoe dermatitis from juvenile plantar dermatosis. Therapeutic suggestions are offered for these entities.

FIRST LINE THERAPIES

■ Await spontaneous resolution	C

Juvenile plantar dermatosis – an 8 year follow-up of 102 patients. Jones SK, English JSC, Forsyth A, Mackie RM. Clin Exp Dermatol 1987;12:5–7.

Of 50 patients traced, the condition had resolved in 38. The mean age of remission was 14.3 years.

SECOND LINE THERAPIES

■ Change to nonocclusive footwear	C
■ Sport avoidance	C
■ Emollients	C
■ Topical corticosteroids	C
■ Rotation of topical agents	C

Juvenile plantar dermatosis in Singapore. Moorthy TT, Rajan VS. Int J Dermatol 1984;23:476–9.

Of 50 patients followed, 28 showed improvement after changing to 'nonocclusive' footwear (six of whom cleared completely). Twenty-two showed no improvement.

Juvenile plantar dermatosis – an 8 year follow-up of 102 patients. Jones SK, English JSC, Forsyth A, Mackie RM. Clin Exp Dermatol 1987;12:5–7.

Evidence levels A Double-blind study B Clinical trial ≥ 20 subjects C Clinical trial < 20 subjects D Series ≥ 5 subjects E Anecdotal case reports

Of 50 patients traced, 22% found simple emollients and 20% found topical corticosteroids helpful; 12% felt that any topical preparation produced some improvement, but only for a limited period. Rotation of emollients and topical corticosteroids may therefore be useful.

Juvenile plantar dermatosis. Graham RM, Verbov JL, Vickers CFH. Br J Dermatol 1987;12:468–70.

White/yellow soft paraffin, impregnated paste bandages and urea-containing emollients helped some patients, though the benefit was often short-lived. Although there was no association with any particular sport, intensive exercise causing skin cracking, soreness, and bleeding was a common complaint; 75% of parents said that a change in footwear had not been helpful.

In contrast to Jones et al. above, only 30% of cases in this series had resolved (mean age 11.8 years), though the ages of the remaining 70% were not stated.

THIRD LINE THERAPIES

■ Zinc oxide/impregnated bandages	C
■ Bed rest/footwear avoidance	E

Juvenile plantar dermatosis – an 8 year follow-up of 102 patients. Jones SK, English JSC, Forsyth A, Mackie RM. Clin Exp Dermatol 1987;12:5–7.

Tar-containing preparations may be helpful.

Juvenile plantar dermatosis. Graham RM, Verbov JL, Vickers CFH. Br J Dermatol 1987;12:468–70.

Occlusion with zinc paste or ichthammol-impregnated bandages were among the most beneficial of treatments.

The aetiology of juvenile plantar dermatosis. Shrank AB. Br J Dermatol 1979;100:641–8.

Bed rest or avoidance of shoes and hosiery for 3 weeks resulted in disease clearance (said to approximate to the time taken to regrow the sweat duct apparatus in the horny layer of the foot).

Juvenile xanthogranuloma

Olivia MV Schofield

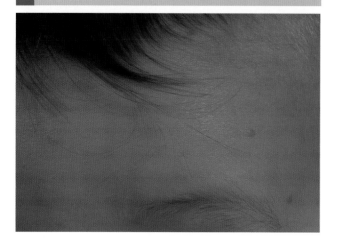

Juvenile xanthogranuloma (JXG) is a benign disorder characterized by solitary or multiple, yellow-red nodules in the skin, and, occasionally, in other organs. The lesions spontaneously regress. It occurs most commonly in infancy and early childhood, but adults may be affected. Treatment is only recommended for systemic lesions if their location interferes with organ function.

MANAGEMENT STRATEGY

The diagnosis of JXG is usually made clinically, but a biopsy is required for atypical clinical variants (giant, plaque-like, paired, clustered, infiltrative, lichenoid, linear, subcutaneous, and intramuscular) and if multiple lesions are present. Unusual histological variants require further examination by immunohistochemistry and electron microscopy. In the most common solitary type (60–80% of all cases), there is a male to female preponderance of 1.5:1 and the usual affected sites are the head, neck, and upper trunk. In the majority of cases no further investigation is required. The lesions will resolve spontaneously within months or years and no follow-up is necessary. A review of systems and general examination is, however, recommended to look for involvement of other sites and to examine for café au lait macules (see below).

Eye involvement

The eye is the most commonly affected extracutaneous site of JXG, and intraocular JXG usually affects the iris. This often presents as an acute red eye due to spontaneous hyphema (hemorrhage into the anterior chamber). The incidence of eye involvement in cutaneous JXG is only 0.2–0.4%, but intraocular JXG can occur without cutaneous disease and can be locally aggressive.

Systemic JXG

There are many reports of extracutaneous involvement occurring with and without cutaneous lesions. After the eye, the subcutis, CNS, lung, liver, and spleen are the commonest sites, but there are reports of every organ system in the body being affected. *As the differential diagnosis is usually neoplasia, it is imperative to determine an accurate diagnosis.* Lesions in extracutaneous sites, like the skin, spontaneously regress and therefore *treatment is only indicated in cases of compromised organ function.*

Triple association of JXG, NF-1, and JMML

The triple association of JXG, neurofibromatosis-1 (NF-1), and juvenile myelomonocytic leukemia (JMML), an aggressive myeloproliferative disorder of childhood, has been reported. There is an increased risk of JMML in children with NF-1. In a population of children with NF-1, the incidence of JMML is 5/10 000 per year. *It is likely that there is an association of JXG with NF-1, but at present there is no evidence to support an increased risk of JMML in individuals with both JXG and NF-1 compared to those with NF-1 alone.*

SPECIFIC INVESTIGATIONS

- In most cases, no specific investigations are required
- Ophthalmological assessment in children under the age of 2 years with multiple lesions
- Full blood count and/or pediatric referral in children with JXG and café au lait macules, NF-1, or a family history of NF-1
- Biopsy in cases with systemic manifestations to confirm diagnosis and avoid unnecessary invasive diagnostic procedures

Radiological and clinicopathological features of orbital xanthogranuloma. Miszkiel KA, Sohaib SAS, Rose GE, et al. Br J Ophthalmol 2000;84:251–8.

Of 150 cases of intraocular JXG, none was identified on routine screening of individuals with cutaneous JXG. Of those children with eye involvement, 92% are under the age of 2 years, and if they have cutaneous lesions these tend to be multiple.

Juvenile xanthogranuloma. Hernandez-Martin A, Baselga E, Drolet BA, Esterley NB. J Am Acad Dermatol 1997;36: 355–67.

Recommendations are made in this review article following assessments of previously reported cutaneous and extracutaneous cases. In general, an awareness of the possibility of extracutaneous involvement is important.

The risk of intraocular juvenile xanthogranuloma: survey of current practices and assessment of risk. Wu Chang M, Frieden IJ, Good W. J Am Acad Dermatol 1996;34:445–9.

A postal survey of pediatric dermatologists (27% response rate) and ophthalmologists (44% response rate) revealed the different incidence of ocular xanthogranuloma presenting to these two groups.

Those children under the age of 2 years with multiple skin lesions have the highest risk of intraocular involvement and should be screened by an ophthalmologist.

Juvenile xanthogranuloma associated with neurofibromatosis-1: 14 patients without evidence of hematologic

malignancies. Cambhiangi SD, Restano L, Caputo R. Pediatr Dermatol 2004;21:97–101.

A retrospective review of 14 individuals affected by JXG and NF-1. The onset of JXG was within the first 2 years of life in 13 patients. Mean follow-up was for 4.3 years (range 1–10 years) in 11 patients and none of these children developed hematologic malignancy during this period.

JXG, NF-1 and JMML: alphabet soup or a clinical issue? Burgdorf WH, Zelger B. Pediatr Dermatol 2004;21:174–6.

An editorial comment and review on this triple association which concludes that there is no evidence to support an increased risk of JMML in children with the combination of JXG and NF-1 compared with those children with NF-1 alone.

FIRST LINE THERAPIES

■ None	E
■ Surgical resection for symptomatic extracutaneous lesions	D
■ Ocular lesions treated with topical or intralesional corticosteroid	D

Juvenile xanthogranuloma: forms of systemic disease and their clinical implications. Freyer DR, Kennedy R, Bostrom BC, et al. J Pediatr 1996;129:227–37.

Surgery can be an effective cure for symptomatic extracutaneous lesions of JXG.

Update on juvenile xanthogranuloma: unusual cutaneous and systemic variants. Wu Chang M. Semin Cutan Med Surg 1999;18:195–205.

In adults, the lesions tend not to resolve spontaneously and can last up to 7 years; excision may therefore be considered appropriate

Early treatment of juvenile xanthogranuloma of the iris with subconjunctival steroids. Casteels I, Olver J, Malone M, Taylor D. Br J Ophthalmol 1993;77:57–60.

Ocular lesions have been successfully treated with topical and intralesional corticosteroids.

SECOND LINE THERAPIES

■ Cutaneous surgery	E
■ Ocular surgery	E
■ Ocular lesions treated with systemic corticosteroids and/or low-dose radiotherapy	E

Giant congenital juvenile xanthogranuloma. Magana M, Vazquez R, Fernandez-Diez J, et al. Pediatr Dermatol 1994; 11:227–30.

Juvenile xanthogranuloma of the oral mucosa. Cohen DM, Brannon RB, Davis LD, Miller AS. Oral Surg 1981;52:513–23.

Excision can be undertaken for cosmetic and diagnostic reasons, but there have been reports of recurrences after complete excisions in both cutaneous and extracutaneous sites.

THIRD LINE THERAPIES

■ Radiotherapy	D
■ Chemotherapy	D

Juvenile xanthogranuloma: forms of systemic disease and their clinical implications. Freyer DR, Kennedy R, Bostrom BC, et al. J Pediatr 1996;129:227–37.

Radiotherapy and chemotherapy, either alone or in combination, have been used in isolated case reports for unresectable or infiltrative lesions, particularly in the CNS.

Juvenile xanthogranuloma of the iris in an adult. Parmley VC, George DP, Fannin LA. Arch Ophthalmol 1998;116:377–9.

A case report of radiotherapy and methotrexate use in a young man with a lesion on his iris.

Kaposi sarcoma

Analisa Vincent Halpern, Steven M Manders

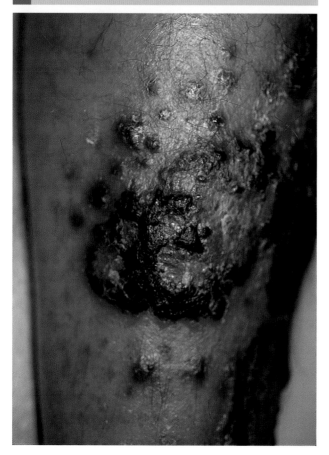

Kaposi sarcoma (KS) is a distinct, often multifocal vascular neoplasm etiologically linked to human herpesvirus-8 (HHV-8). In the USA, epidemic, or AIDS-associated KS is the most common presentation, and the malignancy most often associated with HIV infection. In clinical practice, however, classic, endemic, and immunosuppression-associated KS are also encountered. Although therapy is similar for the three variants, the treatment of epidemic KS is emphasized here.

MANAGEMENT STRATEGY

Therapy of KS is largely viewed as palliative, especially with respect to cutaneous disease. For treatment purposes, patients can be divided into several groups. Limited cutaneous KS is defined as disease in which there are fewer than ten skin lesions, a lack of oral or visceral involvement, and the absence of tumor-associated lymphedema. Treatment options include *cryotherapy, intralesional vinblastine, radiotherapy, alitretinoin gel,* and *interferon* therapy. Because treatment is essentially for cosmesis, side effects such as pigmentary changes and pain become important in therapeutic decisions.

For patients with resistant limited disease, extensive cutaneous involvement, systemic KS, or tumor-associated lymphedema, *cytotoxic chemotherapy in combination with highly active antiretroviral therapy (HAART)* is first line. For epidemic KS, effective antiretroviral therapy can be sufficient by itself to halt progression of disease, and has been found to have a synergistic effect with the *liposomal anthracyclines (pegylated liposomal doxorubicin* or *liposomal daunorubicin), paclitaxel,* and *interferon alfa. Radiotherapy* remains an alternative treatment option for this group of patients.

Treatment of oral lesions is problematic due to inaccessibility to cryotherapy and radiation-induced mucositis. Options include *intralesional vinblastine,* sclerosing agents such as *sodium tetradecyl sulfate,* or systemic treatments.

An increasing number of investigational therapeutics are being explored for the treatment of KS, including anti-angiogenic agents such as TNP 470, orally active matrix metalloproteinase inhibitors, and agents targeting interleukin (IL)-12.

SPECIFIC INVESTIGATIONS

- Serology for HIV, CD4$^+$ T lymphocyte counts, viral load (if HIV positive)
- Complete blood count, renal and hepatic function
- Chest radiograph
- Stool for occult blood

Kaposi's sarcoma. Antman K, Chang Y. N Engl J Med 2000; 342:1027–38.

KS remains the most common AIDS-associated cancer in the USA.

Epidemic Kaposi's sarcoma. Cianfrocca M, Von Roenn JH. Oncology 1998;12:1375–81.

Review of appropriate patient evaluation including thorough history and physical exam and relevant laboratory and imaging studies.

FIRST LINE THERAPIES

■ Cryotherapy	B
■ Intralesional vinblastine	C
■ Radiotherapy	B
■ Alitretinoin gel	A
■ Pegylated liposomal doxorubicin plus HAART	B
■ Paclitaxel	B

Cryotherapy for cutaneous Kaposi's sarcoma (KS) associated with acquired immune deficiency syndrome (AIDS): a phase II trial. Tappero JW, Berger TG, Kaplan LD, et al. J Acquir Immune Defic Syndr 1991;4:839–46.

Treatment was repeated at 3-week intervals, allowing adequate healing time. On average, subjects received three treatments per lesion with a mean follow-up time of 11 weeks (range 6–25 weeks). One treatment consisted of two freeze–thaw cycles, with thaw times ranging from 11 to 60 s per cycle. A 70% cosmetic response rate with duration up to 6 months.

Hypopigmentation and scarring are potential problems in skin types III–VI.

Intralesional vinblastine for cutaneous Kaposi's sarcoma associated with acquired immunodeficiency syndrome. Boudreaux AA, Smith LL, Cosby CD, et al. J Am Acad Dermatol 1993;28:61–5.

Responses were achieved in 88% of treated lesions, but pain and hyperpigmentation are common. Pain was minimized by the addition of bicarbonate buffered lidocaine to the diluent.

Radiotherapy in the management of epidemic Kaposi's sarcoma: a retrospective study of 643 cases. Kirova YM, Belembaogo E, Frikha H, et al. Radiother Oncol 1998;46: 19–22.

An overall 92% response rate was achieved, but treatment of oral lesions frequently led to mucositis.

Phase III vehicle-controlled, multi-centered study of topical alitretinoin gel 0.1% in cutaneous AIDS-related Kaposi's sarcoma. Bodsworth NJ, Bloch M, Bower M, et al; International Panretin Gel KS Study Group. Am J Clin Dermatol 2001;2:77–87.

Response rate was 37% (compared to 7% treated with vehicle).

Marginal response rate and exorbitant cost make the usefulness of this modality questionable. Tretinoin gel (Topical treatment of epidemic Kaposi's sarcoma with all-trans-retinoic acid. Bonhomme L, Fredj G, Averous S, et al. Ann Oncol 1991;2:234–5) may be a reasonable alternative topical retinoid option.

Pegylated liposomal doxorubicin plus highly active antiretroviral therapy versus highly active antiretroviral therapy alone in HIV patients with Kaposi's sarcoma. Martin-Carbonero L, Barrios A, Saballs P, et al; Caelyx/KS Spanish Group. AIDS 2004;18:1737–40.

Randomized study comparing pegylated liposomal doxorubicin plus HAART vs HAART alone showed greater response rate (76 vs 20%, respectively, in the intent-to-treat analysis) in the former group.

These results differ from previous studies showing HAART therapy alone to be effective in regression of KS lesions.

Multicenter trial of low-dose paclitaxel in patients with advanced AIDS-related Kaposi sarcoma. Tulpule A, Groopman J, Saville MW, et al. Cancer 2002;95:147–54.

Phase II trial of 107 patients showed a complete or partial response with or without concomitant protease inhibitor of 59 and 54%, respectively. Grade IV neutropenia was the most common adverse effect (35% of patients).

Two case reports of potentially serious drug–drug interactions occurring in patients on HAART and paclitaxel concomitantly (Potential drug interaction with paclitaxel and highly active antiretroviral therapy in two patients with AIDS-associated Kaposi sarcoma. Bundow D, Aboulafia DM. Am J Clin Oncol 2004;27: 81–4).

SECOND LINE THERAPIES

■ Intralesional interferon	C
■ Subcutaneous or intramuscular interferon	B
■ Interferon plus antiretroviral therapy	B
■ Liposomal anthracyclines (doxorubicin, daunorubicin) as monotherapy	B

Intralesional interferon-alpha and zidovudine in epidemic Kaposi's sarcoma. Dupuy J, Prize M, Lynch G, et al. J Am Acad Dermatol 1993;28:966–72.

Intralesional interferon-alfa (1 million U of interferon-alfa three times weekly for 6 weeks) showed a response rate of 85%, but this was not statistically significant.

Treatment of Kaposi's sarcoma with interferon alpha-2b (Intron A). Volberding PA, Mitsuyasu RT, Golando JP, Spiegel RJ. Cancer 1987;59:620–5.

Response rates up to 45% were noted at high doses (50×10^6 IU/m^2 intravenously). Treatment is contraindicated if severe hepatic dysfunction or peripheral neuropathy is present.

Currently, monotherapy has been largely replaced by combination therapy with antiretroviral agents.

Pegylated-liposomal doxorubicin versus doxorubicin, bleomycin, and vincristine in the treatment of AIDS-related Kaposi's sarcoma: results of a randomized phase III clinical trial. Northfelt DW, Dezube BJ, Thommes JA, et al. J Clin Oncol 1998;16:2445–51.

Liposomal doxorubicin was not only significantly more effective, but had less toxicity than the standard triple chemotherapeutic regimen.

Phase IV study of liposomal daunorubicin (DaunoXome) in AIDS-related Kaposi sarcoma. Rosenthal E, Poizot-Martin I, Saint-Marc T, et al; DNX Study Group. Am J Clin Oncol 2002;25:57–9.

Partial and complete responses in 94 patients were 26.5 and 11.5%, respectively.

Interpretation of the effectiveness of this therapy is confounded because 90% of patients were receiving HAART during the trial.

THIRD LINE THERAPIES

■ Thalidomide	B
■ All-trans retinoic acid, oral	B
■ Liposomal all-trans retinoic acid, intravenous	B
■ Photodynamic therapy	B
■ IM862	B
■ Foscarnet	B
■ 9-cis retinoic acid	B
■ Etoposide	B
■ 3% sodium tetradecyl sulfate	C
■ Matrix metalloproteinase inhibitor COL-3	C
■ Tumor necrosis factor-α/melphalan	D
■ IL-2	E
■ Laser therapy	E
■ Surgical excision	E

Activity of thalidomide in AIDS-related Kaposi's sarcoma. Little RF, Wyvill KM, Pluda JM, et al. J Clin Oncol 2000;18: 2593–602.

At a median dose of 500 mg daily, the response rate was 40%.

A multicenter phase II study of the intravenous administration of liposomal tretinoin in patients with acquired immunodeficiency syndrome-associated Kaposi's sarcoma. Bernstein ZP, Chanan-Khan A, Miller KC, et al. Cancer 2002;95:2555–61.

A thrice weekly dosing schedule (60 mg/m^2 escalating to 120 mg/m^2) was more effective than once a week without any significant difference in toxicity.

All-trans retinoic acid for the treatment of AIDS-related Kaposi's sarcoma: results of a pilot phase II study. Gill PS, Espina BM, Moudgil T, et al. Leukemia 1994;8(suppl 3): s26–32.

Oral all-trans retinoic acid led to a 17% partial response rate.

Photofrin photodynamic therapy for treatment of AIDS-related cutaneous Kaposi's sarcoma. Bernstein ZP, Wilson BD, Oseroff AR, et al. AIDS 1999;13:1697–704.

A clinical response occurred in 96%, but it was often associated with erythema, edema, and necrosis.

Results of a randomized study of IM862 nasal solution in the treatment of AIDS-related Kaposi's sarcoma. Tulpule A, Scadden DT, Espina BM, et al. J Clin Oncol 2000;18:716–23.

IM862 is a dipeptide of L-glutamyl-L-tryptophan initially isolated from the thymus. Administered as intranasal drops, IM862 led to a major response in 36% of patients.

Effect of antiviral drugs used to treat cytomegalovirus end-organ disease on subsequent course of previously diagnosed Kaposi's sarcoma in patients with AIDS. Robles R, Lugo D, Gee L, Jacobson MA. J Acquir Immune Defic Syndr Hum Retrovirol 1999;20:34–8.

In patients being treated for cytomegalovirus with foscarnet, progression of KS was markedly delayed.

9-cis-retinoic acid capsules in the treatment of AIDS-related Kaposi sarcoma: results of a phase 2 multicenter clinical trial. Aboulafia DM, Norris D, Henry D, et al. Arch Dermatol 2003;139:178–86.

Overall response was 19%. Moderate efficacy and substantial toxicity at higher doses limits use.

Phase II evaluation of low-dose oral etoposide for the treatment of relapsed or progressive AIDS-related Kaposi's sarcoma: an AIDS Clinical Trials Group clinical study. Evans SR, Krown SE, Testa MA, et al. J Clin Oncol 2002;20:3236–41.

Overall response rate was 36.1%; neutropenia and opportunistic infections were the most common side effects.

Treatment of oral Kaposi's sarcoma with a sclerosing agent in AIDS patients. A preliminary study. Lucatorto FM, Sapp JP. Oral Surg Oral Med Oral Pathol 1993;75:192–8.

A series of 12 patients with oral lesions showed a high rate of response, but follow-up was brief.

Treatment of oral lesions is often problematic because radiotherapy frequently leads to severe mucositis. Intralesional vinblastine, as well as systemic therapies, offers additional treatment options.

Matrix metalloproteinase inhibitor COL-3 in the treatment of AIDS-related Kaposi's sarcoma: a phase I AIDS malignancy consortium study. Cianfrocca M, Cooley TP, Lee JY, et al. J Clin Oncol 2002;20:153–9.

Eighteen patients received oral COL-3 once daily with an overall response rate of 44%. Most common side effect was dose-related photosensitivity.

Isolated limb perfusion with high-dose tumor necrosis factor-α and melphalan for Kaposi's sarcoma. Lev-Chelouche D, Abu-Abeid S, Merimsky O, et al. Arch Surg 1999;134:177–80.

Extensive symptomatic classic KS was successfully treated, avoiding the need for amputation in four of five patients.

Recombinant interleukin-2 monotherapy for classic Kaposi's sarcoma. Shibagaki R, Kishimoto S, Takenaka H, Yasuno H. Arch Dermatol 1998;134:1193–6.

Weekly intralesional IL-2 led to long-term remission in one patient.

Successful treatment of cutaneous Kaposi's sarcoma by the 585-nm pulsed dye laser. Marchell N, Alster TS. Dermatol Surg 1997;23:973–5.

Pulsed dye laser was found to be effective in a single patient; pulsed CO_2 laser and a diode laser/indocyanine green combination have been used successfully by others.

Local therapy for mucocutaneous Kaposi's sarcoma in patients with acquired immunodeficiency syndrome. Webster GF. Dermatol Surg 1995;21:205–8.

Surgery can occasionally be helpful for isolated lesions, but recurrence is frequent; therefore this modality is of limited value.

Evidence levels A Double-blind study B Clinical trial ≥ 20 subjects C Clinical trial < 20 subjects D Series ≥ 5 subjects E Anecdotal case reports

Kawasaki disease

Warren R Heymann, Ranon Mann, Michael Fisher

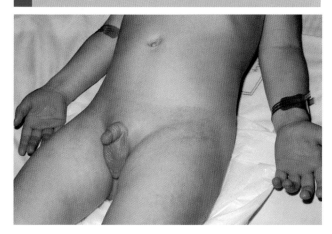

Kawasaki disease primarily affects infants and young children. It is an acute febrile illness characterized by a multi-organ vasculitis and the potential for serious cardiac sequelae. Although the etiology remains unclear, bacterial superantigens may be implicated.

MANAGEMENT STRATEGY

The potential for cardiac complications, including aneurysm formation, myocardial infarction, and sudden death, dictates the need for therapeutic intervention. Therapy in the acute phase, with the goal of controlling acute inflammation and preventing coronary aneurysm formation, consists mainly of *aspirin* and *intravenous gammaglobulin (IVIG)*.

In the acute phase of the disease, aspirin, administered for both its antithrombotic and anti-inflammatory effects, is given at a dose of 80–100 mg/kg daily, in four divided doses. A serum salicylate level of approximately 20–25 mg/dL is desired. After the fever has resolved, at approximately day 14 of the illness, aspirin administration, continued for its antiplatelet effect, is reduced to 3–5 mg/kg as a single daily dose. The optimal salicylate regimen is controversial. There have been no controlled studies to indicate that aspirin reduces the incidence of coronary aneurysm formation.

IVIG, which often leads to rapid defervescence and reduces the potential for cardiac disease, is administered in the acute phase as a single dose of 2 g/kg over 10–12 h. This regimen has been found to be superior to the previously recommended dosing schedule of 400 mg/kg daily over 2 h for four consecutive days.

The most appropriate treatment for patients who fail to respond to IVIG is yet to be determined. Repeat *immune globulin infusions* have been effective in some cases.

Surgical intervention is indicated in cases complicated by significant coronary artery or valvular disease that fail to respond to medical treatment.

SPECIFIC INVESTIGATIONS

- Echocardiography
- Electrocardiography
- Cardiac angiography

Diagnosis, treatment, and long-term management of Kawasaki disease: a statement for health professionals from the Committee on Rheumatic Fever, Endocarditis, and Kawasaki Disease, Council on Cardiovascular Disease in the Young, American Heart Association. Newberger JW, Takahashi M, Gerber MA, et al. Pediatrics 2004;114:1708–33.

A multidisciplinary committee of experts was convened to revise the American Heart Association recommendations for diagnosis, treatment, and long-term management of Kawasaki disease. A new algorithm is presented to aid clinicians in deciding which patients should undergo electrocardiography, receive IVIG treatment, or both. The group also reviews data for children who have had persistent disease despite initial therapy with IVIG, including IVIG retreatment with corticosteroids, tumor necrosis factor-α antagonists, and abciximab.

The ultimate decisions for case management must be made by physicians in light of the particular conditions presented by individual patients.

Guidelines for long-term management of patients with Kawasaki disease. Report from the Committee on Rheumatic Fever, Endocarditis, and Kawasaki Disease, Council on Cardiovascular Disease in the Young, American Heart Association. Dajani A, Taubert K, Takahashi M, et al. Circulation 1994;89:916–22.

Echocardiography is an essential modality for the evaluation and follow-up of coronary artery abnormalities. The initial echocardiogram should be obtained as soon as the diagnosis of Kawasaki disease is suspected. Recommendations for diagnostic testing via echocardiography, electrocardiography, angiography, etc., are given based on the relative risk of myocardial ischemia. The severity of coronary arterial involvement will dictate the long-term evaluation and management of these patients.

FIRST LINE THERAPIES

■ Aspirin (acetylsalicylic acid)	B
■ Immune globulin	B

Probable efficacy of high dose salicylates in reducing coronary involvement in Kawasaki disease. Koren G, Rose V, Lavi S, Rowe R. JAMA 1985;254:767–9.

Patients who received high-dose salicylates (80–180 mg/kg daily) were less likely to develop coronary aneurysms. The study was not randomized and serum salicylate concentrations were not measured.

Aspirin has never been shown via a prospective study to reduce the prevalence of coronary artery aneurysms.

Comparison of low dose aspirin (LDA) vs. high dose aspirin (HDA) as an adjunct to intravenous gamma globulin in the treatment of Kawasaki syndrome. Melish ME, Takahashi M, Shulman ST, et al. Pediatr Res 1992;31:170A.

All patients received immune globulin and either 3–8 mg/kg daily (LDA) or 100 mg/kg daily (HDA) of aspirin until day 14. After day 14, the dose of aspirin administered in both groups was 3–8 mg/kg daily. There was a significantly shorter duration of fever and other indicators of inflammation in the HDA group. There was no difference in coronary artery abnormalities between the groups.

The optimal salicylate regimen in Kawasaki disease is controversial.

The treatment of Kawasaki syndrome with intravenous gamma globulin. Newburger JW, Takahashi M, Burns JC, et al. N Engl J Med 1986;315:341–7.

This study compared the efficacy of two regimens to reduce the frequency of coronary artery aneurysms – 168 children were randomly assigned to receive either aspirin alone (100 mg/kg until day 14 and then 3–5 mg/kg daily) or aspirin and IVIG at a dose of 400 mg/kg daily given over 2 h on four consecutive days; 4% of patients in the aspirin/IVIG group compared to 18% of patients in the group receiving aspirin alone were noted to have coronary artery abnormalities on two-dimensional echocardiography at 7 weeks.

A single intravenous infusion of gamma globulin as compared with four infusions in the treatment of acute Kawasaki syndrome. Newburger JW, Takahashi M, Beiser AS, et al. N Engl J Med 1991;324:1633–9.

Five hundred and forty nine children were randomly assigned to receive gammaglobulin, either as daily infusions of 400 mg/kg for four consecutive days or as a single infusion of 2 g/kg over 10 h. Both treatment groups received aspirin. The single infusion regimen was more effective in reducing both systemic inflammation (mean temperature and duration of fever) and the prevalence of coronary artery abnormalities.

SECOND LINE THERAPIES

■ Systemic corticosteroids	C
■ Immune globulin re-treatment	D

Corticosteroids in the treatment of the acute phase of Kawasaki disease. Shinohara M, Sone K, Tomomasa T, Morikawa A. J Pediatr 1999;135:465–9.

A retrospective, nonrandomized study that suggested a potential role of corticosteroids in the treatment of the acute phase of Kawasaki disease.

Corticosteroid therapy remains controversial. There are conflicting studies as to its potential benefit. Many physicians are reluctant to administer corticosteroids because their use, in an early study, was linked to a high incidence of coronary aneurysms (Kato H, Koike S, Yokoyama T. Kawasaki disease: effect of treatment on coronary involvement. Pediatrics 1979;63:175–9).

Gamma globulin re-treatment in Kawasaki disease. Sundel RP, Burns JC, Baker A, Beiser AS, Newburger JW. J Pediatr 1993;123:657–9.

A retrospective analysis of 13 children with Kawasaki disease who were re-treated with immune globulin due to persistent or recrudescent fever. Within 36 h of one additional treatment, nine patients had resolution of their fever.

Prospective clinical trials are needed to ascertain the appropriate management of initial nonresponders to aspirin/gammaglobulin.

Treatment of immune globulin-resistant Kawasaki disease with pulsed doses of corticosteroids. Wright DA, Newburger JW, Baker A, Sundel RP. J Pediatr 1996;128:146–9.

Four patients with disease resistant to treatment with immune globulin were treated with pulsed methylprednisolone with apparent symptom normalization. The authors caution that these data should be viewed as preliminary.

Controlled studies are needed to determine if pulsed corticosteroids are beneficial in patients who fail to respond to immune globulin.

Pulse methylprednisolone therapy for impending cardiac tamponade in immunoglobulin-resistant Kawasaki disease. Dahlem PG, Rosenstiel IA, Lam J, Kuijpers TW. Intensive Care Med 1999;25:1137–9.

THIRD LINE THERAPIES

■ Ticlopidine	E
■ Pentoxifylline	B
■ Plasma exchange	E
■ Dipyridamole	E
■ Cardiac transplantation	E
■ Coronary artery bypass grafting	B
■ Infliximab	E

Ticlopidine plus aspirin for coronary thrombosis in Kawasaki disease. O'Brien M, Parness IA, Neufeld EJ, et al. Pediatrics 2000;105:1149.

A thrombosed coronary aneurysm that had failed to respond to thrombolytics was successfully treated in a 7-month-old with aspirin and ticlopidine.

Pentoxifylline and intravenous gamma globulin combination therapy for acute Kawasaki disease. Furukawa S, Matsubara T, Umezawa Y, et al. Eur J Pediatr 1994;153:663–7.

In addition to aspirin and immune globulin, patients were randomized in two separate studies to receive either low-dose (10 mg/kg) or high-dose (20 mg/kg) daily pentoxifylline. A reduction in the prevalence of coronary aneurysms was demonstrated in the high-dose group.

Pentoxifylline use for the treatment of Kawasaki disease remains investigational.

Plasma exchange in Kawasaki disease. Takagi N, Kihara T, Yammaguchi S, et al. Lancet 1995;346:1307.

A 4-year-old who failed to respond to immune globulin improved with plasma exchange.

Guidelines for long-term management of patients with Kawasaki disease. Dajani AS, Taubert KA, Takahashi M, et al. Circulation 1994;89:916–22.

For patients at risk of cardiovascular complications, dipyridamole has been used for its antiplatelet effects.

Evidence levels **A** Double-blind study **B** Clinical trial ≥ 20 subjects **C** Clinical trial < 20 subjects **D** Series ≥ 5 subjects **E** Anecdotal case reports

Orthotopic heart transplantation for Kawasaki disease after rupture of a giant coronary artery aneurysm. Koutlas TC, Wernovsky G, Bridges ND, et al. J Thorac Cardiovasc Surg 1997;113:217–8.

A 3-year-old boy received a cardiac transplant during the acute phase of his disease.

Optimal time of surgical treatment for Kawasaki coronary artery disease. Yamauchi H, Ochi M, Fujii M, et al. J Nippon Med Sch 2004;71:279–86.

The authors studied 21 patients with Kawasaki disease and coronary complications who underwent coronary artery bypass grafting (CABG) over a 12-year period. The authors conclude that CABG is successful when completed shortly after the acute onset of disease.

Infliximab as a novel therapy for refractory Kawasaki disease. Weiss JE, Eberhard BA, Chowdhury D, Gottleib BS. J Rheumatol 2004;31:808–10.

A 3-year-old boy with Kawasaki disease and giant coronary artery aneurysms unresponsive to multiple doses of IVIG and methylprednisolone was treated with infliximab. After the first dose he defervesced and his laboratory measures improved.

Keloid scarring

Brian Berman, Deborah Zell,
Ricardo Romagosa

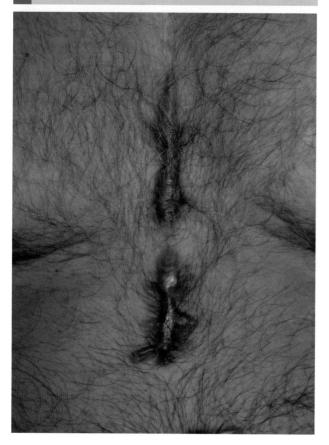

Keloids are dermal hyperproliferative growths with excessive accumulation of extracellular matrix components that may appear in areas of trauma. These scars are characterized by increased collagen and glycosaminoglycan content. In addition to the cosmetic disfigurement and negative psychological impact that keloids may represent to the affected patient, these scars can often be extremely symptomatic with complaints such as pain and pruritus.

MANAGEMENT STRATEGY

The therapeutic options for keloids are numerous and no single therapeutic modality is best for all keloids. The first rule of treatment involves *prevention* and *patient education*. Prevention during surgery by closing all wounds with minimal tension and inflammation is of utmost importance. Non-essential cosmetic surgery should be avoided in those patients known to be predisposed to the formation of keloids. Incision sites in the skin of the mid-chest and skin overlying joints should be avoided, and surgical wounds should parallel skin creases.

Common therapeutic modalities include *occlusive dressings, compression therapy, intralesional corticosteroid injections, intralesional interferon injections, cryosurgery, excision, radiation therapy,* and *laser therapy.*

Intralesional corticosteroids have been the mainstay of treatment. The most commonly used corticosteroid is *triamcinolone acetonide* in concentrations of 10–40 mg/mL

administered intralesionally with a 25–27-gauge needle at 4–6-week intervals. Although topical corticosteroids and topically applied corticosteroid-impregnated tape are used frequently in the treatment of keloids, there are no clear published data to demonstrate efficacy. Occlusive dressings have also been extensively used. *Silicone gel sheets* and *silicone occlusive dressings* have an anti-keloidal effect, which appears to be a result of occlusion and hydration. Pressure devices are thought to induce local tissue hypoxia and have been shown to have a thinning effect on keloids. A novel idea in the treatment of keloids and hypertrophic scars is the use of intralesional interferon. *Interferon-alfa-2b* has been used successfully to decrease scar height and reduce postoperative recurrences. Radiation therapy has been safe and effective in most protocols. Cryosurgical media such as liquid nitrogen affect the microvasculature and cause cell damage via intracellular crystals leading to tissue anoxia. Generally one to three freeze–thaw cycles lasting 10–30 s are used for the desired effect. Treatment may need to be repeated every 20–30 days and is most effective when combined with intralesional corticosteroids. Excision alone yields widely varying results, with recurrence occurring in 45–100%. The *CO$_2$ laser, Nd:YAG, and argon lasers* have been used as destructive modalities in the treatment of keloids. The 585 nm pulsed dye laser has been shown to be effective in decreasing erythema and reduction of symptoms. *Intralesional injection of 5-fluorouracil (5-FU)* has been beneficial for hypertrophic scars and, to a lesser extent, keloids.

SPECIFIC INVESTIGATIONS

- ■ Skin biopsy

Dermatofibrosarcoma protuberans is a unique fibrohistiocytic tumour expressing CD34. Aiba S, Tabata N, Ishii H, et al. Br J Dermatol 1992;127:79–84.

Dermatofibrosarcoma protuberans can be easily misdiagnosed as a keloid. Histopathology may help differentiate the two, but expression of CD34 by tumor cells occurs only in dermatofibrosarcoma protuberans.

FIRST LINE THERAPIES

■ Intralesional corticosteroids	B
■ Occlusive dressing	B
■ Compression	E
■ Intralesional interferon-alfa-2b	B

Experience with difficult keloids. Lahiri A, Tsiliboti D, Gaze NR. Br J Plast Surg 2001;54:633–5.

A retrospective clinical trial of 43 patients (62 keloids) treated with intralesional injections of triamcinolone acetate, cryotherapy, and another intralesional injection of triamcinolone acetate resulted in 12 patients with complete remission, 19 patients with good improvement, and ten patients with some improvement.

Keloids treated with topical injections of triamcinolone acetonide. Immediate and long term results. Kiil J. Scand J Plast Reconstr Surg 1977;11:169–72.

In a prospective clinical trial of 52 patients intralesional injections of triamcinolone acetonide alone resulted in significant flattening and decrease in pruritus in 93% of the

314

keloids. One-third had partial recurrence at 1 year, and at 5 years more than 50% had recurred. All recurrences were successfully treated with further triamcinolone acetonide injections.

An inexpensive self fabricated pressure clip for the ear lobe. Agrawal K, Panda KN, Arumugam A. Br J Plast Surg 1998;51:122–3.

In 26 patients (41 earlobe keloids) self fabricated and inexpensive pressure clips were used for a minimum of 6 months with intralesionally injected triamcinolone acetonide and resulted in 34 ear lobes that have undergone ear boring in follow-up.

Combination of different techniques for the treatment of earlobe keloids. Akoz T, Gideroglu K, Akan M. Aesthetic Plast Surg 2002;26:184.

Nine patients were treated with surgical excision of their earlobe keloids and were followed with a triamcinolone acetonide injection and silicone gel sheets. No recurrences occurred in eight of the nine patients.

Comparison of a silicone gel-filled cushion and silicon gel sheeting for the treatment of hypertrophic or keloid scars. Berman B, Flores F. Dermatol Surg 1999;25:484–6.

Thirty two patients participated and 53% and 36.3% of the patients had a reduction in the keloid volume with the silicone gel cushion and the silicone gel sheeting treatments, respectively.

A controlled clinical trial of topical silicone gel sheeting in the treatment of hypertrophic scars and keloids. Gold MH. J Am Acad Dermatol 1994;30:506–7.

No patient had complete resolution, and more than half had minimal to no improvement. Phase II of the study evaluated the post-excision use of silicone gel sheeting. In the treatment group, of the eight keloids treated, there was a 12% recurrence rate vs 37% of the eight keloids in the excision-only group.

Silicone gel sheeting for the prevention and management of evolving hypertrophic and keloid scars. Fulton JE. Dermatol Surg 1995;21:947–51.

Keloids were reported to have improved in 85% of the 20 cases.

Effects of a water-impermeable, non-silicone-based occlusive dressing on keloids. Bieley HC, Berman B. J Am Acad Dermatol 1996;35:113–14.

A water-impermeable, non-silicone-based occlusive dressing worn continuously for 2 months brought about an average keloid height reduction of 35% in 19 of 21 patients and the majority of patients had reduction in pain, pruritus, and erythema.

Recurrence rates of excised keloids treated with post-operative triamcinolone acetonide injections or interferon alfa-2b injections. Berman B, Flores F. J Am Acad Dermatol 1997;37:755–7.

There was a statistically significant decrease in the recurrence of 124 excised keloids when administering post-excision interferon-alfa-2b (18.7% recurrence) vs excision alone (51.1%), vs treatment with postoperative intralesional triamcinolone (58.4%).

SECOND LINE THERAPIES

■ Intralesional interferon-gamma	C

A controlled trial of intralesional recombinant interferon gamma in the treatment of keloidal scarring. Granstein RD, Rook A, Flotte TJ, et al. Arch Dermatol 1990;126:1295–301.

Six of eight patients had decrease in height of 30.4% compared to 1.1% in control sites; 0.01 mg, 0.1 mg, or diluent was injected into different sites.

As the authors state, further studies are needed to establish the usefulness of this treatment.

Intralesional interferon gamma treatment for keloids and hypertrophic scars. Larrabee WF, East CA, Jaffe HS, et al. Arch Otolaryngol Head Neck Surg 1990;116:1159–62.

Five of the ten study patients had a decrease in their scar size by at least 50% in linear dimensions. The treatment protocol was one treatment per week for 10 weeks. Up to 0.05 mg of interferon-gamma was injected weekly.

THIRD LINE THERAPIES

■ Radiation	B
■ Laser surgery	C
■ Cryosurgery	B
■ Imiquimod	C
■ Intralesional 5-FU	B
■ Topical retinoic acid	B
■ Intralesional bleomycin	B
■ Pulsed light and heat energy device	E
■ Verapamil	B
■ Surgery	C

Treatment of earlobe keloids using the cobalt 60 tele-therapy unit. Malaker K, Zaidi, M, Franka MR. Ann Plast Surg 2003;52:602–4.

Forty seven patients were treated with postoperative Telecobalt external beam radiation and 87.2% of patients had no recurrence at the 6-month follow-up visit.

Treatment of keloids by surgical excision and immediate postoperative single-fraction radiotherapy. Ragoowansi R, Cornes PG, Moss AL, Glees JP. Plast Reconstr Surg 2003;111:1853–9.

In a retrospective study of 80 patients with postoperative single-fraction radiotherapy of 60 kV and 100 kV photon irradiation on the skin and ear respectively, the patients experienced treatment failures at 1 year of six of 64 patients and at 5 years of four of 54 patients.

The treatment of 783 keloid scars by iridium 192 interstitial irradiation after surgical excision. Escarmant P, Zimmermann S, Amar A, et al. Int J Radiat Oncol Biol Phys 1993;26:245–51.

There was a recurrence rate of 21% in 783 keloids treated with follow-up of at least 1 year.

Superficial X-ray therapy in keloid management: a retrospective study of 24 cases and literature review. Norris JEC. Plast Reconstr Surg 1995;95:1051–6.

A retrospective study of superficial X-ray therapy of 24 excised keloids resulted in a recurrence rate of 53% in at least 24 months of follow-up.

Experience with the Nd:YAG laser in the treatment of keloidal scars. Sherman R, Rosenfeld H. Ann Plast Surg 1988;21:231–5.

Improvement was noted in 16 of 17 patients after laser therapy, but no significant follow-up was discussed.

Energy density and numbers of treatment affect response of keloidal and hypertrophic sternotomy scars to the 585-nm flashlamp-pumped pulsed-dye laser. Manuskiatti W, Fitzpatrick RE, Goldman MP. J Am Acad Dermatol 2001; 45:557–65.

Ten patients' keloids were divided into four sections and treated on three sections with 585 nm pulsed dye laser at energy densities of 3, 5, and 7 J/cm^2. Results showed no statistical significant difference in the thickness, erythema, and pliability.

Effect of the 585 nm flashlamp-pumped pulsed dye laser for the treatment of keloids. Paquet P, Hermanns JF, Pierard GE. Dermatol Surg 2001;27:171–4.

Eleven patients were treated with a 585 nm pulsed dye laser and results yielded only minimal effects on the erythema of the keloids.

Treatment of keloid sternotomy scars with 585 nm flashlamp-pumped pulsed-dye-laser. Alster TS, Williams CM. Lancet 1995;345:1198–200.

The 585 nm pulsed dye laser was used to treat 16 patients with sternotomy scars. There was a significant decrease in pruritus, erythema, and scar height in most patients. These results persisted for at least 6 months after treatment.

The effect of carbon dioxide laser surgery on the recurrence of keloids. Norris JEC. Plast Reconstr Surg 1991;87: 44–9.

In this retrospective study, 23 patients had adequate follow-up. One had no recurrence, nine required corticosteroids to suppress recurrence, and 13 were considered to be treatment failures.

Carbon dioxide laser excision of earlobe keloids: a prospective study and critical analysis of existing data. Stern JC, Lucente FE. Arch Otolaryngol Head Neck Surg 1989;115:1107–11.

Of the 23 keloids excised by laser, 17 recurred.

Treatment of keloids and hypertrophic scars with an argon laser. Hulsbergen Henning JP, Roskam Y, Van Gemert MJC. Lasers Surg Med 1986;6:72–5.

Of the 45 patients who participated, only three had over 50% improvement.

Modification of a device and its application for intralesional cryosurgery of old recalcitrant keloids. Zouboulis CC, Rosenberger AD, Forster T, et al. Arch Dermatol 2004;140:1293–4.

In a pilot open study, ten patients with recalcitrant keloids were treated with three to six sessions of intralesional cryosurgery and were followed up over 6 months. Results were 50–100% volume reduction in two patients,

50% volume reduction in five patients, no change in one patient, and progression in two patients.

Intralesional cryotherapy for enhancing the involution of hypertrophic scars and keloids. Har-Shai Y, Amar M, Sabo E. Plast Reconstr Surg 2003;111:1841–52.

Ten patients with 12 hypertrophic scars and keloids were treated with one session of intralesional cryosurgery treatment and there was a 51.4% scar volume reduction with no recurrence at the 18-month follow-up period.

Use of cryosurgery in the treatment of keloids. Rusciani L, Rossi G, Bono R. J Dermatol Surg Oncol 1993;19:529–34.

Sixty five lesions were treated and cryosurgery resulted in complete resolution with no recurrence in 73% of patients after 17–42 months of follow-up.

Outcomes of cryosurgery in keloids and hypertrophic scars. A prospective consecutive trial of case series. Zouboulis CC, Blume U, Buttner P, Orfanos CE. Arch Dermatol 1993;129:1146–51.

Of the 93 patients in the series, 55 had keloids and 38 had hypertrophic scars. Results were reported to be excellent in 32.3%, good in 29.0%, poor in 29.0%, and 9.7% had no response.

Pilot study of the effect of postoperative imiquimod 5% cream on the recurrence rate of excised keloids. Berman B, Kaufman J. J Am Acad Dermatol 2002;47:S209–11.

Thirteen keloids were treated with excision and imiquimod every night for 8 weeks. Ten patients with 11 keloids completed the 6-month study, and there were no recurrences.

Intralesional 5-fluorouracil as a treatment modality of keloids. Nanda S, Reddy BS. Dermatol Surg 2004;30:54–7.

In a prospective, randomized, uncontrolled trial 28 patients were treated with weekly injections of 5-FU for 12 weeks, and at the 24-week follow-up, 70% of the patients had an improvement in keloid size of more than 50%.

Treatment of inflamed hypertrophic scars using intralesional 5-FU. Fitzpatrick RE. Dermatol Surg 1999;25:224–32.

In a retrospective study of 1000 patients with hypertrophic scars and keloids over a 9-year period, the most effective regimen was found to be 0.1 mL of triamcinolone acetonide (10 mg/mL) and 0.9 mL 5-FU (50 mg/mL) injections up to three times a week.

The local treatment of hypertrophic scars and keloids with topical retinoic acid. Janssen de Limpens AMP. Br J Dermatol 1980;103:319–23.

There was a favorable result in 77–79% of the 28 lesions treated. This included a decrease in size or symptoms of scar.

Bleomycin in the treatment of keloids and hypertrophic scars by multiple needle punctures. Espana A, Solano T, Quintanilla E. Dermatol Surg 2001;27:23–7.

Bleomycin was given at a concentration of 1.5 IU/mL to 13 patients using the multiple-puncture method, and seven patients had complete flattening, five patients had highly significant flattening, and one patient had significant flattening.

Evidence levels **A** Double-blind study **B** Clinical trial ≥ 20 subjects **C** Clinical trial < 20 subjects **D** Series ≥ 5 subjects **E** Anecdotal case reports

Treatment of keloid with intralesional bleomycin. Bodokh I, Brun P. Ann Dermatol Venereol 1996;123:791–4.

Of 31 keloids treated with three to five infiltrates within a 1-month period, total regression occurred in 25.

Treatment of a mediastinoscopy-induced keloid with a pulsed light and heat energy device. Levenberg A. Cosmetic Dermatology 2004;17:445–7.

A case report of one patient treated with a non-laser light and heat energy flashlamp device receiving once a week treatments of 30 s intervals for 8 weeks at 5 J/cm^2 (sessions 1–4) and 9 J/cm^2 (sessions 5–8) resulting in the keloid becoming softer, flatter, and erythematous after the first treatment and decreasing in size from 2×0.5 cm to 1.4×0.2 cm.

Combination of surgery and intralesional verapamil injection in the treatment of the keloid. Copcu E, Sivrioglu N, Oztan Y. J Burn Care Rehabil 2004; 25:1–7.

Twenty two patients with keloids were treated with surgical excision and five treatments of verapamil 2.5 mg/mL (doses varied from 0.5 to 5 mL depending on the size of the keloid) over a 2-month period. Patients were evaluated and at the 2-year follow-up, two patients had keloids that had decreased in size from the original lesion, two patients had hypertrophic scars, four patients had pruritus, and one patient had a keloid on the donor site.

Additional studies have been performed using keloid fillet flaps (skin over the keloid was dissected and used as a flap).

Keratoacanthoma

Caroline M Owen, Nicholas R Telfer

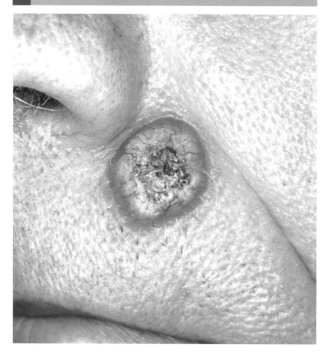

Keratoacanthoma (KA) is a distinctive tumor with characteristic histopathologic and clinical features. It classically presents as a rapidly proliferating, firm, dome-shaped, crateriform nodule. It shares many features of a squamous cell carcinoma (SCC), but is self-healing and can be considered a form of aborted malignancy. Although eventually self-limiting, its growth can be unpredictable and locally destructive, causing problems in management. Lesions are usually solitary and mainly affect sun-exposed sites in patients of middle age and older. Less commonly, lesions may be large (giant KA), progressive with central clearing (KA centrifugum), or multiple (e.g. multiple KA of Ferguson-Smith type, generalized eruptive KA of Grzybowski).

MANAGEMENT STRATEGY

Initial management is directed at making an accurate diagnosis of KA, in particular differentiating it from SCC. Although much research has been directed at the investigation of the differential cytokine profile or ultrastructure of KA and SCC, in practice the diagnosis of KA relies on the correlation between clinical and histopathologic criteria as follows.

A KA classically has three clinical stages:

- proliferative – early rapid growth to form a crateriform nodule;
- fully developed – no growth;
- involutional – the lesion regresses, usually within 4–8 months.

The five most relevant histopathologic criteria when differentiating KA from SCC have been shown to be:

- epithelial lip (in favor of KA);
- sharp outline between tumor and stroma (in favor of KA);

- ulceration (in favor of SCC);
- numerous mitoses (in favor of SCC);
- marked pleomorphism (in favor of SCC).

Accurate assessment of these histopathologic criteria relies upon the provision of an adequate histologic specimen. This should be deep enough to include subcutaneous fat, either by total excision or by transverse biopsy through the center of the lesion.

Once the diagnosis of KA has been established, the aims of treatment are to hasten resolution, prevent destruction of important structures, prevent recurrence, and obtain as favorable a cosmetic outcome as possible. Management therefore depends upon the type of KA, its site, its rate of growth, and whether or not it has previously been treated.

In general, *excision* is the treatment of choice for a small solitary KA because this will remove the lesion, provide an adequate specimen for histologic examination, and generally results in a good cosmetic result. An alternative to this is *transverse biopsy* to provide an adequate histologic specimen followed by *curettage or blunt dissection* of the residual lesion. Recently *topical imiquimod* and *topical 5-fluorouracil* have been used with success. *Argon laser ablation* has also been shown to be an effective treatment of small KA.

If one is sure of the diagnosis and the lesion has been documented as being static or already starting to involute then observation is an option. Obviously any concern that the lesion is not following an involutional pattern makes treatment mandatory.

Large, proliferating lesions for which surgical management is not possible or is likely to result in a poor cosmetic outcome can be treated with *radiotherapy* or *intralesional therapy* (*methotrexate, 5-fluorouracil, interferon-alfa-2a, bleomycin, triamcinolone*).

Multiple KAs have been successfully treated with *oral retinoids* and *intralesional 5-fluorouracil*. Recurrent KA has been shown to respond well to *radiotherapy*, but oral retinoids and *systemic methotrexate* have also been used with success. The level of evidence in the literature for the treatment of KA is poor, consisting mainly of small case series. Without a control group it is very difficult to be sure of the success of any intervention, particularly with a lesion that has a natural history of spontaneous involution.

SPECIFIC INVESTIGATIONS

- Skin biopsy

Keratoacanthoma: a clinico-pathologic enigma. Schwartz RA. Dermatol Surg 2004;30:326–33.

A review of KA with emphasis on clinical and histologic features and a broad overview of management options.

Differentiating squamous cell carcinoma from keratoacanthoma using histopathological criteria. Is it possible? A study of 296 cases. Cribier B, Asch P, Grosshans E. Dermatology 1999;199:208–12.

A study evaluating the reliability of histologic criteria used to distinguish between KAs and SCCs.

Keratoacanthoma observed. Griffiths RW. Br J Plast Surg 2004;57:485–501.

An interesting paper in which 14 patients with a clinical diagnosis of KA were observed with serial photographs every 2 weeks, Mean time to resolution was 27 weeks (range

12–64 weeks). No recurrences occurred during mean follow-up of 3 years 5 months (range from 9 months to 8 years) and all scars were acceptable to the patients. Four further patients were excluded from observational follow-up when there was concern about the growth pattern of the lesions.

Management of small, solitary keratoacanthoma

FIRST LINE THERAPIES

■ Curettage	C
■ Excision	D

Evaluation of curettage and electrodesiccation in the treatment of keratoacanthoma. Nedwich JA. Australas J Dermatol 1991;32:137–41.

Retrospective case series of 111 KAs in 106 patients treated with curettage and electrodesiccation. There were four recurrences after a mean follow-up of 28.5 months.

Treatment of keratoacanthomas with curettage. Reymann F. Dermatologica 1977;155:90–6.

A case series of 47 non-biopsy-proven KAs treated with curettage; there was recurrence in one case during follow-up ranging from 4 months to 5 years (average 32 months).

Keratoacanthomas treated with Mohs' micrographic surgery (chemosurgery). A review of forty-three cases. Larson PO. J Am Acad Dermatol 1987;16:1040–4.

A case series of 43 biopsy-proven KAs in 42 patients treated with Mohs micrographic surgery. There was one recurrence during a 6–24-month follow-up period.

SECOND LINE THERAPIES

■ Topical imiquimod	D
■ Topical 5-fluorouracil	E
■ Argon laser	D

Topical treatment with imiquimod may induce regression of facial keratoacanthoma. Dendorfer M, Oppel T, Wollenberg A, Prinz JC. Eur J Dermatol 2003;13:80–2

Four patients with facial KA (biopsy proven in three) were treated with imiquimod cream 5% on alternate days for 4–12 weeks. Complete regression was seen in all four patients (within 4–6 weeks in three of them). No recurrences occurred during the follow-up of 4–6 months.

Spontaneous regression of keratoacanthoma can be promoted by topical treatment with imiquimod cream. Di Lernia V, Ricci C, Albertini G. J Eur Acad Dermatol Venereol 2004;18:626–9.

Two biopsy-proven facial KAs were treated with imiquimod cream 5% three times per week for one patient and five times per week for the other for 8 weeks. Both resolved completely and remained clear after 1 year of follow-up. Both needed a 1-week rest period off treatment because of erythema, erosion, and crusting at the treatment site.

Topical 5-fluorouracil as primary therapy for keratoacanthoma. Grey RJ, Meland NB. Ann Plast Surg 2000;44:82–5.

Two clinically diagnosed KAs in two patients were treated with 5-fluorouracil 5% once daily for 4 weeks in one and 8 weeks in the other. A rapid response was noted within 3 weeks.

Argon laser treatment of small keratoacanthomas in difficult locations. Neumann RA, Knobler RM. Pharmacol Ther 1990;29:733–6.

Case series of 17 small (<10 mm) histologically proven solitary KAs on the head and neck. These were treated once with argon laser. There was resolution with no scarring in 65% and slight scarring in 35%. There were no recurrences after 2 years of follow-up.

Management of large, rapidly proliferating keratoacanthoma

FIRST LINE THERAPIES

■ Radiotherapy	D
■ Intralesional 5-fluorouracil	D
■ Intralesional methotrexate	D

Treatment of aggressive keratoacanthomas by radiotherapy. Donahue B, Cooper JS, Rush S. J Am Acad Dermatol 1990;23:489–93.

Case series of 29 KAs (eight recurrent after attempted surgical ablation) in 18 patients. Treated with radiotherapy in doses ranging from 3500 cGy in 15 fractions to 5600 cGy in 28 fractions. All lesions regressed completely. Good cosmetic results were reported in 14 patients.

Treatment of keratoacanthomas with intralesional fluorouracil. Odom RB, Goette DK. Arch Dermatol 1978;114:1779–83.

Case series of 14 patients with 26 KAs (12 single and rapidly growing, 14 multiple, none biopsy-proven). Two to five doses of 0.2–0.5 mL 5-fluorouracil 50 mg/mL were injected intralesionally at weekly intervals. Resolution took place with excellent cosmetic results in all but one case. There were no recurrences during a follow-up period of 3–17 months.

Large keratoacanthomas in difficult locations treated with intralesional 5-fluorouracil. Parker CM, Hanke CW. J Am Acad Dermatol 1986;14:770–7.

Case series of five large, facial, biopsy-proven KAs. Two to six intralesional injections of 1–3 mL of 50 mg/mL 5-fluorouracil were given at 1–4-week intervals. Resolution was reported in all five, with no recurrence during follow-up of 18–43 months, but the authors describe a further KA (that had been present for 16 weeks and static for 10) that did not respond, suggesting that intralesional therapy is most appropriate for KAs in the proliferative growth phase.

Treatment of keratoacanthomas with intralesional methotrexate. Melton JL, Nelson BR, Stogh DB, et al. J Am Acad Dermatol 1991;23:1017–23.

Case series of nine solitary KAs, biopsy proven in six. One or two intralesional injections of 0.4–1.5 mL methotrexate (12.5 or 25 mg/mL) resulted in complete resolution with minimal scarring.

Intralesional methotrexate in solitary keratoacanthoma. Cuesta-Romero C, de Grado-Pena J. Arch Dermatol 1998;134:513–14.

Case series of six solitary KAs (four biopsy proven). Between one and four intralesional injections of 0.5–1 mL methotrexate (25 mg/mL) resulted in complete regression with no recurrence during a follow-up period of 10–20 months.

SECOND LINE THERAPIES

■ Intralesional interferon-alfa-2a	D
■ Intralesional bleomycin	D
■ Intralesional triamcinolone	D

Large keratoacanthomas treated with intralesional interferon alfa-2a. Grob JJ, Suzini F, Richard MA, et al. J Am Acad Dermatol 1993;29:237–41.

Case series of six cases of KAs over 2 cm in diameter still in the proliferative growth phase, four of which were biopsy proven. Intralesional interferon-alfa-2a was given at a dose of 3×2–6 million units per week for 3–7 weeks. There was total resolution in five cases, the cosmetic results being excellent in four; surgical scar revision was required in one. There was no recurrence during a follow-up period of 6 months to 3 years.

Treatment of keratoacanthoma with intralesional bleomycin. Sayama S, Tagami H. Br J Dermatol 1983;109:449–52.

Case series of six biopsy-proven KAs. Treatment with one or two injections of 0.2–0.4 mg intralesional bleomycin (1 mg/mL diluted with an equal amount of 0.5% lidocaine) resulted in resolution of the lesion in 2–6 weeks.

Intradermal triamcinolone therapy of keratoacanthomas. McNairy DJ. Arch Dermatol 1964;89:136–40.

Case series of solitary and multiple KAs in ten patients. Sublesional and intralesional injection of triamcinolone 25 mg/mL at 1- or 2-week intervals resulted in involution after 8–78 days.

Management of multiple keratoacanthomas

FIRST LINE THERAPIES

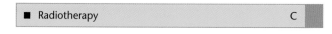

■ Oral etretinate	E
■ Oral isotretinoin	E
■ Intralesional fluorouracil	E

Multiple persistent keratoacanthomas: treatment with oral etretinate. Benoldi D, Alinovi A. J Am Acad Dermatol 1984;10:1035–8.

Two cases of multiple KAs of the Ferguson-Smith type were treated with oral etretinate 1 mg/kg daily, reducing after 8 weeks to a maintenance dose of 0.5–0.75 mg/kg daily. Total clearance was experienced by one patient with follow-up of 1 year; there was partial clearance in the second patient, with follow-up of 6 months.

Etretinate is no longer available. It is anticipated, although not yet proven, that acitretin would have a similar result.

Treatment of multiple keratoacanthomas with oral isotretinoin. Shaw JC, White CR. J Am Acad Dermatol 1986;15:1079–82.

Report of one patient with multiple KAs who was treated with isotretinoin (induction dose 1.5 mg/kg daily). This treatment cleared existing lesions and appeared to prevent recurrences.

Treatment of multiple keratoacanthomas with intralesional fluorouracil. Eubanks SW, Gentry RH, Patterson JW, May DL. J Am Acad Dermatol 1982;7:126–9.

Report of one patient with multiple KAs of the Ferguson-Smith type successfully treated with intralesional 5-fluorouracil.

Management of recurrent keratoacanthoma

FIRST LINE THERAPIES

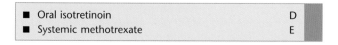

■ Radiotherapy	C

Radiation therapy of giant aggressive keratoacanthomas. Goldschmidt H, Sherwin WK. Arch Dermatol 1993;129:1162–5.

Retrospective case series of 16 large or rapidly growing KAs, 14 of which were recurrent following surgery. They were treated five times weekly with individual doses ranging from 2.5 to 5 Gy (total dose 45–60 Gy). All tumors resolved with satisfactory cosmetic results.

SECOND LINE THERAPIES

■ Oral isotretinoin	D
■ Systemic methotrexate	E

Treatment of solitary keratoacanthomas with oral isotretinoin. Goldberg LH, Rosen T, Becker J, Knauss A. J Am Acad Dermatol 1990;23:934–6.

Case series of 12 biopsy-proven solitary KAs, six primary, six recurrent. Treatment with oral isotretinoin 0.5–1 mg/kg resulted in resolution in nine (four primary, five recurrent) of the 12 cases with a good cosmetic result. None of these lesions recurred during an average follow-up of 12 months.

Keratoacanthomas treated with methotrexate. Kestel JL Jr, Blair DS. Arch Dermatol 1973;108:723–4.

Reports of two biopsy-proven, recurrent KAs. Weekly intramuscular injections of 25 mg methotrexate for either 5 or 8 weeks resulted in complete regression.

Evidence levels   A Double-blind study   **B** Clinical trial ≥ 20 subjects   **C** Clinical trial < 20 subjects   **D** Series ≥ 5 subjects   **E** Anecdotal case reports

Keratosis pilaris and variants

Arash Akhavan, Donald Rudikoff

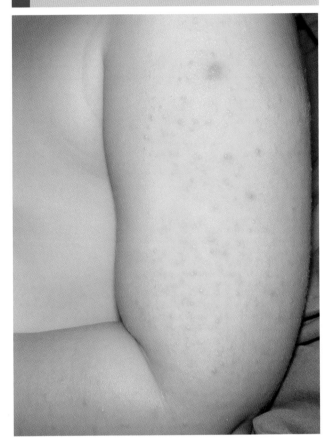

Keratosis pilaris is a common inherited disorder of unknown etiology characterized by hyperkeratosis and keratinous plugging of follicular orifices. It usually becomes apparent during childhood as follicular acuminate papules on the outer aspect of the arms, upper back, anterior surface of the thighs, and, less commonly, on the face and trunk. There is sometimes perifollicular erythema (keratosis pilaris rubra). Variants of keratosis pilaris are described under a host of confusing names, including keratosis pilaris atrophicans (ulerythema ophryogenes), keratosis follicularis spinulosa decalvans (KFSD), and atrophoderma vermiculatum; these are also addressed in this chapter.

MANAGEMENT STRATEGY

Keratosis pilaris is usually asymptomatic and often does not require treatment. This is especially relevant in young children, who are mostly unaware of and unbothered by the condition. Teenagers and adults commonly complain of skin roughness or unsightly cosmetic appearance. Those with extensive or symptomatic involvement often desire treatment, though, even without therapy, the condition often becomes less prominent with increasing age.

Initial treatment involves measures to *decrease excessive skin dryness* that is often worse during winter months. Harsh soaps are to be avoided and bathing should be followed by application of an emollient to damp skin. An abrasive polyester sponge such as Buf-Puf® can be helpful in removing follicular plugs. *Keratolytic agents* such as lactic acid, ammonium lactate, salicylic acid, and urea are the mainstays of treatment used to soften the keratotic papules. Salicylic acid 2% in 20% urea cream or salicylic acid 6% in propylene glycol combines the properties of an emollient with a keratolytic agent. Daily application of one of these compounds by gentle massage with a polyester sponge after showering is particularly helpful. Once adequate relief of symptoms has been achieved, maintenance therapy of weekly or twice-weekly application of 20% urea cream (Carmol 20®) is recommended.

Topical retinoids can be helpful in some cases but can be irritating and expensive if large areas are treated. Lower concentrations of topical tretinoin such as 0.025% cream or 0.01% gel can be used at first. If there is no significant irritation, higher-concentration preparations can be used. Tazarotene 0.05% cream has also been shown to decrease the pruritus, erythema, and roughness of keratosis pilaris in a recent placebo-controlled trial.

If a significant inflammatory component is present, the inflammation can be treated with a *medium potency topical corticosteroid* in an emollient base. If folliculitis is present, a therapeutic trial of *dicloxacillin* or *minocycline* should be given. Once inflammation has abated, corticosteroids are discontinued and keratolytics are introduced. *Oral antihistamines* may have limited value in relieving mild pruritus that sometimes accompanies keratosis pilaris. A 3-month course of oral vitamin A, 50 000 units three times a day, has been advocated for some patients. *Oral isotretinoin* has been helpful in some patients with ulerythema ophryogenes and atrophoderma vermiculatum.

Cutaneous laser therapy has been shown to be helpful treatment for several variants of keratosis pilaris. Pulsed tunable dye laser (PDL) treatment has recently been shown to be a safe and effective treatment for the erythema associated with keratosis pilaris atrophicans. Potassium titanyl phosphate (KTP) laser has been found to be effective in the clearance of keratotic papules and reduction of erythema of keratosis pilaris rubra lesions. Keratosis pilaris spinulosa decalvans has been treated with laser-assisted hair removal using a normal mode, non-Q-switched, high-energy, pulsed ruby laser at fluences of 19–21 J/cm^2 at 6-week intervals. This mode of treatment has been effective in producing persistent reductions of inflammation in this keratosis pilaris variant, albeit at the expense of permanent hair loss in treated areas.

SPECIFIC INVESTIGATIONS

- Serum testosterone levels (in obese females)
- Complete physical examination
- Ophthalmologic examination

Is keratosis pilaris another androgen-dependent dermatosis? Barth JH, Wojnarowska F, Dawber RPR. Clin Exp Dermatol 1988;13:240–1.

In this study of serum testosterone level and body mass index in 78 premenopausal women with hirsutism, hyperandrogenism in the presence of obesity was associated with an increased prevalence and severity of keratosis pilaris.

Keratosis pilaris: skin marker of Hodgkin's disease?
Thomsen K, Nyfors A. Arch Dermatol 1973;107:629–30.

Case report of a patient who suddenly developed keratosis pilaris and was diagnosed with Hodgkin's disease 6 months later. Successful chemotherapy of the Hodgkin's disease was followed by clearance of the skin lesions.

This case may be analogous to cases of acquired ichthyosis reported in association with Hodgkin's disease. On the other hand, keratosis pilaris is very prevalent and can remit spontaneously, so linkage with other conditions and purported responses to therapy of those conditions should be interpreted with care.

Keratosis pilaris atrophicans. One heterogeneous disease or a symptom in different clinical entities? Oranje AP, van Osch LD, Oosterwijk JC. Arch Dermatol 1994;130: 500–2.

Patients with keratosis pilaris atrophicans are reported to have increased incidence of ocular abnormalities, including photophobia, corneal deposits, juvenile cataracts, and corneal dystrophy.

This cogent review clarifies the confusing nosology of keratosis pilaris variants.

FIRST LINE THERAPIES

■ Sodium lactate and urea cream	B
■ Polyester sponge	D
■ Salicylic acid in urea	D
■ Topical corticosteroids	D

Evaluation of a sodium lactate and urea crème to ameliorate keratosis pilaris [Abstract]. Weber TM, Kowcz A, Rizer R. J Am Acad Dermatol 2004;50(suppl 1):47.

A formulation containing sodium lactate and urea was tested on 32 subjects with mild to severe keratosis pilaris. The authors reported progressive, statistically significant improvements in overall condition, skin roughness, and skin tone, at 3, 6, and 12 weeks of use.

Polyester sponge adjunct in acne management. Diamant F. Clin Ther 1980;3:250–3.

Seven patients who used polyester sponges from three times per week to once daily for their keratosis pilaris improved after a mean treatment duration of 7.4 weeks.

Practical management of widespread, atypical keratosis pilaris. Novick NL. J Am Acad Dermatol 1984;11:305–6.

Thirty patients with widespread, atypical or psychologically troubling keratosis pilaris were treated according to a protocol that included prevention of excessive skin drying, application of salicylic acid 2–3% in 20% urea cream using a polyester sponge, and use of emollient-based topical corticosteroids if a prominent inflammatory component was present. All patients reported satisfaction with cosmetic results. Clearing of lesions was noted in 75–100% of cases, with elimination of most lesions achieved within 2–3 weeks of daily therapy.

Keratosis pilaris decalvans non-atrophicans. Drago F, Maietta G, Parodi A, Rebora A. Clin Exp Dermatol 1993;18: 45–6.

Case report of a patient with keratosis pilaris decalvans non-atrophicans with follicular keratotic papules on the limbs and trunk accompanied by loss of body hair. The patient was successfully treated over the course of 3 months with topical emollients and multivitamins. The keratosis pilaris completely disappeared, leaving no scars, and there was complete regrowth of hair.

Traditional methods of treating uncomplicated keratosis pilaris seem to be effective in treating cases of keratosis pilaris decalvans non-atrophicans.

SECOND LINE THERAPIES

■ Topical tazarotene	A
■ Topical tretinoin	D
■ Isotretinoin	E

Tazarotene 0.05% cream for the treatment of keratosis pilaris [Abstract]. Bogle MA, Ali A, Bartel H. J Am Acad Dermatol 2004;50(suppl 1):39.

A randomized, placebo-controlled, double-blind prospective study of tazarotene 0.05% cream for the treatment of keratosis pilaris on the posterior arms of 33 patients reportedly resulted in statistically significant improvement in pruritus, erythema, and roughness of keratosis pilaris lesions.

Natural history of keratosis pilaris. Poskitt L, Wilkinson JD. Br J Dermatol 1994;130:711–13.

This retrospective questionnaire study of 49 patients with keratosis pilaris yielded 14 patients who had benefited from a variety of treatments for keratosis pilaris. Of these patients, eight reported therapy with topical tretinoin cream to be helpful.

Clinical findings, cutaneous pathology, and response to therapy in 21 patients with keratosis pilaris atrophicans. Baden HP, Byers HR. Arch Dermatol 1994;130:469–75.

Twenty-one patients with keratosis pilaris atrophicans were treated with various agents and combinations of agents, including keratolytics, antibiotics, topical corticosteroids, and retinoids, all with very limited response. Treatment of four patients with isotretinoin 1 mg/kg resulted in little or no improvement in three patients and exacerbation of the condition in one patient.

A case of atrophoderma vermiculatum responding to isotretinoin. Weightman W. Clin Exp Dermatol 1998;23: 89–91.

Atrophoderma vermiculatum is a rare variant of keratosis pilaris that results in reticular or honeycomb scarring of the face. In this case report, isotretinoin induced a remission in the inflammatory component of the disease, which was maintained after cessation of treatment.

In severe cases of atrophoderma vermiculatum with significant scarring, a trial of isotretinoin therapy is worthwhile to halt progression of the disease.

Atrophoderma vermiculatum. Case reports and review. Frosch PJ, Brumage MR, Schuster-Pavlovic C, Bersch A. J Am Acad Dermatol 1988;18:538–42.

In this variant of keratosis pilaris, a symmetric worm-eaten or reticular atrophy may result. Dermabrasion may be used to reduce the eventual scarring.

Evidence levels **A** Double-blind study **B** Clinical trial ≥ 20 subjects **C** Clinical trial < 20 subjects **D** Series ≥ 5 subjects **E** Anecdotal case reports

A case of ulerythema ophryogenes responding to isotretinoin. Layton AM, Cunliffe WJ. Br J Dermatol 1993; 129:645–6.

Ulerythema ophryogenes, a variant of keratosis pilaris, begins in the eyebrows as small, discrete, horny, pinhead-sized papules at the hair follicle orifices that spread to the forehead and scalp. Atrophy and alopecia of the eyebrows and scalp may result. There is a variable response to isotretinoin.

THIRD LINE THERAPIES

■ Tetracyclines: oxytetracycline, minocycline	E
■ Long-pulse, non-Q-switched, ruby laser (for keratosis pilaris spinulosa decalvans)	E
■ Pulsed tunable dye laser (for keratosis pilaris atrophicans)	C
■ Potassium titanyl phosphate laser (for keratosis rubra pilaris)	E

Natural history of keratosis pilaris. Poskitt L, Wilkinson JD. Br J Dermatol 1994;130:711–3.

Two patients responding to a retrospective questionnaire stated that treatment with tetracyclines had 'dramatically' improved their keratosis pilaris. The authors warned that the questionnaire did not permit exclusion of possible coincidental acne in these patients and that their reported improvement may have been secondary to the known therapeutic effects of tetracycline on acne. However, tetracyclines are recognized anti-inflammatory agents and this may explain the improvements in keratosis pilaris that are sometimes noted with these agents.

Recalcitrant scarring follicular disorders treated by laser-assisted hair removal: a preliminary report. Chui CT, Berger TG, Price VH, Zachary CB. Dermatol Surg 1999;25:34–7.

A patient with keratosis pilaris spinulosa decalvans of the scalp complicated by recurrent secondary infection was treated with a variety of oral antibiotics and topical corticosteroids with limited success. The patient subsequently underwent five treatments with a normal mode, non-Q-switched, high-energy, pulsed ruby laser at fluences of 19–21 J/cm^2 at 6-week intervals. Eight months after initiation of treatment, significant reduction of inflammation occurred in treated areas, at the expense of a persistent diminution of hair growth.

This is a promising mode of therapy for patients with severe or symptomatic conditions who have not responded to other modes of therapy and are willing to accept permanent hair loss on treated areas as a side effect.

Treatment of keratosis pilaris atrophicans with the pulsed tunable dye laser. Clark SM, Mills CM, Lanigan SW. J Cutan Laser Ther 2000;2:151–6.

All facial areas involved with keratotis pilaris atrophicans in 12 patients were treated with the pulsed dye laser at 585 nm. Patients received two to eight treatments with the laser, with energies ranging from 6.0 to 7.5 J/cm^2. The authors report clinical improvement in all patients, with significant reduction in erythema scores. Significant improvement was not achieved in skin roughness. Treatment was generally well tolerated, with side effects mostly limited to local pain during treatment.

Keratosis rubra pilaris responding to potassium titanyl phosphate laser. Dawn G, Urcelay M, Patel M, Strong AMM. Br J Dermatol 2002;147:822–4.

A 15-year-old girl with erythematous papules on her cheeks, eyebrows, and chin was treated with a potassium titanyl phosphate laser (532 nm) with energy fluence of 12–14 J/cm^2 and pulse width of 510 ms. Both cheeks were treated seven times at 6–8-week intervals, resulting in good cosmetic clearance of keratotic papules and gradual reduction of erythema on her face. During a follow-up period, the patient required two treatments at 4-month intervals, and was happy with her cosmetic result.

Langerhans cell histiocytosis

Anthony Chu

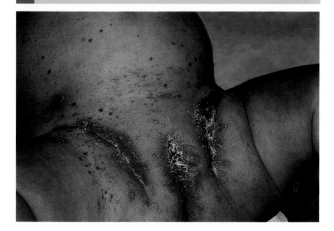

Langerhans cell histiocytosis (LCH) is defined as an accumulation or proliferation of cells bearing the surface phenotype of the epidermal Langerhans cell in various organs of the body, where tissue damage is caused by cytokine production. LCH may occur at any age, but most published data are on childhood disease. Treatment depends on the organs involved and the severity of the disease and is therefore tailored to the individual patient.

MANAGEMENT STRATEGY

Management strategy and prognosis depend on organ involvement. Organs most commonly involved include the bone, skin, lymph nodes, pituitary, liver, lungs, central nervous system (CNS), gastrointestinal tract, spleen, bone marrow, and endocrine system. Patients are staged according to the organ involvement and evidence of organ damage. Organ dysfunction of key organs – liver, lungs, and bone marrow – carries the worst prognosis. Patients are staged as single-system disease (with bone involvement this is further stratified into mono-ostotic and polyostotic bone disease), multisystem disease, and multisystem disease with evidence of organ dysfunction. Although some patients with LCH may undergo spontaneous remission, the disease is unpredictable and many patients progress from single-system disease to multisystem disease. Given this fact, previous suggestions that LCH could be left untreated are now untenable. In single-system bone disease, curettage or *intralesional corticosteroid injections* may lead to resolution. Single-system skin disease may respond to local measures with *topical corticosteroids, topical nitrogen mustard, or psoralen with UVA (PUVA)*. Single-system lung disease may respond to prednisolone at 2 mg/kg daily. In single-system disease that does not respond to these measures, single-system lymph node disease, and multisystem disease without organ dysfunction, systemic treatment with *azathioprine* (2 mg/kg daily) with or without low-dose weekly *methotrexate* (5–10 mg per week) may lead to resolution. In recalcitrant disease or in disease that is multisystem with evidence of organ dysfunction, treatment will depend on the age of the patient. Trials have demonstrated that in pediatric patients, *prednisolone with vinblastine* is the treatment of choice. In adult patients, prednisolone is less effective, other than in lung disease; additionally, patients are very sensitive to the side effect of the drug. In adult patients the responses to vinblastine are poorer and there are more side effects such as peripheral neuropathy. The first line treatment of choice in adult patients is *etoposide*. In pediatric studies the use of maintenance therapy has been shown to reduce the overall morbidity of the disease. Adults often have a more chronic and relapsing course to their disease, and *maintenance therapy with azathioprine* for 1 year should be considered for all patients with multisystem disease. In both children and adults with multisystem disease and organ dysfunction, there remains a small group who do not respond to conventional therapy. In these patients, *2-chlorodeoxyadenosine (2-CDA)* has proven useful and in severe disease, *bone marrow transplantation* has been successful. A number of drugs have been used in various stages of the disease including *trimethoprim–sulfamethoxazole, thalidomide, interferon, retinoids* – but most are anecdotal case reports.

Prior to institution of therapy, a full investigation, as outlined below, must be completed. Long-term morbidity can be correlated to organ involvement or occurs as a direct consequence of treatment. Such morbidities include skeletal deformities, risk of secondary malignancy, endocrine dysfunction, and infertility, particularly with the use of alkylating agents and radiotherapy.

SPECIFIC INVESTIGATIONS

Routine investigations
- Biopsy of organ involved for routine histology with staining for S100 and CD1a or electromicroscopy for Birbeck granules
- Complete and differential blood count
- Erythrocyte sedimentation rate (ESR)
- Liver function tests
- C-reactive protein (CRP)
- Skeletal survey
- Chest radiography

Indicated tests
- CT of the chest if an adult patient who smokes or a child with chest signs or symptoms
- Bronchioalveolar lavage for CD1a+ cells or open lung biopsy if evidence of lung involvement
- Pulmonary function tests in patients with lung disease
- MRI of the brain if skull involvement or localizing CNS signs
- Plasma and urinary osmolality, going on to water deprivation test, if history of polyuria and polydipsia
- CT of the brain and pituitary fossa if evidence of diabetes insipidus
- Full hormone screen if diabetes insipidus is present
- Bone marrow biopsy if there are hematological abnormalities
- Liver CT and biopsy if there is abnormal liver function
- Multiple bowel biopsies if there is evidence of malabsorption or failure to thrive in an infant
- Panorex if gum involvement

Specialised test
- Radioactive CD1a scan

Evidence levels   **A** Double-blind study   **B** Clinical trial ≥ 20 subjects   **C** Clinical trial < 20 subjects   **D** Series ≥ 5 subjects   **E** Anecdotal case reports

Histiocytosis syndromes in children: approach to the clinical and laboratory evaluation of children with Langerhans cell histiocytosis. Broadbent V, Gadner H, Komp DM, Ladisch S. Med Pediatr Oncol 1989;17:492–5.

Multiple organ systems may be involved in patients with LCH. Therefore, the following studies are recommended for all patients at diagnosis: a complete blood count with white blood cell differential, liver function tests, coagulation times (prothrombin time and partial thromboplastin time), chest radiograph, and radiographic skeletal survey (more sensitive than a radionuclide bone scan for detecting bone lesions). A measurement of urine osmolality after overnight water deprivation should also be obtained. Further evaluations, such as pulmonary function tests or brain MRI, should be tailored to patients based on specific presenting signs and symptoms.

A definitive diagnosis can be made by biopsy and identification of Langerhans cells that express CD1a by immunohistochemistry and the finding of Birbeck granules by electron microscopy.

FIRST LINE THERAPIES

Single-system skin disease

■ Topical nitrogen mustard	C
■ PUVA	E

Topical nitrogen mustard: an effective treatment for cutaneous Langerhans cell histiocytosis. Sheehan MP, Atherton DJ, Broadbent V, Pritchard J. J Pediatr 1991;119: 317–21.

Sixteen children with multisystem LCH with severe skin involvement were treated with topical mechlorethamine hydrochloride with rapid clinical improvement. One child developed a contact allergy after use.

Long term follow up of topical mustine treatment for cutaneous Langerhans cell histiocytosis. Hoeger PH, Nanduri VR, Harper JI, et al. Arch Dis Child 2000;82:483–7.

Topical nitrogen mustard (0.02% mechlorethamine hydrochloride mustard) is safe and may eliminate the need for systemic therapy. Follow-up in this study was an average of 8.3 years.

Topical nitrogen mustard is the best studied and most effective topical therapy for cutaneous disease. Contact allergy and the risk of cutaneous carcinogenicity limit its use.

Satisfactory remission achieved by PUVA therapy in Langerhans cell histiocytosis in an elderly patient. Sakai H, Ibe M, Takaahashi H, et al. J Dermatol 1995;23:42–6.

Case report of a 74-year-old man with involvement of the skin and diabetes insipidus treated with topical PUVA for 5 weeks with complete clearing of skin lesions. The endocrinopathy persisted.

Multisystem disease

■ Vinblastine	A
■ Etoposide	B

A randomized trial of treatment for multisystem Langerhans' cell histiocytosis. Gadner H, Grois N, Arico M, et al. J Pediatr 2001;138:728–34.

This randomized controlled trial of 24 weeks of vinblastine (6 mg/m^2 intravenously weekly) or etoposide (150 mg/m^2 daily for 3 days every 3 weeks) and an initial dose of methylprednisolone (30 mg/kg daily for 3 days), recruited 143 untreated children with multisystem Langerhans cell histiocytosis. The two treatments were found to be equally effective with response rates of 58% for vinblastine and 69% for etoposide. Vinblastine is considered safer for use in children.

Etoposide in recurrent childhood Langerhans cell histiocytosis: an Italian cooperative study. Ceci A, De Terlizzi M, Colella R, et al. Cancer 1988;62:2528–31.

Twelve of 18 patients with recurrent LCH had a complete remission after treatment with etoposide.

Treatment of adult Langerhans cell histiocytosis with etoposide. Tsele E, Thomas DM, Chu AC. J Am Acad Dermatol 1992;27:61–4.

Three of three adult patients had a complete response to three or four cycles of etoposide monotherapy.

Langerhans cell histiocytosis in childhood: results from the Italian Cooperative AIEOP-CNR-H.X. '83 study. Ceci A, de Terlizzi M, Colella R, et al. Med Pediatr Oncol 1993;21: 259–64.

Monotherapy with either vinblastine or etoposide is an effective treatment in patients without organ dysfunction.

Etoposide has been consistently shown to be effective in multifocal LCH. However, the small risk of secondary leukemia following treatment in children with etoposide limits its use to the most high-risk pediatric patients.

SECOND LINE THERAPIES

■ Prednisone	B
■ Methotrexate	B
■ 6-mercaptopurine	B
■ 2-CDA	C

Oral methotrexate and alternate-day prednisone for low-risk Langerhans cell histiocytosis. Womer RB, Anunciato KR, Chehrenama M. Med Pediatr Oncol 1995;25:70–3.

Low-risk patients may be successfully treated with prednisone 40 mg/m^2 daily on alternate days and weekly methotrexate 20 mg/m^2. Toxicity is minimal, and recurrences may be treated with the same regimen.

Treatment strategy for disseminated Langerhans cell histiocytosis. Gadner H, Heitger A, Grois N, et al. Med Pediatr Oncol 1994;23:72–80.

One hundred and six patients with disseminated LCH were divided into three groups: group A (multifocal bone disease); group B (soft tissue disease without organ dysfunction); group C (patients with organ dysfunction). All patients received 6 weeks of etoposide, vinblastine, and prednisone, followed by continuation therapy with 1 year of 6-mercaptopurine, vinblastine, and prednisone. Patients in group B also received etoposide during continuation therapy, while those in group C received both etoposide and methotrexate. A complete response was seen in 89% of group A, 91% of group B, and 67% of group C patients.

This study treated patients with 1 year of 'maintenance' chemotherapy, which has not been shown to be superior to the use of intermittent treatment for disease exacerbations.

2-Chlorodeoxyadenosine therapy for disseminated Langerhans cell histiocytosis. Pardanani A, Phyliky RL, Li CY, Tefferi A. Mayo Clin Proc 2003;78:301–6.

Five patients with multisystem LCH were treated with 2-CDA as front line therapy in one patient and as salvage therapy in the remaining four. Three patients achieved complete response and two a partial response.

This confirms the efficacy of 2-CDA in LCH, particularly in patients who have failed to respond on other forms of treatment.

Efficacy of continuous infusion 2-CDA (Cladribine) in pediatric patients with Langerhans cell histiocytosis. Stine KC, Saylors RL, Saccente S, et al. Pediatr Blood Cancer 2004;43:81–4.

Ten children with multiple reactivation of LCH or high-risk disease were treated with 2-CDA. All ten had clinical responses. Seven patients remained disease free for a median of 50 months of follow-up. Three patients needed further drug therapy, but are clinically in remission.

A further study showing the safety and efficacy of this drug in difficult, relapsing or severe LCH.

Development of acute lymphoblastic leukemia in a child after treatment of Langerhans cell histiocytosis: report of one case. Wu JH, Lu MY, Jou ST, Lin DT. Acta Paediatr Taiwan 1999;40:441–2.

The authors report a case of LCH, a localized osteolytic lesion over the metaphysis of the left femur, which was treated with local curettage and chemotherapy with vincristine, prednisone, and 6-mercaptopurine for 8 months. Six years later, the patient had acute lymphoblastic leukemia (ALL).

In their review, only five cases of LCH, including this report, have preceded ALL. The possible association, a reactive process, or a therapy-related process, between LCH and acute leukemia is still unclear at present, and worthy of further study.

THIRD LINE THERAPIES

■ Cytosine arabinoside	C
■ Cyclosporine (ciclosporin)	C
■ Interferon-alfa	D
■ Bone marrow transplantation	D
■ Thalidomide	D
■ 2-deoxycoformycin	E
■ Interleukin-2	E
■ Isotretinoin	E
■ Trimethoprim–sulfamethoxazole	D
■ Radiotherapy	B

Cytosine-arabinoside, vincristine, and prednisolone in the treatment of children with disseminated Langerhans cell histiocytosis with organ dysfunction: experience at a single institution. Egeler RM, de Kraker J, Voute PA. Med Pediatr Oncol 1993;21:265–70.

This combination led to complete remission in 63% of patients with organ dysfunction, and 80% of those without organ dysfunction.

This combination avoids the risk of secondary malignancies associated with etoposide.

Results of treatment of 127 patients with systemic histiocytosis (Letterer–Siwe syndrome, Schüller–Christian syndrome, and multifocal eosinophilic granuloma). Greenberger JS, Crocker AC, Vawter G, et al. Medicine 1981; 60:311–38.

Many patients discussed in this retrospective study achieved remission from local radiation therapy for bone and soft tissue lesions.

Chemotherapy is now generally preferred due to the slight risk of secondary malignancy and because LCH is often a generalized disease and local treatment is thus limited.

Effect of trimethoprim–sulphamethoxazole in Langerhans cell histiocytosis: preliminary observations. Tzortzatou-Stathopoulou F, Xaidara A, Mikraki V, et al. Med Pediatr Oncol 1995;25:74–8.

Patients with single-system disease responded well, while those with multisystem disease had a more limited response.

Cyclosporine A therapy for multisystem Langerhans cell histiocytosis. Minkov M, Grois N, Broadbent V, et al. Med Pediatr Oncol 1999;33:482–5.

Twenty six patients with refractory LCH were treated with cyclosporine alone or in combination with other agents; only one patient had a complete response, and three had a partial response.

Cyclosporine has been effective in only a small number of patients with LCH and remissions tend to be short.

Widespread skin-limited Langerhans cell histiocytosis: complete remission with interferon alpha. Kwong YL, Chan ACL, Chan TK. J Am Acad Dermatol 1997;36:628–9.

Interferon-alfa, either parenteral or intralesional, has been effective in some patients with LCH.

Allogeneic bone marrow transplantation in a patient with chemotherapy-resistant progressive histiocytosis X. Ringden O, Ahstrom L, Lonnqvist B, et al. N Engl J Med 1989;316:733–5.

Several other case reports have documented long-term remissions following bone marrow transplantation. This approach is generally reserved for patients with fulminant disease not responding to chemotherapy.

Successful treatment of adult Langerhans cell histiocytosis with thalidomide. Report of two cases and literature review. Thomas L, Ducros B, Secchi T, et al. Arch Dermatol 1993;129:1261–4.

Several reports document that thalidomide is an effective treatment for LCH, particularly in cutaneous disease. The response is often temporary and there is the risk of neuropathy with prolonged use.

Interleukin-2 therapy of Langerhans cell histiocytosis. Hirose M, Saito S, Yoshimoto T, Kuroda Y. Acta Pediatr 1995;84:1204–6.

Evidence levels   A Double-blind study   B Clinical trial ≥ 20 subjects   C Clinical trial < 20 subjects   D Series ≥ 5 subjects   E Anecdotal case reports

A patient with disseminated LCH achieved a transient remission with intravenous interleukin-2.

Langerhans cell histiocytosis: complete remission after oral isotretinoin therapy. Tsambaos D, Georgiou S, Kapranos N, et al. Acta Derm Venereol 1995;75:62–4.

A patient with single-system skin disease achieved a complete response to oral isotretinoin at 1.5 mg/kg daily for 9 months with no relapse at 5 years.

Successful treatment of two children with Langerhans' cell histiocytosis with 2'-deoxycoformycin. McCowage GB, Frush DP, Kurtzberg J. J Pediatr Hematol Oncol 1996;18: 154–8.

Two patients were treated with the drug at a dose of 4 mg/m^2 given by intravenous push weekly for 8 weeks then continuing every 2 weeks for greater than 21 and 16 months, respectively. Therapy was ongoing at the conclusion of the study. Boeth patients responded to treatment; one patient completely, while the other demonstrated a new, but stable femoral lesion while on treatment. Toxicity was limited to asymptomatic grade III–IV lymphopenia and abnormalities of lymphocyte mitogen responses.

Leg ulcers

Jonathan Kantor, David J Margolis

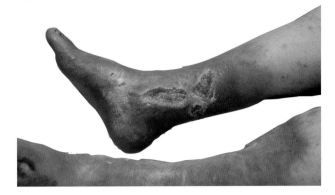

Leg ulcers are a common problem, and affect millions of individuals worldwide. Leg ulcers caused by infection, basal or squamous cell cancer, or pyoderma gangrenosum are discussed elsewhere.

MANAGEMENT STRATEGY

Accurate diagnosis is key in management of these wounds, and therapy is aimed at both mitigating any anatomic abnormalities and optimizing the wound healing environment. When approaching a leg ulcer, it is important to keep a broad differential diagnosis in mind, although the majority may be classified as venous leg ulcers, wounds due to arterial insufficiency, pressure ulcers, or diabetic neuropathic foot ulcers.

Venous ulcers are caused indirectly by ambulatory venous hypertension, most often due to the failure of the calf muscle pump system. Therefore, management hinges on *lower limb compression* and *moist wound dressings*. Elevation of the legs at night and, when necessary, weight reduction, are additional strategies to reduce the impact of venous insufficiency. Other approaches to management include the use of *topical recombinant growth factors*, *skin equivalents* (or cell-based therapies), and *oral pentoxifylline*. Most patients will improve with conservative management (compression and dressings), although compliance with compression therapy (e.g. compression stockings, compression bandages, etc.) may be a challenge. Most of these wounds heal in less than 6 months.

Patients with diabetes mellitus may develop lower extremity wounds. The diabetic neuropathic foot ulcer, which is likely the only wound that is really a direct complication of diabetes, stems from the lower extremity neuropathy that is associated with diabetes and then the unperceived repetitive trauma and pressure from walking leads to the ulcer. Management hinges on optimal control of diabetes, offloading of the affected limb, and moist wound dressings. Other treatment options include recombinant growth factors like recombinant human platelet-derived growth factor (rh-PDGF), and skin equivalents like Apligraf and Graftskin, which may be necessary in order to achieve optimal results. However, recurrent ulcerations and ensuing amputations are a real and serious problem.

SPECIFIC INVESTIGATIONS

- Hemoglobin A1c (glycosylated hemoglobin) measurement
- Clinical testing for neuropathy (e.g. monofilament testing)
- Lower extremity vascular studies, including ankle–brachial index (ABI)
- Skin biopsy may be considered

Effectiveness of the diabetic foot risk classification system of the International Working Group on the Diabetic Foot. Peters EJ, Lavery LA, and the International Working Group on the Diabetic Foot. Diabetes Care 2001;24:1442–7.

A diabetic foot risk classification system was evaluated in a prospective case–control study of 225 patients, which demonstrated that patients with worse glycemic control and neuropathy had a higher incidence of diabetic foot ulcers and amputations.

Effectiveness of Semmes-Weinstein monofilament examination for diabetic peripheral neuropathy screening. Kamei N, Yamane K, Nakanishi S, et al. J Diabetes Complications 2005;19:47–53.

Sensory evaluation using SWME 4.31/2 g at the great toe or the plantar aspect of the fifth metatarsal was the most useful diagnostic test for diabetic peripheral neuropathy, providing 60.0% sensitivity and 73.8% specificity.

Factors predicting lower extremity amputations in patients with type 1 or type 2 diabetes mellitus: a population-based 7-year follow-up study. Hamalainen H, Ronnemaa T, Halonen JP, Toikka T. J Intern Med 1999;246:97–103.

A total of 733 patients were studied and those who required amputations had a lower ABI than those not undergoing amputation.

Nonhealing leg ulcers: a manifestation of basal cell carcinoma. Phillips TJ, Salman SM, Rogers GS. J Am Acad Dermatol 1991;25:47–9.

Seven patients who presented with chronic lower extremity ulcers are discussed; while clinical hints may be present, ultimately biopsy is needed to demonstrate the presence of malignancy in a non-healing wound.

Risk factors associated with the failure of a venous ulcer to heal. Margolis DJ, Berlin JA, Strom BL. Arch Dermatol 1999;135:920–6.

This study of 260 patients demonstrated that several risk factors, identifiable at the initial visit, may be associated with the failure of a venous leg ulcer to heal within 24 weeks of therapy. These include: ulcer size, ulcer duration, ABI of less than 0.8, history of venous ligation or stripping, and history of hip or knee replacement surgery.

FIRST LINE THERAPIES

■ Compression for venous ulcers	A
■ Offloading for diabetic neuropathic ulcers	A

Compression for venous leg ulcers. Cullum N, Nelson EA, Fletcher AW, Sheldon TA. Cochrane Database Syst Rev 2001;(2):CD000265.

This systematic review included 22 trials using a number of different compression methods. Six trials compared compression with no compression, and all demonstrated a clear benefit of compression over no compression.

Off-loading the diabetic foot wound: a randomized clinical trial. Armstrong DG, Nguyen HC, Lavery LA, et al. Diabetes Care 2001;24:1019–22.

Sixty three patients were randomized to different off-loading strategies; those treated with a total contact cast (maximal offloading) had the highest proportion of healed wounds after 12 weeks (89.5% vs 61.4%, p = 0.026).

SECOND LINE THERAPIES

■ Topical rh-PDGF (becaplermin)	A
■ Skin equivalent dressings (Graftskin, Apligraf)	A
■ Oral pentoxifylline	A

Efficacy and safety of a topical gel formulation of recombinant human platelet-derived growth factor-BB (becaplermin) in patients with chronic neuropathic diabetic ulcers. A phase III randomized placebo-controlled double-blind study. Wieman TJ, Smiell JM, Su Y. Diabetes Care 1998;21:822–7.

This multicenter, double-blind, placebo-controlled trial enrolled 382 patients and demonstrated an increase in the proportion of wounds healed after 20 weeks of therapy from 35% with placebo to 50% with becaplermin gel (p = 0.007).

Rapid healing of venous ulcers and lack of clinical rejection with an allogeneic cultured human skin equivalent. Falanga V, Margolis D, Alvarez O, et al. Arch Dermatol 1998;134:293–300.

A randomized controlled trial of human skin equivalent (Graftskin, Apligraf) in 293 patients demonstrated an improvement in the proportion of patients with healed ulcers after 6 months from 49% to 63% (p = 0.02) over compression therapy alone.

The role of Apligraf in the treatment of venous leg ulcers. Dolynchuk K, Hull P, Guenther L, et al. Ostomy Wound Manage 1999;45:34–43.

A study of 240 patients demonstrated a higher proportion of patients healed after 24 weeks with Graftskin plus compression versus compression alone (57% vs 40%).

Pentoxifylline for treating venous leg ulcers. Jull AB, Waters J, Arroll B. Cochrane Database Syst Rev 2000;(2): CD001733.

Nine trials involving 572 patients were included in this Cochrane Review. The relative risk of healing with pentoxifylline versus placebo was 1.41 [95% CI (1.19, 1.66)]. A separate examination only of the trials that compared pentoxifylline plus compression with placebo plus compression also showed a benefit of pentoxifylline therapy with a relative risk of 1.30 [95% CI (1.10, 1.54)].

THIRD LINE THERAPIES

■ Intermittent pneumatic compression	C
■ Oral antibiotic therapy	E
■ Laser	E
■ Therapeutic ultrasound	E
■ Vitamins and minerals	E

Intermittent pneumatic compression for treating venous leg ulcers. Mani R, Vowden K, Nelson EA. Cochrane Database Syst Rev 2001;(4):CD001899.

This review evaluated four randomized controlled trials of intermittent pneumatic compression for the treatment of venous ulcers. Of these, a single trial of 45 patients found a significant benefit in the intermittent pneumatic compression plus standard compression group (versus standard compression alone), with a relative risk of healing of 11.4 [95% CI (1.6, 82)].

Antibiotic treatment for uncomplicated neuropathic forefoot ulcers in diabetes: a controlled trial. Chantelau E, Tanudjaja T, Altenhofer F, et al. Diabet Med 1996;13:156–9.

A total of 44 patients were randomized to either amoxicillin–clavulanic acid or placebo; there was no significant difference in the proportion of wounds healed after 20 days of therapy.

Laser therapy for venous leg ulcers. Flemming K, Cullum N. Cochrane Database Syst Rev 2000;(2):CD001182.

Four trials were included in this systematic review. No significant benefit of laser therapy was demonstrated when the trial results were pooled. One study of combined laser and infrared light suggested a modest benefit in patients with venous ulcers.

Therapeutic ultrasound for venous leg ulcers. Flemming K, Cullum N. Cochrane Database Syst Rev 2000;(4):CD001180.

This review included seven studies, and while some showed a trend toward benefit from ultrasound, there was no statistically significant benefit over sham treatment.

Does oral zinc aid the healing of chronic leg ulcers? A systematic literature review. Wilkinson EA, Hawke CI. Arch Dermatol 1999;134:1556–60.

This review included six trials of zinc therapy, none of which demonstrated a statistically significant benefit of zinc supplementation.

Leiomyoma

Tsui Chin Ling, Ian Coulson

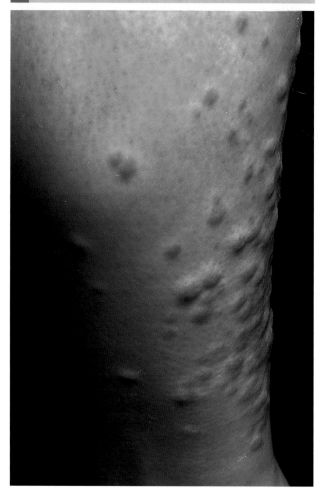

Leiomyomas are rare benign neoplasms of smooth muscle derived from the arrector pili (piloleiomyoma), the scrotal and labial dartos muscle or the smooth muscle of the nipple (dartoic myoma or genital leiomyoma), and vascular walls (angioleiomyoma). The commoner piloleiomyoma may be solitary or multiple, when multiple they may be inherited in an autosomal dominant fashion. Familial multiple leiomyomas may also be associated with uterine leiomyoma (Reed's syndrome). Pain due to muscle contraction may be provoked by cold, touch, or mechanical stimulation. Angioleiomyomas are less frequently symptomatic, and genital leiomyomas are asymptomatic.

MANAGEMENT STRATEGY

Symptomatic solitary lesions are best *excised*. Symptomatic multiple leiomyomas are a therapeutic challenge because of the large area they involve and a reported recurrence rate of 50% after excision. Selective excision of larger painful lesions may be considered. Other methods of therapy are aimed at inhibiting smooth muscle contraction by interfering with local tissue mediators such as norepinephrine (noradrenaline), epinephrine (adrenaline), and acetylcholine. There are reports of success with *doxazosin* (a selective α-1 blocker) 1–4 mg daily, *nifedipine* (a calcium channel

blocker) 10 mg three times daily, *phenoxybenzamine* (a nonselective α blocker) 10 mg twice daily, topical 9% *hyoscine hydrobromide* (an anticholinergic), *nitroglycerine* 0.8–1.6 mg, and simple *analgesics*. Intralesional *botulinum toxin* is an untried but theoretical option. Simple measures such as keeping the affected areas warm should not be forgotten.

Genetic counseling should be offered to all patients with a personal or family history of multiple leiomyomas. In females, particularly those with family history, a gynecologic opinion should be sought to exclude the possible involvement of the uterus ('fibroids'). Menorrhagia may necessitate hysterectomy, and leiomyosarcoma should be excluded. More recently, genetic studies have suggested that germline mutations in the gene encoding fumarate hydratase (an enzyme of the tricarboxylic acid cycle) predispose to multiple cutaneous and uterine leiomyoma syndrome, and occasionally renal cell carcinoma. Analysis for mutations of the fumarate hydratase gene may be helpful in identifying individuals at risk of developing the syndrome.

SPECIFIC INVESTIGATIONS

- Skin biopsy in doubtful cases
- Biochemical assay of fumarate hydratase – the measured activity is very low or absent
- Genetic analysis – for mutations of the fumarate hydratase gene

Tumors with smooth muscle differentiation. Spencer JM, Amonette RA. Dermatol Surg 1996;22:761–8.

The myofibrils in leiomyomas can be highlighted with special stains such as Masson trichrome and phosphotungstic acid–hematoxylin, in which they appear red and purple, respectively. Immunohistochemical techniques demonstrate desmin and actin. Electron microscopic studies show myofilaments.

A well-referenced review article on classification, diagnosis, and treatment of leiomyoma and leiomyosarcoma.

Germline mutations in FH predispose to dominantly inherited uterine fibroids, skin leiomyomata and papillary renal cell cancer. Tomlinson IP, Alam NA, Rowan AJ, et al; Multiple Leiomyoma Consortium. Nat Genet 2002;30:406–10.

The authors show that the gene which predisposes to uterine fibroids, cutaneous leiomyomas, and renal cell carcinoma encodes for fumarate hydratase. This enzyme acts as a tumor suppressor in familial leiomyomas, and its measured activity is very low or absent in tumors from individuals with leiomyomatosis. Mutations of the fumarate hydratase gene are found in the recessive fumarate hydratase deficiency syndrome and in the dominantly inherited susceptibility to multiple cutaneous and uterine leiomyomatosis.

FIRST LINE THERAPY

■ Surgical excision	E

Multiple cutaneous leiomyomas. Report of a case. Tiffee JC, Budnick SD. Oral Surg Oral Med Oral Pathol 1993;76: 716–7.

This is a case report of a 35-year-old man with familial multiple leiomyomas on the face which were surgically excised. Four months following removal, two lesions recurred.

Leiomyomas of the skin. Fisher WC, Helwig EB. Acta Derm Venereol 1963;88:510–20.

The clinical findings and natural course of 54 cutaneous leiomyomas from 38 patients are described. A high recurrence rate of 50% in surgically excised leiomyomas is stated.

SECOND LINE THERAPIES

■ Doxazosin	D
■ Nifedipine	E
■ Phenoxybenzamine	E
■ Topical hyoscine hydrobromide	E
■ Nitroglycerine	E
■ Cryotherapy	E
■ Simple analgesics	E
■ Gabapentin	E

The rarity of the condition means that most publications on therapy are case reports. The therapeutic agents are not consistently effective.

Successful treatment of pain in two patients with cutaneous leiomyomata with the oral alpha-1 adrenoceptor antagonist, doxazosin. Batchelor RJ, Lyon CC, Highet AS. Br J Dermatol 2004;150:775–6.

Two cases of cutaneous leiomyoma are reported. A 52-year-old woman and a 35-year old woman with a long history of leiomyomas were treated with doxazosin 1–4 mg daily with 'dramatic improvement'/complete relief of symptoms. The improvement was sustained in the 52-year-old patient after 6 months. The treatment was well tolerated. Doxasozin is a reversible, selective α-1 blocker, in comparison to phenoxybenzamine, which is unselective.

Pharmacological modulation of cold-induced pain in cutaneous leiomyomata. Archer CB, Whittaker S, Greaves MW. Br J Dermatol 1988;118:255–60.

Two cases of cutaneous leiomyoma are reported. A novel method of pain assessment by cold induction (with an ice cube) is also presented. Several drugs were assessed in both patients by this method: topical 1% phentolamine solution,

9% hyoscine bromide solution, nitroglycerine paste, and 2% lidocaine (lignocaine) gel; sublingual glyceryl trinitrate; and oral phenoxybenzamine, nifedipine, and acetaminophen (paracetamol). One patient appeared to respond only to phenoxybenzamine 10 mg twice daily and the other patient to topical 9% hyoscine bromide. The latter patient also improved with cryotherapy.

Therapy for painful cutaneous leiomyomas. Thompson JA. J Am Acad Dermatol 1985;13:865–7.

A single report of a 24-year-old man with painful multiple leiomyomas treated successfully with nifedipine 10 mg three times daily for 8 months. The dosage was increased to 10 mg four times daily with the onset of cool weather and increase in pain. The physiology of smooth muscle action is explained.

Muscle relaxing agent in cutaneous leiomyoma. Abraham Z, Cohen A, Haim S. Dermatologica 1983;166: 255–6.

A case report of a 21-year-old man with multiple cutaneous leiomyomas who demonstrated a 'dramatic and immediate response' with nifedipine 10 mg three times daily. The pain completely disappeared and there was partial involution of the lesions. The patient was followed up for 5 months.

Multiple cutaneous leiomyomata and erythrocytosis with demonstration of erythropoietic activity in the cutaneous leiomyomata. Venencie PY, Puissant A, Boffa GA, et al. Br J Dermatol 1982;107:483–6.

This is a case report of a 41-year-old woman with leiomyomas who had complete suppression of pain after being placed on phenoxybenzamine but did not respond to nitroglycerine and nifedipine.

Leiomyomatosis cutis et uteri. Engelke H, Christophers E. Acta Derm Venereol (Stockh) 1979;59:51–4.

This is a case report of a female with associated uterine leiomyoma. Skin symptoms responded to oral nitroglycerine 0.8–1.6 mg for acute attacks, as well as nifedipine 20 mg and phenoxybenzamine 60 mg over 2 years of follow-up.

Gabapentin treatment of multiple piloleiomyoma-related pain. Alam M, Rabinowitz AD, Engler DE. J Am Acad Dermatol 2002;46(2 Suppl Case Reports):S27–9.

This is a case report of a 54-year-old female with numerous cutaneous leiomyomas, confirmed histologically, which were present only on the right half of her body. The symptoms of pain responded well to gabapentin 300 mg orally every day for 3 days, twice daily for 3 days, then three times daily for a total of 2 weeks, with near-complete resolution of discomfort. The patient was maintained on the same dose of gabapentin thereafter.

Leishmaniasis

Suhail M Hadi, Haitham Al-Qari

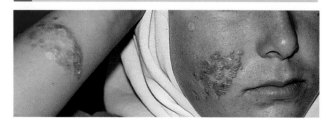

Leishmaniasis is a flagellate protozoan disease caused by many species of the genus *Leishmania*, transmitted by the bite of the infected female phlebotomine sandfly. The disease may be cutaneous (Old and New World), mucocutaneous (espundia) and visceral (kala azar). Generalized, disseminated, cutaneous erysipeloid-like, and mucosal leishmaniasis may be seen in HIV infection and AIDS. There is no single optimal treatment for all forms of cutaneous leishmaniasis. Only the management of cutaneous leishmaniasis is addressed here.

MANAGEMENT STRATEGY

The diagnosis of cutaneous leishmaniasis is established on the basis of a typical lesion, a history of exposure, and demonstration of the parasite (stained smear or culture from the lesion) or positive serology (enzyme-linked immunosorbent assay [ELISA] or indirect fluorescent antibody), which is found in mucocutaneous leishmaniasis only. Polymerase chain reaction (PCR), where available, is highly sensitive. Although the lesions usually heal spontaneously, they leave scars; therefore, treatment is needed to improve the cosmetic outcome.

Pentavalent antimonials are first line therapy. *Meglumine antimoniate* is the drug of choice. It can be given intralesionally with local anesthetic (particularly in children, because of severe pain) or systemically 10 mg/kg daily for 2 weeks. *Leishmania recidivans* requires higher doses for longer periods.

Sodium stibogluconate can be infiltrated into individual lesions 1–2 mL weekly. The drug can be given intramuscularly or intravenously 10 mg/kg daily for 2 weeks for widespread, severe cases.

Most patients develop anorexia, malaise, arthralgia, and myalgia 14 days after treatment; this toxicity is common and appears to be dose related. Other side effects include, cardiotoxicity, acute pancreatitis, mild thrombocytopenia, leucopenia, and elevated liver enzyme levels (aminotransferases).

Amphotericin B has been used in refractory cases (antimony-resistant cases). *Interferon* and *paromomycin* (aminoglycoside antibiotic) reportedly gave encouraging outcomes.

Pentamidine (aromatic diamidine) is effective for diffuse cutaneous leishmaniasis. Hypotension, hypoglycemia, headache, and myalgia are possible side effects of this drug. Both *allopurinol* and *nifurtimox* have antileishmanial activity. *Rifampin* (rifampicin), *trimethoprim–sulfamethoxazole*, *pyrimethamine*, and *metronidazole* have been used with conflicting results.

Cryotherapy or *excision* may be used with other methods. *Immunotherapy using leishmania antigen in BCG* can be tried. Additional treatment methods are presented below.

SPECIFIC INVESTIGATIONS

- Skin biopsy
- Lesional aspirate
- Slit-skin smear
- Culture
- Leishmanin (Montenegro) skin test
- Serology
- PCR for leishmanial DNA

Histology and Giemsa or Brown-Hopps stained aspirates from the periphery of the lesion avoiding the necrotic center (slit-skin smear) may show amastigotes (Leishman–Donovan bodies) inside macrophages with large histiocytes.

Needle aspiration test is useful for papular and nodular lesions using 0.1 mL saline (preservative free) injected through intact skin into the border. The fluid is then aspirated by moving forth and back under the skin while the needle is still inside and then sent for culture.

The gold standard medium for culture of the organisms is Novy-MacNeal-Nicolle (NNN) with positive results in 1–3 weeks or Schneider Drosophila medium, which gives positive results in 1 week (motile promastigotes). In older lesions, culture is considered unreliable because the organisms become scarce and difficult to isolate.

Serological tests play an important role in mucocutaneous and visceral leishmaniasis by detecting antibodies against leishmania.

Value of diagnostic techniques for cutaneous leishmaniasis. Faber WR, Oskam L, van Gool T, et al. J Am Acad Dermatol 2003;49:70–4.

PCR appears to be the most sensitive single diagnostic test. The second most sensitive test for cutaneous leishmaniasis is culture.

Leishmaniasis recidiva cutis in New World cutaneous leishmaniasis. Oliveira-Neto MP, Mattos M, Souza CS, et al. Int J Dermatol 1998;37:846–9.

Detection of leishmanial DNA by PCR was the only positive test in recidivant lesions.

Immunohistochemistry to identify leishmania parasites in fixed tissue. Kenner JR, Aronson NE, Bratthauer GL, et al. J Cutan Pathol 1999;26:130–6.

Isolation of promastigotes by culture is the gold standard. Immunohistochemistry using monoclonal antileishmania antibodies (G2D10) is promising as a good and rapid diagnostic screen for leishmaniasis.

Value of touch preparation (imprints) for diagnosis of cutaneous leishmaniasis. Bahamdan KA, Khan AR, Tallab TM, Mourad MM. Int J Dermatol 1996;35:558–60.

Touch preparation stained with Giemsa is a sensitive method for diagnosis of cutaneous leishmaniasis.

FIRST LINE THERAPIES

Pentavalent antimonials	
■ Meglumine antimoniate	B
■ Sodium stibogluconate antimony	B

A randomized, double-blind study of the efficacy of a 10 or 20 day course of sodium stibogluconate for treatment of cutaneous leishmaniasis in United States military personnel. Wortmann G, Miller RS, Oster C, et al. Clin Infect Dis 2002:1;35:261–7.

Ten days course of sodium stibogluconate (20 mg/kg daily, 19 patients) appears to be less toxic and therapeutically equivalent to the standard 20-day course (19 patients).

Intralesional therapy of American cutaneous leishmaniasis with pentavalent antimony in Rio de Janeiro, Brazil – an area of *Leishmania (V) braziliensis* transmission. Oliveria-Neto MP, Schubach A, Mattos M, et al. Int J Dermatol 1997;36:463–8.

Healing of ulcerative cutaneous lesions and prevention of late mucosal damage were achieved in 80% of patients treated with N-methyl glucamine (74 patients) after 12 weeks with no side effect.

Intralesional treatment of cutaneous leishmaniasis with sodium stibogluconate antimony. Faris RM, Jarallah JS, Khoja TA, Al Yamani MJ. Int J Dermatol 1993;32:610–2.

Healing was achieved in 72% of lesions treated (in 710 patients) and it was as effective as systemic antimonials. Side effects were limited to pain at the site of injection.

A comparative study between sodium stibogluconate BP 88R and meglumine antimoniate in the treatment of cutaneous leishmaniasis. I. The efficacy and safety. (Portuguese) Saldanha AC, Romero GA, Merchan-Hamann E, et al. Rev Soc Bras Med Trop 1999;32:383–7.

One hundred and twenty seven patients with cutaneous leishmaniasis were enrolled in the study – 58 patients were treated with meglumine antimoniate and 69 patients with sodium stibogluconate: 62% of patients were cured with meglumine antimoniate vs 55% with sodium stibogluconate. Headache, myalgia, arthralgia, anorexia, and abdominal pain were seen with sodium stibogluconate.

SECOND LINE THERAPIES

■ Rifampin	A
■ Pentamidine isethionate	C
■ Allopurinol plus low dose meglumine antimoniate	B
■ Azoles	A
■ Cryotherapy	B
■ Hypertonic sodium chloride	D

The role of rifampicin in the management of cutaneous leishmaniasis. Kochar DK, Aseri S, Sharma BV, et al. QJM 2000;93:733–7.

Forty six patients with cutaneous leishmaniasis were enrolled in this double-blind study: 23 received rifampin 600 mg twice daily for 4 weeks and 23 patients received placebo for 4 weeks. Of the rifampin group 73.9% had complete healing of their lesions compared to 4.3% of the placebo group. The difference was statistically significant.

Rifampin is well tolerated with no side effects and is suitable for multiple lesions or if the injectable treatment is not feasible.

Treatment of Old World cutaneous leishmaniasis by pentamidine isethionate. An open study of 11 patients. Hellier I, Dereure O, Tournillac I, et al. Dermatology 2000; 200:120–3.

Pentamidine isethionate (4 mg/kg) was given every other day for three strictly intramuscular injections: 73% of patients responded well with good tolerance. The authors concluded that pentamidine isethionate is effective and safe and can be used as first line treatment for Old World leishmaniasis.

Treatment of cutaneous leishmaniasis with a combination of allopurinol and low-dose meglumine antimoniate. Momeni AZ, Reiszadae MR, Aminjavaheri M. Int J Dermatol 2002;41:441–3.

Treatment was allopurinol 20 mg/kg daily plus low-dose meglumine antimoniate 30 mg/kg daily or meglumine antimoniate 60 mg/kg daily alone for a total 20 days. Of 72 patients with cutaneous leishmaniasis, complete healing occurred in 80.6% of patients on allopurinol and low-dose meglumine antimoniate vs 74.2% of patients on higher-dose meglumine antimoniate. No difference was found between the two groups with respect to side effects.

Fluconazole for the treatment of cutaneous leishmaniasis caused by *Leishmania major*. Alrajhi AA, Ibrahim EA, De Vol EB, et al. N Engl J Med 2002; 346:8915.

A total of 106 patients received fluconazole 200 mg daily and 103 patients received placebo for 6 weeks. Follow-up data were available for 80 and 65 patients, respectively. Healing of lesions was complete in 79% of the fluconazole group and 34% of the placebo group at 3-month follow-up.

Comparative study of the efficacy of oral ketoconazole with intra-lesional meglumine antimoniate (Glucantime®) for the treatment of cutaneous leishmaniasis. Salmanpour R, Handjani F, Nouhpisheh MK. J Dermatolog Treat 2001; 12:159–62.

A total of 96 patients were treated with oral ketoconazole 600 mg daily for adults and 10 mg/kg daily for children for 30 days. This regimen was compared with six to eight biweekly intralesional injections of meglumine antimoniate. Complete clinical cure was achieved in 89% of cases treated with oral ketoconazole and in 72% of cases treated with intralesional meglumine antimoniate.

Treatment of cutaneous leishmaniasis with itraconazole. Randomized double-blind study. Momeni AZ, Jalayer T, Emamjomeh M, et al. Arch Dermatol 1996;132:784–6.

Itraconazole (7 mg/kg daily) was given for a period of 3 weeks. Complete healing was seen in 59% of patients (149 patients). Itraconazole cannot be used as a single agent in the treatment of patients with cutaneous leishmaniasis caused by *Leishmania major*.

Efficacy of cryotherapy and intralesional pentostam in treatment of cutaneous leishmaniasis. Gurei MS, Tatli N, Ozbilge H, et al. J Egypt Soc Parasitol 2000;30:169–76.

Sixty lesions from 42 patients were treated with liquid nitrogen and 73 lesions from 55 patients were treated with intralesional Pentostam®: 92% of lesions treated with intralesional Pentostam® and 78% of lesions treated with liquid nitrogen cryotherapy achieved marked improvement after 3 months.

A new intralesional therapy for cutaneous leishmaniasis with hypertonic sodium chloride solution. Sharquie KE. J Dermatol 1995;22:732–7.

Hypertonic sodium chloride solution injections were given at 7–10-day intervals with a 96% cure rate within 2–6 weeks (comparable to sodium stibogluconate). The treatment is safe, cheap, and effective.

THIRD LINE THERAPIES

■ Gamma interferon	E
■ Hexadecylphosphocholine (miltefosine)	B
■ Imiquimod 5%	C
■ Aminosidine (paromomycin) ointment	A
■ Photodynamic therapy (PDT)	E
■ Direct current electrotherapy	B
■ CO₂ laser	B

Successful treatment of cutaneous leishmaniasis using systemic interferon-gamma. Kolde G, Luger T, Sorg C, Sunderkotter C. Dermatology 1996;192:56–60.

Systemic monotherapy with gamma interferon ($100\,\mu g/m^2$ of body surface daily) given subcutaneously for 28 days can be an effective treatment for complicated cases of human cutaneous leishmaniasis without side effects.

Development status of miltefosine as first oral drug in visceral and cutaneous leishmaniasis. Fischer C, Voss A, Engel J. Med Microbiol Immunol (Berl) 2001;190:85–7.

Miltefosine has been found to induce apoptosis in *Leishmania donovani*. Cure rate for New World cutaneous leishmaniasis was 94% at a dose of 150 mg daily for 3–4 weeks with relative safety and few side effects.

Successful treatment of drug-resistant cutaneous leishmaniasis in humans by the use of imiquimod, an immunomodulator. Arevalo I, Ward B, Miller R, et al. Clin Infect Dis 2001;33:1847–51.

Imiquimod 5% cream was used in combination with meglumine antimoniate (12 patients who had previously not responded to meglumine antimoniate therapy). In combination therapy, the cure rate was 90% at 6-month follow-up period.

Imiquimod kills the intracellular leishmania amastigotes in vitro by activating macrophages to release nitric oxide.

Treatment of cutaneous leishmaniasis with aminosidine (paromomycin) ointment: double-blind, randomized trial in the Islamic Republic of Iran. Bull World Health Organ 2003;81:353–9.

Although spontaneous recovery may occur in half of the cases without treatment, 4 weeks of treatment with paromomycin ointment for uncomplicated cutaneous leishmaniasis due to *Leishmania major* could become the first line treatment. The ointment is useful for single lesions. It was applied twice daily. Four weeks of treatment gave significantly better cure rates (74%) than 2 weeks of treatment (59%). No adverse reactions to the ointment were observed.

Treatment of cutaneous leishmaniasis by photodynamic therapy. Gardlo K, Horska Z, Enk CD, et al. J Am Acad Dermatol 2003;48:893–6.

The efficacy of PDT and paromomycin sulfate were compared in ten lesions of cutaneous leishmaniasis. PDT was given twice weekly and after 12 weeks once weekly for five lesions and paromomycin sulfate was applied once daily to five lesions. All PDT treated lesions and two of five lesions treated with paromomycin sulfate were free of disease clinically and histologically.

Treatment of cutaneous leishmanisis by direct current electrotherapy: the Baghdadin device. Sharquie KE, al-Hamamy H, el-Yassin D. J Dermatol 1998;25:234–7.

One hundred and forty six lesions from 54 patients were treated with weekly sessions of direct current stimulation (5–15 mA for 10 min), which produced total clearance in 95.5% of treated lesions within 4–6 weeks. None of the 21 control lesions showed any sign of improvement after 6 weeks. Of 36 lesions from 15 patients treated with intralesional sodium stibogluconate, 88.9% showed total clearance (not significantly different from the Baghdadin device).

Evaluation of CO₂ laser efficacy in the treatment of cutaneous leishmaniasis. Asilian A, Sharif A, Faghihi G, et al. Int J Dermatol 2004;43:736–8.

One hundred and eighty three lesions from 123 patients were treated with CO_2 laser with a maximum power of 100 W and a pulse width of 0.5–5 s, and 250 lesions from 110 patients were treated with glucantime 50 mg/kg daily for 15 days. The CO_2 laser was 1.12 times more effective than glucantime, with reduction in healing time to 1 month vs 3 months and minor side effects with CO_2 laser (4.5 vs 24%).

Lentigo maligna

John A Carucci, Darrell S Rigel

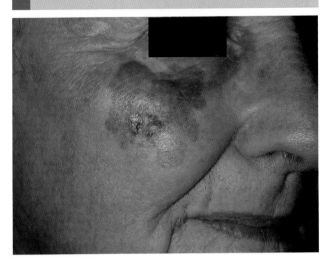

Lentigo maligna (LM) is a form of melanoma in situ affecting sun-exposed areas of the face and neck in older individuals. If left untreated, it can progress to invasive melanoma (lentigo maligna melanoma, LMM). The risk of progression has been reported to range between 2 and 45%.

MANAGEMENT STRATEGY

Successful management of LM depends upon early diagnosis and definitive removal. The differential diagnosis includes macular seborrheic keratosis, pigmented actinic keratosis, and pigmented Bowen's disease. Confirmatory biopsy is necessary prior to definitive treatment. Treatment is primarily surgical although eradication by other modalities may be considered. Patients with a history of LM should have periodic full-body skin examinations by a dermatologist to allow for early detection of recurrence, progression, or second primary skin cancer.

SPECIFIC INVESTIGATIONS

- Skin biopsy and patient evaluation

Diagnosis and treatment of early melanoma. NIH Consens Statement 1992;10:1–26.

Biopsy of sufficient depth is critical for diagnosis and management of pigmented lesions. Punch, saucerization, excision, or incisional biopsy may be acceptable. On microscopic examination, LM is characterized by increased numbers of atypical melanocytes, which may be solitary or arranged in nests, but do not invade the dermis. Evaluation should include personal and family history, complete skin examination, and palpation of regional lymph nodes. Blood tests or imaging studies are not indicated.

FIRST LINE THERAPIES

■ Excision	A
■ Mohs micrographic surgery (MMS)	D
■ Modified Mohs surgery	D
■ Staged excision	D

Diagnosis and treatment of early melanoma. NIH Consens Statement 1992;10:1–26.

Current recommendations are based on the NIH consensus for melanoma in situ, which suggests excision of the lesion or biopsy site with a margin of 0.5 cm of clinically normal skin and layer of subcutaneous tissue. In general, margins of 0.5–1.0 cm are suggested for LM where feasible. Difficulties may arise in determination of clinical margins due to diffuse background sun damage. A Wood's lamp may be useful in defining subclinical extension. Accurate determination of margins is key because LM is likely to recur after inadequate excision.

Mohs micrographic surgery for the treatment of primary cutaneous melanoma. Zitelli JA, Brown C, Hanusa BH. J Am Acad Dermatol 1997;37:236–45.

In this study, 535 patients with 553 melanomas were treated by MMS. The authors report an overall cure rate of over 99% at 5 years. In 83% of cases, tumors were excised with margins of 0.6 cm. Larger lesions on the head, neck, hands, and feet typically required wider margins for clearance. MMS allows for optimal margin control and patient convenience because tumors can be removed and defects repaired in one day in an office setting.

Mohs micrographic excision of melanoma using immunostains. Zalla MJ, Lim KK, Dicaudo DJ, Gagnot MM. Dermatol Surg 2000;26:771–84.

This modification to Mohs technique was developed because difficulties may arise in distinguishing sun-damaged melanocytes from residual LM on frozen sections. Special histologic stains have been used to enhance sensitivity. Zalla et al. reported successful treatment of melanoma by MMS using Melan-A, HMB-45, Mel-5, and S-100. There were no recurrences in 68 patients after a mean follow-up time of 16 months.

Utility of rush paraffin-embedded tangential sections in the management of cutaneous neoplasms. Clayton BD, Leshin B, Hitchcock MG, et al. Dermatol Surg 2000;26: 671–8.

The authors report treatment of 100 patients with melanoma (77 with LM/melanoma in situ, 23 with LMM) with margin control by rush permanent sections to enhance sensitivity. Recurrent LM was noted in one patient and satellite metastasis was noted in one patient with LMM.

A potential disadvantage of relying on 'rush' permanent sections is the amount of time added to each procedure. In addition, the technique depends on off-site tissue processing and interpretation, thus magnifying the possibility of error.

Mohs micrographic surgery for lentigo maligna and lentigo maligna melanoma. A follow-up study. Cohen LM, McCall MW, Zax RH. Dermatol Surg 1998;24:673–7.

A report of successful treatment in 45 patients at 29.2 months with LM and LMM with MMS aided by rush permanent sections. There was one recurrence at 50 months (97% cure rate).

Management of lentigo maligna and lentigo maligna melanoma with staged excision: a follow up. Bub JL, Berg D, Slee A, Odland PB. Arch Dermatol 2004;140:552–8.

The authors report a staged, margin-controlled, vertical-edged excision technique followed by radial sectioning and preparation of paraffin sections. After a mean follow-up of 57 months, 95% of the 59 patients treated were disease free. The average excision margin was 0.55 cm. The use of radial sectioning allowed for more thorough specimen evaluation with relatively narrow margins.

Usefulness of the staged excision for lentigo maligna and lentigo maligna melanoma: the 'square' procedure. Johnson TM, Headington JT, Baker SR, Lowe L. J Am Acad Dermatol 1997;37:758–64.

With this technique, a margin of 0.5–1.0 cm is outlined with angled corners to facilitate processing. A peripheral strip of tissue 2–4 mm wide is excised and processed for evaluation of permanent sections. Residual tumor is subsequently excised in directed fashion based on mapping. There were no recurrences in 35 patients at 2 years.

SECOND LINE THERAPIES

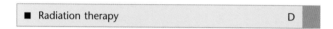

■ Radiation therapy	D

A retrospective study of 150 patients with lentigo maligna and lentigo maligna melanoma and the efficacy of radiotherapy using Grenz or soft X-rays. Farshad A, Burg G, Pannizon R, Dummer R. Br J Dermatol 2002;146:1042–6.

Ninety six patients with LM were treated with Grenz rays. It recurred in five of 96 patients after an average of 46 months. Four patients with recurrent LM were treated with subsequent surgery and one with radiotherapy. No patient with recurrent LM progressed to nodal or distant metastastic disease.

Fractionated radiotherapy of lentigo maligna and lentigo maligna melanoma in 64 patients. Schmid-Wendtner MH, Brunner B, Konz B, et al. J Am Acad Dermatol 2000;43:477–82.

Sixty four patients with LM (42) and LMM (22) were treated with fractionated radiotherapy. There was no recurrence in any of the patients with LM over a mean follow-up of 23 months (range 1–96 months). One of the advantages of this soft X-ray or Miescher's technique is exclusion of underlying bone and minimization of risk of bony necrosis. The potential disadvantage is inadequate depth of penetration.

THIRD LINE THERAPIES

■ Q-switched ruby laser	E
■ Q-switched Nd:YAG laser	D
■ Interferon-alfa	D, E
■ Imiquimod	D
■ Tazarotene	E

Treatment of lentigo maligna with the Q-switched ruby laser. Kauvar ANB, Geronemus R. Lasers Surg Med 1995;48.

Tumor eradication was achieved in three of four patients during 6–24 month follow-up. The fourth patient developed amelanotic LM at 1 month. Q-switched ruby laser may be prone to failure due to inadequate depth of penetration.

Q-switched neodymium:yttrium-aluminum-garnet laser treatment of lentigo maligna. Orten SS, Waner M, Dinehart SM, et al. Otolaryngol Head Neck Surg 1999; 120:296–302.

Eight patients with LM were treated with the Nd:YAG laser. Three patients were treated with both 532 and 1064 nm. Two of these had complete eradication without recurrence at 3.5 years. The other showed a partial response, but died of unrelated causes prior to completion of therapy.

The Nd:YAG laser emits energy at 532 and 1064 nm, which may be especially suited to LM. Melanin has greater absorption at 532 nm whereas the longer wavelength, 1064 nm, may provide deeper penetration.

Intralesional interferon treatment of lentigo maligna. Cornejo P, Vanaclocha F, Polimon I, Del Rio R. Arch Dermatol 2000;136:428–30.

Interferon-alfa is a biological response modifier indicated for adjunctive treatment of high-risk melanoma. The mechanism involves both immunomodulation and direct antiproliferative effects. Successful treatment of 11 LM lesions in ten patients at doses of $3–6 \times 10^6$ IU administered three times weekly is reported, with clearance in all patients after between 12 and 29 doses.

Intralesional interferon for treatment of recurrent lentigo maligna of the eyelid in a patient with primary acquired melanosis. Carucci JA, Leffell DJ. Arch Dermatol 2000;136: 1415–6.

In this case report, clinical and histologic clearance was achieved after a total dose of 39 million units. Toxic effects included fever, chills, and flu-like symptoms and were transient when interferon-alfa was used intralesionally.

Treatment of lentigo maligna with topical imiquimod. Naylor MF, Crowson N, Kuwahara R, et al. Br J Dermatol 2003;149(suppl 66):66–9.

In this study, 30 patients with LM were enrolled in an open-labeled efficacy trial of daily application of imiquimod 5% cream for 3 months. Following treatment, 26 of 28 (93%) evaluable patients showed a 'complete response' based on four quadrant biopsy. No recurrences were seen in 80% of the 26 patients that were followed for 1 year.

Treatment of lentigo maligna with tazarotene 0.1% gel. Chimenti S, Carrozzo AM, Citarella L, et al. J Am Acad Dermatol 2004;50:101–3.

In this series, two elderly patients with facial LM were treated with daily application of tazarotene 0.1% gel for 6–8 months. No recurrence in either patient was observed after follow-up periods of 18 and 30 months. These results should be interpreted with caution considering the relatively short follow-up.

Evidence levels **A** Double-blind study **B** Clinical trial ≥ 20 subjects **C** Clinical trial < 20 subjects **D** Series ≥ 5 subjects **E** Anecdotal case reports

Leprosy (including reactions)

Anne E Burdick, Alyssa M Feiner

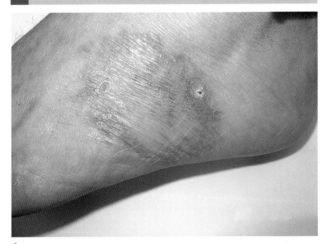

A

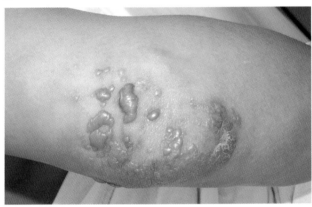

B

Leprosy, also called Hansen's disease (HD) is an infection caused by *Mycobacterium leprae (M. leprae)* that presents as anesthetic asymptomatic skin lesions, which may be hypopigmented macules or erythematous plaques and nodules. Lesions vary in number from a few in limited tuberculoid HD to numerous in diffuse lepromatous HD. Enlarged peripheral nerves (ulnar or greater auricular), absence of sweating, loss of eyebrows and eyelashes, atrophied hand muscles, or claw hand deformities may also be present. Appropriate treatment limits disability due to HD neuropathy and controls disease spread because untreated lepromatous HD patients are the major infectious reservoir. For treatment, the United States National HD Program (US NHDP) and World Health Organization (WHO) classify indeterminate (I), tuberculoid (TT) (Figure A), and borderline tuberculoid (BT) HD with negative slit smears as 'paucibacillary' HD. Midborderline (BB), borderline lepromatous (BL) (Figure B), and lepromatous (LL) HD with positive slit smears are classified as 'multibacillary' HD.

Four reactions may complicate HD. Type 1 reversal reactions (RR) occur in borderline cases (BT, BB, and BL), often during the first 6 months of therapy. Patients may develop erythema, warmth, and edema of preexisting or seemingly resolved HD lesions, hand and foot edema, and painful neuritis of one or more peripheral nerves with new onset anesthesia or motor loss. Nerve weakness or paralysis may result if aggressive treatment is not started promptly. Type 2 erythema nodosum leprosum reactions (ENL) develop in BL and LL patients. ENL is characterized by new crops of tender erythematous papules, plaques, and nodules, often with fever, polyarthralgia, myalgia, malaise, neuritis, and also hand and foot edema. Rarely proteinuria or hematuria occurs. These reactions can occur before, during, or after treatment, and may be difficult to distinguish from relapses.

A downgrading reaction occurs in untreated patients or noncompliant patients on treatment, who experience a shift in their immunity toward the lepromatous end of the HD spectrum. They present with new lesions, fever, and malaise, similar to an RR. Lucio's phenomenon is a rare vasculitic reaction in patients who have untreated Lucio's HD (diffuse lepromatous skin infiltration). It is seen primarily in Mexico and Central America, but has also been reported in the US and other countries. Purpuric tender lesions on the extremities become necrotic and ulcerated.

A 'silent neuropathy' may also develop insidiously in HD patients. This presents with a steady decline in sensory and/or motor function without skin findings. A peripheral neuritis may also develop before, during, or up to several years after treatment is completed.

MANAGEMENT STRATEGY

In 1990, the standard US NHDP *multidrug therapy (MDT) regimen* for paucibacillary HD and multibacillary HD was changed to 1 year for paucibacillary HD and 2 years for multibacillary HD. In 1997, the WHO changed its recommended MDT HD treatment protocols to 6 months for paucibacillary and 1 year for multibacillary regimens.

For paucibacillary HD, the WHO recommends 6 months of daily *dapsone* 100 mg and monthly supervised *rifampin* 600 mg. For paucibacillary patients with a solitary HD lesion, the WHO recommends a single dose of rifampin 400 mg, *ofloxacin* 400 mg, and *minocycline* 100 mg.

The US NHDP treatment regimen for paucibacillary leprosy is 1 year of daily rifampin 600 mg and daily dapsone 100 mg. If active neuritis develops, the NHDP recommends the addition of a third drug, usually *clofazimine*. Patients with pre-existing or subsequent anemia should take lower dapsone doses; the minimal effective dose is 50 mg.

For multibacillary HD, the WHO recommends monthly rifampin 600 mg and clofazimine 300 mg under supervision, and daily dapsone 100 mg and clofazimine 50 mg for 1 year. For multibacillary HD, the NHDP recommendation is 2 years of daily rifampin 600 mg, daily dapsone 100 mg, and daily clofazimine 50 mg. Rifampin is the most bactericidal HD drug available and seems to be more effective when given daily. However, rifampin should be given once a month if a patient is taking prednisone, anticoagulants, and oral contraceptives because rifampin decreases the effectiveness of these drugs. Other recommended alternative HD drugs are *minocycline* 100 mg daily, *ofloxacin* 400 mg daily, *levofloxacin* 500 mg daily, or twice daily *clarithromycin* 500 mg. Clofazimine is a highly effective HD drug when given with dapsone and may prevent or limit ENL reactions. The gray-blue hyperpigmentation of clofazimine may limit patient acceptance and compliance. If clofazimine is refused, the NHDP recommends minocycline 100 mg daily. Some US leprologists treat multibacillary patients with MDT for 2 years as recommended by NHDP, and then continue these patients on dapsone until their slit smears are negative.

Pediatric MDT regimens are the same as adult MDT regimens with doses of dapsone 1 mg/kg daily, rifampin 10 mg/kg daily, and clofazimine 1 mg/kg daily. *Pregnant patients* can be treated with dapsone, clofazimine, and prednisone if necessary. Rifampin, minocycline, and fluoroquinolones are avoided in pregnancy. During *lactation*, standard MDT is used with a minimal risk to the infant.

The NHDP advises that a multibacillary BL or LL patient treated with the previous NHDP regimen of 3 years dapsone and rifampin followed by lifelong daily dapsone should discontinue dapsone if the skin biopsy shows no active disease and the slit smear bacillary index is zero. Multibacillary patients who have taken dapsone monotherapy for 5 or more years should also discontinue dapsone if biopsy and slit smears are negative.

Although a few randomized trials have shown that the BCG (bacillus Calmette-Guérin) vaccine reduces the risk of developing leprosy, the NHDP does not recommend this vaccination. Although physicians in some countries prescribe dapsone to household contacts as chemoprophylaxis, the NHDP does not recommend preventative treatment.

For mild RRs or ENL reactions, nonsteroidal antipyretics and analgesics, such as *ibuprofen* 400 mg three times daily or *aspirin*, are helpful. For a severe RR, *prednisone* 0.5–1.0 mg/kg once or twice daily should be started immediately to prevent motor and sensory damage and given for 3–6 months, then slowly tapered. *Calcium* 600 mg with *vitamin D supplements* twice daily and *alendronate* 70 mg weekly are advised concomitantly with prednisone. *Gabapentin* 100 mg three times daily to a maximum of 600 mg three times daily or *amitriptyline* 50–150 mg nightly may alleviate neuropathic HD pain. *Splinting* the affected limb in a functional position has been advocated, but remains controversial due to a concern for further muscle atrophy. Some leprologists treat patients with severe RRs with *azathioprine* to lower the prednisone dose needed to control the reaction.

For severe RR and ENL reactions, *clofazimine* 100 mg twice or three times daily may be prescribed as an anti-inflammatory agent for 6 weeks and then reduced to 100 mg daily for several months. High doses of clofazimine cause gastrointestinal side effects and rarely megacolon. Thalidomide is of no benefit in RRs. Intestinal parasitic or immune compromising infections may be precipitating factors in patients with chronic ENL.

For severe ENL in men and in women who are postmenopausal, surgically sterilized, or on medroxyprogesterone acetate intramuscularly, *thalidomide* in doses of 100 mg and higher, up to 400 mg, at night is the treatment of choice. Lesions and symptoms resolve within 2–3 days. Thalidomide can be tapered gradually over a period of weeks to months and maintained at 50–100 mg daily. For women of childbearing potential, *prednisone* 0.5–1.0 mg/kg daily is effective and usually prescribed for several months. Once the ENL is controlled, prednisone should be tapered slowly; generally decreasing the daily dose by 5.0 mg every 4–6 weeks. During acute severe ENL, prednisone may be added to thalidomide. Prednisolone is preferable for patients with hepatic disease.

For multibacillary patients who relapse and for paucibacillary patients who relapse with multibacillary disease, the NHDP recommends repeating the 2 year MDT protocol and then continuing dapsone 100 mg for life. For a patient who has completed HD therapy and experiences an RR or ENL reaction requiring prednisone for more than 30 days, the WHO recommends restarting dapsone until the prednisone is discontinued.

Downgrading reactions are treated with HD drugs, as is Lucio's phenomenon. The latter is also treated with *supportive care*. Patients with neuropathy often require periodic neurosensory mapping, special shoes, orthotics, or electromyelograms of affected nerves, as well as podiatry, physical or occupational therapy, ophthalmology, and neurology consultations. Patients with HD neuropathic ulcers require *aggressive wound care, callus debridement, periodic skin biopsies of chronic ulcers to rule out squamous cell carcinoma, bacterial cultures of infected ulcers,* and *X-rays,* and often *bone scans* to rule out osteomyelitis underlying chronic ulcers. Mouse footpad inoculation is rarely performed to rule out drug resistance. An immediate ophthalmology consultation is required if a patient develops iridocyclitis, for which *atropine* and *corticosteroid drops* are prescribed. *Artificial tears* are often recommended for lagophthalmos and decreased lacrimation. Orchitis may accompany a reaction or occur independently and responds well to *prednisone*.

Close follow-up of patients who have completed HD treatment is important. The NHDP recommends every 6 months for at least 5 years for paucibacillary HD and at least 8 years for multibacillary HD. All contacts who lived in the patient's household during the 3 years prior to treatment should be screened for HD: one evaluation for a household contact of a tuberculoid case and annually for at least 5 years for a household contact of a lepromatous case.

The polymerase chain reaction assay (PCR) has been used to detect *M. leprae* in biopsy specimens of patients suspected of having leprosy lesions. Although the PCR for *M. leprae* has been reported to have high sensitivity and specificity in endemic regions, it is usually negative if there are rare or no bacilli identified on Fite-stained sections. In nonendemic populations it is recommended to use the PCR to detect *M. leprae* only for patients who demonstrate acid-fast bacilli on microscopy and have atypical clinical features that may obscure the diagnosis of leprosy.

A reticulum stain may help distinguish sarcoidosis from leprosy because noninfectious conditions tend to preserve the reticulum network and infectious causes tend to destroy this Type III collagen network.

It is sometimes difficult to determine whether a patient is having an RR rather than a relapse. A patient can be determined to have an RR if the new lesions appeared within 1 year of completing treatment (lesions of a relapse occur later), the lesions are edematous and/or painful (lesions of a relapse are asymptomatic), the lesions resolve with prednisone (lesions of a relapse do not), and the lesions develop rapidly within a few days to weeks (lesions of a relapse develop over months).

Evidence levels A Double-blind study   B Clinical trial ≥ 20 subjects   C Clinical trial < 20 subjects   D Series ≥ 5 subjects   E Anecdotal case reports

SPECIFIC INVESTIGATIONS

- Skin biopsy – 4 mm from periphery of lesion; in US send slides to the NHDP for review
- Slit smears – baseline and, if positive, periodically
- Neurosensory testing with nylon filaments, baseline and periodically
- Ophthalmology exam of lepromatous/symptomatic patients, baseline, and occasionally as required
- Glucose-6-phosphate dehydrogenase (G6PD) prior to dapsone
- Liver function tests, baseline and periodically if on rifampin or dapsone
- Complete blood count, baseline and periodically
- Urinalysis, baseline and during ENL
- Pregnancy tests prior to thalidomide and periodically
- Complement, circulating immune complexes, cryoglobulins (Lucio's phenomenon)

National Hansen's Disease Program website. *www.bphc.hrsa.gov/nhdp/*

Resource for the latest US diagnostic and treatment guidelines.

World Health Organization website. *www.who.int/lep/*

Resource for the latest WHO diagnostic and treatment guidelines.

Leprosy. Burdick AE, Frankel S. In: Tropical Dermatology. Tyring S, Lupi O, Hennge U, eds. London: Elsevier; 2005;255–72.

Pathogenesis, clinical evaluation, diagnostic work-up, and therapy reviewed.

Polymerase chain reaction assay for the detection and identification of *Mycobacterium leprae* in patients in the United States. Scollard DM, Gillis TP, Williams DL. Am J Clin Path 1998;109:642–6.

PCR based diagnosis of leprosy in the United States. Williams DL, Scollard DM, Gillis TP. Clin Microbiol Newsl 2003;25:57–61.

Describes indications/limited usefulness of PCR for diagnosing leprosy.

Hansen's disease in a patient with a history of sarcoidosis. Burdick AE, Hendi A, Elgart GW, et al. Int J Lepr Other Mycobact Dis 2000;68:307–11.

Discussion of reticulum stain for distinguishing leprosy and sarcoidosis.

FIRST LINE THERAPIES

■ Antibiotics: rifampin, dapsone, clofazimine	D
■ Nonsteroidal anti-inflammatory drugs (RR and ENL)	E
■ Prednisone (RR and ENL)	D
■ Thalidomide (ENL)	D

Method of leprosy. Joyce MP, Scollard DM. In: Rakel RE, Bope ET, eds. Conn's Current Therapy 2004. Philadelphia: Saunders; 2004;100–5.

Latest treatment guidelines, comparing WHO and US NHDP regimens.

Standards of care for Hansen's disease in the United States. National Hansen's Disease Programs. Louisiana, USA: 2003.

An update on the diagnosis and treatment of leprosy. Moschella SL. J Am Acad Derm 2004;51:417–26.

An excellent clinical review.

Leprosy. Steger JW, Barrett TL. In: Textbook of military medicine: military dermatology. Falls Church, VA Office of the Surgeon General, Dept of Army, USA: 1994;319–54.

The management of leprosy reversal reactions. Britton WJ. Lepr Rev 1998;69:225–34.

Detailed review of corticosteroid doses and duration.

SECOND LINE THERAPIES

■ Minocycline	B
■ Ofloxacin	B
■ Levofloxacin	B
■ Clarithromycin	B

Standards of care for Hansen's disease in the United States. National Hansen's Disease Programs. Louisiana, USA: 2003.

THIRD LINE THERAPIES

■ Gabapentin	E
■ Cyclosporine (ENL and RR)	E
■ Amitriptyline	E
■ Azathioprine	E

Treatment of chronic erythema nodosum leprosum with cyclosporine A produces clinical and immunohistologic remission. Miller RA, Sheri J, Rea TH, Harnisch FP. Int J Lepr 1987;55:441–9.

Two of three multibacillary patients improved with cyclosporine A (6–10 mg/kg) within 2–3 days, allowing the prednisone dose to be decreased.

Leukocytoclastic vasculitis

Jeffrey P Callen

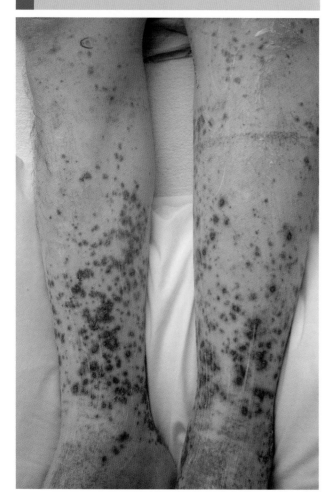

Leukocytoclastic vasculitis (LCV) is a term that defines a histopathological pattern. The clinical disease 'small vessel vasculitis' usually reflects LCV on biopsy examination. LCV is a heterogeneous group of disorders, most often manifested by palpable purpura or urticarial lesions.

MANAGEMENT STRATEGY

Therapy of cutaneous vasculitis depends on whether or not there is clinical or laboratory evidence of internal involvement, the severity of cutaneous disease, and the severity of the systemic disease. Patients with severe systemic necrotizing vasculitis are generally treated with moderate to high doses of *systemic corticosteroids, often with the addition of a cytotoxic agent.*

Patients with acute cutaneous vasculitis in whom there is an identifiable cause such as a drug are treated symptomatically in addition to removing the presumed causative agent. Similarly, patients with Henoch–Schönlein purpura usually have self-limiting disease and are often not given specific treatment. Symptomatic measures include *rest, elevation, gradient support stockings,* and *antihistamines.*

The challenge is to treat the patient who has chronic cutaneous vasculitis in whom there is no easily identifiable cause and who does not have significant systemic involvement. There is often a question regarding the need for therapy because these patients do not have life-threatening disease; however, many of the patients have disease that alters their ability to function normally. Patients may develop small ulcers that can become secondarily infected or may be painful. Patients may not leave their homes because of the psychological distress caused by the presence of purpura. Lastly, patients with urticarial vasculitis complain of itching and burning of their lesions that may result in sleep disturbance. If systemic therapy is considered for disease confined to the skin, then *colchicine* and *dapsone* are often used. *Systemic corticosteroids, methotrexate,* and *azathioprine* have been used in patients refractory to less toxic therapies.

SPECIFIC INVESTIGATIONS

For all patients
- Careful history for drugs and other ingestants
- Skin biopsy for routine microscopy
- Serologic tests for collagen vascular diseases (ANA, rheumatoid factor, anti-Ro/SS-A, etc)
- Serologic tests for infectious diseases (hepatitis C antibody, parvovirus, hepatitis B, etc)
- Chest radiograph

For selected patients
- Skin biopsy for direct immunofluorescence microscopy
- Echocardiography
- Visceral angiography
- Malignancy screening tests

The purpose of evaluation of the patient with cutaneous vasculitis is to identify a cause of the process and assess the presence of systemic involvement. The evaluation begins with a careful history and physical examination, followed by selected testing based upon the acuteness of the process and the findings of the history and physical examination.

Cutaneous vasculitis in children and adults: associated diseases and etiologic factors in 303 patients. Blanco R, Martinez-Taboada VM, Rodriguez-Valverde V, Garcia-Fuentes M. Medicine 1998;77:403–18.

These authors proposed an algorithm for evaluation that differs for children and adults. In children they do not require a skin biopsy for 'humanitarian' reasons. For children, the evaluation includes a blood count, erythrocyte sedimentation rate, urinalysis, stool hematest, and biochemistry profile. For adults, the authors suggest that additional testing include antinuclear antibodies, antineutrophil cytoplasmic antibody, chest radiograph, rheumatoid factor, cryoglobulins, complement levels, hepatitis B surface antigen, and hepatitis C antibody. Subsequent evaluation is directed by additional findings. In children with frequent relapses, suspicion of collagen vascular disease, severe vasculitic syndromes, or hepatic involvement, evaluation should be the same as for adults. Adults with persistent fever, abnormal blood smears, risk for HIV infection, or severe vasculitis should have cultures, echocardiography, hematological evaluation, HIV testing, and when appropriate, visceral angiography and/or biopsy of involved organs.

Evidence levels A Double-blind study B Clinical trial ≥ 20 subjects C Clinical trial < 20 subjects D Series ≥ 5 subjects E Anecdotal case reports

Clinical approaches to cutaneous vasculitis. Gonzalez-Gay MA, Garcia-Porrua C, Pujol RM. Curr Opin Rheumatol 2005;17:56–61.

This is an up-to-date review that details an approach to the patients with small vessel vasculitis and provides a very useful algorithm.

FIRST LINE THERAPIES

■ Observation	D
■ Removal or withdrawal of the causative agent (e.g. drug)	D
■ Colchicine	C
■ Dapsone	E

Management of necrotizing vasculitis with colchicine. Improvement in patients with cutaneous lesions and Behçet's syndrome. Hazen PG, Michel B. Arch Dermatol 1979;115:1303–6.

These authors were the first to note that vasculitis might respond to oral colchicine in an open-label observation of six patients.

Colchicine is effective in controlling chronic cutaneous leukocytoclastic vasculitis. Callen JP. J Am Acad Dermatol 1985;13:193–200.

This open-label study involved 13 patients.

Subsequent work, published only in abstract form, confirmed these initial observations.

Colchicine in the treatment of cutaneous leukocytoclastic vasculitis: results of a prospective, randomized controlled trial. Sais G, Vidaller A, Jucgla A, et al. Arch Dermatol 1995;131:1399–402.

This double-blind, placebo-controlled trial of colchicine failed to demonstrate a positive benefit; however, the colchicine-treated group included all patients who had been previously treated with dapsone and had failed to respond. In addition, there were unequal numbers of patients with hepatitis C-associated disease in each group. Thus the study population included patients with more recalcitrant disease, and there was an inadvertent bias that occurred during the process of randomization.

Sulfone therapy in the treatment of leukocytoclastic vasculitis. Report of three cases. Fredenberg MF, Malkinson FD. J Am Acad Dermatol 1987;16:772–8.

Three patients with LCV limited to their skin were successfully treated with moderate doses of dapsone (100–150 mg daily).

SECOND LINE THERAPIES

■ Systemic corticosteroids	D
■ Immunosuppressive/cytotoxic agents – azathioprine, methotrexate, cyclophosphamide, cyclosporine, mycophenolate mofetil	D

Azathioprine. An effective, corticosteroid-sparing therapy for patients with recalcitrant cutaneous lupus erythematosus or with recalcitrant cutaneous leukocytoclastic vasculitis. Callen JP, Spencer LV, Burruss JB, Holtman J. Arch Dermatol 1991;127:515–22.

Open-label trial involving six patients who had failed to respond to 'less-toxic' therapies.

Prednisone plus azathioprine treatment in patients with rheumatoid arthritis complicated by vasculitis. Heurkens AH, Westedt ML, Breedveld FC. Arch Intern Med 1991;151:2249–54.

These authors studied 28 patients with rheumatoid arthritis-associated vasculitis. Nine patients with severe systemic vasculitis improved with 60 mg of prednisone and 2 mg/kg body weight of azathioprine daily. Nineteen patients with only cutaneous vasculitis entered a randomized controlled study comparing prednisone plus azathioprine treatment vs continuation of a previous regimen. Although measures of both vasculitis and arthritis activity improved to a greater degree in the patients treated with prednisone plus azathioprine in the first 3 months of therapy, and this therapy was associated with a low incidence of relapse of vasculitis, there was no significant difference between the results of the two treatment protocols at the end of the follow-up period.

The authors concluded that the combination was useful only for those patients with severe vasculitis. However, close analysis of their data does suggest that there were lower corticosteroid doses in the azathioprine-treated group.

Low-dose methotrexate therapy for cutaneous vasculitis of rheumatoid arthritis. Upchurch KS, Heller K, Bress NM. J Am Acad Dermatol 1987;17:355–9.

A patient with classic rheumatoid arthritis who developed LCV is described. Low-dose methotrexate produced prompt healing of the skin lesions. After discontinuation of methotrexate, the lesions recurred, with resolution after a second course of the drug.

This is a single case that responded; however, while there are other cases that have responded, there are many examples of patients whose vasculitis was initiated by or was worsened by methotrexate, particularly those with rheumatoid arthritis.

Chronic, recurrent small-vessel cutaneous vasculitis. Clinical experience in 13 patients. Cupps TR, Springer RM, Fauci AS. JAMA 1982;247:1994–8.

The clinical experience in 13 patients with small vessel cutaneous vasculitis limited to the skin is presented. This group of patients is represented by chronic and recurrent isolated cutaneous vasculitis eruptions, absence of disease progression to systemic involvement during long-term follow-up, and relative unresponsiveness to immunosuppressive therapy, including treatment with corticosteroid (prednisone) and cyclophosphamide.

This study suggests that cyclophosphamide therapy is poorly effective and, because of its potential toxicity, should be avoided. Other studies have documented individuals who have responded and individual patients whose disease was presumably induced by the cyclophosphamide. However, patients with severe necrotizing vasculitis, Wegener's granulomatosis, or polyarteritis nodosa should be treated with cyclophosphamide.

THIRD LINE THERAPIES

■ Antihistamines	E
■ Nonsteroidal anti-inflammatory drugs	D
■ Dietary restriction	D
■ Pentoxifylline (oxpentifylline)	E
■ Interferon-alfa	A

Elimination diet in the treatment of selected patients with hypersensitivity vasculitis. Lunardi C, Bambara LM, Biasi D, et al. Clin Exp Rheumatol 1992;10:131–5.

Five patients with hypersensitivity vasculitis were treated with a 3-week elimination diet, followed by open and double-blind challenge tests with specific foods and additives. Four patients achieved a complete remission and one patient experienced great improvement on the elimination diet. In three cases the vasculitis relapsed following the introduction of food additives; in one case with the addition of potatoes and green vegetables (i.e. beans and green peas) and in the last case with the addition of eggs to the diet. The offending foods and additives were subsequently eliminated from the usual diet and no relapses were observed in 2 years of follow-up.

These results show that, in some patients, hypersensitivity vasculitis can be triggered and sustained by food antigens or additives, and possibly treated with an elimination diet.

Leukocytoclastic vasculitis caused by drug additives. Lowry MD, Hudson CF, Callen JP. J Am Acad Dermatol 1994;30:854–5.

A patient with chronic cutaneous LCV in whom the presumed cause was an excipient (a dye) used in the capsule form of lithium carbonate was reported. Elimination of this dye from the patient's diet led to control of her chronic cutaneous vasculitis.

Interferon alfa-2a therapy in cryoglobulinemia associated with hepatitis C virus. Misiani R, Bellavita P, Fenili D, et al. N Engl J Med 1994;330:751–6.

In a prospective, randomized, controlled trial, 53 patients with hepatitis C virus (HCV)-associated type II cryoglobulinemia were studied. A group of 27 patients received recombinant interferon-alfa-2a three times weekly at a dose of 1.5 million units for a week and then 3 million units three times weekly for the following 23 weeks. The 26 control patients did not receive anything apart from previously prescribed treatments. All patients were then followed for an additional 24–48 weeks. After the treatment period, serum HCV RNA was undetectable in 15 of the remaining 25 patients who received interferon-alfa-2a, but in none of the controls. In comparison with the control group, the 15 patients with undetectable levels of HCV RNA in serum had a significant improvement in cutaneous vasculitis ($p = 0.04$) and significant decreases in serum levels of anti-HCV antibody activity ($p = 0.007$), cryoglobulins ($p = 0.002$), IgM ($p = 0.002$), rheumatoid factor ($p = 0.001$), and creatinine ($p = 0.006$). After treatment with interferon-alfa-2a was discontinued, viremia and cryoglobulinemia recurred in all 15 HCV RNA-negative patients. On resumption of treatment, three of four patients had a virologic, clinical, and biochemical response.

In patients with HCV-associated small vessel vasculitis, interferon-alfa may be of benefit.

Synergistic effects of pentoxifylline and dapsone in leucocytoclastic vasculitis. Nurnberg W, Grabbe J, Czarnetzki BM. Lancet 1994;343:491.

A single case is reported.

Chronic leukocytoclastic vasculitis associated with polycythemia vera: effective control with pentoxifylline. Wahba-Yahav AV. J Am Acad Dermatol 1992;26:1006–7.

OTHER THERAPIES

■ α_1-protease inhibitor replacement	E
■ IVIG	D
■ Plasma exchange	E
■ Rituximab	C

Effective treatment with alpha 1-protease inhibitor of chronic cutaneous vasculitis associated with alpha 1-antitrypsin deficiency. Dowd SK, Rodgers GC, Callen JP. J Am Acad Dermatol 1995;33:913–6.

A 49-year-old man with cutaneous vasculitis and α_1-antitrypsin deficiency failed to respond to colchicine, prednisone, and antibiotics, but was controlled by the intermittent administration of α_1-protease inhibitor.

Case report: steroid sparing effect of intravenous gamma globulin in a child with necrotizing vasculitis. Gedalia A, Correa H, Kaiser M, Sorensen R. Am J Med Sci 1995;309:226–8.

A $2\frac{1}{2}$-year-old boy with fever, arthritis, and necrotizing cutaneous vasculitis improved significantly with the administration of prednisone; however, several attempts to diminish the prednisone dose resulted in relapses. The prednisone was successfully tapered and discontinued after intravenous gamma globulin administration.

Plasma exchange in refractory cutaneous vasculitis. Turner AN, Whittaker S, Banks I, et al. Br J Dermatol 1990;122:411–5.

Eight patients with intractable cutaneous LCV were treated with plasma-exchange therapy. Seven improved, five substantially. Four continued to be treated by intermittent plasma exchange for periods of 5–12 years. Apart from one episode of hepatitis B, possibly related to administration of fresh frozen plasma, no major adverse effects have occurred.

Plasma exchange may be useful via the delivery of intravenous immunoglobulin within the fresh frozen plasma. If it were merely 'cleaning' the blood of antigen–antibody complexes, one would presumably require the addition of an immunosuppressive agent.

Nine patients with anti-neutrophil cytoplasmic antibody-positive vasculitis successfully treated with rituximab. Eriksson P. J Intern Med 2005;257:540–8.

This open-label study detailed the author's experience with rituximab, a chimeric monoclonal antibody that depletes CD20+ B-cells, for patients with ANCA+ vasculitis. Several of the patients had cutaneous disease which also improved with this therapy.

Lichen myxedematosus

Avani D Desai, William D James

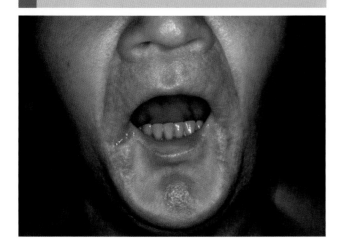

Lichen myxedematosus is a rare, idiopathic cutaneous disorder characterized by the formation of lichenoid papules, nodules, and plaques due to dermal mucin deposition. Infiltration, commonly affecting the face, trunk, and extremities, predisposes to extensive thickening and hardening of the skin, which may become raised, large folds. A severe generalized form of the disease is termed scleromyxedema which is commonly associated with monoclonal IgG λ gammopathy and frequent systemic involvement. Less commonly, some patients exhibit a discrete papular form that tends to remain localized.

MANAGEMENT STRATEGY

Treatment of lichen myxedematosus remains a therapeutic challenge with localized forms having a more favorable prognosis. The absence of any controlled studies concerning the efficiency of different drugs has led to the development of many treatment regimens.

Although the correlation between scleromyxedema with monoclonal gammopathy and multiple myeloma is uncertain, patients with lichen myxedematosus respond favorably to antimetabolites, particularly *melphalan*. Melphalan is an alkylating agent generally prescribed as a pulse regimen of 14 mg four times daily for 4 days every 4–6 weeks or 4 mg four times daily until symptoms resolve; however, its use is limited in localized disease by secondary adverse effects including malignancy and sepsis. Melphalan has also shown beneficial results when used in combination with other therapies, including *plasmapheresis, oral prednisone* 60 mg four times daily for 4–6 weeks with gradual taper, or *autologous stem cell transplant*.

Several other chemotherapeutic agents, including *2-chlorodeoxyadenosine (cladribine)* 0.1 mg/kg for 7 days, *cyclophosphamide* 200 mg four times daily, *cyclosporine* 50–100 mg once daily, *methotrexate* 5 mg per week for 6 months, and *thalidomide* 100 mg once daily have resulted in a demonstrated improvement in several patients with advanced local disease or systemic involvement.

As an alternative to immunosuppressive agents, *isotretinoin* 40 mg twice daily for 4 months has shown favorable responses in several patients including patients with HIV or hepatitis C infection.

Variable anecdotal success has been reported in several patients with the use of *interferon alfa-2b* 6–10 million units subcutaneously three times a week, *high-dose intravenous immunoglobulin, intralesional triamcinolone acetonide, interferon-alfa, psoralen with UVA (PUVA)*, and *extracorporeal photochemotherapy*.

SPECIFIC INVESTIGATIONS

- Serum protein electrophoresis
- Tests for hepatitis C infection
- Tests for HIV infection

Scleromyxedema revisited. Pomann JJ, Rudner EJ. Int J Dermatol 2003;42:31–5.

An abnormal paraprotein, most commonly a monoclonal IgG λ, is found in 80% of patients with scleromyxedema. It does not appear to represent a primary plasma cell dyscrasia, nor is there a consistent association with multiple myeloma.

Lichen myxedematosus associated with chronic hepatitis C. Banno H, Takama H, Nitta Y, et al. Int J Dermatol 2000; 39:212–4.

A high prevalence of hepatitis C virus (HCV) infection associated with lichen myxedematosus is reported – eight of 16 patients displayed liver dysfunction with anti-HCV antibodies.

Updated classification of papular mucinosis, lichen myxedematosus, and scleromyxedema. Rongioletti F, Rebora A. J Am Acad Dermatol 2001;44:273–81.

Fourteen cases of localized lichen myxedematosus in HIV-positive patients have been reported.

FIRST LINE THERAPIES

■ Melphalan	C
■ Systemic corticosteroids	D
■ Plasmapheresis	D

Scleromyxedema. Dinneen AM, Dicken CH. J Am Acad Dermatol 1995;33:37–43.

A review of 17 patients treated with melphalan, revealing improvement of cutaneous symptoms in 12 patients and the development of lethal complications, including hematologic malignancy and sepsis, in nine.

A complete and durable clinical response to high-dose dexamethasone in a patient with scleromyxedema. Horn K, Horn M, Swan J, et al. J Am Acad Dermatol 2004;51: S120–3.

A case of a patient with scleromyxedema successfully treated with high-dose dexamethasone.

Successful treatment of scleromyxedema with plasmapheresis and immunosuppression. Keong CH, Asaka Y, Fukuro S, et al. J Am Acad Dermatol 1990;22:842–4.

Plasmapheresis used in conjunction with immunosuppression (pulse methylprednisolone and cyclophosphamide) caused regression of recalcitrant cutaneous symptoms.

SECOND LINE THERAPIES

■ Isotretinoin/etretinate	D
■ Topical or intralesional corticosteroids	E

Improvement of scleromyxedema associated with isotretinoin therapy. Hisler BM, Savoy LB, Hashimoto K. J Am Acad Dermatol 1991;24:854–7.

A report of scleromyxedema with myopathy showing improvement after treatment with isotretinoin at a dose of 40 mg twice daily.

Discrete papular mucinosis responding to intralesional and topical steroids. Reynolds NJ, Collins CM, Burton JL. Arch Dermatol 1992;128:857–8.

A case of complete response to triamcinolone acetonide and Haelan®, an adhesive polyethylene tape, impregnated with flurandrenolide.

THIRD LINE THERAPIES

■ 2-Chlorodeoxyadenosine	E
■ Cyclophosphamide	E
■ Cyclosporine	E
■ Methotrexate	E
■ Thalidomide	E
■ Autologous stem cell transplantation	E
■ Extracorporeal photophoresis	E
■ Intravenous immunoglobulins	E
■ Interferon-α-2b	E
■ PUVA	E
■ Radiation	E

Chemotherapeutic agents

Treatment of scleromyxedema with 2-chlorodeoxyadenosine. Davis LS, Sanal S, Sangueza OP. J Am Acad Dermatol 1996;35:288–90.

Upon failure to respond to oral prednisone, marked improvement occurred in one patient treated with 2-chlorodeoxyadenosine, a purine analog used mainly in the treatment of lymphoproliferative disorders.

Scleromyxedema: immunosuppressive therapy with cyclophosphamide. Aberer W, Wolff K. Hautarzt 1988;39:277–80.

Monthly high-dose intravenous cyclophosphamide pulse therapy together with prednisone resulted in a dramatic improvement of symptoms.

Successful treatment of intractable scleromyxedema with cyclosporine A. Saigoh S, Tashiro A, Fujita S, et al. Dermatol 2003;207:410–1.

On failing PUVA and oral prednisone, a patient's condition improved rapidly upon starting treatment with cyclosporine A.

Scleromyxedema myopathy: case report and review of the literature. Helfrich DJ, Walker ER, Martinez AJ, Meedsgar TA. Arthritis Rheum 1988;31:1437–41.

Oral prednisone and intravenous methotrexate resulted in improvement of cutaneous and systemic symptoms in one patient.

Treatment of recalcitrant scleromyxedema with thalidomide in 3 patients. Sansbury J, Cocuroccia B, Jorizzo J, et al. J Am Acad Dermatol 2004;51:126–31.

Within 2 months of starting thalidomide treatment, three patients with recalcitrant scleromyxedema displayed marked improvement of cutaneous lesions, joint mobility, and reduction of paraprotein levels.

Complete remission of scleromyxedema following autologous stem cell transplantation. Feasel AM, Donato ML, Duvic M. Arch Dermal 2001;137:1071–2.

Complete resolution was achieved with high-dose pulse dexamethasone, high-dose melphalan, and autologous stem cell transplantation in a patient with rapidly progressive scleromyxedema in whom multiple treatments had previously failed.

Cutaneo-systemic papulosclerotic mucinosis (scleromyxedema): remission after extracorporeal photochemotherapy and corticoid bolus. D'Incan M, Franck F, Kanold J, et al. Ann Dermatol Venereol 2001;128:38–41.

A complete cutaneous therapeutic response was obtained in one patient after twelve extracorporeal photopheresis courses and four pulse treatments of prednisolone.

Intravenous immunoglobulins control scleromyxedema. Righi A, Schiavon F, Jablonska S, et al. Ann Rheum Dis 2002;61:59–61.

Intravenous immunoglobulin has been successfully employed in the treatment of three patients with scleromyxedema.

Scleromyxedema: treatment with interferon alfa. Tschen JA, Chang JR. J Am Acad Dermatol 1999;40:303–7.

One patient who failed to respond to chlorambucil and isotretinoin showed improvement of cutaneous symptoms with interferon-alfa-2b, but little improvement of extracutaneous manifestations.

PUVA treatment of scleromyxoedema. Farr PM, Ive FA. Br J Dermatol 1984;110:347–50.

On failing to respond to cyclophosphamide, treatment with PUVA was commenced in a 60-year-old woman with scleromyxoedema, leading to complete resolution and no recurrence of disease.

Successful management of lichen myxedematosus. Hill TG, Crawford JN, Rogers CC. Arch Dermatol 1976;112:67–9.

A case report of successful treatment with conventional radiation therapy.

Evidence levels **A** Double-blind study **B** Clinical trial ≥ 20 subjects **C** Clinical trial < 20 subjects **D** Series ≥ 5 subjects **E** Anecdotal case reports

Lichen nitidus

Andrew L Wright

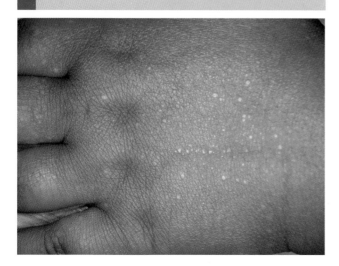

Lichen nitidus is an uncommon idiopathic condition, composed of 1–2 mm diameter flat-topped or domed papules. They usually remain discrete, though they may be grouped. They can occur on any part of the body, but predominantly affect the forearms, penis, abdomen, chest, and buttocks. Palmar lesions may be hemorrhagic.

MANAGEMENT STRATEGY

Lichen nitidus persists for long periods of time, but is generally asymptomatic and *treatment may not be necessary*. No large controlled clinical trials have been reported; most treatments are based on anecdotal reports.

In patients with localized disease, *fluorinated topical corticosteroids* can be successful in clearing lesions. *Antihistamines*, including *astemizole* and *cetirizine*, are reported to have cleared lesions. It should be noted that astemizole has been discontinued because of cardiotoxicity noted with certain drug interactions. It is presumed that safer antihistamines would also be valuable. Generalized lesions have cleared with *psoralen plus UVA (PUVA)* and *acitretin*.

SPECIFIC INVESTIGATIONS

■ Biopsy	

FIRST LINE THERAPIES

■ Topical corticosteroids	E

Successful treatment of lichen nitidus. Wright S. Arch Dermatol 1984;120:155–6.

A 24-year-old woman with a 12-year history of extensive lesions cleared with 1 month's treatment twice daily of 0.05% fluocinonide cream. No recurrence was noted at 12-month follow-up.

SECOND LINE THERAPIES

■ PUVA	E
■ Antihistamines	D
■ Oral retinoids	E
■ Acitretin	E

Treatment of generalised lichen nitidus with PUVA. Randall HW, Sander HM. Int J Dermatol 1986;25:330–1.

A 29-year-old woman with an 8-month history of a generalized eruption was treated with PUVA three times weekly. Lesions cleared after 46 treatments (290 J), and remained clear 5 years later.

Generalised lichen nitidus – a report of two cases treated with astemizole. Ocampo J, Torne R. Int J Dermatol 1989;28:49–51.

Two patients treated with astemizole, a 65-year-old man with a 3-month history and a 48-year-old woman with a 4-month history, were either cleared or dramatically improved with 6–12 days of astemizole 10 mg daily.

Lichen nitidus treated with astemizole. Thio HB. Br J Dermatol 1993;129:342.

A 20-year-old woman with widespread disease responded to astemizole 10 mg daily, after relapsing following a successful course of PUVA. There was no recurrence of lesions at 2-year follow-up.

Association of lichen planus and lichen nitidus – treatment with etretinate. Aram H. Int J Dermatol 1988;27:117.

A 35-year-old woman with a 4-month history cleared with 8 weeks of etretinate 25 mg/50 mg on alternate days. Treatment was stopped 1 month later. There was no recurrence 5 months after completing the treatment.

Treatment of palmoplantar lichen nitidus with acitretin. Lucker GPH, Koopman RJJ, Steijlen PM, Van Der Valik PGM. Br J Dermatol 1994;130:791–3.

A 23-year-old man had a 14-month history of hand and foot involvement that failed to clear with acitretin 50 mg daily, but was reported to have improved significantly on 75 mg daily.

THIRD LINE THERAPIES

■ Itraconazole	E
■ Dinitrochlorobenzene (DNCB)	E
■ Cetirizine dihydrochloride, levamisole	E
■ Isoniazid	E

Treatment of lichen planus and lichen nitidus with itraconazole: reports of six cases. Libow LF, Coots NV. Cutis 1998;62:247–8.

A report of two cases showing partial clearance of lichen nitidus after 2 weeks of itraconazole 200 mg twice daily.

Improvement of lichen nitidus after topical dinitrochlorobenzene application. Kano Y, Otake Y, Shiohara T. J Am Acad Dermatol 1998;39:305–8.

This reports on a patient treated with 0.1% DNCB applied at 2-weekly intervals, following sensitization with 1% DNCB. The lesions were said to have cleared after 7 months of treatment, compared to a control area. Six months after cessation of treatment lesions were said to be recurring in the treated area.

Generalised lichen nitidus in a child – response to cetirizine dihydrochloride/levamisole. Seghal VN, Jain S, Kumar S, et al. Aus J Dermatol 1998;39:60.

A 6-year-old boy with a 6-month history of generalized involvement showed complete regression/healing of lesions over a 4-week period of treatment with cetirizine dihydrochloride 5 mg daily and levamisole 50 mg alternate days for 4 weeks.

Generalised lichen nitidus is successfully treated with an antituberculous agent. Kubota Y, Kirya H, Nakayama J. Br J Dermatol 2002;146:1081–3.

A 10-year old Japanese girl with a 2-year history of lichen nitidus showed almost complete clearance following a 6-month course of oral isoniazid.

Evidence levels A Double-blind study **B** Clinical trial ≥ 20 subjects **C** Clinical trial < 20 subjects **D** Series ≥ 5 subjects **E** Anecdotal case reports

Lichen planopilaris

Eric Berkowitz, Mark G Lebwohl

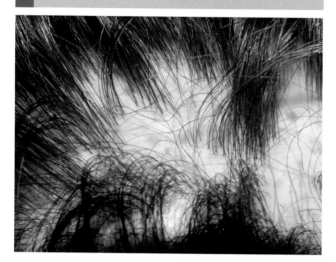

Lichen planopilaris is a clinical syndrome consisting of lichen planus associated with cicatricial scalp alopecia. The condition is more common in women and presents with perifollicular erythema and keratotic plugs at the margins of the expanding alopecia. The follicular involvement is limited to the infundibulum and the isthmus, both demonstrating lichenoid inflammation. The main complications of follicular lichen planus are atrophy and scarring with permanent hair loss.

MANAGEMENT STRATEGY

Therapeutic management for lichen planopilaris is difficult and challenging. However, if the inflammation associated with lichen planopilaris can be controlled in its early stages, follicular units may be preserved and hair regrowth may be possible. For the most part, therapeutic reports are anecdotal. *Oral antihistamines* may be used to control pruritus, while *high potency topical corticosteroids* are used to control the inflammation in early lesions. *Intralesional injections of 3–5 mg/mL of triamcinolone acetonide* are effective in well-developed lesions. *Retinoids* have demonstrated some effect in the treatment of lichen planus and therefore provide a possible alternative to corticosteroid treatment. Additional treatment modalities include the *antimalarials*, in particular hydroxychloroquine if used over months. Other agents that have been reported to work are *cyclosporine* and *mycophenolate mofetil*. There is some rationale for trying biologic agents such as the tumor necrosis factor (TNF) agents for this condition.

SPECIFIC INVESTIGATIONS

- Skin biopsy
- Immunofluorescence studies

Elastic tissue in scars and alopecia. Elston DM, McCollough ML, Warschaw KE, Bergfeld WF. J Cutan Pathol 2000;27:147–52.

This investigation determined that the Verhoeff–van Gieson elastic stain can reliably differentiate scarred from non-scarred dermis and is reliable in distinguishing lichen planopilaris from lupus erythematosus.

Immunofluorescence abnormalities in lichen planopilaris. Ioannides D, Bystryn JC. Arch Dermatol 1992;128:214–6.

Direct immunofluorescence studies were performed on biopsied lesions of patients with lichen planopilaris and lichen planus. All of the lichen planopilaris studies demonstrated abnormal linear deposits of immunoglobin consisting of IgG or IgA restricted to the basement membrane. The biopsies from those with lichen planus demonstrated fibrillar deposits.

These different appearances possibly suggest different disease processes.

FIRST LINE THERAPIES

■ High potency corticosteroids	D
■ Intralesional corticosteroids	C

Lichen planopilaris: report of 30 cases and review of the literature. Chieregato C, Zini A, Barba A, et al. Int J Dermatol 2003;42:342–5.

This clinical trial reports good therapeutic benefit with early treatment with high potency topical steroids. Only four patients did not respond to the therapy and needed other treatments.

Scarring alopecia. Newton RC, Hebert AA, Freese TW, Solomon AR. Dermatol Clin 1987;5:603–18.

High potency topical corticosteroids may be used to control inflammation in early scalp lesions. Intralesional injections with triamcinolone acetonide at concentrations of 3–5 mg/mL are more effective in well-developed lesions. Additionally, oral corticosteroids have been used in short tapering dosages to control severe disease.

SECOND LINE THERAPIES

■ Oral corticosteroids	C
■ Retinoids	C
■ Antimalarials	C

Postmenopausal frontal fibrosing alopecia: a frontal variant of lichen planopilaris. Kossard S, Lee MS, Wilkinson B. J Am Acad Dermatol 1997;36:59–66.

Oral corticosteroids and antimalarials were found to slow the course of lichen planopilaris.

Lichen planopilaris: clinical and pathologic study of forty-five patients. Mehregan DA, Van Hale HM, Muller SA. J Am Acad Dermatol 1992;27(6 Pt 1):935–42.

This large study of 45 patients involved multiple different therapeutic modalities. High potency topical steroids and oral steroids (30–40 mg daily) for 3 months demonstrated the highest success rates.

Oral treatment of keratinizing disorders of skin and mucous membranes with etretinate. Comparative study of 113 patients. Mahrle G, Meyer-Hamme S, Ippen H. Arch Dermatol 1982;118:97–100.

This paper reports the comparative results of the effects of the aromatic retinoid etretinate on various skin disorders.

Retinoids have been found to have a significant impact in cases of lichen planus and therefore have been tried with some success in cases of lichen planopilaris. Isotretinoin may be preferred over acitretin since the latter agent has been associated with hair loss.

THIRD LINE THERAPIES

■ Mycophenolate mofetil	E
■ Griseofulvin	E
■ Cyclosporine	D
■ Tacrolimus	E
■ Thalidomide	E
■ TNF-blocking drugs	E

Treatment of lichen planopilaris with mycophenolate mofetil. Tursen U, Api H, Kaya Y, Ikizoglu G. Dermatol Online J 2004;10:24.

The authors report a case of lichen planopilaris that was successfully treated with mycophenolate mofetil.

Lichen planopilaris [cicatricial (scarring) alopecia] in a child. Sehgal VN, Bajaj P, Srivastva G. Int J Dermatol 2001;40:461–3.

This case report describes the successful treatment of lichen planopilaris using combination therapy with griseofulvin, prednisolone, and topical betamethasone diproprionate lotion.

Short course of oral cyclosporine in lichen planopilaris. Mirmirani P, Willey A, Price V. J Am Acad Dermatol 2003; 49:667–71.

The authors present three patients with recalcitrant lichen planopilaris, unresponsive to hydroxychloroquine, high potency topical steroids, and intralesional steroids, who were treated with cyclosporine. The duration of treatment ranged from 3 to 5 months, with resolution of symptoms, no progression of hair loss, and no evidence of disease activity. One of the patients did have a mild recurrence, which resolved with topical 0.1% tacrolimus in Cetaphil lotion®.

Thalidomide-induced remission of lichen planopilaris. Boyd AS, King LE Jr. J Am Acad Dermatol 2002;47:967–8.

The authors describe the case of a patient who was diagnosed with lichen planopilaris and then treated with hydroxychloroquine, azathioprine, isotretinoin, cyclophosphamide, dapsone, cyclosporine, levamisole, chloroquine, acitretin, methotrexate, clofazamine, and enoxaparin – all without any benefit. The patient was then started on thalidomide 50 mg orally twice a day, with resolution of the symptoms. However, side effects limited the ability to continue the medication. Initially, the patient only complained of fatigue and constipation; however, at 4 months, mild numbness and tingling of the fingers and toes began to develop and the patient experienced significant depression, necessitating discontinuation of the medication.

Thalidomide's mechanism of action in this disorder may involve TNF inhibition, suggesting that medications such as adalimumab, etanercept, or infliximab may be beneficial.

Evidence levels **A** Double-blind study **B** Clinical trial ≥ 20 subjects **C** Clinical trial < 20 subjects **D** Series ≥ 5 subjects **E** Anecdotal case reports

Lichen planus

Mark G Lebwohl

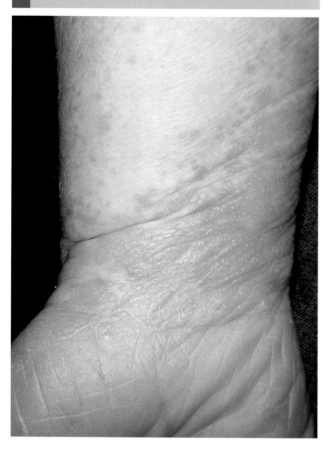

Lichen planus is a pruritic papulosquamous disease with characteristic histopathologic and clinical features. Oral erosive lichen planus, a painful erosive condition that can affect mucous membranes, is addressed on page 444.

MANAGEMENT STRATEGY

Although lichen planus can resolve spontaneously, treatment is usually demanded by patients who can be severely symptomatic. Underlying diseases such as hepatitis C or associated drugs should be sought.

In patients with localized disease, *superpotent corticosteroids* should be applied twice daily for 2–4 weeks. If the response is inadequate, *intralesional injection of corticosteroids* into localized lesions may be beneficial. Topical antipruritic agents containing *menthol, phenol, camphor, lidocaine, pramoxine* or *doxepin hydrochloride* can be useful. *Oral antihistamines* may offer limited benefit in severely pruritic patients. Sedating antihistamines are helpful at bedtime.

Traditionally, patients with extensive lichen planus have been treated with systemic corticosteroids. In recent years *oral metronidazole* has emerged as a safe and effective alternative to systemic corticosteroids: 500 mg twice daily for 20–60 days has proven to be effective in many patients. In patients who do not respond, *oral prednisone* 30–60 mg daily for 2–6 weeks, or its equivalent, tapered over the ensuing 2–6 weeks, is often effective. Unfortunately, even in patients who clear with systemic corticosteroids, relapses are frequent. If patients require more than two courses of high-dose systemic corticosteroids over the span of a few months, alternative treatments should be sought.

Isotretinoin in doses of 10 mg orally twice daily for 2 months has been reported to clear lichen planus in several patients, and *acitretin* 30 mg has also resulted in marked improvement or remission. In refractory cases, *psoralen and UVA (PUVA)* has demonstrated efficacy in the treatment of lichen planus and has been particularly beneficial in the lichen planus-like eruption associated with graft versus host disease. For severe and refractory lichen planus unresponsive to other therapies, immunosuppressive agents including *cyclosporine, mycophenolate mofetil,* or *azathioprine* are often effective.

SPECIFIC INVESTIGATIONS

- Serology for hepatitis B and C
- Liver function tests

Lichen planus and hepatitis C virus: prevalence and clinical presentation of patients with lichen planus and hepatitis C virus infection. Sanchez-Perez J, De Castro M, Buezo GF, et al. Br J Dermatol 1996;134:715–9.

Of 78 patients with lichen planus 20% had anti-hepatitis C virus antibodies.

Lichen planus and chronic active hepatitis. A retrospective survey. Rebora A, Rongioletti F. Acta Derm Venereol 1984; 64:52–6.

Six of 44 patients with lichen planus had abnormal liver function tests and five of the six were found to have chronic active hepatitis on liver biopsy.

Drug-induced lichen planus. Thompson DF, Skaehill PA. Pharmacotherapy 1994;14:561–71.

β-blockers, methyldopa, penicillamine, quinidine, quinine, and nonsteroidal anti-inflammatory agents play a role in the development of lichen planus. There is insufficient evidence to implicate angiotensin-converting enzyme inhibitors, sulfonylurea agents, carbamazepine, gold, lithium, and other drugs.

Many drugs and chemicals have been associated with lichenoid drug eruptions, which can be difficult to distinguish from true lichen planus. In addition to those mentioned above, hepatitis B vaccination, allopurinol, tetracyclines, furosemide, hydrochlorothiazide, isoniazid, and phenytoin are reported to cause lichenoid eruptions.

FIRST LINE THERAPIES

■ Topical corticosteroids	C
■ Intralesional corticosteroids	D
■ Antihistamines	C

Betamethasone-17,21-dipropionate ointment: an effective topical preparation in lichen ruber planus. Bjornberg A, Hellgren L. Curr Med Res Opin 1976;4:212–7.

Patients with lichen planus that had become resistant to betamethasone valerate ointment were treated with betamethasone dipropionate ointment once or twice daily for 2–3 weeks. Fourteen of 19 patients achieved better improvement with betamethasone dipropionate ointment.

Successful treatment of chronic skin diseases with clobetasol propionate and a hydrocolloid occlusive dressing. Volden G. Acta Derm Venereol 1992;72:69–71.

Occlusion of clobetasol propionate lotion led to complete remission of lichen planus in 2.8 weeks.

Although topical and intralesional corticosteroids are first line treatments for lichen planus, their use has been based on multiple anecdotal reports rather than on controlled clinical trials.

Treatment of lichen planus. Oliver GF, Winkelmann RK. Drugs 1993;45:56–65.

Mild lichen planus can be treated with rest, topical corticosteroids with or without wet dressings, or occlusion.

A good review article.

SECOND LINE THERAPIES

■ Metronidazole	C
■ Systemic corticosteroids	C
■ Isotretinoin, acitretin	A
■ Narrowband UVB	C
■ PUVA	C

Oral metronidazole treatment of lichen planus. Büyük AY, Kavala M. J Am Acad Dermatol 2000;43:260–2.

Nineteen patients with lichen planus were treated twice daily with 500 mg oral metronidazole for 20–60 days. Thirteen patients had 80–100% improvement and two additional patients had 50–80% reduction in lichen planus lesions. Only four patients failed to respond.

The safety of oral metronidazole has led many dermatologists to use this treatment as first line therapy for lichen planus.

Intermittent megadose corticosteroid therapy for generalized lichen planus. Snyder RA, Schwartz RA, Schneider JS, Elias PM. J Am Acad Dermatol 1982;6:1089–90.

This is a case report of a 70-year-old man with generalized lichen planus that cleared with 1 g methylprednisolone intravenously in a pulse dose daily for 3 days, each month for 3 months.

Treatment of lichen planus with acitretin. A double-blind, placebo-controlled study in 65 patients. Laurberg G, Geiger JM, Hjorth N, et al. J Am Acad Dermatol 1991;24: 434–7.

Acitretin resulted in marked improvement or remission in 64% of patients compared to 13% of placebo-treated patients in a double-blind trial in 65 subjects. Acitretin doses of 30 mg daily were used, leading to mucocutaneous side effects and hyperlipidemia.

Isotretinoin in doses of 10 mg orally twice daily has been effective in the treatment of oral lichen planus, and anecdotal use suggests efficacy in generalized lichen planus as well. The latter regimen has fewer mucocutaneous side effects than higher doses of acitretin.

Narrowband UVB therapy in the treatment of lichen planus. Saricaoglu H, Karadogan SK, Baskan EB, Tunali S. Photodermatol Photoimmunol Photomed 2003;19:265–7.

Ten patients with lichen planus were treated with narrowband UVB therapy three to four times per week. By the thirtieth session, five patients achieved complete responses and four achieved partial responses. Three of the four with partial responses went on to complete responses over the ensuing weeks.

Bilateral comparison of generalized lichen planus treated with psoralens and ultraviolet A. Gonzalez E, Momtaz-TK, Freedman S. J Am Acad Dermatol 1984;10:958–61.

PUVA demonstrated efficacy for lichen planus in a bilateral comparison study, with five of ten patients clearing completely, another three improving more than 50%, but the remaining two patients worsening. Maintenance treatments were not required to maintain clearing.

Trioxsalen baths plus UV-A in the treatment of lichen planus and urticaria pigmentosa. Väätäinen N, Hannuksela M, Karvonen J. Clin Exp Dermatol 1981;6:133–8.

A modified form of PUVA utilizing UVA exposure following trioxsalen bath has been effective in 16 of 19 treated patients.

Long-term efficacy of PUVA treatment in lichen planus: comparison of oral and external methoxsalen regimens. Helander I, Jansen CT, Meurman L. Photodermatol 1987;4: 265–8.

Good or excellent clearing occurred in ten of 13 patients after eight to 46 bath PUVA treatments compared to five of ten patients after eight to 30 oral PUVA treatments. Examination of patients months after PUVA, however, suggested that treatment might prolong the duration of lichen planus.

Treatment of lichen planus. An evidence-based medicine analysis of efficacy. Cribier B, Frances C, Chosidow O. Arch Dermatol 1998;134:1521–30.

Clinical trials are needed to establish the efficacy of systemic corticosteroids and PUVA.

The authors consider acitretin first line therapy for cutaneous lichen planus.

THIRD LINE THERAPIES

■ Trimethoprim–sulfamethoxazole	E
■ Griseofulvin, itraconazole	E
■ Cyclosporine, FK 506	E
■ Mycophenolate mofetil	E
■ Azathioprine	E
■ Levamisole	E
■ Photodynamic therapy	E
■ Interferon	E
■ 0.1% tacrolimus ointment	E
■ Thalidomide	E
■ UVA1	D

Antimicrobials

Treatment of lichen planus with Bactrim. Abdel-Aal H, Abdel-Aal MA. J Egypt Med Assoc 1976;59:547–9.

Oral trimethoprim–sulfamethoxazole, two tablets twice daily for 5 days, cleared lichen planus within 2 weeks only to have the skin lesions relapse 2 months later. The trimethoprim–sulfamethoxazole was again effective when readministered to patients who experienced relapse.

Histopathological evaluation of griseofulvin therapy in lichen planus: a double-blind controlled study. Sehgal VN,

Bikhchandani R, Koranne RV, et al. Dermatologica 1980;161: 22–7.

Griseofulvin 500 mg daily for 2 months was effective in 18 of 22 patients.

Griseofulvin therapy of lichen planus. Massa MC, Rogers RS III. Acta Derm Venereol 1981;61:547–50.

Griseofulvin was effective for lichen planus in only three of 15 patients.

Treatment of lichen planus and lichen nitidus with itraconazole: reports of six cases. Libow LF, Coots NV. Cutis 1998;62:247–8.

Anecdotally, itraconazole has been effective for isolated cases of lichen planus.

Immunosuppressive agents

Successful treatment of resistant hypertrophic and bullous lichen planus with mycophenolate mofetil. Nousari HC, Goyal S, Anhalt GJ. Arch Dermatol 1999;135: 1420–1.

Mycophenolate mofetil was reported to successfully treat resistant hypertrophic and bullous lichen planus.

Generalized severe lichen planus treated with azathioprine. Verma KK, Sirka CS, Khaitan BK. Acta Derm Venereol 1999;79:493.

Generalized severe lichen planus has been successfully treated with azathioprine.

Treatment of severe lichen planus with cyclosporine. Ho VC, Gupta AK, Ellis CN, et al. J Am Acad Dermatol 1990;22: 64–8.

Oral cyclosporine has been used very effectively in the treatment of severe lichen planus.

Tacrolimus FK 506 is likely to be effective as well. The nephrotoxicity associated with long-term use of both of the latter agents can be avoided if the treatment course is limited to a few months.

Other

Lichen planus treated with levamisole. Shaps RS, Grant JM, Sheard C. J Continuing Education Dermatol 1978; 32(Nov).

Levamisole 150 mg daily on two consecutive days per week for 6 weeks, resulted in improvement of lichen planus in four of six patients.

Treatment of lichen planus of the penis with photodynamic therapy. Kirby B, Whitehurst C, Moore JV, Yates VM. Br J Dermatol 1999;141:765–6.

Photodynamic therapy with δ-aminolevulinic acid has resulted in clearing of isolated lesions of lichen planus.

Successful interferon treatment for lichen planus associated with hepatitis due to hepatitis C virus infection. Lapidoth M, Arber N, Ben-Amitai D, Hagler J. Acta Derm Venereol 1997;77:171–2.

Lichen planus and chronic hepatitis C: exacerbation of the lichen under interferon therapy. Areias J, Velho GC, Cerqueira R, et al. Eur J Gastroenterol Hepatol 1996;8:825–8.

Given the association between lichen planus and hepatitis C, one might expect interferon to benefit both diseases. There are reports of interferon benefiting patients with lichen planus and exacerbating the condition in others.

Recalcitrant erosive flexural lichen planus: successful treatment with a combination of thalidomide and 0.1% tacrolimus ointment. Eisman S, Orteu CH. Clin Exp Dermatol 2004;29:268–70.

A patient with a 12-year history of ulcerated flexural lichen planus refractory to many treatments responded to a combination of topical 0.1% tacrolimus ointment and oral thalidomide followed by tacrolimus ointment alone.

Ultraviolet A1 in the treatment of generalized lichen planus: a report of 4 cases. Polderman MC, Wintzen M, van Leeuwen RL, et al. J Am Acad Dermatol 2004;50:646–7.

Four patients with refractory generalized lichen planus were treated with UVA1 45 J/cm^2 5 days per week for two 4-week treatment periods with a 3-week rest in between. All four patients improved with one of the patients achieving 98% clearance.

Lichen sclerosus

Nuala O'Donoghue, Sallie Neill

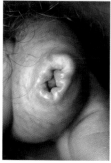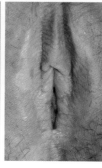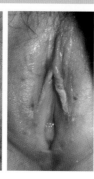

Lichen sclerosus et atrophicus (LSA) was first described as a variant of lichen planus. Some cases are not histologically atrophic, and so the term LSA has now been replaced with lichen sclerosus (LS) alone. LS is a chronic, scarring, lymphocyte-mediated dermatosis that has a predilection for the genital skin. It occurs predominantly in females, and has two peak ages of incidence: one in the prepubertal child and the other in the postmenopausal woman. 5% of cases of anogenital LS may be associated with squamous cell carcinoma (SCC).

MANAGEMENT STRATEGY

The aims of managing LS are to treat the symptoms of itch, burning and pain, heal the cutaneous lesions, reduce further scarring, and to prevent or detect malignant change. The scarring associated with LS in the female may cause loss of the labia minora, sealing over of the clitoral hood and burying of the clitoris. Less commonly there may be introital narrowing (possibly resulting in dyspareunia, and/or difficulties micturating) and the clitoral hood adhesions can result in pseudocyst formation. In young girls painful defecation may be the presenting symptom and *stool softeners* may be required. Scarring in male patients may result in phimosis and meatal stenosis, which may rarely progress to frank obstruction to urinary flow. Both sexes may develop postinflammatory pain syndromes after clinical improvement of the skin lesions (i.e. vestibulodynia, vulvodynia, see page 688), and penile dysesthesia. The symptom of pain does not respond to topical corticosteroids, so treatment includes *topical 5% lidocaine ointment*. Any patient with a chronic genital disorder may develop psychosexual problems and these may need to be addressed.

An *ultrapotent topical corticosteroid* is the first line treatment for LS at any site in either sex, although there have been no randomized controlled trials comparing potency, frequency of application, and duration of treatment. The regimen recommended by the authors for a newly diagnosed case is clobetasol propionate 0.05% ointment, initially once a night for 4 weeks, then on alternate nights for 4 weeks, and for the final third month, twice weekly. If the symptoms return with a drop in the schedule the patient is advised to go back up to the frequency that was effective. A 30 g-tube should last 12 weeks, at which point the patient is reviewed. If the treatment has been successful, the ecchymoses, fissuring, and erosions should have resolved, but the

scarring and some of the hypopigmentation may remain. LS is a disease of relapses and remissions, and topical clobetasol dipropionate is used as required; most patients seem to require 30–60 g annually. Although topical corticosteroids have been demonstrated to improve the symptoms and clinical signs in LS and may obviate the need for a curative *circumcision*, to date there is no evidence to show that their use decreases the risk of developing a SCC.

A *soap substitute* is also recommended, alongside *bland barrier ointments*, particularly if there is any urinary incontinence.

SPECIFIC INVESTIGATIONS

- Biopsy
- Thyroid function tests if clinically indicated

The diagnosis can often be made on clinical grounds. Classically there are white plaques with 'cigarette paper' atrophy in association with purpura, blisters, and erosions. In females the distribution is a figure-of-8 configuration around the vulva and anus. In males, the glans penis and foreskin are usually affected with sparing of the perianal area.

Light microscopic criteria for the diagnosis of early vulvar lichen sclerosus: a comparison with lichen planus. Fung MA, LeBoit PE. Am J Surg Pathol 1998;22:473–8.

Light microscopy classically demonstrates a thinned epidermis with hyperkeratosis, below the dermal-epidermal junction (DEJ) a wide band of homogenized collagen, and a lymphocytic infiltrate beneath this. In early lesions, the inflammatory infiltrate can be close to the DEJ, so differentiation between LS and lichen planus needs to be made: the presence of a psoriasiform lichenoid pattern, epidermotropism, decreased elastic fibers, follicular plugging, a thickened basement membrane, and epidermal atrophy are more suggestive of LS.

Vulval lichen sclerosus: lack of correlation between duration of clinical symptoms and histological appearances. Marren P, Millard PR, Wojnarowska F. J Eur Acad Dermatol Venereol 1997;8:212–6.

Clinicopathological study in 20 untreated patients showing that the inflammatory component of the pathological process was a persistent or recurring phenomenon.

FIRST LINE THERAPIES

■ Ultrapotent topical corticosteroids	A
■ Emollients	E
■ Avoidance of local irritants, including soap substitution	E

Clinical and histologic effects of topical treatments of vulval lichen sclerosus. A critical evaluation. Bracco GL, Carli P, Sonni L, et al. J Reprod Med 1993;38:37–40.

A randomized study on 79 adults, treated for 3 months. Remission of symptoms occurred in 75% of patients treated with 0.05% clobetasol, 20% treated with 2% testosterone, 10% treated with 2% progesterone, and 10% treated with placebo cream.

The treatment of vulval lichen sclerosus with a very potent topical steroid (clobetasol propionate 0.05%) cream. Dalziel KL, Millard PR, Wojnarowska F. Br J Dermatol 1991; 124:461–4.

A 12-week prospective study of 15 patients; twice daily treatment resulted in a marked clinical improvement in all 13 patients who completed the study, maintaining their improvement for up to 22 months of follow-up.

Penile lichen sclerosus et atrophicus treated with clobetasol dipropionate 0.05% cream: a retrospective clinical and histopathological study. Dahlman-Ghozlan K, Hedblad MA, von Krogh G. J Am Acad Dermatol 1999;40:451–7.

Twenty two men treated with clobetasol propionate documented significant improvement in soreness and foreskin tightness.

Clinical features of lichen sclerosus in men attending a department of genitourinary medicine. Riddell L, Edwards A, Sherrard J. Sex Transm Infect 2000;76:311–3.

A case note review of 66 men with LS who were all treated with clobetasol propionate 0.05% cream. Although 12% underwent circumcision and 8% required urethral dilatation, surgery was avoided in the remainder.

Treatment of phimosis with topical steroids in 194 children. Ashfield JE, Nickel KR, Siemens DR, et al. J Urol 2003;169:1106–8.

On referral for circumcision 194 boys with phimosis of unknown cause were treated with a 6-week course of twice daily 0.1% betamethasone ointment to the prepuce. Circumcision was avoided in 87%.

Topical corticosteroids are the standard conservative measure for treating phimosis; 10–15% of these boys have undiagnosed LS.

Treatment of childhood vulvar lichen sclerosus with potent topical corticosteroid. Fischer G, Rogers M. Pediatr Dermatol 1997;14:235–8.

Case series of 11 girls treated with betamethasone dipropionate 0.05%. Eight experienced complete remission after 3 months and three required maintenance therapy with a mild topical corticosteroid.

SECOND LINE THERAPIES

■ Topical tacrolimus	D
■ Circumcision	B
■ Topical tretinoin	B

Successful treatment of anogenital lichen sclerosus with topical tacrolimus. Bohm M, Frieling U, Luger TA, Bonsmann G. Arch Dermatol 2003;139:922–4.

Once daily 0.1% tacrolimus ointment for up to 10 months induced remission in all six patients in this case series, including three children.

Tacrolimus has the theoretical advantage of causing less atrophy than corticosteroids, but may decrease immune surveillance, which is of potential concern in a condition associated with SCC.

Lichen sclerosus et atrophicus causing phimosis in boys: a prospective study with 5-year followup after complete circumcision. Meuli M, Briner J, Hanimann B, Sacher P. J Urol 1994;152:987–9.

Prospective study of 100 boys with phimosis treated with circumcision, 10% of whom were found to have LS. The LS resolved or regressed over 5 years of follow-up.

Surgical treatment of balanitis xerotica obliterans. Campus GV, Ena P, Scuderi N. Plast Reconstr Surg 1984;73: 652–7.

Of 32 symptomatic patients, 13 required circumcision, and six either meatotomy, meatoplasty, or excision and skin grafting. All responded well to surgery, without progression of the disease.

Open study of topical 0.025% tretinoin in the treatment of vulvar lichen sclerosus. One year of therapy. Virgili A, Corazza M, Bianchi A, et al. J Reprod Med 1995;40:614–8.

Once daily tretinoin applied for five days a week for 1 year in this uncontrolled study of 22 patients resulted in 75% having a complete remission of symptoms, as well as a significant improvement in the gross and histological appearance.

Irritancy may be a problem with topical retinoids.

THIRD LINE THERAPIES

■ Pimecrolimus	E

Pimecrolimus for the treatment of vulvar lichen sclerosus. A report of 4 cases. Goldstein AT, Marinoff SC, Christopher K. J Reprod Med 2004;49:778–80.

Three of four patients treated with 1% pimecrolimus cream twice daily for 3 months reported complete resolution of vulval itching and burning. Follow-up for 3 months only.

OTHER THERAPIES

■ Intralesional triamcinolone	D
■ Acitretin	C
■ Topical estrogens	E
■ Oxatomide gel	B
■ Cryosurgery	C
■ Photodynamic therapy with 5-aminolevulinic acid	C
■ CO$_2$ laser vaporization	D
■ Potassium para-aminobenzoate	D
■ Oral stanozolol	D
■ Topical testosterone	B
■ Low-dose UVA1 phototherapy	C
■ Tangential excision	E
■ Oral calcitriol	E

Topical testosterone for lichen sclerosus. Ayhan A, Urman B, Yuce K, et al. Int J Gynecol Obstet 1989;30:253–5.

Uncontrolled study of 23 patients, showing a remission rate of 88% after 6 weeks treatment with 2% testosterone.

Topical testosterone was favored for LS prior to the introduction of clobetasol propionate. Since then, multiple comparative studies (including Bracco et al, see First Line Therapies) do not support its use in LS.

Acitretin in the treatment of severe lichen sclerosus et atrophicus of the vulva: a double-blind, placebo-controlled study. Bousema MT, Romppanen U, Geiger JM, et al. J Am Acad Dermatol 1994;30:225–31.

Fourteen of 22 patients who had been were given acitretin (20–30 mg daily) for 16 weeks noted a decrease in symptoms and signs compared with six of 24 controls.

Lichen simplex chronicus

Larisa Ravitskiy, Erika Gaines Levine, Donald J Baker

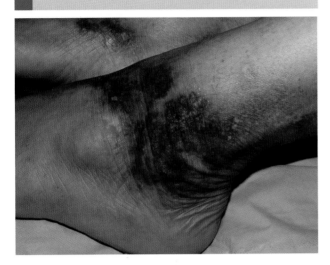

Lichen simplex chronicus (LSC; or neurodermatitis circumscripta) is characterized by pruritic, lichenified plaques that most often occur on the neck, anterior tibias, ankles, wrists, and anogenital region in response to chronic localized scratching or rubbing. Primary LSC evolves on apparently normal skin, whereas secondary LSC is superimposed upon pre-existing dermatoses, especially atopic dermatitis, psoriasis, or dermatophytosis.

MANAGEMENT STRATEGY

The objective of treatment is to remove environmental trigger factors, break the itch–scratch cycle, and treat any underlying cutaneous or systemic disease. Patients' understanding of their role in the itch–scratch cycle is essential if their cooperation in avoiding scratching is to be enlisted, thereby facilitating a more complete and permanent recovery. However, recurrences are frequent and complete resolution often requires multiple approaches to therapy. Environmental trigger factors such as harsh skin care products or bathing regimens, friction, and excessive moisture or dryness should be minimized or eliminated, High-potency *topical corticosteroids*, such as clobetasol, diflorasone, and betamethasone, as creams or ointments, are the initial treatments of choice. The potency and/or frequency of application of topical corticosteroids should be decreased as the lesion resolves to avoid atrophy with their long-term use. Adjunctive therapies such as *doxepin cream* may be introduced if topical corticosteroids are not easily tapered. Occlusion has been found to be a successful aid to therapy because it provides a physical barrier to prevent scratching and permits enhanced and prolonged application of topical medications. *Occlusive plastic film* or hydrocolloid dressings have been used alone or over mid-potency corticosteroids. *Flurandrenolide tape* is very effective as both an occlusive and anti-inflammatory measure and is usually changed once daily, although a short occlusion-free period each day will help minimize the side effects of occlusion therapy. In chronic, difficult cases on the lower leg, an Unna boot (a gauze roll impregnated with zinc oxide) may be applied for up to 1 week, provided there is no concomitant infection of the occluded area. There is a potential role for *calcineurin inhibitors* in the treatment of LSC, though some of these agents can provoke burning and stinging.

Intralesional injections of triamcinolone at weekly intervals can rapidly induce involution. Although often highly effective, repeated injections may cause depigmentation or thinning of the epidermis. Therefore, other therapies should be used if several treatments with intralesional corticosteroids do not clear LSC. Infected areas should not be injected with corticosteroids because of the risk of abscess formation. Secondary infections should be treated with appropriate topical or systemic antibiotics. Intralesional *botulinum toxin* has been reported to offer lasting relief in patients with recalcitrant LSC.

A variety of other therapies have been reported to be effective in the management of LSC. Doxepin cream, *capsaicin cream, or aspirin/dichloromethane solution* are occasionally of value alone, but are probably best used as adjunctive therapy when LSC does not quickly clear with topical or intralesional corticosteroids. *Oral antihistamines* may be useful for their sedative effect on patients who scratch during their sleep. *Cryosurgery* and *surgical excision* have been reported to help some patients with nodular neurodermatitis. In more severe or recalcitrant conditions, *psychotherapy* and/or the use of *psychopharmacologic agents* may be needed for sustained improvement. *Benzodiazepines, amitriptyline, pimozide,* and *doxepin* have been used to treat neurotic excoriations and severe neurodermatitis (see page 431). *Acupuncture* and *electroacupuncture* are labor intensive, but have been effective in treating some cases of LSC. Neurodermatitis has improved with habit-reversal *behavioral therapy* and *hypnotherapy* in certain individuals.

SPECIFIC INVESTIGATIONS

- ■ Skin biopsy with periodic acid-Schiff (PAS) stain

LSC that is atypical in appearance or poorly responsive to therapy should be biopsied and cultured to look for pre-existing dermatoses and underlying cutaneous malignancy or infection. The presence of lice or scabies infestation should be excluded. Patch testing may be useful, especially in patients whose biopsy is suggestive of allergic contact dermatitis. In particularly refractory or unusual cases, systemic disease and malignancy should be ruled out.

FIRST LINE THERAPIES

■ Topical corticosteroids	A
■ Occlusion – flurandrenolide tape	C
■ Intralesional corticosteroids	C

A double-blind, multicenter trial of 0.05% halobetasol propionate ointment and 0.05% clobetasol 17-propionate ointment in the treatment of patients with chronic, localized atopic dermatitis or lichen simplex chronicus. Datz B, Yawalkar S. J Am Acad Dermatol 1991;25:1157–60.

In 127 patients with chronic, localized atopic dermatitis or LSC, healing was reported in 65.1% of those treated with halobetasol propionate ointment (a superpotent group I topical corticosteroid) compared with 54.7% of those treated with clobetasol propionate (a weaker group I topical corticosteroid). Success rates, early onset of therapeutic effect, and adverse effects were similar in the two treatment groups.

A review of two controlled multicenter trials comparing 0.05% halobetasol propionate ointment to its vehicle in the treatment of chronic eczematous dermatoses. Guzzo CA, Weiss JS, Mogavero HS, et al. J Am Acad Dermatol 1991;25: 1179–83.

Two vehicle-controlled, double-blind studies were performed: a paired comparison study in 124 patients and a parallel group study in 100 patients. In both studies, treatments were applied twice daily for 2 weeks. Severity scores and patient ratings favored halobetasol propionate over the vehicle treated group. Global assessments showed complete resolution or marked improvement for 83% of patients using halobetasol propionate vs 28% using vehicle. The study concluded that 0.05% halobetasol propionate is highly effective and well tolerated with rapid action and a high degree of clearing.

Group I topical corticosteroids should not be used for more than 2 weeks. They are therefore best combined with adjuvant therapies such as topical doxepin cream.

A double-blind, multicenter, parallel-group trial with 0.05% halobetasol propionate ointment versus 0.1% diflucortolone valerate ointment in patients with severe, chronic atopic dermatitis or lichen simplex chronicus. Brunner N, Yawalkar S. J Am Acad Dermatol 1991;25:1160–3.

One hundred and twenty patients with chronic, localized atopic dermatitis or LSC were studied. Success rates and early onset of therapeutic effect were reported in a higher percentage of patients treated with halobetasol propionate ointment vs diflucortolone valerate ointment.

Flurandrenolone tape in the treatment of lichen simplex chronicus. Bard JW. J Ky Med Assoc 1969;67:668–70.

Of the 18 patients in the study, ten used flurandrenolone tape and eight used a topical corticosteroid preparation without occlusion. Lasting remissions were seen in 70% of those using the tape vs 25% of those using topical corticosteroids without occlusion. Duration of therapy is not mentioned.

The use of occlusion with topical corticosteroids is considered a treatment of choice for LSC despite the lack of adequate clinical trials.

Local infiltration of triamcinolone acetonide suspension in various skin conditions. Shah CF, Pandit DM. Indian J Dermatol Venereol 1971;37:231–4.

Fifteen of 17 patients with LSC experienced fair to complete improvement with up to three injections of triamcinolone acetonide suspension (10 mg/mL).

Corticosteroid injections are considered first line therapy despite the lack of adequate controlled clinical trials.

SECOND LINE THERAPIES

■ Doxepin cream	B
■ Capsaicin cream	E
■ Cryosurgery	E

The antipruritic effect of 5% doxepin cream in patients with eczematous dermatitis. Doxepin Study Group. Drake LA, Millikan LE. Arch Derm 1995;131:1403–8.

A multicenter double-blind trial conducted to evaluate the safety and antipruritic efficacy of 5% doxepin cream in patients with LSC (n = 136), nummular eczema (n = 87), or contact dermatitis (n = 86). Patients treated with doxepin vs vehicle had significantly greater pruritus relief. Of doxepin-treated patients, 60% experienced relief from pruritus within 24 h, with a response rate of 84% by the end of the study.

Treatment of prurigo nodularis, chronic prurigo and neurodermatitis circumscripta with topical capsaicin. Tupker RA, Coenraads PJ, van der Meer JB. Acta Derm Venereol 1992;72: 463.

In this small, open study, two patients with corticosteroid-unresponsive neurodermatitis circumscripta were treated with 0.25% capsaicin, applied five times daily, resulting in flatter lesions and marked relief of itching.

Cryosurgical treatment of nodular neurodermatitis with Refrigerant 12. McDow RA, Wester MM. J Derm Surg Oncol 1989;15:621–3.

This case report presents a 42-year-old male patient with an 8-month history of a persistent nodular, pruritic lesion, diagnosed clinically as neurodermatitis. Cryosurgery with Refrigerant 12 yielded successful clinical and esthetic results.

THIRD LINE THERAPIES

■ Ketotifen	C
■ Acupuncture	C
■ Electroacupuncture	C
■ Botulinum toxin	D
■ Aspirin	A
■ Psychotherapy	D
■ Hypnosis	E
■ Psychopharmacotherapy	E
■ Plum-blossom needle	E
■ Surgical excision	E

Effectiveness of ketotifen in the treatment of neurodermatitis in childhood. Kikindjanin V, Vukaviic T, Stevanocvic V. Dermatol Monatsschr 1990;176:741–4.

Seventeen children with neurodermatitis were treated with ketotifen, a mast cell stabilizer, at a dosage of 1 mg twice daily. Alleviation of the itching occurred within 2 weeks and the patients became itch free after 20 days on average. Skin lesions cleared between 7 and 9 months of treatment.

Acupuncture treatment of 139 cases of neurodermatitis. Yang Q. J Tradit Chin Med 1997;17:57–8.

Acupuncture was used to treat 96 patients with localized neurodermatitis and 43 patients with generalized neurodermatitis. A course of treatment was 10 days, and 3–5-day rest periods were given in between multiple courses of therapy. An 81% cure rate and 14% improvement rate was reported, but the number of courses of therapy and long-term follow-up were not specified.

Acupuncture and electroacupuncture (where acupuncture needles are stimulated with low-voltage, high-frequency stimulation) may be used to reduce the proinflammatory neuropeptide

Evidence levels **A** Double-blind study **B** Clinical trial ≥ 20 subjects **C** Clinical trial < 20 subjects **D** Series ≥ 5 subjects **E** Anecdotal case reports

state in pruritic and inflamed skin, and thereby promote a more normal state of neuropeptide homeostasis.

Treatment of 86 cases of local neurodermatitis by electro-acupunture (with needles inserted around diseased areas). Liu JX. J Tradit Chin Med 1987;7:67.

Electroacupuncture was used to treat 86 cases of localized neurodermatitis. Patients received multiple courses of daily therapy for 10 days, with 3–5-day rest periods in between courses; 88% of patients were cured and 11% of patients were improved. However, the number of courses of therapy and long-term follow-up were not specified.

Botulinum toxin type A injection in the treatment of lichen simplex: An open pilot study. Heckmann M, Heyer G, Brunner B, Plewig G. J Am Acad Dermatol 2002;46:617–9.

Four patients received 20 units of botulinum toxin type A (100 units/mL) per 2×2 cm^2 area of LSC plaque; 1 week after the injection there was a noticeable reduction in pruritus levels. Three patients were free of itching and one had over 50% reduction in itching. After 12 weeks, three patients remained asymptomatic.

The effect of topically applied aspirin on localized circumscribed neurodermatosis. Yosipovitch G, Sugeng M, Chan YH, et al. J Am Acad Dermatol 2001;45:910–3.

In this double-blind, crossover, placebo-controlled study, 29 patients with LSC were randomized to receive aspirin/dichloromethane solution treatment followed by placebo or vice versa. In the aspirin/dichloromethane treatment group 46% achieved a significant response; 12% of the placebo group achieved a comparable improvement.

The behavioral treatment of neurodermatitis through habit-reversal. Rosenbaum MS, Ayllon T. Behav Res Ther 1981;19:313–8.

Four patients with neurodermatitis received a single treatment session in which they learned to substitute a competing response for their urges to scratch. There was a rapid reduction in scratching in all patients. At 6 months, scratching had been eliminated in one patient and markedly reduced in three patients.

Brief hypnotherapy of neurodermatitis: a case with 4-year followup. Lehman RE. Am J Clin Hypn 1978;21:48–51.

One patient with extensive neurodermatitis was treated with eight sessions of hypnotherapy. She was clear within 2 weeks after her last session, and remained clear at 4-year follow-up.

Improvement of chronic neurotic excoriations with oral doxepin therapy. Harris BA, Sherertz EF, Flowers FP. Int J Dermatol 1987;26:541–3.

Two patients with chronic neurotic excoriations had improvement in symptoms and in clinical signs of their skin condition within several weeks of oral doxepin (30–75 mg daily).

Neurodermatitis treated by plum-blossom needle. Zhong MQ. J Tradit Chin Med 1984;4:265–8.

Forty one cases of neurodermatitis were treated with plum-blossom needling with a 54% cure rate and 44% improvement rate. The average number of courses was 25–40 sessions and long-term follow-up was incomplete.

Plum-blossom needling uses a small hammer with multiple fine needles, which are lightly tapped against the skin to produce the desired effects.

Nodular lichen simplex of the scrotum treated by surgical excision. Porter WM, Bewley A, Dinneen M, et al. Br J Dermatol 2001;144:343–6.

Two patients with nodular LSC of the scrotum were treated by surgical excision of LSC plaques with remission lasting over 12 months.

Linear IgA bullous dermatosis

Neil J Korman

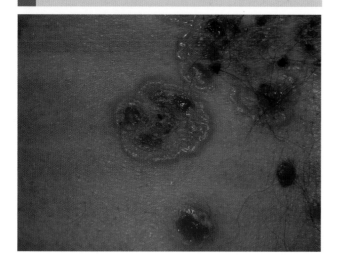

Linear IgA bullous dermatosis is an acquired autoimmune blistering disease of the skin and mucous membranes. The skin lesions consist of papulovesicles or blisters and may have an arcuate pattern with a 'cluster of jewels' grouping of blisters along with urticarial plaques. Involvement of the oral mucous membranes is common and ocular involvement, with subsequent scarring of the conjunctiva, may uncommonly occur. Although originally believed to be a distinct entity, it is now clear that chronic bullous disease of childhood is the childhood counterpart of adult linear IgA bullous dermatosis. Direct immunofluorescence studies demonstrate that all patients have linear IgA deposits at the epidermal basement membrane zone and the diagnosis of linear IgA bullous dermatosis is dependent upon this finding. The target antigens involved are 97 kD and, less commonly, 290 kD. The 97 kD antigen is an anchoring filament protein that is part of the 180 kD bullous pemphigoid antigen-2, and antibodies directed against the 290 kD protein represent an IgA response directed against type VII collagen. Several reports stress the association with ulcerative colitis. Drug-induced disease is a well-recognized entity, and vancomycin is the most commonly implicated agent.

MANAGEMENT STRATEGY

If drug-induced disease is considered, the suspect trigger drug must be withdrawn. Treatment of linear IgA bullous dermatosis is dictated by the severity of disease and the areas of involvement. All patients should be evaluated by an ophthalmologist to ensure the absence of ocular disease. Because linear IgA bullous dermatosis tends to be chronic it is important to be aware of the potential not only for short-term, but also long-term toxicities in any treatment used. In addition, treatment of children with chronic bullous disease of childhood (the childhood counterpart of linear IgA bullous dermatosis of adults) requires special consideration to ensure that any medications used have no specific contraindications in children.

The majority of patients with disease limited to the skin will respond well to treatment with *dapsone* and this is the first line therapy for patients with linear IgA bullous dermatosis. Dapsone generally works quite rapidly, with responses often occurring in the first few days of starting the drug. Dapsone is most effective for the skin lesions of linear IgA bullous dermatosis, with the mucous membrane lesions being more resistant.

Due to a dose-related oxidant stress on normal ageing red blood cells, all patients treated with dapsone will experience some degree of hemolysis that is usually dosage dependent. A reduction of approximately 2–3 g of hemoglobin is often observed. As long as this decrease is relatively gradual and patients have no history of cardiovascular disease or anemia, this is usually well tolerated. It is important to measure levels of glucose-6-phosphate dehydrogenase (G6PD) in patients to be treated with dapsone because those with a deficiency in this enzyme can develop severe hemolysis. Methemoglobinemia, which is also dosage dependent, occurs in most patients, but is usually asymptomatic. More worrisome toxicities include bone marrow suppression and even agranulocytosis, which usually occurs early in the course of therapy, and a dapsone-induced neuropathy, which occurs more commonly in patients treated for several years with more than 200 mg daily of dapsone. Less commonly, hepatitis, nephritis, pneumonitis, erythema multiforme, and the dapsone hypersensitivity syndrome have all been reported.

For those patients who fail to achieve satisfactory control of their disease with dapsone as first line therapy, it is often of value to add *systemic corticosteroids*. This combination of dapsone and prednisone is considered second line therapy. The dosage of prednisone required is often in the 20–40 mg daily range. Often the addition of prednisone will not only cause significant clinical improvement, but it may also allow the dosage of dapsone to be decreased, thereby minimizing its potential toxicity.

Other viable second line therapies include *colchicine, sulfapyridine,* and the combination of *tetracycline* and *niacinamide*: sulfapyridine at doses of approximately 1–3 g daily and colchicine has been reported to be beneficial at doses of 1.0–1.5 mg daily. The combination of tetracycline and niacinamide, usually at doses of 1.5 g of niacinamide and 2 g of tetracycline, has been used with success. Tetracycline should not be used in children under 9 years of age because it can permanently stain teeth.

Third line therapies include *sulfamethoxypyridazine, dicloxacillin, erythromycin, mycophenolate mofetil, azathioprine, cyclosporine, methotrexate, interferon alfa,* and *intravenous immunoglobulin (IVIG)*. Toxicity profiles and financial considerations favor using either erythromycin, dicloxacillin or sulfamethoxypyridazine prior to treatment with the immunosuppressive agents or IVIG.

SPECIFIC INVESTIGATIONS

- Skin biopsy of blister for histology
- Perilesional skin biopsy for direct immunofluorescence
- Indirect immunofluorescence
- Consider G6PD level before dapsone use
- Consider thiopurine methyl transferase estimation before azathioprine use
- Ophthalmology consult

Evidence levels A Double-blind study   B Clinical trial ≥ 20 subjects   C Clinical trial < 20 subjects   D Series ≥ 5 subjects   E Anecdotal case reports

Linear IgA disease in adults. Leonard JN, Haffenden GP, Ring NP, et al. Br J Dermatol 1982;107:301–16.

A clinicopathological study of mucosal involvement in linear IgA disease. Kelly SE, Frith PA, Millard PR, et al. Br J Dermatol 1988;119:161–70.

Cicatrizing conjunctivitis as predominant manifestation of linear IgA bullous dermatosis. Webster GF, Raber I, Penne R, et al. J Am Acad Dermatol 1994;30:355–7.

Chronic bullous disease of childhood, childhood cicatricial pemphigoid, and linear IgA disease of adults. A comparative study demonstrating clinical and immunopathologic overlap. Wojnarowska F, Marsden RA, Bhogal B, Black MM. J Am Acad Dermatol 1988;19:792–805.

The above are excellent reviews of the clinical and immunological features of linear IgA bullous dermatosis.

Vancomycin-induced linear IgA bullous dermatosis. Baden LA, Apovian C, Imber MJ, Dover JS. Arch Dermatol 1988;124:1186–8.

Litt's Drug Eruption Reference Manual, 10th edn (New York: Taylor and Francis; 2004) implicates acetaminophen, aldesleukin, amiodarone, ampicillin, atorvastatin, candesartan, captopril, carbamazepine, cefamandole, ceftriaxone, co-trimoxazole, cyclosporine, diclofenac, furosemide, glyburide, granulocyte-macrophage colony stimulating factor (GM-CSF), ibuprofen, interferon-alfa, lithium, metronidazole, naproxen, penicillins, phenytoin, piroxicam, rifampin, sulfamethoxazole, and vancomycin as drug triggers for linear IgA disease. The extent of disease may sometimes simulate toxic epidermal necrolysis.

The diagnosis of linear IgA bullous dermatosis requires routine histologic studies as well as direct and indirect immunofluorescence studies. Once the diagnosis is confirmed, laboratory studies to be obtained will depend upon the specific treatment anticipated.

FIRST LINE THERAPIES

■ Dapsone	C

Linear IgA dapsone responsive bullous dermatosis. Wojnarowska F. J R Soc Med 1980 73:371–3.

One of the first reports of this condition and response to dapsone. Since then, most series have demonstrated dapsone as the most effective first line monotherapy.

SECOND LINE THERAPIES

■ Dapsone and prednisone	D
■ Sulfapyridine	C
■ Colchicine	D
■ Tetracycline and niacinamide	E

Linear IgA bullous dermatosis: successful treatment with colchicine. Arum H. Arch Dermatol 1984;120:160–1.

Successful treatment of chronic bullous dermatosis of childhood with colchicine. Zeharia A, Hodak E, Mukamel M, et al. J Am Acad Dermatol 1994;30:660–1.

Colchicine as a novel therapeutic agent in chronic bullous dermatosis of childhood. Banodkar DD, Al-Suwaid AR. Int J Dermatol 1997;36:213–6.

Treatment of linear IgA bullous dermatosis of childhood with colchicine. Ang P, Tay YK. Pediatr Dermatol 1999;16:50–2.

In total there are 11 reports of colchicine use in both adults and children.

Treatment of linear IgA bullous dermatosis: successful treatment with tetracycline and nicotinamide. Peoples D, Fivenson DP. J Am Acad Dermatol 1992;26:498–9.

Treatment of pemphigus and linear IgA dermatosis with nicotinamide and tetracycline. Chaffins ML, Collison D, Fivenson DP. J Am Acad Dermatol 1993;28:998–1001.

Sublamina densa-type linear IgA bullous dermatosis successfully treated with oral tetracycline and niacinamide. Yomoda M, Komani A, Hashimoto T. Br J Dermatol 1999;141:608–9.

There are four reports of successful use of 2 g of tetracycline and 1.5 g of nicotinamide daily in adults only.

THIRD LINE THERAPIES

■ Sulfamethoxypyridazine	E
■ Dicloxacillin	E
■ Erythromycin	E
■ Methotrexate	E
■ Interferon-alfa	E
■ Mycophenolate mofetil	E
■ Azathioprine	E
■ Cyclosporine	E
■ IVIG	E

Sulphamethoxypridazine for dermatitis herpetiformis, linear IgA disease, and cicatricial pemphigoid. McFadden JP, Leonard JN, Powles AV, et al. Br J Dermatol 1989;121:759–62.

Reports of sulfamethoxypyridazine (0.25–1.5 g daily) use as monotherapy in four patients with linear IgA disease who were intolerant of dapsone.

Treatment of chronic bullous dermatosis of childhood with oral dicloxacillin. Skinner RB, Totondo CK, Schneider MA, et al. Pediatr Dermatol 1995;12:65–6.

Chronic bullous disease of childhood: successful treatment with dicloxacillin. Siegfried EC, Sirawan S. J Am Acad Dermatol 1998;39:797–800.

Mixed immunobullous disease of childhood: a good response to antimicrobials. Powell J, Kirtschig G, Allen J, et al. Br J Dermatol 2001;144:769–74.

Linear IgA disease: successful treatment with erythromycin. Cooper SM, Powell J, Wojnarowska F. Clin Exp Dermatol 2002;27:677–9.

Antibiotic use has been largely in childhood disease and is a reasonable option due to low toxicity.

Treatment of linear IgA bullous dermatosis of childhood with mycophenolate mofetil. Farley-Li J, Mancini AJ. Arch Dermatol 2003;139:1121–4.

Successful treatment of linear IgA bullous dermatosis with mycophenolate mofetil. Glaser R, Sticherlin M. Acta Derm Venereol 2002;82:308–9.

The adult dose used is usually 1–2 g twice daily.

Methotrexate and cyclosporine are of value in the treatment of adult linear IgA disease. Burrows NP, Jones RR. J Dermatol Treat 1992;3:31–3.

Linear IgA disease: successful treatment with cyclosporine. Young HS, Coulson IH. Br J Dermatol 2000;143:204–5.

Therapy-resistant blistering responding to cyclosporine 4 mg/kg daily.

Interferon alpha for linear IgA bullous dermatosis. Chan LS, Cooper KD. Lancet 1992;340:425.

Linear IgA bullous dermatosis in a patient with chronic renal failure: response to intravenous immunoglobulin therapy. Khan IU, Bhol KC, Ahmed AR. J Am Acad Dermatol 1999;40:485–8.

High-dose intravenous immune globulin is also effective in linear IgA disease. Kroiss MM, Vogtt T, Landthaler M, Stolz W. Br J Dermatol 2000;142:582–4.

Linear IgA bullous disease limited to the eye: response to intravenous immunoglobulin therapy. Letko E, Bhol K, Foster CS, Ahmed AR Ophthalmology 2000;107:1524–8.

IVIG therapy decreased the titer of circulating antibodies and induced a remission in this patient.

Successful treatment of linear IgA disease with salazosulphapyridine and intravenous immunoglobulins. Goebeler M, Seitz C, Rose C, et al. Br J Dermatol 2003;149:912–4.

Upper aerodigestive tract complications in a neonate with linear IgA bullous dermatosis. Gluth MB, Witman PM, Thompson DM. Int J Pediatr Otorhinolaryngol 2004;68:965–70.

A newborn with skin involvement had life-threatening respiratory compromise from disease affecting the larynx, subglottis, trachea, and esophagus. Management with both tracheostomy and gastrostomy tube placement was necessary. Treatment included systemic corticosteroids, dapsone, and IVIG.

Most patients treated receive 400 mg/kg IVIG daily for 5 days during each cycle of therapy.

Evidence levels **A** Double-blind study **B** Clinical trial ≥ 20 subjects **C** Clinical trial < 20 subjects **D** Series ≥ 5 subjects **E** Anecdotal case reports

Lipodermato-sclerosis

Tania J Phillips, Bahar Dasgeb

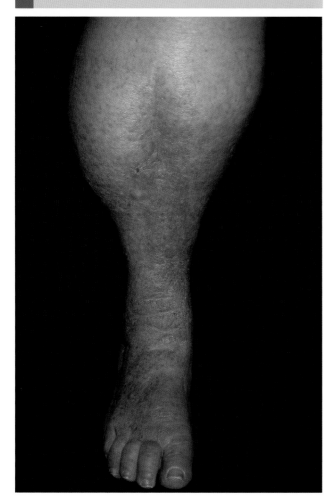

Lipodermatosclerosis (LDS) consists of a progressive fibrotic process of the skin and subcutaneous fat induced by chronic venous insufficiency. LDS usually presents as an indurated fibrotic region surrounding venous ulcers above the medial malleolus on the lower legs. The diagnosis of LDS is based on clinical findings. It more often affects female, elderly, patients who have a high body mass index and venous insufficiency. Pain is the most consistent presenting symptom. Two stages of LDS have been described: acute LDS and chronic LDS. The acute form of LDS is usually painful, tender, and slightly indurated. Often clinicians mistake the acute form of LDS for cellulitis, phlebitis, erythema nodosum, inflammatory morphea, or panniculitis. The chronic variant, which is strongly associated with venous insufficiency, is densely indurated and less painful than the acute form. In its late stages, chronic LDS alters the shape of the leg, making it look like an inverted bottle or bowling pin with extreme fibrosis and sclerosis in the dermis and subcutaneous tissue. It may be associated with hyperpigmentation.

MANAGEMENT STRATEGY

The current treatment of choice is the *combination of stanozolol and compression therapy*. Compression therapy helps increase venous return. Often patients with acute LDS find compression therapy painful; in this case stanozolol is used alone. Stanozolol is contraindicated in patients with uncontrolled hypertension and heart failure. *Pentoxifylline* is a helpful alternative that stimulates fibrinolysis, but may adversely affect the gastrointestinal tract. *Niacin* has some fibrinolytic properties and has been used for the disorder. Other treatments such as *antibiotics, anti-inflammatory agents, antimetabolites, and long term cimetidine* have been proposed. *Surgical approaches* include *subfascial perforator endoscopic surgery (SEPS), surgical correction of superficial venous reflux, ultrasound therapy*, and *complete excision of LDS followed by split-thickness skin graft repair*.

SPECIFIC INVESTIGATIONS

- Biopsy
- Duplex ultrasound
- Laser Doppler scanning
- Ultrasound indentometry
- Capillary microscopy

The clinical spectrum of lipodermatosclerosis. Kirsner RS, Pardes JB, Eaglstein WH, et al. J Am Acad Dermatol 1993; 28:623–7.

In most cases biopsy is not warranted because the diagnosis of LDS is based on clinical findings; 50% of biopsy sites do not heal and may become chronically ulcerated.

Lipodermatosclerosis: the histologic spectrum with clinical correlation to the acute and chronic forms. Hurwitz D, Kirsner RS, Falanga V, Elgard GW. J Clin Pathol 1996;23:78.

If deemed necessary, an incisional biopsy should be taken at the edges of the lesion with primary wound closure. Biopsy specimens from patients with acute LDS showed little epidermal change or capillary proliferation in papillary dermis. However, there were significant changes in the subcutis where there was lobular and septal panniculitis. In addition, eosinophils, fibrin thrombi, and purpura were seen. Biopsy specimens from patients with chronic LDS showed significant dermal change, which are often associated with venous insufficiency. These included capillary proliferation, hemosiderin deposition, and fibrosis. Epidermal hypertrophy and fibrosis were also detected in subcutaneous tissue in chronic disease. Patients who had both chronic and acute LDS showed overlap of the above features.

Duplex venous imaging: role for a comprehensive lower extremity examination. Badgett DK, Comerota MC, Khan MN, et al. Ann Vasc Surg 2000;14:73–6.

Results of duplex scanning of 205 lower extremities with varices: 106 not previously operated and 99 previously operated for varicose veins. Egeblad K, Baekgaard N. Ugeskr Laeger 2003:3016–8.

Color Duplex ultrasound scanning has been shown to accurately detect the specific location of lower extremity venous insufficiency that often leads to LDS.

Quantifying fibrosis in venous disease: mechanical properties of lipodermatosclerosis and healthy tissue. Geyer MJ, Brienza DM, Chib V, Wang J. Adv Skin Wound Care 2004; 17:131–42.

A novel ultrasound indentometry method was used to quantify fibrotic tissue in LDS. This noninvasive technique can be used as a method to quantify fibrosis in venous disease.

Excision of lipodermatosclerotic tissue: an effective treatment for non-healing venous ulcer. Ahnlide I, Bjellerup M, Akesson H. Acta Derm Venereol 2000;80:28–30.

In this study of seven cases, laser Doppler scanning showed that there is an increase in blood flow in lipodermatosclerotic skin. This increased flow decreased after operation and removal of the affected area.

Microangiopathy in chronic venous insufficiency: quantitative assessment by capillary microscopy. Howlader MH, Smith PD. Eur J Vasc Endovasc Surg 2003;26:325–31.

Capillary microscopy was used to assess patients with chronic venous disease and normal controls. Advanced venous disease (LDS and healed ulcer) was associated with a decreased number of capillaries and increased capillary convolution compared to healthy control subjects.

FIRST LINE THERAPIES

■ Compression therapy	A
■ Stanozolol	B
■ Compression therapy plus stanozolol	B
■ HR (0-[betahydroxymethyl]-rutosides)	B

The clinical spectrum of lipodermatosclerosis. Kirsner RS, Pardes J, Eaglstein WH, Falanga VJ. Am Acad Dermatol 1993;28:623–7.

Traditionally LDS has been treated with compression therapy with graded stockings or elastic bandages. The authors suggest open-toe and below-the-knee graded stockings, with 30–40 mmHg pressure around the ankle. Some stockings come with the zipper in the back, which makes them easier for elderly patients to use. Patients with acute LDS, however, often have too much pain to be able to use compression stockings; in these patients, stanozolol, at a dose of 2 mg twice daily, was found to dramatically decrease pain and tenderness.

Graduated compression stockings reduce lipodermatosclerosis and ulcer recurrence. Vandongen YK, Stacey MC. Phlebology 2000;25:33–7.

A randomized controlled trial of 150 patients showed that elastic stockings alone can improve the skin changes of LDS and lower the rate of ulcer recurrence.

Removal of dermal edema with class I and II compression stockings in patients with lipodermatosclerosis. Gniadecka M, Karlsmark T, Bertram A. J Am Acad Dermatol 1998;39:966–70.

In this study, high-frequency ultrasonography demonstrated that low levels of compression, class I (18–26 mmHg) in LDS are as effective as class II (26–36 mmHg) in the removal of dermal edema. Light compression may be a useful modality for patients with chronic venous insuffi-

ciency and LDS who are not candidates for high compression therapy.

Venous lipodermatosclerosis: treatment by fibrinolytic enhancement and elastic compression. Burnand K, Clemenson G, Morland M, et al. BMJ 1980;280:7–11.

From this study of 23 patients, Burnand et al. suggest that stanozolol (5 mg twice a day) and elastic stockings be used together. Stanozolol has been shown to reduce extravascular fibrin and induration, and relieve the pain, tenderness, and hyperpigmentation associated with LDS.

Patients taking stanozolol should be carefully monitored for excessive fluid retention, hirsutism, acne, liver function, and plasma fibrinogen concentration. Stanozolol is contraindicated in patients with uncontrolled hypertension or congestive heart failure.

HR (Paroven, Venoruton; 0-(beta-hydroxyethyl)-rutosides) in venous hypertensive microangiopathy. Incandela L, Belacaro G, Renton S et al. J Cardiovasc Pharmacol Ther 2002;7(suppl):S7–10).

HR (Paroven-Venoruton; 0-[betahydroxyethyl]-rutosides) decreased signs and symptoms of chronic venous insufficiency and LDS.

SECOND LINE THERAPIES

■ Pentoxifylline	C
■ Total triterpenic fraction of *Centella asiatica* (TTFCA)	C
■ Superficial venous surgery	B

Pentoxifylline in the treatment of venous leg ulcer. Babarino C. Curr Med Res Opin 1992;12:547–51.

Pentoxifylline for treating venous leg ulcer. Jull AB, Waters J, Arroll B. Cochrane Database Syst Rev 2002(1): CD001733.

Pentoxifylline is a dimethylxanthine derivative that increases red blood cell flexibility and alters fibroblast physiology. In addition, it stimulates fibrinolysis and changes fibroblast activity. The dose of 400 mg of oral pentoxifylline taken three times daily may be increased to 800 mg three times daily if no improvement occurs.

Pentoxifylline is a good alternative in those intolerant to stanozolol. Side effects include nausea, dizziness, heartburn, and, occasionally, vomiting.

Effect of total triterpenic fraction of *Centella asiatica* in venous hypertension microangiopathy. Cesarone MR, Belcaro G, De Sanctis et al. Angiology 2001;52(suppl 2): S15–8.

TTFCA was reported to improve signs and symptoms of venous insufficiency. Lipodermatosclerosis was not specifically measured.

Comparison of surgery and compression with compression alone in chronic venous ulceration (ESCHAR study): randomized controlled trial. Barwell JR, Davis CE, Deacon J, et al. Lancet 2004;363:1854–9.

Surgical correction of superficial venous reflux reduced 12 months ulcer recurrence, compared to treatment with compression alone.

The effects on LDS were not specifically mentioned in this study, but it might reasonably be expected to improve with correction of reflux.

THIRD LINE THERAPIES

■ Niacin	E
■ Cimetidine	E
■ Subfascial perforator endoscopic surgery (SEPS)	E
■ Ultrasound	E
■ Excision of lipodermatosclerotic tissue	E
■ Antibiotics	E

Lipid lowering and enhancement of fibrinolysis with niacin. Holvoet P, Collen D. Circulation 1995;92:698–9.

Niacin, taken at the dose of 100–150 mg, three to five times a day, has been shown to help treat the hyperlipidemia that is often associated with LDS. In large doses, it causes vasodilation and stimulates fibrinolysis. It also decreases uric acid excretion and alters glucose tolerance.

Niacin is another alternative for patients who cannot tolerate stanozolol.

Pathogenesis of lipodermatosclerosis of venous disease: the lesson learned from eosinophilic fasciitis. Naschitz JE, Yashurum D, Schwartz H. Cardiovascular Surg 1993;1: 524–9.

The authors propose that long-term cimetidine therapy has widespread beneficial results in lipodermatosclerosis. However, there has not been much supporting evidence in the literature for this.

Early benefit of subfascial endoscopic perforator surgery (SEPS) in healing venous ulcer. Sparks SR, Ballard JL, Bergan JJ, Killeen JD. Ann Vasc Surg 1997;11:367–73.

SEPS can be helpful in treating LDS in patients who do not heal with traditional methods. The perforating veins are ligated to ameliorate venous hypertension, which usually perpetuates the LDS.

No other data have been published.

Hypodermatitis sclerodermiformis. Rowe L, Cantwell A. Arch Dermatol 1982;118:312–4.

Rowe and Cantwell used ultrasound to treat six patients and found promising results in four of them. Treatments were given two to three times weekly for a month or two and were repeated after rest for a month, or more.

This study was not randomized, blinded, or placebo controlled. No confirmatory studies have been published.

Excision of lipodermatosclerotic tissue: an effective treatment for non-healing venous ulcer. Ahnlide I, Bjellerup M, Akesson H. Acta Derm Venereol 2000;80:28–30.

From this small, uncontrolled study, Ahnlide et al. suggest that excision of lipodermatosclerotic tissue can help heal venous ulcers, because the lipodermatosclerotic area impedes the healing process. Laser Doppler scanning showed increased basal blood flow in lipodermatosclerotic skin, which normalized after surgery.

Local microcirculation in chronic venous incompetence and leg ulcer. Fagrell B. Vasc Surg 1979;13:217–25.

Although the number of capillaries is reduced in venous incompetence, those remaining are dilated and tortuous, causing increased blood flow to the region. This impairs healing. Thus removal of the lipodermatosclerotic tissue, together with skin grafting, can help the healing process in recalcitrant venous ulcers.

Hypodermatitis sclerodermiformis and unusual acid-fast bacteria. Cantwell A, Kelso D, Rowe L. Arch Dermatol 1979; 115:449–52.

There is little evidence to support the use of antibiotics, anti-inflammatory agents, and antimetabolites.

Livedo reticularis

Ruwani P Katugampola,
Andrew Y Finlay

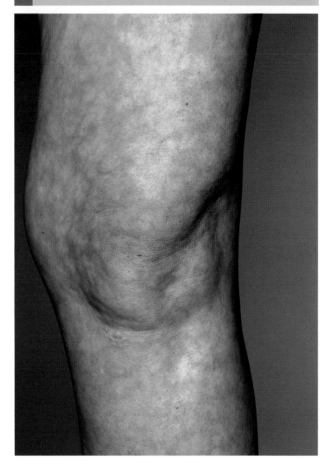

Livedo reticularis (LR) is a net-like mottled violaceous discoloration of the skin secondary to dilatation and stagnation of blood within dermal capillaries. The unaffected normal colored islands of skin are the areas where blood supply is sufficient; in the network areas the supply is insufficient. This commonly occurs on the legs, arms and trunk, but can be diffuse, and is more pronounced following exposure to cold. Livedo reticularis can be physiological (cutis marmorata) or can occur as a primary phenomenon (idiopathic LR) or secondary to a number of diseases that cause dermal vessel wall thickening and/or lumen occlusion, such as systemic lupus erythematosus, polyarteritis nodosa, the antiphospholipid syndrome (see page 50), cryoglobulinemia, and cholesterol emboli. Idiopathic LR may be congenital (cutis marmorata telangiectatica congenita), or associated with painful ulcers (livedoid vasculopathy, see page 366) or with cerebrovascular involvement (Sneddon's syndrome).

MANAGEMENT STRATEGY

The etiology of physiological and primary LR is unknown, and no definitive treatment is available. The management of primary LR depends on the presence of associated ulcers, anomalies (congenital form), and systemic involvement (Sneddon's syndrome). In secondary LR, the underlying cause needs to be identified and treated.

Physiological LR, which occurs in healthy children and adults in response to cold weather, is diffuse, mild, temporary, and usually asymptomatic. No specific treatment is required for this condition except *avoidance of cold exposure* and protection from cold exposure with *warm clothing* and *re-warming* the affected area.

Cutis marmorata telangiectatica congenita is rare and presents at birth or soon after birth. A small proportion of affected children have associated congenital anomalies such as hemangiomas, glaucoma, limb atrophy, cardiac malformations, or psychomotor retardation that need to be identified and referred for appropriate specialist care. The LR in these children usually disappears spontaneously or markedly improves with age.

Patients with Sneddon's syndrome are at risk of cerebrovascular disease and may benefit from *antithrombotic treatment*. The timing of such treatment is debated because LR may precede the neurological events by up to 10 or more years. Advice regarding other risk factors predisposing to cerebrovascular events, such as smoking, obesity, hypertension, and oral contraceptives, is important.

Although a number of agents including *antiplatelet therapy, danazol, pentoxifylline* and *systemic corticosteroids* have been used to treat ulcers associated with LR, no single agent has been shown to completely resolve the LR itself.

SPECIFIC INVESTIGATIONS

- Skin biopsies for microscopy and direct immunofluorescence (adults)
- Full blood count and renal function
- Antinuclear antibody, rheumatoid factor, antineutrophil cytoplasmic antibodies
- Cryoglobulin level
- Anticardiolipin antibodies
- Coagulation screen
- Serum lipid profile

A detailed history followed by physical examination is essential, especially in diagnosing Sneddon's syndrome, identifying congenital anomalies in infants, and excluding secondary causes of LR. The histology of LR is non-inflammatory thickening of dermal vessel walls with eventual occlusion of the lumen.

Diagnostic impact and sensitivity of skin biopsies in Sneddon's syndrome. A report of 15 cases. Wohlrab J, Fischer M, Wolter M, Marsch WC. Br J Dermatol 2001; 145:285–8.

Deep 4 mm punch biopsies from the central white part of the LR demonstrated a sensitivity of 27% with one biopsy, 53% with two biopsies, and 80% with three biopsies of diagnosing Sneddon's syndrome in clinically suspected cases. The authors concluded that the positive histology was important for commencing prophylaxis of cerebrovascular events in patients initially presenting with LR.

The spectrum of livedo reticularis and anticardiolipin antibodies. Asherson RA, Mayou SC, Merry P, et al. Br J Dermatol 1989;120:215–21.

In this retrospective study of 65 patients with LR (idiopathic and secondary), 28 anticardiolipin antibody-positive patients were compared with 37 anticardiolipin antibody-negative patients. There was a statistically significant

Evidence levels A Double-blind study B Clinical trial ≥ 20 subjects C Clinical trial < 20 subjects D Series ≥ 5 subjects E Anecdotal case reports

increase in the incidence of strokes, transient ischemic attacks, venous thrombosis, fetal loss, and valvular heart disease in the anticardiolipin-positive patients compared with anticardiolipin-negative patients.

FIRST LINE THERAPIES

■ Aspirin (Sneddon's syndrome)	D

Sneddon's syndrome: generalized livedo reticularis and cerebrovascular disease – importance of hemostatic screening. Devos J, Bulcke J, Degreef H, Michielsen B. Dermatology 1992;185:296–9.

Two cases of Sneddon's syndrome are described, one of whom was shown to have twice the normal level of tissue plasminogen activator antigen, fourfold the normal level of plasminogen activator-inhibitor, abnormal thrombin time, and elevated levels of factor XII during a neurological event. Aspirin was commenced at 300 mg daily with normalization of the hemostatic parameters after 4 months of treatment and freedom from neurological symptoms at 10 months.

There was no change in the patient's LR with aspirin treatment.

SECOND LINE THERAPIES

■ Psoralen plus UVA (PUVA)	D
■ Pentoxifylline plus methylprednisolone	E

Livedo reticularis and livedoid vasculitis responding to PUVA therapy. Choi HJ, Hann SK. J Am Acad Dermatol 1999;40:204–7.

Two patients with ulcers due to livedoid vasculitis of the lower legs resistant to treatment with other systemic treat-ment including aspirin, prednisolone, and pentoxifylline, were treated with systemic PUVA using methoxsalen. Only the lower legs were exposed to UVA, initially with $4\,J/cm^2$ three times a week and subsequent $1\,J/cm^2$ increments. No significant ulcers had recurred at 3 and 6 months follow-up of the two patients after the last treatment.

Improvement in the discoloration of the skin affected by LR was noted in one of the patients at completion of PUVA treatment.

Widespread livedoid vasculopathy. Marzano AV, Vanotti M, Alessi E. Acta Derm Venereol 2003;83:457–60.

A 37-year-old woman with widespread LR and recurrent painful ulcers on all limbs, trunk, and scalp was treated with both intravenous methylprednisolone 80 mg daily for 5 days, followed by intramuscular and subsequent tapering oral dose to 32 mg daily and with pentoxifylline 400 mg twice daily for 2 months. There was a marked clinical improvement within 2 weeks of treatment and the intensity of the LR faded but did not completely resolve.

THIRD LINE THERAPIES

■ Simvastatin	E

Livedo reticularis caused by cholesterol embolization may improve with simvastatin. Finch TM, Ryatt KS. Br J Dermatol 2000;143:1319–20.

A 69-year-old man with LR without ulceration of the legs extending to the lower abdomen due to cholesterol embolization failed to respond to low-dose aspirin and a low-fat diet. Fasting serum cholesterol was 6.9 mmol/L (normal < 6.5 mmol/L) and serum triglyceride was normal. Three months after initiation of simvastatin 10 mg daily his serum cholesterol decreased to 4.9 mmol/L with an associated reduction in extent and prominence of the LR.

Livedoid vasculopathy

Bethany R Hairston, Mark D P Davis

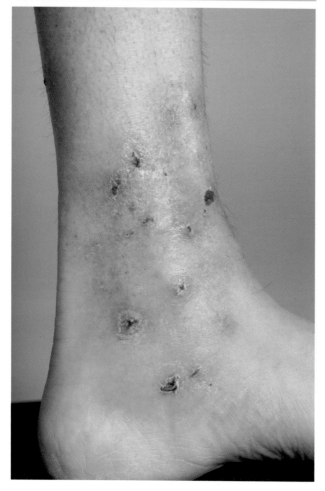

Livedoid vasculopathy, or livedoid vasculitis, is a painful ulcerative condition of the lower extremities with characteristic clinical and histopathologic features. The lesions of atrophie blanche, a term once synonymous with the disease, are typically present on the lower extremities and are characterized by smooth, porcelain-white lesions surrounded by punctate telangiectasia and hyperpigmentation. Central, shallow ulceration is often present. This condition is difficult to treat and often recalcitrant to therapy.

MANAGEMENT STRATEGY

Appropriate diagnosis of livedoid vasculitis is necessary before treatment options can be considered. Histologic identification of the characteristic segmental hyalinized appearance of the dermal blood vessels is important to exclude other causes of lower extremity ulcerative disease. Increasing numbers of reports suggest that the disease has a procoagulant predisposition, with both hereditary and acquired hypercoagulable states.

Typically shallow and numerous, the ulcerations in livedoid vasculopathy are painful and slow healing. *Wound care* is an important facet of treatment. Excellent *dressings and* *topical products* are available to treat chronic ulcerative diseases, and selection depends on the moisture content of the wound and the possibility of superinfection. *Topical and oral antibiotics* may be beneficial, and wounds should be cultured to determine appropriate sensitivity to medications. *Pain management* is also essential.

Because of the potential procoagulant mechanisms involved in disease etiology, medical therapy has traditionally centered on prevention and treatment of dermal vessel thrombosis and improvement of vascular perfusion. Medical management has included *aspirin (acetylsalicylic acid)*, *niacin (nicotinic acid)*, *pentoxifylline*, *dipyridamole*, *warfarin*, *danazol*, and *ketanserin*. Systemic corticosteroids are not considered a primary therapy; however, some patients' conditions have improved with immunosuppressants in combination therapy. *Psoralen with UVA (PUVA)* has also been used. Patients with livedoid vasculopathy recalcitrant to traditional management have been treated with *minidose heparin, subcutaneous low-molecular-weight heparin injections, intravenous iloprost (a prostacyclin analogue), intravenous immunoglobulin (IVIG)*, and a *tissue-type plasminogen activator (tPA)*.

SPECIFIC INVESTIGATIONS

- Skin biopsy – including routine histology and direct immunofluorescence
- Wound and tissue cultures
- Laboratory studies – hemogram, serum homocysteine, cryoglobulin, anticardiolipin antibody, R506Q of factor V Leiden and 20210G/A of protein C levels, biological activity and antigen levels of protein C and S, functional and immunologic levels of antithrombin III protein, and detection of lupus anticoagulant
- Noninvasive venous and arterial function testing – continuous wave Doppler, venous duplex imaging, plethysmography, and transcutaneous oximetry

Livedo vasculitis (the vasculitis of atrophie blanche): immunohistopathologic study. Schroeter AL, Diaz-Perez JL, Winkelmann RK, Jordan RE. Arch Dermatol 1975;111: 188–93.

Histologic and direct immunofluorescent studies that distinguish livedo vasculitis from other forms of cutaneous vasculitis are presented.

Homocysteinemia and livedoid vasculitis. Gibson GE, Li H, Pittelkow MR. J Am Acad Dermatol 1999;40:279–81.

The mean homocysteine level in women with livedoid vasculitis (8.7 μmol/L [SD 3.1 μmol/L]) was significantly higher than the mean for female controls (7.0 mmol/L [SD 2.9 mmol/L]) (p = 0.03), indicating a possible association between plasma homocysteine levels and the small vessel thrombotic vasculopathy.

The authors of this study acknowledge that a major shortcoming was that the control group was not age-matched. This is relevant because the homocysteine level increases with age. In this report the mean age of patients with livedoid vasculitis was nearly 56 years compared to 38 years of age in the control group.

Livedoid vasculitis: a manifestation of the antiphospholipid syndrome? Acland KM, Darvay A, Wakelin SH, Russell-Jones R. Br J Dermatol 1999;140:131–5.

Evidence levels **A** Double-blind study **B** Clinical trial ≥ 20 subjects **C** Clinical trial < 20 subjects **D** Series ≥ 5 subjects **E** Anecdotal case reports

Four patients with ulcerative livedoid vasculitis were described, all of whom had associated elevated anticardiolipin antibody levels, but no other evidence of systemic disease.

Livedo (livedoid) vasculitis and the factor V Leiden mutation: additional evidence for abnormal coagulation. Calamia KT, Balabanova M, Perniciaro C, Walsh JS. J Am Acad Dermatol 2002;46:133–7.

A case of livedo vasculitis with the factor V Leiden mutation is described.

Livedoid vasculopathy associated with heterozygous protein C deficiency. Boyvat A, Kundakci N, Babikir MO, Gurgey E. Br J Dermatol 2000;143:840–2.

Livedoid vasculopathy in association with protein C deficiency is described in one patient.

Atrophie blanche: a disorder associated with defective release of tissue plasminogen activator. Pizzo SV, Murray JC, Gonias SL. Arch Pathol Lab Med 1986;110:517–9.

Plasma from eight patients with atrophie blanche was analyzed for release of vascular tPA before and after venous occlusion. The average plasma level of releasable tPA was only 0.03 IU/mL compared with 0.70 IU/mL for 118 healthy controls.

FIRST LINE THERAPIES

■ Wound care (including bed rest and leg elevation)	D
■ Aspirin	D
■ Dipyridamole	D

Atrophie blanche: a clinicopathological study of 27 patients. Yang LJ, Chan HL, Chen SY, et al. Changgeng Yi Xue Za Zhi 1991;14:237–45.

Twenty seven patients were reviewed with respect to mean age at onset, disease duration, natural course, and clinical morphology. Thirteen patients responded to local wound care, bed rest, and low-dose aspirin plus dipyridamole as treatment for the first attack or recurrent episodes.

Antiplatelet therapy in atrophie blanche and livedo vasculitis. Drucker CR, Duncan WC. J Am Acad Dermatol 1982;7:359–63.

Seven patients with abnormal platelet function in vitro had clinical improvement after treatment with dipyridamole and aspirin.

SECOND LINE THERAPIES

■ Pentoxifylline	E
■ Danazol	D

Pentoxifylline (Trental) therapy for the vasculitis of atrophie blanche. Sauer GC. Arch Dermatol 1986;122:380–1.

Six patients with livedoid vasculopathy treated with pentoxifylline had improved or healed ulcerations in 2–3 months. They remained free of ulcers as long as pentoxifylline was continued, but ulcers recurred when the drug was stopped.

Low-dose danazol in the treatment of livedoid vasculitis. Hsiao GH, Chiu HC. Dermatology 1997;194:251–5.

Six of seven patients treated with low-dose danazol (200 mg daily orally) had rapid cessation of new lesion formation, prompt reduction in pain, and healing of active ulceration.

Livedoid vasculitis with anticardiolipin antibodies: improvement with danazol. Wakelin SH, Ellis JP, Black MM. Br J Dermatol 1998;139:935–7.

A patient with livedoid vasculitis was found to have anticardiolipin antibodies. The ulcerations were recalcitrant to conventional first and second line therapies. She responded to danazol in combination with initially high-dose systemic corticosteroids.

THIRD LINE THERAPIES

■ Low-molecular-weight heparin	E
■ Vitamin K antagonists (fluindione, warfarin)	E
■ Minidose heparin	E
■ IVIG	C
■ tPA	C
■ Iloprost	E
■ Sulfapyridine	C
■ Ketanserin	E
■ PUVA	C
■ Hyperbaric oxygen	E

Treatment of livedoid vasculopathy with low-molecular-weight heparin: report of 2 cases. Hairston BR, Davis MD, Gibson LE, Drage LA. Arch Dermatol 2003;139:987–90.

Two patients with livedoid vasculopathy recalcitrant to conventional first and second line therapies had a beneficial response to subcutaneous injections of low-molecular-weight heparin.

Difficult management of livedoid vasculopathy. Frances C, Barete S. Arch Dermatol 2004;140:1011.

Fourteen of 16 patients treated with either low-molecular-weight heparin or a vitamin K antagonist (fluindione) had more effective results than with antiplatelet drugs. One patient responded partially to aspirin and dipyridamole; the remaining patient responded to no treatments.

The authors recommend that the benefit–risk ratio, cost, and quality of life be considered when prescribing either low-molecular-weight heparin or vitamin K antagonists.

Minidose heparin therapy for vasculitis of atrophie blanche. Jetton RL, Lazarus GS. J Am Acad Dermatol 1983;8:23–6.

One patient with severe livedoid vasculitis had a complete remission when treated with minidose heparin sodium injections.

Pulsed intravenous immunoglobulin therapy in livedoid vasculitis: an open trial evaluating 9 consecutive patients. Kreuter A, Gambichler T, Breuckmann F, et al. J Am Acad Dermatol 2004;51:574–9.

The efficacy and safety of IVIG were investigated in nine patients with livedoid vasculitis that was refractory to other treatment modalities in seven of them. Vast improvement in erythema, healing of ulceration, and pain was noted in all patients.

Tissue plasminogen activator for treatment of livedoid vasculitis. Klein KL, Pittelkow MR. Mayo Clin Proc 1992;67: 923–33.

In a prospective study, six patients who had non-healing ulcers caused by livedoid vasculitis, and in whom numerous conventional therapies had failed, were treated with a low-dose tPA. In five of the six patients, dramatic improvement with almost complete healing of the ulcers occurred during hospitalization. Several were maintained with warfarin therapy after their inpatient treatment.

Livedoid vasculopathy with combined thrombophilia: efficacy of iloprost. (French) Magy N, Algros MP, Racadot E, et al. Rev Med Interne 2002;23:554–7.

One patient with lupus anticoagulant and factor V (Leiden) gene mutation had a dramatic and effective response to intravenous iloprost after unsuccessful anti-coagulant therapy.

Clinical studies of livedoid vasculitis (segmental hyalinizing vasculitis). Winkelmann RK, Schroeter AL, Kierland RR, Ryan TM. Mayo Clin Proc 1974;49:746–50.

Clinical, laboratory, and histologic studies of 37 patients with livedoid vasculitis were presented. Treatment options were discussed, including niacin, which was effective because of the inhibiting effect of nicotinate on the contraction of vascular smooth muscle of the skin. Nine of 12 patients had sustained remission of their livedoid vasculopathy. Rest and wet-dressing therapy produced short remissions, and some patients responded to sulfapyridine (six of 11) or guanethidine (three of eight treated). Corticosteroids, sympathectomy, and forms of chemotherapy were not successful.

Clinical profile and treatment outcome of livedoid vasculitis: a case series. Lee SS, Ang P, Tan SH. Ann Acad Med Singapore 2003;32:835–9.

Conventional therapy was unsuccessful in six patients with livedoid vasculitis, including four patients treated with pentoxifylline and two with aspirin. Combination therapy with immunosuppressants, including prednisolone, colchicine, and azathioprine, yielded better results in this study.

Chronic leg ulceration with livedoid vasculitis, and response to oral ketanserin. Rustin MH, Bunker CB, Dowd PM. Br J Dermatol 1989;120:101–5.

A patient with a 6-year history of recalcitrant painful ulcerations due to livedoid vasculitis healed rapidly after treatment with oral ketanserin.

Livedoid vasculitis responding to PUVA therapy. Lee JH, Choi HJ, Kim SM, et al. Int J Dermatol 2001;40:153–7.

Eight patients treated with systemic PUVA had rapid cessation of new lesion formation, notable symptom relief, and complete healing of primary lesions without unacceptable side effects.

Intractable livedoid vasculopathy successfully treated with hyperbaric oxygen. Yang CH, Ho HC, Chan YS, et al. Br J Dermatol 2003;149:647–52.

Hyperbaric oxygen, an effective method of treating ischemic wounds, was effective for two patients with painful livedoid vasculopathy.

Evidence levels **A** Double-blind study **B** Clinical trial ≥ 20 subjects **C** Clinical trial < 20 subjects **D** Series ≥ 5 subjects **E** Anecdotal case reports

Lyme borreliosis

Sian Jones, Fran Wallach

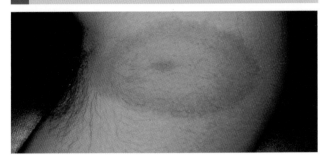

(Picture courtesy of Vijay K Sikand MD, East Lyme, CT)

Lyme disease is a multisystem illness caused by spirochetes of the genus *Borrelia*. In the USA, the disease is caused by *B. burgdorferi*. Different borrelial species may be responsible for illness in Europe and Asia, resulting in somewhat different clinical presentations. Depending upon the stage of the illness, infection may be limited to the skin or involve the nervous, cardiac, and musculoskeletal systems. The disease was first described in 1977 after a geographic clustering of purported juvenile rheumatoid arthritis in Lyme, Connecticut was linked to a tick vector. Today, Lyme disease is the most common vector-borne disease in the USA and is endemic in the Northeast, Upper Midwest, and Northwest. In the Northeast, the *Ixodes scapularis* tick transmits *B. burgdorferi*, whereas *I. pacificus* transmits the spirochete on the West Coast. Ninety percent of Lyme disease in the USA occurs in 10 states in the Northeastern and Great Lakes regions.

Mice and deer make up the major animal reservoir of *B. burgdorferi*. *Ixodes* ticks feed once in each of the three stages of their 2-year life cycle. The eggs hatch in the spring. Larvae feed in summer, acquiring *B. burgdorferi* from their preferred host and reservoir, the white-footed mouse. The following spring, the larvae molt into nymphs, which again feed off the white-footed mouse. The nymphs mature into adult ticks, which feed and mate in fall and winter, usually on the white-tailed deer. *B. burgdorferi* is passed back and forth between ticks and their hosts. Humans are most often infected as accidental hosts in the spring and summer, when the nymphs are actively feeding.

MANAGEMENT STRATEGY

Routine antimicrobial prophylaxis or serologic tests after a tick bite are *not* recommended. Some experts recommend antibiotic prophylaxis for patients bitten by *I. scapularis* ticks that have been attached for more than 36 h if the exposure is in an endemic area. This recommendation is based on data that showed that a single 200 mg dose of doxycycline prevented 87% of Lyme borreliosis infections if administered within 72 h of the tick bite. Often, however, accurate and detailed exposure history is not available. People who have had a tick exposure should be monitored for up to 30 days for occurrence of skin lesions or temperature elevation >38°C. People who develop skin lesions or other symptoms within 1 month after removing attached ticks should be assessed for acute Lyme disease.

The best method for preventing infection with *B. burgdorferi* is to avoid tick-infested areas. If exposure to ticks is unavoidable, then persons should wear light-colored clothing and long pants that are tucked into socks to prevent ticks from readily finding exposed skin. Daily inspection of the entire body also can be beneficial, since ticks removed within 24–36 h of attachment are unlikely to transmit the spirochete. Tick and insect repellents with DEET applied to skin and clothing provide further protection. *Ixodes* ticks are very small: larvae are less than 1 mm in size and adult females are 2–3 mm in size. Ticks found on persons should be removed with tweezers by pulling on the mouth apparatus of the tick close to the skin; taking care not to leave parts of the embedded tick behind.

Lyme disease generally occurs in stages, with different clinical symptoms and signs at each stage. Antimicrobial therapy can be separated into oral and intravenous regimens, depending upon the stage and site of infection.

Localized early disease

Erythema migrans, also known as erythema chronicum migrans (ECM), starts as an erythematous papule and becomes an annular, flat, erythematous, minimally tender lesion with partial central clearing at the site of tick bite. The erythema migrans lesion appears 3–30 days after spirochete inoculation in the vast majority of persons diagnosed with Lyme disease. The erythema migrans lesion can be accompanied by fever and regional lymphadenopathy. Untreated erythema migrans usually fades within 3–4 weeks. Administration of *doxycycline* 100 mg twice daily or *amoxicillin* 500 mg three times daily for 14–21 days is recommended for early localized or early disseminated Lyme disease associated with erythema migrans. Doxycycline is relatively contraindicated during pregnancy or lactation and for children younger than 8 years of age. Doxycycline has the advantage of treating unrecognized human granulocytic ehrlichiosis, which is transmitted by the same *Ixodes* tick vector as *B. burgdorferi*, and can co-infect the patient along with Lyme disease in the eastern USA. Alternative therapies include *cefuroxime axetil* 500 mg orally twice daily, which should be reserved for people who are allergic or intolerant to amoxicillin or doxycycline.

Early disseminated infection

Over the course of several weeks after initial infection, early dissemination of the spirochete occurs via blood or lymphatics to many sites. Secondary annular skin lesions can occur which resemble primary erythema migrans but are generally smaller. Other common symptoms include fever, lethargy, myalgias, headache, and mild neck stiffness. Virtually any organ system can be affected. Patients may present with cardiac conduction block, iritis or uveitis, aseptic meningitis (lymphocytic pleocytosis in CSF), Bell's palsy, other cranial neuropathies, or peripheral neuritis. In adults, *intravenous ceftriaxone* 2 g daily for 14–28 days is recommended as a first line agent for Lyme disease associated with neurologic involvement or advanced cardiac conduction disturbances. *Intravenous penicillin G* at 18–24 million units each day (divided into 4-hourly doses) is an acceptable alternative. Temporary pacing may be required for patients with high-degree AV block; however, insertion of a permanent pacer is not necessary as conduction defects resolve spontaneously. Lyme arthritis can be treated successfully with oral or intravenous antibiotics. Doxycycline 100 mg twice daily or amoxicillin 500 mg three times daily for 28 days is recommended for patients with Lyme arthritis.

Late infection

Stage 3 infection typically occurs months to years after initial infection. Symptoms include chronic arthritis predominantly involving the knees, chronic sensory peripheral neuropathy, and a subacute encephalopathy characterized by memory loss, mood changes, and sleep disturbance. A dermatologic finding associated with advanced Lyme disease is *acrodermatitis chronica atrophicans*, a violaceous discoloration and swelling of involved skin, usually at the site of a former tick bite, that over time becomes atrophic. Acrodermatitis chronica atrophicans is rarely seen in the USA, but is not infrequent in Europe, where it is associated with infection by *B. afzelii*, which is endemic in parts of Europe.

Chronic arthritis without neurologic disease may be treated with either a 28-day oral or a 2-week parenteral antibiotic regimen. Recurrent arthritis after an oral regimen can be retreated with an oral or parenteral regimen. Persistent arthritis despite appropriate antibiotics occurs in 10% of patients in the USA. Chronic arthritis appears to be immunologically mediated and is most common in individuals with the HLA-DR4 haplotype. Multiple repeated courses of antibiotics are unhelpful. However, symptomatic treatment with nonsteroidal agents or, in severe cases, arthroscopic synovectomy may provide relief.

Chronic CNS or peripheral nervous system disease should be treated with a parenteral regimen for 14–28 days.

SPECIFIC INVESTIGATIONS

- Positive ELISA with confirmatory Western blot provides supportive evidence

Recommendations for test performance and interpretation from the Second International Conference on Serologic Diagnosis of Lyme disease. [Anonymous]. MMWR Morb Mortal Wkly Rep 1995;44:590–1.

Guidelines for laboratory evaluation in the diagnosis of Lyme disease. American College of Physicians. [Anonymous]. Ann Intern Med 1997; 127:1106–8.

Laboratory evaluation in the diagnosis of Lyme disease. Tugwell P, Dennis DT, Weinstein A, et al. Ann Intern Med 1997;127:1109–23.

Lyme disease is diagnosed clinically. According to criteria of the Centers for Disease Control (CDC), a diagnosis of early Lyme disease can be made by the presence of erythema migrans in a patient residing in an area endemic for Lyme disease, since serology may be negative at presentation with erythema migrans. Later stages of Lyme disease require clinical signs of disseminated disease and laboratory evidence of infection. A positive culture for *B. burgdorferi* is strong evidence of Lyme disease infection. However, spirochetes are uncommonly isolated except from culture of an erythema migrans lesion. Immunologic tests are available but are only useful in the context of strong clinical suspicion. Serologic testing for Lyme disease is a two-step process. An ELISA should be followed by Western blot testing for all positive ELISAs, to rule out false positive reactions. In persons with symptoms persisting for more than 1 month, an isolated positive IgM for Lyme is likely a false positive, as patients should have developed an IgG response by this time. In diagnosing neuroborreliosis, a CSF:serum ratio of *B. burgdorferi* IgG of >1 suggests intrathecal antibody production. Polymerase chain reaction has shown sensitivities of 80–85% in synovial fluid, but there are much fewer data on sensitivity in CSF specimens.

FIRST LINE THERAPIES

Localized early disease
- Doxycycline 100 mg twice daily for 14–21 days (contraindicated in pregnancy, children <8 years)   A
- Amoxicillin 500 mg three times daily for 14–21 days   A

Neurologic involvement or advanced cardiac conduction block
- Ceftriaxone 2 g i.v. daily for 14–28 days   B
- Penicillin G 18–24 million units daily (divided into 4-hourly doses) for 14–28 days   B

Lyme arthritis
- Doxycycline 100 mg twice daily for 28 days   B
- Amoxicillin 500 mg three times daily for 28 days   B

Chronic neurologic Lyme disease
- Ceftriaxone 2 g i.v. daily for 14–28 days   B
- Penicillin G 18–24 million units daily (in 4-hourly divided doses) for 14–28 days   B

Chronic Lyme arthritis
- Doxycycline 100 mg twice daily for 28 days   B
- Amoxicillin 500 mg three times daily for 28 days   B
- If an oral regimen fails, it is reasonable to use parenteral therapy with ceftriaxone or penicillin G   B

Prophylaxis with single-dose doxycycline for the prevention of Lyme disease after an *Ixodes scapularis* tick bite. Nadelman RB, Nowakowski J, Fish D, et al; Tick Bite Study Group. N Engl J Med 2001;345:79–84.

In this study, 482 were randomized to receive 200 mg doxycycline or placebo within 72 h of removal of an *I. scapularis* tick. One of 235 subjects (0.4%) who received doxycycline, as compared with 8 of 247 (3.2%) who received placebo, developed an erythema migrans lesion. No asymptomatic seroconversions occurred nor did any subject develop extracutaneous Lyme disease. Prophylaxis was 87% efficacious; however, more gastrointestinal symptoms occurred in the doxycycline group.

Amoxicillin plus probenecid versus doxycycline for treatment of erythema migrans borreliosis. Dattwyler RJ, Volkman DJ, Conaty SM, et al. Lancet 1990;336:1404–6.

Seventy-two adults with early Lyme disease were randomized to either amoxicillin 500 mg three times daily or doxycycline 100 mg twice daily for 3 weeks. Both groups had 100% cure rates of their erythema migrans lesions and were asymptomatic after a 6-month follow-up period.

Evidence levels   A Double-blind study   B Clinical trial ≥ 20 subjects   C Clinical trial < 20 subjects   D Series ≥ 5 subjects   E Anecdotal case reports

Duration of antibiotic therapy for early Lyme disease. Wormser GP, Ramanathan R, Nowakowski J, et al. Ann Intern Med 2003;138:697–704.

In this study, 180 patients with erythema migrans were randomized to receive 10 days of oral doxycycline, with or without a single intravenous dose of ceftriaxone, or 20 days of oral doxycycline. The complete response rate at 30 months was similar in all groups: 83.9% in the 20-day doxycycline group, 90.3% in the 10-day doxycycline group, and 86.5% in the doxycycline–ceftriaxone group (p > 0.2). Diarrhea occurred more frequently in the ceftriaxone group.

Two controlled trials of antibiotic treatment in patients with persistent symptoms and a history of Lyme disease. Klempner MS, Hu LT, Evans J, et al. N Engl J Med 2001; 345:85–92.

Patients with persistent symptoms after previously treated documented Lyme disease were randomized to receive either intravenous ceftriaxone 2 g daily for 30 days followed by oral doxycycline 200 mg daily for 60 days, or matching placebos. This study was halted after a planned interim analysis of the first 107 patients enrolled indicated that the study would be unlikely to reveal a significant difference in outcome between the groups.

SECOND LINE THERAPIES

Localized early disease	
■ Cefuroxime axetil 500 mg twice daily for 14–28 days	B
■ Erythromycin 250 mg orally four times daily for 14–28 days	B
■ Azithromycin 500 mg daily for 7 days	B
Neurologic involvement or advanced cardiac conduction block	
■ Doxycycline 100 mg twice daily for 14–28 days	B

Comparison of cefuroxime axetil and doxycycline in the treatment of early Lyme disease. Nadelman RB, Luger SW, Frank E, et al. Ann Intern Med 1992;117:273–80.

A randomized, multicenter, investigator-blinded clinical trial treated 123 patients with erythema migrans for 20 days with either cefuroxime axetil 500 mg twice daily (n = 63) or doxycycline 100 mg twice daily (n = 60). Cure or improvement was achieved in 51 of 55 (93%) evaluable patients treated with cefuroxime axetil and in 45 of 51 (88%) patients treated with doxycycline. At 1 year post-treatment, the percentage of patients who achieved a satisfactory outcome was comparable between the two treatment groups. Cefuroxime was associated with more diarrhea than was doxycycline and is more costly than doxycycline or amoxicillin.

Treatment of the early manifestations of Lyme disease. Steere AC, Hutchinson GJ, Rahn DW, et al. Ann Intern Med 1983;99:22–6.

During 1980 and 1981, the authors compared antibiotic regimens in 108 adult patients with early Lyme disease. Erythema migrans lesions and associated symptoms improved faster in patients treated with penicillin or tetracycline than in those given erythromycin. None of 39 patients given tetracycline developed major late complications (meningoencephalitis, myocarditis, or recurrent attacks of arthritis), compared with 3 of 40 given penicillin and 4 of 29 given erythromycin. Based on this study and similar studies, erythromycin is considered less efficacious than first line drugs.

Azithromycin compared with amoxicillin in the treatment of erythema migrans. A double-blind, randomized, controlled trial. Luft BJ, Dattwyler RJ, Johnson RC, et al. Ann Intern Med 1996;124:785–91.

In this study, 246 adult patients with erythema migrans lesions were randomized to treatment with either amoxicillin 500 mg three times daily for 20 days or azithromycin 500 mg once daily for 7 days. Those treated with amoxicillin were more likely than those treated with azithromycin to achieve complete resolution of disease at day 20 (88% for amoxicillin compared with 76% for azithromycin; p = 0.024). More azithromycin recipients (16%) than amoxicillin recipients (4%) had relapses.

VACCINE

■ Lyme disease vaccine	A

DNA vaccine expressing a fusion product of outer surface proteins A and C from *Borrelia burgdorferi* induces protective antibodies suitable for prophylaxis but not for resolution of Lyme disease. Wallich R, Siebers A, Jahraus O, et al. Infect Immun 2001;69:2130–6.

Lymerix®, a recombinant outer surface protein A vaccine, was approved for use in December 1998 and was shown to be effective at preventing, but not treating, Lyme disease. In clinical trials, efficacy of Lymerix® in preventing definite cases of disease varied from 76% to 92%. However, the vaccine was withdrawn from the market in February 2002 due to poor sales.

Lymphangioma circumscriptum

Sandeep H Cliff, Peter S Mortimer

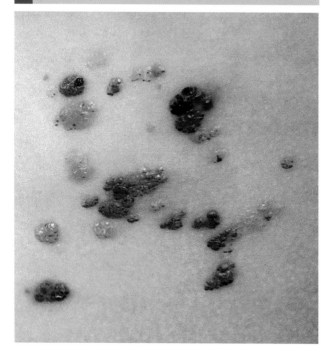

The term 'lymphangioma' should be confined to benign neoplastic or hamartomatous proliferations of lymph vessels that do not communicate with the normal lymph conducting system. Lymphangioma circumscriptum is characterized by subcutaneous lymphatic cisterns communicating through dilated channels with superficial thin-walled vesicles on the skin surface. These vesicles may be up to 5 mm in diameter and typically contain lymph, but not infrequently contain red blood cells.

'Acquired lymphangioma' may develop following surgery or radiation of the lymphatic network. This condition represents dilatation of existing normal cutaneous lymphatics (lymphangiectasia) due to backpressure and is therefore not a true lymphangioma.

MANAGEMENT STRATEGY

The main indications for treating this condition are cosmetic as well as controlling complications such as infection, hemorrhage, and pain. If the condition is asymptomatic then a 'watch and wait' policy is advised. Intervention can disturb the lymphangioma, causing progression or complications. To be certain of 'cure' one needs to remove not only the superficial component but, more importantly, the deeper lymphatic cisterns. Treatments therefore involve either *surgical destruction* of lesions and/or *laser ablation*. However, as there is no reliable means of ensuring that the deeper lymph sacs have been removed, there is a well-documented high recurrence rate with all but the most aggressive treatments.

All other treatments are palliative, seeking to control symptoms (i.e. improve pain or cosmetic disability and reduce lymphorrhea [lymph seepage]). Limited excision runs the risk of the subsequent development of new surface lymphangiomas. *Electrocautery, cryotherapy,* and *CO₂ laser* have been used to 'seal' weeping lymphangiomas and reduce the risk of infection. Evidence of efficacy is derived from a series of published cases with no controlled trials. Injection sclerotherapy using intralesional *doxycycline* or *Picibanil (OK-432)* has been reported as helpful.

Pain may result from either a rise in pressure within the lymphangioma, due presumably to a build-up of lymph, or from hemorrhage or infection. Treatment of infection is by *penicillin V (phenoxymethylpenicillin)* 500 mg four times daily for 6 weeks (authors' recommendation). If infection is persistent or recurrent, long-term treatment with penicillin V 500 mg twice daily for 1 year is advised. External pressure using *elastic hosiery* may be helpful for weeping lymphangiomas on a limb, but discomfort may be a problem.

SPECIFIC INVESTIGATIONS

- Lymphangiography
- MRI

Lymphangiography and surgery in lymphangioma of the skin. Edwards JM, Peachey RDG, Kinmonth JB. Br J Surg 1972;59:36–41.

Lymphangiography has been carried out on patients with lymphangioma circumscriptum and shows the presence of a normal lymphatic network surrounding these sacs. It also confirms the absence of any communication between the sacs and the normal lymphatic network.

Magnetic resonance imaging in the evaluation of lymphangioma circumscriptum. McAlvany JP, Jorizzo JL, Zanolli D, et al. Arch Dermatol 1993;129:194–7.

MRI may prove useful prior to surgery to limit the risk of recurrence. However, smaller lymphatic cisterns are frequently not reliably visible with MRI.

FIRST LINE THERAPIES

■ Leave undisturbed	D
■ Surgery	D
■ Control of infection	D

Lymphangioma circumscriptum. Mordehai J, Kurzbart E, Shinbar D, et al. Pediatr Surg Int 1998;13:208–10.

Reports on two children with lymphangioma circumscriptum treated with wide local excision. One child required four repeat excisions and at the time of the report was still awaiting further surgery for recurrences. The other child had no recurrences at 2-year follow-up.

Surgical management of lymphangioma circumscriptum. Browse NL, Whimster I, Stewart G, et al. Br J Surg 1986;73: 585–8.

Small lesions (less than 7 cm in diameter) are potentially curable. Large lesions (> 7 cm in diameter on the skin) treated by radical excision resulted in recurrence in four of 20 patients.

SECOND LINE THERAPIES

■ Electrocautery	D
■ CO_2 laser	D
■ Superficial X-rays	E
■ Cryotherapy	D
■ Injection sclerotherapy	D

A case of lymphangioma circumscriptum. Noyes AWF. Br Med J 1993;1:1159.

Superficial destruction of lesions with electrocautery is effective, but as expected, there is a high recurrence rate. However, electrocautery may produce temporary relief of leakage of lymph by sclerosing the vessels.

Carbon dioxide laser vaporisation of lymphangioma circumscriptum. Bailin PL, Kantor GR, Wheeland RG. J Am Acad Dermatol 1986;14:257–62.

Describes the use of the CO_2 laser (10 600 nm) to vaporize the vesicles of lymphangioma circumscriptum in seven patients. The authors accept that the purpose was not to destroy the deeper component, but to deal with the superficial lesions. They conclude that the recurrence rate is lower than with other destructive techniques because the CO_2 laser destroys the superficial lymphatic vessels and seals the communicating channels. Follow-up at 1 year showed recurrences in two of five patients.

The laser may be a useful treatment modality for this notoriously treatment-resistant condition. However, one should be cautious because follow-up is short.

Recalcitrant breast lymphangioma circumscriptum treated by UltraPulse carbon dioxide laser. Haas AF, Narurkar VA. Dermatol Surg 1998;24:893–5.

The use of the newer high energy short-pulsed CO_2 laser is described for persistent lymphangioma circumscriptum, which was recurrent despite two previous surgical treatments.

Laser modalities are usually effective initially, but due to the nature of the lesion, recurrence is almost inevitable.

Successful control of lymphangioma circumscriptum by superficial x-rays. O'Cathail S, Rostom AY, Johnson ML. Br J Dermatol 1985;113:611–5.

Describes a patient with lymphangioma circumscriptum treated successfully with superficial radiotherapy. It was noted that time to response was long (12 months), but treatment was effective with no recurrence reported at time of publication.

With any cutaneous radiotherapy one cannot be certain of the long-term effects with respect to the development of non-melanoma skin cancer. To date, there have been no reports of this developing in patients treated with radiotherapy for lymphangioma circumscriptum.

Radiotherapy is a useful treatment for lymphangioma circumscriptum: a report of two patients. Denton AS, Baker-Hines R, Spittle MF. Clin Oncol 1996;8:400–1.

A report of two cases, which although unsuitable for excision, were treated successfully by radiotherapy. The authors consider radiotherapy an effective treatment for unresectable lesions or for patients who are unwilling to consider surgery.

Successful results of treatment with solid carbon dioxide. Arch Dermatol Syph 1946;54:202–4.

Cryodestruction of lymphangioma circumscriptum has been widely employed to destroy superficial vesicles. There are recurrences, but they may be delayed or occur at different sites due to scarring induced by the cryogen.

Percutaneous sclerotherapy of lymphangiomas. Molitch HL, Unger ES, Witte CL, van Sonnenberg E. Radiology 1995;194:343–7.

Successful treatment using intralesional doxycycline sclerotherapy in five patients.

Lymphangioma circumscriptum treated with pulsed dye laser. Lai CH, Hanson SG, Mallory SB. Pediatr Dermatol 2001;18:509–10.

A child with symptomatic lymphangioma circumscriptum is described in which hemorrhage was a feature. This responded well to treatment with the 585 nm pulsed dye laser. This laser may be considered in patients in whom hemorrhage is a feature in the lymphatic vesicles.

Lymphedema

Geover Fernandez, Giuseppe Micali, Robert A Schwartz

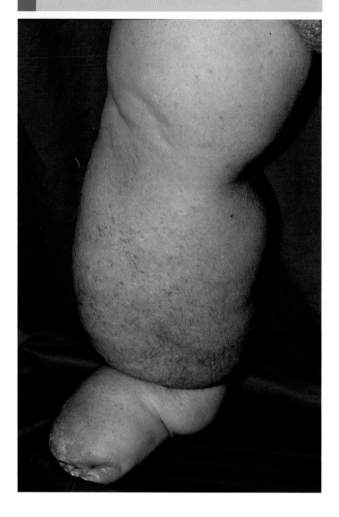

Lymphedema is a chronic, sometimes debilitating condition, characterized clinically by its brawny, non-pitting edema. It is due to the accumulation of protein-rich lymph in interstitial spaces, caused by ineffective lymphatic drainage. Lymphedema is classified into primary and secondary forms. Primary lymphedema is caused by a developmental malformation of the lymphatic system. Primary congenital lymphedema (Milroy disease) is an uncommon autosomal dominant disorder due, in some families, to missense mutations that interfere with vascular endothelial growth factor receptor-3 signaling, resulting in abnormal lymphatic vascular function. Primary lymphedema may be further classified by age of onset into congenital lymphedema, lymphedema praecox, and lymphedema tarda. Secondary lymphedema is usually due to blockage or destruction of otherwise normal lymph channels. In the United States the most common causes are compression by tumor, surgical manipulation, or radiation damage. Worldwide, the most common cause is filariasis. Acquired lymphedema may predispose to an aggressive type of angiosarcoma, best documented postmastectomy, and known as the Stewart-Treves syndrome. Chronic lymphedema may result in verrucous and proliferative changes resembling elephant skin (elephantiasis).

MANAGEMENT STRATEGIES

Lymphedema must be distinguished from edema of cardiac, hepatic, and renal origin. Lymphoscintigraphy (isotope lymphography) is a first line imaging modality to evaluate and diagnose disorders of the lymphatic vasculature. The treatment options for lymphedema are basically the same. A *medical, conservative approach* is the standard of treatment for lymphedema. The main management strategy is to *reduce stagnation of protein-rich lymph in the extravascular tissue* and to *improve the outflow of lymphatic circulation.*

Complete decongestive therapy represents a superb treatment plan. It is a four-component therapeutic modality composed of *multilayer compression bandage, manual lymphatic drainage, skin care,* and *exercise.* Patients should be encouraged to use compression bandage or garments continuously during the day, as well as leg elevation. *Pneumatic compression pumps* were widely utilized to control lymphedema, but due to the poor outcome as a monotherapy, their current use has been limited. Medications, such as *diuretics,* have shown limited or no effect on lymphedema. *Meticulous skin care and hygiene* may prevent secondary bacterial and fungal infections. At the earliest sign of infection, *topical and systemic antibiotics* should be administered to prevent sepsis. This is especially important because recurrent infections may lead to further lymphatic injury.

Surgical approaches are reserved for cases recalcitrant to conservative management. *Microsurgical lymphaticovenous implantation* combined with decongestive therapy has yielded excellent results. *Excisional surgical therapy* has been performed to reduce limb size and to improve mobility in chronic advanced cases of lymphedema.

SPECIFIC INVESTIGATIONS

- ■ Lymphoscintigraphy
- ■ MRI
- ■ CT

Advances in imaging of lymph flow disorders. Witte CL, Witte MH, Unger EC, et al. Radiographics 2000;6:1697–719.

Excellent review article illustrating multiple clinical cases in which lymphoscintigraphy, MRI, and CT were useful in the evaluation and diagnosis of patients with primary or secondary lymphedema. The advantages and limitations of each imaging modality are reviewed.

FIRST LINE THERAPIES

■ Decongestive lymphatic therapy	B

The effectiveness of complete decongestive physiotherapy for the treatment of lymphedema following groin dissection for melanoma. Hinrichs CS, Gibbs JF, Driscoll D, et al. J Surg Oncol 2004;85:187–92.

Small cohort study showing significant reduction of lymphedema in patients treated with complete decongestive physiotherapy following lymph node groin dissection for melanoma.

Evidence levels A Double-blind study **B** Clinical trial ≥ 20 subjects **C** Clinical trial < 20 subjects **D** Series ≥ 5 subjects **E** Anecdotal case reports

The effect of complete decongestive therapy on the quality of life of patients with peripheral lymphedema. Weiss JM, Spray BJ. Lymphology 2002;35:46–58.

Study showing significant improvement in the quality of life of 36 patients with lymphedema following complete decongestive therapy. However, improvement of quality of life did not necessarily correlate with limb volume reduction.

SECOND LINE THERAPIES

■ Pneumatic compression therapy	B

Decongestive lymphatic therapy for patients with breast carcinoma-associated lymphedema. A randomized, prospective study of a role for adjunctive intermittent pneumatic compression. Szuba A, Achalu R, Rockson SG. Cancer 2002;95:2260–7.

Prospective randomized study of 23 patients comparing decongestive lymphatic therapy alone vs decongestive lymphatic therapy plus intermittent pneumatic compression. Intermittent pneumatic compression proved effective as an adjunctive therapy to decongestive therapy.

THIRD LINE THERAPIES

■ Surgery	B

Follow-up study of upper limb lymphedema patients treated by microsurgical lymphaticovenous implantation (MLVI) combined with compression therapy. Yamamoto Y, Horiuchi K, Sasaki S, et al. Microsurgery 2003;23:21–6.

Follow-up study of 18 patients treated by microsurgical lymphaticovenous implantation combined with compression therapy shows favorable results in 78% of patients. Average follow-up was 2 years.

Microsurgical techniques for lymphedema treatment: derivative lymphatic-venous microsurgery. Campisi C, Boccardo F. World J Surg 2004;28:609–13.

Of the 447 patients followed, 380 (85%) have been able to discontinue the use of conservative measures, with an average follow-up of more than 7 years and average reduction in excess volume of 69%. There was an 87% reduction in incidence of cellulitis after microsurgery.

One of the main problems of microsurgery for lymphedema is the discrepancy between the excellent technical possibilities and the subsequently insufficient reduction of the lymphedematous tissue fibrosis and sclerosis. Improved results can be expected with operations performed early, during the first stages of lymphedema.

Lymphocytoma cutis

Fiona J Child, Sean J Whittaker

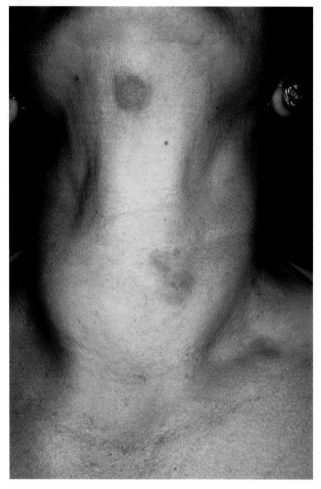

Lymphocytoma cutis is an entity encompassing a spectrum of benign B cell lymphoproliferative diseases that share clinical and histopathologic features. Various stimuli can induce lymphocytoma cutis, but in most cases the cause is not known. It is more common in females, with a three-to-one female-to-male ratio. Most cases are characterized by localized, erythematous, plum-colored nodules and plaques, which may be difficult to distinguish from cutaneous B cell lymphoma. Less frequently the generalized form may present with multiple miliary papules measuring a few millimeters in diameter.

MANAGEMENT STRATEGY

A skin biopsy for histopathology and immunohistochemistry is required to confirm the diagnosis, though the distinction between lymphocytoma cutis and cutaneous B cell lymphoma may be difficult on both clinical and histopathologic evaluation. There are no agreed histologic criteria, but features that suggest lymphocytoma cutis include well-formed, nonexpanded, reactive germinal centers, the majority of the infiltrate consisting of small round lymphocytes with a B:T cell ratio of less than 3:1, and polytypic expression of κ and λ light chains. Another feature is the presence of numerous tingible body macrophages within the lymphoid follicles. Molecular analysis of the immunoglobulin heavy chain gene has shown that a significant proportion harbor B cell clones, which suggests that many cases previously thought to be lymphocytoma cutis represent indolent low-grade primary cutaneous B cell lymphomas (PCBCL). Therefore, in cases with a detectable B cell clone a careful evaluation to exclude systemic disease (a thorough clinical examination, thoraco-abdomino-pelvic CT scan, and bone marrow biopsy) is required with adequate long-term follow-up.

A history of possible stimuli that are known to cause lymphocytoma cutis should be sought and include *Borrelia burgdorferi* infection, trauma, vaccinations, allergy hyposensitization injections, ingestion of drugs, arthropod bites, acupuncture, gold pierced earrings, tattoos, treatment with leeches (*Hirudo medicinalis*) and post-herpes zoster scars. The majority of cases, however, are of unknown etiology.

The course of the disease varies, but tends to be chronic and indolent. Some lesions may resolve spontaneously without treatment. There is no therapy of proven value for lymphocytoma cutis, with only anecdotal case reports and small series reported in the literature.

If a cause can be identified, the causative agent should be removed. If infection with *B. burgdorferi* is suspected, treatment with appropriate *antibiotics (amoxicillin* 500–1000 mg three times daily or *doxycycline* 100 mg two to three times daily for a period of at least 3 weeks) should be initiated.

Localized disease can be treated by simple *excision* and may respond to *intralesional injection of corticosteroids, local irradiation,* or *intralesional interferon-alfa.* More widespread (generalized) disease is traditionally treated with *oral antimalarials,* most commonly *hydroxychloroquine* (maximum dose 6.5 mg/kg daily); however, lesions may fail to respond to treatment or may recur following cessation of therapy. Other treatment modalities include *subcutaneous interferon-alfa* and *oral thalidomide.* Effective responses to destructive therapies including *cryotherapy* and the *argon laser* have been reported. A subtype of generalized lymphocytoma cutis may be exacerbated by light, and therefore *sun avoidance* and the use of *sun block* is important.

SPECIFIC INVESTIGATIONS

- Serology for *B. burgdorferi*
- Skin biopsy for histology, immunophenotype, and immunoglobulin gene analysis
- Patch testing (if a possible contact allergen is suspected)

The spirochetal etiology of lymphadenosis benigna cutis solitaria. Hovmark A, Asrink E, Olsson I. Acta Derm Venereol 1986;66:479–84.

Of ten patients investigated, four reported a previous tick bite. Positive *Borrelia* serology was found in six of nine patients and spirochetes were cultivated from one of two skin biopsies.

Lymphadenosis benigna cutis resulting from *Borrelia* infection (*Borrelia* lymphocytoma). Albrecht S, Hofstadter MD, Artsob H, Chaban RT. J Am Acad Dermatol 1991;24:621–5.

Evidence levels **A** Double-blind study **B** Clinical trial ≥ 20 subjects **C** Clinical trial < 20 subjects **D** Series ≥ 5 subjects **E** Anecdotal case reports

A child who developed lymphocytoma cutis on her ear following a tick bite 6 months previously had positive *Borrelia* serology and a *Borrelia*-like organism was identified in skin biopsy sections. The lesion regressed during a 2-month course of penicillin V.

Cutaneous lymphoid hyperplasia and cutaneous marginal zone lymphoma: comparison of morphologic and immunophenotypic features. Baldassano MF, Bailey EM, Ferry JA, et al. Am J Surg Pathol 1999;23:88–96.

Histologic and immunophenotypic features of 14 cases of lymphocytoma cutis and 16 cases of cutaneous marginal zone lymphoma are compared.

Differential diagnosis of cutaneous infiltrates of B lymphocytes with follicular growth pattern. Leinweber B, Colli C, Chott A, et al. Am J Dermatopathol 2004;26:4–13.

Histopathological, immunophenotypic, and molecular features of *B. burgdorferi*-associated lymphocytoma cutis, primary cutaneous follicle center cell lymphoma, and primary cutaneous marginal zone lymphoma were compared. Features that favored lymphocytoma cutis were the presence of tingible body macrophages, strong proliferation rate of follicular cells, BCL2-negative follicular cells, and the absence of monoclonality.

Borrelia burgdorferi-associated lymphocytoma cutis: clinicopathologic, immunophenotypic, and molecular study of 106 cases. Colli C, Leinweber B, Müllegger R, et al. J Cutan Pathol 2004;31:232–40.

One hundred and six cases of *B. burgdorferi*-associated lymphocytoma cutis, in a region endemic for *Borrelia* spp. infection, were studied retrospectively. The most common sites affected were the earlobe, genital area, and nipple (these locations may be due to the predilection for cooler body sites by *B. burgdorferi* spirochetes). In some cases the histopathologic, immunophenotypic, and molecular features were misleading, and it was concluded that integration of all data is necessary to obtain the correct diagnosis.

Clonal rearrangements of immunoglobulin genes and progression to B cell lymphoma in cutaneous lymphoid hyperplasia. Wood GS, Ngan BY, Tung R, et al. Am J Pathol 1989;135:13–9.

In this study, five of 14 cases of cutaneous lymphoid hyperplasia exhibited a clonal immunoglobulin rearrangement by Southern blot analysis. One of these five cases evolved into a diffuse large B cell lymphoma during a 2-year follow-up period, suggesting that monoclonal populations may exist in some cases of cutaneous lymphoid hyperplasia, and these may represent a subgroup more likely to evolve into lymphoma.

Immunophenotypic and genotypic analysis in cutaneous lymphoid hyperplasias. Hammer E, Sangueza O, Suwanjindar P, et al. J Am Acad Dermatol 1993;28:426–33.

Of 11 cases with histologic and immunophenotypic features of lymphocytoma cutis, clonal rearrangements were detected in two patients, both of whom subsequently developed B cell lymphoma.

Polymerase chain reaction analysis of immunoglobulin gene rearrangement analysis in cutaneous lymphoid hyperplasias. Bouloc A, Delfau-Larue M-H, Lenormand B, et al. Arch Dermatol 1999;135:168–72.

Twenty four patients with a diagnosis of lymphocytoma cutis according to clinical, histopathologic, and immunophenotypic criteria underwent polymerase chain reaction (PCR) analysis of the immunoglobulin heavy chain gene using DNA from lesional skin. In one of 24 patients a B cell clone was detected. A polyclonal result was obtained in the other patients.

Cutaneous B cell lymphomas are known to have a relatively high false-negative rate using PCR due to somatic hypermutation, which affects the variable region of the immunoglobulin heavy chain gene and may prevent primer binding. The number of false-negative results may be reduced by using multiple primer sets for different parts of the variable region. This paper only used one set of primers and therefore the detection of only one B cell clone may be a significant underestimate.

Lymphomatoid contact reaction to gold earrings. Fleming C, Burden D, Fallowfield M, Lever R. Contact Dermatitis 1997;37:298–9.

A rare entity characterized by nodules at sites of piercing with gold jewelry and the histologic features of lymphocytoma cutis. Patch tests to gold sodium thiosulfate are positive.

FIRST LINE THERAPIES

Localized	
■ Excision	E
■ Topical corticosteroids	E
■ Intralesional corticosteroids	E
■ Oral antibiotics (if positive *Borrelia* serology)	E
Generalized	
■ Antimalarials	E
■ Sun avoidance and sunblock (for light-exacerbated cases)	E

Treatment of cutaneous pseudolymphoma with hydroxychloroquine. Stoll DM. J Am Acad Dermatol 1983;8:696–9.

A case report of a 40-year-old woman with generalized lymphocytoma cutis that cleared with 400 mg hydroxychloroquine daily.

A study of the photosensitivity factor in cutaneous lymphocytoma. Frain-Bell W, Magnus IA. Br J Dermatol 1971;84:25–31.

Patients with lymphocytoma and associated light sensitivity are reported and previous cases reviewed.

Pseudolymphoma occurring in a tattoo. Kahofer P, El Shabrawi-Caelen L, Horn M, et al. Eur J Dermatol 2003;13:209–12.

A 34-year-old woman with a nodular infiltrate limited to the red areas of a tattoo is described. Topical treatment with corticosteroids was not successful so a total excision of the lesion was performed.

SECOND LINE THERAPIES

Localized	
■ Superficial radiotherapy	E
■ Intralesional interferon-alfa	E
■ Argon laser	E
■ Cryotherapy	D

Cutaneous lymphoid hyperplasia: results of radiation therapy. Olson LE, Wilson JF, Cox JD. Radiology 1985;155: 507–9.

Four cases of lymphocytoma cutis were treated with radiation therapy. Over a follow-up period of 8 months to 7 years there were no recurrences.

Local orthovolt radiotherapy in primary cutaneous B-cell lymphoma. Pimpinelli N, Vallecchi C. Skin Cancer 1999;14: 219–24.

Data from 115 patients with PCBCL showed a 98.2% complete remission rate and a median disease-free period of 55 months; recurrences were mostly limited to the skin. In view of the difficulties in distinguishing between PCBCL and lymphocytoma cutis, many groups have used superficial radiotherapy in cases of lymphocytoma cutis, though evidence remains anecdotal.

In our experience lymphocytoma cutis is relatively radioresistant compared with PCBCL.

Role of the argon laser in treatment of lymphocytoma cutis. Wheeland RG, Kantor GR, Bailin PL, Bergfeld WF. J Am Acad Dermatol 1986;14:267–72.

The argon laser improved cosmetic appearance and alleviated symptoms of lymphocytoma cutis, but failed to provide complete histological clearing in a young man who had failed to respond adequately to initial therapy with hydroxychloroquine.

Lymphocytoma cutis: a series of five patients successfully treated with cryosurgery. Kuflik AS, Schwartz RA. J Am Acad Dermatol 1992;26:449–52.

Five patients with lymphocytoma cutis underwent therapy with liquid nitrogen to individual lesions with a single cycle of 15–20 s per lesion with complete clinical resolution of all lesions treated within 3–6 weeks.

THIRD LINE THERAPIES

Generalized	
■ Subcutaneous interferon-alfa-2b	E
■ Thalidomide	E

Spiegler-Fendt type lymphocytoma cutis: a case report of two patients successfully treated with interferon alpha-2b. Hervonen K, Lehtinen T, Vaalasti A. Acta Derm Venereol 1999;79:241–2.

Two men, who had generalized lymphocytoma cutis and had failed to respond to other therapies, were treated with subcutaneous interferon-alfa-2b 2.5 MU three times a week with complete resolution of all lesions by 3 months. However, lesions recurred in both men between 6 and 23 months following completion of treatment.

Treatment of cutaneous lymphoid hyperplasia with thalidomide: report of two cases. Benchikhi H, Bodemer C, Fraitag S, et al. J Am Acad Dermatol 1999;40:1005–7.

Two cases of lymphocytoma cutis involving the nose that showed complete regression following treatment with thalidomide for 3 months at a dose of 100 mg once daily for 2 months and 50 mg once daily for the third month. There was no recurrence at 36 and 31 month follow-up, respectively.

Evidence levels **A** Double-blind study   **B** Clinical trial ≥ 20 subjects   **C** Clinical trial < 20 subjects   **D** Series ≥ 5 subjects   **E** Anecdotal case reports

Lymphogranuloma venereum

Patrice Morel

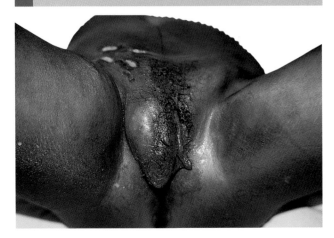

Lymphogranuloma venereum (LGV) is a sexually transmitted disease caused by the serovars L1, L2, or L3 of *Chlamydia trachomatis*. It accounts for 2–10% of genital ulcer disease in some areas of Africa and India. Inguinal lymphadenopathy and coloproctitis are the most frequent clinical manifestations in developed countries. Outbreaks of LGV among homosexual men with proctitis have recently been observed in Western Europe (Rotterdam and Paris).

MANAGEMENT STRATEGY

Antibiotic treatment of LGV is necessary:

- to prevent the spread of the infection that may lead to a painful inflammation and infection of the inguinal and/or femoral lymph nodes (buboes), rectal and perirectal complications with proctitis followed by abscesses, fistulas, strictures, and genital elephantiasis;
- to prevent transmission to sex partners;
- to prevent the co-transmission of HIV.

Because LGV is caused by *C. trachomatis*, treatments with *doxycycline* or *erythromycin* for 21 days is the most recommended regimen. Antibiotic treatment cures the ongoing infection and prevents further tissue damage. Patients should be followed clinically until signs and symptoms have resolved. Buboes may require *aspiration* through intact skin to relieve the inguinal pain and to prevent the formation of ulcerations. The late complications of LGV may necessitate *surgical repair* after antibiotic treatment is complete.

Patients with HIV infection should be treated according to the same regimen. Anecdotal evidence suggests that LGV infection in HIV-positive patients may require prolonged therapy and that resolution might be delayed.

Sex partners of patients who have LGV should be examined, tested for urethral or cervical chlamydial infection, and treated if they had sexual contact with the patient during the 30 days preceding the onset of symptoms in the patient.

SPECIFIC INVESTIGATIONS

- Chlamydial serology
- Culture

Genital ulcer disease: accuracy of clinical diagnosis and strategies to improve control in Durban, South Africa. O'Farrel N, Hoosen AA, Coetzee KD, Van Den Ende J. Genitourin Med 1994;70:7–11.

There is a relatively poor degree of clinical suspicion for LGV in countries endemic for chancroid, donovanosis, and LGV. In Durban, the accuracy of a clinical diagnosis of LGV was 66% in men and 40% in women.

A cluster of lymphogranuloma venereum among homosexual men in Rotterdam with implications for other countries in Western Europe. Gotz HM, Ossewaarde JM, Nieuwenhuis RF, et al. Ned Tijdschr Geneeskd 2004;148: 441–2.

The authors report 15 cases of LGV among male homosexuals. Most patients presented with proctitis and some with constipation. Similar cases were recently observed in Paris. Evaluation of gastrointestinal syndromes that might have been sexually transmitted should include appropriate diagnostic procedures (e.g. anoscopy or sigmoidoscopy) and microbiologic testing for *C. trachomatis*, syphilis, herpes, *Neisseria gonorrhoeae*, and common enteric pathogens that can be sexually transmitted (CDC-2004).

Isolation in endothelial cell cultures of *Chlamydia trachomatis* LGV (serovar L2) from a lymph node of a patient with suspected cat scratch disease. Maurin M, Raoult D. J Clin Microbiol 2000;38:2062–4.

The histology of the lymph nodes in LGV is not pathognomonic. Cat scratch disease is the most frequent differential diagnosis in developed countries.

Lymphogranuloma venereum: 27 cases in Paris. Scieux C, Barnes R, Bianchi A, et al. J Infect Dis 1989;160:662–8.

Definitive diagnosis is made by isolation and identification of *C. trachomatis* biovar LGV from tissue, lymph node aspirates, and/or rectal biopsy specimens.

Lymphogranuloma venereum: biopsy, serology and molecular biology. Kellock DJ, Barlow R, Suvarna SK, et al. Genitourin Med 1997;73:399–401.

The specificity of cell culture for *C. trachomatis* serovar L1–3 is excellent, but its sensitivity is only about 50%. Microimmunofluorescence titers are usually high (> 1/512), but this test has broad cross-reaction with other *C. trachomatis* serovars. The whole inclusion immunofluorescence test is more specific. A rise of 1/64 or greater with LGV complement fixation tests is seen in 50% of patients. This response, in conjunction with the elevated whole inclusion immunofluorescence test, is indicative of LGV. The polymerase chain reaction may provide an accurate laboratory diagnosis of LGV in low-prevalence areas.

FIRST LINE THERAPIES

■ Doxycycline 100 mg orally twice daily for 21 days	B

Sexually transmitted diseases. Treatment guidelines – 2002. Centers for Disease Control and Prevention. MMWR Recomm Rep 2002;51(RR-6):1–78.

Doxycycline is the preferred treatment. Erythromycin is the alternative regimen. The activity of azithromycin against *C. trachomatis* suggests that it may be effective. Successful treatments with azithromycin (1.0 g orally once weekly for 3 weeks) were reported.

SECOND LINE THERAPIES

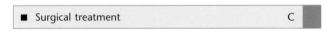

■ Erythromycin base 500 mg orally four times daily for 21 days	B
■ Tetracycline 500 mg orally four times daily for 21 days	B
■ Aspiration of buboes	B

Lymphogranuloma venereum. Becker LE. Int J Dermatol 1976;15:26–33.

Buboes should not be surgically incised and drained or allowed to spontaneously rupture. If the bubo becomes fluctuant and rupture seems likely, the bubo should be aspirated with a large syringe using an 18- or 19-gauge needle. The bubo should be entered through normal skin, preferably superiorly, and not directly through the involved skin to decrease the possibility of sinus tract formation.

Incision and drainage versus aspiration of fluctuant buboes in the emergency department during an epidemic of chancroid. Ernst AA, Marvez-Valls E, Martin DH. Sex Transm Dis 1995;22:217–20.

These authors consider that incision and drainage is an effective method for treating fluctuant buboes and may be preferable to traditional needle aspiration considering the frequency of required re-aspirations.

We do not agree completely with the conclusion of this study involving cases of chancroid and LGV. We think that incision and drainage may delay the recovery, facilitate a bacterial superinfection, and increase the risk for developing chronic lymphocutaneous fistulae.

THIRD LINE THERAPIES

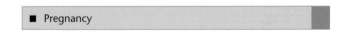

■ Surgical treatment	C

Problematic ulcerative lesions in sexually transmitted diseases: surgical management. Parkash S, Radhakrishna K. Sex Transm Dis 1986;13:127–33.

Anatomic changes resulting from chronic infection are not amenable to antibiotic therapy and may require surgical repair, although the patient should always receive a course of antibiotics first.

SPECIAL CONSIDERATIONS

■ Pregnancy	

Pregnant and lactating women should be treated with the erythromycin regimen. Infection with LGV in infants born to infected women has not been addressed in the literature.

Evidence levels **A** Double-blind study **B** Clinical trial ≥ 20 subjects **C** Clinical trial < 20 subjects **D** Series ≥ 5 subjects **E** Anecdotal case reports

Lymphomatoid papulosis

Jacqueline M Junkins-Hopkins,
Alain H Rook, Carmela C Vittorio

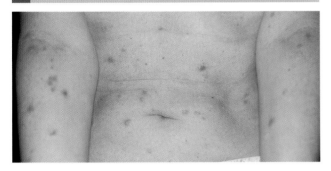

Lymphomatoid papulosis (LyP) is a distinct subset of CD30⁺ lymphoproliferative disorders defined by characteristic histopathology, which includes a variable infiltrate of CD30⁺ lymphocytes, in conjunction with a history of recurrent, self-healing papulonodules. The papules and nodules evolve into a crusted or necrotic stage, which often heal with a scar. LyP can affect any age group, having been reported in patients as young as 11 months of age, and typically persists for years to decades. Approximately 10–20% of patients with LyP may present with or develop a lymphoid malignancy, such as mycosis fungoides (MF – cutaneous T cell lymphoma [CTCL], see page 415), CD30⁺ lymphoma, and Hodgkin's and non-Hodgkin's lymphomas. Patients with LyP may also have a slight risk of developing a non-hematologic neoplasm. Although LyP may not represent a malignant lymphoma from the outset, the same clone has been documented in patients with LyP and MF, and patients with LyP may progress to CD30⁺ lymphoma, supporting the concept that LyP lies on a spectrum of CTCL. Clinical and histologic overlap may also be seen with LyP and pityriasis lichenoides et varioliformis acuta (PLEVA, see page 498).

MANAGEMENT STRATEGY

Most importantly, the management of LyP begins with understanding the natural course of this disease. It was recently proposed that LyP be defined as a recurrent, self-healing (remission of every individual lesion), papulo-nodular eruption, with histology suggesting CTCL. The latter includes histology with CD30⁺ cells resembling the Reed–Sternberg cells of Hodgkin's disease, admixed with inflammatory cells (LyP type A), histology simulating MF (LyP type B), and cohesive sheets of CD30⁺ cells (LyP type C). A diagnosis of LyP should be reserved for patients without constitutional symptoms, hepatosplenomegaly, or lymphadenopathy. Patients with these findings should undergo a hematologic evaluation and CT scanning to exclude systemic lymphoma. It also important to differentiate LyP from primary CD30⁺ lymphoma, though this may be difficult because there is much clinical and histologic overlap, including the feature of spontaneous regression. While some have used criteria such as lesions greater than

2–3 cm in diameter that do not involute, and/or histology showing sheets of CD30⁺ cells extending into the subcutaneous fat to favor CD30⁺ lymphoma, some patients do not fit well into either category. Such borderline LyP-CD30 lymphoma cases have similar biologic behavior as LyP, and can be managed as such.

Once the diagnosis of LyP is firmly established, treatment should be tailored to the disease burden because most of the modalities currently available do not alter the natural course of LyP, nor do they prevent the development of extracutaneous lymphomas. Treatment should be reserved for symptomatic or scarring disease. There may be some response to topical *corticosteroids*, but this does not induce remission. Other alternatives, such as *tetracycline* and *acyclovir*, have anecdotally been associated with clearance, but these options cannot replace those discussed below. In cosmetically bothersome cases, *low-dose methotrexate* or *8-methoxypsoralen with UVA (PUVA)* are appropriate first line treatment modalities. Patients may respond to as little as 5 mg/week of methotrexate, but may require 15–20 mg/week. A response can be seen within the first few weeks of treatment and include the development of fewer lesions, shortening of the life cycle of the individual lesions, and an induction of remission while on the drug. PUVA is a valuable treatment, but conventional UVB is of less benefit. Large lesions that take longer than 6 weeks to clear can be treated with local radiotherapy or excision. This is also an accepted treatment for CD30⁺ lymphoma, should the diagnosis be equivocal. Various other forms of therapy that are beneficial in MF may also be useful in clearing lesions of LyP, including topical *carmustine (BCNU)*, topical *mechlorethamine (nitrogen mustard)*, and biologic agents such as *interferon-α* and *interferon-γ*. Retinoids are also beneficial. In particular, the retinoid X receptor agonist bexarotene has been associated with clearing of LyP lesions, with diminished recurrences, at doses of 150–300 mg daily. In our experience, topical bexarotene in a region of localized disease prevented recurrence of the condition. LyP can persist for decades, requiring careful consideration of treatment side effects and continued monitoring for the development of lymphoma. Multi-agent chemotherapy is not indicated, despite histologic features that may suggest CD30⁺ lymphoma.

SPECIFIC INVESTIGATIONS

- Biopsy and histologic review to confirm the diagnosis
- Exclusion of constitutional ('B') symptoms and clinically detectable hepatosplenomegaly or lymphadenopathy
- Consider staging procedures for LyP type C, including chest, thoracic, abdominal, and pelvic CT and bone marrow evaluation
- Ongoing surveillance for a lymphoproliferative neoplasm

Spectrum of primary cutaneous CD30 (Ki-1)-positive lymphoproliferative disorders. A proposal for classification and guidelines for management and treatment. Willemze R, Beljaards RC. J Am Acad Dermatol 1993;28:973–80.

This review stresses the spectrum of CD30⁺ lymphoproliferative disease, and offers guidelines for management. Typical cases of LyP, including those with type C histology, do not require staging procedures if there is a normal physical examination and review of systems. However, one might consider a staging work-up if there is histology that overlaps with CD30 lymphoma. Close, long-term follow-up is required for all subtypes. Typical LyP requires either no treatment or PUVA, topical mechlorethamine, topical carmustine, or low-dose methotrexate. Prompt improvement and disease-free intervals are easily achieved, but relapse occurs after discontinuation of treatment, with rare permanent remissions.

Lymphomatoid papulosis. Reappraisal of clinicopathologic presentation and classification into subtypes A, B, and C. El Shabrawi-Caelen L, Kerl H, Cerroni L. Arch Dermatol 2004;140:441–7.

A retrospective review of 85 patients with LyP documented histologic overlap between the subtypes A, B, and C and between type B and MF. The authors also stress the tight overlap with LyP and CD30 lymphoma. A variety of clinical–histopathologic presentations of LyP, including those with histology showing follicular mucinosis, syringotropism, vesicle formation, MF-like band-like infiltrates, and associated keratoacanthoma were discussed.

CD30/Ki-1-positive lymphoproliferative disorders of the skin – clinicopathologic correlation and statistical analysis of 86 cases: a multicentric study from the European Organization for Research and Treatment of Cancer Cutaneous Lymphoma Project Group. Paulli M, Berti E, Rosso R, et al. J Clin Oncol 1995;13:1343–54.

Four clinicopathologic categories of CD30+ lymphoproliferative disease are defined: LyP, anaplastic large cell lymphoma (ALCL), nonanaplastic CD30 lymphoma, and borderline LyP and ALCL (spontaneous resolution, but borderline histology). The latter category emphasizes the difficulty in differentiating some cases of LyP from CD30+ lymphoma. The prognosis was excellent and similar to LyP in this borderline group.

Primary and secondary cutaneous CD30+ lymphoproliferative disorders: a report from the Dutch Cutaneous Lymphoma Group on the long-term follow-up data of 219 patients and guidelines for diagnosis and treatment. Bekkenk MW, Geelen FAMJ, van Voorst Vader PC, et al. Blood 2000;95:3653–61.

In this plenary paper, the authors propose guidelines for the diagnosis and treatment of patients with CD30+ lymphoproliferative disorders based on long-term follow-up of 219 patients, 118 of whom had LyP (type A, type B, and type C; 4% had tumors) They routinely staged all patients with type C LyP, which included physical examination, routine examination for blood morphology, blood chemistry, chest radiography, CT of the thorax, abdomen, and bone marrow biopsy. No extracutaneous disease was found. Fifty two of the 118 patients received no treatment or topical corticosteroids. The remainder received a variety of standard treatments, none of which were associated with complete, sustained remission. Nineteen per cent developed an associated lymphoma (only one with LyP C). Induction of remission of the secondary lymphoma with chemotherapy or total electron beam therapy had no effect on the natural course of LyP. The calculated risk for extracutaneous disease was 4% at 10 years.

The t(2;5)-associated p80 NPM/ALK fusion protein in nodal and cutaneous CD30+ lymphoproliferative disorders. Su LD, Schnitzer B, Ross CW, et al. J Cutan Pathol 1997; 24:597–603.

The chromosomal translocation t(2;5) and subsequent expression of ALCL tyrosine kinase (ALK) is often identified in nodal CD 30+ lymphoma. The authors found 24 cases of LyP to stain negative for this antibody.

Utilization of this test may potentially play a role in evaluating for secondary skin involvement by a CD30+ lymphoid infiltrate in cases of LyP type C.

CD30+ cutaneous lymphoproliferative disorders: the Stanford experience in lymphomatoid papulosis and primary cutaneous anaplastic large cell lymphoma. Liu HL, Hoppe RT, Kohler S, et al. J Am Acad Dermatol 2003;49: 1049–58.

In 31 of 56 cases with LyP, a higher than previously reported associated coexisting hematolymphoid malignancy (61% with one or more) was noted. Most of the patients with malignancy had MF, which was noted to occur before, during, or after the diagnosis of LyP. Some had two hematolymphoid malignancies. Three progressed to ALCL, with an interval time ranging from 77 to 152 months. The overall 5- and 10-year survival of patients with LyP was 100 and 92%, respectively, and none died of their LyP. Those who developed ALCL had a favorable course. LyP subtype did not predict the risk of developing an associated malignancy. Treatment included observation (most patients), topical corticosteroids, low-dose methotrexate, phototherapy, mechlorethamine ointment, and radiation. Two inadvertently received multi-agent chemotherapy, which did not alter the course of the disease.

The higher association with malignancy may represent selection bias.

Increased risk of lymphoid and nonlymphoid malignancies in patients with lymphomatoid papulosis. Wang HH, Myers T, Lach LJ, et al. Cancer 1999;86:1240–5.

Six of 57 (10.5%) of patients with LyP and one of 67 (1.5%) of matched controls followed for 8 years developed a nonlymphoid malignancy (lung, breast, and pancreatic carcinoma, and neuroblastoma). Two patients and no controls developed MF and ALCL. The calculated relative risk was 3.11 for nonlymphoid malignancies and 13.33 for malignant lymphomas in patients with LyP. There was no significant difference in survival between the two groups. The risk of developing a malignancy was not associated with the subtype of LyP, previous malignancy, or past radiation treatment, but it was significantly associated with advanced age (63 years vs 43 years at entry into the study).

Single cell analysis of CD30+ cells in lymphomatoid papulosis demonstrates a common clonal T-cell origin. Steinhoff M, Hummel M, Anagnostopoulos L, et al. Blood 2002;100:578–84.

The large CD30+ cells in LyP represent a single clone, while the CD 30− cells are polyclonal.

Assessment for clonality will not help to differentiate borderline cases of LyP and ALCL or MF.

Lymphomatoid papulosis associated with mycosis fungoides: a study of 21 patients including analyses for clonality. Zackheim H, Jones C, LeBoit PE, et al. J Am Acad Dermatol 2003;49:620–3.

Of 54 patients with LyP, 39% had MF. LyP preceded (67%), followed (19%), or was concurrent with (14%) a diagnosis of MF – 95% had type A LyP. Of those checked (seven patients) 100% had an identical clone in MF and LyP lesions.

FIRST LINE THERAPIES

■ Therapy not required	B
■ PUVA	B
■ Low-dose methotrexate	B
■ Topical corticosteroids	E

Primary and secondary cutaneous CD30[+] lymphoproliferative disorders: a report from the Dutch Cutaneous Lymphoma Group on the long-term follow-up data of 219 patients and guidelines for diagnosis and treatment. Bekkenk MW, Geelen FAMJ, van Voorst Vader PC, et al. Blood 2000;95:3653–61.

In patients with relatively few and nonscarring LyP lesions, active treatment is not necessary.

PUVA-treatment in lymphomatoid papulosis. Wantzin GL, Thompsen K. Br J Dermatol 1982;107:687–90.

Four patients with classic LyP and one with 1–2 cm tumors were treated with PUVA, 51–124 J/cm^2 and 481 J/cm^2, respectively. There was a decrease in the number of lesions and shortening of the life cycle of each individual lesion to 1 week from 3–6 weeks. Remission was attained in one patient.

Methotrexate is effective therapy for lymphomatoid papulosis and other primary cutaneous CD30[+] lymphoproliferative disorders. Vonderheid EC, Sajjadian A, Kadin ME. J Am Acad Dermatol 1996;34:470–81.

A 20-year experience of methotrexate therapy in 45 patients with LyP, CD30[+] lymphoma, and borderline cases is reviewed. Patients responded within 4 weeks to doses ranging from 15–20 mg weekly, with a slightly better initial response noted with intramuscular rather than oral dosing. Maintenance doses were given at 10–14-day intervals (range 7–28 days). Twenty nine per cent had concomitant MF, requiring other therapies (mechlorethamine hydrochloride, carmustine, standard UV therapy, and PUVA), which offered some additional benefit, but the relative effectiveness was less than with methotrexate. LyP and CD30[+] lymphoma responded similarly. Diminished responsiveness, suggesting resistance to methotrexate, was noted in three patients. Severe exacerbations were noted upon abrupt drug discontinuation.

This is an effective modality that many consider first line therapy for symptomatic disease, but because remission is rare, there are limitations for long-term treatment with methotrexate.

Lymphomatoid papulosis: successful weekly pulse superpotent topical corticosteroid therapy in three pediatric patients. Paul MA, Krowchuk DP, Hitchcock MG, Jorizzo JL. Pediatr Dermatol 1996;13:501–6.

Three children with LyP were treated with halobetasol or clobetasol propionate twice daily for 2–3 weeks, followed by weekly pulsed application, resulting in complete resolution of nearly all cutaneous lesions. Adjuvant intralesional triamcinolone was used for three ulcerated lesions.

Although this modality is unlikely to alter the disease course, it is a reasonable treatment approach because it has a relatively low complication profile.

SECOND LINE THERAPIES

■ Topical mechlorethamine (nitrogen mustard)	B
■ Topical carmustine	C
■ Acyclovir	E
■ Topical bexarotene	C

Long-term efficacy, curative potential, and carcinogenicity of topical mechlorethamine chemotherapy in cutaneous T cell lymphoma. Vonderheid EC, Tan ET, Kantor AF, et al. J Am Acad Dermatol 1989;20:416–28.

Seven patients with LyP, and 17 patients with concomitant LyP and MF were treated with 10–20 mg of mechlorethamine dissolved in 40–60 mL water, and applied once daily to the entire skin surface except for the genitalia. Therapy was continued until at least 2 weeks after complete clearance of lesions. Four of the seven with LyP achieved a complete response, with one achieving a complete response for more than 8 years of follow-up. A slightly increased risk in the squamous and basal cell carcinomas, Hodgkin's disease, and colon cancer was noted.

A common side effect of mechlorethamine therapy is an allergic hypersensitivity reaction. There may be a decreased incidence of contact allergy to mechlorethamine when prepared in an ointment base.

Topical carmustine therapy for lymphomatoid papulosis. Zacheim HS, Epstein EH, Crain WR. Arch Dermatol 1985; 121:1410–4.

Seven patients with LyP were treated with once daily total skin applications of topical carmustine, prepared by dissolving a 100 mg vial of carmustine in 50 mL of 95% (or absolute) ethanol; 5 mL (10 mg) was added to 60 mL of water and applied with a 2-inch paintbrush after showering. Total doses ranged from 280 to 1180 mg. Local treatment of individual lesions after the total skin course included twice daily application of 2 or 4 mg/mL of 95% ethanol. All patients had a rapid reduction in the number and size of lesions. Lesions cleared faster and did not scar with maintenance local therapy, but remission was not seen. Rare widespread, persistent telangiectases were noted.

Bexarotene is a new treatment option for lymphomatoid papulosis. Krathen RA, Ward S, Duvic M. Dermatology 2003;206:142–7.

Topical bexarotene gel used in patients with less than 10% body surface area involved with LyP was associated with more rapid disappearance, less necrosis, and a reduction in the number of new lesions.

Acyclovir in lymphomatoid papulosis and mycosis fungoides. (Letter) Burg G, Klepzig K, Kaudewitz P, et al. JAMA 1986;256:214–5.

Two of five patients with LyP noted regression of lesions within 10 days with acyclovir intravenously at 15 mg/kg daily. Response to oral treatment seemed to correlate with the serum level achieved.

THIRD LINE THERAPIES

■ Oral bexarotene	C
■ Recombinant interferon	C
■ Radiotherapy	E
■ Topical methotrexate	E

Bexarotene is a new treatment option for lymphomatoid papulosis. Krathen RA, Ward S, Duvic M. Dermatology 2003;206:142–7.

Oral doses of bexarotene, initiated at 300 mg/m^2 daily were associated with more rapid disappearance, less necrosis, and a reduction in the number of new lesions. One of three patients with oral therapy had a complete response. Oral bexarotene was found to be helpful in tapering methotrexate in one patient.

Bexarotene is often used in conjunction with thyroxine and oral fenofibrate and/or atorvastatin because of frequently seen hypothyroidism and hyperlipidemia.

Lymphomatoid papulosis: response to treatment with recombinant interferon alfa-2b. (Letter) Proctor SJ, Jackson GH, Lennard AL, Marks J. J Clin Oncol 1992;10:170.

Recombinant interferon-alfa-2b 1 mU injected intralesionally three times in 1 week completely cleared lesions less than 0.5 cm im diameter. Larger lesions required three to ten injections. Maintenance with thrice weekly 3 mU subcutaneous doses appeared to reduce recurrences.

This anecdotal report suggests that, similar to MF, biologic modalities may play a role in the treatment of symptomatic LyP lesions.

Therapeutic use of interferon-alpha for lymphomatoid papulosis. Schmuth M, Topar G, Illersperger B, et al. Cancer 2000;89:1603–10.

Four of five patients receiving subcutaneous interferon-alfa, 3–15 million international units three times per week for a 12–13-month course, had a complete response at 6-week follow-up. All noted some response. Two had rapid recurrences after discontinuing short-term interferon-alfa

(5–7 months), but one had a complete response when long-term therapy was then instituted (17 months). Only one of six controls achieved spontaneous remission.

Interferon-alfa is one of the few therapies that has shown potential for altering the course of LyP. Its benefit is associated with long-term treatment courses, but the side effect profile for low-dose interferon-alfa is low, allowing a prolonged treatment course.

Ki-1 lymphoproliferative disorders: management with radiation therapy. Kaufmann TP, Coleman M, Nisce LZ. Cancer Invest 1997;15:91–7.

Two patients with multiple lesions consistent with LyP or CD30$^+$ borderline lesions were treated with local radiation. Most lesions received 3000 cGy in 3 weeks, with a complete response achieved in all lesions. One of the lesions cleared after 1200 cGy. Size, depth, and time of disease detection may impact radiation dosing.

Topical methotrexate for lymphomatoid papulosis. Bergstrom JS, Jaworsky C. J Am Acad Dermatol 2003;49: 937–9.

A 71-year-old man with LyP with 1–2.0 cm lesions responding to 12.5 mg methotrexate orally per week self-treated himself with a home concoction of this medication when recurrence occurred upon discontinuation of the medication. The topical methotrexate was prepared by moistening a 2.5 mg tablet with tap water and rubbing it on the bandage until the gauze turned orange. Application of the medication-soaked bandage to newly formed lesions daily (approximately one-third of a tablet or 0.83 mg) resulted in regression of the lesions within 2–3 days. The lesions rarely lasted more than 1 week and achieved a size that was much smaller than prior to treatment (5–10 mm). Scarring was avoided, but the clinical course was not altered.

This report is an innovative approach using a medication that has known efficacy in treating LyP, yet a limiting complication profile. The bioavailability of methotrexate in tap water is not known, and it is possible that the patient is achieving enough systemic absorption to clear his lesions. Further investigation is needed.

Malignant atrophic papulosis (Degos' disease)

James R Wharton, Clay J Cockerell

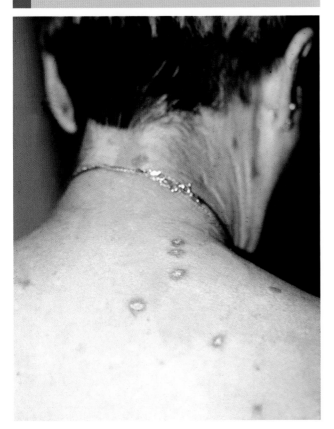

Malignant atrophic papulosis (MAP) is a potentially fatal multiorgan vasculopathy, characterized in the skin by porcelain-white atrophic papules with peripheral telangiectatic erythema, which often precedes multiorgan involvement. The etiology is uncertain and some studies suggest a defect in the fibrinolytic process, genetic influences, or possibly a viral etiology. Treatment is often ineffective.

MANAGEMENT STRATEGY

Initial reports of MAP showed poor outcomes. The condition has been stereotyped as being refractory to treatment and universally fatal. More recent reports stress that heredity, disorders of coagulation, or infectious causes may play a role in at least some cases of MAP, and that not all cases are fatal. There is no uniformly effective therapy. Due to the rarity of MAP, no controlled studies have been performed evaluating therapy; most evidence comes from anecdotal case reports. The disorder is characterized histologically by vasculitis and thrombosis. This pattern has led to initial treatments with *fibrinolytics* and *anticoagulants* such as aspirin, heparin, and dipyridamole. Prednisone has been used in some instances, although there is no rational pathophysiologic basis for its use. Indeed, prednisone has been associated with intestinal perforation.

Disease progression while undergoing therapy often necessitates more aggressive measures with *immunosuppressive agents* such as cyclosporine, cyclophosphamide, tacrolimus, and azathioprine. Management is directed at preventing thrombotic complications in critical organs such as the gastrointestinal tract, brain, lungs, and eyes. Often, surgical intervention is required to deal with secondary thrombotic complications.

The pathognomonic cutaneous eruption of MAP is typified by recurrent, asymptomatic crops of erythematous papules that evolve into porcelain-white macules with a peripheral erythematous, telangiectatic, macular to slightly elevated rim. The eruption has a tendency toward being distributed more proximally than distally and may involve mucosal membranes. Cutaneous lesions may predate internal involvement by months to years in some patients. Recognition of the premonitory skin manifestations allows potential intervention before critical organ involvement has occurred. Initially, up to one-third of patients may present with only skin involvement. The gastrointestinal tract is the most frequent site of internal involvement, with almost half of all patients affected. Intestinal infarcts often are heralded by bleeding, nausea, abdominal pain, vomiting, diarrhea, ileus, or malabsorption. CNS involvement may present with headache or localizing neurologic symptoms. Other commonly affected organs include the lungs, heart, eyes, and oral cavity. Sepsis from peritonitis is the leading cause of death, followed by CNS bleeds, and involvement of the pleura or pericardium. A high mortality still exists for patients within the first 2–3 years of diagnosis. No predictive factors exist that determine whether a patient will have only cutaneous involvement.

Diseases such as lupus, systemic sclerosis, panniculitis, and Creutzfeldt–Jakob disease have been known to mimic MAP clinically and should be excluded. Some authors have theorized that MAP may even be a reaction pattern seen in some forms of lupus. Histologically, MAP may also overlap with connective tissue diseases. Common features include a vacuolar interface dermatitis with a perivascular lymphocytic infiltrate, basement membrane smudging, a thin epidermis, dermal sclerosis, and a characteristic mucinous degeneraration and deposition.

SPECIFIC INVESTIGATIONS

- Complete physical examination with attention to the skin, gastrointestinal tract, nervous system, lungs, and heart
- Skin biopsy of any suspicious lesions
- Imaging studies as dictated by symptoms
- Coagulation studies
- Complete blood count
- Liver functions
- Renal functions
- Stool guiaic
- Endoscopy (if symptomatic)
- Antinuclear antibodies
- Antiphospholipid antibodies
- Anticardiolipin antibodies
- Protein C and S levels
- Lupus anticoagulant

Acute abdominal pain as a leading symptom for Degos' disease (malignant atrophic papulosis). Lankisch M, Scolapio J, Fleming C. Am J Gastroenterol 1999;94:1098–9.

Lesions resembling malignant atrophic papulosis in a patient with dermatomyositis. Tsao H, Busam K, Barnhill RL, Haynes HA. J Am Acad Dermatol 1997;36:317–9.

Absence of antiphospholipid and anti-endothelial cell antibodies in malignant atrophic papulosis: a study of 15 cases. Assier H, Chosidow O, Piette JC, et al. J Am Acad Dermatol 1995;33:831–3.

Malignant atrophic papulosis (Degos' disease) involving three generations of a family. Katz S, Mudd B, Roenigk H. J Am Acad Dermatol 1997;37:480–4.

Three members with definite disease and three with probable disease over three generations, combined with multiple familial clusterings in the literature, suggest a possible genetic influence.

FIRST LINE THERAPIES

■ Heparin	E
■ Coumadin (warfarin)	E
■ Aspirin	E
■ Dipyridamole	E

Malignant atrophic papulosis. Degos R. Br J Dermatol 1979; 100:21–35.

Numerous clinical manifestations have been reported and can affect the skin, mucosa, gastrointestinal tract, viscera, and CNS, and may require surgical intervention or fibrinolytic therapy. Anticoagulants have shown the most favorable responses.

Malignant atrophic papulosis: treatment with aspirin and dipyridamole. Stahl D, Thomsen K, Hou-Jensen K. Arch Dermatol 1978;114:1687–9.

A case report of a patient in whom treatment with aspirin 0.5 g twice daily and dipyridamole 50 mg three times daily arrested the development of both cutaneous lesions and systemic symptoms. Discontinuation of therapy resulted in no relapses 4 months post therapy.

Malignant atrophic papulosis in an infant. Torrelo A, Sevilla J, Mediero I, et al. Br J Dermatol 2002;146:916–8.

A 7-month-old female with cutaneous lesions, vomiting, and poor weight gain was treated successfully with aspirin 12 mg/kg daily and dipyridamole 4 mg/kg daily in three divided doses.

SECOND LINE THERAPIES

■ Phenformin	E
■ Ethylestrenol	E
■ Nicotine patches	E
■ Lansoprazole (for gastrointestinal ulceration)	E
■ Cyclosporine	E

Effect of fibrinolytic treatment in malignant atrophic papulosis. Delaney TJ, Black MM. Br Med J 1975;3:415.

The further development of cutaneous disease was halted in a 42-year-old female patient placed on phenformin 50 mg twice daily and ethylestrenol 2 mg four times daily. Withdrawal of therapy resulted in relapse that responded to reinstitution of therapy.

Penile ulceration in fatal malignant atrophic papulosis (Degos' disease). Thompson KF, Highet AS. Br J Dermatol 2000;143:1320–2.

A fatal outcome in a patient who initially presented with penile ulceration and was treated with aspirin and dipyridamole, but could not tolerate the therapy. Cyclosporine resulted in clinical improvement. Neurologic and gastrointestinal symptoms developed and lansoprazole resulted in healing of gastric ulceration. Atrial fibrillation and pleuritic pain were treated with heparin, with clinical improvement. Continued symptoms prompted trials of tacrolimus, prednisolone, azathioprine, and cyclophosphamide, without success.

A case of malignant atrophic papulosis successfully treated with nicotine patches. Kanekura T, Uchino Y, Kanzaki T. Br J Dermatol 2003;149:660–2.

Nicotine patches that released 5 mg every 24 h were applied daily and resulted in clearing of skin lesions. Three weeks after withdrawal of the patches, lesions recurred and again responded to therapy. The patient had no systemic involvement.

THIRD LINE THERAPIES

■ Azathioprine	E
■ Cyclophosphamide	E
■ Tacrolimus	E

Malignant atrophic papulosis of Degos. Report of a patient who failed to respond to fibrinolytic therapy. Howsden SM, Hodge SJ, Herndon JH, Freeman RJ. Arch Dermatol 1976;112:1582–8.

A 21-year-old female died of complications from MAP after therapy with phenformin, ethylestrenol, aspirin, niacin, and low-molecular-weight dextran.

There are many such reports in the literature noting therapies that are proven either inconsistent, ineffective, or too dangerous to recommend their routine use.

Benign familial Degos disease worsening during immunosuppression. Powell J, Bordea C, Wojnarowska J, et al. Br J Dermatol 1999;141:524–7.

A 61-year-old woman with Degos' disease underwent a cadaveric kidney transplant. Her condition worsened with the use of prednisolone, azathioprine, and cyclosporine.

[An autopsy case of Degos' disease with ascending thoracic myelopathy]. Sugai F, Sumi H, Hara Y, et al. Rinsho Shinkeigaku 1998;38:1049–53. In Japanese.

Aggressive therapies, including pulsed-dose methylprednisolone and cyclophosphamide, were not successful in this 44-year-old man with Degos' disease complicated by thoracic transverse myelopathy, with the patient ultimately succumbing to respiratory failure.

Evidence levels **A** Double-blind study **B** Clinical trial ≥ 20 subjects **C** Clinical trial < 20 subjects **D** Series ≥ 5 subjects **E** Anecdotal case reports

Malignant melanoma

Jackie M Tripp, Alfred W Kopf

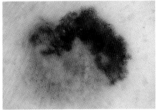 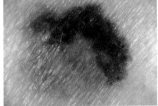

A   **B**

Melanoma is the leading cause of death among all cutaneous diseases in the USA. It is estimated that 59 580 new cases of invasive melanoma will be diagnosed and 7770 will die of this cancer in the year 2005. The principal management of primary cutaneous melanoma is surgical.

MANAGEMENT STRATEGY

Certain markers help to identify individuals at higher risk for melanoma. Among these markers are skin phototype I or II, history of intermittent sunburns, and a personal or family history of dysplastic nevi and/or melanoma.

Helping both physicians and patients in early detection are the *ABCD signs of melanoma* (Asymmetry of the lesion, Border irregularity, Color variability, Diameter > 6 mm). *Dermoscopy* supplements clinical features as a noninvasive technique, but the gold standard for establishing the diagnosis of melanoma is *biopsy and histologic examination*. The ideal biopsy of a suspected primary cutaneous melanoma is a complete full-thickness excision with at least a 2 mm margin of normal-appearing surrounding skin. If in toto excision is not practical, full-thickness in parte biopsy usually suffices. Measurement of Breslow tumor thickness is an important determinant of patient management and prognosis. In addition, the histologic status of the sentinel lymph node (SLN) has been shown to be a prognostic factor even more dominant than tumor thickness.

Important in the management of melanoma is *primary prevention* (risk reduction) and *secondary prevention* (early detection). Educating the public about the risks of sun exposure is a crucial part of primary prevention. Secondary prevention involves teaching high-risk patients about the ABCD signs and how to perform total body self-examinations. The NIH stresses the importance of screening programs and regular skin examinations by health professionals.

Staging of melanoma is crucial because it not only assigns patients into well-defined risk groups, but it also aids in clinical decision making and in comparing treatment results. In 2001 the American Joint Committee on Cancer released the final version of their cancer staging system for cutaneous melanoma. Significant changes from the previous staging system include upstaging patients when ulceration is present and describing nodal metastases in histologic terms so as to take into account information gleaned from SLN biopsies.

The primary treatment for stage IA (invasive melanoma up to 1 mm thick without ulceration and without Clark level IV invasion) melanoma is *wide local excision*. Total excision of primary melanoma with wide margins offers the best chance for cure.

Management of stage IB (< 1 mm thick but with ulceration or Clark level IV invasion) and stage II (> 1 mm thick, but without nodal disease) melanomas includes wide local excision, but also involves discussing *SLN biopsy* with the patient.

Sentinel lymph node (SLN) biopsy is an important diagnostic procedure in the work-up of melanoma. The SLN is detected by preoperative lymphoscintigraphy followed by intraoperative injection of a blue dye and/or a radiocolloid around the primary lesion. Once removed, the SLN is examined for melanoma, and if positive, represents a significant negative prognostic indicator. Selecting which patients should undergo a SLN biopsy is a critical decision and there is much debate as to the minimal tumor thickness requiring this procedure. The National Comprehensive Cancer Network suggests that SLN biopsy be discussed with patients in those with melanomas at least 1 mm in thickness or in those with ulceration or invasion to the reticular dermis. If the SLN is histologically positive, a *selective lymphadenectomy* is usually recommended. The overall effect of selective lymphadenectomy following a positive SLN has yet to show survival benefit.

Elective lymphadenectomy involves removal of regional lymph nodes without preceding clinical or microscopic evidence of nodal metastases. One large study demonstrated that this procedure increases the survival rate in certain subgroups of patients with melanoma (those with ulceration and those with tumor thicknesses between 1 and 2 mm). However, it did not show improved overall survival in all patients with melanoma. This procedure, which results in significant morbidity, remains controversial.

For those who have stage III (evidence of either microscopic or macroscopic nodal disease) melanoma, in addition to wide local excision with nodal dissection, the only adjuvant therapy approved by the FDA at this time is high-dose *interferon-alfa-2b*. (Interferon is also approved by the FDA for stage IIB and IIC disease.) Some studies have shown that interferon may increase the relapse-free interval, but there is no clear evidence that this treatment improves overall survival. Alternatively to receiving interferon, patients with stage III disease may either be observed or entered into a clinical trial.

For patients with clinically positive lymph nodes, a diagnostic nodal biopsy (e.g. fine-needle biopsy) is recommended and, if positive, a *therapeutic lymphadenectomy* is performed.

Traditionally, patients with satellitosis or in-transit metastases on an extremity have been candidates for treatment with *isolated limb perfusion (ILP)* with chemotherapeutic agents (the most successful of which is melphalan) or immunomodulatory agents.

Stage IV (distant metastases) melanoma has a very poor prognosis, with patients demonstrating less than 5% 5-year survival. For those in whom only a solitary metastasis can be found, *resection of the metastasis* may be feasible. Generally, at this stage, the treatment options are limited and not very effective. No randomized controlled trials have demonstrated a significant survival advantage for any of the stage IV therapies. *Chemotherapy, radiation, and immunotherapy* are some of the options available for such patients. Chemotherapy with *dacarbazine (DTIC)*, which has an approximate 20% response rate, is commonly employed. Treatment with immunotherapy (e.g. interleukin-2) has also yielded some positive results but more double-blind, controlled studies are needed. Radiation may be used as primary treatment for lentigo maligna and as palliation in metastatic melanoma. Lastly, clinical trials are ongoing assessing vaccine therapies, but as of yet none have shown an impact on survival.

SPECIFIC INVESTIGATIONS

- Biopsy of primary site
- Sentinel lymph node biopsy
- Laboratory and imaging studies (chest radiograph, CT, MRI, PET scans)
- Family history of melanoma and/or dysplastic nevi
- Total cutaneous exam and clinical examination for metastases
- Dermoscopy

Final version of the American Joint Committee on Cancer staging system for cutaneous melanoma. Balch CM, Buzaid AC, Soong SJ, et al. J Clin Oncol 2001;19:3635–48.

This paper describes the revised staging system for cutaneous melanoma. This revised system takes into account the presence of ulceration in the primary cutaneous melanoma as well as the histology of the SLN(s). Accurate staging is important in clinical decision making and in comparing treatment results between different centers.

Technical details of intraoperative lymphatic mapping. Morton DL, Wen DR, Wong JH, et al. Arch Surg 1992; 127:392–9.

This was the first description of intraoperative lymphatic mapping to identify the first node in the lymphatic watershed that drains the site of the melanoma. A total of 223 patients with either stage I or stage II melanoma were evaluated.

Reassessing the role of lymphatic mapping and sentinel lymphadenectomy in the management of cutaneous malignant melanoma. Perrott RE, Glass LF, Reintgen DS, Fenske NA. J Am Acad Dermatol 2003;49:567–88.

This is an excellent review of the technical aspects of SLN biopsy as well as an update on the current controversies surrounding this procedure.

Multi-institutional melanoma lymphatic mapping experience: the prognostic value of sentinel lymph node status in 612 stage I or II melanoma patients. Gershenwald JE, Thompson W, Mansfield PF, et al. J Clin Oncol 1999;17: 976–83.

A total of 612 patients with primary cutaneous melanoma who had SLN biopsy were reviewed retrospectively. In these patients, SLN status was the most significant prognostic factor with respect to disease-free survival.

National Comprehensive Cancer Network. Clinical practice guidelines in oncology. V.1.2004. Online. Houghton AN, Colt DG. Available: *http://www.nccn.org/ professionals/physician_gls/PDF/melanoma.pdf* 25 Sept 2004.

The extent of initial work-up is controversial. Most agree that chest radiography and blood work are not necessary for stage IA disease. For stage IB and stage II melanomas, a baseline chest radiograph and lactate dehydrogenase are optional because they are insensitive and nonspecific, but they are indicated for stage III and IV melanomas. Other imaging studies such as CT, MRI and/or PET scans should be performed as indicated by symptoms, signs and/or lab values. These guidelines also discuss frequency of follow-up visits and appropriate follow-up tests both of which depend on the stage of the melanoma as well as other risk factors.

Atlas of dermoscopy. Marghoob AA, Braun R, Kopf AW, eds. London: Parthenon Publishing; 2004.

This clinician-oriented atlas is an up-to-date multi-authored text dealing with virtually every aspect of dermoscopy.

FIRST LINE THERAPIES

■ Surgical excision	B
■ Selective lymphadenectomy	C
■ Follow-up	C

Narrow excision (1-cm margin). A safe procedure for thin cutaneous melanoma. Veronesi U, Cascinelli N. Arch Surg 1991;126:438–41.

The WHO trial included 612 patients with primary melanomas that were 2 mm thick or less, that were excised using margins of either 1 or 3 cm. There were no differences in overall survival rates between the two groups, nor were there any statistically significant differences in local recurrence. The five local recurrences that did occur, however, were from lesions that were between 1 and 2 mm thick. Due to this non-statistically significant trend, the effectiveness of 1 cm margins for melanomas 1–2 mm deep has remained somewhat controversial. Nonetheless, the authors recommend 1 cm margins of excision for melanomas less than 2 mm thick.

Long-term results of a prospective surgical trial comparing 2 cm vs. 4 cm excision margins for 740 patients with 1–4 mm melanomas. Balch CM, Soong SJ, Smith T, et al. Ann Surg Oncol 2001;8:101–8.

The Intergroup Melanoma Surgical Trial included 468 patients with stage I melanoma with a thickness between 1 and 4 mm. Surgical margins of either 2 cm or 4 cm were used. The two groups showed no significant differences in survival or local recurrences, demonstrating the safety of using 2 cm margins in melanomas up to 4 mm in thickness.

Excision margins in high-risk malignant melanoma. Thomas JM, Newton-Bishop J, A'Hern R, et al. N Engl J Med 2004;350:757–66.

A randomized clinical trial with 900 subjects comparing 1-cm and 3-cm margins in high risk tumors (thickness 2 mm or greater). The median follow-up was 60 months. A 1-cm margin of excision was associated with a significantly increased risk of locoregional recurrence. There were 128 deaths attributable to melanoma in the group with 1-cm margins, as compared with 105 in the group with 3-cm margins but overall survival was similar in the two groups.

Evidence levels **A** Double-blind study **B** Clinical trial ≥ 20 subjects **C** Clinical trial < 20 subjects **D** Series ≥ 5 subjects **E** Anecdotal case reports

Guidelines of care for primary cutaneous melanoma. Sober AJ, Chuang TY, Duvic M, et al. J Am Acad Dermatol 2001;45:579–86.

For melanoma in situ and for primary melanoma thicker than 4 mm, there are no large prospective randomized studies examining appropriate margins. This American Academy of Dermatology task force recommends taking margins of 0.5 cm for melanoma in situ, and at least 2 cm for melanomas thicker than 4 mm. They also suggest, in agreement with WHO guidelines, 1 cm margins for melanomas with a depth of invasion less than 2 mm, and 2 cm margins for melanomas more than, or equal to, 2 mm deep.

Long-term results of a multi-institutional randomized trial comparing prognostic factors and surgical results for intermediate thickness melanomas (1.0 to 4.0 mm). Intergroup Melanoma Surgical Trial. Balch CM, Soong S, Ross MI, et al. Ann Surg Oncol 2000;7:87–97.

Previous prospective studies showed that elective lymphadenectomy did not benefit all patients. This trial included 740 patients. The results suggest that elective lymphadenectomy may benefit certain subgroups of patients, specifically those with primary lesions 1–2 mm thick, those without ulcerated tumors, and those younger than 60 years of age.

As elective lymphadenectomy falls out of favor due to high morbidity and limited therapeutic value, selective lymphadenectomy is rapidly gaining acceptance. However, despite the proved efficacy in identifying the SLN, a large prospective trial looking at the effect of selective lymphadenectomy on survival is lacking. The Multicenter Selective Lymphadenectomy Trial and Florida Melanoma Trial are both in progress and the results should tell us more about the impact this treatment has on survival.

Utility of follow-up tests for detecting recurrent disease in patients with malignant melanoma. Weiss M, Loprinzi CL, Creagan ET, et al. JAMA 1995;274:1703–5.

The frequency of follow-up after melanoma resection is controversial. However, it is known that most recurrences of primary melanoma are discovered by history and/or physical exam. In this retrospective study of 261 patients with resected local and regional nodal melanoma, chest radiography first diagnosed about 6% of those with recurrence.

Despite that, the authors claimed that routine chest radiographs, along with routine blood work, were of limited value in the postoperative follow-up of patients with resected intermediate- and high-risk melanomas.

SECOND LINE THERAPIES

■ Immunotherapy	B
■ Chemotherapy	B
■ Regional isolation perfusion	B

Interferon alfa therapy for malignant melanoma: a systematic review of randomized controlled trials. Lens MB, Dawes M. J Clin Oncol 2002;20:1818–25.

This review looked at all the randomized controlled studies examining interferon-alfa therapy. One trial showed benefit to overall survival, and two showed benefit in disease-free survival. However, taking all the studies into account, it was concluded that interferon-alfa demonstrated no clear benefit on overall survival in patients with melanoma.

Palliative therapy of disseminated malignant melanoma: a systematic review of 41 randomised clinical trials. Eigentler TK, Caroli UM, Radny P, Garbe C. Lancet Oncol 2003;4:748–59.

Dacarbazine remains the standard treatment for distant disease. None of the combination regimens have yet to demonstrate a significant survival advantage in randomized controlled studies.

Management of in-transit melanoma of the extremity with isolated limb perfusion. Fraker DL. Curr Treat Options Oncol 2004;5:173–84.

The primary use of ILP is in the treatment of satellitosis and in-transit metastasis. ILP involves very high doses of chemotherapeutic agents, usually melphalan, administered through either femoral, iliac, or axillary vessels to isolated anatomic regions. Reports have shown that the addition of tumor necrosis factor to melphalan may improve response rates, but no clear benefit has been demonstrated.

THIRD LINE THERAPIES

■ Radiation therapy	B
■ Mohs micrographic surgery	B

Radiotherapy for melanoma. Ang KK, Geara FB, Byers RM, Peters LJ. In: Balch CM, Houghton AN, Sober AJ, Soong S, eds. Cutaneous melanoma. Philadelphia: JB Lippincott; 1998:389–401.

Radiation is rarely used for the primary treatment of melanoma (except in certain cases of facial lentigo maligna melanoma).

This chapter offers an excellent review of radiation treatment for melanoma, discussing studies examining radiotherapy as a palliative treatment for cutaneous, subcutaneous, osseous, and brain metastases.

Mohs micrographic surgery for the treatment of primary cutaneous melanoma. Zitelli JA, Brown C, Hanusa BH. J Am Acad Dermatol 1997;37:236–45.

In this large study, 535 patients with cutaneous melanoma of various thicknesses were treated with Mohs micrographic surgery. After being divided into groups, depending on the thickness of the melanoma, the results were compared to historical controls that were treated with standard wide-margin surgical excision. The patients in this trial showed 5-year survival and metastatic rates that were equal to or better than historic controls.

With the lack of a randomized prospective study, this trial can only suggest the possible advantages of Mohs surgery over standard excisional surgery in the treatment of primary cutaneous melanoma.

Mastocytoses

Nicholas A Soter

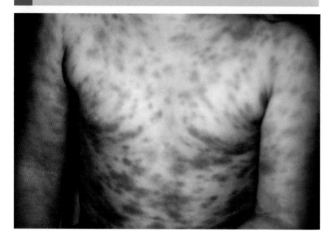

Mastocytoses are a group of disorders of mast cell proliferation that may exhibit both cutaneous and systemic features. The most frequent site of organ involvement in individuals with any form of mastocytosis is the skin. Cutaneous forms include urticaria pigmentosa (shown here), mastocytoma, diffuse and erythrodermic cutaneous mastocytosis, and telangiectasia macularis eruptiva perstans. The cutaneous forms of mastocytosis may be present with or without systemic manifestations. Only the treatment of the cutaneous features will be discussed.

MANAGEMENT STRATEGY

An important aspect of therapy of the cutaneous lesions of mastocytosis is avoidance of triggering factors, which include temperature changes, friction, physical exertion, ingestion of alcohol, the use of nonsteroidal anti-inflammatory agents or opiate analgesics, and emotional stress. Of concern is the possibility of anaphylaxis after stings by *Hymenoptera* spp., which may occur even in patients receiving venom immunotherapy.

A history seeking systemic features should be undertaken, as well as a physical examination to determine the types of skin lesions and to seek lymphadenopathy and hepatosplenomegaly. The presence of specific systemic manifestations will dictate the type of specialty physician to whom a referral should be made.

A skin biopsy should be obtained in all individuals with cutaneous lesions. Increased numbers of mast cells are recognized with metachromatic stains, such as Giemsa's reagent or toluidine blue. A complete blood count with differential analysis, a blood chemistry profile that includes liver function tests, and a blood tryptase level should be obtained in all patients with cutaneous lesions except in those with mastocytomas. If there are abnormalities of the complete blood count, a bone marrow examination should be obtained. Plasma histamine levels are not useful to screen patients. 24-hour urine levels of mast cell mediators may be obtained in patients with systemic features. Abdominal imaging studies provide a noninvasive means to assess the lymph nodes, liver, and spleen. In patients with bone pain, a ^{99}Tc bone scan is useful. Osteoporosis may be detected by bone density analysis.

In many cases, cutaneous mastocytoma may involute spontaneously; it is rarely described in adults. Childhood urticaria pigmentosa spontaneously regresses in approximately 50% of cases and urticaria pigmentosa in older adults in 10%. Diffuse and erythrodermic cutaneous mastocytosis usually resolves spontaneously between the ages of 15 months and 5 years. Urticaria pigmentosa that appears in adults and telangiectasia macularis eruptiva perstans tend to be chronic conditions.

Most of the therapeutic reports have been in patients with urticaria pigmentosa and, to a lesser degree, in diffuse and erythrodermic cutaneous mastocytosis. The major therapeutic measure is the administration of *oral H1 antihistamines* to alleviate pruritus and whealing. The use of antihistamines that interfere with the HERG K^+ channel and cause cardiac arrhythmias should be avoided. *Oral disodium cromoglycate* has been efficacious in some individuals. The role and efficacy of topical high-potency corticosteroid preparations with plastic-film occlusion or hydrocolloid dressings, of psoralens and ultraviolet A (PUVA) photochemotherapy, and UVA1 phototherapy have not been subjected to controlled clinical trials or remain anecdotal. There is no therapy that will eradicate the mast cells in the cutaneous lesions.

SPECIFIC INVESTIGATIONS

- Blood tryptase levels
- 24-hour urine histamine, histamine metabolites, and prostaglandin metabolites
- Bone marrow examination

The α form of human tryptase is the predominant type present in blood at baseline in normal subjects and is elevated in those with systemic mastocytosis. Schwartz LB, Sakai K, Bradford TR, et al. J Clin Invest 1995;96:2702–10.

Most patients with mastocytosis and systemic disease had total blood tryptase (α and β tryptase) levels that were higher than 20 ng/mL. Those patients with levels less than 20 ng/mL had only cutaneous manifestations.

Elevated blood tryptase levels appear to be useful in differentiating patients with systemic disease from those with cutaneous disease.

Improved diagnosis of mastocytosis by measurement of the major urinary metabolite of prostaglandin D$_2$. Morrow JD, Guzzo C, Lazarus G, et al. J Invest Dermatol 1995;104:937–40.

The major urinary metabolite of prostaglandin D$_2$, PGD-M (9α, 11β-dihydroxy-15-oxo-2,3,18,19-tetranorprost-5-ene-1,20-dioic acid) is a more sensitive biochemical diagnostic indication of systemic mastocytosis than are histamine and its metabolite NT-methylhistamine.

Elevation of these mast cell products does not reliably differentiate purely cutaneous from systemic mastocytosis and they should not be routinely obtained. These tests are neither more sensitive nor specific than the measurement of blood total tryptase.

Hematopathology of the bone marrow in pediatric cutaneous mastocytosis: a study of 17 patients. Kettelhut BV, Parker RI, Travis WD, Metcalfe DD. Am J Clin Pathol 1989; 91:558–62.

Evidence levels **A** Double-blind study **B** Clinical trial ≥ 20 subjects **C** Clinical trial < 20 subjects **D** Series ≥ 5 subjects **E** Anecdotal case reports

In children with urticaria pigmentosa or diffuse cutaneous mastocytosis, eosinophilia and focal increased numbers of mast cells were observed. The focal mast cell aggregates that consist of nodular collections of fusiform mast cells associated with lymphocytes and eosinophils that occur in adults with urticaria pigmentosa and systemic mastocytosis were not seen.

Bone marrow aspirates with biopsies in adult or pediatric cutaneous mastocytosis should be restricted to individuals with changes in the complete blood count, organomegaly, or alterations in other organ systems. Some investigators recommend a bone marrow aspirate and biopsy in all patients with adult-onset disease.

FIRST LINE THERAPIES

■ H$_1$ antihistamines	A
■ H$_2$ antihistamines	D
■ Disodium cromoglycate	A

A double-blind, placebo-controlled, crossover trial of ketotifen versus hydroxyzine in the treatment of pediatric mastocytosis. Kettelhut BV, Berkebile C, Bradley D, Metcalfe DD. J Allergy Clin Immunol 1989;83:866–70.

In six children with urticaria pigmentosa and two with diffuse cutaneous mastocytosis, hydroxyzine alleviated pruritus (in seven) or the formation of bullae (in five). Ketotifen alleviated pruritus (in one) or the formation of bullae (in three).

A double-blind cross-over study of the effect of ketotifen in urticaria pigmentosa. Czarnetzki BM. Dermatologica 1983;166:44–7.

In ten adult patients with urticaria pigmentosa, a statistically significant reduction in pruritus (p < 0.01) and whealing (p < 0.025) was found with the use of ketotifen 1.0 mg twice daily.

This H$_1$ antihistamine with sedative side effects has additional antiallergy activities, but is not available in the USA.

Comparison of azelastine and chlorpheniramine in the treatment of mastocytosis. Friedman BS, Santiago ML, Berkebile C, Metcalfe DD. J Allergy Clin Immunol 1993; 92:520–6.

In a double-blind, randomized, crossover trial in 13 subjects with urticaria pigmentosa and systemic mastocytosis, the administration of both azelastine and chlorpheniramine (chlorphenamine) for 4 weeks was associated with a decrease in pruritus.

Comparison of the therapeutic efficacy of cromolyn sodium with that of combined chlorpheniramine and cimetidine in systemic mastocytosis: results of a double-blind clinical trial. Frieri M, Alling DW, Metcalfe DD. Am J Med 1985;78:9–14.

Five of six patients had less pruritus and four of six had less urticaria while receiving chlorpheniramine and cimetidine. There was no beneficial effect in those receiving disodium cromoglycate.

Systemic mastocytosis treated with histamine H$_1$ and H$_2$ receptor antagonists. Gasior-Chrzan B, Falk ES. Dermatology 1992;184:149–52.

In a single patient with telangiectasia macularis eruptiva perstans and systemic mastocytosis, there was improvement in pruritus, erythema, and urticaria after the administration of cyproheptadine and cimetidine.

Cimetidine in systemic mastocytosis. Berg MJ, Bernhard H, Schentag JJ. Drug Intell Clin Pharm 1981;15:180–3.

An adult with systemic disease received treatment with cyproheptadine, Lomotil (diphenoxylate–atropine), and cimetidine. Prompt recurrence of gastrointestinal and dermatological symptoms occurred after stopping the cimetidine. The drug was restarted in 3 days and the symptoms subsided.

In systemic mastocytosis H$_2$ antagonists can play an additional role in reducing gastric hyperacidity.

Oral disodium cromoglycate in the treatment of systemic mastocytosis. Soter NA, Austen KF, Wasserman SI. N Engl J Med 1979;301:465–9.

In a double-blind, crossover study in five patients with systemic mastocytosis and urticaria pigmentosa, in 15 of 18 trials, oral disodium cromoglycate ameliorated pruritus and whealing.

Urticaria pigmentosa: clinical picture and response to oral disodium cromoglycate. Czarnetzki BM, Behrendt H. Br J Dermatol 1981;105:563–7.

In a crossover study in three children and ten adults with urticaria pigmentosa with or without systemic features, the administration of oral disodium cromoglycate was associated with improvement in pruritus and, to a lesser extent, whealing.

Urticaria pigmentosa treated with oral disodium cromoglycate. Lindskov R, Wantzin GL, Knudsen L, Søndergaard I. Dermatologica 1984;169:49–52.

In three of four patients with urticaria pigmentosa, the oral administration of disodium cromoglycate was associated with a decrease in pruritus and whealing as assessed by a diminution in dermographism.

Bullous urticaria pigmentosa (cutaneous mastocytosis) and sodium cromoglycate therapy. Acta Derm Venereol 1982;61:572–5.

The appearance of bullae in urticaria pigmentosa stopped in two infants after the administration of oral disodium cromoglycate.

Treatment of bullous mastocytosis with disodium cromoglycate. Welch EA, Alper JC, Bogaars H, Farrell DS. J Am Acad Dermatol 1983;19:349–53.

A decrease in pruritus, whealing response, and blister formation occurred in two infants with diffuse and erythrodermic cutaneous mastocytosis with bullae who were treated with oral disodium cromoglycate.

SECOND LINE THERAPIES

■ Topical corticosteroid with plastic-film occlusion or hydrocolloid dressings	C
■ Oral PUVA photochemotherapy	D
■ Psoralen baths plus UVA photochemotherapy	D
■ UVA1 phototherapy	D

Treatment of urticaria pigmentosa with corticosteroids. Barton J, Lavker RM, Schechter NM, Lazarus GS. Arch Dermatol 1985;121:1516–23.

In six patients with urticaria pigmentosa, topical application of betamethasone dipropionate ointment 0.05% under occlusion for 8 hours daily for 6 weeks was associated with an absence of pruritus and Darier's sign. All patients remained clear of lesions at a mean follow-up time of 11.5 months (range 9–15 months).

Urticaria pigmentosa: systemic evaluation and successful treatment with topical steroids. Guzzo C, Lavker R, Roberts LJ II, et al. Arch Dermatol 1991;127:191–6.

In seven of nine adult patients with urticaria pigmentosa, the topical application of betamethasone dipropionate ointment 0.05% under occlusion overnight to one-half of the body for 6 weeks was associated with resolution of the lesions, with a maximum response within 3–12 weeks after the cessation of treatment. Lesions began to recur between 6 and 9 months after completing therapy. Re-treatment for 6 months followed by once-weekly application of betamethasone dipropionate ointment under occlusion kept the patients clear of lesions with the longest follow-up time of 2.5 years.

Treatment of urticaria pigmentosa by corticosteroids applied under a hydrocolloid dressing. Taylor G, Wojnarowska F, Chia Y, Kennedy C. Eur J Dermatol 1993; 3:276–8.

In a single adult with urticaria pigmentosa treated with clobetasol propionate 0.05% under a hydrocolloid dressing once weekly for 6 weeks, there was a reduction in pruritus and fading of hyperpigmentation that has lasted for 18 months.

The appropriate method for using topical corticosteroids in patients with urticaria pigmentosa needs to be determined in controlled trials.

Mastocytoma: topical corticosteroid treatment. Mateo JR. J Eur Acad Dermatol Venereol 2001;15:492–94.

Four infants aged between 2.5 and 6 months with mastocytomas were treated with twice-daily applications of clobetasol propionate 0.05% for 6 weeks and on alternate days for 6 weeks with tapering for a total treatment for 6 months. At the end of treatment there were residual macules with atrophy.

PUVA-treatment of urticaria pigmentosa. Christophers E, Hönigsmann H, Wolff K. Br J Dermatol 1978;98:701–2.

In ten patients with urticaria pigmentosa who were treated with PUVA photochemotherapy four times a week for six to 57 treatments, whealing after physical trauma could no longer be produced and pruritus was relieved. Relapses occurred after 3–6 months.

Photochemotherapy (PUVA) in the treatment of urticaria pigmentosa. Vella Briffa D, Eady RAJ, James MP, et al. Br J Dermatol 1983;109:67–75.

In eight patients with urticaria pigmentosa treated with PUVA photochemotherapy twice weekly for 15 to 69 exposures, the amount of pruritus and whealing was reduced. The disease tended to relapse once the treatment was discontinued.

Short- and long-term effectiveness of oral and bath PUVA therapy in urticaria pigmentosa and systemic mastocyto-

sis. Godt O, Proksch E, Streit V, Christophers E. Dermatology 1997;195:35–9.

In 20 patients with urticaria pigmentosa treated with PUVA photochemotherapy, improvement in pruritus was seen in eight of 15. Darier's sign was suppressed in seven and reduced in eight patients. There was follow-up for 18 years; 25% showed improvement for more than 5 years. Bath PUVA photochemotherapy with 8-methoxypsoralen was without effect. The success of PUVA photochemotherapy lasted from only a few weeks to more than 10 years.

Trioxsalen baths plus UV-A in the treatment of lichen planus and urticaria pigmentosa. Väätäinen N, Hannuksela M, Karvonen J. Clin Exp Dermatol 1981;6:133–8.

In five patients with urticaria pigmentosa treated with trioxsalen baths plus UVA, pruritus and the tendency to whealing decreased. Results could be maintained with maintenance therapy at 2–4-week intervals.

Photochemotherapy of dominant, diffuse, cutaneous mastocytosis. Smith ML, Orton PW, Chu H, Weston WL. Pediatr Dermatol 1990;7:251–5.

In three infants and one child with diffuse cutaneous mastocytosis treated with oral PUVA photochemotherapy twice weekly for 3–5 months, there was decreased pruritus, decreased blister formation, and a less thick skin with persistence of dermographism.

High-dose UVA1 for urticaria pigmentosa. Stege H, Schöpf E, Ruzicka T, Krutman J. Lancet 1996;347:64.

In four adult patients with urticaria pigmentosa treated with a daily dose of 130 J/cm^2 of UVA1 phototherapy five times a week for 2 weeks, pruritus was controlled and urinary histamine decreased to normal levels. There were no relapses with follow-up times of 10–23 months.

Medium- versus high-dose ultraviolet A1 therapy for urticaria pigmentosa: a pilot study. Gobello T, Mazzanti C, Sordi D, et al. J Am Acad Dermatol 2003;49:679–84.

In 12 patients with urticaria pigmentosa, treatment with both medium-dose (60 J/cm^2) for 15 days and high-dose (130 J/cm^2) for 10 days UVA1 was associated with decreased pruritus, with a decrease in the number of mast cells, and a change in the number of lesions over a 6-month period.

The appropriate method and schedules for the use of oral and bath PUVA photochemotherapy, UVA1 phototherapy, and even UVB phototherapy should be determined by controlled trials.

THIRD LINE THERAPIES

■ Interferon-alfa	D
■ Leukotriene-receptor inhibitor	E
■ Cyclosporine	E
■ Nifedipine	E
■ Hydrocolloid dressings	E
■ Surgical excision	E
■ Flashlamp-pumped pulsed dye laser	E
■ Electron beam radiation	E
■ Imatinib mesylate	E

Treatment of urticaria pigmentosa using interferon alpha. Kolde G, Sunderkötter C, Luger TA. Br J Dermatol 1995; 133:91–4.

Evidence levels **A** Double-blind study **B** Clinical trial ≥ 20 subjects **C** Clinical trial < 20 subjects **D** Series ≥ 5 subjects **E** Anecdotal case reports

In six patients with urticaria pigmentosa, the subcutaneous injection of interferon-alfa in various doses and frequencies up to 12 months was associated with a decrease in pruritus, but there was no reduction in the number of skin lesions.

Leukotriene-receptor inhibition for the treatment of systemic mastocytosis. Tolar J, Tope WD, Neglia JP. N Engl J Med 2004;350:735–6.

In a 2-month-old boy with systemic mastocytosis and skin lesions, wheezing, and hepatomegaly, when montelukast 0.25 mg/kg twice daily was not given, wheezing and cutaneous vesicles reappeared and subsided when the drug was re-administered.

The leukotriene-receptor inhibitors should be evaluated in mastocytosis in a controlled trial.

Response to cyclosporin and low-dose methylprednisolone in aggressive systemic mastocytosis. Kurosawa M, Amano H, Kanbe N, et al. J Allergy Clin Immunol 1999; 103:S412–20.

In a single adult man with aggressive systemic mastocytosis with urticaria pigmentosa, the administration of cyclosporine (100 mg daily) and methylprednisolone 4 mg daily was associated with control of pruritus and a reduction in the extent of urticaria pigmentosa.

This single anecdotal report does not allow assessment of the effect of cyclosporine.

Urticaria pigmentosa responsive to nifedipine. Fairley JA, Pentland AP, Voorhees JJ. J Am Acad Dermatol 1984;11: 740–3.

In a single adult woman with urticaria pigmentosa, the administration of nifedipine 10 mg three times daily was associated with a decrease in urtication of the skin lesions.

Flushing due to solitary cutaneous mastocytoma can be prevented by hydrocolloid dressings. Yung A. Pediatr Dermatol 2004;21:262–4.

In an 8-week-old boy, a double-layer hydrocolloid dressing reduced the shearing forces and prevented flushing.

Solitary mastocytoma in an adult: treatment by excision. Ashinoff R, Soter NA, Freedberg IM. J Dermatol Surg Oncol 1993;19:487–8.

In a 33-year-old woman, a solitary mastocytoma was excised.

Treatment of telangiectasia macularis eruptiva perstans with the 585-nm flashlamp-pumped dye laser. Ellis DL. Dermatol Surg 1996;22:33–7.

In a 10-year-old girl with telangiectasia macularis eruptiva perstans treated with a 585 nm flashlamp-pumped pulsed dye laser with concomitant oral antihistamines, the lesions resolved completely with one treatment, but 70% of the lesions recurred by 14 months.

The efficacy of lasers in the treatment of various forms of cutaneous skin lesions of mastocytosis at this time remains unknown.

Treatment of telangiectasia macularis eruptiva perstans with total electron beam radiation. Monahan TP, Petropolis AA. Cutis 2003;71:357–9.

In a 60-year-old man with telangiectasia macularis eruptiva perstans treated with 4000 cGy in 40 fractionated treatments, both pruritus and cutaneous lesions resolved with a 1-year follow-up.

Complete remission with imatinib mesylate (Glivec) of an idiopathic hypereosinophilic syndrome associated with a cutaneous mastocytosis after failure of interferon-alpha. Pottier P, Planchon B, Grossi O. Rev Med Interne 2003;24:542–6.

Imatinib mesylate is for systemic use and is currently not recommended for cutaneous disease.

Melasma

Christopher E M Griffiths

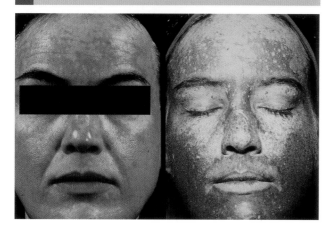

Melasma, also known as chloasma, is a condition of macular hyperpigmentation occurring predominantly in women. The commonest affected site is the face, presenting as several recognizable patterns, namely: central involving the forehead, cheeks, chin, and upper lip; malar; and mandibular. Melasma is usually symmetric and has an irregular 'moth-eaten' border. The condition may also manifest on the extensor aspect of the forearms either in isolation or accompanying facial melasma. Examination under Wood's light or black light commonly accentuates the area of skin affected by melasma, making it easier to identify and monitor during treatment. Histologically, there are three forms of melasma contingent on the predominant distribution of melanin: epidermal, dermal, and mixed epidermal and dermal. It is commonly accepted that epidermal melasma is the more responsive to therapy.

The etiology and pathomechanisms of melasma are poorly understood. There is a definite relationship to high estrogen states, namely pregnancy (sometimes referred to as the mask of pregnancy) and the oral contraceptive pill. There is some evidence that hormone replacement therapy may contribute to the development of melasma in some individuals. Usually, melasma resolves spontaneously postpartum or on stopping the oral contraceptive pill. There are some reports of melasma or a melasma-like condition occurring as an irritant response to cosmetics. Melasma often occurs idiopathically. It most commonly affects women of Latin American or Far East Asian descent and may be familial. In black women, a melasma-like condition occurs on the malar eminences, although it is uncertain as to whether this is true melasma or a separate clinical entity.

MANAGEMENT STRATEGY

The diagnosis of melasma is usually straightforward, given the clinical features described above. If the woman is pregnant, reassurance that melasma will usually fade postpartum is important; if she is taking the oral contraceptive pill, it may be advisable to switch to a low-estrogen 'mini pill' or preferably to another form of contraception. As all cases of melasma are most obvious during the summer months (i.e. at times of high ultraviolet light intensity), because of extensive sun-induced pigment darkening, advice about sun avoidance and use of a broad-spectrum sunblock, particu-

larly one that blocks UVA, is probably the best strategy. It is important to counsel patients about the risks of UVA exposure, even if sitting in a car, as UVA penetrates window glass. There is some evidence that hormone replacement therapy may be an underreported trigger of melasma.

As an adjunct to sun avoidance, specific topical therapies include 2–4% *hydroquinone*, 0.05–0.1% all-trans *retinoic acid*, and 10–20% *azelaic acid* creams, applied daily for 1–6 months. Newer, less-well-documented topical therapies include *kojic acid*, *liquiritin*, and *N-acetyl-4-S-cysteaminylphenol*. There is increasing evidence that combination therapies are of more benefit than monotherapy and that *laser therapy* and *clinical peels*, including glycolic acid and Jessner's, may be effective in resistant cases. Overall, treatment is unsatisfactory and topical therapies need to be adhered to rigorously if success is to be achieved.

SPECIFIC INVESTIGATIONS

- Thyroid function tests

Association of melasma with thyroid autoimmunity and other thyroidal abnormalities and their relationship to the origin of the melasma. Lufti RJ, Fridmanis M, Misiumas AL, et al. J Clin Endrocinol Metab 1985;61:28–31.

In 84 patients with melasma, the frequency of thyroid disorders (58.3%) was four times greater than that in the control group. The most sensitive test was for microsomal thyroid autoantibodies.

FIRST LINE THERAPIES

■ Hydroquinone	A
■ Tretinoin	A
■ Adapalene	A
■ Triple combination	A
■ 'Kligman cream'	B

[Double blind clinical study of the treatment of melasma with azelaic acid versus hydroquinone]. Piquero Martin J, Rothe de Arocha J, Beniamini Loker D. Med Cutan Ibero Lat Am 1988;16:511–4. In Spanish.

This double-blind comparative study in 60 subjects for 24 weeks found that 20% azelaic acid cream is no different in efficacy from 4% hydroquinone.

Topical tretinoin (retinoic acid) improves melasma. A vehicle-controlled, clinical trial. Griffiths CEM, Finkel LJ, Ditre CM, et al. Br J Dermatol 1993;129:415–21.

Thirteen (68%) of 19 women treated once daily with 0.1% tretinoin cream for 40 weeks showed significant clinical improvement in melasma as compared with one (5%) of 19 women treated with vehicle cream used in conjunction with a SPF-15 sunscreen. A good controlled trial using a variety of assessment measures – clinical, colorimetry, and histology.

Topical retinoic acid (tretinoin) for melasma in black patients. A vehicle-controlled clinical trial. Kimbrough-Green CK, Griffiths CEM, Finkel LJ, et al. Arch Dermatol 1994; 130: 727–33.

Using a novel assessment measure for melasma – the Melasma Area Severity Index (MASI) – this study found that

Evidence levels A Double-blind study B Clinical trial ≥ 20 subjects C Clinical trial < 20 subjects D Series ≥ 5 subjects E Anecdotal case reports

40 weeks' treatment with once-daily 0.1% tretinoin cream produced 32% improvement in melasma, as compared with 1% improvement with vehicle. Melasma in black patients is under-researched and poorly defined.

Adapalene in the treatment of melasma: a preliminary report. Dogra S, Kanwar AJ, Parsad D. Int J Dermatol 2002; 29:539–40.

Fourteen weeks of once daily application of adapalene 0.1% gel produced significant improvement in melasma, equivalent to 0.05% tretinoin cream, in this 'split-face' comparative study of 15 Indian women.

Efficacy and safety of a new triple combination agent for the treatment of facial melasma. Taylor S, Torok H, Jones T, et al. Cutis 2003;72:67–72.

Two multicenter, double-blind, randomized, 8-week studies in 641 patients with moderate to severe facial melasma treated once daily with either a triple combination product containing fluocinolone acetonide 0.01%, 4% hydroquinone, and 0.05% tretinoin cream, or any of the three possible combinations of two of its active ingredients. At 8 weeks, 77% of patients receiving the triple combination were significantly improved. This improvement was significantly better than any of the dual-therapy groups.

Intermittent therapy for melasma in Asian patients with combined topical agents (retinoic acid, hydroquinone and hydrocortisone): clinical and histological studies. Kang WH, Chan SC, Lee S. J Dermatol 1998;25:587–96.

Four months of twice-weekly application of a formula containing 0.1% tretinoin, 5% hydroquinone, and 1% hydrocortisone in 25 Korean women achieved good clinical results and was less irritating than daily use.

A new formula for depigmenting human skin. Kligman AM, Willis I. Arch Dermatol 1975;111:40–8.

First description of 'Kligman cream', a combination of 0.1% tretinoin, 5.0% hydroquinone, and 0.1% dexamethasone in hydrophilic ointment.

SECOND LINE THERAPIES

■ Azelaic acid	A
■ Liquiritin	A

Topical liquiritin improves melasma. Amer M, Metwalli M. Int J Dermatol 2000;39:299–301.

Controlled, split-face trial of twice-daily liquiritin cream or vehicle for 4 weeks in 20 women.

Liquiritin is a flavinoid derived from licorice.

Double-blind comparison of azelaic acid and hydroquinone in the treatment of melasma. Verallo-Rowell VM, Verallo V, Graupe K, et al. Acta Derm Venerol Suppl (Stockh) 1989;143:58–6l.

Comparison of twice-daily use of either 20% azelaic acid cream or 2% hydroquinone cream over 24 weeks, used in conjunction with a broad-spectrum sunscreen, in patients of Indo-Malay-Hispanic origin. Improvement occurred in 73% of azelaic acid treated patients, compared with 19% of hydroquinone patients, indicating that 20% azelaic acid is superior to 2% hydroquinone.

THIRD LINE THERAPIES

■ Kojic acid	B
■ N-acetyl-4-S-cysteaminylphenol	D
■ Glycolic acid peel	A
■ Jessner's solution	D
■ Laser(s)	C

The combination of glycolic acid and hydroquinone or kojic acids for the treatment of melasma and related conditions. Garcia A, Fulton JE. Dermatol Surg 1996;22: 443.

Thirty-nine patients were treated with glycolic acid/kojic acid on one side of the face and glycolic acid/hydroquinone on the other. There was no significant difference in improvement between the two sides.

N-acetyl-4-S-cysteaminylphenol as a new type of depigmenting agent for the melanoderma of patients with melasma. Jimbow K. Arch Dermatol 1991;127:1528–34.

Small, open study using a new depigmenting agent, a phenolic thioether, N-acetyl-4-S-cysteaminylphenol. Improvement was achieved in all 12 patients treated daily for 4 weeks using an oil-in-water emulsion preparation. Apparently, this agent is apparently less irritating than hydroquinone and is specific for melanocytes

Glycolic acid peels in the treatment of melasma among Asian women. Lim JT, Tham SN. Dermatol Surg 1997;23: 177–9.

Ten Asian women were treated with twice-daily applications of a cream containing 10% glycolic acid and 2% hydroquinone to the whole face, and glycolic acid peels every 3 weeks to one-half of the face, for 26 weeks. All patients used SPF-15 sunscreen. Improvement was achieved with the glycolic acid/hydroquinone cream, and this was enhanced by additional glycolic acid peels.

Treatment of melasma with Jessner's solution versus glycolic acid: a comparison of clinical efficacy and evaluation of the predictive ability of Wood's light examination. Lawrence N, Cox SE, Brody HJ. J Am Acad Dermatol 1997; 36:589–93.

Eleven women were treated initially with 0.05% tretinoin cream once daily for 1–2 weeks, then the right side of the face was peeled using 70% glycolic acid and left side was peeled using Jessner's solution. Patients underwent a total of three peels, 1 month apart. After peeling, the whole face was treated with 0.05% tretinoin cream and 4% hydroquinone. Results showed no difference between the two peels.

An impression that superficial peels hasten response to topical treatment.

Erbium:YAG laser resurfacing for refractory melasma. Manaloto RM, Alster T. Dermatol Surg 1999;25:121–3.

Ten women with melasma refractory to therapy with bleaching creams and chemical peels underwent treatment with an erbium:YAG laser (2.94 μm) at 5.1–7.6 J/cm^2 energy. Marked improvement was seen in all 10 women, but all exhibited postinflammatory hyperpigmentation 3–6 weeks post treatment.

Only recommended when all else fails.

The removal of cutaneous pigmented lesions with the Q-switched ruby laser and the Q-switched neodymium: yttrium-aluminium-garnet laser. A comparative study. Tse Y, Levine VJ, McClain SA, Ashinoff R. J Derm Surg Oncol 1994;20:795–800.

Both lasers are equally but moderately effective for treatment.

Combined ultrapulse CO_2 laser and Q-switched Alexandrite laser compared with Q-switched Alexandrite laser alone for refractory melasma: split-face design. Angsuwarangsee S, Polnikorn N. Dermatol Surg 2003;29: 59–64.

A small study (n = 6) showed that combination laser was better than the Q-switched Alexandrite laser alone.

Evidence levels **A** Double-blind study **B** Clinical trial ≥ 20 subjects **C** Clinical trial < 20 subjects **D** Series ≥ 5 subjects **E** Anecdotal case reports

Miliaria

Periasamy Balasubramaniam,
Warren R Heymann

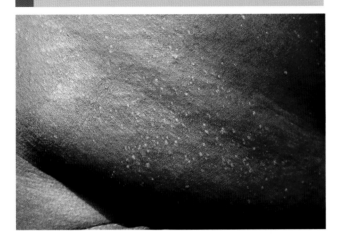

Miliaria (subtypes miliaria rubra, miliaria crystallina, and miliaria profunda) is a transient eruptive disorder of retained sweat in the occluded eccrine duct at various levels. Miliaria rubra is the commonest type and clinically presents as itchy papulovesicles with a surrounding collar of erythema. Miliaria crystallina appears as clear sweat-filled tiny vesicles, and the rare miliaria profunda presents with tiny white papules. Histologically the eccrine duct occlusion is at the level of stratum malpighii, stratum corneum, and dermal–epidermal junction or dermis, respectively. (Fox–Fordyce disease, also known as apocrine miliaria, is discussed on page 233.)

MANAGEMENT STRATEGY

Miliaria is generally a benign condition caused by excessive sweating due to high environmental temperature or pyrexia, and is often exacerbated by tight clothing and high humidity. Because the condition is common and transient, patients are likely to seek medical care for treatment of itching or if there are any complications. The management of miliaria begins with the *removal of the inciting factors,* so most of the literature has focused on identifying causative agents and there is no strong evidence for the treatment options.

Miliaria rarely poses diagnostic difficulties. Neonates are likely to present with lesions in the neck and intertriginous areas or as diaper dermatitis. In most cases the history of fever or heavy blanketing is available and a simple explanation of causative factors with advice on avoidance should be adequate. Adults often develop miliaria during travel and military service in the tropics or with heavy exercise. Gradual exposure helps to acclimatize to a hot and humid environment, but this may take a few months. *Loose fitting clothing and cool showering* may minimize the symptoms. Mild cases may benefit from the use of light powders like *cornstarch or baby talcum powder.* In the use of any topical lotion, cream, or powder, care must be taken to ensure that the product applied does not occlude the skin, further exacerbating the condition. In the case of severe itching, *antihistamines, cold packs,* and *topical corticosteroids* may be used. *Oatmeal baths* have been anecdotally reported to provide relief. However, all these measures will prove ineffective if the sweating is not reduced. All cases will respond to *air-conditioning, exposure of the involved skin* and use of *antipyretics,* in appropriate circumstances. Miliaria profunda has been reported to respond to *oral retinoids* and *anhydrous lanolin.*

Miliaria may be complicated by superinfection. If infection occurs, it should be treated with *systemic antibiotics* aimed at staphylococci as the likely pathogen. Clinicians should make patients aware that anhidrosis in the area of the eruption may occur and persist up to 3 weeks (or sometimes even longer) after the onset of lesions, and increased heat retention may occur if a large surface area was initially affected. Thus, patients at risk of heat exhaustion or heat stroke should take precautions to remain in air-conditioned environments during hot weather. A biopsy may be helpful in atypical cases of miliaria.

SPECIFIC INVESTIGATIONS

- None usually required

In atypical cases
- Microbiology – swab for bacteria and yeasts
- Histology

Nonneoplastic disorders of the eccrine glands. Wenzel FG, Horn TD. J Am Acad Dermatol 1998;38:1–7.

The histology and pathophysiology of eccrine sweat ducts are reviewed, as are normal and abnormal sweat content and formation. The erythematous macule or papule of miliaria rubra occurs with an obstruction of the sweat duct at the level of the stratum malpighii. In the case of miliaria crystallina the disruption is in the stratum corneum, and with miliaria profunda, at or beneath the dermal–epidermal junction.

Duct disruption, a new explanation of miliaria. Shuster S. Acta Derm Venereol 1997;77:1–3.

A hypothesis is presented that ascribes miliaria crystallina to mechanical disruption of the eccrine duct, rather than the commonly accepted pathogenesis of duct plugging. This disruption is attributed to UV irradiation causing a split between upper epidermal cells and stratum corneum.

The role of extracellular polysaccharide substance produced by *Staphylococcus epidermidis* in miliaria. Mowad CM, McGinley KJ, Foglia A, Leyden JJ. J Am Acad Dermatol 1995;33:729–33.

The ability of various strains of coagulase-negative staphylococci to induce miliaria under an occlusive dressing as well as microbiologic, histologic, and immunostaining features were evaluated. *Staphylococcus epidermidis* was the only strain that induced miliaria. The authors conclude that periodic acid-Schiff (PAS)-positive extracellular polysaccharide substance (EPS) produced by *S. epidermidis* plays a central role in the pathogenesis of miliaria by obstructing sweat delivery.

The pathogenesis of miliaria rubra: role of the resident microflora. Holzle E, Kligman AM. Br J Dermatol 1978;99: 117–37.

The degree of miliaria rubra and anhidrosis induced in 55 subjects was shown to be directly correlated with the density of resident flora present on occluded areas of skin, as measured by detergent scrub and culture.

A historical overview of research into the pathogenesis of miliaria rubra is included.

Miliaria crystallina in an intensive care setting. Haas N, Martens F, Henz BM. Clin Exp Dermatol 2004;29:32–4.

Two cases of miliaria crystallina occurring in an intensive care setting are presented. The authors hypothesize that the mechanism is secondary to transient poral closure due to the drugs used in the intensive care setting.

FIRST LINE THERAPIES

■ Prevention	D
■ Frequent showering	E
■ Cornstarch powder	E
■ Air conditioning	B
■ Oatmeal baths	E
■ Topical antiseptics	E
■ Antipyretics	E

Miliaria rubra of the lower limbs in underground miners. Donoghue AM, Sinclair MJ. Occup Med (Lond) 2000;50: 430–3.

Case series of 25 miners working in a hot and humid environment who developed miliaria. Symptoms resolved after 4 weeks of sedentary duties in the air-conditioned areas. This report also analyzed the coexisting dermatological conditions in these patients.

Diseases of the eccrine sweat glands. Hurley HJ. In: Bolognia JL, Jorizzo JL, Rapini RP, eds. Dermatology. Philadelphia: Mosby; 2003:578–9.

Cornstarch or other light powders may be used to absorb moisture and minimize the maceration that cause the early changes needed for the development of miliaria.

Diseases of the eccrine sweat glands. Hurley HJ. In: Moschella SL, Hurley HJ, eds. Dermatology. Philadelphia: WB Saunders; 1992:1526–30.

Regular showering to remove salt and bacteria may be helpful in the case of miliaria profunda.

Treatment of diaper dermatitis. Boiko S. Dermatol Clin 1999;17:235–40.

If care is not taken to distinguish miliaria from other forms of 'generic' diaper dermatitis, the condition can be worsened by treatment. As most over-the-counter diaper rash products contain zinc oxide or petrolatum, indiscriminate use of such products can exacerbate miliaria by further occluding eccrine ducts. Oatmeal baths have been recommended only anecdotally as a soothing treatment.

Heat-related illnesses. Khosla R, Guntupalli KK. Crit Care Clin 1999;15:251–63.

Wearing loose fitting clothing and avoiding heavy creams or powders may prevent miliaria. In the event that miliaria does form, chlorhexidine cream or lotion, with or without

salicylic acid, can be applied. Antipyretics can be used to lower the temperature of a febrile patient with miliaria. If any signs of superinfection on miliaria develop systemic antibiotics may be given.

An outbreak of occupational dermatosis in an electronics store. Koh D. Contact Dermatitis 1995;32:327–30.

In an electronic store 21% of employees who worked in the non air-conditioned area developed miliaria whereas only 11% of the employees who worked in the air-conditioned area were affected.

SECOND LINE THERAPIES

■ Topical corticosteroids	E
■ Systemic antibiotics	E

Miliaria rubra. Stearns JA. In: Dambro MR, ed. Griffith's 5-minute Clinical Consult. Philadelphia: Lippincott, Williams & Wilkins; 2000:688–9.

For relief of pruritus, 0.1% betamethasone twice daily for 3 days may be applied over the affected area. In the event of superimposed infection, an antistaphylococcal agent such as dicloxacillin (flucloxacillin) 250 mg four times daily for 10 days may be used.

Prickly heat. In: Rosen P, ed. Emergency Medicine. Concepts and Clinical Practice. 4th edn. St Louis: Mosby; 1998:992.

If a case of miliaria rubra becomes pustular, oral erythromycin has been shown to be helpful. During the most acute phase of miliaria rubra, chlorhexidine lotion or cream can be used as an antibacterial agent, with salicylic acid 1% three times daily over small areas to aid in desquamation.

THIRD LINE THERAPIES

■ Anhydrous lanolin/isotretinoin	E
■ Ascorbic acid	B

Miliaria profunda. Kirk JF, Wilson BB, Chun W, Cooper PH. J Am Acad Dermatol 1996;35:854–6.

This case report describes a 23-year-old man with miliaria profunda, successfully treated with anhydrous lanolin and isotretinoin, after a poor response to topical corticosteroids. Characteristic features, pathogenesis, histopathology, and treatment are discussed.

The effects of administration of ascorbic acid in experimentally induced miliaria and hypohidrosis in volunteers. Hindson TC, Worsley DE. Br J Dermatol 1969;81:226–7.

Miliaria and hypohidrosis were induced in 36 subjects, half of whom were given 1 g daily of ascorbic acid and half a placebo, beginning on the day of wrapping the skin with polythene occlusion. The ascorbic acid group developed less severe miliaria and hypohidrosis, had quicker healing of visible lesions, and notable improvement in hypohidrosis at 1 week, compared to the placebo group.

Evidence levels   **A** Double-blind study   **B** Clinical trial ≥ 20 subjects   **C** Clinical trial < 20 subjects   **D** Series ≥ 5 subjects   **E** Anecdotal case reports

Molluscum contagiosum

Dermot B McKenna, E Claire Benton

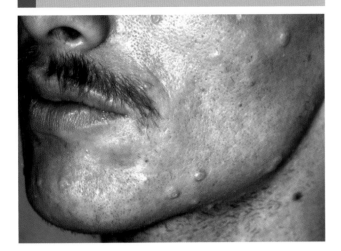

Molluscum contagiosum (MC) is a common self-limiting poxvirus infection of the skin and occasionally mucous membranes. Lesions occur in children, usually on the trunk and body folds, and in young adults, if sexually transmitted, in the genital region. They typically present as multiple, 1–10 mm in diameter, discrete, pearly-white or flesh-colored, umbilicated papules. They may be surrounded by an eczematous reaction, which disappears on resolution of the infection. Mollusca may be very extensive and recalcitrant to treatment in all forms of cell-mediated immunosuppression, especially patients with AIDS.

MANAGEMENT STRATEGY

There is no specific antiviral treatment for MC. Both physical and chemical destructive methods, as well as topical and systemic immunostimulatory therapies have been tried, but only a few have been subjected to the rigours of placebo-controlled studies – important in a condition that has a high spontaneous resolution rate.

The choice of therapy will depend on the age and immune status of the patient as well as the number and location of the lesions. In immunocompetent patients with few lesions it is reasonable to await *spontaneous resolution*, which will usually occur within a few months. Secondarily infected MC may need *topical antiseptic or antibiotic* treatment to minimize the risk of atrophic scarring. Active intervention may be justified for cosmetic reasons or to hasten resolution to prevent autoinoculation or transmission of the virus to close contacts. *Avoiding communal bathing and restricting the sharing of towels* should also help prevent the spread of infection to others.

A commonly used and inexpensive treatment is the *manual extrusion of individual lesions* using gloved fingers or fine forceps. This has proved more effective than *cryotherapy* applied every 3–4 weeks. *Curettage and electrodesiccation* of larger lesions may result in scarring and also requires pain alleviation, especially in children, by the prior application of a eutectic mixture of local anesthetics (lidocaine and prilocaine cream). Topically applied caustic agents have been used with variable results. Good success rates are reported with *topical application of 40% silver nitrate paste, 0.5% podophyllotoxin, and 10% povidone–iodine with 50% salicylic acid*. A useful alternative is *5% acidified nitrite, applied nightly with 5% salicylic acid under occlusion*. Significant scarring has been documented both with *potassium hydroxide and phenol* and the latter is no longer recommended. Although *cantharidin* has proved to be an effective treatment, it is not readily available in the UK and is not currently recommended by the Food and Drug Administration. The topical immune response modifier *imiquimod* has been shown to be effective in two placebo-controlled studies. In patients with AIDS, both 1% imiquimod and *topical cidofovir 3%*, a competitive inhibitor of DNA polymerase, have proved successful for treating MC. Recovery of immune function with *highly active antiretroviral therapy (HAART)* may also result in the resolution of MC in these patients.

SPECIFIC INVESTIGATIONS

- Methylene blue staining of a smear to look for molluscum bodies or histopathology of a curetted specimen

This is only required when the diagnosis is in any doubt.

FIRST LINE THERAPIES

■ Await spontaneous resolution	B
■ Manual extrusion with gloved fingers or fine forceps	B

The natural history of molluscum contagiosum in Fijian children. Hawley TG. J Hygiene 1970;68:631–2.

Although the individual lesions of MC last 6–8 weeks, by autoinoculation the total duration of infection may be up to 8 months.

Scarring in molluscum contagiosum: comparison of physical expression and phenol ablation. Weller R, O'Callaghan CJ, MacSween RM, White MI. BMJ 1999;319:1540.

There was no difference in overall efficacy of the two methods, but phenol resulted in significantly more scarring.

SECOND LINE THERAPIES

■ Topical 5% applied acidified nitrite co-applied with 5% salicylic acid	A
■ Topical 40% silver nitrate paste	B
■ Topical 0.5% podophyllotoxin	B
■ Topical 10% povidone–iodine and 50% salicylic acid	B
■ Cryotherapy	C

Molluscum contagiosum effectively treated with a topical acidified nitrite, nitric oxide liberating cream. Ormerod AD, White MI, Shah SAA, Benjamin N. Br J Dermatol 1999;141: 1051–3.

Double-blind study in 30 children of sodium nitrite 5% co-applied nightly with 5% salicylic acid resulted in a cure rate of 75% compared to 21% with salicylic acid alone.

Treatment of molluscum contagiosum with silver nitrate paste. Niizeki K, Hashimoto K. Pediatr Dermatol 1999;16: 395–7.

In 389 patients topical 40% silver nitrate paste was applied after 2% lidocaine jelly; 70% cleared after one application, 97.7% after three applications. Treatment was well tolerated and no scarring was reported. It was easier to apply compared to a 40% aqueous solution of silver nitrate.

Podophyllotoxin in the treatment of molluscum contagiosum. Deleixhe-Mauhin F, Piérard-Franchimont C, Piérard GE. J Dermatol Treat 1991;2:99–101.

Twenty four patients applied 0.5% podophyllotoxin solution daily. All cleared after less than 15 applications without side effects, apart from mild irritation.

Molluscum contagiosum treated with iodine solution and salicylic acid plaster. Ohkuma M. Int J Dermatol 1990;29: 443–5.

Povidone–iodine solution, 10%, and 50% salicylic acid plaster applied daily to MC in 20 patients was significantly more effective than either agent used alone with a mean duration to clearance of 26 days and with no adverse effects.

Molluscum contagiosum in children – evidence based treatment. White MI, Weller R, Diack P. Clin Exp Dermatol 1997;22:51.

Study comparing the efficacy and potential for scarring of manual extrusion, cryotherapy, and topical phenol.

Manual extrusion was more effective than cryotherapy. Phenol was associated with significant scarring and is not recommended for treating MC.

THIRD LINE THERAPIES

Physical destruction	
■ Curettage with EMLA®	C
■ Electrodesiccation	C
■ Pulsed dye laser	C
■ Photodynamic therapy (PDT)	D
■ Application of duct tape	E
Topical therapy	
■ 10% potassium hydroxide solution	B
■ Topical 1–5% imiquimod	A
■ Cantharidin	C
■ Australian lemon myrtle	C
■ Topical cidofovir	E
■ Tretinoin	E
Systemic therapy	
■ Cimetidine	D
■ Interferon-alfa – subcutaneous	E

Treatment of molluscum contagiosum using a lidocaine/prilocaine cream (EMLA) for analgesia. de Waard-van der Speck FB, Oranje AP, Lillieborg S, et al. J Am Acad Dermatol 1990;23:685–8.

Double-blind study in 83 children showed efficacy of EMLA cream applied for less than 60 min in reducing pain of curettage, though no comment on clearance rates.

Curettage of molluscum contagiosum in children: analgesia by topical application of a lidocaine/prilocaine cream (EMLA® cream). Rosdahl L, Edmar B, Gisslen H, et al. Acta Derm Venereol 1988;68:149–53.

EMLA® cream provided effective local anesthesia for the curettage of MC in 55 children.

Treatment of molluscum contagiosum with the pulsed dye laser over a 28-month period. Hancox JG, Jackson J, McCagh S. Cutis 2003;71:414–6.

All treated lesions in 43 patients resolved and in 15 of them no further lesions developed after two treatments

Treatment of molluscum contagiosum with the 585-nm pulsed dye laser. Hughes PS. Dermatol Surg 1998;24:229–30.

Almost all lesions in a child cleared with one treatment.

Photodynamic therapy for molluscum contagiosum infection in HIV-coinfected patients: review of 6 cases. Moiin A. J Drugs Dermatol 2003;6:637–9.

Treatment of six patients with 5-aminolevulinic acid (ALA) and PDT resulted in a reduction in lesion count and severity.

The successful use of ALA-PDT in the treatment of recalcitrant molluscum contagiosum. Gold MH, Boring MM, Bridges TM, Bradshaw VL. J Drugs Dermatol 2004;3:187–90.

Case report of successful treatment with ALA–PDT of molluscum contagiosum in a patient with HIV infection.

Use of duct tape occlusion in the treatment of recurrent molluscum contagiosum. Lindau MS, Munar MY. Pediatr Dermatol 2004;21:609.

Case report of well tolerated and successful home therapy of multiple MC used over 2 months

Treatment of molluscum contagiosum with potassium hydroxide: a clinical approach in 35 children. Romiti R, Ribeiro AP, Grinblat BM, et al. Pediatr Dermatol 1999;16: 228–31.

Potassium hydroxide solution, 10%, was applied twice daily until lesions underwent inflammation or ulceration. Of 35 children, 32 cleared with a mean treatment period of 30 days. Hypertrophic scarring occurred in one patient, while pigmentary change was observed in nine others.

Treatment of molluscum contagiosum in males with an analogue of imiquimod 1% cream: a placebo controlled, double-blind study. Syed TA, Goswami J, Ahmadpour OA, Ahmad SA. J Dermatol 1998;25:309–13.

One hundred male patients applied either the analogue cream or placebo to their mollusca three times daily for 5 days each week for 1 month; 82% cleared with active treatment compared to 16% of those using placebo. The treatment was well tolerated.

Treatment of molluscum contagiosum with imiquimod 5% cream. Skinner RB. Arch Dermatol 2002;47(suppl);221–4.

Five patients treated for up to 8 weeks with 5% imiquimod cream showed complete resolution of multiple MC.

Comparison (with references) of the various treatment modalities available.

Effectiveness of imiquimod cream 5% for treating childhood molluscum contagiosum in a double blind

Evidence levels **A** Double-blind study **B** Clinical trial ≥ 20 subjects **C** Clinical trial < 20 subjects **D** Series ≥ 5 subjects **E** Anecdotal case reports

randomised pilot trial. Theos AU, Cummins R, Silverberg NB, Paller AS. Cutis 2004;74:134–8.

Complete clearance of MC occurred in 33% of 12 children compared with 11% of the vehicle-only group.

Experience in treating molluscum contagiosum in children with imiquimod 5% cream. Bayerl C, Feller G, Goerdt S. Br J Dermatol 2003;149(suppl 66):25–9.

Three times weekly application for 16 weeks in 15 children gave complete remission in two and partial remission in nine; side effects included burning, redness, and itching.

Recalcitrant molluscum contagiosum in an HIV-afflicted male treated successfully with topical imiquimod. Brown CW, O'Donoghue M, Moore J, Tharp M. Cutis 2000;65:363–6.

Imiquimod cream, 5%, cleared recalcitrant lesions in a patient.

Combination topical treatment of molluscum contagiosum with cantharidin and imiquimod 5% in children: a case series of 16 patients. Ross GL, Orchard GC. Aust J Dermatol 2004;445:100–2.

Sixteen children were treated with one application of cantharidin followed by topical imiquimod nightly for up to 5 weeks. Twelve of 16 showed over 90% clearance of MC.

Childhood molluscum contagiosum: experience with cantharidin therapy in 300 patients. Silverberg NB, Sidbury R, Mancini AJ. J Am Acad Dermatol 2000;43:503–7.

A retrospective study of topical cantharidin applied to nonfacial MC for 4–6 h was complicated by the use of other concurrent therapies. Of 300 children, over 90% cleared after a mean of 2.1 treatments; 90% of children experienced blistering at the treated site, but none developed bacterial infections.

Essential oil of Australian lemon myrtle (*Backhousia citriodora*) in the treatment of molluscum contagiosum. Burke BE, Baillie JE, Olson RD. Biomed Pharmacother 2004; 58:245–7.

Once daily application of a 10% solution of *Backhousia citriodora* gave over 90% reduction in lesions in nine of 16 children compared with none of 16 in the control group (vehicle alone).

Topical cidofovir. A novel treatment for recalcitrant molluscum contagiosum in children infected with human immunodeficiency virus 1. Toro JR, Wood LV, Patel NK, et al. Arch Dermatol 2000;136:983–5.

Topical 3% cidofovir applied daily for 5 days per week for 8 weeks cleared previously recalcitrant lesions in two children.

Topical cidofovir for severe molluscum contagiosum. Davies EG, Thrasher A, Lacey K, Harper J. Lancet 1999;353: 2042.

Topical cidofovir for 3 weeks was effective in clearing mollusca in a 12-year-old boy with Wiskott–Aldrich syndrome.

Venereal herpes-like molluscum contagiosum: treatment with tretinoin. Papa CM, Berger RS. Cutis 1976;18:537–40.

Twice-daily application of 0.1 or 0.05% tretinoin cleared mollusca in two patients.

Treatment of molluscum contagiosum with oral cimetidine: clinical experience in 13 patients. Dohil M, Prenderville JS. Pediatr Dermatol 1996;13:310–2.

Patients were treated with a 2-month course at a dose of 40 mg/kg daily, with clearance reported in all children who completed the course.

Inefficiency of oral cimetidine for non-atopic children with molluscum contagiosum. Cunningham BB, Paller AS, Garzon M. Pediatr Dermatol 1998;15:71–2.

Response of MC to cimetidine may be better in atopic compared to nonatopic children.

Interferon alpha treatment of molluscum contagiosum in immunodeficiency. Hourihane J, Hodges E, Smith J, et al. Arch Dis Child 1999;80:77–9.

Molluscum contagiosum in two children with combined immunodeficiency cleared with subcutaneous interferon-alfa.

Molluscum contagiosum. Recent advances in pathogenetic mechanisms and new therapies. Smith KJ, Skelton H. Am J Clin Dermatol 2002;3:536–45.

A good review paper.

Resolution of disseminated molluscum contagiosum with highly active anti-retroviral therapy (HAART) in patients with AIDS. Calista D, Boschini A, Landi G. Eur J Dermatol 1999;9:211–3.

Three patients with recalcitrant MC cleared 6 months after commencing HAART.

Resolution of severe molluscum contagiosum on effective anti-retroviral therapy. Horn CK, Scott GR, Benton EC. Br J Dermatol 1998;138:715–7.

Severe molluscum infection in a patient with HIV disease largely disappeared after treatment of the HIV infection with ritonavir and lamivudine.

Morphea

Bernice R Krafchik

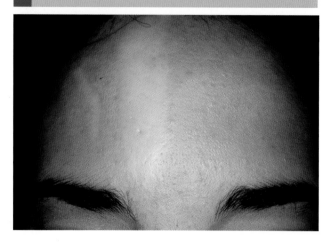

Morphea is a rare connective tissue disease affecting the skin and subcutaneous tissue. Occasionally underlying tissue such as muscle, fascia, and bone may be involved. Clinically, the disease affects children and adults, may be limited or widespread, and undergoes spontaneous resolution within about 3–5 years, though some cases may be active for up to 10 years and the disease may be recurrent. The condition is mainly classified into plaque, generalized, and linear varieties, but there are many more subgroups. Morphea may cause serious cosmetic defects (skin atrophy, hyper-pigmentation, hypopigmentation) and physical disability, due to secondary muscle atrophy and interference with bone growth.

MANAGEMENT STRATEGY

Morphea is difficult to treat, though in recent years new therapies have emerged. It is difficult to assess treatment modalities because there is a tendency for the disease to become inactive spontaneously without intervention. Once fibrosis occurs no medical intervention is helpful and surgery may be considered to correct the defect. *Topical corticosteroids* (fluorinated, medium potency, and hydrocorti-sone) may be useful during the initial inflammatory stage, though controlled clinical trials are not available. *Intra-lesional triamcinolone* (5 mg/mL every 4 weeks for a total of 3 months) may improve linear morphea involving the scalp and forehead (en coup de sabre). *Topical calcipotriene* 0.005% ointment twice a day under occlusion for 3 months has been used with success in active morphea. *Psoralen plus UVA (PUVA)-bath photochemotherapy* may be effective for wide-spread plaque and linear morphea. Patients are immersed for 20 min in a warm water bath containing 1 mg/L of methoxsalen. This is followed by irradiation with UVA, 0.2–0.5 J/cm² for a maximum of 1.2–3.5 J/cm² to a mean cumulative dose of 41.1 J/cm². More recently, it has been shown that *low-dose UVA alone* (20 J/cm² for a total of 600 J/cm²) may clear or improve severe disease. *Low-dose methotrexate*, 15–25 mg per week, may halt progression of the disease. Children with severe disabling morphea showed improvement with methotrexate, 0.3–0.6 mg/kg per week until the disease becomes inactive and then con-tinued for a year before tapering; this is combined with pulsed *intravenous methylprednisolone* (30 mg/kg for 3 days, monthly) for a total period of 3 months.

Oral calcitriol has been shown to be effective in localized morphea. However, unlike topical calcipotriene, this drug may have a pronounced effect on calcium metabolism. *Physical therapy* is extremely helpful in preventing and treating contractures.

SPECIFIC INVESTIGATIONS

- No diagnostic tests
- Skin biopsy (if diagnosis is in doubt)
- MRI and ultrasound of affected areas to rule out underlying involvement

Skin imaging with high frequency ultrasound – prelimi-nary results. Szymanska E, Nowicki A, Mlosek K, et al. Eur J Ultrasound 2000;12:9–16.

It has always been difficult to assess the skin changes in patients with morphea. This study using high-frequency ultrasound demonstrated the skin changes that occurred in patients with morphea following treatment for their disease.

FIRST LINE THERAPIES

■ Topical corticosteroids	E
■ Intralesional corticosteroids	E
■ Topical calcipotriene	C
■ Topical imiquimod	E
■ Topical tacrolimus	E

Topical calcipotriene for morphea/linear scleroderma. Cunningham BB, Landells IDR, Langman C, et al. J Am Acad Dermatol 1998;39:211–5.

Calcipotriene is a synthetic derivative of vitamin D3. Twelve patients with biopsy-documented active morphea or linear scleroderma were treated with calcipotriene ointment (0.005%) for 3 months. All patients showed improvement, including decrease in erythema, telangiectasis, and depig-mentation. The ointment was well tolerated and there were no laboratory alterations in calcium metabolism.

A double-blind, placebo-controlled trial will be necessary to confirm the above findings, though the results of this open clini-cal trial appear encouraging.

Use of imiquimod cream 5% in the treatment of localized morphea. Man J, Dytoc MT. J Cutan Med Surg 2004;8:166–9. Epub 2004 May-Jun.

These authors treated a patient with morphea with 5% imiquimod and considered that this therapy led to soften-ing of the lesions. They imply that the interferon might inter-fere with the profibrotic cytokines.

Obviously this is one case report and other studies with more patients will be needed to confirm these findings.

Topical tacrolimus in the treatment of localized sclero-derma. Mancuso G, Berdondini RM. Eur J Dermatol 2003;13: 590–2.

This report involved treating two patients with the calcineurin inhibitor 0.1% twice a day with softening of the skin.

Evidence levels   **A** Double-blind study   **B** Clinical trial ≥ 20 subjects   **C** Clinical trial < 20 subjects   **D** Series ≥ 5 subjects   **E** Anecdotal case reports

Although these results are encouraging, it might be prudent to wait with this therapy until the scare regarding cancers has been resolved.

SECOND LINE THERAPIES

■ PUVA	B
■ PUVA-bath photochemotherapy	C
■ UVA	C
■ UVA1	B

UVA/UVA1 phototherapy and PUVA photochemotherapy in connective tissue diseases and related disorders: a research based review. Breuckmann F, Gambichler T, Altmeyer P, Kreuter A. BMC Dermatol 2004;4:11.

These authors systematically review the literature on UVA/UVA1 and PUVA therapy in various skin conditions including morphea. They conclude that significant softening of the skin occurs with all modalities used. High-dose UVA1 was of more benefit than low-dose treatment.

Different low doses of broad-band UVA in the treatment of morphea and systemic sclerosis. El-Mofty M, Mostafa W, El-Darouty M, et al. Photodermatol Photoimmunol Photomed 2004;20:148–56.

Sixty three patients with both progressive systemic sclerosis and morphea were tested with various strengths of UVA. The results after using 5 and 10 J/cm² were as good as using 20 J/cm². This is a relatively easy treatment because many centers have UVA.

Ultraviolet A1 phototherapy. Dawe RS. Br J Dermatol 2003;148:626–37.

This review highlights the efficacy of using both low- and high-dose UVA1 therapy in various forms of morphea and included the report of one case where there was a marked softening of the skin in a 16-year-old with pansclerotic morphea.

Phototherapy for scleroderma: biologic rationale, results, and promise. Fisher GJ, Kang S. Curr Opin Rheumatol 2002; 14:723–6.

These authors analyze the results of UVA1 therapy and point out that the machine and equipment required for UVA1 is very expensive whereas UVA seemed to produce similar improvement with and without the addition of oral or bath psoralen.

Ultraviolet A sunbed used for the treatment of scleroderma. Oikarinen A, Knuutinen A. Acta Derm Venereol 2001;81:432–3.

A letter describing the use of a UVA sunbed, its effect on softening the skin of patients with morphea, and comparing it with the expensive modality of using UVA1.

Low dose broad-band UVA in morphea using a new method for evaluation. El-Mofty M, Zaher H, Bosseila M, et al. Photodermatol Photoimmunol Photomed 2000;16: 43–9.

In this open trial of broadband UVA, 12 patients with morphea were treated with 20 J/cm² three times per week for 20 sessions. Softening of skin lesions and reduction in concentration of collagen on skin biopsy were reported.

Low-dose UVA phototherapy for treatment of localized scleroderma. Kerscher M, Volkenandt M, Gruss C, et al. J Am Acad Dermatol 1998;38:21–6.

Low-dose UVA, in the range of 340–400 nm, was given to 20 patients with severe localized scleroderma for a total exposure of 600 J/cm² over a period of 12 weeks. Two patients with subcutaneous localized scleroderma did not respond to UVA. Clearance or marked improvement was noted in 90% of the treated patients. Histopathologic findings correlated well with clinical results.

UVA1, while not widely available, is emerging as an effective therapy for morphea.

THIRD LINE THERAPIES

■ Methotrexate	C
■ Methotrexate plus pulsed prednisolone	C
■ Oral calcitriol	C
■ Cyclosporine	E
■ Surgery	E

Low-dose methotrexate in the treatment of widespread morphea. Seyger MMB, van den Hoogen FHJ, de Boo T, et al. J Am Acad Dermatol 1998;39:220–5.

Nine patients, all adult, with widespread morphea were treated with oral methotrexate, 15 mg per week for a 24-week period. Six patients showed improvement in the score for skin induration, while three patients had no benefit. There were no serious adverse reactions.

Because spontaneous improvement occurs in morphea, a prospective double-blind, placebo-controlled study will be necessary to justify the use of methotrexate in this disease.

Methotrexate and corticosteroid therapy for pediatric localized scleroderma. Uziel Y, Feldman BM, Krafchik BR, et al. J Pediatr 2000;136:91–5.

Ten patients, mean age 6.8 years, with active localized scleroderma of 4 years' mean duration were treated with methotrexate and intravenous methylprednisolone for a 3-month period. Nine patients responded to therapy and treatment was generally well tolerated.

Methotrexate has been shown to be effective in the treatment of juvenile rheumatoid arthritis. Its use in childhood morphea will have to be evaluated by a future controlled trial and probably will be restricted to severe, disabling disease.

Treatment of linear scleroderma with oral 1,25-dihydroxy-vitamin D3 (calcitriol) in seven children. Elst EF, Van Suijlekom-Smit LW, Oranje AP. Pediatr Dermatol 1999;16: 53–8.

Seven children with linear scleroderma were treated with oral calcitriol. Five showed good to excellent improvement. No side effects were observed including no changes in the urinary calcium/creatinine ratio. Calcitriol has been shown to have a dose-dependent effect on fibroblast proliferation and collagen synthesis, and also has immunoregulatory activities.

Calcitriol may have a pronounced effect on calcium metabolism, so patients should be carefully monitored for calcium, inorganic phosphate, creatinine, and urea in serum and urine.

Good response of linear scleroderma in a child to ciclosporin. Strauss RM, Bhushan M, Goodfield MJ. Br J Dermatol 2004;150:790–2.

A 12-year-old child with rapidly expanding linear morphea was first treated with clobetasol twice a day. Because there was little improvement in her condition, cyclosporine 3 mg/kg daily was added to the regimen, with rapid improvement and softening of the lesion on her thigh. This took 4 months to occur. The treatment was stopped and there was no recurrence in 1 year. The authors talk about the effect of cyclosporine on interfering with the cytokine IL-2, which is increased in activated lymphocytes.

Treatment of coup de sabre deformity with porous polyethylene implant. Copcu E. Plast Reconstr Surg 2004;113: 758–9.

In this article a porous polyethylene implant was used to correct an en coup de sabre defect with excellent results. This highlights the future role of surgery to correct the severe cosmetic disabilities that are sometimes encountered in facial lesions of morphea.

This chapter is dedicated to the memory of Raul Fleischmajer who wrote this chapter for the first edition of Treatment of Skin Disease: Comprehensive Therapeutic Strategies.

Mucous membrane pemphigoid

Alison J Bruce, Roy S Rogers III

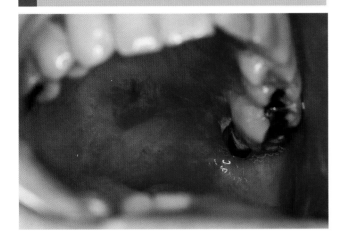

Mucous membrane pemphigoid is a relatively rare, chronic, subepidermal, immune-mediated, vesiculobullous disease. It is seen most commonly in older age groups and affects the oral and ocular mucosa most frequently. Other areas that may be involved include mucosal surfaces such as the nose, throat, and esophagus; skin such as the scalp, face, and extremities; and the umbilicus and anogenital areas.

MANAGEMENT STRATEGY

Mucous membrane pemphigoid may be localized or extensive. Localized forms include:

- gingival pemphigoid, the pemphigoid type of desquamative gingivitis;
- oral pemphigoid;
- ocular pemphigoid.

Localized disease is more amenable to therapeutic control. Some patients with localized disease may develop more extensive disease while others can be treated into remission.

Extensive disease involves several sites including oral, ocular, and other mucosal surfaces; scalp, face, and extremities; and the umbilical and anogenital surfaces. Extensive disease is more difficult to control, particularly if the disease process is rapidly progressive.

Systemic corticosteroids are considered to be the first line of therapy for mucous membrane pemphigoid, particularly the extensive type. *Immunosuppressive agents* such as *azathioprine* and *cyclophosphamide* have been used as adjunctive corticosteroid-sparing therapy with benefit. *Dapsone* and the related *sulfapyridine* (*sulphapyridine*) have been used for pemphigoid with excellent efficacy.

Systemic corticosteroids are administered in doses of 1–2 mg/kg body weight and continued in the larger doses until the disease process is quiescent. At the outset of therapy, an anti-inflammatory immunosuppressive agent such as azathioprine or cyclophosphamide is started in doses of 1.5–2.5 mg/kg body weight. This dose is continued

as the systemic corticosteroids are tapered in anticipation of monotherapy in 6–12 months. Azathioprine is less toxic than cyclophosphamide and is the first choice for disease that is progressing slowly. A blood level of the enzyme thiopurine methyl transferase (TPMT), which allows the clinician to assess the risk of neutropenia, should be obtained before using azathioprine. *Mycophenolate mofetil* may prove to have similar efficacy, but is expensive. Cyclophosphamide is indicated when the disease process is progressing rapidly.

Dapsone and sulfapyridine are useful in the treatment of pemphigoid diseases. Dapsone is indicated for localized disease or slowly progressing extensive disease. A red blood cell level of the enzyme, glucose-6-phosphate dehydrogenase (G6PD), should be obtained before using dapsone. Dapsone causes a hemolytic anemia, and so dosing is begun at 25 mg daily for 3 days, increasing by 25 mg daily every third day to 100 mg daily for 7 days to allow the bone marrow to adapt to the hemolytic insult. The dose of dapsone may be increased to 125 mg daily in a single daily dose and maintained at 125–150 mg daily for 12 weeks. Most patients with localized or slowly progressive extensive mucous membrane pemphigoid will respond in 12 weeks. If disease control is inadequate at 12 weeks, systemic corticosteroids plus immunosuppressive drug therapy should be commenced.

Dapsone can be effective in maintenance therapy when the systemic corticosteroids have been tapered and discontinued and the anti-inflammatory immunosuppressive agents are providing control of the disease. Dapsone therapy can be instituted as azathioprine or cyclophosphamide is tapered and discontinued.

Some patients with localized mucous membrane pemphigoid can be tapered off all medications eventually, though most patients with extensive mucous membrane pemphigoid will require long-term therapy.

Other anti-inflammatory agents such as *tetracycline* and *niacinamide* have minimal significant side effects, but are not always helpful except in patients with minimal or localized disease. Topical therapy with *high-potency corticosteroids* and/or *tacrolimus* may be adequate in patients with disease localized to the gingivae.

For those patients with rapidly progressive, extensive or treatment-resistant mucous membrane pemphigoid, *intravenous immunoglobulin (IVIG)* therapy may be necessary. *Subconjunctival mitomycin C* has been evaluated for recalcitrant eye disease.

SPECIFIC INVESTIGATIONS

- Blood G6PD enzyme level
- Blood TPMT enzyme level
- Direct immunofluorescence testing of mucosal biopsy specimens
- Serum for indirect immunofluorescence to determine antibody titer, and for use on salt-split skin to determine antibody location
- Baseline and follow-up laboratory testing

Bullous and cicatricial pemphigoid: clinical, histopathologic and immunopathologic correlations. Person JR, Rogers RS III. Mayo Clin Proc 1977;52:54–66.

Most patients with mucous membrane pemphigoid have linear deposition of immunoglobulins and/or complement at the basement membrane zone in mucosal and cutaneous biopsy specimens. Few patients have circulating anti-basement membrane zone antibodies. A positive test is necessary to classify a subepithelial vesiculobullous disease as pemphigoid.

The sensitivity and specificity of direct immunofluorescence testing in disorders of mucous membranes. Helander SD, Rogers RS III. J Am Acad Dermatol 1994;30: 65–75.

The diagnosis of mucous membrane pemphigoid is established by direct immunofluorescence study of mucous membrane biopsy specimens.

A pharmacogenetic basis for safe and effective use of azathioprine and other thiopurine drugs in dermatologic patients. Snow JL, Gibson LE. J Am Acad Dermatol 1995;32: 114–6.

Discussion of genetic variation in TPMT activity and the efficacy of azathioprine as well as side effect profile of azathioprine therapy.

Sulfones and sulfonamides in dermatology today. Lang PJ Jr. J Am Acad Dermatol 1979;1:479–94.

An excellent review of the use of dapsone and sulfonamides in dermatology.

Dapsone therapy of cicatricial pemphigoid. Rogers RS III, Mehregan DA. Semin Dermatol 1988;7:201–5.

Detailed review of use of dapsone in the treatment of mucous membrane (cicatricial) pemphigoid including dosing regimens and monitoring for toxicity.

FIRST LINE THERAPIES

■ Systemic corticosteroids	B
■ Immunosuppressive agents: azathioprine and cyclophosphamide	B
■ Dapsone and sulfapyridine	B
■ Intralesional corticosteroids for recalcitrant lesions	D

Cicatricial pemphigoid. Fleming TE, Korman NJ. J Am Acad Dermatol 2000;43:571–91.

An excellent review on the clinical spectrum, pathology and treatment of cicatricial pemphigoid.

Cicatricial pemphigoid. Ahmed AR, Rogers RS III. J Am Acad Dermatol 1991;24:987–1001.

Extensive discussion of pharmacological approaches to the treatment of mucous membrane pemphigoid including topical and systemic therapy.

Management of the immunobullous disorders. I. Pemphigoid. Huilgol SC, Black MM. Clin Exp Dermatol 1995;20: 189–201.

Discussion of therapeutic options including immunosuppressive agents.

Cicatricial pemphigoid: diagnosis and treatment. Nyuyen QD, Foster CS. Int Ophthalmol Clin 1996;36:41–60.

Overview of ocular mucous membrane pemphigoid including differential diagnosis, laboratory evaluation, and medical and surgical management.

Dapsone therapy of cicatricial pemphigoid. Rogers RS III, Mehregan DA. Semin Dermatol 1988;7:201–5.

Discussion of use of dapsone and/or sulfapyridine in the management of mucous membrane pemphigoid. Discussion of long-term outcome.

Mucous membrane pemphigoid. Rogers RS III. In: Dyall-Smith D, Marks R, eds. Dermatology at the Millennium. London: Parthenon Publishing; 1997:654–8.

An extension of the previous study by Rogers and Mehregan 1988 with more patients and longer follow-up.

The first international consensus on mucous membrane pemphigoid: definition, diagnostic criteria, pathogenic factors, medical treatment, and prognostic indicators. Chan LS, Ahmed AR, Anhalt GJ, et al. Arch Dermatol 2002;138:370–9.

A panel of 26 experts review mucous membrane pemphigoid in detail including consensus recommendations on treatment.

SECOND LINE THERAPIES

■ Other immunomodulatory agents	D
■ Mycophenolate mofetil	E
■ IVIG therapy	B

Desquamative gingivitis: preliminary observations with tetracycline treatment. Roubeck BA, Lind PO, Thrane PS. Oral Surg Oral Med Oral Pathol 1990;69:694–7.

Tetracycline therapy had a beneficial effect in localized disease.

Treatment of cicatricial pemphigoid with tetracycline and niacinamide. Poskitt L, Wojnarowska F. Br J Dermatol 1995;132:784–9.

Tetracycline and nicotinamide (niacinamide) had a beneficial effect in some patients.

Treatment of cicatricial pemphigoid with mycophenolate mofetil as a steroid-sparing agent. Megahed M, Schiedeberg S, Becker J, et al. J Am Acad Dermatol 2001;45:256–9.

Three patients treated with mycophenolate mofetil and prednisolone responded well to therapy. None of them showed relapse of the disease for a follow-up period of 6–14 months after complete cessation of mycophenolate mofetil and prednisolone.

Consensus statement on the use of intravenous immunoglobulin therapy in the treatment of autoimmune mucocutaneous blistering diseases. Ahmed AR, Dahl MV. Arch Dermatol 2003;139:1051–9.

Detailed guidelines on the use of IVIG for immunobullous disease.

Intravenous immunoglobulin therapy for ocular cicatricial pemphigoid. Foster CS, Ahmed AR. Ophthalmology 1999; 106:2136–43.

Experience with ten patients with ocular cicatricial pemphigoid resistant to standard therapy. Clinical deterioration was arrested in all ten patients.

Evidence levels   **A** Double-blind study   **B** Clinical trial ≥ 20 subjects   **C** Clinical trial < 20 subjects   **D** Series ≥ 5 subjects   **E** Anecdotal case reports

THIRD LINE THERAPIES

■ Plasmapheresis	E
■ Anti-tumor necrosis factor-α (etanercept)	E
■ Thalidomide	E
■ Topical tacrolimus	E
■ Subconjunctival mitomycin C injections (for ophthalmologist use)	C

Plasmapheresis therapy for bullous pemphigoid. Goldberg NS, Robinson JK, Roenigk Jr HH, et al. Arch Dermatol 1985;121:1484–5.

A case of antiepiligrin cicatricial pemphigoid successfully treated by plasmapheresis. Hashimoto Y, Suga Y, Yoshiike T, et al. Dermatology 2000;201:58–60.

A single report of the ocular lesions of cicatricial pemphigoid being arrested by combining corticosteroids and immunosuppressives with double filtration plasmapheresis.

Treatment of recalcitrant cicatricial pemphigoid with the tumor necrosis factor alpha antagonist etanercept. Sacher C, Rubbert A, Konig C, et al. J Am Acad Dermatol 2002;46:113–5.

A single patient with longstanding cicatricial pemphigoid responds to etanercept.

Thalidomide therapy for cicatricial pemphigoid. Duong DJ, Moxley RT 3rd, Kellman RM, et al. J Am Acad Dermatol 2002;47(suppl 2):S193–5.

A single patient responded to thalidomide monotherapy.

Topical tacrolimus treatment for cicatricial pemphigoid. Günther C, Wozel G, Meurer M, et al. J Am Acad Dermatol 2004;50:325–6.

Daily application of tacrolimus 0.1% to genital lesions allowed gradual tapering of systemic prednisone in a patient intolerant of other systemic immunosuppressives.

Subconjunctival mitomycin C for the treatment of ocular cicatricial pemphigoid. Donnenfeld ED, Perry HD, Wallerstein A, et al. Ophthalmology 1999;106:72–8.

A prospective evaluation of the efficacy of treating ocular cicatricial pemphigoid with subconjunctival mitomycin C (0.25 mL of 0.2 mg/mL mitomycin C) to the superior and inferior bulbar conjunctivae in nine patients. Each patient's least affected eye was used as a control. Eight of nine patients showed quiescence of their ocular cicatricial pemphigoid in the treated eye based on serial evaluation of conjunctival cicatrization and grading of conjunctival erythema. Five of the nine untreated eyes showed progression of the conjunctival disease.

Mycetoma: eumycetoma and actinomycetoma

Wanda Sonia Robles

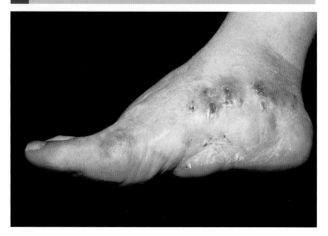

Mycetomas (Madura foot) are defined as chronic subcutaneous infections caused by fungi or actinomycetes that have the ability to form granules or grains. The infections are known as eumycetomas when produced by fungi, and actinomycetomas when produced by actinomycetes. The organisms gain entry into the dermis or subcutaneous tissue through traumatic implantation from the natural environment, as they occur as saprophytes in soil or on plants. The infections are characterized by the formation of large aggregates of fungal or actinomycete filaments in the form of grains within abscesses in subcutaneous tissue. The abscesses usually discharge onto the skin surface through sinuses but may also involve contiguous structures, especially the bone, where they can cause chronic osteomyelitis. The disease is more common in tropical and subtropical countries and affects mainly agricultural workers. Actinomycetoma infections with *Nocardia* species are more common in Central America and Mexico. Eumycetomas due to *Madurella mycetomatis* as well as actinomycetomas due to *Streptomyces somaliensis* are more common in Sudan and the Middle East.

MANAGEMENT STRATEGY

Treatment of mycetomas is difficult, and management varies from a very conservative approach to chemotherapy and surgery. Effective treatment for actinomycetoma is available; however, treatment of eumycetoma is often very difficult. As eumycetoma infection is quite indolent and seldom life threatening, conservative management is often appropriate. Treatment is then symptomatic, with *relief of pain* and *applications of dressings* to affected areas, particularly the sinuses. If chemotherapy is considered, many different antifungal drugs have been used with varying degrees of success. Actinomycetoma responds quite well to treatment with *trimethoprim–sulfamethoxazole* or *diamino-diphenyl-sulfone*, alone or in combination. If the condition is particularly severe or unresponsive to these treatments, *amikacin* should be a consideration, especially if there is a risk of spread to adjacent organs. Surgical procedures are seldom used for treatment of actinomycetoma. Eumycetoma, however, offers quite a treatment challenge. A combination of chemotherapy and surgical excision is usually advisable. For a small lesion, surgical procedures alone may be all that is required. A range of antifungal drugs have been used for eumycetoma. *Ketoconazole* at the dose of 100–400 mg daily has been effective, and in other cases, responses have been seen with *amphotericin B*, either in conventional formulation or in lipid systems. Chemotherapy should be continued for at least 3–4 months and, in some cases, long-term treatment for over a year may be necessary. *Itraconazole* has also been reported as useful in treatment of eumycetoma, with considerable clinical improvement after 6 months of treatment. *Surgery* is the ultimate method of eradicating eumycetoma but this may require amputation or other mutilating excision.

SPECIFIC INVESTIGATIONS

- Direct microscopy
- Culture
- Histopathology

The diagnosis of mycetoma is confirmed by the demonstration and identification of grains in lesions. It is important to differentiate eumycetoma, which responds poorly to chemotherapy, from actinomycetoma, which responds well; the identification of the organism therefore has prognostic and treatment implications. Within the range of organisms causing eumycetoma there are also differences in response. Infections caused by *M. mycetomatis* are reported to respond to ketoconazole in about 50–60% of cases. In order to get a good specimen, an intact pustule should be identified. This is gently pierced with a sterile needle. Most of the content is extruded and spread onto a glass slide. The granules are visualized by direct microscopy in 5–10% potassium hydroxide. Culture is best carried out using conventional media such as Sabouraud's agar for primary isolation. Deep surgical biopsy is advisable for histopathology. A superficial biopsy is often inadequate, mainly because the amount of material is usually insufficient to identify grains. However, histology can also be performed on grains extracted from the lesions and fixed immediately.

FIRST LINE THERAPIES

■ Trimethoprim–sulfamethoxazole	C
■ Ketoconazole	C

Treatment of eumycetoma and actinomycetoma. Welsh O, Salinas MC, Rodriquez MA. Curr Top Med Mycol 1995;6: 47–71.

A good review article. Trimethoprim–sulfamethoxazole, alone or in combination with dapsone, is considered the treatment of choice for actinomycetoma. Surgery is unnecessary. Combination treatment with chemotherapy and surgery is advised for eumycetoma, the drug of choice being ketoconazole at the dose of 400 mg daily. This is especially recommended for eumycetoma caused by *M. mycetomatis*. Response to itraconazole is variable, and fluconazole has been mostly unsuccessful.

Management of mycetoma in West Africa. Develoux M, Dieng MT, Kane A, Ndiaye B. Bull Soc Pathol Exot 2003; 96:376–82.

A good review paper that highlights the need for good assessment of the extent of the lesion, assessment of bone involvement, and identification of etiologic agents. For eumycetoma patients, treatment with ketoconazole or itraconazole in combination with surgery is recommended. For actinomycetoma, antibiotic therapy according to the etiologic agent is the management of choice.

Mycetoma: a thorn in the flesh. Fahal AH. Trans R Soc Trop Med Hyg 2004;98:3–11.

Also a review of the condition in an area of prevalence. These patients highlight the clinical similarities between eumycetoma and actinomycetoma infections, although actinomycetoma has a more rapid course. Therapeutic advice is combined antibiotic treatment for actinomycetoma and aggressive surgical treatment in combination with antifungal agents for eumycetoma.

Treatment of eumycetoma with ketoconazole. Venugopal PV, Venugopal TV. Australas J Dermatol 1993;34:27–9.

The authors report 10 patients treated with oral ketoconazole 400 mg daily for 8–24 months. In eight of these patients, the foot was affected, and *M. mycetomatis* was responsible for four of the infections. The drug was reported to have been tolerated well, with no adverse reactions. Six patients had a complete cure, and there was no evidence of recurrence during follow-up, which ranged from 3 months to 2 years.

Mycetoma caused by *Madurella mycetomatis*: a neglected infectious burden. Ahmed AO, van Leeuwen W, Fahal A, et al. Lancet Infect Dis 2004;4:566–74.

A good review article on developments in the clinical, epidemiologic, and diagnostic management of Madurella mycetomatic eumycetoma.

Mycetoma: 130 cases. Dieng MT, Sy MH, Diop BM, et al. Ann Dermatol Venereol 2003;130:16–9.

This is a report of 130 cases of mycetoma in Senegal from 1983 to 2000. The treatment approach was medical intervention for patients with actinomycetoma and surgical treatment for patients with eumycetoma. This paper also highlights the remarkable long duration of the disease before presentation.

Mycetoma. Hay RJ, Mahgoub ES, Leon G, et al. J Med Vet Mycol 1992;30(suppl 1):41–9.

A good review article. The correct approach for treatment of patients with mycetoma is a combination of surgery and chemotherapy.

Ketoconazole in the treatment of eumycetoma due to *Madurella mycetomii*. Mahgoub ES, Gumaa SA. Trans R Soc Trop Med Hyg 1984;78:376–9.

A clinical trial with ketoconazole in which 13 patients were treated. Five of them were reported as completely cured and four showed improvement. The daily dose was 400 or 300 mg for those who were cured. The patients who showed only improvement were treated with 200 mg daily.

Nocardia, nocardiosis and mycetoma. Boiron P, Locci R, Goodfellow M, et al. Med Mycol 1998;36(suppl 1):26–37.

A review article. Sulfonamide-based treatment is considered effective. Optimal treatment, however, may be guided by the use of susceptibility tests of clinical isolates.

Case report: *Nocardia asteroides* mycetoma. Lum CA, Vadmal MS. Ann Clin Lab Sci 2003;33:329–33.

Case report of a primary cutaneous *N. asteroides* infection in an immunocompetent individual. This was successfully treated with trimethoprim–sulfamethoxazole.

Madura foot: atypical finding and case presentation. Foltz KD, Fallat LM. J Foot Ankle Surg 2004;43:327–31.

A case report of actinomycetoma successfully treated with surgical resection and long-term antibiotic treatment. This report is interesting in that it shows that surgical intervention may be necessary in some cases of actinomycosis infection, not just in eumycetomas.

SECOND LINE THERAPIES

■ Itraconazole	E
■ Itraconazole and flucytosine	E
■ Amphotericin B	E

Mycetoma. Fahal AH, Hassam MA. Br J Surg 1992;79: 1138–41.

A review article. Extensive surgical excision of the affected area and sometimes limb amputation is considered as first line treatment for mycetoma. Medical treatment alone and in combination with surgery is discussed.

With present availability of newer antifungal drugs, surgical procedures should be considered as second line therapies.

Eumycetoma due to *Madurella mycetomatis* acquired in Jamaica. Fletcher CL, Moore MK, Hay RJ. Br J Dermatol 2001;145:1018–21.

Case report of a female patient who spent her childhood in Jamaica and had been resident in the UK for 20 years before presentation. This patient was successfully treated with itraconazole.

[Black-grain eumycetoma due to *Madurella grisea*. A report of 2 cases]. Machado LA, Rivitti MC, Cuce LC, et al. Rev Inst Med Trop Sao Paulo 1992;34:569–80. In Portuguese.

Report of two cases of black-grain eumycetoma caused by *M. grisea*. Treatment with itraconazole for a period of 3 months was unsuccessful in both cases.

This further supports the observation that not all eumycetomas respond well to treatment with itraconazole. It may also imply that a longer period of treatment is necessary to obtain a good response.

***Scedosporium* infection in immunocompromised patients: successful use of liposomal amphotericin B and itraconazole.** Barbaric D, Shaw PJ. Med Pediatr Oncol 2001;37:122–5.

A report of five cases of *Scedosporium* infection in immunosuppressed patients. Three of these patients died despite treatment with various combinations of amphotericin B and itraconazole. Two patients were successfully treated with liposomal amphotericin B and itraconazole.

Cutaneous infection due to *Scedosporium apiospermum* in an immunosuppressed patient. Chaveiro MA, Vieira R, Cardoso J, Afonso A. J Eur Acad Dermatol Venereol 2003;17:47–9.

A case report of cutaneous infection by *S. apiospermum* in a patient with rheumatoid arthritis and diabetes mellitus treated with cyclosporine and corticosteroids. Successful treatment was achieved with itraconazole 400 mg daily for 3 months.

Improvement of eumycetoma with itraconazole. Resnik BI, Burdick AE. J Am Acad Dermatol 1995;33:917–9.

A case report of treatment of a eumycetoma in an 18-year-old patient. This improved significantly after 6 months of treatment with itraconazole, initially at a dose of 100 mg daily, increased to 200 mg daily after 2 months.

Atypical eumycetoma caused by *Phialophora parasitica* successfully treated with itraconazole and flucytosine. Hood SV, Moore CB, Cheesbrough JS, et al. Br J Dermatol 1997;136:953–6.

A case of eumycetoma caused by *P. parasitica* in a healthy British female resident. Surgical excision in combination with itraconazole 400 mg daily failed to give her improvement, but she responded to treatment with itraconazole 400 mg in combination with flucytosine at the dose of 1 g three times daily for 12 months.

First report of mycetoma caused by *Arthrographis kalrae*: successful treatment with itraconazole. Degavre B, Joujoux JM, Dandurand M, Guillot B. J Am Acad Dermatol 1997;37:318–20.

Report of a case of a mycetoma affecting the hand that was successfully treated with itraconazole 400 mg daily for 4 months.

Madura foot in the UK: fungal osteomyelitis after renal transplantation. O'Riordan E, Dento J, Taylor PM, et al. Transplantation 2002;73:151–3.

Case report of an immunosuppressed Asian patient who developed pain in the right great toe and was diagnosed with gout. Two weeks later, he developed a discharging sinus on his toe and the diagnosis of eumycetoma by *M. grisea* was made. It failed to respond to treatment with both itraconazole and amphotericin B, for which amputation of the toe was required.

THIRD LINE THERAPIES

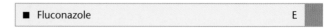

■ Fluconazole	E

Fluconazole in the therapy of tropical deep mycoses. Gugnani HC, Ezeanolue BC, Khalil M, et al. Mycoses 1995; 38:485–8.

Two patients with eumycetoma were successfully treated with fluconazole.

Evidence levels **A** Double-blind study **B** Clinical trial ≥ 20 subjects **C** Clinical trial < 20 subjects **D** Series ≥ 5 subjects **E** Anecdotal case reports

Mycobacterial (atypical) skin infections

Sanjay Agarwal, John Berth-Jones

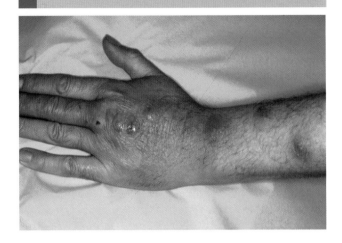

Swimming pool (fish tank) granuloma

Fish tank granuloma is an infection of the skin caused by *Mycobacterium marinum*. It is characterized by asymptomatic nodules, commonly on hands and elbows, which may spread in a sporotrichoid fashion. It occurs after minor trauma in people who come in contact with the organism. The most common sources of infection are tropical fish aquariums and swimming pools.

MANAGEMENT STRATEGY

No controlled trials have been conducted, probably due to the paucity of cases. A literature review revealed that 66 of 92 reported cases had been successfully treated with various *antimicrobials*. Antibiotic therapies fall into three main classes: *rifampin (rifampicin) plus ethambutol or isoniazid; tetracyclines like minocycline;* and *co-trimoxazole*. The mean duration of treatment in various reports ranges between 6 weeks and 5 months. No statistical difference in efficacy between these treatments has been demonstrated. Lesions can often be effectively treated by *simple excision,* but occasionally this seems to result in a prolonged period of infection. *Heat treatment* of the infected area may have an adjunctive role according to some authors.

In addition, the self-limiting nature of the disease makes the evaluation of the therapeutic regimens difficult.

The second line treatments described below have been so designated because there is relatively little published information about them. The third line treatments are probably best regarded as 'adjunctive' to the others.

SPECIFIC INVESTIGATIONS

- Histology
- Culture
- Polymerase chain reaction (PCR) to detect mycobacterial DNA

Histology shows noncaseating granulomas. Culture of the biopsy specimen yields pigmented colonies of *M. marinum*. In culture-negative cases, PCR systems can provide rapid and sensitive detection of mycobacterial DNA in formalin-fixed, paraffin-embedded specimens. In-vitro sensitivity studies have not been uniformly predictive of clinical response to the antibiotics. Although they do not have a routine role in directing initial treatment, they may be useful in resistant cases.

Polymerase chain reaction based detection of *Mycobacterium tuberculosis* in tissues showing granulomatous inflammation without demonstrable acid-fast bacilli. Hsiao PF, Tzen CY, Hsiu-Chin Chen HC, Su HY. Int J Dermatol 2003;42:281–6.

A total of 38 specimens were analyzed with two different primers targeting the gene encoding for 16S ribosomal RNA and IS6110; 18 of these were diagnosed as *M. tuberculosis* and four as atypical mycobacteria.

FIRST LINE THERAPIES

Minocycline 100–200 mg once daily for 6–12 weeks	D
Rifampin 600 mg and ethambutol 1.2 g daily for 3–6 months	D
Co-trimoxazole two to three tablets twice daily for 6 weeks	D

Mycobacteria marinum infection of the skin in Japan. Hiroko A, Hiroshi N, Ryukichi N. J Dermatol 1984;11:37–42.

Seventy five cases of *M. marinum* infection were reviewed. Chemotherapy, thermotherapy, and surgery have been used as treatment in Japan. Rifampin was the most frequently used drug and was effective alone within an average of 14 weeks. Minocycline alone was effective in 6 weeks. In-vitro sensitivity testing suggested that minocycline was more effective than antituberculosis drugs. Minocycline was recommended as the drug of choice.

Review article based on several reports in Japanese dermatological journals.

Fish tank granuloma in a 14 month old girl. Speight EL, Williams HC. Pediatr Dermatol 1997;14:209–12.

Case report of a child who responded well to a 6-month course of rifampin 100 mg daily despite in-vitro sensitivity tests reporting resistance to rifampin.

Therapy of *Mycobacterium marinum* infections. Use of tetracyclines vs rifampin. Donta ST, Smith PW, Levitz RE, Quintiliani R. Arch Intern Med 1986;146:902–4.

A description of a series of four cases that did not respond to tetracyclines. A prompt response to combination therapy with rifampin 300 mg twice daily and ethambutol 800–1200 mg daily was noted.

The authors recommended antibiotic sensitivity testing as helpful in guiding therapy.

Aquarium-borne *M. marinum* skin infection. Huminer D. Arch Dermatol 1986;122:698–703.

This is a case report and review of the English language literature of 44 cases. The authors concluded that co-trimoxazole two tablets twice daily for 6 weeks or rifampin 600 mg daily and ethambutol 800 mg daily for 16 weeks were the drugs of choice.

The successful treatment of tropical fish tank granuloma (*Mycobacterium marinum*) with co-trimoxazole. Black MM, Eykyn SJ. Br J Dermatol 1977;97:689–92.

A description of a series of three cases that responded to co-trimoxazole two tablets twice daily. The duration of treatment varied from 6 weeks to 3 months.

SECOND LINE THERAPIES

■ Ciprofloxacin 500 mg with clarithromycin 250 mg twice daily for 4 months	E
■ Rifabutin 600 mg with clarithromycin 500 mg twice daily and ciprofloxacin 500 mg twice daily	E

Antibiotic treatment of fish tank granuloma. Laing RB. J Hand Surg [Br] 1997;22:135–7.

A series of three cases is described. The authors concluded that, in the light of the low toxicity profile, the combination of ciprofloxacin 500–1000 mg daily and clarithromycin 250–500 mg twice daily offers a useful alternative to existing treatments, particularly in patients who require protracted therapy. The duration of treatment varied from 8 weeks to 12 weeks, depending on the clinical response. The authors suggest that rifabutin 600 mg may also prove valuable in cases that fail to respond to conventional antibiotic treatment.

THIRD LINE THERAPIES

■ Simple excision	E
■ Curettage and electrodesiccation	E
■ Incision and drainage	E
■ Heat therapy by gloves, hot water, or heated armlet	E

Tropical fish tank granuloma. Keckzes K. Br J Dermatol 1974;91:709.

A case report describing *M. marinum* infection of the upper limb that was successfully treated with co-trimoxazole two tablets twice daily and thermotherapy for 6 months. Heat therapy involved a polythene-covered, insulated, electrically heated armlet, which was worn for 12–16 hours each day (temperature not specified).

Infections with *Mycobacterium marinum*. Jolly WH Jr, Seabury JH. Arch Dermatol 1972;106:32–6.

Thirty one cases of culture-proven infections with *M. marinum* in the New Orleans area were studied. Various modes of therapy including chemotherapy and surgery were employed. Excision or curettage and electrodesiccation or both resulted in cure in 13 patients.

The authors recommended surgery as the treatment of choice for cutaneous infection with M. marinum.

Mycobacterium kansasii

Mycobacterium kansasii most commonly causes pulmonary disease; skin lesions are rare. The route of entry is usually through a minor injury. Most reported cases have occurred in people who are immunocompromised. The gross morphology of such lesions varies greatly and can be verrucous, nodular, or sporotrichoid. In the USA, the organism is endemic in Texas, Louisiana, the Chicago area, and California.

MANAGEMENT STRATEGY

As cutaneous infection with *M. kansasii* is rare no firm treatment guidelines have been recommended. Although conventional combination chemotherapy with *antituberculous drugs* is effective, the choice of treatment should be determined by in-vitro sensitivity.

SPECIFIC INVESTIGATIONS

■ Culture of tissue for mycobacteria

FIRST LINE THERAPIES

■ Antituberculous drugs with kanamycin 500 mg intramuscularly three times a week	E
■ Minocycline 100–200 mg daily for 16 weeks	E

Cutaneous *Mycobacterium kansasii* infection presenting as cellulitis. Rosen T. Cutis 1983;31:87–9.

The report describes a renal transplant patient who developed a cellulitis-like lesion on the leg and periarticular soft tissue swelling due to *M. kansasii*. Rifampin 600 mg daily and isoniazid 300 mg daily were initiated. Due to liver function abnormalities, isoniazid was substituted with ethambutol 400 mg twice a day. Subsequently kanamycin 500 mg intramuscularly three times a week was added. Three months of therapy with rifampin, ethambutol, and kanamycin resulted in clearing of the skin and periarticular lesions.

A sporotrichoid-like *Mycobacterium kansasii* infection of the skin treated with minocycline hydrochloride. Dore N, Collins JP, Mankiewicz E. Br J Dermatol 1979;101: 75–9.

A sporotrichoid-like *M. kansasii* infection of the skin responded to minocycline hydrochloride therapy. The patient received minocycline 50 mg four times daily for 6 weeks. Subsequently the dose was reduced to 100 mg daily for a further ten weeks and resulted in complete resolution of the cutaneous lesions.

Cutaneous *Mycobacterium kansasii* infection associated with a papulonecrotic tuberculid reaction. Callahan EF,

Licata AL, Madison JF. J Am Acad Dermatol 1997;36: 497–8.

Treatment with isoniazid 300 mg daily, rifampin 600 mg daily, and ethambutol 1200 mg daily for 9 months resulted in complete clearing of all cutaneous lesions.

Mycobacterium fortuitum complex (injection abscess)

Mycobacterium fortuitum, *Mycobacterium chelonei*, and *Mycobacterium abscessus* are generally grouped together to form the *Mycobacterium fortuitum* complex. Cutaneous lesions due to *M. fortuitum* complex usually occur after surgery, percutaneous catheter insertion, or accidental inoculation. Dark red nodules develop with abscess formation and clear fluid drainage. Disseminated disease occurs most commonly in immunosuppressed hosts.

MANAGEMENT STRATEGY

Organisms of the *M. fortuitum* complex should be individually identified and in-vitro sensitivity tests should be performed prior to the initiation of chemotherapy. Susceptibility testing is recommended because of subspecies variability and even variability within subgroups. Both *M. fortuitum* and *M. chelonei* are resistant to most antituberculous drugs except *kanamycin* and *amikacin*; *M. fortuitum* is more susceptible to *amikacin*, *cefoxitin*, *ciprofloxacin*, and *imipenem*; *M. abscessus* is usually sensitive to *amikacin*, *cefoxitin*, and *clarithromycin*; *tobramycin* and *clarithromycin* are more effective than amikacin in the treatment of *M. chelonei*. The wide variability in antibiotic sensitivity means that each case must be considered individually. For persistent nonhealing cutaneous lesions, *wide excisional surgery* with delayed closure or skin grafting can be undertaken. The duration of therapy can vary from 6 weeks to 7 months and is dictated by clinical and microbiological response.

SPECIFIC INVESTIGATIONS

- Histology
- Culture of infected tissue
- PCR for species identification

Histology reveals polymorphonuclear microabscess and granuloma formation with foreign body-type giant cells. Acid-fast bacilli may be demonstrated in the microabscesses. Diagnosis is usually confirmed by culture. PCR systems can also be used for diagnosis and species identification in selected cases.

Atypical cutaneous mycobacteriosis diagnosed by polymerase chain reaction. Collina G, Morandi L, Lanzoni A, Reggiani M. Br J Dermatol 2002;147:781–4.

This articles reports two cases where *M. chelonae* and *M. fortuitum* were identified by PCR from tissue samples.

FIRST LINE THERAPIES

■ Amikacin 300–400 mg intravenously twice daily plus doxycycline 100 mg three times daily	D
■ Sulfamethoxazole 50 mg/kg daily for 3–6 months	D
■ Clarithromycin 500 mg twice daily	D
■ Minocycline 100–200 mg daily	E

Clinical usefulness of amikacin and doxycycline in the treatment of infection due to *M. fortuitum* and *M. chelonae*. Dalovisio JR, Pankey GA, Wallace RJ, Jones DB. Rev Infect Dis 1981;3:1068–74.

A series of ten cases. The authors suggest that amikacin 300–400 mg twice daily and doxycycline 100 mg three times daily are the drugs of choice in this condition. Conventional antituberculous drugs have no place in the treatment of these infections. The authors further recommended that antimicrobial therapy should be prolonged (up to 7 months) and combined with surgical debridement.

The clinical presentation, diagnosis, and therapy of cutaneous and pulmonary infection due to the rapidly growing mycobacteria, *M. fortuitum* and *M. chelonae*. Wallace RJ. Clin Chest Med 1989;10:419–29.

An excellent review article.

Sulfonamide activity against *Mycobacterium fortuitum* and *Mycobacterium chelonei*. Wallace RJ, Jones DB, Wiss K. Rev Infect Dis 1981;3:898–904.

Forty eight clinical strains of *M. fortuitum* and 15 clinical strains of *M. chelonei* were evaluated for susceptibility to sulfonamides, including trimethoprim–sulfamethoxazole (TMP–SMZ). Six patients with disease due to rapidly growing mycobacteria were treated with sulfonamides, and all showed a good response to therapy. Sulfonamides may be the treatment of choice for infections due to *M. fortuitum* and offer potential for the therapy of disease due to *M. chelonei*.

Resistant cutaneous infection caused by *Mycobacterium chelonei*. Fenske NA, Millns JL. Arch Dermatol 1981;117: 151–3.

A case report and review of the literature. The authors describe a case of *M. chelonei* that was resistant to most antituberculous drugs. Minocycline 100 mg twice a day resulted in healing of ulcerations in 8 weeks. Discontinuation of therapy 6 months later was followed by marked recrudescence with ulceration in 1 week. Reinstitution of minocycline resulted in substantial remission, but not eradication of the infection.

Development of resistance to clarithromycin after treatment of cutaneous *Mycobacterium chelonae* infection. Driscoll MS, Tyring SK. J Am Acad Dermatol 1997;36:495–6.

A case report and review of the literature. Initially the patient was prescribed minocycline 100 mg twice daily and advised to apply heat to the affected leg. There was no response and the treatment was changed to clarithromycin 500 mg twice daily. After 7 weeks the lesions had regressed and the treatment was discontinued. Two months later the nodules had recurred and erythromycin 400 mg three times daily was commenced. There was no response after 3 months. Subsequently, ciprofloxacin and azithromycin were tried without any response. The authors recommended that treatment should be combined with clarithromycin and a second agent chosen on the basis of antibiotic testing.

Clinical trial of clarithromycin for cutaneous (disseminated) infection due to *Mycobacterium chelonae*. Wallace RJ, Tanner D, Brennan PJ. Ann Intern Med 1993;119:482–6.

Fourteen patients (ten with disseminated disease) were treated with at least 3 months of therapy with clarithromycin 500 mg twice daily. All patients had excellent response to therapy. The mean duration of therapy was 6.8 months (range 4.5–9 months).

Evidence levels **A** Double-blind study **B** Clinical trial ≥ 20 subjects **C** Clinical trial < 20 subjects **D** Series ≥ 5 subjects **E** Anecdotal case reports

Mycosis fungoides

Jeremy R Marsden, Sajjad F Rajpar

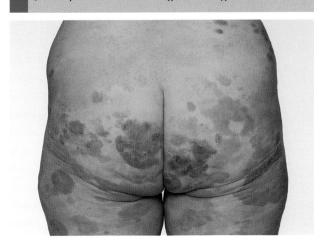

Cutaneous T cell lymphomas (CTCL) are a group of disorders characterized by malignant clonal proliferation of T lymphocytes. The most frequent CTCL is mycosis fungoides (MF), which has an estimated annual incidence of 0.5 per 100 000 population. The prevalence is much higher due to the relatively good prognosis. MF most commonly presents in the sixth decade and is slightly more common in males and blacks. Poikiloderma atrophicans vasculare and parapsoriasis en plaque are generally considered to be early MF and so are grouped with this disorder for the purposes of management. Prognosis, mortality, and choice of treatment are related to disease stage, which can be classified as follows:

- Stage 1. Patches and plaques involving less (1A) or more (1B) than 10% of the skin.
- Stage 2. As stage 1, with nonmalignant lymphadenopathy (2A) or cutaneous tumors (2B).
- Stage 3. Erythroderma.
- Stage 4. Malignant infiltration of lymph nodes (4A) or viscera (4B).

MANAGEMENT STRATEGY

Management starts with accurate diagnosis. Confirmation by skin biopsies is essential; frequently these need to be multiple to avoid sampling error, and may need to be repeated if equivocal in the face of continuing clinical suspicion. The key finding is epidermal invasion by abnormal lymphoid cells with a convoluted 'cerebriform' nucleus.

With the possible exception of very early disease, there is no evidence that MF is curable. Progression is often very slow or even absent; consequently, the aim of treatment is safe, effective control of symptoms. Patients with skin lymphoma should ideally be managed by a team including a dermatologist, a histopathologist familiar with skin lymphoma, and a radiation oncologist. This approach minimizes the risk of management error.

Studies claiming to cure patients with very early MF are flawed by having inadequate controls and diagnostic criteria that would not be considered adequate today. While the possibility of cure in very early stage 1A MF cannot be excluded, this has not been proved. Nonetheless, it is

reasonable to consider curative *local radiotherapy* for localized or limited disease, since this can be given with little morbidity.

The objectives of treatment, therefore, are to control symptoms, to slow progression, or both. Many patients will require treatment changes to induce or maintain a response, and many need treatment combinations. In stage 1 MF this can be achieved with *emollients*, but may require *potent topical corticosteroids* or *photochemotherapy (PUVA)*, with a good chance of complete response (CR). As disease stage advances, so treatment becomes less likely to produce CR but can still provide very effective control. Thus, in stage 2 MF, many patients will respond to combinations of topical treatment as before with PUVA, or to PUVA plus *retinoids* or PUVA plus *interferon-α-2a*. Local radiotherapy is very effective in controlling persistent plaques or tumors, and total skin electron beam (TSEB) therapy is a good option when skin involvement is widespread and refractory to other approaches.

Topical chemotherapy (nitrogen mustard and BCNU) is used in the management of stage 1 and 2 MF in some centers in the USA, but is not as widely used in the UK. There are concerns about the safety of topical chemotherapy both in terms of its long-term carcinogenicity in a disease that usually progresses slowly, and in terms of environmental exposure to others. Whether or not these anxieties are justified, there are no published approved guidelines for the safe use of topical chemotherapy in MF, and until these are available, its use is likely to remain limited.

The above treatments are of little value for stage 3 MF. Patients may progress from earlier stages or present de novo. The principal symptom is severe and persistent itch, and this is remarkably unresponsive to treatment. The rash frequently improves with *low-dose methotrexate*, although response is often slow. The diagnosis of Sézary syndrome should be confirmed by demonstrating >5% Sézary cells per 100 circulating lymphocytes and a T cell clone in blood in the presence of erythroderma. Sézary syndrome patients may be stage 3 to 4B. *Extracorporeal photopheresis (ECP)* has been used for over 12 years for Sézary syndrome; despite this, no randomized controlled trial has been done, and reports of its efficacy are inconsistent, with case series often including patients in whom a circulating clone has not been confirmed. Though some improvement often does occur, its effect on survival is unclear. Durable CRs have been reported, however, and ECP clearly warrants further investigation.

Chemotherapy with *deoxycoformycin* is associated with significant improvement in over 50% of patients, though this rarely lasts for more than 12–18 months. Other high-dose single-agent regimens such as fludarabine are less effective. Combination chemotherapy, e.g. with CHOP, offers no therapeutic advantage and is associated with a very significant risk of neutropenic sepsis and opportunistic infections such as *Pneumocystis* can occur even months after completion of treatment.

In stage 4 MF, survival is limited; responses to combination chemotherapy are rarely complete, and, as above, are associated with significant risk, but may offer the best chance of improvement. Prompt relapse following treatment is common. The best-tried approach is *CHOP* at two-thirds of the normal dosage, and there are other lymphoma regimens that may offer a similar compromise between safety and efficacy. Local radiotherapy is useful for bulky nodal disease and symptomatic skin lesions. This group may be suitable for phase 1 trials of new chemotherapeutic agents, and for new approaches such as allogeneic stem cell transplantation. Effective palliation requires consideration of common symptoms such as nausea, constipation, pain, anorexia, and depression.

SPECIFIC INVESTIGATIONS

- Histology
- Hematology, differential white cell count and film
- T cell receptor (TCR) gene analysis (skin and peripheral blood)
- HTLV-1 serology

Joint British Association of Dermatologists and U.K. Cutaneous Lymphoma Group guidelines for the management of primary cutaneous T-cell lymphomas. Whittaker SJ, Marsden JR, Spittle M, Russell Jones R; British Association of Dermatologists; U.K. Cutaneous Lymphoma Group. Br J Dermatol 2003;149:1095–107.

Management of cutaneous lymphoma. Russell-Jones R, Spittle MF. Baillières Clin Haematol 1996;9:756–7.

All patients should have skin biopsies with immunophenotyping and TCR gene analysis using polymerase chain reaction both on the skin and peripheral blood: this is rarely abnormal in blood in stage 1A MF, but T cell clonality is found in 60% of cases of 1B disease and with increasing frequency as disease stage progresses. All patients should have a full blood count, differential, and film with Sézary cell count together with CD4 and CD8 counts, indices of liver and renal function, and lactate dehydrogenase. HTLV-1 is associated with CTCL-like skin lesions, and serology should be done to exclude this as a cause. If lymph nodes are clinically abnormal, they should be biopsied, and examined for histology, immunophenotype, and TCR gene analysis as the skin. Although evidence suggests that MF is a systemic disease even when skin involvement is limited, these staging investigations rarely detect further disease in clinical stage 1A MF, and infrequently in clinical stage 1B. Patients with clinical stage 2A disease and above require a CT scan of the thorax and abdomen, and bone marrow aspirate and trephine. Tests should only be repeated on the basis of clinical evidence of progression, particularly since the radiation dose from a CT scan is significant.

FIRST LINE THERAPIES

Stage 1 MF	
■ Emollients	E
■ Topical corticosteroids	B
■ PUVA or UVB	B
■ Topical chemotherapy	B
Stage 2 MF	
As above plus:	
■ Local radiotherapy	B
■ Interferon-α-2a	B

It is common to combine treatments; for instance, a patient receiving PUVA for stage 1B MF may respond well but develop a tumor on the nonexposed scalp requiring local radiotherapy. However, care should be used with drug combinations for which there are few or no published safety data.

Clinical stage 1A (limited patch and plaque) mycosis fungoides. A long term outcome analysis. Kim YH, Jensen RA, Watanabe GL. Arch Dermatol 1996;132:1309–13.

In a study of 122 patients with stage 1A MF and mean follow-up of 9.8 years, only 11 progressed and three died from their disease. Seventy-three received topical mechlorethamine with 68% CR, and 34 TSEB with 97% CR. Despite these differences in treatment outcome, survival was similar in the two groups. Actuarial survival was no different from a matched normal population.

A randomized trial comparing combination electron-beam radiation and chemotherapy with topical therapy in the initial treatment of mycosis fungoides. Kaye FJ, Bunn PA, Steinberg SM, et al. N Engl J Med 1989;321:1784–90.

It is clear from this randomized trial of 103 patients that early aggressive treatment with TSEB and combination chemotherapy produces greater response rates than conservative treatment, but, crucially, this does not translate into longer disease-free or overall survival.

Topical steroids for mycosis fungoides – experience in 79 patients. Zackheim HS, Kashani-Sabet M, Amin S. Arch Dermatol 1998;134:949–54.

In this prospective uncontrolled study, 63% of 51 stage 1A patients and 25% of 28 stage 1B patients achieved a CR. Partial response (PR) occurred in 31% of stage 1A and 57% of stage 2A patients. Post-treatment biopsies in 7 of 39 patients with clinical CR appeared to confirm pathologic CR. Median follow-up was 9 months. Comparison with data for topical mechlorethamine suggests a lower rate of CR with corticosteroids. There were no major adverse effects.

There is no evidence that topical corticosteroids cure MF. Consequently, there are no data showing that CR is a necessary or even desirable endpoint; if the control of itch is the main treatment objective, then whether or not appearance improves may be only of secondary relevance. Further, many of the CRs were transient. However, treatment is safe, and experience suggests that topical corticosteroids offer a good compromise between efficacy and safety for the treatment of patches and plaques. A trial comparing corticosteroids with emollient placebo would be helpful.

PUVA treatment of erythrodermic and plaque type mycosis fungoides; a ten year follow up study. Abel EA, Sendagorta E, Hoppe RT, Hu CH. Arch Dermatol 1987;123:897–901.

Results following PUVA are presented on 29 patients, 19 of whom were pretreated with topical chemotherapy or TSEB. Fifteen were stage 1 or 2A, 10 were stage 3, and four were stage 4A. Seventeen patients cleared, including seven with erythroderma, in about 5 months, but the stage 3 patients tolerated only small UVA doses. Most had relapsed by 22 months despite maintenance treatment, but the majority cleared again with PUVA. Two patients developed disseminated herpes simplex.

Ultraviolet-B phototherapy for early stage cutaneous T-cell lymphoma. Ramsay DL, Lish KM, Yalowitz CB, Soter NA. Arch Dermatol 1992;128:931–3.

This retrospective uncontrolled study involved 26 patients with stage 1A MF and eight with stage 1B disease. UVB treatment was given three times weekly, starting at 50–60% of the minimal erythema dose (MED). Twenty-five patients achieved remission after a median treatment period of 5 months (range 1–33). Eighteen had maintenance treatment, with a median remission duration of 22 months. Five patients relapsed, two on treatment. UVB was well tolerated. Patients with infiltrated plaques did not respond.

Both PUVA and UVB are effective in MF. There is more experience with PUVA, and most patients with stage 1 MF will clear; it is less effective in thick plaques and does not work in tumors, but rather surprisingly can work well in stage 3 MF. In general, the earlier the stage, the longer the remission. As maintenance treatment has not been shown to prolong remission, PUVA often does not need to be continued for more than 12–16 weeks. Treatment can be repeated and still be effective, but, as with many of the treatments used for MF, it is unknown whether this prolongs survival.

Topical mechlorethamine therapy for early stage mycosis fungoides. Ramsay DL, Halperin PS, Zeleniuch-Jacquotte A. J Am Acad Dermatol 1988;19:684–91.

In a prospective study, 67 of 117 patients achieved CR using topical mechlorethamine daily until remission, then with a reducing frequency for a further 2 years. Patients with patches cleared in a median of 6.5 months, those with plaques in 41 months; and of those with tumors, only 4 of 10 cleared, in a median 39 months. Among patients with patches, 44% relapsed in a median of 66 months; 61% with plaques relapsed in 44 months, and 100% with tumors relapsed within 8 months.

Long-term efficacy, curative potential, and carcinogenicity of topical mechlorethamine chemotherapy in cutaneous T cell lymphoma. Vonderheid EC, Tan ET, Kantor AF, et al. J Am Acad Dermatol 1989;20:416–28.

This retrospective review of 331 patients identified 25 CRs lasting more than 8 years in 116 patients with stage 1A or stage 1B MF; 22 of 37 patients with stage 3 MF also had a CR. However, there is uncertainty of pathologic diagnosis in some patients who had a durable CR. CRs lasting more than 8 years were also described in nine patients with stage 2 or stage 3 MF, where we know cure is very unlikely. There were significant increases in risk of squamous cell carcinoma, basal cell carcinoma, Hodgkin's disease, and colon cancer, and maintenance treatment was continued for at least 3 years.

Topical nitrogen mustard, 10 mg in 60 mL water, or as ointment, is effective in stage 1 and 2 MF. As with PUVA, earlier stage disease responds more quickly and for longer. Both treatments are carcinogenic, so maintenance treatment is probably best avoided. Topical BCNU is also effective, causes much less contact allergic dermatitis, and appears to work more quickly; each treatment is limited to 3–4 weeks because of the risk of myelosuppression, which may be cumulative. Claims that topical chemotherapy can cure MF are unconfirmed. Guidelines for safe use of topical chemotherapy are not available; it is therefore difficult to recommend this treatment approach.

Interferon alfa 2a in the treatment of cutaneous T cell lymphoma. Olsen EA, Rosen ST, Vollmer RT, et al. J Am Acad Dermatol 1989;20:395–407.

Twenty-two patients with all stages of CTCL were treated with either 3 MU or 36 MU interferon-α-2a daily for 10 weeks, then maintenance for 9.5 months. Three of eight responded to the lower dose, and 11 of 14 to the higher dose, but 86% of this latter group needed dose reductions. Remissions lasted 4–27.5 months. In the lower-dose group, dose escalation increased responses. Mean time to CR was 5.4 months.

Phase II trial of intermittent high-dose recombinant interferon alfa-2a in mycosis fungoides and the Sézary syndrome. Kohn EC, Steis RG, Sausville EA, et al. J Clin Oncol 1990;8:155–60.

Twenty-four patients with advanced, pretreated MF were given very-high-dose pulsed interferon, 10 MU/m² on day 1, then 50 MU/m² for days 2–5, every 3 weeks; after the first four cycles, stable and partially responding patients underwent dose escalation to twice the starting dose. Seven patients had responses, but only one was complete. Dose increments did not increase responses.

Interferon alpha-2a in cutaneous T cell lymphoma. Vegna ML, Papa G, Defazio D, et al. Eur J Haematol 1990;45 (suppl 52):32–5.

In 23 patients with CTCL, lower doses of interferon-α-2a produced at least 80% response rates in stage 1–2 MF, but only 57% in stage 4A.

There are no adequately powered randomized controlled trials of interferon in the treatment of MF. However, a large number of open studies have been done, and the drug clearly is effective, often as much as chemotherapy. Patients with stage 1 or 2 disease respond best, and many require only 3 MU of interferon-α-2a three times weekly; there is little evidence that larger doses are more effective, and they are more toxic. Treatment needs to be continued for a minimum of 6 months to establish a response, and thereafter for 12–18 months or longer to maintain it. Flu-like symptoms and leukopenia are common adverse effects. The former often improve in the first few weeks of treatment; the latter normally recovers promptly on drug withdrawal. Interferon can usually be reintroduced at a lower dose with careful monitoring. Liver function also needs to be checked during treatment.

Interferon alfa-2a combined with phototherapy in the treatment of cutaneous T-cell lymphoma. Kuzel TM, Gilyon K, Springer E, et al. J Natl Cancer Inst 1990;82:203–7.

Fifteen patients with CTCL, including nine with stage 1 and four with stage 2, were treated with relatively high doses of interferon-α-2a, 6–30 MU, and PUVA, each three times weekly. Twelve patients achieved CR and two PR, with a median duration of nearly 2 years.

Photochemotherapy alone or combined with interferon alpha-2a in the treatment of cutaneous T-cell lymphoma. Roenigk HH Jr, Kuzel TM, Skoutelis AP, et al. J Invest Dermatol 1990;95(6 suppl):198S–205S.

Eighty-two patients with MF or parapsoriasis were treated with PUVA: 51 cleared and 31 of these relapsed during follow-up. In addition, 15 patients with more advanced disease were also treated with 6–30 MU interferon-α-2a, and 12 cleared. Median duration of response was 23 months.

There are two other small uncontrolled studies claiming to show that interferon plus PUVA is better. However, it is unclear whether these results are better than for PUVA alone, and a randomized trial is needed. Moreover, to clarify whether combinations really are additive or synergistic requires definition of the dose–response curve for each treatment.

Stage 3 MF	
■ Interferon-α-2a	B
■ Low-dose methotrexate	B
■ ECP	B
■ PUVA	C

Low-dose methotrexate to treat erythrodermic cutaneous T-cell lymphoma: results in twenty-nine patients. Zackheim HS, Kashani-Sabet M, Hwang ST. J Am Acad Dermatol 1996;34:626–31.

In this retrospective study, 29 patients with erythrodermic CTCL were treated with methotrexate 5–12.5 mg weekly for 2–129 months; 70% had at least 10% Sézary cells, but in only 2 of 11 patients was bone marrow histology abnormal. Forty-one percent of patients achieved CR and 17% PR. The median duration of response was 31 months. Response was unrelated to Sézary cell count or presence of lymphadenopathy. Toxicity was moderate, including lung fibrosis in two patients and myelosuppression in three. Median survival was 8.4 years.

These are interesting data, but the definition of erythrodermic CTCL lacks precision in the study. For instance, only 13 had skin biopsies diagnostic of CTCL; the rest were suggestive or consistent with the diagnosis. None had a T cell clone identified, only 2 of 11 had bone marrow involvement. Median survival was surprisingly long. Nonetheless, this does seem to be a potentially useful treatment and should be investigated further.

Treatment of cutaneous T-cell lymphoma by extracorporeal photochemotherapy. Edelson R, Berger C, Gasparro F, et al. N Engl J Med 1987;316:297–303.

Twenty-four of 29 patients with erythrodermic CTCL responded to ECP, as defined by a reduction of >25% in the product of erythema and involved skin surface area; nine patients had a CR, as defined by a >75% reduction; three of eight patients with patch/plaque/tumor MF responded. Only 11 of 37 patients had a T cell clone.

Extracorporeal photopheresis in Sézary syndrome: no significant effect in the survival of 44 patients with a peripheral blood T-cell clone. Fraser-Andrews E, Seed P, Whittaker S, Russell-Jones R. Arch Dermatol 1998;34:1001–5.

A retrospective analysis of outcome in 44 patients with Sézary syndrome defined by erythroderma, >10% Sézary cells, a T cell clone, and skin histology showing CTCL. Twenty-nine patients had ECP, and their survival was no different from 15 patients who did not receive ECP.

There are several small, open studies of ECP, but it is still unclear exactly how effective ECP is, which patients might benefit, whether it is effective in the adjuvant setting, and whether claims that it prolongs survival are true. A randomized, controlled trial is urgently required.

Stage 4 MF As for stages 2 and 3 plus:	
■ Combination chemotherapy	B
■ Radiotherapy to lymph nodes	E

Systemic therapy of cutaneous T-cell lymphomas (mycosis fungoides and the Sézary syndrome). Bunn PA, Hoffman SJ, Norris D, et al. Ann Intern Med 1994;121:592–602.

Data exist for a large number of cytotoxic agents in MF; responses are obtained in about 65% of cases, and are complete in 30%. No single drug stands out as preferable; methotrexate is well studied and seems effective even in low dose without folinic acid rescue. Alternatives include purine analogues, vincristine, etoposide, bleomycin, and cisplatin. Response rates are higher (80%, 40% CR) with combination chemotherapy, but it is unlikely that this translates into

greater clinical benefit. CHOP is widely used, but is frequently associated with neutropenic sepsis; this is a particular risk in patients with ulcerated tumors, and in erythrodermic MF, when normal T cell numbers may be profoundly reduced. To minimize this risk, the dose should be reduced by a third, and suitable prophylaxis provided against opportunistic infection.

MF is often chemoresponsive, especially in patients who are not heavily pretreated – the problem is maintaining the response, which is frequently short lived.

SECOND LINE THERAPIES

Stage 1 MF	
■ Retinoids plus PUVA	B
■ Interferon-α-2a	B

Retinoids plus PUVA (RePUVA) and PUVA in mycosis fungoides, plaque stage. Thomsen K, Hammar H, Molin L, Volden G. Acta Derm Venereol 1989;69:536–8.

This small study shows that the response rate is not increased by combining PUVA with etretinate, probably because response rates to PUVA alone are so high. The total PUVA dose was reduced.

Retinoids – isotretinoin is the most studied – are effective in MF, but are often not well tolerated and seem most useful when combined with other treatments such as PUVA so that the cumulative dose can be reduced. They may also have a place in helping to maintain remission, though any direct cancer-protective effect in MF is unproven.

Stage 2 MF As for stage 1 plus:	
■ Low-dose methotrexate	B
■ TSEB radiotherapy	B

Electron beam treatment for cutaneous T-cell lymphoma. Jones GW, Hoppe RT, Glatstein E. Hematol Oncol Clin North Am 1995;9:1057–76.

These data on nearly 1000 patients show that up to 50% with stage 1A MF have still not relapsed up to 20 years following TSEB.

The data on 'cure' following TSEB have the same limitations as those following topical chemotherapy, and require a higher level of proof.

Stage 3 MF As for stage 2 plus:	
■ TSEB radiotherapy	B
■ Chlorambucil plus prednisolone	E
■ Radiotherapy to lymph nodes	E

Experience with total skin electron beam therapy in combination with extracorporeal photopheresis in the management of patients with erythrodermic (T4) mycosis fungoides. Wilson LD, Jones GW, Kim D, et al. J Am Acad Dermatol 2000;43:54–60.

A retrospective, nonrandomized series of 44 patients with erythrodermic MF treated with TSEB alone (n = 23) or in combination with ECP (n = 21). CR was achieved in 32 of the 44 patients following TSEB; among these, the 2-year overall survival was 63% in the 17 patients who received only TSEB and 88% for the 15 patients who received TSEB + ECP.

From these data, TSEB does seem to be effective in stage 3 MF, although others disagree. This series includes patients from 1974 who do not meet current diagnostic criteria; whether ECP adds benefit is unclear, since the study was not randomized.

Management of cutaneous lymphoma. Russell-Jones R, Spittle MF. Baillières Clin Haematol 1996;9:756–7.

There are few published data to support the use of chlorambucil and prednisolone in CTCL, but experience clearly indicates their value in other low-grade non-Hodgkin's lymphomas. Treatment is cyclical to minimize the risk of myelosuppression.

Stage 4 MF	
■ Purine analogues	B
■ Denileukin diftitox (DAB-IL2)	B

Experimental therapies in the treatment of cutaneous T cell lymphoma. Foss FM, Kuzel TM. Hematol Oncol Clin North Am 1995;9:1127–37.

Deoxycoformycin, fludarabine, and 2-chlorodeoxyadenosine are all effective in CTCL, and were used in the hope that T-cell-specific cytotoxicity would improve the therapeutic index; however, toxicity is significant, and responses often short lived. There is, however, quite good evidence to support the use of deoxycoformycin in stage 3 MF.

Pivotal phase III trial of two dose levels of denileukin diftitox for the treatment of cutaneous T-cell lymphoma. Olsen E, Duvic M, Frankel A, et al. J Clin Oncol 2001;19: 376–88.

DAB-IL2 is a new biologic that targets diphtheria toxin to the interleukin-2 receptor. This phase III study involved 71 patients with stage 1B to stage 4A CTCL that was CD25-positive. There was a 10% CR and 20% PR. The median duration of response was 6.9 months.

DAB-IL2 has now been licensed in the USA for CTCL; recent reports suggest that toxicity is tolerable. Further data are required to define its place in treatment.

THIRD LINE THERAPIES

Stage 1A MF	
■ Topical bexarotene	B
Stage 1B MF	
■ TSEB radiotherapy	B
Stage 1B and stage 2A MF	
■ Oral bexarotene	B
■ Topical bexarotene	B
Stage 2B and stage 3 MF	
■ Single-agent chemotherapy	B
■ Reduced-dose combination chemotherapy	B
■ Oral bexarotene	B
Stage 4 MF	
■ Reduced-dose combination chemotherapy	B
■ Oral bexarotene	B
■ Bone marrow transplantation	D

Phase 1 and 2 trial of bexarotene gel for skin-directed treatment of patients with cutaneous T-cell lymphoma. Breneman D, Duvic M, Kuzel T, et al. Arch Dermatol 2002;138:325–32.

Sixty-seven patients with stage 1A to 2A CTCL used this topical retinoid in incremental doses. There was a 21% CR and 42% PR. The median time to relapse was 23 months.

Phase 2 and 3 clinical trial of oral bexarotene (Targretin capsules) for the treatment of refractory or persistent early-stage cutaneous T-cell lymphoma. Duvic M, Martin AG, Kim Y, et al. Arch Dermatol 2001;137:581–93.

This study investigated 58 patients with stage 1A to stage 2A CTCL which had proved resistant to PUVA, UVB, TSEB irradiation, or topical chemotherapy. Oral bexarotene at a dose of 300 mg/m^2 produced 50% or greater improvement in 54% of patients. Both response rates and side effects were dose-related.

Bexarotene is effective and safe for treatment of refractory advanced-stage cutaneous T-cell lymphoma: multinational phase II–III trial results. Bexarotene Worldwide Study Group. J Clin Oncol 2001;19:2456–71.

This trial included 94 patients with stage 1B to stage 4B CTCL. There was a 45–55% overall response rate, with a mean response duration of 9.8 months.

Bexarotene is a novel retinoid that interacts specifically with the RXR receptor and promotes apoptosis of malignant T cells. Median time to response is 16 weeks and median time to relapse is 43 weeks. The response is dose-related and a daily dose of 300 mg/m^2 optimizes the risk:benefit ratio. Side effects include hypertriglyceridemia (75%) and central hypothyroidism (20%). Both are easily managed with statins, fibrates (excluding gemfibrozil, which can raise bexarotene levels, resulting in even higher triglycerides), and thyroxine. Side effects are reversible on ceasing therapy.

Efficacy for all stages of CTCL, including refractory disease and Sézary syndrome, has been demonstrated. The favorable side-effect profile and the ease of oral administration facilitate outpatient use. Bexarotene is thus gaining an increasing important role in CTCL management; however, its relatively high cost (approximately £1700 per month) may present a barrier to use for some.

Allogeneic hematopoietic stem cell transplantation for advanced mycosis fungoides: evidence of a graft versus tumour effect. Burt RK, Guitart J, Traynor A, et al. Bone Marrow Transplant 2000;25:111–13.

Allogeneic stem cell transplants can be curative in hematological cancer, but the associated myeloablative conditioning is very toxic. However, efficacy is partly mediated by a graft versus tumor effect, and early results suggest that durable engraftment and good responses can be achieved with much less aggressive conditioning regimens.

Autologous bone marrow transplantation produces responses in MF of only short duration, but this new approach raises the possibility of greater efficacy and much reduced toxicity. This is important, since toxicity from current conditioning regimens makes them unsuitable for use in those over 40.

Myiasis

Robert G Phelps, Jianyou Tan

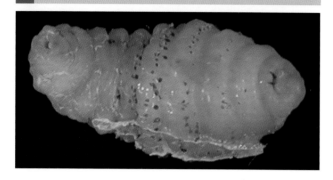

Myiasis refers to the infestation of human and animal tissue by the larval or pupal stages of flies (Diptera). Numerous species can be involved and clinical presentations include nodules, ulcers, creeping eruption, and contamination of a wound (wound myiasis). The goal of therapy is complete removal of larvae from the areas involved and the prevention of future infestation.

MANAGEMENT STRATEGY

Ultimately, the management goal should be limitation of exposure to larvae. At the beginning of the 20th century, myiasis was a major public health problem and a major economic problem, often affecting livestock. Simple improvements in hygiene and wound care have largely eliminated this. Nevertheless reports of human infection continue, including nosocomial outbreaks.

As many cases of myiasis are acquired during travel to endemic areas, the traveler should be warned about the risk, especially in Central and South America and parts of Africa. Individuals traveling to rural areas should be *covered at all times* with long-sleeved garments and hats. At night, *sleeping under a mosquito net* is appropriate. *Insect repellents* may also be useful. *Clothing should be hot ironed and dried* appropriately to remove any residual eggs.

To prevent wound myiasis *simple antisepsis* is usually adequate. Wounds should be adequately cleaned and irrigated at appropriate intervals and have proper dressings. Patients with any type of wound should never be permitted to sleep outside and, if in an indoor or hospital environment, the windows should never be opened.

Once infestation has occurred, therapy consists of *removal of all larvae* with minimal trauma to the organisms. Simple infiltration of the area with lidocaine and *surgical removal* usually suffices when few organisms are present. Care must be taken to extract the larvae whole otherwise a considerable foreign body reaction may ensue. If there is secondary pyogenic infection, this should be treated with appropriate antibiotics.

SPECIFIC INVESTIGATIONS

- Detailed travel history
- Morphologic identification of the parasite

Case report: myiasis – the botfly boil. Pallai L, Hodge J, Fishman SJ, Millikan LE, Phelps RG. Am J Med Sci 1992; 303:245–8.

Most of the reported cases of myiasis in the continental US have been of the *Dermatobia hominis* type. Endemic foci include Belize, Costa Rica, and Brazil.

Cutaneous myiasis. In: Alexander JO. Arthropods and Human Skin. New York: Springer-Verlag; 1984:88–113.

Scanning electron microscopy studies of sensilla and other structures of adult *Dermatobia hominis* (L. Jr., 1781) (Diptera: Cuterebridae). De Fernandes FF, Chiarini-Garcia H, Linardi PM. J Med Entomol 2004;41:552–60.

Molecular identification of two species of myiasis-causing Cuterebra by multiplex PCR and RFLP. Noel S, Tessier N, Angers B, et al. Med Vet Entomol 2004;18:161–6

The fly larvae should be extracted whole and specific identification attempted. Each larva, however, may molt and have several instars, each with a slightly different morphology. This can complicate identification. The adult fly should be identified as well, if possible. It is advisable to consult an entomologist in more difficult cases. Scanning electron microscopy and molecular studies by multiplex polymerase chain reaction (PCR) may be helpful in identifying some species.

FIRST LINE THERAPIES

■ Surgical removal with local anesthesia	E

Myiasis. Millikan LE. Clin Dermatol 1999;17:191–5.

The authors describe their preferred approach: surgically excise the organism with lidocaine anesthesia and close the wound primarily. This gives the optimal cosmetic result. Alternatively, the lidocaine can be used to forcibly extrude the larvae under pressure.

In a surgical approach, care should be taken to avoid lacerating the larvae because retained larval parts may precipitate a foreign body reaction. The larva of D. hominis *is anchored in subcutaneous tissue, making manual removal difficult.*

SECOND LINE THERAPIES

■ Bacon therapy	E
■ Pork fat therapy	E
■ Vaseline® therapy	E

Alternatives to bacon therapy. Biggar RJ. JAMA 1994;271: 901–2.

The authors try smothering the larva using Vaseline® over the wound. The larva emerges spontaneously.

Traditional methods encourage the larva to exit on its own, taking advantage of its requirement for oxygen by using various occlusive dressings to suffocate it. This is very important in areas where clean surgical removal is not possible.

Bacon therapy and furuncular myiasis. Brewer TF, Wilson ME, Gonzalez E, Flesenstein D. JAMA 1993;270: 2087–8.

Evidence levels **A** Double-blind study **B** Clinical trial ≥ 20 subjects **C** Clinical trial < 20 subjects **D** Series ≥ 5 subjects **E** Anecdotal case reports

Multiple strips of raw bacon were placed over the nodule with the fat occluding the central punctum. Within 3 h, the larvae migrated sufficiently into the bacon fat to be grasped with toothed tweezers and gently removed. This treatment is both inexpensive and nontraumatic. The covering should not be restrictive (e.g. nail polish) because this may asphyxiate the larvae without causing them to migrate out of the skin.

Dermal myiasis: the porcine lipid cure. Sauder DN, Hall RP, Wurster CF. Arch Dermatol 1981;117:681–2.

Pork fat was placed on the lesions and then covered with an occlusive tape. The emerging larvae were teased out with forceps.

THIRD LINE THERAPIES

■ Systemic ivermectin	E
■ Topical ivermectin	E
■ Chloroform/ether	E

Cutaneous myiasis: review of 13 cases in travelers returning from tropical countries. Jelinek T, Nothdurft HD, Reider N, Loscher T. Int J Dermatol 1995;34:624–6.

Use of ivermectin in the treatment of orbital myiasis caused by _Cochliomyia hominivorax_. De Tarso P, Pierre-Filho P, Minguuini N, et al. Scand J Infect Dis 2004;36:503–5.

Ivermectin is a broad-spectrum antiparasitic agent that stimulates and increases the receptor affinity of γ-aminobutyric acid (GABA). A single dose of ivermectin (200 μg/kg) was used for infestation with _Hypoderma lineatum_, and led to spontaneous migration of the maggots. A case of orbital myiasis caused by _C. hominivorax_ was successfully treated similarly with oral ivermectin.

Myiasis: successful treatment with topical ivermectin. Victoria J, Trujillo R, Barreto M. Int J Dermatol 1999;38: 142–4.

Four patients presented with traumatic myiasis caused by _C. hominivorax_, each infested with 50–100 larvae. A single topical treatment with 1% ivermectin in a propylene glycol solution was directly applied to the affected area. The topical solution was left for 2 h, followed by gentle washing with normal saline or sterile water. Within 1 h almost all the larvae stopped moving and by 24 h all had died.

Flies and myiasis. Elgart ML. Dermatol Clin 1990;8:237–44.

Application of chloroform, chloroform in light vegetable oil, or ether, with removal of the larvae under local anesthesia, is advocated for wound myiasis.

Myxoid cyst

David de Berker

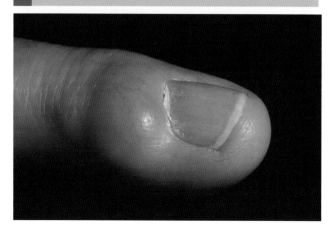

Myxoid cysts are also known as digital mucus cysts or pseudocysts and represent a ganglion of the distal interphalangeal joint. They arise in different forms in soft tissues above or distal to the distal interphalangeal joint. Most typically, they are found as a translucent nodule on the dorsum of the digit.

MANAGEMENT STRATEGY

Myxoid cysts contain gelatinous material that has escaped from the distal interphalangeal joint. Treatment can involve removal of the material combined with measures to prevent further escape from the joint. *Simple drainage* through an incision can achieve the first, but normally there is relapse with further synovial fluid in the myxoid cyst within a few weeks. Measures to prevent accumulation of further fluid are directed at reducing joint pathology or blocking the pathway of escape of fluid. The first category includes the use of *injected triamcinolone*, which might reduce synovial inflammation and pressure of fluid within the joint, and also, *surgery* for osteophytes. Osteophytes appear to weaken the joint capsule and possibly contribute to joint pathology and synovial fluid production. Their removal is associated with resolution of the myxoid cyst.

Blockage of the path of fluid escape is achieved by a range of traumatic and scarring procedures. The challenge is to produce an effective scar over the joint without excess morbidity or a long-term nail dystrophy.

A practical blend of morbidity, complexity of treatment, and efficacy is to employ *cryosurgery* in the first instance. This is best used with a distal block with plain lidocaine or bupivacaine. The cyst is then incised and drained. Two 20-s freezes with liquid nitrogen are given with a complete thaw in between. The wound is dressed over the next 2 weeks. This results in success in about 50% of cases involving fingers. Those that fail can be re-treated in the same way or proceed to surgery. Morbidity is least when there is precise surgery to the path of joint fluid escape. This can be identified by methylene blue injection into the joint and then raising a flap in a distal to proximal path, containing the cyst in the roof of the flap. The pathway is dyed and can be tied with absorbable ligature. The flap is sutured back in place and success is reported as 94% in the fingers. In some instances patient preference or medical considerations may mean that surgery is the first line therapy.

SPECIFIC INVESTIGATIONS

- Transillumination
- Pricking and expression of gelatinous material
- MRI

Transillumination is a useful clinical aid. Where there is diagnostic doubt, simple incision can be helpful to demonstrate gelatinous material. Alternatively, high-resolution ultrasound or MRI can be employed. The first can only help define whether the structure is cystic or not. The latter provides better anatomical definition and allows location of the pedicle communicating between the cyst and joint in over 80% of cases.

MR imaging of digital mucoid cysts. Drapé JL, Idy Peretti I, Goettmann S. Radiology 1996;200:531–6.

FIRST LINE THERAPIES

■ Cryosurgery	B
■ Repeated puncture	D
■ Laser therapy	C
■ Sclerosant	C

Myxoid cysts of the finger: treatment by liquid nitrogen spray cryosurgery. Dawber RPR, Sonnex T, Leonard J, Ralphs I. Clin Exp Dermatol 1983;8:153–7.

Fourteen patients were treated with two 30-s freezes and no evacuation of the cyst. Follow-up was between 14 and 40 months with an 86% cure rate. One patient had a significant nail dystrophy as a long-term complication.

Removal of the overlying cyst or evacuation of the contents might reduce the dose of cryosurgery needed.

Specific indications for cryosurgery of the nail unit. Kuflik EG. J Dermatol Surg Oncol 1992;18:702–6.

Forty nine patients were treated with a range of single cryosurgical doses, from 20 to 30 s using open spray and 30 to 40 s using the cryoprobe. This was combined with curettage in 23 and simple de-roofing in the remainder. There was resolution in 63% over the follow-up period of 1–60 months.

A simple technique for managing digital mucous cysts. Epstein E. Arch Dermatol 1979;115:1315–16.

Repeated puncture of myxoid cysts in 40 patients led to resolution in 72% after two to five treatments, but no follow-up period is given.

Treatment of digital myxoid cysts with carbon dioxide laser vaporization. Huerter CJ, Wheeland RG, Bailin PL, Ratz JL. J Dermatol Surg Oncol 1987;13:723–7.

Carbon dioxide laser cured ten patients with follow-up of 35 months.

Treatment of mucoid cysts of fingers and toes by injection of sclerosant. Audebert C. Dermatol Clin 1989;7:179–81.

The sclerosant sodium tetradecyl sulphate (3%) was injected into the myxoid cyst in 15 patients. 'A few drops' was used at each injection. Four needed a second injection

Evidence levels A Double-blind study   **B** Clinical trial ≥ 20 subjects   **C** Clinical trial < 20 subjects   **D** Series ≥ 5 subjects   **E** Anecdotal case reports

and one a third. The result was resolution in all cases, although the period of follow-up was not reported.

There is a chance of producing painful necrosis of the nail fold, but this is seldom extensive. The theoretical complication of sclerosant entering the joint does not appear to occur.

SECOND LINE THERAPIES

■ Surgery	B

Marginal osteophyte excision in treatment of mucous cysts. Eaton RG, Dobranski AI, Littler JW. J Bone Joint Surg 1973;55A:570–4.

Forty four patients with surgery entailing tracing of communication between cyst and joint, excision of cyst, and in some instances, surgery to the osteophytes, provided success in 43 of 44 patients, with follow-up of between 6 months and 10 years.

There is a theoretical possibility of operating on the osteophytes alone, leaving the cyst in place and allowing it to involute once the precipitating pathology has been removed.

Etiology and treatment of the so called mucous cyst of the finger. Kleinert HE, Kutz JE, Fishman JH, McCraw LH. J Bone Joint Surg 1972;54:1455–8.

Similar surgery, but with less emphasis on osteophyte debridement, resulted in success for all of 36 patients followed for between 12 and 18 months postoperatively.

Surgical treatment of myxoid cysts guided by methylene blue joint injection. de Berker D, Lawrence C. Br J Dermatol 1998;139(suppl 51):72.

Tracing the communication between joint and cyst with methylene blue and then ligating it with absorbable suture, resulted in cure in 29 of 31 patients followed for 8–15 months. In this procedure excision of the lesion was not required.

Ganglion of the distal interphalangeal joint (myxoid cyst): therapy by identification and repair of the leak of joint fluid. de Berker D, Lawrence C. Arch Dermatol 2001;137: 607–10.

A study of 54 patients utilized methylene blue dye injected into the distal interphalangeal joint for identification of the communication between the joint and cyst. A skin flap was designed around the cyst. The communication was sutured and the flap was replaced with no tissue excision. In 89% of patients the communication was identified. At 8 months, 48 patients remained cured with no visible scarring. Myxoid cysts of the toes had a higher relapse rate than those of the fingers.

THIRD LINE THERAPIES

■ Infrared photocoagulation	C
■ Flurandrenolone tape	D

The most likely course of action after failure of surgery is either to repeat the surgery or modify the surgical approach to include osteophyte surgery if these were not treated in the first instance. If a CO_2 laser is available, this might also be chosen, given the good results reported in the small published series. Alternatively, sclerosant could be used although again, multiple treatments could be anticipated.

Myxoid cysts treated by infra-red photocoagulation. Kemmett D, Colver GB. Clin Exp Dermatol 1994;19:118–20.

Infrared photocoagulation employs broad-spectrum radiation from a specialized source, delivering a metered destructive dose. In a series of 14 patients, 12 had resolution after one treatment and re-treatment cured a further one patient. There was some notching of the nail fold in three.

Treatment of myxoid cyst with flurandrenolone tape. Ronchese F. R I Med J 1970;57:154–5.

After the failure of electrodesiccation, five patients were treated with corticosteroid tape for 2–3 months and reported success in all during a follow-up of 2–3 years.

Necrobiosis lipoidica

Abdul Hafejee, Ian Coulson

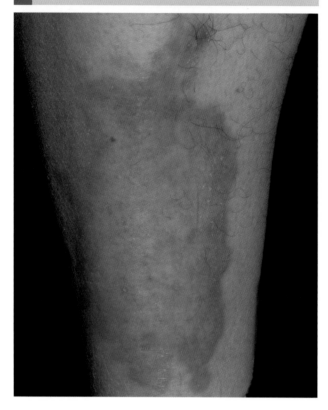

A complication in 1 in 300 diabetics, though sometimes unassociated with glucose intolerance, this granulomatous and ultimately atrophic pretibial eruption may ulcerate, and is rarely complicated by squamous cell carcinoma.

MANAGEMENT STRATEGY

It is essential to encourage patients to *desist from smoking and avoid trauma* to the affected shins that may transform an unsightly plaque into a painful, recalcitrant ulcer. The progression of new lesions may be halted by intralesional or occluded *potent topical corticosteroids* applied to the margins of the lesions. Once atrophy has developed there is little that will reverse this, though *topical retinoids* may be tried. Telangiectasia is often marked and has been treated with *pulsed dye laser*. Extensive lesions may justify trials of *nicotinamide* or *prednisolone*. *Antiplatelet therapy* in the form of either *aspirin, dipyridamole, or ticlopidine* has its enthusiasts, though responses are inconclusive. Topical *psoralen and UVA (PUVA)* has received recent interest and may arrest progression and improve the appearance. A *variety of systemic anti-inflammatory and immunosuppressive agents* have received recent attention, *including mycophenolate mofetil, fumaric acid esters, cyclosporine, antimalarials and infliximab*.

The chronically ulcerated lesion is a challenge; *antibiotics* deal with secondary infection and appropriate dressings are required and growth factors such as *becaplermin* and *granulocyte-macrophage colony stimulating factor (GM-CSF)* may accelerate healing. As diabetics may have coexisting large vessel atherosclerosis that may contribute to ulceration, noninvasive arterial studies or angiography need to be considered if clinically indicated. Venous hypertension may also contribute to the localization and ulceration of necrobiosis. Excision and grafting may transform the patient's quality of life.

Work with the diabetologist to *optimize diabetic control*.

SPECIFIC INVESTIGATIONS

- 2-hour postprandial glucose
- Skin biopsy
- Consider angiography or venous circulation studies
- Consider a biopsy to exclude sarcoidosis, which may mimic necrobiosis lipoidica (NL), or if clinical features suggest the rare development of squamous cell carcinoma

Bilateral squamous cell carcinomas arising in long-standing necrobiosis lipoidica. Beljaards RC, Groen J, Starink TM. Dermatologica 1990;180:96–8.

Carcinoma cuniculatum arising in necrobiosis lipoidica. Porneuf M, Monpoint S, Barneon G, et al. Ann Dermatol Venereol 1991;118:461–4.

Although rare, squamous cell carcinomas may complicate any condition in which papillary dermal scarring is appreciable.

Unilateral necrobiosis lipoidica of the ischemic limb – a case report. Naschitz JE, Fields M, Isseroff H, Wolffson V, Yeshurun D. Angiology 2003;54:239–42

A possible ischemic pathogenesis of NL emerges from a case of unilateral large vessel arteriosclerotic ischaemia with ipsilateral NL.

The author has experience of a severely ulcerated area of NL that only started to heal after disobliteration of severe femoropopliteal atheroma

FIRST LINE THERAPIES

■ Stop smoking and optimize diabetic control	C
■ Intralesional or topical corticosteroids under occlusion	D

Necrobiosis lipoidica diabeticorum: association with background retinopathy, smoking, and proteinuria. A case controlled study. Kelly WF, Nicholas J, Adams J, Mahmood R. Diabet Med 1993;10:725–8.

Stop smoking and control diabetes mellitus with vigilance. Fifteen diabetics with NL were each matched with five control subjects with diabetes mellitus. Background retinopathy, proteinuria, and smoking were all more common with NL. No differences were noted between those with NL and controls in the prevalence of vascular disease and neuropathy. Glycosylated hemoglobin concentrations were higher in patients with NL.

Granuloma annulare and necrobiosis lipoidica treated by jet injector. Sparrow G, Abell E. Br J Dermatol 1975;93: 85–9.

Three of five cases of NL underwent complete resolution and one had partial improvement with 5 g/mL triamcinolone injection to the edges of lesions. No serious complications of this type of treatment were observed.

Treatment of psoriasis and other dermatoses with a single application of a corticosteroid left under a hydrocolloid occlusive dressing for a week. Juhlin L. Acta Derm Venereol 1989;69:355–7.

A 0.1% betamethasone alcoholic lotion under a hydrocolloid dressing was an effective, well-tolerated treatment, and three applications only were required.

SECOND LINE THERAPIES

■ Systemic corticosteroids	D
■ Aspirin and dipyridamole	C
■ Ticlopidine	D
■ Nicotinamide	D
■ Clofazimine	D
■ Topical PUVA	D

Necrobiosis lipoidica: treatment with systemic corticosteroids. Petzelbauer P, Wolff K, Tappeiner G. Br J Dermatol 1992;126:542–5.

Oral methylprednisolone was given to six patients with nonulcerating NL for 5 weeks; in all there was cessation of disease activity in the 7-month follow-up period. Initial dosage was 1 mg/kg daily for 1 week then 40 mg daily for 4 weeks, followed by tapering and termination in 2 weeks. All, including the diabetics, tolerated the treatment well. There was no improvement in atrophy. Benefit was maintained at the end of the 7-month follow-up period.

Careful monitoring of blood glucose is mandatory in all diabetic patients with NL treated with systemic corticosteroids.

Ulcerating necrobiosis lipoidica effectively treated with pentoxifylline. Noz KC, Korstanje MJ, Vermeer BJ. Clin Exp Dermatol 1993;18:78–9.

Ulcerated NL healed completely within 8 weeks of administration of 400 mg pentoxifylline twice daily.

Healing of necrobiotic ulcers with antiplatelet therapy. Correlation with plasma thromboxane levels. Heng MC, Song MK, Heng MK. Int J Dermatol 1989;28:195–7.

NL in diabetics has been considered to be a cutaneous manifestation of diabetic microangiopathy. Seven diabetic patients with necrobiotic ulcers of recent onset that healed after administration of 80 mg/day of acetylsalicylic acid and 75 mg three times daily of dipyridamole had elevated thromboxane levels. Healing was associated with depression of the elevated thromboxane levels in all seven patients.

Treatment of necrobiosis lipoidica with low-dose acetylsalicylic acid. A randomized double-blind trial. Beck HI, Bjerring P, Rasmussen I, et al. Acta Derm Venereol 1985;65:230–4.

No response was seen with the use of 40 mg acetylsalicylic acid daily for 24 weeks despite documented platelet aggregation inhibition.

A randomized double blind comparison of an aspirin dipyridamole combination versus a placebo in the treatment of necrobiosis lipoidica. Statham B, Finlay AY, Marks R. Acta Derm Venereol 1981;61:270–1.

Fourteen patients with a clinical and histologic diagnosis of NL were treated in a double blind control study with either an aspirin–dipyridamole combination or a matching placebo for an 8-week period. None of the patients in the aspirin–dipyridamole group showed a significant improvement.

Necrobiosis lipoidica treated with ticlopidine. Rhodes EL. Acta Derm Venereol 1986;66:458.

When 33 patients were given an unstated dose of this antiplatelet agent, NL cleared in nine and improved in 17. The author warns that cases of agranulocytosis have been reported with ticlopidine.

High dose nicotinamide in the treatment of necrobiosis lipoidica. Handfield-Jones S, Jones S, Peachey R. Br J Dermatol 1988;118:693–6.

An open study of high-dose nicotinamide in the treatment of 15 patients with NL. Of 13 patients who remained on treatment for more than 1 month, eight improved. A decrease in pain, soreness, and erythema and the healing of ulcers if present, was noted. There were no significant side effects, particularly with respect to diabetic control. Lesions tended to relapse if treatment was stopped.

Clofazimine – therapeutic alternative in necrobiosis lipoidica and granuloma annulare. Mensing H. Int J Dermatol 1989;28:195–7.

Ten patients with NL were treated with clofazimine 200 mg orally daily. Six of ten patients responded; three of the responders achieved complete remission of the dermatosis. All the patients treated had reddening of the skin, but this was reversible after the end of therapy, as were the other side effects (i.e. diarrhea and dryness of the skin).

Topical PUVA treatment for necrobiosis lipoidica. McKenna DB, Cooper EJ, Tidman MJ. Br J Dermatol 2000; 143:71.

Four of eight patients with NL responded favorably to topical PUVA using a 0.15% methoxsalen emulsion, with weekly treatments, starting with 0.5 J/cm^2 with 20% dose incremental increases until erythema developed at the edge of the lesions. The mean number of treatments administered was 39.

THIRD LINE THERAPIES

■ Topical retinoids	E
■ Cyclosporine	E
■ Heparin	E
■ Chloroquine	E
■ Mycophenolate mofetil	E
■ Infliximab	E
■ Fumaric acid esters	D
■ Promogran™ for ulceration	E
■ GM-CSF for ulceration	D
■ Becaplermin for ulceration	E
■ Pulsed dye laser for telangiectasia	E
■ Surgery for ulceration	E

Necrobiosis lipoidica treated with topical tretinoin. Heymann WR. Cutis 1996;58:53–4.

A case is presented in which atrophy was diminished by the application of topical tretinoin.

Persistent ulcerated necrobiosis lipoidica responding to treatment with cyclosporin. Darvay A, Acland KM, Russell-Jones R. Br J Dermatol 1999;141:725–7.

Two patients with severe ulcerated NL. Ulceration healed completely after 4 months of cyclosporine therapy, and both patients have remained free of ulceration since. Effective doses were between 3 and 5 mg/kg daily. Three other reports of the effective use of cyclosporine therapy in ulcerated NL now exist.

Minidose heparin therapy for vasculitis of atrophie blanche. Jetton RL, Lazarus GS. J Am Acad Dermatol 1983;8:23–6.

The authors speculate that subcutaneous heparin 5000 IU twice daily may help NL because it helped the vasculitis associated with atrophie blanche. A subsequent letter informs that perilesional low-dose heparin has been successfully used in NL by Russian dermatologists.

Necrobiosis lipoidica diabeticorum treated with chloroquine. Nguyen K, Washenik K, Shupack J. J Am Acad Dermatol 2002;46(2 Suppl Case Reports):S34–6.

Single report of the first case of successful treatment of NL with oral chloroquine

Successful treatment of ulcerated necrobiosis lipoidica with mycophenolate mofetil. Reinhard G, Lohmann F, Uerlich M, et al. Acta Derm Venereol 2000;80:312–13.

A 61-year-old woman with NL for over 30 years was started on mycophenolate mofetil 0.5 g twice daily and lesions regressed within 4 weeks. The dose was reduced to 0.5 g over the next 4 months then stopped. Within 14 days of stopping mycophenolate mofetil the ulceration recurred.

Infliximab: a promising new treatment option for ulcerated necrobiosis lipoidica. Kolde G, Muche JM, Schulze P, et al. Dermatology 2003;206:180–1.

A 33-year-old man with insulin-dependent diabetes mellitus and ulcerated NL was treated with infliximab monotherapy 5 mg/kg infusions each month. By the second infusion, the ulceration had healed, but subsequent infusions were stopped due to the development of miliary tuberculosis. The NL did not recur on stopping infliximab.

Clearance of necrobiosis lipoidica with fumaric acid esters. Gambichler T, Kreuter A, Freitag M, et al. Dermatology 2003;207:422–4.

A 50-year-old woman with a 15-year history of recalcitrant NL was treated with Fumaderm initial (30 mg dimethylfumarate) starting at one tablet daily increased at weekly intervals up to three tablets daily. After the third week, Fumaderm (120 mg dimethylfumarate) was started at one tablet daily and increased to a maximum dose of two tablets daily. After 6 months of treatment the NL had resolved apart from skin atrophy. Remission was maintained in a subsequent 6-month follow-up period.

The management of hard-to-heal necrobiosis with Promogran. Omugha N, Jones AM. Br J Nurs 2003;15(suppl):S14–20.

Single case study with nonhealing ulcerated NL of 3 years' duration. Treatment with a new protease modulating matrix (freeze dried matrix composed of collagen and oxidized regenerated cellulose) resulted in complete healing of the ulcer after 8 weeks, where other dressing regimens had failed to affect healing over a period of 2.5 years.

Healing of chronic leg ulcers in diabetic necrobiosis lipoidica with local granulocyte-macrophage colony stimulating factor treatment. Remes K, Ronnemaa T. J Diabetes Complications 1999;13:115–18.

Topical recombinant human GM-CSF healed two patients with ulcerated NL within 10 weeks. A decrease in the size of the ulcers was already evident after the first topical applications. The ulcers have remained healed for more than 3 years.

Becaplermin and necrobiosis lipoidicum diabeticorum: results of a case control pilot study. Stephens E, Robinson JA, Gottlieb PA. J Diabetes Complications 2001;15:55–6.

Five patients with type 1 diabetes mellitus and NL were treated with topical becaplermin gel (recombinant platelet-derived growth factor). The index patient had ulcerated NL, and this healed. Three of the five patients with nonulcerated NL reported subjective improvement in sensation and lightening of color of the lesions. However, serial photographs and measurements over the 5-month treatment period showed no significant change in the size of the treated areas.

Necrobiosis lipoidica diabeticorum treated with the pulsed dye laser. Moreno-Arias GA, Camps-Fresneda A. J Cosmet Laser Ther 2001;3:143–6.

A single report of the successful eradication of unsightly telangiectasia, a prominent feature of mature NL.

The surgical treatment of necrobiosis lipoidica diabeticorum. Dubin BJ, Kaplan EN. Plast Reconstr Surg 1977;60:421–8.

Seven cases treated by excision of the lesions down to the deep fascia, ligation of the associated perforating blood vessels, and the use of split-skin grafts to cover the defects. There were no recurrences.

Evidence levels A Double-blind study **B** Clinical trial ≥ 20 subjects **C** Clinical trial < 20 subjects **D** Series ≥ 5 subjects **E** Anecdotal case reports

Necrolytic migratory erythema

Larisa Ravitskiy, Steven M Manders

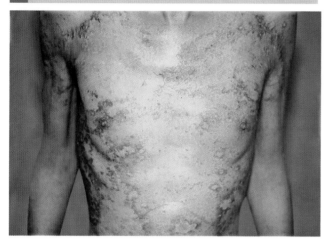

Necrolytic migratory erythema (NME) is a cutaneous reaction pattern, classically associated with a pancreatic islet-cell neoplasm, diabetes mellitus, weight loss, anemia, and hyperglucagonemia as part of the glucagonoma syndrome. In the absence of glucagonoma, NME has also been reported with glucagon infusion-dependent states as well as hepatic disease, gluten-sensitive enteropathy, pancreatic insufficiency, and other malabsorptive or malnutritional states. These cases may be related to zinc, amino acid, and essential fatty acid deficiencies.

MANAGEMENT STRATEGY

Treatment of the underlying disease is the preferred therapy for NME. In the setting of glucagonoma, *surgical excision* of the tumor is the treatment of choice, though curative resection is possible in only a minority due to frequent metastasis. Chemotherapy, primarily with *dacarbazine* and *streptozocin*, is a frequent albeit not very successful adjunctive therapy. *Octreotide*, a long-acting somatostatin analogue, alone or in combination with *interferon-α*, is useful in the treatment of metastases or inoperable tumors. Some patients with NME secondary to glucagonoma have had improvement of skin lesions after intravenous infusions of *amino acids* and *fatty acids*.

The occurrence of NME in the absence of glucagonoma should direct focus toward nutritional deficiencies encountered in hepatic disease, celiac disease, Crohn's disease, enteropathies, and chronic pancreatitis. Deficiency in *amino acids*, *essential fatty acids*, or *zinc* should be corrected.

SPECIFIC INVESTIGATIONS

- Serum glucagon
- Serum zinc, amino acids, total protein, albumin, essential fatty acid levels
- Hemoglobin/hematocrit
- Serum glucose
- Serum liver function tests
- Abdominal CT scan, endoscopic ultrasound, celiac angiography

Islet cell tumors of the pancreas: the medical oncologist's perspective. Brentjens R, Saltz L. Surg Clin North Am 2001; 81:527–42.

An excellent review of surgical, chemotherapeutic, and other treatment options of neuroendocrine tumors of the pancreas.

Pancreatic endocrine tumors: the search goes on. Doppman JL. N Engl J Med 1992;326:1770–2.

Transabdominal ultrasound and CT scan are recommended as the initial studies for detecting pancreatic endocrine tumors larger than 2 cm in diameter. If these studies are negative, pancreatic arteriography and endoscopic ultrasonography may be helpful.

Necrolytic migratory erythema without glucagonoma in patients with liver disease. Marinkovich MP, Botella R, Datloff J, Sangueza OP. J Am Acad Dermatol 1995;32:604–9.

In the absence of glucagonoma, hepatocellular dysfunction and hypoalbuminemia appear to be the most common factors associated with NME. NME may be a cutaneous marker for various liver diseases associated with malnutrition and low-protein states.

FIRST LINE THERAPIES

■ Tumor resection	B
■ Somatostatins	C

Diagnosis and treatment of malignant pancreatic endocrine tumor. Wang L, Zhao YP, Lee CI, Liao Q. Chin Med Sci J 2004;19:130–3.

Retrospective analysis of 36 cases of malignant pancreatic endocrine tumors. Surgical removal of primary tumor and resectable hepatic metastases were curative. Adjunct chemotherapy was employed.

Clinical experience in diagnosis and treatment of glucagonoma syndrome. Zhang M, Xu X, Shen Y, et al. Hepatobiliary Pancreat Dis Int 2004;3:473–5.

Postoperative resolution of NME was achieved within 1 week of surgical resection of a solitary pancreatic tumor.

Somatostatin analogues in the treatment of endocrine tumors of the gastrointestinal tract. Arnold R, Wied M, Behr TH. Expert Opin Pharmacother 2002;3:643–56.

A comprehensive review of somatostatin-based therapies.

SECOND LINE THERAPIES

■ Intravenous amino acid infusion	D
■ Zinc replacement	D
■ Essential fatty acid supplementation	D

Necrolytic migratory erythema and zinc deficiency. Sinclair SA, Reynolds NJ. Br J Dermatol 1997;136:783–5.

Several patients with inflammatory bowel disease or alcoholic cirrhosis with NME-like eruptions and low zinc levels had resolution of their rash following zinc supplementation.

Peripheral amino acid and fatty acid infusion for the treatment of necrolytic migratory erythema in the glucagonoma syndrome. Alexander KE, Robinson M, Staniec M, Gluhy RG. Clin Endocrinol 2002;57:827–31.

Long-term intermittent peripheral intravenous administration of amino acids and fatty acids led to significant improvement in NME symptoms.

THIRD LINE THERAPIES

■ Gluten-free diet	E
■ Pancreatic enzyme replacement	E
■ Dacarbazine	D

Necrolytic migratory erythema: a report of three cases. Thorisdottir K, Camisa C, Tomecki KJ, Bergfeld WF. J Am Acad Dermatol 1994;30:324–9.

NME associated with nutritional deficiencies in a patient with inadequate pancreatic enzymes resolved with vitamin and mineral supplementation and remained clear with pancreatic enzyme supplementation. Noncompliance with avoidance of dietary gluten in a patient with NME secondary to gluten-sensitive enteropathy led to cutaneous flares, which resolved with reinstitution of adherence to the diet.

Successful treatment of glucagonoma-related necrolytic migratory erythema with dacarbazine. van der Loos TLJM, Lambrecht MC, Lambers JCCA. J Am Acad Dermatol 1987;16:468–72.

Intravenous dacarbazine led to prolonged remission of NME in a patient with surgically incurable glucagonoma.

Evidence levels **A** Double-blind study **B** Clinical trial ≥ 20 subjects **C** Clinical trial < 20 subjects **D** Series ≥ 5 subjects **E** Anecdotal case reports

Neurofibromatosis, type 1

Erum N Ilyas, Rhonda E Schnur

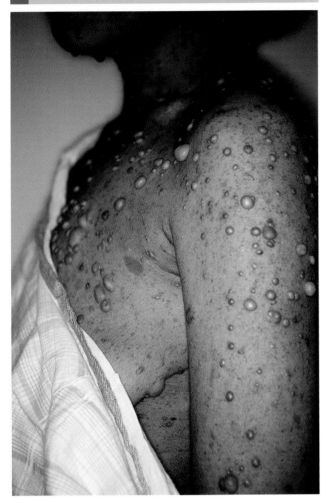

Type I neurofibromatosis (NF1) is an autosomal dominant neurocutaneous disorder with highly variable expression. NF1 is caused by changes in the neurofibromin gene on chromosome 17; the neurofibromin protein is a GTPase-activating protein that negatively regulates Ras protein signal transduction, limiting cell growth and malignant transformation. Neurofibromas may be benign subcutaneous lesions or deeper, larger, plexiform tumors that follow nerves and/or extend into deeper bony and visceral structures; malignant peripheral nerve sheath tumors (MPNSTs) may develop in deeper lesions.

MANAGEMENT STRATEGY

The diagnosis of NF1 is established by well-defined clinical criteria. The sensitivity of mutation analysis varies depending upon the techniques utilized, but is improving. The nature of the mutation may impact prognosis; large deletions or null mutations are detected in a higher percentage of patients with MPNSTs.

Currently, there is no proven medical therapy to prevent or treat neurofibromas. *Ketotifen* has been used for pain,

tenderness, and pruritus. Otherwise, treatment is limited to *surgery*. For benign neurofibromas, cosmetic concerns or discomfort are indications for removal. Most neurofibromas are small and can be removed by simple excision by scalpel or punch biopsy. Although there is little morbidity, surgery is not practical for large tumor burdens.

A wire loop connected to a *monopolar diathermy* machine can be used in the cutting mode to treat up to hundreds of small lesions. Healing is by secondary intention, hemostasis is readily obtained, and cosmetic outcome is good. *CO_2 laser vaporization* has been used for small tumors (< 1 cm) with healing by secondary intention or for larger tumors in conjunction with primary closure. Hundreds of tumors can be removed in one outpatient session under local anesthesia. Unfortunately, surgery is not curative; lesions may continue to progress, requiring repeated procedures.

Treatment of plexiform neurofibromas is particularly challenging because these tumors are often highly vascular and invasive. Symptomatic lesions are evaluated by MRI because of their risk for evolution into MPNSTs. Unexplained pain or rapid growth within a plexiform neurofibroma, and areas displaying necrosis or an unusual appearance on imaging studies merit biopsy to exclude malignant transformation. cDNA gene expression profiling may be used in the future to help distinguish benign from premalignant and malignant lesions.

Nonsurgical treatments for plexiform neurofibromas and MPNSTs are under investigational study. This new generation of therapeutic agents includes *angiogenesis inhibitors* and *anti-inflammatory agents* that inhibit cell growth and induce apoptosis. Drugs that target Ras signal transduction or limit Ras post-translational processing, such as farnesyl transferase inhibitors, look promising.

SPECIFIC INVESTIGATIONS

- Complete cutaneous and ocular exams (with slit-lamp) of patient and first degree relatives
- MRI of brain, optic nerves, and spinal cord if patient is symptomatic
- MRI of deep or changing plexiform neurofibromas
- Biopsy of changing or suspicious lesions
- Radiographs if osseous involvement is suspected
- DNA analysis

Recent advances in neurofibromatosis type 1. Arun D, Gutmann DH. Curr Opin Neurol 2004;17:101–5.

This is a comprehensive basic science and clinical overview of NF1.

Medical management of neurofibromatosis 1: a cross-sectional study of 383 patients. Drappier JC, Khosrotehrani K, Zeller J, et al. J Am Acad Dermatol 2003;49:440–4.

A study highlighting the importance of clinical examination and the lack of utility of screening tests for complications of NF1 in a mostly adult patient group.

Molecular profiles of neurofibromatosis type 1-associated plexiform neurofibromas: identification of a gene expression signature of poor prognosis. Lévy P, Vidaud D, Leroy K, et al. Clin Cancer Res 2004;10:3763–71.

Reverse transcription-polymerase chain reaction of cells from plexiform neurofibromas may be used to screen for acquired genetic changes that mark malignant transformation.

Constitutional NF1 mutations in neurofibromatosis 1 patients with malignant peripheral nerve sheath tumors. Kluwe L, Friedrich RE, Peiper M, et al. Hum Mutat 2003;22:420.

The risk of malignant transformation may be particularly high in patients with gene deletions.

Exhaustive mutation analysis of the NF1 gene allows identification of 95% of mutations and reveals a high frequency of unusual splicing defects. Messiaen LM, Callens T, Mortier G, et al. Hum Mutat 2000;15:541–55.

Combinations of mutation detection techniques, usually including protein truncation, are now utilized to increase mutation detectability, but are costly and labor intensive.

FIRST LINE THERAPIES

■ Surgical excision	C
■ CO₂ laser	C
■ Diathermy	E

The role of surgery in children with neurofibromatosis. Neville HL, Seymour-Dempsey K, Slopis J, et al. J Pediatr Surg 2001;36:25–9.

This is a large study of 249 pediatric patients with NF1 and NF2. Fifty (48 with NF1) had surgery – 14 of the 50 had malignancies, and eight underwent multiple resections. Both surgical and postoperative management are reviewed.

Carbon dioxide laser for removal of multiple cutaneous neurofibromas. Moreno JC, Mathoret C, Lantieri L, et al. Br J Dermatol 2001;144:1096–8.

CO₂ laser under general anesthesia was used to treat hundreds of cutaneous neurofibromas in 13 patients with NF1 with minimal morbidity. Flat, smooth depigmented scars resulted. Most patients who had previous surgical excisions considered the CO₂ laser scars to be as acceptable as those obtained with surgery.

An operation for the treatment of cutaneous neurofibromatosis. Roberts AHN, Crockett DJ. Br J Plast Surg 1985; 38:292–3.

Rapid removal of multiple cutaneous neurofibromas was performed using a wire loop held in diathermy forceps connected to a monopolar diathermy machine. Five patients with an average of 243 lesions were treated. They were hospitalized for 2–7 days and healed completely within 3 weeks.

SECOND LINE THERAPIES

■ Ketotifen	B

A controlled multiphase trial of ketotifen to minimize neurofibroma-associated pain and itching. Riccardi VM. Arch Dermatol 1993;129:577–81.

Ketotifen, 2–4 mg daily, decreased itching, pain, and tenderness associated with neurofibromas in 52 patients with sustained long-term efficacy and minimal side effects.

THIRD LINE THERAPIES

■ Farnesyl transferase inhibitors	E
■ Retinoids	E
■ Thalidomide	C
■ Sulindac derivatives	E
■ Three-dimensional conformal radiotherapy	E
■ Other agents	E

Plexiform neurofibromas in NF1: toward biologic-based therapy. Packer RJ, Gutmann DH, Rubenstein A, et al. Neurology 2002;58:1461–70.

An excellent review of potential therapeutic approaches based on the molecular biology of NF1.

Hyperactive Ras as a therapeutic target in neurofibromatosis type 1. Weiss B, Bollag G, Shannon K. Am J Med Genet 1999;89:14–22.

Potential NF1 therapies are proposed based on the normal function of neurofibromin as a negative regulator of Ras signal transduction. Agents include farnesyl transferase inhibitors (affect post-translational RAS processing) and MEK-mitogen-activated protein kinase inhibitors (affect the downstream effector pathway). Cell differentiation inducers (e.g. retinoids), inhibitors of growth factors, and angiogenesis inhibitors (e.g. thalidomide) may also be useful.

Protein farnesyltransferase inhibitors. Ayral-Kaloustian S, Salaski EJ. Curr Med Chem 2002;9:1003–32.

A recent review of farnesyl transferase inhibitors. In addition to targeting Ras, they may also inhibit angiogenesis and induce apoptosis.

Isolated plexiform neurofibroma: treatment with three-dimensional conformal radiotherapy. Robertson TC, Buck DA, Schmidt-Ullrich R, et al. Laryngoscope 2004; 114:1139–42.

Case report in which a plexiform neurofibroma of the tongue was treated with three-dimensional conformal radiotherapy, with only mild xerostomia as a side effect.

Phase I study of thalidomide for the treatment of plexiform neurofibroma in neurofibromatosis 1. Gupta A, Cohen BH, Ruggieri P, et al. Neurology 2003;60:130–2.

Twelve patients with severe plexiform neurofibromas were treated for 1 year with thalidomide (1–4 mg/kg daily). Although only four patients showed small decreases in tumor size, seven had symptomatic improvement (e.g. decreased pain and paresthesia) with minimal side effects.

Sulindac derivatives inhibit cell growth and induce apoptosis in primary cells from malignant peripheral nerve sheath tumors of NF1-patients. Frahm S, Kurtz A, Kluwe L, et al. Cancer Cell Int 2004;17;4:4.

Results in two primary cell lines from patients with NF1 suggest that this class of anti-inflammatory compounds may be of therapeutic benefit for MPNSTs.

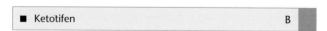

Evidence levels **A** Double-blind study **B** Clinical trial ≥ 20 subjects **C** Clinical trial < 20 subjects **D** Series ≥ 5 subjects **E** Anecdotal case reports

Neurotic excoriation

John Koo, Anjeli Krishnan

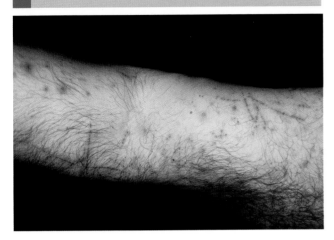

Neurotic excoriation refers to a psychodermatologic condition in which patients participate in compulsive skin picking or scratching of normal skin or skin with minor surface irregularities. This, in turn, can cause self-inflicted skin ulcers, abscesses, or scars that can ultimately become disfiguring. Neurotic excoriations has been associated with both obsessive–compulsive disorder (in the anxiety disorder spectrum) as well as borderline personality disorder, and is thought to be related to emotional stress; in addition, depression may be a common underlying psychopathology. Treatment strategies may vary depending upon the individual patient or clinician because there is a lack of evidence in the medical literature as to a systematic approach to these patients.

MANAGEMENT STRATEGY

Prior to diagnosing a patient with neurotic excoriation, it is important to first rule out other psychodermatologic disorders, such as dermatitis artefacta (which is often associated with damage done with objects other than just fingernails, secrecy about the etiology of skin lesions, as well as a potentially demanding and manipulative personality) and delusions of parasitosis (which is associated with delusional thinking, particularly the absolute belief in the presence of parasites infesting the skin). These two conditions may respond to other forms of therapy. Because neurotic excoriation is primarily a psychiatric disorder, psychopharmacology is the most effective line of therapy. The condition may be associated with several psychopathologic states, including anxiety, stress, depression, and psychosis. As such, pharmacologic agents directed toward these conditions can be of benefit. Broadly speaking, however, neurotic excoriation is probably best treated with *doxepin* (a tricyclic antidepressant) as a first line treatment. There is not a sufficient number of clinical trials demonstrating its efficacy in this condition, but the authors believe it is useful due to its antidepressant as well as antihistaminic activity, which may be critical in breaking the itch–scratch cycle. Doxepin is usually started at 10–25 mg at bedtime, with a gradual increase in the dose of 10–25 mg per week until the patient is taking up to 100 mg every evening, which is the typical effective dose,

particularly if the underlying psychopathology is major depression. If the patient requires even higher dosages, a maximum of up to 300 mg daily of doxepin may be used, provided there are no side effects. Doxepin can prolong the QT interval, so a screening ECG is recommended for patients over the age of 55 years or any patient with a past history of cardiac dysrhythmia. Sedation, weight gain, and orthostatic hypotension are other potential side effects.

Selective-serotonin reuptake inhibitors (SSRIs), antidepressants that include *fluoxetine*, *sertraline*, and *fluvoxamine*, have also been shown in several reports to be effective for neurotic excoriations. These have better safety profiles than doxepin and are less associated with sedation and cardiac conduction abnormalities. There has even been a recent case report that *paroxetine*, another SSRI, improved a case of neurotic excoriations. Other tricyclic antidepressants, such as *clomipramine* and *amitriptyline* and various *benzodiazepines* are third line therapies that should only be considered if the patient does not respond to the more conventional treatments outlined above or cannot tolerate the side effects. *Pimozide*, a traditional antipsychotic, *olanzapine*, an atypical antipsychotic, and *naltrexone*, an opioid antagonist, may also play a role for some patients in treating neurotic excoriations, especially if the underlying pathology involves psychosis.

Treating associated infection and pruritus through the prudent use of *antibiotics and antihistamines (oral or topical)*, respectively, and using *topical corticosteroids* may provide additional symptomatic benefit for patients with neurotic excoriations. Finally, *psychotherapy* and *cognitive behavioral techniques*, including aversion therapy and habit reversal treatments have been reported in certain cases to be effective for this disorder, though a lack of substantial evidence should render this an adjunctive therapy at best. There have been two very recent case reports of the efficacy of *cognitive psychotherapy with laser irradiation* of disfiguring skin lesions. As mentioned previously, neurotic excoriations is primarily a psychiatric disorder, so close follow-up with a primary care physician and a psychiatrist (if the patient is willing) may help to maintain lasting remission.

SPECIFIC INVESTIGATIONS

Close follow-up with a primary care physician or psychiatrist is recommended due to a high incidence of co-morbid psychiatric conditions.

Psychogenic excoriation. Clinical features, proposed diagnostic criteria, epidemiology and approaches to treatment. Arnold LM, Auchenbach MB, McElroy SL. CNS Drugs 2001;15:351–9.

A recent review article outlines the clinical features of neurotic excoriations, as well as co-morbid psychiatric conditions, treatments demonstrated to be effective, and potential criteria for its diagnosis.

Characteristics of 34 adults with psychogenic excoriation. Arnold LM, McElroy SL, Mutasim DF, et al. J Clin Psychiatry 1998;59:509–15.

Patients with neurotic excoriations have a high prevalence of concurrent psychiatric illnesses such as mood disorders (68%), anxiety disorders (41%), somatoform disorders (21%), substance abuse (12%), and eating disorders (12%).

Neurotic excoriations and dermatitis artefacta. Koblenzer CS. Dermatol Clin 1996;14:447–55.

A good review article.

Dermatology and conditions related to obsessive–compulsive disorder. Stein DJ, Hollander E. J Am Acad Dermatol 1992;26:237–42.

Patients with neurotic excoriations often have obsessive–compulsive symptoms and therefore may respond to specific therapies aimed at this type of disorder.

FIRST LINE THERAPIES

■ Doxepin	E

Psychopharmacology for dermatologic patients. Koo J, Gambla C. Dermatol Clin 1996;14:509–24.

Describes in further detail the use of doxepin in neurotic excoriations.

Improvement of chronic neurotic excoriations with oral doxepin therapy. Harris BA, Sherertz EF, Flowers FP. Int J Dermatol 1987;26:541–3.

Case report of two patients who responded to doxepin 30 mg and 75 mg daily.

SECOND LINE THERAPIES

■ Fluoxetine	A
■ Sertraline	B
■ Fluvoxamine	C

A double-blind trial of fluoxetine in pathologic skin picking. Simeon D, Stein DJ, Gross S, et al. J Clin Psychiatry 1997;58:341–7.

Fluoxetine was started at 20 mg daily and increased by 20 mg per week up to a maximum dose of 80 mg daily. Improvements in the treatment arm were statistically significant (based on an intent-to-treat analysis) at 6 weeks with an average dose of 55 mg daily. This trial is limited by a small sample (ten patients in study arm and 11 in placebo arm), a high drop-out rate (40% in the fluoxetine group), and a study period of only 10 weeks, but the study did substantiate earlier case reports.

Sertraline in the treatment of neurotic excoriations and related disorders. Kalivas J, Kalivas L, Gilman D, Hayden CT. Arch Dermatol 1996;132:589–90.

Sertraline was started at 25–50 mg daily and titrated upward to 100–200 mg daily as necessary with improvements seen in 19 of 28 patients (68%) at an average of 4 weeks.

An open clinical trial of fluvoxamine treatment of psychogenic excoriation. Arnold LM, Mutasim DF, Dwight MM, et al. J Clin Psychopharmacol 1999;19:15–18.

Fluvoxamine was started at 25–50 mg daily and increased by up to 50 mg per week to a maximum dose of 300 mg daily for 12 weeks. Although all 14 subjects demonstrated significant improvements in six of eight self-reported scales, the seven subjects who completed the study (50%) had improvements in only two of eight self-reported scales.

THIRD LINE THERAPIES

■ Paroxetine	E
■ Clomipramine	E
■ Amitriptyline	E
■ Benzodiazepines	E
■ Pimozide	E
■ Olanzapine	E
■ Naltrexone	E
■ Psychotherapy	D
■ Cognitive behavioral therapy	E

Paroxetine in a case of psychogenic pruritus and neurotic excoriations. Biondi M, Arcangeli T, Petrucci RM. Psychother Psychosom 2000;69:165–6.

This is one case report demonstrating success with this SSRI. The medication was chosen based on the personality of the patient and was thought to work secondary to its anticompulsive activity.

Neurotic excoriations: a review and some new perspectives. Gupta MA, Gupta AK, Haberman HF. Compr Psychiatry 1986;27:381–6.

A case report of successful treatment using clomipramine 50 mg every evening for 6 months.

Neurotic excoriations: a personality evaluation. Fisher BK, Pearce KI. Cutis 1974;14:251–4.

Successful treatment using amitriptyline 50–75 mg daily was reported.

Neurotic excoriations. Fisher BK. Can Med Assoc J 1971; 105:937–9.

This is a case report on the success of various benzodiazepines prior to the availability of SSRIs.

A psychosomatic approach to the management of recalcitrant dermatoses. Levy SW. Psychosomatics 1963;4:334–7.

This is a case report on the success of various benzodiazepines prior to the availability of SSRIs. In general, benzodiazepines may be useful only if anxiety is the primary cause of neurotic excoriations.

Clinical experience with pimozide: emphasis on its use in post-herpetic neuralgia. Duke EE. J Am Acad Dermatol 1983;8:845–50.

This case report primarily demonstrates the efficacy of pimozide (2 mg two or three times daily) in the treatment of postherpetic neuralgia (eight patients) and neurotic excoriations (two patients).

Olanzapine may be an effective adjunctive therapy in the management of acne excoriée: a case report. Gupta MA, Gupta AK. J Cutan Med Surg 2001;5:25–7.

This is a recent case report on the success of olanzapine, an atypical antipsychotic, for neurotic excoriations.

Naltrexone for neurotic excoriations. Smith KC, Pittelkow MR. J Am Acad Dermatol 1989;20:860–1.

This article discusses reported efficacy of naltrexone for neurotic excoriations.

Psychotherapeutic strategy and neurotic excoriations. Fruensgaard K. Int J Dermatol 1991;30:198–203.

Evidence levels A Double-blind study   B Clinical trial ≥ 20 subjects   C Clinical trial < 20 subjects   D Series ≥ 5 subjects   E Anecdotal case reports

This article reports a positive impact of goal-directed psychotherapy for 22 patients followed over a period of approximately 5 years for neurotic excoriations.

Treatment of facial scarring and ulceration resulting from acne excoriée with 585-nm pulsed dye laser irradiation and cognitive psychotherapy. Bowes LE, Alster TS. Dermatol Surg 2004;30:934–8.

Two case reports of successful treatment of acne excoriee with a pulsed dye laser to improve the appearance of scars and ulcers as well as cognitive psychotherapy to maintain improvement.

Acne excoriée – a case report of treatment using habit reversal. Kent A, Drummond LM. Clin Exp Dermatol 1989; 14:163–4.

This is a case report on the success of habit reversal, a cognitive behavioral technique, for neurotic excoriations.

The behavioral treatment of neurodermatitis through habit reversal. Rosenbaum MS, Ayllon J. Behav Res Ther 1981;19:313–8.

This article reports a response to habit reversal therapy for neurodermatitis in three patients.

Treatment of neurodermatitis by behavior therapy: a case study. Ratcliffe R, Stein N. Behav Res Ther 1968;6:397–9.

This is a case report in which neurodermatitis secondary to neurotic excoriation improved in a 22-year old woman by aversion therapy, a cognitive behavioral technique.

Nevoid basal cell carcinoma syndrome

Katina Byrd-Miles, Gary L Peck

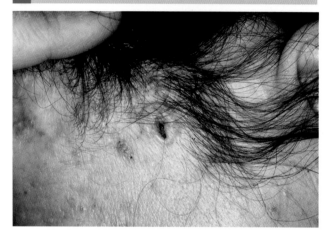

Nevoid basal cell carcinoma syndrome (NBCCS) is associated with a variety of neoplasms and skeletal anomalies with more than 50% of affected patients exhibiting multiple basal cell carcinomas (BCCs), palmar and plantar pits, odontogenic keratocysts, rib abnormalities, and calcification of the falx cerebri. Other neoplasms include medulloblastomas and ovarian fibromas. The chromosomal defect in this autosomal dominant disease is mapped to chromosome 9q22.3-31, resulting in a mutation of the patched gene, which functions as a tumor suppressor gene. The PTCH protein operates in the hedgehog signal transduction pathway and inhibits the activity of smoothened protein. Dysregulation of this transmembrane protein favors subsequent tumor formation.

MANAGEMENT STRATEGY

Affected individuals often present with multiple primary BCCs that pose a therapeutic challenge. The goal of therapy is to achieve adequate cancer control while minimizing cosmetic disfigurement. Therapy should also include *emotional support* and *genetic counseling*. The treatment of BCCs in NBCCS is similar to that of sporadic BCC and includes *surgical excision, Mohs' micrographic surgery (MMS), electrodesiccation and curettage, cryosurgery, topical chemotherapy, topical immunomodulation, photodynamic therapy (PDT), the use of lasers,* and *chemoprevention.* Although BCC occurs in sunlight-protected areas in NBCCS, measures to protect against sun exposure are essential. In the past 3 years, most of the medical literature regarding the nonsurgical treatment of BCC has focused on PDT, the use of lasers, topical immunomodulation with imiquimod, and combination of various therapies.

SPECIFIC INVESTIGATIONS

- Radiologic studies
- Biopsy of lesions
- Genetic studies

Radiologic images in dermatology: nevoid basal cell carcinoma syndrome. Mirowski GW, Liu AA, Parks ET, Caldemeyer KS. J Am Acad Dermatol 2000;43:1092–3.

Radiologic procedures may be performed to detect the various skeletal and soft tissue anomalies associated with this disorder including odontogenic keratocysts, lamellar calcification of the falx cerebri, macrocephaly, cleft lip and/or palate, rib and vertebral anomalies, and short fourth metacarpal.

A novel polymorphism in the PTC gene allows easy identification of allelic loss in basal cell nevus syndrome lesions. Zedan W, Robinson PA, High AS. Diagn Mol Pathol 2001;10:41–5.

A C/T polymorphism of the PTC gene has been identified and a PTC allelic loss has been demonstrated in NBCCS-associated BCC and keratocysts as well as sporadic BCC.

Nevoid basal cell carcinoma syndrome. Gorlin RJ. Dermatol Clin 1995;13:113–23.

UV-specific p53 and PTCH mutations in sporadic basal cell carcinoma of sun exposed skin. Ratner D, Peacocke M, Zhang H, et al. J Am Acad Dermatol 2001;44:293–7.

Update on familial cancer syndromes and the skin. Tsao H. J Am Acad Dermatol 2000;42:939–69.

FIRST LINE THERAPIES

■ Surgical management	B
■ Mohs' micrographic surgery	B
■ Protection against radiation exposure	C

Assessment and surgical treatment of basal cell skin cancer. Goldberg DP. Clin Plas Surg 1997;24:673–86.

Surgical excision, with a 2–5 mm margin of normal skin depending on tumor size, has a cure rate as high as 95–99% for primary tumors. Low-risk sporadic BCCs located on the neck, trunk, and extremities are associated with recurrence rates of 1–10%, while BCCs on the ear, nasolabial groove, scalp, or forehead exhibit higher recurrence rates. BCCs associated with NBCCS have a predilection to involve the embryonic cleft areas of the face including eyelids, periorbital, and midfacial regions. MMS, rather than simple surgical excision, is recommended for deeply invading tumors, recurrent tumors, tumors with poorly defined margins or infiltrating histologic growth patterns, or tumors involving cartilage or bone. Extensive surgery for multiple lesions may require general anesthesia. If a skin graft is required for closure, it should be remembered that BCC can occur within the graft in patients with NBCCS and complicate future surgery.

Advantages of surgical excision over electrodesiccation and curettage, cryosurgery, and other techniques include a healing time of 1–2 weeks, a cosmetically pleasing linear scar which in most cases improves with time, and verification of the histologic margins.

Guidelines for the management of BCC. Telfer NR, Colver GB, Bowers PW. Br J Dermatol 1999;141:415–23.

MMS is a technique that limits destruction of normal skin while effectively treating BCC and is associated with low recurrence rates and an overall 5-year cure rate of 99%. It is the treatment of choice for high-risk BCCs, such as those located on the eyelids, nose, lips, and ears, and those exhibiting infiltrative, morpheic, and micronodular growth patterns. The greatest advantage of the procedure is the maximal preservation of normal skin in cosmetically important areas such as the face, high-functioning areas such as hands and feet, and in aggressive tumors in immunosuppressed patients.

The nevoid basal cell carcinoma syndrome: sensitivity to the ultraviolet and x-ray irradiation. Frentz G, Munch-Petersen B, Wulf HC, et al. J Am Acad Dermatol 1987;17:637–43.

Radiation therapy should be avoided because patients with NBCCS develop BCC as a consequence of radiotherapy within 6 months to 3 years, in contrast to the usual 20–30-year lag period for radiation-induced tumors seen in patients with sporadic BCC.

SECOND LINE THERAPIES

■ Electrodesiccation and curettage	B

Combined curettage and excision: a treatment method for primary basal cell carcinoma. Johnson TM, Tromovitch TA, Swanson NA. J Am Acad Dermatol 1991;24:613–7.

This therapy is appropriate for smaller primary BCCs less than 2 cm in size, and located in low-risk recurrence areas such as the neck, trunk, and extremities. When used to treat non-aggressive primary lesions, the 5-year cure rate approaches 97%. Curettage and electrodesiccation should not be performed on recurrent tumors because scar tissue from the initial procedure interferes with the textural contrast needed for successful treatment with this technique. This procedure should also be avoided when tumors are large, exhibit a histologic infiltrative subtype, when the tumors are invading fat or other soft tissues, when they involve adnexal structures, and when large tumors are located in high-risk areas of the midface and periorbital region.

With the multiplicity and high recurrence rate of tumors in NBCCS, electrodesiccation and curettage is certainly a therapeutic option, but should be employed after careful consideration of recurrence and location and tumor size.

THIRD LINE THERAPIES

■ Imiquimod	A
■ CO$_2$ laser	C
■ PDT	C
■ Cryosurgery	B
■ Retinoids	C
■ 5-Fluorouracil (5-FU)	E
■ Interferon	C
■ Dermabrasion	E
■ Paclitaxel	E

The use of imiquimod 5% cream for the treatment of superficial basal cell carcinomas in a basal cell nevus syndrome patient. Kagy MK, Amonette R. Dermatol Surg 2000;26:577–9.

Imiquimod 5% cream for the treatment of superficial basal cell carcinomas: results from two phase III, randomized, vehicle-controlled studies. Geisse J, Caro I, Lindholm J, et al. J Am Acad Dermatol 2004;50:722–33.

Imiquimod is an immunomodulatory drug that is a Toll-like receptor 7 agonist that stimulates monocytes/macrophages and dendritic cells to produce interferon-α and other cytokines to stimulate cell-mediated immunity and has been approved in the treatment of genital and perianal warts. More recently, numerous studies have demonstrated the efficacy of imiquimod in the treatment of superficial BCC, warranting FDA approval for this specific purpose. Two identical, randomized, vehicle-controlled 6-week studies using imiquimod to treat superficial BCC demonstrated histologic clearance rates of 79 and 82%. A 6-week, five times a week therapy regimen is recommended. Kagy et al. achieved complete regression of multiple, superficial, non-facial BCC in a patient with NBCCS with imiquimod 5% cream, but the therapy was poorly tolerated by this patient. Reported local side effects include itching, burning, pain, and flu-like symptoms.

Gorlin syndrome: the role of the carbon dioxide laser in-patient management. Grobbelaar AO, Horlock N, Gault DT. Ann Plast Surg 1997;39:366–73.

Grobbelaar et al. report using a CO$_2$ laser to treat multiple tumors rapidly and successfully, resulting in complete destruction without recurrence at 26-month follow-up. CO$_2$ laser is a promising modality for treating multiple BCCs with the advantages of a 2–3 week healing time, minimal postoperative pain, and acceptable cosmetic results. Side effects include postoperative erythema lasting up to 3 months as well as hypo- and hyperpigmentation.

Recent research presents CO$_2$ lasers as an effective therapy for patients with multiple BCCs in whom complete surgical excision and other treatment modalities are impractical. This therapy is most effective when used in combination with other treatment modalities.

Microscopically controlled surgical excision combined with ultrapulse CO$_2$ vaporization in the management of a patient with the nevoid basal cell carcinoma syndrome. Krunic AL, Viehman E, Madani S, Clark RE. J Dermatol 1998;25:10–2.

Krunic et al. used an ultrapulse CO$_2$ laser in combination with MMS to treat large plaque tumors and reported no recurrence of the treated areas at 15-month follow-up.

Full-face carbon dioxide laser resurfacing in the management of a patient with the nevoid basal cell carcinoma syndrome. Doctoroff A, Oberlender SA, Purcell SM. Dermatol Surg 2003;29:1236–40.

A CO$_2$ laser was used to treat a 32-year-old woman with multiple BCCs on the face that were not amenable to other surgical modalities. Two months after the procedure, she presented with two BCCs on the face, which were treated with MMS. At 10-month follow-up, she presented with four BCCs on the face, which were treated with MMS. Imiquimod successfully removed one of the tumors, which was located on her nose.

Photodynamic therapy of multiple nonmelanoma skin cancers with verteporfin and red light-emitting diodes: two-year results evaluating tumor response and cosmetic outcomes. Lui H, Hobbs L, Tope WD, et al. Arch Dermatol 2004;140:26–32.

Clearance rates of 93% and a complete response rate of 95% at 24-month follow up when using intravenous verteporfin and a red light emitting diode (688 nm) at a light dose of 180 J/cm^2 permitting activation of the drug within deep portions of the tumor.

Photodynamic therapy using topical methyl aminolevulinate vs surgery for nodular basal cell carcinoma: results of a multicenter randomized prospective trial. Rhodes LE, de Rie M, Enström Y, et al. Arch Dermatol 2004;140:17–23.

Topical methyl aminolevulinate in the treatment of nodular BCC in conjunction with a noncoherent red light (570–670 nm) at 75 J/cm^2 achieved a complete response of 91% with a tumor-free rate of 83% at 12 months. Benefits of this therapy include the capability to treat large and multiple tumors and being typically nonscarring. Side effects include photosensitivity, which can last for several months, as well as localized treatment site pain, burning/stinging, and erythema. The use of phototherapy in children has been associated with poor response and scarring.

PDT, which has been employed for a range of malignancies, involves the use of a photosensitizing agent intravenously, intralesionally, or topically. Upon exposure to visible light, the photosensitizing agent is activated, producing oxygen species that preferentially accumulate for longer periods of time in malignant cells, which are then selectively destroyed by a phototoxic reaction. The light source for PDT is often derived from a laser of appropriate wavelength as dictated by the photosensitizer used. Many studies have found that PDT is most appropriate for superficial BCCs and for those with multiple BCCs in low-risk areas when surgical options are impractical.

Cryosurgery for cutaneous malignancy: an update. Kuflik EG. Dermatol Surg 1997;23:1081–7.

Cryosurgery is best suited for superficial noninfiltrating tumors with well-defined borders. Cryosurgery is not effective for morpheaform or infiltrating histologic subtypes, recurrent lesions, or deeply penetrating or very aggressive tumors. Advantages of this procedure include its effectiveness in treating large superficial tumors, tumors that are fixed to cartilage, and lesions located within a burn scar. This therapy also provides an alternative for high-risk surgical patients such as the elderly and those with coagulopathy or with a pacemaker. Cryosurgery should be avoided in people of color and those with cryoglobulinemia. Reported cure rates are as high at 98.4% with a 5-year cure rate of 99% for primary tumors.

Cryosurgery and topical fluorouracil: a treatment method for widespread basal cell epithelioma in basal cell nevus syndrome. Tsuji T, Otake N, Nishimura M. J Dermatol 1993;20:507–13.

Combined therapy with cryosurgery and topical 5% 5-FU was more effective in producing complete clinical and histologic clearance of BCC in a patient with NBCCS than either modality used alone.

Treatment and prevention of basal cell carcinoma with oral isotretinoin. Peck GL, DiGiovanna JJ, Sarnoff DS, et al. J Am Acad Dermatol 1988;19:176–85.

Prevention of skin cancer in xeroderma pigmentosum with the use of oral isotretinoin. Kraemer K, DiGiovanna JJ, Moshell A, Peck GL. N Engl J Med 1988;318:1633–7.

Peck et al studied the use of isotretinoin in patients with NBCCS and in patients with multiple BCCs secondary to excessive sun exposure or arsenic exposure. Isotretinoin at the dose of 4.5 mg/kg daily induced complete remission in 10% of the tumors and the authors concluded that the risk of toxicity outweighed the benefit. Lower doses of 1.5 mg/kg daily were chemopreventive. Chemopreventive benefit was observed in three patients who were treated with doses as low as 0.5 mg/kg daily for 2–8 years. When treatment was discontinued, new BCCs appeared, emphasizing the importance of maintenance therapy. Similar chemopreventive effects of isotretinoin were observed in patients with xeroderma pigmentosum. The lowest effective chemopreventive dosage in xeroderma pigmentosum varied from 0.5 to 1.5 mg/kg daily.

Common side effects of systemic retinoids include mucocutaneous toxicity, hypertriglyceridemia, and teratogenicity.

Effectiveness of isotretinoin in preventing the appearance of basal cell carcinomas in basal cell nevus syndrome. Goldberg LH, Hsu SH, Alcalay J. J Am Acad Dermatol 1989;21:144–5.

Isotretinoin 0.4 mg/kg daily reduced the number of new BCCs in a patient with NBCCS, but the patient's twin with NBCCS treated with isotretinoin at 0.2 mg/kg daily had four times as many new lesions.

Etretinate treatment of the nevoid basal cell carcinoma syndrome: therapeutic and chemopreventive effect. Hodak E, Ginzburg A, David M, Sandbank M. Int J Dermatol 1987;26:606–9.

Partial or complete regression was observed in 76% of existing BCCs and the arrest of new tumor formation in a patient with NBCCS treated with etretinate initially at 1.0 mg/kg daily and later at 0.7 mg/kg daily for 13 months.

Nevoid basal cell carcinoma syndrome: combined etretinate and surgical treatment. Sanchez-Conejo-Mir J, Camacho F. J Dermatol Surg Oncol 1989;15:868–71.

This report describes complete clinical regression in 26% of BCCs in a patient with NBCCS treated with etretinate (1 mg/kg daily for 3 months); moreover, no new tumors developed during a 9-month period when 0.5 mg/kg daily was employed.

Beneficial effect of low-dose systemic retinoid in combination with topical tretinoin for the treatment and prophylaxis of premalignant and malignant skin lesions in renal transplant recipients. Rook AH, Jaworsky C, Nguyen T, et al. Transplantation 1995;59:714–9.

Topical tretinoin (0.025–0.05%) was effective in preventing skin cancer when used in combination with oral etretinate (10 mg daily) in renal transplant patients with multiple actinic keratoses and a history of multiple squamous cell carcinomas per year.

Long-term therapy with low-dose isotretinoin for prevention of basal cell carcinoma: a multicenter clinical trial.

Isotretinoin Basal Cell Carcinoma Study Group. Tangrea JA, Edwards BK, Taylor PR, et al. J Natl Cancer Inst 1992; 84:328–32.

Oral isotretinoin used as monotherapy at a low dose of 10 mg daily given for 3 years to patients with a history of sporadic BCC was ineffective in preventing new tumors.

Long-term management of basal cell nevus syndrome with topical tretinoin and 5-fluorouracil. Strange PR, Lang PG. J Am Acad Dermatol 1992;27:842–5.

The topical retinoid, tretinoin, has been shown to exhibit cancer chemopreventive benefit. Strange et al. report successful treatment of a child with NBCCS for 10 years with 0.1% tretinoin and 5% 5-FU creams. The authors state that hundreds of superficial BCCs initially present disappeared with the combination therapy, leaving less that 20 BCCs at any given time with no growth of these remaining tumors. They concluded that the regimen was both therapeutic and tumor-suppressive and had an excellent safety profile as developmental or laboratory abnormalities were not noted.

Topical 5% 5-FU has been used to treat sporadic superficial BCC as well as BCC associated with NBCCS. Studies to date yield conflicting results of the effectiveness of 5-FU in the treatment of NBCCS. As previously mentioned, 5-FU is more effective in promoting complete tumor clearance in NBCCS when combined with another treatment modality such as cryosurgery or tretinoin.

Widespread basal cell carcinoma of the scalp treated by dermabrasion. Melandri D, Carruthers A. J Am Acad Dermatol 1992;26:270–1.

A patient with multiple confluent BCCs on the scalp developed recurrent BCC despite numerous surgical and MMS procedures. The entire scalp underwent dermabrasion with complete healing within 6–7 days and only one recurrent BCC within 6 years.

Intralesional interferon therapy for basal cell carcinoma. Cornell RC, Greenway HT, Tucker SB, et al. J Am Acad Dermatol 1990;23:694–700.

Different treatment modalities for the management of a patient with the nevoid basal cell carcinoma syndrome. Kopera D, Cerroni L, Fink-Puches R, Kerl H. J Am Acad Dermatol 1996;34:937–9.

Failure of interferon alfa and isotretinoin combination therapy in the nevoid basal cell carcinoma syndrome. Sollitto R, DiGiovanna J. Arch Dermatol 1996;132:94–5.

To date, intralesional interferon to treat BCC has been used largely for investigational purposes. Its use is limited by its high cost and side effect profile of flu-like symptoms. More studies are required to determine the effectiveness and clinical usefulness of intralesional interferon in NBCCS. In a number of studies, however, intralesional interferon has been shown to cause regression in nodulo-ulcerative and superficial lesions.

In the study by Cornell et al. a patient with BCC not associated with NBCCS received three intralesional injections per week for 3 weeks of 1.5 million IU of interferon-alfa-2b, resulting in a complete regression in 81% of the lesions at 1 year with excellent cosmetic effects. Kopera et al. administered the same dosing and time schedule of intralesional interferon-alfa-2b to a patient with NBCCS and noted only a reduction in size and flattening of the lesions, and subsequently treated the patient with CO_2 laser. Kopera et al. therefore, concluded that interferon-alfa-2b is inadequate to eradicate BCC in NBCCS. Sollitto et al. combined isotretinoin 2 mg/kg daily and intralesional interferon-alfa, with clearance in only one of three lesions at the end of 7 weeks in a patient with NBCCS.

Successful treatment of an intractable case of hereditary basal cell carcinoma syndrome with paclitaxel. Sobky E, Reem A, Kallab AM, et al. Arch Dermatol 2001;137:827–8.

A 54-year-man with NBCCS was treated with 19 cycles of the chemotherapeutic agent paclitaxel. The treatment was well tolerated without any toxicity. At 16-month follow-up most of his preexisting lesions had healed without scarring. The BCCs that were still present were clinically regressing and no new BCCs were noted.

Nevus sebaceus

Robert Burd

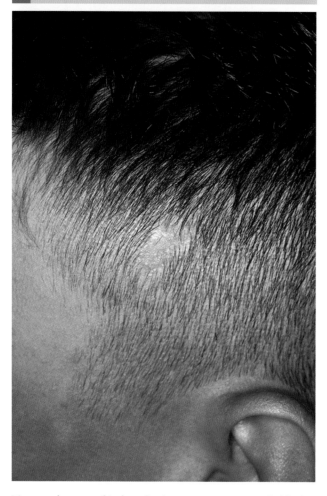

Nevus sebaceus of Jadassohn is a common congenital lesion that occurs predominantly on the face and scalp. Initially, it appears as a well-defined waxy, yellow-red plaque devoid of hair. During puberty the lesion thickens and may become verrucous. Treatment is aimed at providing the correct diagnosis and managing the cosmetic implications of this lesion.

MANAGEMENT STRATEGY

A clinical diagnosis can usually be made easily. It is also recognized that nevus sebaceus may eventually develop a variety of both benign and malignant tumors within it. The most common malignant tumor is a basal cell carcinoma (BCC), the most frequent benign tumor being a trichoblastoma. The risk of malignant transformation within a nevus sebaceus is unknown. In an attempt to determine the malignant potential, a number of series of nevus sebaceus have been retrospectively examined; they show a marked discrepancy in the frequency of tumor development. The more recent studies have shown that malignant transformation is a very rare event, with many previously misdiagnosed BCCs actually been shown to be trichoblastomas on re-examination. Previously it was standard practice to advise *prophylactic excision* of nevus sebaceus. However, in the light of recent evidence this should be reconsidered and now the

cosmetic implications of treatment need to be weighed against those of the lesion and its very small malignant potential.

It is also important to recognize that rarely an extensive or linear nevus sebaceous may arise in conjunction with central nervous system abnormalities such as epilepsy and mental retardation, ocular pathology, and skeletal defects – the linear nevus sebaceus syndrome.

Naevus sebaceous: a report of 140 cases with special regard to the development of secondary tumours. Wilson Jones E, Heyl T. Br J Dermatol 1970;82:99–117.

A total of nine BCCs were found in this series of 140 cases of nevus sebaceus.

Tumors arising in nevus sebaceus: a study of 596 cases. Cribier B, Scrivener Y, Grosshans E. J Am Acad Dermol 2000;42:263–8.

A large retrospective analysis of 596 cases of nevus sebaceus. Two BCCs were found. The authors sought especially to differentiate BCC from trichoblastoma. They found 28 lesions that had previously been misdiagnosed as BCC, but were subsequently considered to have typical features of trichoblastomas. No other malignancies were found and the authors thus urge caution in the prophylactic removal of nevus sebaceus from children.

Basaloid neoplasms in nevus sebaceous. Kaddu S, Schaeppi H, Kerl H, Soyer HP. J Cutan Pathol 2000;27: 327–37.

A series of 316 cases of nevus sebaceus examined for basaloid neoplasms specifically looking for features of BCC and trichoblastoma. Of the 24 basaloid neoplasms found, 22 had typical features of trichoblastoma while only two had features of BCC.

Trichoblastoma is the most common neoplasm developed in nevus sebaceous of Jadassohn: a clinicopathological study of a series of 155 cases. Jaqueti G, Requena L, Sanchez Yus E. Am J Dermatopathol 2000;22:108–18.

A retrospective study of 155 cases. No malignant neoplasms were found in this series. The commonest tumors found were trichoblastomas and therefore early excision to prevent malignancy was inappropriate.

SPECIFIC INVESTIGATIONS

■ Biopsy

If the diagnosis is in any doubt, histologic examination of a skin biopsy will reveal typical histology. During childhood the sebaceous glands are underdeveloped, but the presence of incompletely differentiated hair structures should allow the diagnosis to be made. After puberty the large numbers of mature sebaceous glands and epidermal hyperplasia make the diagnosis straightforward.

FIRST LINE THERAPIES

■ Surgical excision	E
■ Observation	D

Historically, prophylactic surgical excision of nevus sebaceus has been the preferred method of treatment. For small lesions,

Evidence levels A Double-blind study   B Clinical trial ≥ 20 subjects   C Clinical trial < 20 subjects   D Series ≥ 5 subjects   E Anecdotal case reports

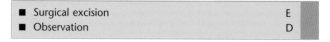

especially on the scalp, the cosmetic consequences of excision are minimal. For larger lesions and those on the face, the cosmetic consequences following surgery may be considerable. Recent histopathological studies have indicated that the risk of malignant transformation is low, especially in children, and that clinical follow-up may be more appropriate.

Nevus sebaceous: clinical outcome and consideration for prophylactic excision. Chun K, Vazquez M, Sanchez JL. Int J Dermatol 1995;34:538–41.

Of 225 cases of nevus sebaceus only nine neoplasms were identified; all were benign. Of these nine, six were removed for prophylactic or cosmetic reasons and in only three cases were the neoplasms suspected clinically.

Should nevus sebaceous of Jadassohn in children be excised? A study of 757 cases, and literature review. Santibanez-Gallerani A, Marshall D, Duarte AM, et al. J Craniofac Surg 2003;14:658–60.

In a retrospective analysis of 757 cases of nevus sebaceus excised from children 16 years or younger, no cases of BCC were identified.

SECOND LINE THERAPIES

■ Curettage and cautery	E
■ Cryotherapy	E
■ Laser resurfacing	E
■ Photodynamic therapy	E

When surgery is declined or the results of surgery are considered to outweigh the benefits, a variety of other techniques may be employed. These techniques may improve the appearance of the lesion, but will not remove deeper elements and therefore continued observation is advised.

Photodynamic therapy for nevus sebaceous with topical δ-aminolevulinic acid. Dierickx CC, Goldenhersh M, Dwyer P, et al. Arch Dermatol 1999;135:637–40.

A single case report of photodynamic therapy using 20% δ-aminolevulinic acid and laser light at 630 nm. Following 13 treatment sessions a good cosmetic result was seen, and this was maintained for 16 months.

Linear nevus sebaceous of Jadassohn treated with the carbon dioxide laser. Ashinoff R. Pediatric Dermatol 1993; 10:189–91.

A single case report of cosmetic improvement of a nevus sebaceus on the nose of a 10-year-old boy following resurfacing with a CO_2 laser.

Onchocerciasis

Michele E Murdoch

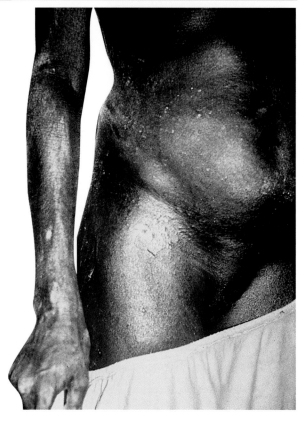

Onchocerciasis is a major tropical parasitic infection caused by the filarial worm *Onchocerca volvulus* and is transmitted by blood-sucking *Simulium* spp. blackflies, which breed near fast-flowing rivers. The disease is endemic in 28 countries in sub-Saharan Africa; small foci also exist in the Yemen and Central and Southern America (Mexico, Guatemala, Ecuador, Colombia, Venezuela, and Brazil). Worldwide, there are an estimated 17.7 million infected cases. The first manifestation of infection is usually intense pruritus and subsequently a wide variety of acute and chronic skin and eye changes develop.

MANAGEMENT STRATEGY

The socioeconomic consequences of onchocerciasis are most marked in hyperendemic areas in sub-Saharan Africa. Globally, approximately 270 000 people are blind and 500 000 have significant visual loss directly as a consequence of onchocerciasis. A multi-country study in Africa revealed that 42% of the adult population in endemic villages suffered from pruritus and 28% of the population had onchocercal skin lesions.

The global control of onchocerciasis hinges on strategies to reduce the level of disease in endemic areas until it is no longer a significant public health problem. Three Regional Programmes have been established to coordinate control. The Onchocerciasis Control Programme (OCP, 1974–2002) successfully used *aerial larviciding* of rivers in West Africa to control the vector blackfly and more recently it has distributed *ivermectin* to control any recrudescence. The Oncho-

cerciasis Elimination Programme in the Americas (OEPA, 1991–2007) aims to eliminate clinical manifestation of onchocerciasis and interrupt transmission of disease altogether using 6-monthly mass ivermectin therapy. The largest programme, the African Programme for Onchocerciasis Control (APOC), which commenced in 1995 and is planned to continue until 2009, comprises large-scale annual distribution of ivermectin in 18 non-OCP countries. Ivermectin is a safe, effective microfilaricide (i.e. it kills the immature larval stages of filarial worms), but as it does not kill the adult worms when given annually, treatment has to be repeated throughout the life span of the adult worm (10–14 years). A few months after dosing with ivermectin, the numbers of microfilariae in the skin gradually increase back towards pre-treatment levels so a single dose of ivermectin per year may not completely interrupt transmission.

Recently, *Wolbachia* spp. symbiotic endobacteria have been identified as essential for the filarial worms' fertility and they offer novel targets for mass treatment. Additional treatment with *doxycycline* to sterilize the worms may thus enhance ivermectin-induced suppression of microfilaridermia and is a promising basis for blocking transmission (Onchocerciasis. Hoerauf A, Büttner DW, Adjei O, Pearlman E. BMJ 2003;326:207–10).

Onchocerciasis and lymphatic filariasis commonly coexist and current integrated control programmes employ repeated *annual mass treatment of endemic communities with ivermectin and albendazole.*

SPECIFIC INVESTIGATIONS

- Skin snips
- Other parasitological forms of diagnosis
  - Detection of intraocular microfilariae using a slit lamp
  - Demonstration of adult worms by collagenase digestion of excised nodules
- Full blood count (for eosinophilia)
- Mazzotti test
- Diethylcarbamazine (DEC) patch test
- Future investigative tools
  - Serodiagnosis
  - Polymerase chain reaction (PCR)

WHO Expert Committee on Onchocerciasis. Third Report. World Health Organization. World Health Organ Tech Rep Ser 1987;752:114–9.

It should be remembered that skin snips and other parasitological methods of assessment may fail to detect prepatent and early or light infections.

Onchocerciasis and its control. Report of a WHO Expert Committee on onchocerciasis control. World Health Organization. World Health Organ Tech Rep Ser 1995;852:46.

The Mazzotti test should only be used when onchocerciasis is suspected, but microfilariae cannot be demonstrated in the skin or eyes (i.e. the person is likely to be lightly infected). A single oral dose of 50 mg of DEC is given and the patient is observed for the effects of microfilarial death such as itching, papular rash, and lymphadenitis, which may develop after 1–24 h. The test is contraindicated in heavily infected individuals because severe reactions can occur, including pulmonary edema and collapse.

Evidence levels A Double-blind study B Clinical trial ≥ 20 subjects C Clinical trial < 20 subjects D Series ≥ 5 subjects E Anecdotal case reports

Improved immunodiagnostic tests to monitor onchocerciasis control programmes – a multicenter effort. Ramachandran CP. Parasitol Today 1993;9:77–9.

A specific serological diagnostic test for onchocerciasis is not routinely available at present, but it is anticipated that such a tool will become available in the future using a cocktail of recombinant *O. volvulus* antigens. Antibody-based diagnostic tests are not routinely used in endemic areas because of limited access to labs capable of performing these tests.

Antibody detection tests for *Onchocerca volvulus*: comparison of the sensitivity of a cocktail of recombinant antigens used in the indirect enzyme-linked immunosorbent assay with a rapid-format antibody card test. Rodriguez-Pérez MA, Dominguez-Vázquez A, Méndez-Galván J, et al. Trans R Soc Trop Med Hyg 2003;97:539–41.

Recently, a rapid format immunochromatography test (ICT) has been developed and compared with an ELISA using three recombinant antigens in a Mexican population. The sensitivities of the ELISA and ICT were 97 and 86%, respectively.

Polymerase chain reaction-based diagnosis of *Onchocerca volvulus* infection: improved detection of patients with onchocerciasis. Zimmerman PA, Guderian RH, Aruajo E, et al. J Infect Dis 1994;169:686–9.

PCR-based assays to detect the repetitive DNA sequence known as O-150 (found only in *O. volvulus*) in skin snips show 100% species specificity and 100% sensitivity. The PCR method is more sensitive than skin snipping in patients with low intensities of infection.

Detection of *Onchocerca volvulus* infection by O-150 polymerase chain reaction analysis of skin scratches. Toé L, Boatin BA, Adjami A, et al. J Infect Dis 1998;178:282-5.

Unlike skin snipping, detection of parasite DNA in skin scrapings is minimally invasive, painless, and presents no risk for the transmission of blood-borne diseases.

Although PCR tests are expensive and require considerable laboratory expertise, newer 'DNA detection test strips' are a rapid and low-tech tool for potential future use in endemic countries.

DEC patch test

This 'Mazzotti patch test' assesses the local reaction to 10% DEC in Nivea® cream or Nivea® milk.

Detection of *Onchocerca volvulus* infection in low prevalence areas: a comparison of three diagnostic methods. Boatin BA, Toé L, Alley ES, et al. Parasitology 2002;125:545–52.

Where prevalence is low, PCR and the DEC patch test are more sensitive than skin-snipping, which has a low sensitivity.

FIRST LINE THERAPIES

■ Ivermectin	A
■ Ivermectin combined with doxycycline	B

The effects of ivermectin on onchocercal skin disease and severe itching: results of a multicentre trial. Brieger WR,

Awedoba AK, Eneanya CI, et al. Trop Med Int Health 1998;3:951–61.

The effects of ivermectin were assessed in 3-monthly, 6-monthly, and annual doses in 4072 villagers in forest zones of Ghana, Nigeria, and Uganda who underwent interviews and clinical examinations at baseline and at five follow-up visits. Reactive skin lesions were categorized as acute papular onchodermatitis, chronic papular onchodermatitis, and lichenified onchodermatitis. From 6 months onwards, there was a 40–50% reduction in the prevalence of severe itching after ivermectin treatment compared with the placebo group. Also, a greater decrease in prevalence and severity of reactive skin lesions over time was seen in those receiving ivermectin. The differences between the various ivermectin treatment regimens were not significant.

A trial of a three-dose regimen of ivermectin for the treatment of patients with onchocerciasis in the U.K. Churchill DR, Godfrey-Faussett P, Birley HDL, et al. Trans R Soc Trop Med Hyg 1994;88:242.

As ivermectin is also thought to suppress embryogenesis in adult worms, the efficacy of three doses of ivermectin given at monthly intervals was studied to determine whether such a regimen could lead to a greater suppression of microfilaridermia. Thirty three patients (of whom 27 were European) with onchocerciasis were treated with a single dose of 150–200 μg/kg ivermectin and observed in hospital for 72 h. Second and third doses of ivermectin were given as outpatients 1 and 2 months later, respectively. Patients were followed up at 3-, 6-, and 12-monthly intervals after the last dose of ivermectin. The patients with positive skin snips prior to treatment were compared with patients given a single dose of ivermectin in a previous study (Godfrey-Faussett P et al., 1991, see below). Relapses occurred slightly less frequently after three doses.

In contrast to studies in West Africa where reactions to ivermectin are rare, 17 patients (52%) had reactions to ivermectin. The authors therefore recommend that the first dose of ivermectin for lightly infected expatriates is given in hospital.

The treatment of lightly infected expatriates with onchocerciasis is therefore a single dose of 150–200 μg/kg ivermectin with observation in hospital for 72 h, followed by two subsequent doses at monthly intervals. If there is a recurrence of itching, a typical rash, or eosinophilia, the individual may require further doses of ivermectin at 6–12-monthly intervals.

Ivermectin in the treatment of onchocerciasis in Britain. Godfrey-Faussett P, Dow C, Black ME, Bryceson ADM. Trop Med Parasitol 1991;42:82–4.

Thirty one patients with early, light infection were treated with a single dose of 150–200 μg/kg ivermectin. Those who relapsed were re-treated after an interval of not less than 5 months. Approximately two-thirds relapsed within 1 year. A similar pattern was seen after the second dose. A single dose of ivermectin, repeated every 3–6 months as necessary, was considered to be the treatment of choice for patients in nonendemic areas, lightly infected with *O. volvulus*. One-third of such patients may be cured with each treatment.

Effects of standard and high doses of ivermectin on adult worms of *Onchocerca volvulus*: a randomised controlled trial. Gardon J, Boussinesq M, Kamgno J, et al. Lancet 2002;360:203–10.

Ivermectin, given at 150 µg/kg at intervals of 0.5–3.0 months is known to cause slight but significant increased mortality of adult worms. In this randomized study of 657 Cameroonian patients with onchocerciasis, 3-monthly treatment with ivermectin killed more female adult worms than annual treatment. There was no difference between standard (150 µg/kg) and high-dose schedules (800 µg/kg).

The feasibility of large-scale 3-monthly ivermectin treatment in endemic areas and its likely greater effect in reducing transmission have still to be determined.

An investigation of persistent microfilaridermias despite multiple treatments with ivermectin, in two onchocerciasis-endemic foci in Ghana. Awadzi K, Boakye DA, Edwards G, et al. Ann Trop Med Parasitol 2004;98:231–49.

Some individuals in endemic areas have persistent microfilaridermia despite nine treatments with ivermectin. In this open, case–control study of 21 'suboptimal' responders, seven amicrofilaridermic responders and 14 ivermectin-naïve subjects, the results revealed that the persistent microfilaridermias are mainly due to nonresponsiveness of the adult female worms, raising the possibility that the worms have developed resistance to ivermectin.

Adverse systemic reactions to treatment of onchocerciasis with ivermectin at normal and high doses given annually or three-monthly. Kamgno J, Gardon J, Gardon-Wendel N, et al. Trans R Soc Trop Med Hyg 2004;98:496–504.

In Cameroon, after the first dose, ivermectin 150 µg/kg given at 3-monthly intervals was associated with a reduced risk of reactions (especially edematous swellings, pruritus, and back pain) compared with standard annual treatment doses of 150 µg/kg. High doses of ivermectin (800 µg/kg) at annual and 3-monthly intervals caused subjective ocular symptoms.

Endosymbiotic bacteria in worms as targets for a novel chemotherapy in filariasis. Hoerauf A, Volkmann L, Hamelmann C, et al. Lancet 2000;355:1242–3.

Activity of doxycycline against endosymbiotic *Wolbachia* spp. bacteria and fertility of adult female worms was assessed by examination of excised subcutaneous onchocercal nodules in 22 Ghanian individuals treated with doxycycline 100 mg daily for 6 weeks and 14 untreated controls. Immunohistology with an antibody to bacterial heat shock protein-60 was used to assess presence or absence of *Wolbachia* spp. and the morphology of female worms was examined. In addition PCR reactions using first endobacterial primers and second nematode primers were performed. None of the treated worms had usual bacterial loads and there was total suppression of normal embryonic worm development during early oocyte/morula stages, while nodules from untreated controls showed normal embryogenesis.

Depletion of Wolbachia endobacteria in *Onchocerca volvulus* by doxycycline and microfilaridermia after ivermectin treatment. Hoerauf A, Mand S, Adjei O, et al. Lancet 2001;357:1415–6.

The Ghanian participants in this study were not randomized because this was not acceptable to the village elders. Instead, the first 55 patients were allocated to ivermectin and doxycycline and the next 33 to ivermectin alone.

Doxycycline 100 mg daily was given from the start of the study for 6 weeks. Subgroup A (31 doxycycline-treated and 24 controls) was given ivermectin 2.5 months after the start of the study and subgroup B (24 doxycycline-treated and nine controls) 6 months after the onset of the study. The results suggested a complete block in worm embryogenesis for at least 18 months after treatment with ivermectin and doxycycline.

The principle of targeting *Wolbachia* spp. in combination with ivermectin offers the potential of interrupting transmission. Shorter anti-*Wolbachia* spp. regimens (either with other antibiotics or combinations) are needed for mass treatment of endemic areas.

A combination of doxycycline (100 mg daily for 6 weeks) plus ivermectin is now advisable for individuals leaving an onchocerciasis-endemic area for a long time.

SECOND LINE THERAPIES

■ Albendazole	A

Albendazole in the treatment of onchocerciasis: double-blind clinical trial in Venezuela. Cline BL, Hernandez JL, Mather FJ, et al. Am J Trop Med Hyg 1992;47:512–20.

Forty nine individuals with onchocerciasis (26 treated and 23 controls) were treated with a 10-day course of albendazole (400 mg daily) or placebo. Patients with baseline microfilarial densities over 5 mf/mg skin showed a significant decrease in microfilarial densities at 12 months in the albendazole-treated group. Albendazole was well tolerated and is believed to interfere with embryogenesis in adult *O. volvulus* worms.

The co-administration of ivermectin and albendazole – safety, pharmacokinetics and efficacy against *Onchocerca volvulus*. Awadzi K, Edwards G, Duke BOL, et al. Ann Trop Med Parasitol 2003;97:165–78.

In a randomized double-blind, placebo-controlled trial in 44 male patients with onchocerciasis in Ghana, the co-administration of ivermectin (200 µg/kg) with albendazole (400 mg) did not offer any advantage over ivermectin alone.

The safety, tolerability and pharmacokinetics of levamisole alone, levamisole plus ivermectin, and levamisole plus albendazole, and their efficacy against *Onchocerca volvulus*. Awadzi K, Edwards G, Opoku NO, et al. Ann Trop Med Parasitol 2004;98:595–614.

Levamisole (2.5 mg/kg) given alone or with albendazole (400 mg) had little effect on *O. volvulus*. Co-administration of ivermectin (200 µg/kg) with levamisole was no more effective than ivermectin alone.

OTHER THERAPIES

■ Suramin	
■ Future therapies	
– New macrofilaricides	

Thirty-month follow-up of sub-optimal responders to multiple treatments with ivermectin, in two onchocerciasis-endemic foci in Ghana. Awadzi K, Attah SK, Addy ET, et al. Ann Trop Med Parasitol 2004;98:359–70.

Evidence levels **A** Double-blind study **B** Clinical trial ≥ 20 subjects **C** Clinical trial < 20 subjects **D** Series ≥ 5 subjects **E** Anecdotal case reports

A macrofilaricide is a drug that can kill adult parasite worms and hence a single course of treatment is potentially curative. Suramin is a macrofilaricide and a microfilaricide, but unfortunately a course of suramin requires weekly intravenous infusions and may cause serious adverse effects including nephrotoxicity. After the use of ivermectin became widely established, the only indications for suramin were: the curative treatment of selected individuals in areas without transmission and that of individuals leaving an endemic area; and severe hyper-reactive onchodermatitis unresponsive to repeated treatments with ivermectin.

In this paper Awadzi et al. propose the use of suramin under hospital supervision in selected individuals with onchocerciasis who are resistant to multiple doses of ivermectin. The treatment regimen proposed was a total adult dose of 5.0 g (72.5–84.7 mg/kg) over 6 weeks.

The antiparasitic moxidectin: safety, tolerability, and pharmacokinetics in humans. Cotreau MM, Warren S, Ryan JL, et al. J Clin Pharmacol 2003;43:1108–15.

As there is now a considerable risk of the development of ivermectin resistance, there is an urgent need to find a safe macrofilaricide suitable for large-scale field use. Molecules chemically related to known antiparasitic drugs are currently being evaluated. Moxidectin is already in use in veterinary medicine, and studies in animal models suggest that it is a potential macrofilaricidal agent. This preliminary study in healthy human male volunteers revealed that moxidectin is safe and well tolerated between the doses of 3 and 36 mg.

Oral lichen planus

Alison J Bruce, Roy S Rogers III

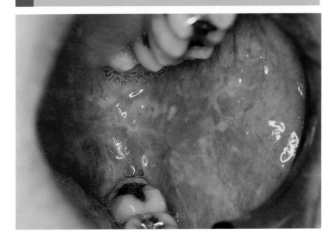

Oral lichen planus (OLP) is a common disease of the oral mucosa with a reported incidence equivalent to that of psoriasis. Unlike cutaneous lichen planus, the disease remains chronic with a fluctuant course and few complete remissions. Clinical variants range from asymptomatic reticulated lesions to debilitating erosive disease necessitating treatment. Extraoral involvement is frequent and sites include genital mucosa, esophagus, eyes, ears, scalp, and nails.

MANAGEMENT STRATEGY

OLP seldom achieves spontaneous remission and patients should anticipate a chronic course with intermittent acute exacerbations. Therapy is tailored to control of symptoms because no curative treatment exists. Asymptomatic patients do not require treatment.

The overall lifetime risk of developing squamous cell carcinoma in association with lichen planus is in the order of 1% and patients should be followed annually. Although there are no confirmatory data, it seems likely that the erosive forms of disease are associated with a higher risk of malignancy, and control of severe erosive disease is appropriate both to alleviate symptoms and reduce this theoretical risk. Patients who are asymptomatic between flares may require treatment only for acute episodes.

Provocative factors such as irritant foods, mechanical trauma, and tobacco use should be avoided, and dental plaque and calculus controlled. Allergies to dental metals have been implicated as a causative factor in OLP and in patients with severe or refractory disease, particularly that adjacent to fillings, patch testing to dental materials should be undertaken. If positive allergens are identified, serious consideration should be given to removal of the offending dental restoration. (In our experience, patients with strong positive reaction on patch testing, and disease most severe in tissues contiguous to the offending dental metal, improve greatly with removal of the dental restoration.)

For mild localized disease with infrequent flares, *high-potency topical corticosteroids* should be applied three to four times daily to affected areas for 2–4 weeks or until symptomatic control is achieved and then gradually tapered. We favor topical fluocinonide gel.

Topical immunosuppressants such as *tacrolimus* are proving to be highly effective in patients with both mild and moderate disease, as well as for the management of other mucosal sites. Tacrolimus 0.1% should be applied three to four times daily to affected areas. The response may be rapid, within 2–3 weeks, and once the acute flare is controlled the regimen should be gradually tapered to the lowest dosing regimen that keeps the disease quiescent. The patient should be aware that this is an off-label indication and the medication is labeled 'for external use only'.

Patients can use *palliative mouthwashes* for symptom control irrespective of disease severity. Various combinations of antihistamines, coating agents, and anesthetics can be compounded. We typically use an elixir of diphenhydramine and Maalox®, occasionally with the addition of viscous lidocaine if necessary.

Patients with more severe flares usually respond to *oral prednisone* 40–60 mg daily tapered over 3–6 weeks, or the use of *intralesional corticosteroids* injected submucosally. This use of corticosteroids is appropriate for acute flares, but is not suitable for maintenance therapy in patients with more frequent attacks or severe involvement, and these patients should be considered for systemic anti-inflammatory therapies.

Retinoids, both topically and systemically, have been reported as therapeutically beneficial, though not reliably so. Anecdotally, topical retinoids are more helpful with localized gingival disease. *Systemically administered acitretin 25–50 mg daily has been used for OLP. Hydroxychloroquine* may also be of benefit.

For control of severe OLP, or in patients with involvement of mucosal sites such as the esophagus or eyes, systemic immunosuppressives may be indicated such as *azathioprine* or *mycophenolate mofetil* along with aggressive local therapy. *Cyclosporine* has been reported to be of benefit both topically and as a systemic agent, but the former mode of delivery is too costly for practical use. Recently, use of the *308 nm excimer laser* has been reported, but data are limited.

Intercurrent candidiasis should be suspected in patients who have had good control of the disease and have a sudden deterioration.

SPECIFIC INVESTIGATIONS

- Biopsy for hematoxylin and eosin and direct immunofluorescence testing
- Annual follow-up for monitoring with biopsy of suspicious or atypical areas
- Hepatitis serologies (no longer routine)
- Patch testing in patients with dental restorations and lichenoid tissue changes adjacent to restorations

The sensitivity and specificity of direct immunofluoresence testing in disorders of mucous membranes. Helander SD, Rogers RS III. J Am Acad Dermatol 1994;30:65–75.

The authors report that the gingivae represent the best site for obtaining an immunofluorescence biopsy specimen in patients with OLP. The clinical and histological appearances of gingival lesions are often nondiagnostic and a biopsy for immunofluorescence showing characteristic shaggy fibrinogen deposition at the basement membrane zone is helpful in establishing the diagnosis of OLP.

Evidence levels **A** Double-blind study **B** Clinical trial ≥ 20 subjects **C** Clinical trial < 20 subjects **D** Series ≥ 5 subjects **E** Anecdotal case reports

The clinical features, malignant potential, and systemic associations of oral lichen planus: a study of 723 patients. Eisen DR. J Am Acad Dermatol 2002;46:207–14.

Although an association between hepatitis infection and OLP has been previously reported, this association may depend on geographic factors. Based on the findings in this large series, routine hepatitis screening in Western European and American patients is not warranted. Oral squamous cell carcinoma developed in six of 723 patients (0.8%), in keeping with the previously reported risk.

Relevant contact sensitivities in patients with the diagnosis of oral lichen planus. Yiannias JA, el-Azhary RA, Hand JH, et al. J Am Acad Dermatol 2000;42:177–82.

In 46 patients with lichenoid lesions and a diagnosis of OLP, 17 had positive reactions to metals – 14 of these patients reacted to gold, and within this group, ten were thought to be clinically relevant in the development of OLP. Four patients' symptoms resolved after removal of the gold filling.

Lichenoid contact stomatitis: is inorganic mercury the culprit? Rogers RS III, Bruce AJ. Arch Dermatol 2004;140: 1524–5.

FIRST LINE THERAPIES

■ Topical corticosteroids	B
■ Topical tacrolimus	C
■ Intralesional corticosteroids	E

Topical corticosteroids in association with miconazole and chlorhexidine in the long-term management of atrophic-erosive oral lichen planus: a placebo-controlled and comparative study between clobetasol and fluocinonide. Carbone M, Conrotto D, Carrozzo M, et al. Oral Dis 1999; 5:44–9.

Systemic and topical corticosteroid treatment of oral lichen planus: a comparative study with long-term follow-up. Carbone M, Goss E, Carrozzo M, et al. J Oral Pathol Med 2003;32:323–9.

Two groups of patients treated with either topical clobetasol alone or after initial systemic prednisone yielded similar results, suggesting that topical high-potency corticosteroid therapy remains suitable, easy, and cost-effective.

Higher-potency preparations seem to be more effective than mid-potency corticosteroids, and should be used initially to achieve control, and then tapered. The use of topical corticosteroids is based on many heterogeneous trials with variation in design and response criteria.

Intralesional triamcinolone (10–20 mg/mL) diluted 1:1 with lidocaine can be highly effective for severe erosive lesions. These can be repeated 4–6-weekly until control is achieved.

The clinical manifestations and treatment of oral lichen planus. Eisen DR. Dermatol Clin 2003;21:79–89.

An excellent review article with stepwise approach to therapy.

Long-term efficacy and safety of topical tacrolimus in the management of ulcerative/erosive oral lichen planus. Hodgson TA, Sahni N, Kaliakatsou F, et al. Eur J Dermatol 2003;13:466–70.

Topical tacrolimus in the treatment of symptomatic oral lichen planus: a series of 13 patients. Rozycki TW, Rogers RS III, Pittelkow MR, et al. J Am Acad Dermatol 2002; 46:27–34.

Several publications document the efficacy of tacrolimus in controlling erosive OLP. It appears to provide rapid control in the majority of patients with minimal side effects. No randomized controlled trials exist to date.

Response of oral lichen planus to topical tacrolimus in 37 patients. Byrd JA, Davis MDP, Bruce AJ, et al. Arch Dermatol 2004;140:715–20.

SECOND LINE THERAPIES

■ Systemic corticosteroids	C
■ Topical retinoids	C
■ Systemic retinoids	A
■ Hydroxychloroquine	C
■ Systemic immunosuppressives (azathioprine, mycophenolate mofetil)	B

Topical retinaldehyde treatment in oral lichen planus and leukoplakia. Boisnic S, Licu D, Ben Slama L, et al. Int J Tissue React 2002;24:123–30.

Seventeen patients were treated with 0.1% retinaldehyde gel, which showed good clinical efficacy.

Treatment of lichen planus with acitretin: a double-blind, placebo-controlled study in 65 patients. Laurberg G, Geiger JM, Hjorth N, et al. J Am Acad Dermatol 1991; 24:434–7.

Treatment of oral erosive lichen planus with systemic isotretinoin. Camisa C, Allen CM. Oral Surg Oral Med Oral Pathol 1986;62:393–6.

Treatment of lichen planus: an evidence-based medicine analysis of efficacy. Cribier B, Frances C, Chosidow O. Arch Dermatol 1998;134:1521–30.

Systemic isotretinoin treatment of oral and cutaneous lichen planus. Woo TY. Cutis 1985;35:390–1.

These studies show the efficacy of acitretin 30 mg daily in management of cutaneous lichen planus. Etretinate (25–50 mg daily), isotretinoin (0.5 mg/kg daily), and tretinoin (10–30 mg daily) have also had some degree of success in treating cutaneous lichen planus. Woo's study showed two patients successfully treated with oral isotretinoin that responded rapidly. Camisa and Allen had five of six patients slightly improved in 8 weeks on oral isotretinoin 10–60 mg daily.

Hydroxychloroquine sulfate (Plaquenil) improves oral lichen planus: an open trial. Eisen D. J Am Acad Dermatol 1993;28:609–12.

Nine of ten patients had an excellent response to hydroxychloroquine 200–400 mg daily as monotherapy for 6 months. Three of six patients with erosions at baseline had complete healing. Pain relief and reduced erythema were usually observed after 1–2 months of therapy, but erosions required 3–6 months of treatment before they resolved. There were no adverse effects.

A prospective study of findings and management in 214 patients with oral lichen planus. Silverman Jr S, Gorsky M, Lozada-Nur F, et al. Oral Surg Oral Med Oral Pathol Oral Radiol Endod 1991;72:665–70.

Azathioprine may be effective for OLP. Initial doses of 50 mg daily can be initiated and advanced to 100–150 mg daily if indicated, recognizing that clinical response is slow and may require 3–6 months of therapy before maximal benefit is achieved.

New and emerging therapies for diseases of the oral cavity. Popovsky JL, Caisa C. Dermatol Clin 2000;18:113–25.

Mycophenolate mofetil is emerging as a new and effective therapy for OLP. Doses of 2–3 g daily may be needed to achieve control. The response and side effect profile are similar to azathioprine, but the drug is considerably more costly.

THIRD LINE THERAPIES

■ Cyclosporine	D
■ Sulodexide	D
■ Phenytoin	D
■ Thalidomide	E
■ Laser	D

Severe lichen planus clears with very low-dose cyclosporine. Levell NJ, Munro CS, Marks JM. Br J Dermatol 1992;127:66–7.

Because of potential toxicity, systemic cyclosporine should be reserved for refractory cases and used for limited duration. Topical cyclosporine is prohibitively expensive, but in unusual cases a small amount of the 100 mg/mL solution can be used as a mouthwash one to three times daily. Reports on the efficacy of topical cyclosporine are varied.

Oral erosive/ulcerative lichen planus: preliminary findings in an open trial of sulodexide compared with cyclosporine (ciclosporin) therapy. Femiano F, Gombos F, Scully C. Int J Dermatol 2003;42:308–11.

A heparinoid, sulodexide, administered systemically may be more effective than topical cyclosporine.

Lichen planus: treatment of thirty cases with systemic and topical phenytoin. Bogaert H, Sanchez E. Int J Dermatol 1990;29:157–8.

Two of four cases with oral lesions cleared with phenytoin.

Effective treatment of oral erosive lichen planus with thalidomide. Camisa C, Popovsky JL. Arch Dermatol 2000; 136:1442–3.

A single report of oral erosive LP unresponsive to prednisolone and many other immunosuppressive agents, resolving with thalidomide over 12 months (initially 50 mg daily, increasing to 100 mg daily), with recurrence on discontinuation.

Treatment of oral lichen planus with the 308-nm UVB excimer laser – early preliminary results in eight patients. Kollner K, Wimmershoff M, Landthaler M, et al. Lasers Surg Med 2003;33:158–60.

Six of eight patients treated with this laser technique showed clinical improvement; two had complete remission.

Orf

Jane C Sterling

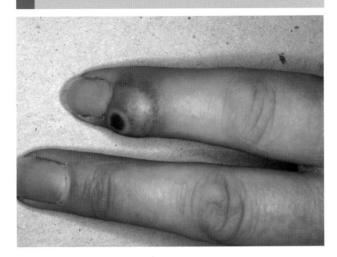

Orf is an infection by a parapoxvirus, which causes inflammation and necrosis of the skin at the site of viral entry. It is predominantly an occupational disease because the orf virus is carried by sheep and occasionally goats.

MANAGEMENT STRATEGY

Orf is a self-limiting viral disease and *treatment is usually not necessary*. The immune response to the virus will usually result in resolution of the disease within 2–7 weeks without any specific treatment. There is no available treatment that is specifically antiviral for the orf virus and no human vaccine has been produced. Treatment is usually only indicated if there is secondary bacterial infection or immunosuppression. Erythema multiforme can be triggered by orf infection.

Various treatments have been reported anecdotally. *Idoxuridine, surgery,* and *cryotherapy* have been suggested to reduce the time to healing. For immunosuppressed individuals, infection with orf may result in a more persistent infection or giant orf. In such cases, interventional treatment is warranted. Surgery may be performed to remove the bulk of the infected tissue. Idoxuridine, *cidofovir,* and cryotherapy have also been reported to improve time to healing or to clear persistent infection. *Interferon* has shown some potential benefit.

SPECIFIC INVESTIGATIONS

- Electron microscopy of scrapings from lesion
- Biopsy

Diagnosis is usually clinical, but can be confirmed by the above investigations if required.

The structure of the orf virus. Nagington J, Newton A, Horne RW. Virology 1964;23:461–72.

The ultrastructural description of the orf virus.

Orf. Report of 19 human cases with clinical and pathological observations. Leavell UW, McNamara MJ, Muelling R, et al. JAMA 1968;204:109–16.

Detailed description of clinical and histological features of 19 cases of orf infection. Defines six stages of infection. Over half the lesions healed within 5 weeks.

FIRST LINE THERAPIES

- No specific treatment usually necessary

For most patients, treatment of this virus infection is unnecessary because natural clearance will occur.

Orf. Report of 19 human cases with clinical and pathological observations. Leavell UW, McNamara MJ, Muelling R, et al. JAMA 1968;204:109–16.

Lymphangitis and lymphadenopathy occurred in three of 19 cases.

Awareness of the risk of secondary bacterial infection is important.

SECOND LINE THERAPIES

■ Surgery	D
■ Cryotherapy	E
■ Idoxuridine	E
■ Cidofovir	E
■ Interferon	E

Orf nodule: treatment with cryosurgery. Candiani JO, Soto RG, Lozano OW. J Am Acad Dermatol 1993;29:256–7.

A healthy female with orf received a single treatment with liquid nitrogen (two freeze–thaw cycles) and the lesion healed in 2 weeks.

A case of ecthyma contagiosum (human orf) treated with idoxuridine. Hundkaar S. Dermatologica 1984;168:207.

The orf lesion of a healthy female was treated with 40% idoxuridine in dimethylsulfoxide three times daily for 6 days. The lesion healed in under 4 weeks.

Parapoxvirus orf in kidney transplantation. Peeters P, Sennasael J. Nephrol Dial Transplant 1998;13:531.

A large lesion on the thumb recurred after excisional surgery. After 40% idoxuridine topically, further surgery, and repeated cryotherapy, the lesion resolved.

'Giant' orf of finger in a patient with a lymphoma. Savage J, Black MM. Proc Roy Soc Med 1972;65:28–30.

A patient who had received chemotherapy developed an enlarging orf lesion on one finger. Amputation of the finger was performed.

Giant orf in a patient with chronic lymphocytic leukaemia. Hunskaar S. Br J Dermatol 1986;114:631–4.

A large palmar orf lesion was excised and small local recurrences treated with 40% idoxuridine.

A case of human orf in an immunocompromised patient treated successfully with cidofovir cream. Geerinck K, Lukito G, Snoeck R, et al. J Med Virol 2001;64:543–9.

An immunosuppressed renal transplant patient developed a persistent giant orf lesion. Treatment with 1%

cidofovir cream daily for five cycles of 5 days of treatment alternating with five rest days plus debridement as necessary led to full resolution of the lesion.

Recurrent orf in an immunocompromised host. Tan ST, Blake GB, Chambers S. Br J Plast Surg 1991;44:465–7.

A tumor-like orf lesion in an immunosuppressed patient was unresponsive to surgery and idoxuridine. Temporary improvement occurred after 2 weeks of daily intralesional interferon of 1 million IU per injection with clearance following repeat surgery with subcutaneous interferon (1 million IU daily).

Evidence levels A Double-blind study **B** Clinical trial ≥ 20 subjects **C** Clinical trial < 20 subjects **D** Series ≥ 5 subjects **E** Anecdotal case reports

Palmoplantar keratoderma

Ravi Ratnavel

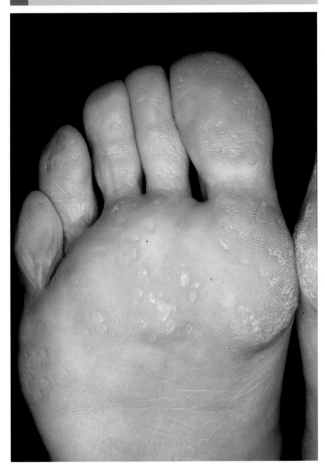

Palmoplantar keratodermas (PPKs) consist of a heterogeneous group of disorders characterized by thickening of the palms and soles. The condition may be subdivided into hereditary keratodermas, acquired forms, and syndromes with PPK as an associated feature of a specific dermatosis.

MANAGEMENT STRATEGY

PPK may be localized to the hands and feet or develop as part of a more generalized skin disorder. It is important to establish its morphology and the presence of any associated ectodermal disease at sites other than the palms and soles when making a diagnosis. Biopsy may be necessary to distinguish between some hereditary forms of PPK. PPK can be associated with infections (dermatophytes, human papillomavirus, HIV, syphilis, and scabies), drugs (arsenic exposure), and internal malignancy, or may be a cutaneous manifestation of systemic disease (myxedema, diabetes mellitus, or cutaneous T cell lymphoma). Hyperkeratosis of the palms and soles can also be a feature of eczema, psoriasis, and cutaneous T cell lymphoma.

The treatment of PPK is difficult. Most therapeutic options produce only short-term improvement and are frequently compounded by unwanted adverse effects. Treatment options range from simple measures such as salt-water soaks with paring and topical keratolytics to systemic retinoids and reconstructive surgery with total excision of the hyperkeratotic skin followed by grafting.

In patients with limited disease, *topical keratolytics* containing salicylic acid, lactic acid, or urea in a suitable base may be tried. Examples include 5–10% salicylic acid, 10–40% propylene glycol, or 10% lactic acid in aqueous cream or a combination therapy using 10% urea and 5% lactic acid in aqueous cream to be applied twice daily. These formulations can be made up on an individual basis or the closest proprietary product prescribed. The efficacy of these agents may be increased by occlusion at night. *Topical retinoids* such as tretinoin (0.01% gel and 0.1% cream) may also be tried; treatment is often limited by skin irritation. *Potent topical corticosteroids*, such as clobetasol propionate 0.05%, with or without keratolytics are occasionally of value in inflammatory PPK. *5-fluorouracil*, 5%, has produced dramatic results in spiny keratoderma, but its use in other keratodermas has not been evaluated.

The efficacy of the *oral retinoids* in keratoderma is well established. Good responses have been seen in mal de Meleda, Papillon-Lefèvre syndrome, and erythrokeratoderma variabilis. In some types of PPK, hyperesthesia may limit usefulness or practicality of treatment with retinoids. The risk of bone toxicity should also be carefully assessed against the benefits of treatment in patients on long-term therapy. Yearly radiologic bone monitoring is recommended and intermittent therapy should be prescribed whenever possible. The optimal dosage of acitretin is between 25 and 35 mg daily in adults or 0.7 mg/kg daily in children, which may be adjusted after 4 weeks of therapy.

Psoralen plus UVA (PUVA) therapy or *Re-PUVA* (synergistic combination of oral retinoids and PUVA) may be effective in PPK secondary to psoriasis or eczema. In oculocutaneous tyrosinemia (an autosomal recessive condition characterized by focal palmoplantar keratosis, corneal ulceration, and mental retardation), *dietary restriction of phenylalanine and tyrosine* has led to resolution of PPK. *Oral administration of 1-α, 25-dihydroxyvitamin D_3* and *topical calcipotriol* ointment have been reported to be effective. Regular chiropody, careful selection of footwear, and treatment of secondary fungal infections is an integral part of management of all PPK. *Surgical or laser dermabrasion* is an option for some patients, with potential amelioration of symptoms and improved penetration of topical agents.

For severe refractory PPK *excision and skin grafting* may be considered. Excision should remove the hyperkeratotic skin, including dermis, epidermis, and subcutis to prevent any risk of recurrence.

SPECIFIC INVESTIGATIONS

- Scrapings for mycology
- Thyroid function tests

An epidemiologic investigation of dermatologic fungus infections in the northernmost county of Sweden (Norbotten) 1977–81. Gamborg Nielson P. Mykosen 1984;27: 203–10.

In a 5-year survey of dermatophyte infections in Norbotten the frequency of dermatophytosis among patients with hereditary PPK was shown to be 35%, corresponding to a prevalence of 36.7%. The predominant feature of dermatophytosis in patients with hereditary PPK was scaling and fissuring. Treatment improved the clinical signs after 2–3 months.

Hereditary palmoplantar keratoderma and dermatophytosis in the northernmost county of Sweden (Norbotten). Gamborg Nielson P. Acta Derm Venereol Suppl (Stockh) 1994;188:1–60.

In relatives of the original propositi, dermatophytosis was found in 65% of men, 22% of women, and 21% of children, resulting in a total frequency of 36.2%. Statistically, it was proven that *Trichophyton mentagrophytes* occurred more often in patients with hereditary PPK. Vesicular eruptions along the hyperkeratotic border occurred significantly more often in patients with dermatophytosis and were considered pathognomonic of secondary dermatophytosis.

Palmoplantar keratoderma in association with myxoedema. Hodak E, David M, Feuerman EJ. Acta Derm Venereol 1986;66:354–5.

A patient with myxedema and intractable PPK showed improvement after treatment with thyroid replacement therapy. The possibility of a causal relationship between hypothyroidism and PPK was questioned.

Severe palmar keratoderma with myxoedema. Tan OT, Sarkany I. Clin Exp Dermatol 1977;2:287–8.

A patient with myxedema and PPK showed rapid improvement in PPK after thyroxine treatment.

FIRST LINE THERAPIES

■ Topical keratolytics	B
■ Topical retinoids	B

Vitamin A acid in the treatment of palmoplantar keratoderma. Gunther SH. Arch Dermatol 1972;106:854–7.

Nine patients with PPK were treated with retinoic acid 0.1% in petroleum jelly and all improved within 4 months. Permanent remission ensued in two patients. Recurrence was observed in the majority of cases 8 weeks after the withdrawal of treatment. This was avoided by the topical application of vitamin A acid once or twice weekly.

Topical treatment of keratosis palmaris et plantaris with tretinoin. Touraine R, Revuz J. Acta Derm Venereol Suppl (Stockh) 1975;(suppl 74):152–3.

Six patients were treated for 2 months with either tretinoin 0.1% lotion or 0.05% cream. Improvement was seen in most patients. Better results were achieved with the use of occlusive dressings, mechanical paring prior to topical application, or when a higher concentration of topical tretinoin was used (0.3%).

SECOND LINE THERAPIES

■ Systemic retinoids	A

The treatment of keratosis palmaris et plantaris with isotretinoin. A multicenter study. Bergfeld WF, Derbes VJ, Elias PM, et al. J Am Acad Dermatol 1982;6:727–31.

Five of six patients with PPK were safely and effectively treated with isotretinoin with dramatic clearing of the keratoderma within the first 4 weeks of therapy. The mean dose was 1.95 mg/kg daily, with a mean duration of therapy of 113 days.

Acitretin in the treatment of severe disorders of keratinisation. Results of an open study. Blanchet-Bardon C, Nazzaro VV, Rognin C, et al. J Am Acad Dermatol 1991; 24:983–6.

An open, noncomparative study to evaluate the clinical response of patients with nonpsoriatic disorders of keratinization to acitretin and to establish the optimal dosage for efficacy and tolerance. Thirty three patients with ichthyoses, PPK, or Darier's disease were treated for 4 months. Most patients showed marked improvement. The optimal acitretin dosage providing the best efficacy with minimal side effects varied from patient to patient. The mean daily dose ($\pm$ SD) was 27 $\pm$ 11 mg in adults and 0.7 $\pm$ 0.2 mg/kg in children.

A controlled study of comparative efficacy of oral retinoids and topical betamethasone/salicylic acid for chronic hyperkeratotic palmoplantar dermatitis. Capella GL, Fracchiolla C, Frigerio E, Altomare G. J Dermatolog Treat 2004;15:88–93.

A single-blind, matched-sample investigation was carried out in 42 patients with chronic hyperkeratotic palmoplantar dermatitis, who were administered acitretin 25–50 mg daily for 1 month, which was controlled vs a conventional topical treatment (betamethasone/salicylic acid ointment). Acitretin was significantly better than the conventional treatment after 30 days (two sided p < 0.0001). The authors suggested that acitretin should be considered a first choice treatment

Acitretin in the treatment of mal de Meleda. Van de Kerkhof PC, Dooren-Greebe RJ, Steijlen PM. Br J Dermatol 1992;127:191–2.

Two patients with mal de Meleda treated with acitretin experienced a marked reduction of PPK. The optimal dosage was found to be between 10 and 30 mg daily. Higher dosages resulted in hyperesthesia. Discontinuation of acitretin resulted in relapse within days.

Keratoderma climactericum (Haxthausen's disease): clinical and laboratory findings and etretinate treatment in 10 patients. Deschamps P, Leroy D, Pedailles S, Mandard JC. Dermatologica 1986;172:258–62.

Etretinate 0.7–0.8 mg/kg daily brought about partial or total remission of hyperkeratosis in ten cases of keratoderma climactericum.

Mutilating palmoplantar keratoderma successfully treated with etretinate. Wereide K. Acta Derm Venereol 1984;64: 556–9.

Three patients with mutilating keratodermas were successfully treated with oral etretinate. All had constriction of one or more digits with impending pseudoamputation. Treatment resulted in disappearance of the pseudoainhum and normalization of the digital blood circulation.

It is assumed that acitretin would provide a similar outcome.

Evidence levels **A** Double-blind study **B** Clinical trial ≥ 20 subjects **C** Clinical trial < 20 subjects **D** Series ≥ 5 subjects **E** Anecdotal case reports

THIRD LINE THERAPIES

■ Reconstructive surgery with total excision of hyperkeratotic skin followed by grafting	C
■ Topical calcipotriol	E
■ Oral vitamin D3 analogues	E
■ Topical corticosteroids with or without keratolytics	E
■ PUVA or Re-PUVA	D
■ Dermabrasion	E
■ CO_2 laser	B
■ 5-fluorouracil	E
■ Tyrosine-restricted diet in oculocutaneous keratoderma	E

Plastic surgery in the management of palmoplantar keratoderma (palmoplantar neoplasty). Farina R. Aesthetic Plast Surg 1987;11:249–53.

Five cases of PPK were treated successfully by grafting skin taken from the calves and thighs.

Surgical treatment of epidermolytic hereditary palmoplantar keratoderma. Tropet Y, Zultak M, Blanc D, Laurent R, Vichard P. J Hand Surg [Am] 1989;14:143–9.

A patient with epidermolytic PPK was successfully treated by excision and skin grafting.

Surgical correction of pseudo-ainhum in Vohwinkel syndrome. Pisoh T, Bhatia A, Oberlin C. J Hand Surg [Br] 1995;20:338–41.

Successful surgical correction of constricting rings in a patient with Vohwinkel syndrome.

Surgical correction of hyperkeratosis in the Papillon-Lefevre syndrome. Peled IJ, Weinrauch L, Cohen HA, Wexler MK. J Dermatol Surg Oncol 1981;7:142–3.

A patient with Papillon-Lefèvre syndrome underwent successful surgical correction of hyperkeratosis of the palms.

Topical calcipotriol in the treatment of epidermolytic palmoplantar keratoderma of Vorner. Lucker GP, Van de Kerkhof PC, Steijlen PM. Br J Dermatol 1994;130:543–5.

A patient with hereditary epidermolytic PPK of Vorner was successfully treated with topical calcipotriol.

Efficacy, tolerability, and safety of calcipotriol ointment in disorders of keratinisation. Results of a randomized, double blind vehicle-controlled, right/left comparative study. Kragballe K, Steijlen PM, Ibsen HH, et al. Arch Dermatol 1995;131:556–60.

Twenty patients with PPK showed no therapeutic benefit with topical calcipotriol.

Improvement of palmoplantar keratoderma of nonhereditary type (eczema tyloticum) after oral administration of 1 alpha 25-dihydroxyvitamin D3. Katayama H, Yamane Y. Arch Dermatol 1989;125:1713.

A patient with acquired PPK was successfully treated with oral 1α,25-dihydroxyvitamin D, 0.5 μg daily for 3 months, with no side effects.

Oral psoralen photochemotherapy (PUVA) of hyperkeratotic dermatitis of the palms. Mobacken H, Rosen K, Swanbeck G. Br J Dermatol 1983;109:205–8.

PUVA was found to be effective in five patients with chronic hyperkeratotic dermatitis of the palms.

Dermabrasion of the hyperkeratotic foot. Daoud MS, Randle HW, Yarborough JM. Dermatol Surg 1995;21:243–4.

A patient with acquired PPK treated with dermabrasion and then 2% crude coal tar and 5% salicylic acid in petrolatum showed no evidence of recurrence after 6 months. The indications for dermabrasion include dry, fissured hyperkeratotic heels, psoriatic keratoderma before PUVA therapy, punctate keratoderma, and generalized keratoderma.

Methods and effectiveness of surgical treatment of limited hyperkeratosis with CO_2 laser. Babaev OG, Bashilov VP, Zakharov AK. Khirurgiia (Mosk) 1993;4:74–9.

Five hundred and two patients with limited hyperkeratosis were treated with a favorable clinical effect. Recurrences were noted in only 4% of cases.

Dietary management of oculocutaneous tyrosinemia in an 11 year old child. Ney D, Bay C, Scheider JA, et al. Am J Dis Child 1983;137:995–1000.

An 11-year-old girl with oculocutaneous tyrosinemia with plantar keratosis and keratitis demonstrated resolution of her keratitis and improvement of her plantar keratosis with dietary restriction of phenylalanine and tyrosine to less than 100 mg/kg.

Palmoplantar pustulosis

Carolina Talhari, Thomas Ruzicka, Helger Stege

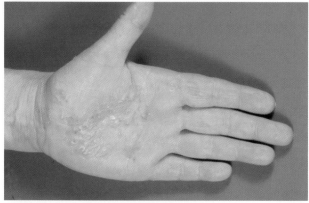

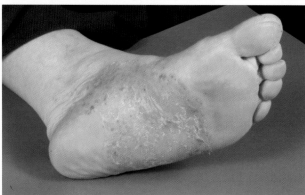

Palmoplantar pustulosis (PPP) is a distinct entity characterized by a chronic and relapsing vesiculopustular eruption of the palms and soles. Its relationship to psoriasis vulgaris is controversial.

MANAGEMENT STRATEGY

PPP is a common, recalcitrant, and difficult-to-treat condition. Association with thyroid disease, arthropathies (pustulosis palmoplantaris with osteoarthritis sternoclavicularis), and diabetes mellitus should be investigated.

In patients with only mild manifestations of PPP, *topical corticosteroids under occlusion* should be tried at first. *Psoralen with UVA (PUVA)* treatment, either with topical or systemic psoralen, is usually very effective. However, the response is slower than in psoriasis vulgaris. The efficacy of *tetracycline* (250 mg twice daily) and *clomocycline* (170 mg once daily) has been confirmed by well-controlled studies. Clomocycline is no longer available on the market.

Oral retinoids have been successfully used in the treatment of PPP. Etretinate at a daily dose of 1 mg/kg for 8 weeks was effective in clearing the skin and suppressing the formation of new pustules in patients with PPP in a randomized placebo–control study. Acitretin, which replaced etretinate in many countries, is equally effective in similar initial doses (0.5 mg/kg daily). *Oral low-dose cyclosporine* at (2.5–5 mg/kg daily) was also confirmed to be effective. Due to its side-effects, the patients under cyclosporine therapy must undergo monthly clinical and laboratory investigations, significantly for kidney function and blood pressure. Once major improvement is achieved, the drug can be withdrawn and topical treatment with corticosteroids can be used.

Several other approaches have been reported for the treatment of PPP. *Methotrexate* in weekly oral doses of 25 mg may be used for severe forms. The utilization of oral and intralesional corticosteroids in the treatment of PPP is not recommended due to their multiple cutaneous and systemic side effects when administrated for prolonged periods. A rebound with worsening of pustulation after the withdrawal of corticosteroids may occur. Some patients, however, may show improvement with *high doses of prednisolone. Colchicine, clofazimine, itraconazole, granulocyte colony stimulating factor (G-CSF)* and *superficial X-ray therapy* have been reported to be clinically effective in the treatment of PPP. Nevertheless, superficial X-ray therapy may be not indicated for young patients due to its carcinogenic property. Hydroxyurea has also employed for the treatment of PPP, but does not improve the disease.

Despite the lack of reports concerning the use of *tumor necrosis factor-α inhibitors* in PPP, we believe that these drugs are a promising therapeutic option for the treatment of the disease.

SPECIFIC INVESTIGATIONS

- Thyroid function tests
- Screen for arthropathy
- Screen for diabetes mellitus
- Exclude SAPHO (synovitis, acne, pustulosis, hyperostosis, and osteitis) syndrome

Thyroid disease in pustulosis palmoplantaris. Agner T, Sindrup JH, Höier-Madsen M, et al. Br J Dermatol 1989;121: 487–91.

Thyroid disease was demonstrated in 53% of the patients with PPP compared to 16% in the matched control group.

Frequency of skeletal disease, arthro-osteitis, in patients with pustulosis palmoplantaris. Jurik AG, Ternowitz T. J Am Acad Dermatol 1988;18:666–71.

Five of 14 patients with PPP showed symptoms and both clinical and radiographic signs of skeletal disease.

Skeletal involvement in pustulosis palmoplantaris with special reference to the sterno-costo-clavicular joints. Hradil E, Gentz CF, Matilainen T, et al. Acta Derm Venereol 1988;68:65–73.

Skeletal scintigraphy was performed in 73 patients with PPP with 16 of them demonstrating an increased isotope uptake in the sternocostoclavicular area. Nine of these 16 patients had local symptoms.

Glucose tolerance in pustulosis palmaris et plantaris. Uehara M, Fujigaki T, Hayashi S. Arch Dermatol 1980;116: 1275–6.

Of 41 patients with PPP, eight exhibited a diabetic pattern and 20 demonstrated a borderline pattern in the glucose tolerance test.

SAPHO syndrome: a long-term follow-up study of 120 cases. Hayem G, Bouchaud-Chabot A, Benali K, et al. Semin Arthritis Rheum 2000;29:332–34.

Among the 102 patients who were prospectively followed up, a significant association of PPP with axial osteitis was found.

FIRST LINE THERAPIES

■ Oral retinoids	A
■ Tetracycline, clomocycline	A
■ PUVA	B
■ Topical corticosteroids	E

A randomized trial of etretinate (Tigason®) in palmoplantar pustulosis. Foged E, Holm P, Larsen PO, et al. Dermatologica 1983;166:220–3.

Fifty patients with PPP were treated with either oral etretinate (1 mg/kg daily) or placebo for 8 weeks. Eighteen of 20 patients on etretinate showed good or moderate response, while six of 21 patients on placebo showed similar results.

Acitretin has supplanted etretinate as the retinoid of choice for this condition.

Pustulosis palmaris et plantaris. Thomsen K, Osterbye P. Br J Dermatol 1973;89:293–6.

Forty patients with PPP received oral tetracycline 250 mg twice daily or placebo in three periods of 4 weeks each. Tetracycline resulted in marked improvement in 42 of 59 courses, while placebo had a similar result in 20 courses.

A double-blind trial of clomocycline in the treatment of persistent palmoplantar pustulosis. Ward J, Corbett M, Hanna MJ. Br J Dermatol 1976;95:317–22.

Forty patients with PPP received 3 months each of clomocycline (170 mg once daily) and placebo in a random order. Twenty two did not respond to any treatment, 15 showed significant improvement with clomocycline, two improved on placebo, and one improved on both treatments.

A controlled trial of photochemotherapy for persistent palmoplantar pustulosis. Murray D, Corbett MF, Warin AP. Br J Dermatol 1980;102:659–63.

Clearing or much improvement of one randomly selected side occurred in 21 of 22 patients with bilaterally symmetrical PPP treated with 20 oral PUVA treatments. Later on, 13 of 17 patients treated with topical PUVA on the side that had previously been used as a control showed complete clearing or much improvement.

Pustulosis palmoplantaris and chronic eczematous hand dermatitis. Rosen K. Acta Derm Venereol 1988;S137.

Although potent topical corticosteroids are considered a first line treatment for mild PPP, this study demonstrated that only one-third of the patients treated with this approach showed partial remission of the pustulation.

The use of topical corticosteroids in the treatment of PPP has been based on multiple anecdotal reports. A good review article.

SECOND LINE THERAPIES

■ Cyclosporine	A

Cyclosporine in the treatment of palmoplantar pustulosis. A randomized, double-blind, placebo-controlled study. Reitamo S, Erkko P, Remitz A, et al. Arch Dermatol 1993;129:1273–79.

Seventeen of 19 patients with PPP treated with cyclosporine (2.5 mg/kg daily) showed a significant reduction of formation of new pustules. Among 19 patients who received placebo, only four were classified as responders.

THIRD LINE THERAPIES

■ Hydroxyurea	A
■ Radiotherapy	B
■ Colchicine	B
■ Methotrexate	B
■ Clofazimine	B
■ Oral corticosteroids	B
■ Intralesional corticosteroids	D
■ Itraconazole	E
■ G-CSF	E
■ Tumor necrosis factor-α inhibitors	E

Pustulosis palmaris et plantaris treated with hydroxyurea. Hattel T, Sondergaard J. Acta Derm Venereol 1974;54:152–4.

Thirteen patients received hydroxyurea (1.5 g daily) and placebo, each for 3 weeks. No significant difference in the scores for severity of disease was seen between hydroxyurea and placebo.

Superficial X-ray therapy in the treatment of palmoplantar pustulosis. Fairris GM, Jones DH, Mack DP, et al. Br J Dermatol 1984;111:499–502.

Nine symmetrical, paired sites of three patients with PPP were randomly given a dose of 100 rad (1 Gy) of conventional superficial X-ray treatment at 50 kV or a placebo dose. This modality of treatment showed little or no therapeutic effect upon PPP.

The effect of Grenz ray therapy on pustulosis palmoplantaris. Lindelof B, Beitner H. Acta Derm Venereol 1990;70:529–31.

One side of the body of 15 patients with PPP was randomly assessed and treated with 4 Gy of Grenz rays 10 kV on six occasions at intervals of 1 week. The lesions on the other side received stimulated treatment and served as a control. The treated side showed moderate response, but no lesions healed completely.

Treatment of pustulosis palmaris et plantaris with oral doses of colchicine. Takigawa M, Miyachi Y, Uehara M, et al. Arch Dermatol 1982;118:458–60.

Thirty two patients were given twice daily 1–2 mg of oral colchicine for 1–4 weeks. Maintenance dosage was 0.25–0.5 mg twice daily for 1–6 weeks. Thirteen patients showed complete clearing of pustulation, 14 patients demonstrated remarkable improvement, one patient did not respond and four discontinued treatment because of side effects.

Pustulosis palmaris et plantaris treated with methotrexate. Thomsen K. Acta Derm Venereol 1971;51:397–400.

Twenty five patients were given methotrexate in weekly oral doses of 25 mg for 2 months. Only eight patients responded satisfactorily to methotrexate.

Clofazimine-enhanced phagocytosis in pustulosis palmaris et plantaris. Molin L. Acta Derm Venereol 1975;55: 151–3.

Oral clofazimine (400 mg daily) was given to 27 patients for 3–4 months, followed by a maintenance daily dosage of 200–300 mg. After 6 months of therapy, 21 patients showed a significant improvement, four demonstrated a mild improvement, and in two the therapy had no effect.

The treatment of pustular dermatoses of the extremities with oral triamcinolone. Robinson TWE. Br J Dermatol 1966;78:158–60.

Thirty three patients with a history of recurrent intractable pustular eruptions were treated with oral triamcinolone (6 mg daily). The dose was shortly reduced to 3 mg daily over a 4-month period. Twenty four patients responded satisfactorily (12 with 6–24 months of treatment and 12 with 6–36 months).

Treatment of palmoplantar pustulosis with intralesional triamcinolone injections. Goette DK, Morgan AM, Fox BJ, et al. Arch Dermatol 1984;120:319–23.

Five patients with PPP were treated with intralesional injections of 3.3–5.0 mg/mL of triamcinolone acetonide. Clearing of symptoms and lesions at the site of injection was observed within 24 h after the procedure and lasted 3–6 months.

Itraconazole as a new treatment for pustulosis palmaris et plantaris. Mihara M, Hagari Y, Morimura T, et al. Arch Dermatol 1998;134:639–40.

Seven patients were treated once daily with 100 mg oral itraconazole for 2–6 weeks. Maintenance daily dosages were 50 mg for four patients and 100 mg and 50 mg alternately for two patients. One patient continued to take the initial dosage of 100 mg for 6 months. All patients showed marked improvement, but relapses were seen when the drug was discontinued.

Successful treatment of pustulosis palmaris et plantaris with granulocyte colony stimulating factor (G-CSF) in a patient with hereditary neutropenia. Hino M, Yamane T, Kuwaki T, et al. Int J Hematol 1998;68:453–6.

One patient with hereditary neutropenia and PPP showed improvement of the skin lesions with 5 μg/kg daily of G-CSF.

Successful treatment of acrodermatitis continua of Hallopeau by the tumour necrosis factor-alpha inhibitor infliximab (Remicade). Mang R, Ruzicka T, Stege H. Br J Dermatol 2004;150:379–80.

One patient with acrodermatitis continua of Hallopeau, considered by most authors as a variant of pustular palmoplantar psoriasis, showed complete clearance of the pustules after 23 infusions of infliximab. The initial dose was 3 mg/kg, followed by 4 mg/kg (21 infusions).

Addition of low-dose methrotexate to infliximab in the treatment of a patient with severe, recalcitrant pustular psoriasis. Barland C. Arch Dermatol 2003;139:949–50.

A patient with recalcitrant pustular psoriasis of the palms and soles was successfully treated with a combination of infliximab (10 mg/kg, two infusions) and methotrexate (7.5 mg weekly). The lesions were virtually absent within 2 weeks of treatment.

The last two case reports mentioned above showed good response of diseases related to PPP to a tumor necrosis factor-α inhibitor.

Evidence levels   **A** Double-blind study   **B** Clinical trial ≥ 20 subjects   **C** Clinical trial < 20 subjects   **D** Series ≥ 5 subjects   **E** Anecdotal case reports

Panniculitis

Robert A Allen, Richard L Spielvogel

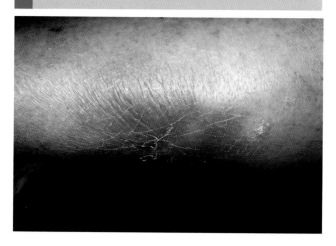

Panniculitis is a collective term for a group of inflammatory diseases that involve the subcutaneous fat. Most types present with tender dermal and subcutaneous papules, nodules, and plaques. The panniculitides are subdivided into groups based upon where the predominant amount of inflammation is seen on a skin biopsy, either in intralobular septa or within the fat lobule itself. Erythema nodosum is the most common form of panniculitis and is discussed on page 204. While erythema nodosum involves mainly the septal tissue between fat lobules, almost all other forms of panniculitis primarily involve the fat lobule. The differential diagnosis of lobular panniculitis includes infectious panniculitis, lupus profundus, Weber–Christian disease (WCD), nodular vasculitis (erythema induratum), pancreatic panniculitis, α_1-antitrypsin (A1AT) deficiency panniculitis, cytophagic histiocytic panniculitis (CHP)/forms of subcutaneous T cell lymphoma, and the childhood forms of panniculitis.

MANAGEMENT STRATEGY

A skin biopsy is helpful to determine whether the inflammation is primarily septal or lobular. The type of biopsy should be a large punch or an incisional specimen. This should be performed if the history and physical signs do not support a diagnosis of erythema nodosum or a subcutaneous infection. If infection is in the differential diagnosis, a small piece of the biopsy should be sent to microbiology for Gram stain and culture for bacteria, mycobacteria, and fungi. If a mycobacterial infection is in the differential diagnosis, the specimen should be grown at 24, 30, 37, and 42°C. Treatment for proven infectious causes should be based on antibiotic sensitivity testing if possible.

A work-up for lupus may be performed if this diagnosis is suspected. Lupus profundus occurs in 2–5% of cases of systemic lupus erythematosus (SLE) and it tends to have a chronic course that does not involve internal organs. It is often painful, with skin lesions showing overlying signs of discoid lupus erythematosus. In contrast to erythema nodosum, its distribution is usually on the trunk and proximal extremities. Laboratory studies should include antinuclear antibody (ANA), dsDNA, ssDNA, SSA, SSB, chemistry profile, and a complete blood count (CBC). A biopsy for direct immunofluorescence should be ordered to confirm the diagnosis in cases without classical histopathology. The first line treatment is *antimalarials,* with or without *systemic corticosteroids*, and *sunscreens.*

The diagnosis of WCD is one of exclusion. It is the idiopathic form of chronic lobular panniculitis without vasculitis. Patients are usually intermittently febrile. Several studies have documented other causes of panniculitis when cases of WCD are re-inspected for infection, pancreatic disease, and erythema nodosum. The work-up should include an erythrocyte sedimentation rate, liver function studies, amylase and lipase to rule out pancreatic panniculitis, and A1AT levels. Treatment is variable and commonly requires trials of several agents before a suitable response is obtained. *Corticosteroids*, *dapsone*, and *tetracycline* are all reported to help in some cases. *More aggressive immunosuppression* may be required.

A work-up for causes of vasculitis can also be undertaken. If cultures for mycobacteria are negative (erythema induratum) or if a rapid diagnosis is required, the tissue may be sent for mycobacterial DNA by polymerase chain reaction (PCR). Treatment usually consists of *potassium iodide, colchicine, corticosteroids,* or *antimalarials.* Polyarteritis nodosa can also occur in the panniculus. However, it tends to spare veins in the biopsy specimens and has systemic involvement.

Pancreatic panniculitis can occur with any form of pancreatic tissue necrosis, including pancreatitis, pancreatic duct stricture, or pancreatic carcinoma. It is important to note that abdominal symptoms may be absent. Serum amylase and lipase levels should be measured because they are frequently elevated. A CBC with differential should be ordered to look for eosinophilia, which occurs in 60% of patients. Imaging with MRI is helpful to look for a pancreatic malignancy. The condition only resolves with treatment of the underlying cause of pancreatic inflammation.

A1AT panniculitis results from deficiency of this enzyme, which leads to chronic inflammation in the subcutaneous fat because lipase, elastase, and other enzymes are not neutralized. An elastic tissue stain of the biopsy may be helpful to show the decreased elastic tissue and lobular or septal panniculitis characteristic of this entity. Treatment consists of *enzyme replacement, dapsone, colchicine,* or *liver transplantation* to permanently replace the missing enzyme.

Cytophagic histiocytic panniculitis features tender subcutaneous nodules along with fever, hepatosplenomegaly, pancytopenia, and liver dysfunction. It has been associated with viral infections (mainly Epstein–Barr) and hematologic malignancies. Histopathologic specimens show 'bean-bag' cells, which are giant cells engulfing lymphocytes, neutrophils, and erythrocytes. Absence of immunoperoxidase staining with CD56 on the skin biopsy may portend a better clinical outcome. Treatment consists of *treating any underlying malignancy,* possibly with *bone marrow transplant.* If malignancy is ruled out, cyclosporine is usually effective.

The physical forms of panniculitis, such as those resulting from cold exposure, foreign body, or factitial creation, usually resolve by *removing the offending trigger* or surgical removal of the foreign body. This is similar to panniculitis caused by the use of silicone or paraffin that had been used for cosmetic purposes. Panniculitis can also occur in infants. It is manifested as sclerema neonatorum or as subcutaneous fat necrosis of the newborn (see page 637). The latter condition usually resolves spontaneously, but may be complicated by hypercalcemia. Sclerema neonatorum may be fatal.

SPECIFIC INVESTIGATIONS

- Skin biopsy for routine microscopy
- Skin biopsy for culture and sensitivity (routine, mycobacterial, fungal)
- Skin biopsy for PCR
- Skin biopsy for immunoperoxidase and gene rearrangement studies
- ANA and other rheumatologic serologic tests
- Serum A1AT
- Serum lipase and amylase
- Abdominal MRI

There are no specific investigations for panniculitis other than an adequate skin biopsy containing abundant fat. Further investigation should be based on history and physical findings.

Lupus panniculitis

FIRST LINE THERAPIES

■ Antimalarials	E
■ Systemic or intralesional corticosteroids	E

Systemic lupus erythematosus presenting as panniculitis (lupus profundus). Diaz-Jouanen E, DeHoratius RJ, Alarcon-Segovia D, Messner RP. Ann Intern Med 1975;82: 376–9.

A case study in which five of six patients improved after adding hydroxychloroquine to their systemic corticosteroid regimens.

Connective tissue panniculitis. Winkelmann RK, Padilha-Goncalves A. Arch Dermatol 1980;116:291–4.

Case report of a patient obtaining remission with hydroxychloroquine 200 mg twice daily and systemic corticosteroids. However, she developed SLE. A second patient on hydroxychloroquine was cleared of the condition after failing to respond to nonsteroidal anti-inflammatory drugs (NSAIDs), potassium iodide, and corticosteroids.

Lupus erythematosus panniculitis (profundus). Maciejewski W, Bandmann HJ. Acta Derm Venereol Suppl (Stockh) 1979;59:109–12.

Case report of a patient diagnosed with lupus profundus with direct immunofluorescence and treated with chloroquine.

Lupus erythematosus presenting as panniculitis. Verbov JL, Borrie PF. Proc R Soc Med 1971;64:28–9.

A case report of the condition clearing in one patient with hydroxychloroquine 200 mg twice daily.

Treatment of chronic discoid lupus erythematosus with intralesional triamcinolone. Rowell NR. Br J Dermatol 1962;74:354–7.

One patient with lupus profundus and 27 patients with discoid lupus erythematosus were treated with intralesional triamcinolone, 10 mg/mL and the condition in 27 of the 28 cleared or was clearing. All patients had failed to respond to antimalarials. The condition cleared in the lupus profundus patient.

SECOND LINE THERAPIES

■ Topical corticosteroids under occlusion	E

Lupus erythematosus profundus treated with clobetasol propionate under a hydrocolloid dressing. Yell JA, Burge SM. Br J Dermatol 1993;128:103.

A single case of a cure with clobetasol under hydrocolloid dressing occlusion, changed weekly. The patient responded after 1 month.

THIRD LINE THERAPIES

■ Gold	E
■ Bismuth	E

Lupus erythematosus profundus. Arnold HL Jr. Arch Dermatol 1956;73:14–26.

One patient had a partial response to intravenous gold followed by bismuth sodium thioglycollate.

Weber–Christian disease

FIRST LINE THERAPIES

■ Tetracycline	E
■ Nonsteroidal anti-inflammatory agents	E
■ Systemic or intralesional corticosteroids	E

Panniculitis responsive to high dose tetracycline. Sturman SW. Arch Dermatol 1975;111:533–4.

One patient presented with fever, splenomegaly, and panniculitis that responded to tetracycline, but recurred with two taperings. Finally, high-dose tetracycline (1 g four times daily) achieved remission. An infectious work-up did not find a causative organism.

Weber–Christian disease. Analysis of 15 cases and review of the literature. Panush RS, Yonker RA, Dlesk A, et al. Medicine (Baltimore) 1985;64:181–91.

Twelve of 13 patients with WCD improved with various therapies: 80% received corticosteroids, 33% NSAIDs, 40% antimalarials, and one patient methotrexate; 27% of patients received azathioprine after failing to respond to corticosteroids.

Panniculitis (Rothmann–Makai), with good response to tetracycline. Chan HL. Br J Dermatol 1975;92:351–4.

One patient responded well to low-dose tetracycline.

Evidence levels **A** Double-blind study **B** Clinical trial ≥ 20 subjects **C** Clinical trial < 20 subjects **D** Series ≥ 5 subjects **E** Anecdotal case reports

SECOND LINE THERAPIES

■ Heparin	E
■ Cyclosporine	E
■ Azathioprine	E
■ Antimalarials	E
■ Methotrexate	E

Ocular and adnexal changes associated with relapsing febrile non-suppurative panniculitis (Weber–Christian disease). Frayer WC, Wise RT, Tsaltas TT. Trans Am Ophthalmol Soc 1968;66:233–42.

A case report of a patient remission with heparin.

Successful treatment of Weber–Christian disease by cyclosporin A. Usuki K, Kitamura K, Urabe A, Takaku F. Am J Med 1988;85:276–8.

One patient who had failed to respond to prednisone and had persistent fever achieved a remission with intravenous cyclosporine followed by a change to oral therapy. The patient was disease free at 7 months.

Azathioprine-induced remission in Weber–Christian disease. Hotta T, Wakamatsu Y, Matsumura N, et al. South Med J 1981;74:234–7.

A woman with subcutaneous nodules was originally diagnosed with dermatomyositis. After failing to respond to prednisolone and NSAIDs for 5 months, the diagnosis was changed to WCD. Azathioprine 150 mg daily resulted in clearing with minimal side effects (leukopenia). She flared upon tapering to 50 mg daily, but was stabilized at 100 mg daily for 2 years.

Weber–Christian disease. Analysis of 15 cases and review of the literature. Panush RS, Yonker RA, Dlesk A, et al. Medicine (Baltimore) 1985;64:181–91.

Twelve of 13 patients with WCD improved with various therapies: 80% received corticosteroids, 33% NSAIDs, 40% antimalarials, and one patient methotrexate; 27% of patients received azathioprine after failing to respond to corticosteroids.

THIRD LINE THERAPIES

■ Cyclophosphamide	E
■ Thalidomide	E
■ Skin grafting	E

Cyclophosphamide-induced remission in Weber–Christian panniculitis. Kirch W, Duhrsen U, Hoensch H, Ohnhaus E. Rheumatol Int 1985;5:239–40.

One patient with WCD failed to respond to hydroxychloroquine and prednisone. Cyclophosphamide led to rapid improvement.

Weber–Christian disease with nephrotic syndrome. Srivastava RN, Mayekar G, Anand R, Roy S. Am J Dis Child 1974;127:420–1.

A 5-year-old boy presented with nephrotic syndrome and WCD panniculitis. He improved initially with prednisone. However, cyclophosphamide 50 mg on alternate days with prednisone 30 mg daily was added after a flare. This resulted in rapid correction of the proteinuria and resolution of the panniculitis over the next 9 months.

Thalidomide in Weber–Christian disease. [Letter] Eravelly J, Waters MF. Lancet 1977;1:251.

A single patient was controlled with high-dose corticosteroids, but flared when tapering; she responded to thalidomide 300 mg daily. She was able to stop her corticosteroids and taper off the thalidomide after 13 weeks. She was disease free at 13 months.

A review of the concept of Weber–Christian panniculitis with a report of five cases. Macdonald A, Feiwel M. Br J Dermatol 1968;80:355–61.

A case report of two patients who healed after skin grafting after failing to improve with prednisone, antimalarials, and NSAIDs.

Nodular vasculitis

FIRST LINE THERAPIES

■ NSAIDs	E
■ Potassium iodide	D
■ Treat underlying tuberculosis	B

Neutrophilic vascular reactions. Jorizzo JL, Solomon AR, Zanolli MD, Leshin B. J Am Acad Dermatol 1988;19:983–1005.

A review article in which nodular vasculitis is one of the causes of necrotizing vasculitis. NSAIDs may benefit some symptoms, such as serum sickness-like features, but do not help cutaneous lesions.

Potassium iodide in the treatment of erythema nodosum and nodular vasculitis. Horio T, Imamura S, Danno K, Ofuji S. Arch Dermatol 1981;117:29–31.

A case study in which 11 of 51 patients had nodular vasculitis. Seven of these 11 patients responded within 2 weeks to potassium iodide 300 mg three times daily.

Treatment of erythema nodosum and nodular vasculitis with potassium iodide. Schulz EJ, Whiting DA. Br J Dermatol 1976;94:75–8.

Sixteen of 17 patients responded to potassium iodide, usually with relief of symptoms within 2 days. The average duration of therapy was 3 weeks. The daily dose ranged from 360 to 900 mg.

Successful treatment of erythema induratum of Bazin following rapid detection of mycobacterial DNA by polymerase chain reaction. Degitz K, Messer G, Schirren H, et al. Arch Dermatol 1993;129:1619–20.

A single case of diagnosis and treatment of tuberculosis with isoniazid, rifampin (rifampicin), and ethambutol.

PCR has revolutionized the diagnosis of mycobacterial disease, confirming the long-held suspicion that many tuberculids may be due to residual mycobacterial antigens.

Erythema induratum of Bazin. Cho KH, Lee DY, Kim CW. Int J Dermatol 1996;35:802–8.

A retrospective study of 32 patients with proven erythema induratum of Bazin. All improved with triple therapy, but four of 32 relapsed and subsequently cleared.

Diagnosis and treatment of erythema induratum (Bazin). Feiwel M, Munro DD. Br Med J 1965;1:1109–11.

Twelve patients were diagnosed with erythema induratum secondary to tuberculosis and all responded well to two- to three-drug therapy, streptomycin, para-aminosalicylic acid 12.5 mg daily, and isoniazid 200–260 mg daily for 9 months.

SECOND LINE THERAPIES

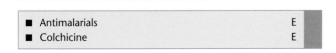

■ Antimalarials	E
■ Colchicine	E

Chloroquine-induced remission of nodular panniculitis present for 15 years. Shelley WB. J Am Acad Dermatol 1981;5:168–70.

One patient responded to chloroquine 250 mg daily within 1 month after failing to respond to various therapies for nodular panniculitis. These included corticosteroids, NSAIDs, and tetracycline.

Cutaneous necrotizing vasculitis. Lotti T, Comacchi C, Ghersetich I. Int J Dermatol 1996;35:457–74.

Oral colchicine, by inhibiting neutrophil chemotaxis, in doses of 0.6 mg twice daily, may be helpful in chronic forms of the disease.

THIRD LINE THERAPIES

■ Gold	E

Nodular vasculitis (erythema induratum): treatment with auranofin. Shaffer N, Kerdel FA. J Am Acad Dermatol 1991; 25:426–9.

One patient with nodular vasculitis responded to oral gold 3 mg twice daily and improved after 3 weeks. She had previously failed to respond to prednisone, colchicine, D-penicillamine, sulindac, and bumetanide (a loop diuretic) for suspected erythema nodosum.

Pancreatic panniculitis

FIRST LINE THERAPIES

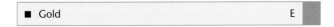

■ Treat underlying pancreatic problem	E

Resolution of panniculitis after placement of pancreatic duct stent in chronic pancreatitis. Lambiase P. Am J Gastroenterol 1996;91:1835–7.

One patient with pancreatitis secondary to alcohol presented with chest pain and tender skin nodules on the shins. After a skin biopsy showed panniculitis, he was diagnosed with pancreatitis without abdominal pain, but with a high amylase. A stent was placed to correct a stricture in the pancreatic duct, leading to resolution of the symptoms and skin lesions within 1 month.

Panniculitis caused by acinous pancreatic carcinoma. Heykarts B, Anseeuw M, Degreef H. Dermatology 1999;198: 182–3.

One patient with skin nodules was found to have acinar pancreatic carcinoma upon surgical resection. She was initially unresponsive to high-dose corticosteroids and methotrexate, but the skin lesions resolved slowly after the resection. Subsequently, metastases were found in the right liver and the patient failed to respond to ledorvain and fluorouracil.

SECOND LINE THERAPIES

■ Octreotide	E

Liquefying panniculitis associated with acinous carcinoma of the pancreas responding to octreotide. Hudson-Peacock MJ, Regnard CFB, Farr PM. J R Soc Med 194;87: 361–2.

One patient presented with increasing numbers of painful leg nodules secondary to poorly differentiated adenocarcinoma. She failed to respond to prednisolone, but octreotide 50 µg twice daily subcutaneously halted skin nodule progression. However, despite the therapy, the patient died 3 weeks later.

Cytophagic histiocytic panniculitis

FIRST LINE THERAPIES

■ Treat underlying T cell lymphoma (chemotherapy)	E
■ Prednisone	E
■ Cyclosporine (if T cell lymphoma ruled out)	E

Cytophagic histiocytic panniculitis and subcutaneous panniculitis-like T-cell lymphoma: report of 7 cases. Marzano AV, Berti E, Paulli M, Caputo R. Arch Dermatol 2000;136:889–96.

A report of seven cases of CHP. Five patients had subcutaneous T cell lymphoma and died after failing to respond to various chemotherapeutic agents. One patient has done well with prednisone for 13 months and the other living patient has done well with systemic corticosteroids, cyclophosphamide, and dapsone for 36 years.

Successful treatment of cytophagic histiocytic panniculitis with modified CHOP-E. Cyclophosphamide, adriamycin, vincristine, prednisone, and etoposide. Matsue K, Itoh M, Tsukuda K, et al. Am J Clin Oncol 1994;17:470–4.

One patient with CHP received eight courses of modified CHOP-E every 3 weeks and has obtained a remission that has lasted 2 years.

Cytophagic histiocytic panniculitis. Case report with resolution after treatment. Alegre VA, Fortea JM, Camps C, Aliaga A. J Am Acad Dermatol 1989;20:875–8.

One patient with CHP for 2 months with an extensive work-up was treated with cyclophosphamide, vincristine, doxorubicin, and prednisone for nine cycles and achieved a cure. The authors recommend early, aggressive treatment.

Cytophagic histiocytic panniculitis – a syndrome associated with benign and malignant panniculitis: case comparison and review of the literature. Craig AJ, Cualing H, Thomas G, et al. J Am Acad Dermatol 1998;39:721–36.

A case report of two patients who presented with CHP. One responded to prednisone 1 mg/kg daily and cyclosporine 15 mg/kg daily and responded well enough to be discharged home. However, he developed fatal septicemia 1 month later. An autopsy revealed no malignancy, but extensive *Aspergillus* sp. infection. Patient 2 presented with T cell lymphoma and CHP and died during chemotherapy with cyclophosphamide, mitoxantrone, prednisone, and vincristine, and X-ray therapy.

Subcutaneous panniculitic T-cell lymphoma in children: response to combination therapy with cyclosporine and chemotherapy. Shani-Adir A, Lucky AW, Prendiville J, et al. J Am Acad Dermatol 2004; 50(2 Suppl):S18–22.

A case report of two adolescents with CHP and subcutaneous T cell lymphoma who symptomatically responded to cyclosporine (5 and 12 mg/kg daily) with a decrease in fever and subcutaneous nodules. Complete remission was achieved in one patient with subsequent chemotherapy.

Successful treatment of severe cytophagic histiocytic panniculitis with cyclosporine A. Ostrov BE, Athreys BH, Eichenfield AH, Goldsmith DP. Semin Arthritis Rheum 1996;25:404–13.

A 16-year-old patient who presented with CHP initially responded to prednisone 2 mg/kg daily. A flare occurred and cyclosporine 4 mg/kg daily was instituted. A remission followed, but she was left with permanent hypothyroidism. She has remained disease free for 6 years after discontinuing the cyclosporine.

SECOND LINE THERAPIES

■ Bone marrow transplantation	E
■ Potassium iodide	E
■ Dapsone	E
■ Cyclophosphamide	E
■ Irradiation (total body)	E

Effective high-dose chemotherapy followed by autologous peripheral blood stem cell transplantation in a patient with the aggressive form of cytophagic histiocytic panniculitis. Koizumi K, Sawada K, Nishio M, et al. Bone Marrow Transplant 1997;20:171–3.

One patient with CHP secondary to an aggressive T cell lymphoma was treated with cyclophosphamide, doxorubicin, vincristine, prednisolone, etoposide, and granulocyte-macrophage colony stimulating factor (GM-CSF), and achieved a remission after three cycles (every 2 weeks). He was subsequently treated with autologous bone marrow transplant and remained disease free for 1 year.

Cytophagic histiocytic panniculitis is not always fatal. White JW Jr, Winkelmann RK. J Cutan Pathol 1989;16:137–44.

One patient with CHP was treated with potassium iodide and achieved a remission for 15 years. Another patient achieved remission with prednisone and was disease free at 28 years.

Successful treatment of a patient with subcutaneous panniculitis-like T-cell lymphoma with high-dose chemotherapy and total body irradiation. Mukai HY, Okoshi Y, Shimizu S, et al. Eur J Haematol 2003;70:413–6.

One patient with CHP and subcutaneous T cell lymphoma achieved a remission after three courses of CHOP chemotherapy, followed by high dose chemotherapy and total body irradiation with autologous stem cell transplant. He remained disease free at 2 years.

α_1-Antitrypsin deficiency panniculitis

FIRST LINE THERAPIES

■ Doxycycline	E
■ Dapsone	D
■ A1AT concentrate if emergent	E

Use of anti-collagenase properties of doxycycline in treatment of alpha 1-antitrypsin deficiency panniculitis. Humbert P, Faivre B, Gibey R, Agache P. Acta Derm Venereol 1991;71:189–94.

Three patients with recurrent A1AT panniculitis were treated with doxycycline 200 mg daily for 3 months. All achieved clearing within 8 weeks. After this period, two of the three were able to stop the medicine while the other was maintained on 100 mg daily. The authors speculate that this was due to the anticollagenase effect of the drug.

Clinical and pathologic correlations in 96 patients with panniculitis, including 15 patients with deficient levels of alpha 1-antitrypsin. Smith KC, Su WP, Pittelkow MR, Winkelmann RK. J Am Acad Dermatol 1989;21:1192–6.

Fifteen of 96 patients had A1AT panniculitis. Five of six of those treated with dapsone responded.

Panniculitis associated with severe alpha 1-antitrypsin deficiency. Treatment and review of the literature. Smith KC, Pittelkow MR, Su WP. Arch Dermatol 1987;123:1655–61.

One patient with A1AT deficiency failed to respond to prednisone, but did respond to dapsone 75 mg daily and an infusion of A1AT concentrate weekly. The patient was able to have split-thickness skin grafting after 2 weeks. Another patient had poor responses to chloroquine, azathioprine, and prednisone, but improved on the dapsone and A1AT inhibitor concentrate.

Protease-inhibitor deficiencies in a patient with Weber–Christian panniculitis. Bleumink E, Klokke HA. Arch Dermatol 1984;120:936–40.

One patient with tender leg nodules of A1AT panniculitis failed to respond to tetracycline, but did respond to dapsone 50 mg daily. She did have a few minor recurrences while on long-term dapsone therapy.

Treatment of alpha1-antitrypsin-deficiency panniculitis with minocycline. Ginarte M, Roson E, Peteiro C, Toribio J. Cutis 2001;68:27–30.

The condition cleared with minocycline 100 mg twice daily in one patient who was unable to tolerate treatment with dapsone or systemic corticosteroids. She was maintained on a dose of 100 mg once daily.

SECOND LINE THERAPIES

■ A1AT concentrate	E
■ Liver transplant	E
■ Potassium iodide	E
■ Plasmapheresis	E
■ Cyclophosphamide	E
■ Colchicine	E
■ Prednisone	E

Alpha 1-antitrypsin deficiency-associated panniculitis: resolution with intravenous alpha 1-antitrypsin administration and liver transplantation. O'Riordan K, Blei A, Rao MS, Abecassis M. Transplantation 1997;63:480–2.

Two patients with homozygous deficiency were treated with A1AT replacement. One patient received a liver transplant and was cured. The other was treated with intravenous A1AT and was clear while on this medicine. She had a relapse when her free A1AT level fell below 50 µg/100 mL of serum.

Treatment of alpha-1-antitrypsin deficiency, massive edema, and panniculitis with alpha-1 protease inhibitor. Furey NL, Golden RS, Potts SR. Ann Intern Med 1996 15;125:699.

A patient with red thigh nodules was found to have A1AT deficiency panniculitis. The patient failed to respond to doxycycline and received α_1-protease inhibitor concentrate 60 mg/kg with great improvement within 24 h.

Atlantic Provinces Dermatology Association Society Meeting, May 3, 1986. Miller RAW, cited by Ross JB. J Can Dermatol Assoc 1986:13–7.

One patient with A1AT deficiency panniculitis failed to respond to prednisone and azathioprine, but responded after dapsone, potassium iodide, and plasmapheresis two to three times a week.

Cyclophosphamide therapy for Weber–Christian disease associated with alpha 1-antitrypsin deficiency. Strunk RW, Scheld WM. South Med J 1986;79:1425–7.

One patient with A1AT deficiency panniculitis failed to respond to prednisone 80 mg daily and heparin intravenously (given for suspected deep vein thrombosis). Cyclophosphamide was added at 150 mg daily with a good response. The prednisone was tapered over 2 months and the cyclophosphamide was discontinued after 14 months. The patient had been disease free for 2 years after stopping the cyclophosphamide.

Necrotic panniculitis with alpha-1 antitrypsin deficiency. Viraben R, Massip P, Dicostanzo B, Mathieu C. J Am Acad Dermatol 1986;14:684–7.

A patient with A1AT panniculitis with necrotic plaques on the flanks and thighs failed to respond to lincomycin, prednisolone, colchicine, and cyclophosphamide. Rapid improvement followed plasma exchange infusions of 8 L once daily for 8 weeks.

Familial occurrence of alpha 1-antitrypsin deficiency and Weber-Christian disease. Breit SN, Clark P, Robinson JP, et al. Arch Dermatol 1983;119:198–202.

A report of two cases of A1AT panniculitis. Patient 1 responded to dexamethasone 5 mg intravenously every 6 h. After 2 weeks he developed gas pain and an abdominal ileus. The dexamethasone was tapered to 6 mg four times daily and cyclophosphamide 200 mg daily was added. After 9 months the cyclophosphamide was discontinued, followed by the corticosteroids 3 months later. The patient has remained disease free for 2 years except for small lesions at the sites of trauma. The brother of patient 1 had a similar attack and received 0.5 mg of colchicine three times daily and dicloxacillin. The lesions resolved after 2 weeks and treatment was stopped 1 week later.

Deficiencia de alda-1-antitripsina en la panniculitis de Weber-Christian. [Abstract] Olmos L, Superby A, Lueiro M. Actas Dermato-Sifilograficas 1981;72:371–6.

One patient had resolution of panniculitis with prednisone. It also flared upon tapering.

Severe panniculitis caused by homozygous ZZ alpha 1-antitrypsin deficiency treated successfully with human purified enzyme (Prolastin). Chowdhury MM, Williams EJ, Morris JS, et al. Br J Dermatol 2002;147:1258–61.

Life-threatening panniculitis and skin necrosis in one patient was cleared with Prolastin (human purified enzyme) and prednisolone. She cleared on a dose 100 mg/kg every 6 days after being started on 60 mg/kg. She remained clear on a maintenance regimen of 6 g once weekly.

THIRD LINE THERAPIES

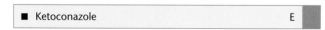

■ Ketoconazole	E

Panniculitis associated with histoplasmosis and alpha 1-antitrypsin deficiency. Pottage JC Jr, Trenholme GM, Aronson IK, Harris AA. Am J Med 1983;75:150–3.

A patient with nodules on the legs was found to have A1AT deficiency and histoplasmosis, which was diagnosed after exploratory thoracotomy and culture of lymph nodes. He received ketoconazole 400 mg daily for 6 months and was clear for another 9 months.

Paracoccidioido-mycosis (South American blastomycosis)

Wanda Sonia Robles

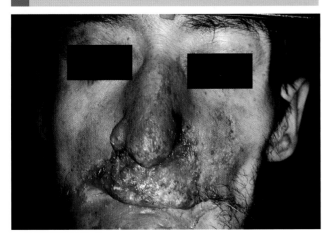

Paracoccidioidomycosis is a chronic granulomatous, primary pulmonary fungal infection caused by the dimorphic fungus *Paracoccidioides brasiliensis*. The condition may affect skin, mucous membranes, lymph nodes, and other internal organs. The disease has been reported from many Latin American countries but is commonest in Brazil, where it is particularly prevalent in the state of São Paulo. It is also seen regularly in Colombia, Argentina, Ecuador, Peru, and Venezuela and less often in other parts of Central and South America. There are no reports of the infection from other continents.

MANAGEMENT STRATEGY

Itraconazole is the drug of choice in the treatment of most cases of paracoccidioidomycosis; it has been found to produce good results with 3–6 months of treatment. Long-term follow-up is required, however, as relapse rates are unknown. *Ketoconazole* is an alternative. *Amphotericin B* is the drug of choice in those patients who have rapidly progressive or severe infection. *Fluconazole* appears to be effective in experimental studies, but the results of clinical trials are not available to date.

SPECIFIC INVESTIGATIONS

- Direct microscopy of sputum or exudates in potassium hydroxide
- Culture
- Histology
- Serological test
- Serology for HIV/AIDS (where relevant)

Paracoccidioidomycosis associated with human immuno-deficiency virus infection. Report of 10 cases. Silva-

Vergara ML, Teixeira AC, Curi VG, et al. Med Mycol 2003;41:259–63.

Report of 10 cases of paracoccidioidomycosis in HIV-infected patients. However, the authors concluded that the frequency of paracoccidioidomycosis in HIV-infected individuals is not known to be different from that reported in non-HIV individuals.

FIRST LINE THERAPIES

■ Itraconazole	C
■ Ketoconazole	C

Randomized trial with itraconazole, ketoconazole and sulfadiazine in paracoccidioidomycosis. Shikanai-Yasuda MA, Benard G, Higaki Y, et al. Med Mycol 2002;40:411–7.

A randomized controlled trial involving 42 patients with active paracoccidioidomycosis, to compare the effectiveness of itraconazole, ketoconazole, and sulfadiazine in the treatment of the condition.

There was no evidence of superiority of any one regimen over the others in the clinical and serologic responses.

A case of paracoccidioidomycosis: experience with long-term therapy. Borgia G, Reynaud L, Cerini R, et al. Infection 2000;28:119–20.

Case report of a 61-year-old male patient from Venezuela who developed pulmonary lesions with evidence of bone infection. Once the diagnosis of infection by *Paracoccidioides brasiliensis* had been established, treatment was initiated with itraconazole 400 mg daily, reduced to 200 mg daily after 2 months. Complete remission was observed after 2 years of chemotherapy.

SECOND LINE THERAPIES

■ Amphotericin B	E
■ Terbinafine	E
■ Sulfamethoxazole–trimethoprim	E

Paracoccidioidomycosis: a clinical and epidemiological study of 422 cases observed in Mato Gross do Sul. Paniago AM, Aguiar JI, Aguiar ES, et al. Rev Soc Bras Med Trop 2003;36:455–9.

In terms of treatment, this paper shows that in endemic areas of paracoccidioidomycosis patients may benefit from treatment with sulfamethoxazole–trimethoprim.

Paracoccidioidomycosis in children: clinical presentation, follow-up and outcome. Pereira RM, Bucaretchi F, Barison Ede M, et al. Rev Inst Med Trop Sao Paulo 2004;46:127–31.

This paper focuses on the main features of paracoccidioidomycosis in children. It advocates sulfamethoxazole–trimethoprim as first line treatment for the infection.

Chronic paracoccidioidomycosis in a female patient in Austria. Mayr A, Kirchmair M, Rainer J, et al. Eur J Clin Microbiol Infect Dis 2004;23:916–9.

Case report of a female patient who was misdiagnosed as having tuberculosis. Once the correct diagnosis had been established, antifungal therapy was commenced with amphotericin B for 10 days and this was followed by voriconazole 200 mg daily for 3 months. The patient was originally from Cuba and this is an imported case of the condition.

Paracoccidioidomycosis case report: cure with amphotericin B and triple sulfa. Washburn RG, Bennet JE. J Med Vet Mycol 1986;24:235–7.

Case report of a male patient with paracoccidioidomycosis successfully treated with 2.5 g of amphotericin B and a 3-year course of sulfa. The patient is reported free of disease after 12 years of follow-up.

Failure of amphotericin B colloidal dispersion in the treatment of paracoccidioidomycosis. Dietze R, Flowler VG Jr, Steiner TS, et al. Am J Trop Med Hyg 1999;60:837–9.

Small clinical trial involving four adults with the juvenile form of paracoccidioidomycosis who were treated with amphotericin B colloidal dispersion at the dose of 3 mg/kg daily for at least 28 days. Although patients initially responded clinically, all four relapsed within 6 months of treatment.

Possible reasons for failure include dose, duration of therapy, and reduced efficacy of the lipid formulation.

Paracoccidioidomycosis (South American blastomycosis) successfully treated with terbinafine: first case report. Ollague JM, de Zurita AM, Calero G. Br J Dermatol 2000; 143:188–91.

Report of a 63-year-old male patient who developed a skin infection in perianal, perineal and scrotal areas, which proved to be due to paracoccidioidomycosis. Initial treatment was carried out with trimethoprim–sulfamethoxazole, with no clinical improvement. This was followed by a trial of terbinafine 250 mg twice daily for 6 months. There was rapid resolution of all lesions and the patient was clinically well without evidence of infection 2 years after completion of treatment.

Osteomyelitis caused by *Paracoccidioides brasiliensis* in a child from the metropolitan area of Rio de Janeiro. Nogueira SA, Guedes AL, Wanke B, et al. J Trop Pediatr 2001;47:311–5.

A report of a 7-year-old girl who developed osteomyelitis, misdiagnosed and treated as bacterial infection. She was successfully treated with amphotericin B.

Case report: severe juvenile type paracoccidioidomycosis with hepatitis C. Pellegrino A, de Capriles CH, Magaldi S, et al. Am J Trop Med Hyg 2003;68:301–3.

Case report of a 34-year-old male with a history of hepatitis C who developed severe paracoccidioidomycosis successfully treated with amphotericin B and itraconazole.

Fatal disseminated paracoccidioidomycosis in a two-year-old child. Pereira RM, Tresoldi AT, da Silva MT, Bucaretchi F. Rev Inst Med Trop Sao Paulo 2004;46:37–9.

This is a case report of a 2-year-old child who developed severe multisystem paracoccidioidomycosis and died despite prompt initiation of treatment with intravenous sulfamethoxazole–trimethoprim.

THIRD LINE THERAPIES

The use of glucan as immunostimulant in the treatment of paracoccidioidomycosis. Meira DA, Pereira PC, Marcondes-Machado J, et al. Am J Trop Med Hyg 1996;55: 496–503.

In this clinical trial, a group of 10 patients, nine of them reportedly severely infected with *Paracoccidioides brasiliensis*, received glucan (β-1,3 polyglucose) as an immunostimulant intravenously once weekly for 1 month, followed by monthly doses of 10 mg over a period of 11 months; this was used in conjunction with antifungal drugs. The control group, which consisted of eight moderately infected patients, was treated with only the antifungal agents. Patients who received glucan, despite being more seriously ill, showed a more favorable response to therapy.

Evidence levels **A** Double-blind study **B** Clinical trial ≥ 20 subjects **C** Clinical trial < 20 subjects **D** Series ≥ 5 subjects **E** Anecdotal case reports

Parapsoriasis

Alex Milligan, Rosie Davis

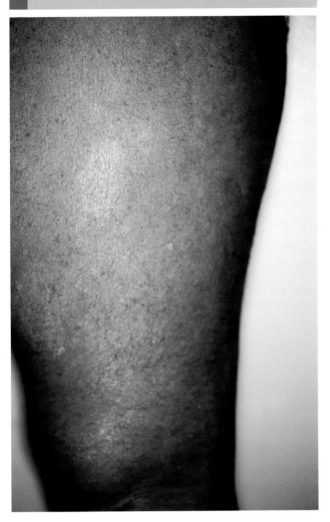

The diagnosis parapsoriasis, even as an umbrella term, continues to cause diagnostic difficulties and there is still debate as to whether the variants described in this chapter are in fact precursors of cutaneous T cell lymphomas. This chapter covers the entities small plaque parapsoriasis (SPP: chronic superficial scaly dermatitis; persistent superficial dermatitis; digitate dermatosis; xanthoerythroderma perstans) and large plaque parapsoriasis (LPP: parakeratosis variegata; retiform parapsoriasis; atrophic parapsoriasis; poikilodermatous parapsoriasis). Confusingly parapsoriasis en plaque has been used for either SPP or LPP.

Other conditions sometimes grouped under the banner of parapsoriasis are pityriasis lichenoides et varioliformis acuta (PLEVA), pityriasis lichenoides chronica, and lymphomatoid papulosis. These are covered on pages 498, 496, and 381.

Small plaque parapsoriasis

SPP consists of fixed small scaly erythematous plaques, which are asymptomatic or only mildly itchy and occur mainly on the trunk. The lesions sometimes appear to run in lines parallel to the ribs (hence the name 'digitate dermatosis'). SPP runs a chronic, indolent, and benign course.

MANAGEMENT STRATEGY

Diagnosis of parapsoriasis is made on clinical grounds, with histology supporting the clinical impression, especially when early cutaneous T cell lymphoma is in the differential diagnosis. Patches of LPP are larger than 5 cm in diameter, and often 10 cm or larger, distinguishing them from SPP, which is characterized by lesions smaller than 5 cm.

If malignancy is considered in the differential diagnosis, T cell receptor gene rearrangement studies are more likely to demonstrate monoclonality in cutaneous T cell lymphoma, though monoclonality is not entirely sensitive nor specific for the latter diagnosis. Repeat studies may be warranted if progression to cutaneous T cell lymphoma is suspected.

While some advocate unaggressive therapies, such as *topical corticosteroids*, for parapsoriasis, the potential for progression to cutaneous lymphoma in patients with LPP justifies the use of *psoralen with UVA (PUVA). Sunlight, broadband UVB,* and *narrowband UVB* have been used successfully as well, particularly for SPP.

SPECIFIC INVESTIGATIONS

- ■ The diagnosis is principally made on clinical findings
- ■ Histology is nonspecific
- ■ TCR gene rearrangement studies

Clonal T cell receptor gamma-chain gene rearrangement by PCR-based GeneScan analysis in the skin and blood of patients with parapsoriasis and early-stage mycosis fungoides. Klemke CD, Dippel E, Dembinski A, et al. J Pathol 2002;197:348–54.

Although studies have shown T cell clonality in both skin and peripheral blood, monoclonality is neither easily demonstrable nor thought to be a prerequisite for diagnosis.

FIRST LINE THERAPIES

■ Emollients, tar, topical corticosteroids	E
■ PUVA	C
■ Narrowband UVB	C
■ UVA/UVB	E

Treatments with emollients, topical tar, and topical corticosteroid is cited in books, and appear effective in clinical practice. There have been no studies or case reports to back this up and these treatments are therefore unreferenced.

Treatment of parapsoriasis and mycosis fungoides: the role of psoralen and long-wave ultraviolet light A (PUVA). Powell FC, Spiegel GT, Muller SA. Mayo Clin Proc 1984;59:538–46.

Seven patients with SPP had complete clearance with as few as 15 treatments (84 J/cm^2) of standard PUVA. Three patients experienced some recurrence at follow-up (mean of

13 months) and one of these patients was then successfully treated with topical corticosteroid.

Narrowband (311-nm) UV-B therapy for small plaque parapsoriasis and early-stage mycosis fungoides. Hofer A, Cerroni L, Kerl H, Wolf P. Arch Dermatol 1999;35:1377–80.

Fourteen patients with SPP were treated with narrowband UVB, three to four times weekly for 5–10 weeks. Complete response was achieved after an average of 20 exposures. All patients then relapsed after an average of 6 months and topical corticosteroid therapy was effective at producing a second clearance in an unspecified number of patients with parapsoriasis.

Home ultraviolet phototherapy of early mycosis fungoides: preliminary observations. Milstien H, Vonderheid E, Van Scott E, Johnson W. J Am Acad Dermatol 1982;6: 355–62.

Three patients with SPP were treated with home UV therapy (UVA and UVB source) for 3–18 months. Complete response was achieved after 6–7 months in the patients treated for the longer time period. Partial response was observed in the patient treated for only 3 months.

Balneophototherapy in small plaque parapsoriasis – four case reports. Gambichler T, Manke-Heimann A. J Eur Acad Dermatol Venereol 1998;10:179–81.

Four patients were treated for 4 weeks with salt-water baths and UV radiation. Clearance of over 90% was achieved and sustained for 8–12 weeks following therapy.

SECOND LINE THERAPIES

■ Topical nitrogen mustard	E

Topical carmustine (BCNU) for mycosis fungoides and related disorders: a 10-year experience. Zackheim HS, Epstein EH Jr, McNutt NS, et al. J Am Acad Dermatol 1983;9:363–74.

One patient with SPP was treated with carmustine as a subgroup of the study. A variety of treatment regimens were used and not individually specified. Complete response was achieved at follow-up, but the duration is not specified.

Large plaque parapsoriasis

Like SPP, the trunk is mainly affected, but the lesions are larger, atrophic, and even poikilodermatous, with a red or yellow-orange color.

SPECIFIC INVESTIGATIONS

■ Skin biopsy	
■ TCR gene rearrangement studies	

The diagnosis is suggested clinically. Histology can vary from a mild dermatitis to epidermal atrophy, lichenoid changes at the dermoepidermal junction, and a band-like lymphocytic infiltrate in the papillary dermis.

Progression to T cell lymphoma can occur. T cell clonality can be demonstrated in some patients.

Large plaque parapsoriasis: clinical and genotypic correlations. Simon M, Flaig MJ, Kind P, et al. J Cutan Pathol 2000;27:57–60.

TCR gene rearrangement status was assessed in 12 patients. Six of 12 patients showed a clonal T cell population, one of whom developed cutaneous T cell lymphoma after a follow-up of 8 years. The other five patients showed no such progression after follow-up of 2–21 years. The authors conclude that TCR gene rearrangement status has no prognostic significance and does not allow distinction of LPP and early mycosis fungoides.

The nosology of parapsoriasis. Lambert WC, Everett MA. J Am Acad Dermatol 1981;5:373–95.

Of 129 cases of LPP 11% developed mycosis fungoides over a follow-up period ranging from 1 to 64 years.

Parapsoriasis and mycosis fungoides: the Northwestern University experience, 1970 to 1985. Lazar AP, Caro WA, Roenigk HH, Pinski KS. J Am Acad Dermatol 1989;21: 919–23.

Of 89 patients with LPP, 30% developed mycosis fungoides. The follow-up period was not specified.

FIRST LINE THERAPIES

■ PUVA	C
■ PUVA with 4,6,4′-trimethylangelicin (TMA)	E

Photochemotherapy in cutaneous T cell lymphoma and parapsoriasis en plaque. Long-term follow-up in forty-three patients. Rosenbaum MM, Roenigk HH Jr, Caro WA, Esker A. J Am Acad Dermatol 1985;13:613–22.

Seven patients with LPP were included as part of the above study. They were treated with oral psoralens and ultraviolet A. Complete response was achieved in all seven patients though the total dosages of PUVA are not stated. Average follow-up for all 43 patients was 38.4 months (range 4–67 months) and during that time relapse was observed in five out of the seven patients with LPP.

Because cutaneous T cell lymphoma is in the differential diagnosis of LPP, and PUVA is effective for both conditions, this therapy is useful in patients in whom it is difficult to distinguish between the two conditions.

Treatment of a case of mycosis fungoides and one of parapsoriasis en plaque with topical PUVA using a monofunctional furocoumarin derivative, 4,6,4′-trimethylangelicin. Morita A, Takashima A, Nagai M, Dall'Acqua F. J Dermatol. 1990;17:545–9.

A single patient with LPP was treated with 0.1% TMA topical lotion (a monofunctional psoralen), followed 2 h later with UVA light. Clearance was achieved after nine treatments with 24 J/cm². A control area did not have the topical TMA applied to it and clearance was not obtained even after 20 treatments.

SECOND LINE THERAPIES

■ Topical nitrogen mustard	E

Topical carmustine (BCNU) for mycosis fungoides and related disorders: a 10-year experience. Zackheim HS, Epstein EH Jr, McNutt NS, et al. J Am Acad Dermatol 1983;9:363–74.

One patient with LPP was treated with carmustine as a subgroup of the larger study. Initially complete response was achieved, but at follow up (unknown duration), a partial response was observed. A variety of treatment regimens were used and not individually specified.

Evaluation of a one-hour exposure time to mechlorethamine in patients undergoing topical treatment. Foulc P, Evrard V, Dalac S, et al. Br J Dermatol 2002; 147:926–30.

Three patients with large plaque psoriasis were included in this study. One patient stopped treatment due to side effects and two of the three resulted in complete remission. The mechlorethamine regimen, however, varied between the four centers included in the study and is not specified for the individual patient.

Usefulness of topical chemotherapy is limited by the development of contact dermatitis. In addition, the incidence of squamous cell carcinoma of the skin is dramatically increased in patients treated with topical nitrogen mustard and PUVA.

THIRD LINE THERAPIES

■ Topical 2-4-dinitrochlorobenzene	E

Successful treatment of parapsoriasis en plaques with 2-4-dinitrochlorobenzene. Mandrea E. Arch Derm 1971;103: 560–1.

A single patient with LPP was treated topically with twice daily 1% 2-4-dinitrochlorobenzene in equal parts with olive oil and propylene glycol. The patient developed a painful, erythematous reaction and the treatment was stopped; 18 months later the skin remained clear.

Paronychia

Richard B Mallett

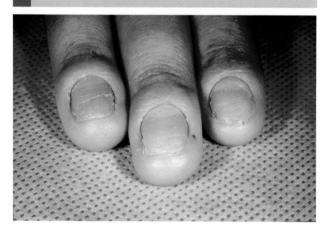

(Picture courtesy of Dr M J Majors)

Paronychia is characterized by inflammation of the proximal and/or lateral nailfolds, the fingers being more commonly affected than the toes. Acute paronychia is a painful pyogenic infection occurring after injury or minor trauma and is characteristically caused by *Staphylococcus aureus*, although anaerobic organisms are also found.

Chronic paronychia presents as tender erythema of the nailfolds with thickening of the tissues, loss of the cuticle, and subsequent dystrophy of the nail. Repetitive microtrauma and exposure to water, irritants and allergens resulting in a dermatitis with subsequent colonization by yeasts, and secondary bacterial infection are causative factors in chronic paronychia, one of the commonest nail disorders. Paronychia with pseudo-pyogenic granuloma may occur with systemic retinoids, antiretroviral drugs such as indinavir or lamivudine, the anti-epidermal growth factor antibody cetuximab, and gefitnib, an epidermal growth factor inhibitor.

MANAGEMENT STRATEGY

Acute paronychia requires urgent effective treatment to prevent damage to the nail matrix. If the infection is superficial and pointing, then *incision and drainage* without anesthesia is possible. Infection is often due to *S. aureus*, but β-hemolytic streptococci and anaerobic organisms may also be found. A swab for bacterial culture and antibiotic sensitivity must be taken and a *broad-spectrum antibiotic* covering both aerobic and anaerobic organisms given. *Warm compresses with an astringent* (e.g. aluminum acetate lotion, if available) can help reduce edema and provide a hostile environment for bacteria. For deeper infections, antibiotic treatment should be started immediately, and if there has been no marked clinical improvement after 48 h, *surgical treatment* undertaken. Under local anesthesia, the proximal third of the nail plate is removed and a gauze wick is laid under the proximal nailfold to allow drainage.

Chronic paronychia is a dermatitis often associated with wet work – in domestics, cooks, bartenders, fishmongers, etc. – and may be exacerbated by contact irritants or allergens. Immediate sensitivity to fresh foods can be a factor. In children, thumb sucking may initiate the condition. Eczema or psoriasis may predispose to chronic paronychia, as may poor peripheral circulation. Microtrauma, including overzealous manicuring of the cuticle, is also important. The middle and index fingers of the right hand and middle finger of the left hand are most commonly affected, but any finger may be involved. Inflammation with bolstering of the nailfold and loss of the cuticle opens a space between the nailfold and the nail plate, which commonly becomes infected with yeast, especially *Candida* species, and a wide range of other microorganisms. Acute exacerbations due to bacterial infection may occur. Successful treatment relies on protection of the affected fingers from water, irritants, allergens, and trauma, together with anti-inflammatory treatment with moderately potent or potent *topical corticosteroids*. Swabs for yeast and bacteria should be taken, *anticandidal preparations* can be useful, and antibiotic preparations may also be needed. Treatment should be continued until the inflammation has subsided and the cuticle has reformed and reattached to the nail plate (3 months or more). Applying 80% phenol with a toothpick to the groove under the proximal nailfold may encourage reattachment. Warm compresses for 10 minutes with an astringent lotion may help acute exacerbations. For frequent acute episodes, *intralesional or systemic corticosteroids plus systemic antibiotics* for a week may be useful. In cases where conservative management fails, surgery or *low-dose superficial radiotherapy* may be considered.

Drug-induced pseudo-pyogenic granulomatous paronychia responds to daily topical 2% *mupirocin* with *clobetasol propionate* ointment.

SPECIFIC INVESTIGATIONS

- Skin swabs
- Open patch tests

Anaerobic paronychia. Whitehead SM, Eykyn SJ, Phillips I. Br J Surg 1981;68:420–2.

Swabs were taken from 116 acute paronychias. Anaerobes or mixed aerobes and anaerobes were isolated in 30%. Of 81 paronychias with aerobic organisms only, *S. aureus* was isolated in 69%.

Chronic paronychia. Short review of 590 cases. Frain-Bell W. Trans St John's Hosp Dermatol Soc 1957;38:29–35.

On culture, *Candida albicans* was grown in 70% and bacteria, including *S. aureus*, in 10%.

An excellent overview.

Role of foods in the pathogenesis of chronic paronychia. Tosti A, Guerra L, Morelli R, et al. J Am Acad Dermatol 1992;27:706–10.

Nine of 20 food handlers with chronic paronychia had positive reactions to 20-minute open patch tests with suspected fresh foods, including wheat flour, egg, chicory, and tomatoes.

FIRST LINE THERAPIES

Acute	
■ Amoxicillin with clavulinic acid	E
■ Surgical drainage	E
Chronic	
■ Topical corticosteroid preparations	B
■ Topical econazole lotion four times daily	B
■ Topical clotrimazole drops	E
■ Topical clindamycin solution	E
Drug-induced periungual granuloma	
■ Mupirocin and clobetasol propionate	E

Paronychia: a mixed infection, microbiology and management. Brook I. J Hand Surg [Br] 1993;18:358–9.

Culture from 61 patients with paronychia showed a mixture of both aerobic and anaerobic bacteria in 49%. The combination of amoxicillin with clavulinic acid is suggested as first line treatment for acute bacterial paronychia, together with appropriate surgical drainage.

Nail surgery and traumatic abnormalities. Haneke E, Baran R, Brauner GJ. In: Baran R, Dawber RP, eds. Diseases of the Nails and their Management, 2nd edn. Oxford: Blackwell Scientific; 1994:408.

For acute paronychia, under local anesthesia the proximal third of the nail plate is removed and a wick laid under the proximal nailfold.

Topical steroids versus systemic antifungals in the treatment of chronic paronychia: an open, randomized double-blind and double dummy study. Tosti A, Piraccini BM, Ghetti E. J Am Acad Dermatol 2002;47:73–6.

An open, randomized, double-blind trial of oral itraconazole, oral terbinafine, and topical methylprednisolone aceponate. Patients were treated for 3 weeks and observed for a further 6 weeks. Of 48 nails treated with methylprednisolone aceponate, 41 (85%) were improved or cured at the end of the study, compared with only 30 of 57 (53%) with itraconazole and 29 of 64 (45%) with terbinafine.

The management of superficial candidiasis. Hay RJ. J Am Acad Dermatol 1999;40(6 pt 2):S35–42.

The central role of *Candida* in chronic paronychia is debatable, and other factors such as irritant or allergic dermatitis may play a role. Therefore, as well as polyenes or imidazoles, concomitant use of a topical corticosteroid is a logical approach.

Comparison of the therapeutic effect of ketaconazole tablets and econazole lotion in the treatment of chronic paronychia. Wong ESM, Hay RJ, Clayton YM, Noble WC. Clin Exp Dermatol 1984;9:489–96.

A randomized trial comparing oral ketaconazole 200 mg once daily versus topical econazole lotion 2 mL four times daily in 24 patients with chronic paronychia and positive cultures for *Candida* species. All patients were also advised to wear rubber gloves for wet work and to dry hands thoroughly, and told not to push back the nailfold or wear nail varnish. There was no significant difference between the two treatments, suggesting that topical econazole lotion is suitable for first line treatment of chronic paronychia in the presence of *Candida* infection.

Diseases of the nails in infants and children: paronychia. Silverman RA. In: Callen JP, Dhal MV, Golitz LE, et al, eds. Advances in Dermatology. Volume 5. Chicago: Year Book; 1990:164–5.

Clotrimazole drops several times a day should inhibit fungal growth. Topical clindamycin solution applied to the fingers several times daily kills bacteria, has a bitter taste to discourage finger sucking, and has an alcohol–propylene glycol vehicle that dries out residual moisture. Side effects from oral absorption of these medications have not been reported.

Paronychia associated with antiretroviral therapy. Tosti A, Piraccini BM, D'Antuono A, et al. Br J Dermatol 1999;140:1165–8.

Six cases of periungual pseudo-pyogenic granuloma induced by indinavir, lamivudine, and zidovudine responded to daily applications of clobetasol propionate and mupirocin.

SECOND LINE THERAPIES

Chronic	
■ 15% Sulfacetamide in 50% spirit	E
■ Nystatin ointment	E
■ 4% Thymol in chloroform	E
■ Intralesional or systemic corticosteroids and antibiotics	E

Management of disorders of the nails. Samman PD. Clin Exp Dermatol 1982;7:189–94.

Chronic paronychia can be treated with 15% sulfacetamide in 50% spirit applied frequently. Sulfacetamide is both antifungal and antibacterial.

A good overview of nail disease.

Treatment of chronic paronychia. Vickers HR. Br Med J 1979;2:1588.

A nystatin-containing ointment should be worked into the affected nailfold every time the patient is going to get the hands wet, for at least 6 weeks.

Paronychia and onycholysis, aetiology and therapy. Wilson JW. Arch Dermatol 1965;92:726–30.

Thymol has both bactericidal and antifungal properties. Apply 4% thymol in chloroform to the nailfold and allow to penetrate by capillary action. Application should be three times daily and, additionally, immediately after immersion in water.

Fungal and other infections. Hay RJ, Baran R, Haneke E. In: Baran R, Dawber RP, eds. Diseases of the Nails and their Management, 2nd edn. Oxford: Blackwell Scientific; 1994:119–20.

For frequent acute exacerbations of chronic paronychia, intralesional or systemic corticosteroids plus either erythromycin 1 g daily or tetracycline 1 g daily for a week is recommended.

THIRD LINE THERAPIES

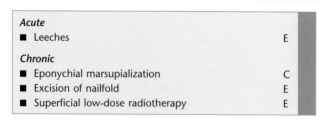

Acute	
■ Leeches	E
Chronic	
■ Eponychial marsupialization	C
■ Excision of nailfold	E
■ Superficial low-dose radiotherapy	E

Thumb paronychia treated with leeches. Graham CE. Med J Austr 1992;156:512.

Acute paronychia successfully treated with leeches while trekking in Tasmania.

Eponychial marsupialization and nail removal for surgical treatment of chronic paronychia. Bednar MS, Lane LB. J Hand Surg [Am] 1991;16:314–7.

Twenty-eight fingers with chronic paronychia were treated with marsupialization of the dorsal roof of the proximal nailfold plus complete or partial removal of the nail in those patients with associated nail abnormality. Post-operative treatment was with hydrogen peroxide soaks and oral antibiotics for 5–14 days. Twenty-seven of 28 fingers were cured.

Surgical treatment of recalcitrant chronic paronychia of the fingers. Baran R, Bureau H. J Dermatol Surg Oncol 1981;7:106–7.

Description of the technique of simple excision of the affected nailfold without the need for marsupialization.

How we treat paronychia. Fliegelman MT, Lafayette GO. Postgrad Med 1970;48:267–8.

For recalcitrant cases of chronic paronychia, triamcinolone can be injected into the affected nailfold. For the most severe cases, a course of low-dose superficial radiotherapy may be given.

Evidence levels **A** Double-blind study **B** Clinical trial ≥ 20 subjects **C** Clinical trial < 20 subjects **D** Series ≥ 5 subjects **E** Anecdotal case reports

Parvovirus infection

Robert Burd

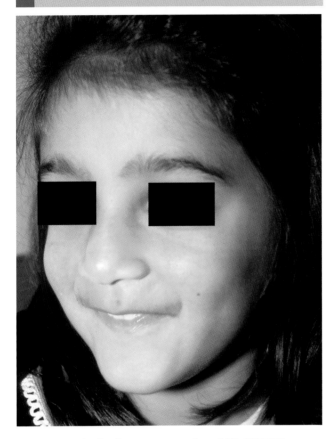

Infection with the human parvovirus B19 (HPB19) causes erythema infectiosum, the 'fifth' of the classic childhood exanthems. The infection may be asymptomatic, there being no rash in up to 50% of people. Erythema infectiosum usually affects school-aged children between 5 and 15 years. There is a short prodrome of fever, malaise, and pharyngitis. The classic features of the exanthem are the 'slapped cheek' sign together with circumoral pallor and an evanescent macular, reticulated or 'lace-like' rash over the trunk and proximal limbs. The rash may last for up to 4 weeks and subsequently may recur following sun exposure. In patients with a predisposing hematological condition infection with HPB19 may cause a transient aplastic crisis. Chronic infection is rarely encountered in immunosuppressed patients.

MANAGEMENT STRATEGY

Erythema infectiosum is typically a self-resolving exanthem, so in the majority of cases, *supportive care and reassurance* are all that are required; however, the clinician should be aware of a variety of rare atypical presentations of HPB19 infection.

The rash is immune complex-mediated so patients are assumed to be no longer infectious by the time that it appears. Once a clinical diagnosis has been made parents can be reassured and advised on simple supportive meas-ures such as antipyretics, fluids, and simple emollients for the rash. In the majority of immunocompetent patients the condition is self-resolving.

Infection with HPB19 is known to be the cause of a variety of other cutaneous manifestations. The most common is an acral, so-called 'glove and stocking' petechial eruption. This eruption may be seen together with the 'slapped cheek' sign; it can also be seen in isolation. More recently, it has been reported that infection with HPB19 is associated with the development of the cutaneous signs of various connective tissue disorders, in particular dermato-myositis and a lupus erythematosus-like condition.

In older patients, especially middle-aged women, the infection may cause arthritis. This may accompany the rash, but often follows it. Often the arthritis is also self-resolving and *nonsteroidal anti-inflammatory drugs (NSAIDs)* may be given for symptomatic relief. Occasionally the arthritis may lead a more chronic course. HPB19 has also been implicated in the development of juvenile rheumatoid arthritis.

HPB19 is extremely tropic for erythroblasts. In predis-posed individuals with either an underlying hemolytic state, actively bleeding, or iron deficiency, HPB19 infection can cause a transient aplastic crisis. In addition to anemia, there may be moderate neutropenia and thrombocytopenia. Usually the anemia is self-limiting but *transfusion* may be indicated if severe. In immunocompromised patients chronic HPB19 infection can result in chronic anemia due to a pure red cell aplasia. This can be rapidly treated with com-mercial *immunoglobulin infusion*. Potentially fatal marrow necrosis rarely occurs in very young children. Severe cases of aplastic anemia that do not respond to intravenous immunoglobulin may be cured by undergoing *bone marrow transplantation*.

Pregnant ladies who are in contact with children with parvovirus infection are advised to have their own immu-nity checked because of the rare complication of 'hydrops fetalis'. In immunosuppressed patients, HPB19 infection may have more serious consequences. In the absence of an appropriate immune response the infection can become chronic. This may lead to more profound red cell aplasia and may require *immunoglobulin infusions*, which are often cura-tive. In refractory cases, *interferon therapy* may be helpful.

Infection with HPB19 has also been identified as a cause of chronic fatigue syndrome, central nervous system vas-culitis, and liver failure. Immunoglobulin infusions have been useful in managing rare complications including chronic fatigue syndrome.

SPECIFIC INVESTIGATIONS

- ■ Hematology (complete blood count)
- ■ Serology

IgM antibodies to HPB19 indicate recent infection. IgG antibodies to HPB19 indicate past exposure and may be positive in over half the adult population.

A typical clinical appearance together with supportive serology is sufficient to establish the diagnosis in the major-ity of cases. In at-risk patients or those who have symptoms of anemia a full blood count will establish whether there is any significant level of anemia requiring transfusion.

It is possible to detect virus DNA, both in the blood and lesional skin, using polymerase chain reaction techniques.

This may be of use if investigating an atypical presentation of HPB19 infection.

Parvovirus B19. Young NS, Brown KE. N Engl J Med 2004;350:586–97.

A comprehensive review of HPB19 infection.

The cutaneous manifestations of human parvovirus B19 infection. Magro CM, Dawood MR, Crowson N. Hum Pathol 2000;31:488–97.

A description of the cutaneous manifestations of a series of 14 patients who were shown to have antecedent HPB19 infection with positive serology and/or B19 genome in skin samples.

FIRST LINE THERAPIES

■ Reassurance	E
■ Antipyretics (e.g. acetaminophen [paracetamol], ibuprofen)	E

Acute and chronic parvovirus infection. Young NS. In: Schlossberg D, ed. Current Therapy of Infectious Diseases, 2nd edn. St Louis: Mosby; 2001:610–2.

The majority of children require no specific therapy and parents can be reassured that the rash will resolve with time. Simple supportive therapies may be used during this time.

SECOND LINE THERAPIES

■ NSAIDs	E
■ Systemic corticosteroids	E
■ Blood transfusion	E

Human parvovirus infection: rheumatic manifestations, angioedema, C1 esterase inhibitor deficiency, ANA positivity and possible onset of systemic lupus erythematosus. Fawaz-Estrup F. J Rheumatol 1996;23:1180–5.

A series of nine adult patients with serological evidence of acute or recent HPB19 infection and polyarthralgia/polyarthritis. All patients responded to NSAIDs, though one patient also required pulsed intravenous methylprednisolone for a lupus-like illness.

In older children and adults the arthralgia/arthritis may be severe enough to warrant treatment with a NSAID. In the majority of cases the joint symptoms settle within a few days or weeks.

Parvoviruses and bone marrow failure. Brown KE, Young NS. Stem Cells 1996;14:151–63.

In patients with underlying hemolytic disorders, infection with HPB19 is the primary cause of a transient aplastic crisis, which may require transfusion. In immunocompromised patients, persistent infection may manifest as pure red cell aplasia and chronic anemia.

THIRD LINE THERAPIES

■ Immunoglobulin infusion	D
■ Bone marrow transplantation	E
■ Interferon-α/β	E

Persistent B19 parvovirus infection in patients infected with human immunodeficiency virus type 1 (HIV-1): a treatable cause of anaemia in AIDS. Frickhofen N, Abkowitz J, Safford M, et al. Ann Intern Med 1990;113:926–33.

A series of seven patients who were HIV positive with persistent HPB19 infection and anemia. Six patients were treated with intravenous immunoglobulin and showed rapid reduction in serum virus concentrations and subsequent resolution of their anemia. Two patients relapsed but again responded to further immunoglobulin.

Successful intravenous immunoglobulin therapy in 3 cases of parvovirus B19-associated chronic fatigue syndrome. Kerr JR, Cunniffe VS, Kelleher P, et al. Clin Infect Dis 2003;36:e100–6.

Three patients with chronic fatigue syndrome secondary to persistent parvovirus B19 infection were successfully treated with intravenous immunoglobulin therapy at a dosage of 400 mg/kg daily for 5 days.

Successful bone marrow transplantation for severe aplastic anaemia in a patient with persistent human parvovirus B19 infection. Goto H, Ishida A, Fujii H, et al. Int J Hematol 2004;79:384–6.

A single case of a previously immunocompetent 9-year-old girl with persistent HPB19 infection and aplastic anemia treated with a bone marrow transplant from an HLA-identical sibling donor.

Initial and innate responses to viral infections – pattern setting in immunity or disease. Biron CA. Curr Opin Microbiol 1999;2:374–81.

Endogenous interferon-α/β can help control the magnitude of the innate response to viral infections.

There is evidence that interferons-α and β enhance the immune reaction to virus-infected cells; this may be useful in exceptional circumstances in patients with chronic parvovirus infection.

Pediculosis

Charlot Grech, Mark G Lebwohl

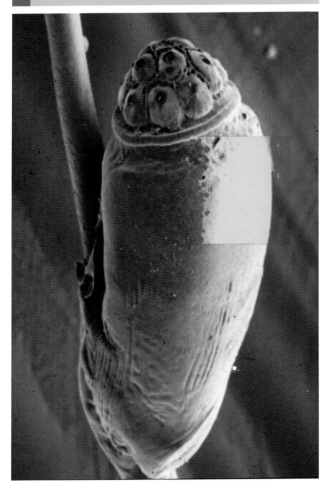

Lice are wingless, dorsoventrally flattened, blood-sucking insects that are obligate ectoparasites of birds and mammals. Pediculosis is an infestation by *Pediculosis capitis* (head louse), *Pediculosis humanus* (body louse), or *Phthirus pubis* (pubic or crab louse). The bites of lice are painless and can rarely be detected. The clinical signs and symptoms are the result of the host's reaction to the saliva and anticoagulant injected into the dermis by the louse at the time of feeding. Depending on the degree of sensitivity and previous exposure, the feeding sites produce red macules or papules hours to days after feeding. An acute wheal may develop as an immediate reaction. Pruritus is the most common symptom of any type of pediculosis.

Pediculosis capitis

MANAGEMENT STRATEGY

All children and adults in the household should be examined. Some authors treat only those individuals found to be infested, while others suggest routinely *treating the entire family* simultaneously; this author concurs with the latter.

Families should be instructed in contact tracing that is listing people likely to have had head-to-head contact with the infected members during the previous 4–6 weeks. These people should then perform detection combing to check for live lice and be treated if necessary.

There are a number of *insecticides* available that kill both head lice and their eggs. All are neurotoxic (acetylcholinesterase inhibitors) to the lice, but young eggs do not possess a nervous system and may survive a single treatment. *Two treatments should therefore be given, 7 days apart.* Insecticides should not be applied more than once a week for 3 weeks at a time. The minimal volume required for a single application is usually 50–60 mL (depending on the product and hair density). Any concurrent bacterial infection should be treated with the appropriate antibiotic. In patients with scalp dermatitis only water-based insecticides should be used because the alcoholic ones will sting the open skin.

Following therapy, infested individuals should put on clean clothes and should *machine-wash and dry (hot cycle) all clothing, bed linens, towels, and any headgear. Combs and brushes should be washed in hot water or coated with a pediculicide for about 15 min and then washed. Floors and furniture should be vacuumed.*

SPECIFIC INVESTIGATIONS

- Examination for nits and lice

FIRST LINE THERAPIES

■ Permethrin 1% cream rinse	A
■ Malathion 0.5% lotion	B
■ Carbaryl 0.5% lotion	B

American Academy of Pediatrics guidelines for the prevention and treatment of head lice infestation. Frankowski BL. Am J Manag Care 2004;10:S269–72.

Resistance to permethrin 5% and lindane has emerged, whereas malathion 0.5% remains approximately 98% ovicidal, and resistance has not been a problem.

The guidelines point out that malathion is flammable and can cause serious adverse effects if ingested, but there have been very few cases of malathion toxicity. The guidelines also criticize 'no-NIT' policies in schools stating that this overresponse to pediculosis is out of proportion to its medical significance.

Efficacy of a reduced application time of Ovide lotion (0.5% malathion) compared to Nix creme rinse (1% permethrin) for the treatment of head lice. Meinking TL, Vicaria M, Eyerdam DH, et al. Pediatr Dermatol 2004;21: 670–4.

In this investigator-blinded study, a 20-min application of 0.5% malathion was significantly more pediculicidal and ovicidal (98%) than 1% permethrin (55%) applied for 8–12 h.

Carbaryl lotions for head lice – new laboratory tests show variation in efficacy. Burgess I. Pharm J 1990;245:159–61.

Comparative efficacy of treatments for pediculosis capitis infestations. Meinking TL, Taplin D, Kalter DC, Eberle MW. Arch Dermatol 1986;122:267–71.

In-vitro comparisons. Before the development of widespread resistance to current medications, alcohol-based lotions containing terpene fragrances (Carylderm® [carbaryl] and Suleo-M® [malathion] lotions) had greater ovicidal activity than those without terpenes (Prioderm® [malathion]). Malathion lotion was demonstrated to be a highly effective, rapid-acting pediculicide and an excellent ovicide. The permethrin crème rinse was less ovicidal than the liquids and lotions.

Shampoo formulations have low ovidical activity and may not kill lice. They are no longer recommended.

Permethrin. Taplin D, Meinking TL. Curr Probl Dermatol 1996;24:255–60.

Five controlled clinical trials conducted between 1983 and 1993 treated a total of 2148 patients. Permethrin 1% (Nix® crème rinse) rendered 98% of patients free from head lice and viable eggs 2 weeks after a single treatment. It was superior to 1% lindane shampoo (77%) and two synergized natural pyrethrin products. This also demonstrated a marked difference in efficacy between two products with the same amount of active ingredients but in different vehicles (Rid® lotion vs R&C® shampoo [58% vs 16%]).

SECOND LINE THERAPIES

■ Lindane 1% shampoo	B
■ Topical ivermectin	B
■ Oral ivermectin	B
■ Oral co-trimoxazole	C
■ Topical crotamiton	B
■ Topical petrolatum	D

Topical application of ivermectin for human ectoparasites. Youssef MY, Sadaka HA, Eissa MM, el Ariny AF. Am J Trop Med Hyg 1995;53:652–3.

This study treated 50 patients with scabies and 25 patients with head lice with topical ivermectin as a liquid form in a concentration of 0.8% weight to volume dilution using 15–25 mL for each patient. All patients treated for head lice were cured, clinically and parasitologically, within 48 h after a single topical application. No topical formulation of ivermectin is currently available.

Efficacy of ivermectin for the treatment of head lice. Glaziou P, Nyguyen LN, Moulia-Pelat JP, et al. Trop Med Parasitol 1994;45:253–4.

In this study, 26 patients with head lice received a single dose of oral ivermectin 200 μg/kg body weight in an open fashion. On day 14 after treatment, 20 had responded (77%).

Oral therapy of pediculosis capitis with cotrimoxazole. Shashindran CH, Gandhi IS, Krishnasamy S, Ghosh MN. Br J Dermatol 1978;98:699.

Twenty patients were treated with varying doses of co-trimoxazole. The minimal effective dose of co-trimoxazole in pediculosis was found to be one tablet twice daily for 3 days. Two courses of co-trimoxazole spaced 10 days apart will eradicate the infestation without requiring any external application. Neither trimethoprim nor sulfamethoxazole is effective when given alone.

A single application of crotamiton lotion in the treatment of patients with pediculosis capitis. Karacic I, Yawalkar SJ. Int J Dermatol 1982;21:611–13.

A single application of 10% crotamiton lotion cured 96% of the 49 patients treated for pediculosis capitis. Only 4% of patients needed a second application.

Treatment resistant head lice: alternative therapeutic approaches. Schachner LA. Pediatr Dermatol 1997;14:409–10.

This article makes reference to the 'Dr Schachner's petrolatum shampoo' where 30–40 g of standard petrolatum is massaged on the entire surface of the hair and scalp. It is left overnight with a shower cap over the scalp and hair. Diligent shampooing is usually necessary for at least the next 7–10 days to remove the residue. The working hypothesis is that viscous petrolatum clogs both the respiratory spiracles of the adult louse, blocking efficient exchange of air, as well as the holes in the operculum of the head louse nit. This deprives the young nymph of the air exchange it needs for survival and to expel itself from the nit.

THIRD LINE THERAPIES

■ Combination permethrin and trimethoprim/sulfamethoxazole	B
■ Citronella to repel head lice	A
■ Oral thiabendazole	B

Head lice infestation: single drug versus combination therapy with one percent permethrin and trimethoprim/sulfamethoxazole. Hipolito RB, Mallorca FG, Zuniga-Macaraig ZO, et al. Pediatrics 2001;107:E30.

Children were treated with either 1% permethrin creme rinse, oral trimethoprim/sulfamethoxazole, or a combination of both treatments; 79.5% of children were free of lice or nits at 2 weeks in the group treated with permethrin creme rinse. Of children treated with oral trimethoprim/sulfamethoxazole, 83% were clear at 2 weeks compared to 95% clearing of children treated with both agents.

The addition of oral trimethoprim/sulfamethoxazole appears to enhance the efficacy of topical pediculicides such as permethrin.

Repellency of citronella for head lice: double-blind randomized trial of efficacy and safety. Mumcuoglu KY, Magdassi S, Miller J, et al. Isr Med Assoc J 2004;6:756–9.

In this double-blind, placebo-controlled study, 12% of children treated with a slow-release citronella formulation were infested with lice compared to 50.5% of those treated with placebo. The only side effects were unpleasant odor in 4.4% and slight itching and burning in 1% of children.

Treatment of pediculosis capitis with thiabendazole: a pilot study. Namazi MR. Int J Dermatol 2003;42:973–6.

Oral thiabendazole 20 mg/kg was administered twice daily for 1 day and repeated at day 10; 91% of subjects improved and 61% had complete responses. Nausea and dizziness were reported in four of 23 patients.

Evidence levels   A Double-blind study   B Clinical trial ≥ 20 subjects   C Clinical trial < 20 subjects   D Series ≥ 5 subjects   E Anecdotal case reports

Pediculosis pubis

MANAGEMENT STRATEGY

The insecticide should be applied to infested and adjacent hairy areas with particular attention to the mons pubis and perianal regions. Only aqueous preparations should be used. In hairy individuals, the application should include the thighs, trunk, and axillary hair due to their frequent involvement. Treatment should be repeated after an interval of 7–10 days. All sexual contacts should be treated simultaneously and following treatment fresh underclothing, nightwear and bed linen should be used; these items should be machine washed and dried.

FIRST LINE THERAPIES

■ Carbaryl 1% in an aqueous vehicle	B
■ Malathion 0.5% in an aqueous vehicle or 1% cream shampoo	B
■ Lindane 1% shampoo	B

Scabies and pediculosis pubis: an update of treatment regimens and general review. Wendel K, Rompalo A. Clin Infect Dis 2002;35(Suppl 2):S146–51.

Although resistance to topical permethrin, lindane, or pyrethrins with piperonyl butoxide has been reported in head lice, these agents have remained effective in the treatment of pubic lice.

Treatment of pediculosis pubis. Kalter DC, Sperber J, Rosen T, Matarasso S. Arch Dermatol 1987;123:1315–19.

Pyrethroids have only limited efficacy.

Pediculosis ciliaris. Chin GN, Denslow GT. J Pediatr Ophthalmol Strabismus 1978;15:173–5.

This article is a case report and review of the various treatments of eyelash infection with the pubic louse. Mechanical removal, epilation of eyelashes, cryotherapy, thick application of petrolatum twice daily for 2 weeks, yellow mercuric oxide ointment, and physostigmine ointment (popular with ophthalmologists) have all been reported. A child was treated with a 1% permethrin cream rinse, applied to the eyelashes on a cotton swab and rinsed 10 min later. A course of co-trimoxazole or tetracycline is usually effective. The safest treatment is petrolatum.

Pediculosis corporis

MANAGEMENT STRATEGY

Therapy consists of proper hygiene, use of clean clothes and bedding, and a head-to-toe treatment with 5% permethrin cream or lotion left for 8–14 h. In mass eradication, permethrin or malathion dusting powder should be used and all clothing and bedding fumigated or discarded as hazardous waste.

FIRST LINE THERAPIES

■ Attention to hygiene	C
■ 5% permethrin cream or lotion	E

Pemphigus

Carlos H Nousari, Grant J Anhalt

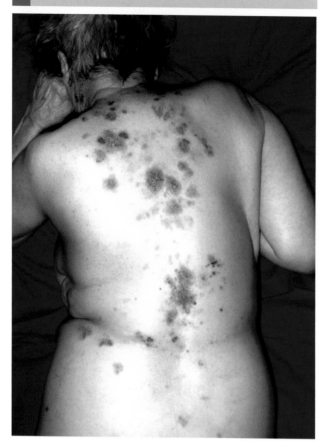

The term 'pemphigus' is applied to a group of autoimmune mucocutaneous blistering disorders defined by the presence of pathogenic autoantibodies against desmosomal adhesion molecules. There are three immunopathologically distinct subsets of pemphigus: vulgaris, foliaceus, and paraneoplastic. The risks of morbidity and mortality vary greatly between each subset, and treatment is therefore individualized.

MANAGEMENT STRATEGY

The treatment of pemphigus is different from that of most other skin diseases because it is an autoimmune disease in which the epidermis is merely the 'target'. Animal studies have clearly shown that if enough autoantibody reaches the skin, blistering will occur, and this damage cannot be prevented by inhibition of inflammatory events or even pretreatment with high doses of *systemic corticosteroids*. The primary goal in all forms of pemphigus must be reducing the synthesis of autoantibodies by the immune system; topical treatment of the mucous membranes or skin has no net effect on the course of the disease. Some temporary reduction of pain or inflammation can occur with *topical corticosteroids or intralesional injections or corticosteroids*, but these will not be discussed for this reason.

The unique immunologic mechanism of each subset of pemphigus dictates some variation in individual therapeutic regimens. Other factors complicate the management, and include the following.

1. Circulating autoantibodies have a degradative half-life of about 3 weeks. Lasting improvement can only occur with reduction of both existing and newly produced antibody, so improvement occurs very slowly unless the antibodies are physically removed by *plasmapheresis* or their catabolism is increased by administration of high doses of exogenous *normal human immunoglobulin (IVIG)*.
2. Pemphigus is notorious in its persistence. Spontaneous permanent remissions typically do not occur, and remissions and relapses are common. Most people require some form of treatment for life.
3. Only a small repertoire of drugs are effective at reducing autoantibody synthesis, and the most effective of those, *cyclophosphamide*, has potential toxicities that cause concern to many treating physicians and can restrict the appropriate use of this drug.
4. All forms of pemphigus are rare, and this prohibits the execution of large, controlled trials. The literature discussing therapeutic regimens is dominated by small series and case reports, which is a weak evidence base for the design of rational treatment. However, we do have excellent animal models of this disease, and have a good understanding of the pathophysiology from these studies, which are instrumental in designing our approach to treatment.

Treatment consists of four basic steps.

1. Systemic corticosteroids alone.
2. Corticosteroids plus an antimetabolite such as *azathioprine* or *mycophenolate mofetil*.
2a. Step 2 with the additional use of IVIG or *rituximab*.
3. Corticosteroids plus cyclophosphamide.
4. Corticosteroids plus cyclophosphamide plus short-term plasmapheresis.

The commitment to the use of cyclophosphamide is a serious one. This drug is extremely effective, but use of this alkylating agent is accompanied by a long-term increased risk of leukemia, lymphoma, and bladder cancer, as well as the risk of sterility in younger patients. The use of newer agents such as IVIG and rituximab is being explored as a way to avert having to use cyclophosphamide.

A number of drugs have been reported to be beneficial in small series or case reports, but these lack a clear rationale for their use because they have no known mechanism(s) by which they can effectively inhibit new antibody synthesis, and should not be employed. This list includes tetracycline and niacin (nicotinamide), methotrexate, dapsone, and gold. A recent well-performed randomized trial also showed no corticosteroid-sparing benefit with the use of cyclosporine, so its use in pemphigus vulgaris is not recommended, though it still has a role in the treatment of paraneoplastic pemphigus (see Cyclosporine, page 477).

SPECIFIC INVESTIGATIONS

- Skin biopsy for routine microscopy
- Skin biopsy for direct immunofluorescence
- Serum for indirect immunofluorescence
- Malignancy screening tests in patients with paraneoplastic pemphigus

Making sense of antigens and antibodies in pemphigus.
Anhalt GJ. J Am Acad Dermatol 1999;40:763–6.

Accuracy of indirect immunofluorescence testing in the diagnosis of paraneoplastic pemphigus. Helou J, Allbritton J, Anhalt GJ. J Am Acad Dermatol 1995;32:441–7.

The diagnosis of pemphigus must be established by fulfilling three criteria; without documentation of all three, the diagnosis is not certain. These criteria are:

- the appropriate clinical features;
- histologic changes showing acantholysis of affected epithelium;
- demonstration of IgG autoantibodies on the cell surface of affected epithelium or detection of antigen-specific autoantibodies in the blood.

Pemphigus vulgaris is characterized by progressively evolving fragile blisters and erosions. Oral involvement essentially 'always' occurs and is the major point to differentiate pemphigus vulgaris from pemphigus foliaceus. Histologic changes include suprabasilar acantholysis and cell surface-bound IgG. Circulating autoantibodies are specific for desmoglein 3 alone when lesions are restricted to the mouth, and for both desmoglein 3 and 1 when cutaneous lesions are present in addition to oral lesions. Definition of the specificity of desmoglein autoantibodies can be reliably gained by enzyme-linked immunosorbent assay (ELISA).

In pemphigus foliaceus mucosal lesions 'never' occur; this is the major clinical feature to differentiate it from pemphigus vulgaris. Cutaneous lesions are more superficial scaling erosions. Immunopathologic studies reveal subcorneal acantholysis and tissue-bound and circulating anti-desmoglein 1 antibodies.

Paraneoplastic pemphigus occurs in the context of the following lymphoproliferative disorders: non-Hodgkin's lymphoma, chronic lymphocytic leukemia, Castleman's disease, thymomas, and retroperitoneal sarcomas. Intractable mucositis with lichenoid erosions is the most constant clinical finding. Polymorphous cutaneous involvement with lesions that resemble erythema multiforme, pemphigus, pemphigoid, or lichenoid eruptions are observed. Histology can show suprabasilar acantholysis or interface/lichenoid changes. The key diagnostic finding is the presence of antibodies against desmoglein 3 and 1, and additional autoantibodies against epithelial plakin proteins such as desmoplakin, envoplakin, and periplakin. These antiplakin autoantibodies can be defined by immunoblotting or immunoprecipitation techniques, or inferred by their reactivity with murine bladder epithelium by immunofluorescent techniques.

FIRST LINE THERAPIES

Pemphigus vulgaris and foliaceus.

■ Systemic corticosteroids	B

Pemphigus: a 20 year review of 107 patients treated with corticosteroids. Rosenberg FR, Sanders S, Nelson CT. Arch Dermatol 1976;112:962–70.

The first line therapy for all forms of pemphigus is systemic corticosteroids. Corticosteroids work relatively quickly and are relatively safe when used at appropriate doses for limited periods of time. In the past, regimens employing rapidly accelerating doses of corticosteroids were employed, but these should no longer be used. The major cause of morbidity and mortality in pemphigus is the use of very high doses of corticosteroids and the consequent complications. The use of doses greater than 1 mg/kg daily of prednisone is associated with unacceptable risks. Initial treatment should start at 1 mg/kg daily (lean body weight), and a good clinical response, defined by resolution of the majority of existing lesions and absence of newly developing lesions, should be evident within 2–3 months. The dose should then be reduced to 40 mg daily and subsequently tapered over 6–9 months, ideally to a maintenance dose of 5 mg every other day. Tapering can be accomplished by reduction of the prednisone by an average of 10 mg per month initially, and 5 mg per month later. There are some advantages to beginning an alternate dose regimen at 40 mg daily, so that monthly reductions would ideally be 40/20 mg alternate days, 40/0 mg, 30/0 mg, 20/0 mg, 15/0 mg, and 10/0 mg, and then 5/0 mg alternate days for maintenance.

The use of a second line therapy is indicated if, during this ideal prednisone taper, the patient develops or is anticipated to develop significant corticosteroid side effects, the disease does not improve sufficiently to allow continuous tapering, or the disease flares.

Monthly pulse corticosteroids have been suggested as a less toxic alternative to daily oral therapy, but pemphigus is a very persistent autoimmune disease that usually requires more consistent daily or alternate day dosing to achieve suppression.

The potential development of corticosteroid-induced osteopenia must be monitored by bone mineral density studies (DEXA scan) at institution of therapy and annually thereafter. In patients without a history of renal calculi, prophylaxis with the use of *supplemental calcium* 1500 mg daily and *vitamin D* 400–800 IU daily is required. In patients with osteopenia or osteoporosis, additional therapies may include *hormonal replacement* (estrogen/progesterone for women and raloxifen for women in whom estrogens are contraindicated [e.g. history of breast carcinoma]), *exogenous testosterone* for men with low serum levels of this hormone, *bisphosphonates* such as alendronate, and *intranasal calcitonin*.

In pemphigus vulgaris, therapy as outlined should commence in all patients once the diagnosis is confirmed. Even in cases with limited oral lesions, the disease will progress unless treated with systemic agents, and palliative therapy with topical agents or intralesional injections just delays definitive therapy. There is clinical evidence that early intervention with definitive treatment leads to a better long-term outcome.

In pemphigus foliaceus, not every patient requires immediate treatment. Some patients have very limited and smoldering disease, and can therefore benefit from some palliative treatment such as topical corticosteroids.

In paraneoplastic pemphigus, the disease is usually relentlessly progressive, and the immediate institution of systemic corticosteroids and a second line treatment is justified. If a patient has an associated benign lymphoproliferative disorder such as thymoma, hyaline vascular Castleman's disease, or sarcoma, complete surgical removal should be attempted. Complete resection of such tumors can result in a prolonged remission of the disease.

SECOND LINE THERAPIES

■ Mycophenolate mofetil	B
■ Azathioprine	C
■ High-dose IVIG	C
■ Rituximab	D

Treatment of pemphigus vulgaris and foliaceus with mycophenolate mofetil. Mimouni D, Anhalt GJ, Cummins DL, et al. Arch Dermatol 2003;139:739–42.

Forty two patients were treated with mycophenolate mofetil, 1.5 g twice daily, and standard prednisone therapy. Complete clinical remission was defined as achieving no new lesions with prednisone doses less than 10 mg daily. This was achieved in 70% of patients with pemphigus vulgaris and 55% of patients with pemphigus foliaceus. Therapy was discontinued in only two cases due to adverse effects – one secondary to febrile neutropenia and one for gastrointestinal intolerance.

For pemphigus vulgaris and foliaceus, two effective antimetabolite immunosuppressive drugs are azathioprine and mycophenolate mofetil. Mycophenolate has an excellent safety profile, but it is very expensive. Azathioprine appears to be equally effective and is much cheaper, but has much more frequent toxicities. These drugs are added to the systemic corticosteroids, if the indications for their use are met. Once their beneficial effect is observed, the corticosteroids should be progressively tapered, while the second agent is used at full doses for up to 2–3 years to induce a durable remission. For both drugs, the doses required are greater than those needed to control other cutaneous diseases because only at high doses does one observe the required inhibition of the synthesis of autoantibodies by B cells.

Mycophenolate mofetil should be used at a total dose of 35–45 mg/kg daily, given in divided doses twice daily. Onset of action is slow, and remissions are observed in responders after 2–12 months of therapy. Monitoring of complete blood count and liver enzymes should be performed monthly, but cytopenias and hepatotoxicity are usually not observed. Some lymphopenia without neutropenia is common, but has no adverse consequences and can correlate with a good clinical effect. Some nausea and diarrhea can occur, but improve with dosage reduction.

Azathioprine in the treatment of pemphigus vulgaris. A long term follow-up. Aberer W, Wolff-Schreiner EC, Stingl G, Wolff K. J Am Acad Dermatol 1987;16:527–33.

Azathioprine is given in a single daily dose of 3–4 mg/kg. At this dose, there is a risk of neutropenia, thrombocytopenia, hepatotoxicity, and severe or debilitating nausea. Monitoring should consist of complete blood count and liver enzymes, initially every 2 weeks. Patients with thiopurine methyltransferase deficiency (TPMT) cannot metabolize the drug effectively and can develop severe pancytopenia during the first 2 months of therapy. Late effects include elevation of liver enzymes and drug fever. The drug also requires 6–8 weeks of therapy before its effect on the disease can be judged. The drug is quite effective, but even if one screens patients for TPMT deficiency before starting treatment, the incidence of side effects is greater than with mycophenolate. It is still a useful second line agent for those who cannot afford mycophenolate. There is also concern that exposure to this drug can increase one's lifetime risk of leukemia or lymphoma, but the risk is very much less than that associated with the use of alkylating agents.

High-dose intravenous immune globulin for the treatment of autoimmune blistering diseases. Harman KE, Black MM. Br J Dermatol 1999;140:865–74.

Treatment of pemphigus with intravenous immunoglobulin. Bystryn JC, Jiao D, Natow S. J Am Acad Dermatol 2002: 358;358–63.

Both studies used IVIG in addition to treatment with prednisone and immunosuppressive therapy. IVIG produced a rapid reduction of circulating autoantibody levels, which was accompanied by significant clinical improvement in some cases.

High-dose IVIG can be used for acute control of active pemphigus. This treatment seems to accelerate the catabolism of the autoantibody and reduce circulating levels as effectively as plasmapheresis. It is generally safe and well tolerated, but has some risk. A small number of patients can develop thrombotic complications such as deep venous thrombosis or stroke. It is enormously expensive (as much as $12 000 per treatment for a 70 kg patient), and may lose its effectiveness after repeated treatment cycles. It can be given intravenously at a dose of 2 g/kg body weight, infused in divided doses over 2–5 days monthly.

IVIG may have a role to play in acute control when plasmapheresis is not indicated and in those patients who are not good candidates for alkylating agents. The use of IVIG for extended periods to induce a remission is more controversial and requires better data.

Treatment of refractory pemphigus vulgaris with rituximab (anti-CD20 monoclonal antibody). Dupuy A, Viguier M, Bedane C, et al. Arch Dermatol 2004;140:91–6.

Three cases of refractory pemphigus responded to the additional use of rituximab, two with complete remission, one partial. CD20[+] B cells were depleted for 6–10 months, and their reappearance in the circulation correlated with a relapse in two cases, necessitating a second course of the drug. Bacterial infections occurred in two cases.

Depletion of CD20[+] B cells by the use of anti-CD20 monoclonal antibody is emerging as a potentially powerful tool in many autoimmune diseases. CD20 is not expressed on pre-B cells or plasma cells, so it is not profoundly immunosuppressive, and the effect only lasts 6–10 months, as the CD20[+] cells regenerate. Toxicity is minimal, but the addition of the drug to patients already exposed to corticosteroids and immunosuppressive drugs increases the risk of infection, including one fatal case of Pneumocystis carinii pneumonia (PCP). PCP prophylaxis should be considered. The drug can cause rapid reduction of autoantibody levels in even severely affected cases, with initial case reports recording often dramatic recoveries.

THIRD LINE THERAPIES

■ Cyclophosphamide	B
■ Cyclophosphamide plus plasmapheresis	E
■ Chlorambucil	D

Dexamethasone-cyclophosphamide pulse therapy for pemphigus. Pasricha JS, Khaitan BK, Raman RS, Chandra M. Int J Dermatol 1995;34:875–82.

Alkylating agents such as cyclophosphamide have a profound effect on inhibition of autoantibody synthesis, and are the most effective agents for inducing a remission. They also have very significant potential toxicities, which restrict their use to third line therapy.

Cyclophosphamide is the preferred agent because any neutropenia associated with its use is predictable in onset, and withdrawal of the drug results in rapid recovery of neutrophils (within 1 week to 10 days). There are four ways to administer the drug:

1. Daily orally at 2.5 mg/kg. A single morning dose is followed by aggressive fluid consumption throughout the day to rinse metabolites from the bladder and prevent hemorrhagic cystitis. Weekly complete blood counts and urinalysis are required. With this use, a durable remission can be obtained after 18–24 months of therapy in almost all cases. This exposure probably increases the patient's lifetime risk of leukemia, lymphoma, or bladder cancer by as much as 5–10% over the normal population. This risk is appreciated some 20–30 years after treatment. Such treatment can also cause sterility in young patients.

2. Monthly intravenous pulses at a dose of 750 mg/m² body surface area. Monthly intravenous administration reduces the risk of hemorrhagic cystitis, but this intermittent use is not as effective in suppressing the disease.

3. Monthly intravenous administration with lower dose oral daily maintenance. This can also be very effective in inducing a remission.

4. Single, very high-dose immunoablative therapy. *This experimental treatment is effective in many autoimmune diseases.* It employs a dose of intravenous cyclophosphamide of 200 mg/kg, given over 4 days, which induces profound marrow aplasia. Upon recovery, the patients often enjoy a durable remission. *Its potential role in all forms of pemphigus is being explored.*

Synchronization of plasmapheresis and pulse cyclophosphamide therapy in pemphigus vulgaris. Euler HH, Loffler H, Christophers E. Arch Dermatol 1987;123:1205–10.

Plasmapheresis is the only method by which one can rapidly reduce autoantibody levels, and is used in patients with very extensive and accelerated disease. Its use involves a total of six high-volume removals (3–3.5 L per removal, three times weekly for two consecutive weeks). This must be combined with the concomitant use of systemic corticosteroids and oral cyclophosphamide. If these drugs are not used, the reduction of autoantibodies removes feedback inhibition to the autoimmune B cells, and causes a rebound flare of the disease. This can be blunted only by alkylating agents due to their preferential toxicity to rapidly proliferative B cells. This causes the induction of a durable remission, though cyclophosphamide must still be used at full doses for 18–24 months to harden that remission.

The use of chlorambucil with prednisone in the treatment of pemphigus. Shah N, Green AR, Elgart GW, Kerdel F. J Am Acad Dermatol 2000;42:85–8.

In patients who develop hemorrhagic cystitis from cyclophosphamide, chlorambucil can be substituted.

Chlorambucil is more difficult to use because the cytopenias induced by it are more unpredictable and may take months to resolve.

Cyclosporine

Ineffectiveness of cyclosporine as an adjuvant to corticosteroids in the treatment of pemphigus. Ioannides D, Chrysomallis F, Bystryn JC. Arch Dermatol 2000;868:505–6.

Thirty three consecutive patients hospitalized with pemphigus vulgaris (n = 29) or foliaceus (n = 4) were randomized to receive either prednisolone or prednisolone plus cyclosporine, 5 mg/kg daily. The groups were similar in terms of disease severity, and demographics. The addition of cyclosporine produced no change in the response to treatment or the total dose of corticosteroid administered. Complications were, however, more common in those patients that received cyclosporine.

Although there are anecdotal cases reporting benefit from the use of cyclosporine, this well-performed study with an impressive number of cases is good evidence that the drug should not be used in pemphigus vulgaris and foliaceus. There is still good anecdotal evidence that cyclosporine may have a role to play in the management of paraneoplastic pemphigus, a disease with a much more complex pathophysiology.

Perforating dermatoses

Sarah Hodulik, Robert Carruthers, Mark G Lebwohl

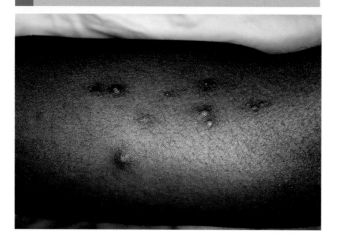

The perforating dermatoses are a varied group of conditions which are characterized by the transepidermal elimination of dermal material. Four primary conditions are included in the discussion of the perforating disorders:

- Reactive perforating collagenosis, which is characterized by the transepidermal elimination of collagen
- Elastosis perforans serpiginosa (EPS), characterized by transepidermal extrusion of elastic material.
- Perforating folliculitis, in which epidermal perforation involves hair follicles.
- Kyrle's disease, in which dermal connective tissue perforates through the epidermis.

MANAGEMENT STRATEGY

Definitive diagnosis of the perforating disorders depends on the demonstration of transepidermal elimination on skin biopsy. Differentiation between the different forms of perforating disorders can be accomplished by Masson trichrome stains for collagen (reactive perforating collagenosis), Verhoeff–van Gieson stains for elastic tissue (EPS), and step-sectioning to look for hair follicles (perforating folliculitis). Differentiation between these various disorders may be important since EPS is associated with other diseases such as pseudoxanthoma elasticum, Down syndrome, osteogenesis imperfecta, Ehlers–Danlos syndrome, Rothmund–Thomson syndrome, Marfan syndrome, and penicillamine treatment. Management of the perforating diseases involves determination of underlying etiologies. Most often, conditions like diabetes mellitus and renal failure will be known to the patient who presents with perforating skin lesions. When the underlying cause is not apparent, serum chemistry for renal and liver function tests and glucose tolerance test may be helpful.

Once the diagnosis of underlying diseases is ascertained, treatment is directed at associated symptoms. Pruritus can be managed initially with *topical* or *intralesional corticosteroids*, *topical anesthetics and menthol*, as well as *oral antihistamines*, but the latter agents are usually not sufficiently effective. Minimizing pruritus is important because many of the perforating disorders typically exhibit a Koebner phenomenon, meaning that lesions develop in traumatized or scratched skin. Topical antipruritic agents such as menthol, phenol, or camphor, and topical anesthetics such as lidocaine (lignocaine) and pramocaine are useful. *Topical doxepin hydrochloride* or oral antihistamines may also be of some benefit. Trimming the fingernails to minimize trauma to the skin and avoidance of scratching are key elements of treatment. *Topical tretinoin* and *topical tazarotene* have been shown to be effective for some patients. In patients with renal disease, *UVB* is dramatically effective for pruritus and has been reported to benefit perforating skin lesions as well. If UVB, narrowband UVB, and topical retinoids are ineffective, *oral retinoids* or *allopurinol* can be tried.

SPECIFIC INVESTIGATIONS

- Skin biopsy with Masson trichrome stains and Verhoeff–van Gieson stains
- Serum BUN, creatinine, ALT, AST, alkaline phosphatase, bilirubin, uric acid
- Serum glucose or glucose tolerance test
- Serum parathyroid hormone level
- Thyroid function tests

Reactive perforating collagenosis associated with diabetes mellitus. Poliak SC, Lebwohl MG, Parris A, Prioleau PG. N Engl J Med 1982;306:81–4.

Reactive perforating collagenosis was found in three of 15 dialysis patients with diabetes mellitus. Typical lesions are described in six patients, all of whom had severe diabetes with retinopathy. Five of the six had chronic renal disease.

Acquired reactive perforating collagenosis. Report of six cases and review of the literature. Faver IR, Daoud MD, Su SP. J Am Acad Dermatol 1994;30:575–80.

Reactive perforating collagenosis was associated with hyperparathyroidism, hypothyroidism, liver disorders, and neurodermatitis in six patients.

FIRST LINE THERAPIES

■ Tretinoin 0.1%	E
■ Tazarotene gel 0.1%	E
■ UVB	E

Successful treatment of reactive perforating collagenosis with tretinoin. Cullen SI. Cutis 1979;23:187–91,193.

A 25-year-old woman with reactive perforating collagenosis failed to improve with numerous topical and systemic medications, with the exception of tretinoin 0.1% cream, which effectively reduced the number of lesions.

Tazarotene is an effective therapy for elastosis perforans serpiginosa. Outland JD, Brown TS, Callen JP. Arch Dermatol 2002;138:169–71.

A report of two patients with EPS who responded to daily treatment with 0.1% tazarotene gel. A 22-year-old woman had been treated unsuccessfully with liquid nitrogen cryotherapy, topical tretinoin, oral isotretinoin, and CO$_2$ laser surgery. A 56-year-old woman had failed to respond to

Evidence levels **A** Double-blind study **B** Clinical trial ≥ 20 subjects **C** Clinical trial < 20 subjects **D** Series ≥ 5 subjects **E** Anecdotal case reports

cryotherapy, corticosteroids, tretinoin, and triamcinolone acetonide. Both patients were treated with tazarotene. The skin condition of the 22-year-old greatly improved and that of the 56-year-old moderately improved.

[Acquired reactive collagen disease in the adult: successful treatment with UV-B light]. Vion E, Frenk E. Hautarzt 1989;40:448–50. In German.

A 77-year-old woman with reactive perforating collagenosis and severe pruritus responded to phototherapy with UVB. Both the pruritus and skin lesions improved.

UVB is a well-established modality for uremic pruritus. Since many patients with perforating diseases have associated renal failure, UVB phototherapy may dramatically benefit pruritus and reduce the number of skin lesions.

SECOND LINE THERAPIES

■ Allopurinol	D
■ Narrowband UVB	E
■ Isotretinoin	E
■ PUVA	E
■ Acitretin	E

Acquired reactive perforating collagenosis in a non-diabetic hemodialysis patient: successful treatment with allopurinol. Iyoda M, Hayashi F, Kuroki A, et al. Am J Kidney Dis 2003;42:E11–3.

A 59-year-old man with end-stage renal failure and acquired reactive perforating collagenosis, who had been unresponsive to treatment with topical steroids and oral antihistamines, was given 100 mg daily of oral allopurinol and skin lesions cleared within 2 months.

Treatment of acquired reactive perforating collagenosis with allopurinol. Querings K, Balda BR, Bachter D. Br J Dermatol 2001;145:174–6.

A 57-year-old woman with diabetes mellitus and acquired reactive perforating collagenosis was successfully treated with allopurinol. Treatment with topical corticosteroids, antihistamines, and UVB phototherapy had failed to resolve the patient's skin condition. Within 2 weeks of introduction of 100 mg daily of oral allopurinol, skin lesions improved; following 7 weeks of treatment, lesions completely cleared.

Several case reports have now documented improvement of reactive perforating collagenosis with allopurinol treatment in patients with or without hyperuricemia.

Reactive perforating collagenosis: a condition that may be underdiagnosed. Satchell AC, Crotty K, Lee S. Australas J Dermatol 2001;42:284–7.

Three patients with diabetes mellitus were treated for reactive perforating collagenosis.

A 73-year-old woman was treated with 0.5% phenol with 10% glycerine in sorbolene cream. After 1 month of treatment, itch resolved and skin lesions diminished in number and size.

A 75-year-old woman responded to treatment with narrowband UVB. The patient received phototherapy three times per week for 2 months, with resolution of lesions. When the condition recurred 6 months later, it again cleared with 3 months of narrowband UVB.

A 58-year-old woman who did not respond to corticosteroids, antihistamines, UVB, or PUVA was successfully treated with oral acitretin. Treatment with 25 mg daily of acitretin resolved itch and cleared skin lesions.

Kyrle's disease. Effectively treated with isotretinoin. Saleh HA, Lloyd KM, Fatteh S. J Fla Med Assoc 1993;80:395–7. Erratum in J Fla Med Assoc 1993;80:467.

A 63-year-old patient with Kyrle's disease and chronic renal failure was treated with oral isotretinoin for 13 weeks. Cutaneous lesions cleared completely.

Reactive perforating collagenosis responsive to PUVA. Serrano G, Aliaga A, Lorente M. Int J Dermatol 1988;27:118–9.

A 21-year-old woman with a 10-year history of reactive perforating collagenosis was treated with PUVA four times per week. Improvement was noted in 2 weeks. Lesions stopped developing after completion of PUVA therapy (326 J/cm^2 total) and no new lesions were noted in over a year of post-treatment observations.

THIRD LINE THERAPIES

■ 0.5% Phenol with 10% glycerine in sorbolene	E
■ Surgical debridement	E
■ Cryotherapy	E
■ Ultrapulse laser	E
■ Doxycycline	E
■ Transcutaneous electrical nerve stimulation (TENS)	E

Successful treatment of acquired reactive perforating collagenosis with doxycycline. Brinkmeier T, Schaller J, Herbst RA, Frosch PJ. Acta Derm Venereol 2002;82:393–5.

An 87-year-old woman with acquired reactive perforating collagenosis responded to treatment with oral doxycycline 100 mg daily for 2 weeks. Within 5 days of initiation of doxycycline, new skin lesions ceased to form, and within 10 days of treatment, most lesions had healed.

A new treatment for acquired reactive perforating collagenosis. Oziemski MA, Billson VR, Crosthwaite GL, et al. Australas J Dermatol 1991;32:71–4.

A single patient with reactive perforating collagenosis was successfully treated with surgical debridement and split skin grafting of the affected areas.

Because skin lesions are often numerous, surgical removal and skin grafting may be impractical.

Elastosis performans serpiginosa: treatment with liquid nitrogen. Tuyp EJ, McLeod WA. Int J Dermatol 1990;29:655–6.

Liquid nitrogen was applied with a cotton-tipped applicator for approximately 10 s on six occasions over 7 months. Lesions of EPS disappeared and did not return.

Localized idiopathic elastosis perforans serpiginosa effectively treated by the coherent ultrapulse 5000C aesthetic laser. Abdullah A, Colloby PS, Foulds IS, Whitcroft I. Int J Dermatol 2000;39:719–20.

Portions of lesions of EPS were treated by laser, with complete clearing of treated sites but no changes in untreated sites.

Response of elastosis perforans serpiginosa to pulsed CO$_2$, Er:YAG, and dye lasers. Saxena M, Tope WD. Dermatol Surg 2003;29:677–8.

A 17-year-old male presenting with EPS on the neck was treated with CO$_2$ laser (UltraPulse 5000C) on the right neck and erbium:YAG laser (UltraFine; Coherent) on the left neck. Only mild improvement of EPS was achieved and subtle atrophic scarring occurred on the area treated with the CO$_2$ laser. The patient then received pulsed dye laser therapy on both sides of the neck, resulting only in minimal improvement of EPS.

Treatment of pruritis of reactive perforating collagenosis using transcutaneous electrical nerve stimulation. Chan LY, Tang WY, Lo KK. Eur J Dermatol 2000;10:59–61.

A 47-year-old woman and an 85-year-old woman, each of whom had failed to respond to treatment with topical steroids and antihistamines, received TENS therapy for 1 hour daily over the course of 3 weeks. Skin lesions cleared within 3 months of treatment for both patients.

Evidence levels **A** Double-blind study **B** Clinical trial ≥ 20 subjects **C** Clinical trial < 20 subjects **D** Series ≥ 5 subjects **E** Anecdotal case reports

Perioral dermatitis

John Berth-Jones, Sheila M Clark, Catriona A Henderson

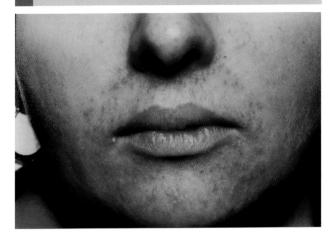

Perioral dermatitis is an eruption of inflammatory papules (and sometimes pustules) on the chin, perioral areas, and nasolabial folds, characteristically sparing the skin immediately adjacent to the vermilion border. It is usually seen in young adult females but also occurs in childhood. The development of perioral dermatitis is frequently preceded by intentional or inadvertent application of potent topical corticosteroids to the facial skin. A similar eruption involving the eyelids and periorbital skin has been termed periocular dermatitis.

Although sometimes described as a variant of rosacea, perioral dermatitis is distinguished from this disease by its distribution, by the relatively monomorphic appearance of the lesions, by the absence of flushing and telangiectasia, and by its tendency to occur in younger patients.

MANAGEMENT STRATEGY

Many cases are associated with the use of potent topical corticosteroids, and withdrawal of this medication is the most important measure in this group. Patients must be warned that the condition may initially flare after this maneuver. If the flare proves intolerable, initial use of a less potent topical corticosteroid can often be helpful. Systemic tetracyclines are also frequently employed and a range of other modalities are used less frequently.

SPECIFIC INVESTIGATIONS

No investigation is routinely required.

FIRST LINE TREATMENT

■ Withdrawal of topical corticosteroids	B
■ Oral tetracyclines	B

Complications of topical hydrocortisone. Guin JD. J Am Acad Dermatol 1981;4:417–22.

Perioral dermatitis developed following use of topical hydrocortisone.

Although usually associated with the use of potent topical corticosteroids, this case suggests that even hydrocortisone may induce perioral dermatitis.

Perioral dermatitis: aetiology and treatment with tetracycline. Macdonald A, Feiwel M. Br J Dermatol 1972;87:351–9.

Tetracycline 250 mg given three times daily for a week, then twice daily for 2–3 months, proved highly effective in this series of 29 cases.

Perioral dermatitis in renal transplant recipients maintained on corticosteroids and immunosuppressive therapy. Adams SJ, Davison AM, Cunliffe WJ, Giles GR. Br J Dermatol 1982;106:589–92.

A report of five cases where perioral dermatitis developed in patients on oral corticosteroids that could not be discontinued. A 2-month course of doxycycline was effective.

SECOND LINE TREATMENTS

■ Topical tetracycline	B
■ Topical erythromycin	B
■ Oral erythromycin	E
■ Topical metronidazole	C
■ Topical azelaic acid	D
■ Oral isotretinoin	E

Topical tetracycline in the treatment of perioral dermatitis. Wilson RG. Arch Dermatol 1979;115:637.

Topical tetracycline, applied twice daily, proved highly effective in this series of 30 patients. Twenty-four cleared completely after 5–28 days.

A topical erythromycin preparation and oral tetracycline for the treatment of perioral dermatitis: a placebo-controlled trial. Weber K, Thurmayr R, Meisinger A. J Dermatol Treat 1993;4:57–9.

A comparison of the response to topical erythromycin (33 patients), oral tetracycline (35 patients), and placebo (31 patients). Oral tetracycline and topical erythromycin were comparable in efficacy and both were superior to placebo.

Topical therapy for perioral dermatitis. Bikowski JB. Cutis 1983;31:678–82.

Six cases cleared on topical erythromycin.

Identical twins with perioral dermatitis. Weston WL, Morelli JG. Pediatr Dermatol 1998;15:144.

Two cases responded to oral erythromycin.

Topical metronidazole in the treatment of perioral dermatitis. Veien NK, Munkvad JM, Nielsen AO, et al. J Am Acad Dermatol 1991;24:258–69.

A prospective, randomized, double-blind trial in 109 patients. Both groups improved but 1% metronidazole cream applied twice daily was less effective than oxytetracycline 250 mg twice daily over 8 weeks.

Topical metronidazole gel (0.75%) for the treatment of perioral dermatitis in children. Miller SR, Shalita AR. J Am Acad Dermatol 1994;31:847–8.

Three children with perioral or periocular eruptions were treated with topical metronidazole gel (0.75%) twice daily.

Significant improvement was observed after 2 months. Complete resolution occurred after 14 weeks.

Azelaic acid as a new treatment for perioral dermatitis: results from an open study. Jansen T. Br J Dermatol 2004; 151:933–4.

Ten cases were treated with topical 20% azelaic acid cream applied twice daily. Complete clearing was reported in all cases after 2–6 weeks. The cream was well tolerated.

Perioral dermatitis with histopathologic features of granulomatous rosacea: successful treatment with isotretinoin. Smith KW. Cutis 1990;46:413–5.

Isotretinoin was used successfully in a resistant case.

Peutz–Jeghers syndrome

Mordechai M Tarlow, Adam S Stibich, Robert A Schwartz

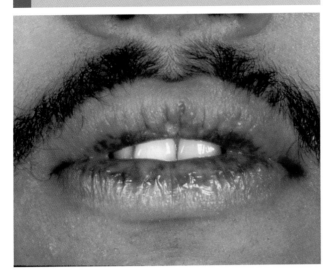

Peutz–Jeghers syndrome (PJS) is one of the more common hereditary polyposis syndromes and is characterized by gastrointestinal polyps and obstruction as well as periorificial pigmentation.

MANAGEMENT STRATEGY

The pigmented macules of PJS are typically periorificial, especially around the mouth, eyes, and anus. The hands, feet, and oral mucosa may also be transiently involved in early years. The histology of the hyperpigmented macule is characterized by basal layer hyperpigmentation. A normal number of melanocytes is present. The genetic abnormality associated with this autosomal dominant disorder is a germline mutation of the STK11/LKB1 gene, located at 19p13.3, as well as a more recently identified second PJS disease locus at 19q13.4; genetic testing is not required for a diagnosis, but may aid in unclear cases, as well as in genetic counseling of at-risk family members.

In patients with PJS the management strategy is to educate about visceral complications, provide genetic counseling, and reassure that the cutaneous macules are benign in nature and that after puberty one can expect an improvement of the non-labial macules. In some cases the pigmented facial lesions are psychologically unacceptable to the patient. In these individuals there are few options, almost all of which deal with the use of *laser surgery* for correction. This treatment is prefaced by the fact that these lesions are a marker of a syndrome that may include recurrent intussusceptions, gut bleeding, and a variety of visceral anomalies and extraintestinal malignancies. Symptomatology usually begins between the ages of 10 and 30 years, but any child with recurrent unexplained abdominal pain should be evaluated for an intussusception, a medical emergency associated with PJS. Thus, removal of cutaneous macules may hide this clinical valuable clue in a critical and compromising situation. Gastrointesti-

nal evaluation is a key in the management of patients with PJS.

The *ruby laser (Q-switched and short pulsed)* has been used for the treatment of labial macules. The response to treatment is excellent; no sequelae or recurrences are usually noted. No anesthesia is required and no wound care is necessary with this laser. This suggests that ruby laser therapy is safe and a suitable approach for the treatment of labial macules in children with PJS.

The *CO₂, alexandrite, and argon lasers* have also been shown to be effective in the treatment of the labial macules of PJS. Cosmetic results of their use have been found to be excellent. *Intense pulsed light* has been shown to be very effective as well.

Cryosurgery can be used, but does not fully eliminate the macules and may leave a hypopigmented spot. Trichloroacetic acid may not produce total resolution. Surgical excision, electrodesiccation, and dermabrasion commonly result in incomplete removal, scarring, or changes in normal pigmentation. Thus, these treatments give suboptimal results.

SPECIFIC INVESTIGATIONS

- ■ Histology (if diagnosis is in question)
- ■ Gastrointestinal evaluation
- ■ Genetic testing (in some cases)

The labial melanotic macule. Weathers DR, Corio RL, Crawford BE, et al. Oral Surg Oral Med Oral Pathol 1976;42: 196–205.

Fifty five cases are reported of this variety of melanotic lesion of the lips, which is well known but not well described.

On the basis of follow-up information obtained and the histopathologic character of the lesions, this entity is benign and does not, in our opinion, have any malignant potential.

Peutz–Jeghers syndrome. McGarrity TJ, Kulin HE, Zaino RJ. Am J Gastroenterol 2000;95:596–604.

A comprehensive review article on the intestinal as well as the extraintestinal manifestations of PJS. A management scheme of the non-cutaneous aspects is included.

Although the non-dermatologic aspects of this disease are typically in the realm of the internist and gastroenterologist, this review allows the dermatologist to offer additional patient education. It discusses all aspects, including history of the disease and genetic testing.

Peutz–Jeghers syndrome: genetic screening. Leggett BA, Young JP, Barker M. Expert Rev Anticancer Ther 2003;3: 518–24.

A review of PJS and genetic screening.

Diagnostic and predictive genetic testing is now possible in many families due to the identification of causative mutations in the serine/threonine kinase (STK)-11 (also known as the LKB1) gene. Such testing has now entered routine clinical practice and will allow early recognition of the condition in young, at-risk family members.

Genetic testing for polyposis: practical and ethical aspects. Jarvinen HJ. Gut 2003;52(suppl 2):ii19–22.

This review delineates possible pitfalls and benefits of genetic testing as well as an appropriate approach to minimize misunderstanding and anxiety.

Peutz–Jeghers syndrome: confirmation of linkage to chromosome 19p13.3 and identification of a potential second locus, on 19q13.4. Mehenni H, Blouin JL, Radhakrishna U, et al. Am J Hum Genet 1997;61:1327–34.

This paper confirms the location of the most prevalent mutation in PJS to be the LKB1/STK11 gene at location 19p13.3 and identifies an additional locus.

This study highlights the limitation of genetic testing because PJS has not been associated with the LKB1/STK-11 gene in every case. The second gene on 19q13.4 has since been confirmed in an additional study.

Genotype–phenotype correlations in Peutz-Jeghers syndrome. Amos CI, Keitheri-Cheteri MB, Sabripour M, et al. J Med Genet 2004;41:327–33.

Mutations in the STK-11 gene were found in 69% of probands with PJS. Individuals with missense mutations had a significantly delayed time to onset of first polypectomy and of other symptoms compared to those with either truncating mutations or no detectable mutation.

This study suggests that genetic analysis may be of value beyond diagnosis of PJS.

FIRST LINE THERAPIES

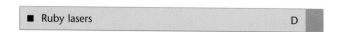

■ Ruby lasers	D

Q-switched ruby laser treatment of labial lentigos. Ashinoff R, Geronemus RG. J Am Acad Dermatol 1992;27: 809–11.

The Q-switched ruby laser causes selective damage to pigmented cells in the skin. This laser, which has a wavelength of 694 nm and a pulse duration of 40 ns, has shown very promising results in the treatment of both amateur and professional tattoos. Fewer data are available on its ability to treat benign pigmented lesions of the skin. Three patients who had labial lentigines were treated with the Q-switched ruby laser, and dramatic clearing occurred after one or two treatments with a fluence of $10 \, J/cm^2$.

Q-switched ruby laser treatment of labial lentigines in Peutz–Jeghers syndrome. DePadova-Elder SM, Milgraum SS. J Dermatol Surg Oncol 1994;20:830–2.

The authors report successful treatment with the Q-switched ruby laser and consider it the treatment of choice for these lesions.

Q-switched ruby laser treatment of mucocutaneous melanosis associated with Peutz–Jeghers syndrome. Chang CJ, Nelson JS. Ann Plast Surg 1996;36:394–7.

The Q-switched ruby laser produces clinically significant fading of mucocutaneous melanosis in association with PJS without the complications often seen with other therapeutic modalities.

Successful treatment of mucosal melanosis of the lip with normal pulsed ruby laser. Hanada K, Baba T, Sasaki C, Hashimoto I. J Dermatol 1996;23:263–6.

In this study, six Japanese patients with labial melanosis of PJS were successfully treated with the pulsed ruby laser.

The therapy achieved rapid results without producing changes in mucosal texture or recurrence after operation.

Effective removal of certain skin pigment spots (lentigines) using the Q-switched ruby laser. (Dutch) Njoo MD, Westerhof W. Ned Tijdschr Geneeskd 1997;141:327–30.

In 15 patients, Q-switched ruby laser treatment was applied to solar lentigines, labial lentigines (two), segmental lentigines (two), and lentigo simplex (one). The light energy ranged from 3 to $10 \, J/cm^2$. In 11 of 15 patients, one treatment session sufficed to remove the lesion completely.

In the cases described, Q-switched ruby laser was a successful treatment for lentigines. For macules of this nature, Q-switched ruby laser is preferred above conventional forms of therapy such as cryotherapy, chemical peeling, and abrasion.

Ruby laser therapy for labial lentigines in Peutz–Jeghers syndrome. Kato S, Takeyama J, Tanita Y, Ebina K. Eur J Pediatr 1998;157:622–4.

Ruby laser therapy of labial lentigines in two children with PJS is described. The response to treatment was excellent and no sequelae or recurrence of the lesions were noted.

This work suggests that ruby laser therapy is safe and a suitable approach for the treatment of labial melanotic macules in children with PJS.

Q-switched ruby laser treatment of tattoos and benign pigmented lesions: a critical review. Raulin C, Schonermark MP, Greve B, Werner S. Ann Plast Surg 1998;41:555–65.

An excellent review on the applications of the Q-switched ruby laser, with emphasis on its particular attractiveness in removing pigmented lesions in precarious anatomic regions such as the lips and eyelids.

SECOND LINE THERAPIES

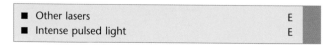

■ Other lasers	E
■ Intense pulsed light	E

Treatment of labial lentigos in atopic dermatitis with the frequency-doubled Q-switched Nd:YAG laser. Akita H, Matsunaga K, Fujisawa Y, Ueda H. Arch Dermatol 2000;136: 936–7.

Treatment of Peutz–Jeghers lentigines with the carbon dioxide laser. Benedict LM, Cohen B. J Dermatol Surg Oncol 1991;17:954–5.

The authors report a successful outcome in the treatment of these lentigines with the CO_2 laser.

Treatment of pigmentation of the lips and oral mucosa in Peutz–Jeghers syndrome using ruby and argon lasers. Ohshiro T, Maruyama Y, Nakajima H, Mima M. Br J Plast Surg 1980;33:346–9.

Three patients with punctate pigmented spots on the lips and oral mucosa accompanying PJS were successfully treated with ruby and argon lasers.

The basic principles of laser treatment, the characteristics of the different laser systems, and the skin reaction to ruby and argon lasers are discussed.

Q-switched Alexandrite laser in the treatment of pigmented macules in Laugier–Hunziker syndrome.

Evidence levels A Double-blind study B Clinical trial ≥ 20 subjects C Clinical trial < 20 subjects D Series ≥ 5 subjects E Anecdotal case reports

Papadavid E, Walker NP. J Eur Acad Dermatol Venereol 2001;15:468–9.

Two patients with pigmented macules on their lips were treated with the Q-switched alexandrite laser.

Laugier–Hunziker syndrome presents with similar macules to those in PJS, but there are no associated gastrointestinal abnormalities. In this report one patient cleared with initial treatment, and one required repeat treatment for a relapse prior to complete clearance.

Treatment of facial lentigines in Peutz–Jeghers syndrome with intense pulsed light source. Remington BK, Remington TK. Dermatol Surg 2002;28:1079–81.

A case report of a series of 12 treatment sessions resulting in complete clearance; most resolved with a single course and a few required a second.

This report offers a viable alternative to laser treatment.

Physical urticarias, aquagenic pruritus, and cholinergic pruritus

*Clive E H Grattan, Sam Gibbs,
Frances Lawlor*

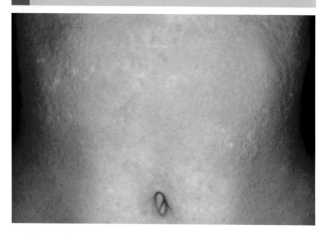

Physical urticarias

Clive E H Grattan, Sam Gibbs

About 25% of patients with chronic urticaria have a definable physical trigger that distinguishes them from those with ordinary urticaria and urticarial vasculitis. Physical urticarias are defined by the predominant stimulus that brings them out reproducibly (Table 1). More than one physical stimulus elicits urticaria in some patients, and physical urticarias can overlap with ordinary urticaria.

MANAGEMENT STRATEGY

Pharmacologic

The clinical presentation of the physical urticarias may vary considerably in severity, so drug management should be guided more by the degree of disability and impairment in quality of life than by the specific diagnosis. For instance, cholinergic urticaria may result in occasional mild exercise-induced whealing, more extensive urticaria with angioedema, or, very rarely, anaphylaxis. The milder forms may require little more than explanation, *avoidance of situations likely to trigger an attack*, and an occasional dose of *antihistamine*, while a very severe attack involving anaphylaxis would require emergency treatment with *intramuscular epinephrine (adrenaline)*. Very acute presentations of physical urticaria may require short courses of *oral corticosteroids* (e.g. prednisolone 30–40 mg daily for 5 days) in addition to regular treatment with antihistamines, which are the cornerstone of management for all patterns. A range of other interventions can be tried if there is little or no response to antihistamines, although the evidence supporting their use is often poor.

Nonpharmacologic

The triggering physical stimulus should be avoided where possible. Aspirin and food additives have been implicated in exacerbations of some physical urticarias, but exclusion diets have little role in the management of most cases.

SPECIFIC INVESTIGATIONS

- ■ Physical challenge tests
- ■ Blood tests (cryoproteins, IgE)

With the exceptions of testing for cryoglobulins, cold agglutinins, and cryofibrinogens in secondary cold urticaria and specific IgE in food- and exercise-induced anaphylaxis, routine laboratory investigations are unnecessary and should not be undertaken.

Urticaria. Dreskin SC, ed. Immunol Allergy Clin North Am 2004;24(2).

A good recent review of the diagnosis, pathogenesis, and treatment of physical urticarias.

Physical urticaria: classification and diagnostic guidelines. An EAACI position paper. Kontou-Fili K, Borici-Mazi R, Kapp A, et al. Allergy 1997;52:504–13.

A comprehensive review of classification, presentation, and testing for physical urticarias. Standardized challenge protocols should be observed whenever possible.

Cold urticaria syndromes: historical background, diagnostic classification, clinical and laboratory characteristics, pathogenesis and management. Wanderer AA. J Allergy Clin Immunol 1990;85:965–81.

A well-referenced review of cold urticaria and its investigation.

Food-dependent exercise-induced anaphylaxis. Kidd JM, Cohen SH, Sosman AJ, Fink JN. J Allergy Clin Immunol 1983;71:407–11.

Anaphylaxis may rarely result from exercise after a heavy food load or eating certain foods for which specific IgE can be demonstrated by skin prick or RAST testing.

Reactions to aspirin and food additives in patients with chronic urticaria, including the physical urticarias. Doeglas HMG. Br J Dermatol 1975;93:135–43.

Aspirin sensitivity was demonstrated in 52% of cholinergic urticaria patients and 43% of those with delayed pressure urticaria. Exacerbations of these physical urticarias were also demonstrated after challenge with food additives (including tartrazine and sodium benzoate) in some patients with proven aspirin sensitivity.

FIRST LINE THERAPIES

- ■ Nonsedating ('second generation') antihistamines   A
- ■ Classical sedating antihistamines and drugs with antihistaminic properties   A

Therapeutic effects of cetirizine in delayed pressure urticaria: clinicopathological findings. Kontou-Fili K,

Table 1 Classification of physical urticarias by the eliciting stimulus (in approximate reducing frequency of occurrence).

Symptomatic dermographism	Stroking or rubbing the skin
Cholinergic urticaria (pale, papular wheals with red flares)	Rise in core temperature and other causes of sweating (exercise, hot baths, spicy food, and stress)
Cold urticaria	Rewarming of skin after cooling (localized or systemic)
Delayed pressure urticaria	Sustained perpendicular pressure
Solar urticaria	Ultraviolet or visible solar radiation
Localized heat urticaria	Local heat contact
Adrenergic urticaria (red papular wheals with surrounding pallor)	Emotional stress
Aquagenic urticaria	Local water contact at any temperature
Exercise-induced anaphylaxis (sometimes a variant of cholinergic urticaria)	Exercise
Food and exercise-induced anaphylaxis	Exercise following a heavy food load or eating specific foods
Vibratory angioedema	Vibration

Table 2 Examples of non- and mildly sedating antihistamines.

Acrivastine	Nonsedating, three-times-daily dosing
Cetirizine	Mildly sedating, once-daily dosing
Levocetirizine	(the active enantiomer of cetirizine)
Fexofenadine	Nonsedating, once-daily dosing
Loratadine	Nonsedating, once-daily dosing
Desloratadine	(the active metabolite of loratadine)
Mizolastine	Nonsedating, once-daily dosing

Although they have not been compared against each other in a systematic way for the different patterns of physical urticaria, these drugs are probably all of similar efficacy. Cetirizine is notable for its inhibitory effects on eosinophil migration, which may be of additional benefit in delayed pressure urticaria. Mizolastine is contraindicated with drugs that inhibit cytochrome P450 oxidation, prolongation of the QT interval, and in heart failure.

Maniatakou G, Demaka P, et al. J Am Acad Dermatol 1991; 24:1090–3.

Double-blind, placebo-controlled study in 11 patients, showing a reduction in weight-induced wheal area and lesional eosinophil numbers on cetirizine 10 mg three times daily.

The use of cetirizine above the licensed dose appears to be beneficial for this indication.

A comparison of new nonsedating and classical antihistamines in the treatment of primary acquired cold urticaria. Villas-Martinez F, Contreras FJ, Lopez-Cazana JM, et al. J Invest Allergol Clin Immunol 1992;2:258–62.

Randomized, double-blind study showing cetirizine, loratadine, cyproheptadine, and ketotifen were equally effective at suppression of symptoms and wheal reduction; however, more side effects were experienced with cyproheptadine.

Comparison of cinnarizine, cyproheptadine, doxepin and hydroxyzine in treatment of idiopathic cold urticaria: usefulness of doxepin. Neittaanmäki H, Myöhänen T, Fräki JE. J Am Acad Dermatol 1984;11:483–9.

A double-blind sequential study, with 2-week treatment periods in the first phase (n = 10) and 1-week treatment periods in the second phase (n = 12), in which all treatments inhibited the wheal response to local ice challenge, and doxepin offered the best subjective improvement.

The sedating and anticholinergic effects of sedating antihistamines are such that they have been largely superseded by second generation nonsedating antihistamines for most purposes.

Effect of ketotifen treatment on cold-induced urticaria. St-Pierre JP, Kobric M, Rackham A. Ann Allergy 1985;55:840–3.

A placebo-controlled, double-blind, crossover study in 11 patients with primary cold urticaria, in which ketotifen increased the threshold duration for ice-induced whealing and was more effective than placebo on a 4-point scale.

Classical sedating antihistamines, doxepin, and the mast-cell stabilizing antihistamine ketotifen have been extensively studied for cold urticaria in particular, but are probably no more effective than the more modern nonsedating equivalents.

SECOND LINE THERAPIES

Symptomatic dermographism

■ H2 receptor antagonists	A
■ PUVA	C

The effect of H1 and H2 histamine antagonists on symptomatic dermographism. Matthews CNA, Boss JM, Warin RP, Storari F. Br J Dermatol 1979;101:57–61.

Ten patients were randomized to sequential 2-week periods of cimetidine 400 mg four times daily plus chlorphenamine (chlorpheniramine) 4 mg four times daily or either active treatment alone. Chlorphenamine plus cimetidine produced a greater reduction in the wheal and flare response to a standard stroking stimulus than did chlorphenamine alone, and higher global improvement scores. Cimetidine alone appeared to worsen the subjective assessments.

In dermographic urticaria H2 receptor antagonists have a small but therapeutically irrelevant additional effect compared with H1 antagonists alone. Sharpe GR, Shuster S. Br J Dermatol 1993;129:575–9.

In this double-blind, crossover study, 19 patients were randomized to treatment with cetirizine 10 mg at night plus either ranitidine 150 mg twice daily or placebo. There was an increase in whealing threshold with additional H2 blockade, but no subjective benefit.

The effect of psoralen photochemotherapy (PUVA) on symptomatic dermographism. Logan RA, O'Brien TJO, Greaves MW. Clin Exp Dermatol 1989;14:25–8.

Five of 14 patients treated with oral PUVA experienced a useful reduction in itching after 4 weeks of treatment but there was no difference in whealing threshold between covered and exposed skin when tested with a standardized stroking stimulus.

Cholinergic urticaria

■ Danazol	A

Beneficial effects of danazol on symptoms and laboratory changes in cholinergic urticaria. Wong E, Eftekhari N,

Greaves MW, Milford Ward A. Br J Dermatol 1987;116: 553–6.

Seventeen male patients were treated with danazol 200 mg three times daily in a double-blind crossover study, with sustained improvement in the number of exercise-induced wheals over 12 weeks. Levels of protease inhibitors increased over this period but declined to baseline within 1 month of stopping treatment. Anabolic steroids should only be considered for severe cholinergic urticaria not responding adequately to antihistamines, because of their potential for virilizing effects and hepatotoxicity.

Cholinergic pruritus, erythema and urticaria. A disease spectrum responding to danazol. Berth-Jones J, Graham-Brown RAC. Br J Dermatol 1989;121:123–7.

A male patient responded well to danazol 200 mg three times daily. The improvement in symptoms was accompanied by an increase in the serum level of the antiprotease α_1-antichymotrypsin.

This drug should be reserved for severe cases and avoided during pregnancy, since it is hepatotoxic and teratogenic.

Cold urticaria

■ Cold tolerance	C
■ Terbutaline with aminophylline	B
■ Leukotriene receptor antagonists	E

Cold urticaria: a clinico-therapeutic study in 30 patients; with special emphasis on cold desensitization. Henquet JM, Martens BPM, van Volten WA. Eur J Dermatol 1992;2: 75–7.

Cold desensitization in four patients with severely disabling cold urticaria resulted in symptom-free follow-up ranging from 4 to 14 years. Induction of cold tolerance took 1–2 weeks.

Patients had to take cold showers (around 15°C) for 5 min twice a day to maintain the tolerance, so this approach is not for the faint-hearted.

Treatment of cold urticaria. Husz S, Tóth-Kása I, Kiss M, Dobozy A. Int J Dermatol 1994;33:210–3.

Thirty-seven of 42 patients with primary cold urticaria responded to terbutaline 5 mg three times daily for 1 week initially, then 2.5 mg three times daily, with aminophylline 150 mg three times daily for 6 weeks in an open study. Beta agonists and aminophylline may reduce mast cell 'releasability' but palpitations, tachycardia, and tremor were common side effects in this study.

Improvement of cold urticaria by treatment with the leukotriene receptor antagonist montelukast. Hani N, Hartmann K, Casper C, et al. Acta Derm Venereol 2000;80: 229.

A case report of a patient with acquired cold contact urticaria responding subjectively and objectively to montelukast 10 mg daily after only 4 days.

It is not clear whether montelukast was given as monotherapy or in combination with an antihistamine.

Treatment of acquired cold urticaria with cetirizine and zafirlukast in combination. Bonadonna P, Lombardi C, Senna G, et al. J Am Acad Dermatol 2003;49:714–6.

Two patients with severe cold contact urticaria improved subjectively and objectively on a combination of cetirizine 10 mg once daily and zafirlukast 20 mg twice daily. Combination therapy was better than either drug alone.

Further studies are required to clarify what place (if any) leukotriene receptor antagonists have in the management of antihistamine-unresponsive urticaria.

Delayed pressure urticaria

■ Leukotriene receptor antagonists	B
■ Sulfasalazine	E
■ Dapsone	D

Oral corticosteroids are often used for the management of severe delayed pressure urticaria since antihistamines are usually ineffective, but adverse effects from long-term administration are common and alternative therapies should be used whenever possible.

Efficacy of montelukast, in combination with loratadine, in the treatment of delayed pressure urticaria. Nettis E, Pannafino A, Cavallo E, et al. J Allergy Clin Immunol 2003; 112:212–3.

Objective pressure rechallenge after 15 days showed montelukast 10 mg once daily with loratadine 10 mg once daily was more effective than either drug alone in a small randomized study.

This encouraging early report needs confirmation with a larger study. Clinical experience with montelukast in delayed pressure urticaria is often disappointing.

Chronic sulfasalazine therapy in the treatment of delayed pressure urticaria and angioedema. Engler RJM, Squire E, Benson P. Ann Allergy Asthma Immunol 1995;74:155–9.

Two patients with disabling pressure-induced wheals, requiring oral corticosteroids, cleared with 2–4 g daily of sulfasalazine and were able to maintain the improvement off corticosteroids.

Potential side effects include bone marrow depression and hypersensitivity reactions, so patients need careful monitoring.

Delayed pressure urticaria. Successful treatment of 5 cases with dapsone. Gould DJ, Campbell D, Dayani A. Br J Dermatol 1991;125(suppl 38):25.

Five patients with confirmed delayed pressure urticaria cleared on dapsone 50 mg daily and four relapsed on stopping.

This preliminary report has not been published as a full paper and remains to be confirmed.

Solar urticaria

■ Induction of tolerance	D
■ Plasmapheresis	E
■ Cyclosporine	E

The management of idiopathic solar urticaria. Bilsland D, Ferguson J. J Dermatol Treatment 1991;1:321–3.

The use of PUVA desensitization, with or without preceding UVA radiation, is reviewed briefly.

Studies on the mechanism of clinical tolerance in solar urticaria. Keahey TM, Lavker RM, Kaidbey KH, et al. Br J Dermatol 1984;110:327–8.

Evidence levels **A** Double-blind study **B** Clinical trial ≥ 20 subjects **C** Clinical trial < 20 subjects **D** Series ≥ 5 subjects **E** Anecdotal case reports

Studies of graded whole body exposures to UVA in three patients indicated that tolerance may be due to an increase in the mast cell degranulation threshold.

UVA rush hardening for the treatment of solar urticaria. Beissert S, Ständer H, Schwarz T. J Am Acad Dermatol 2000; 42:1030–2.

Protection was achieved within 3 days of exposing three patients to multiple incremental UVA irradiations at 1-h intervals. Rush hardening with UVA did not cause sunburn reactions and provided protection against visible light and UVB-induced urticaria in two of the three patients.

Solar urticaria – effective treatment by plasmapheresis. Duschet P, Leyen P, Schwarz T, et al. Clin Exp Dermatol 1987;12:185–8.

A refractory period of at least 12 months followed a single treatment with 3 L plasmapheresis.

Cyclosporin A therapy for severe solar urticaria. Edström DW, Ros AM. Photodermatol Photoimmunol Photomed 1997;13:61–3.

A clinically useful reduction in sensitivity to visible or UV light occurred while taking cyclosporine at 4.5 mg/kg daily, but the symptoms recurred within 1–2 weeks of stopping treatment. The authors suggest that this treatment might be appropriate for severe disease when other treatments have failed, especially in countries where treatment is necessary only for a few months during summer.

Adrenergic urticaria

■ β blockers	E

Adrenergic urticaria: a new form of stress-induced hives. Shelley WA, Shelley ED. Lancet 1985;ii:1031–2.

Two cases of a distinctive pattern of stress-induced urticaria associated with increased plasma epinephrine (adrenaline) and norepinephrine (noradrenaline) concentrations responding to propanolol. The clinical presentation and response to a β blocker usually distinguishes adrenergic from cholinergic urticaria.

THIRD LINE THERAPIES

■ Topical corticosteroids	D
■ Epinephrine (adrenaline) cream	E
■ Stanozolol	D
■ Intravenous immunoglobulins	D
■ Cyclosporine	E

The effects of topical steroids on delayed pressure urticaria. Barlow RJ, Macdonald DM, Kobza Black A, Greaves MW. Arch Dermatol Res 1995;287:285–8.

The hypothesis that local application of a very potent topical corticosteroid under occlusion could reduce pressure-induced whealing, possibly through a reduction in mast cell numbers, was confirmed in six patients.

It is difficult to see how this observation is likely to be useful therapeutically because of the potential risks of skin atrophy and systemic absorption of topically applied corticosteroid.

Dyspareunia and vulvodynia: unrecognised manifestations of symptomatic dermographism. Lambiris A, Greaves MW. Lancet 1997;349:28.

Marked relief of pruritus and swelling was achieved by application of 2% epinephrine (adrenaline) cream to the vulval area as required, in conjunction with a systemic antihistamine.

Familial cold urticaria. Investigation of a family and response to stanozolol. Ormerod AD, Smart L, Reid TMS, Milford-Ward A. Arch Dermatol 1993;129:343–6.

Three of eight patients of a family with cold urticaria responded to stanozolol 5 mg twice daily, but the condition relapsed within days of stopping therapy. Familial cold urticaria has a different pathogenesis to primary or secondary cold urticaria and is very rare.

Anabolic steroids should not be offered for acquired cold urticaria.

Effect of high-dose intravenous immunoglobulin in delayed pressure urticaria. Dawn G, Urcelay M, Ah-Weng A, et al. Br J Dermatol 2003;149:836–40.

Three of eight patients went into remission after one or more infusions of intravenous immunoglobulin at 2 g/kg and two improved, but confirmation of pressure-induced wheals by objective testing was not done and all patients had associated ordinary chronic urticaria. It was not clear whether the benefit of treatment was mainly on the pressure urticaria component or the ordinary urticaria, which has been reported before.

Cold urticaria responding to systemic ciclosporin. Marsland AM, Beck MH. Br J Dermatol 2003;149:214.

One patient with acquired cold contact urticaria of over a year's duration and unresponsive to antihistamines improved within a week of starting cyclosporine at 3 mg/kg daily and the improvement was maintained at 1.7 mg/kg daily. It was not stated what happened on stopping treatment.

There is currently no good evidence that acquired cold contact urticaria is an autoimmune disease, so the use of immunomodulating drugs should be regarded as speculative and of unproven benefit.

Aquagenic pruritus

Frances Lawlor

Aquagenic pruritus is diagnosed when itching, prickling, burning, buzzing, or other skin discomfort, which may be intense, is provoked by contact with water. There are no visible skin changes. The sensation is associated with feelings of anger, irritability, or depression in approximately half the patients. The symptoms are provoked at any water temperature and degree of salinity. These occur within minutes rather than hours and start either during a bath or shower or soon afterwards. The discomfort may be present for between 10 min and 2 h. Any part of the body may be affected. Patients may also itch when the ambient temperature changes. Spontaneous remission is rare. The pathogenesis of the condition is not clear.

MANAGEMENT STRATEGY

Other chronic skin diseases must be ruled out by taking a full history and by clinical examination, particularly aquagenic pruritus of the elderly manifesting as xerosis, and other physical urticarias (i.e. cold urticaria, aquagenic urticaria, cholinergic urticaria, dermatographism, and vibratory angioedema). Direct questioning is necessary about cold-induced symptoms and whealing, water-induced whealing or syncope, exercise-, heat-, or emotion-induced symptoms and whealing, and friction-induced itching and whealing. The well-recognized 'bath itch' which occurs in approximately 40% of patients with polycythemia rubra vera must be ruled out before aquagenic pruritus is diagnosed. Rarely, other hematological abnormalities have also been associated. Occasionally, antimalarial drugs have induced an aquagenic pruritus-like picture in patients with lupus erythematosus. When the diagnosis is reached, it is important to explain that aquagenic pruritus is a recognized skin condition, which, while very unpleasant and difficult to manage, has no immediate implications with regard to the patient's general health. It may help the sufferer to realize that he or she is not mentally unstable. Therapy is usually based on the use of *antihistamines, adding sodium bicarbonate to the water*, and *phototherapy*.

SPECIFIC INVESTIGATIONS

- Complete blood count (repeated yearly)
- Leukocyte alkaline phosphatase (repeated yearly)
- Water induction

FIRST LINE THERAPIES

■ Explanation	E
■ Minimally sedating antihistamine	C
■ Sodium bicarbonate added to bath water	D

Aquagenic pruritus. Greaves MW, Black AK, Eady RAJ, Coutts A. Lancet 1981;282:2008–11.

Aquagenic pruritus. Steinman HK, Greaves MW. J Am Acad Dermatol 1985;13:91–6.

Aquagenic pruritus: pharmacological findings and treatment. Greaves MW, Handfield-Jones SE. Eur J Dermatol 1992;2:482–4.

Antihistamines are used by these authors in the management of aquagenic pruritus. The treatment of this condition is difficult. There is no consensus regarding the first line treatment as the response of each patient is individual and no single treatment is effective in all cases; however, it would seem reasonable to start by advising a minimally sedating antihistamine 2 h before the bath or shower on a regular basis. Patients may have a good response to antihistamines. Not all patients respond to antihistamine treatment, however, and of those who do, the response may consist of a diminution rather than an abolition of symptoms.

Baking soda baths for aquagenic pruritus. Bayoumi AHM, Highet AS. Lancet 1986;11:464.

[Idiopathic aquagenic pruritis treated with the addition of sodium bicarbonate to bath water]. Meunier L, Levy A, Costes Y, Meynadier J. Presse Med 1988;19:262. In French.

Aquagenic pruritus treatment with sodium bicarbonate and evidence for a seasonal form. Bircher AJ. J Am Acad Dermatol 1989;21:817

Aquagenic pruritus may respond to the addition of sodium bicarbonate to the bath water. Advice about the amount of sodium bicarbonate to be added varies. In those who have responded, 200 g, 100 g, and 25 g have been added. The most practical approach might be to start with approximately 200 g per bath, and if there is a satisfactory response, to decrease gradually to a level which continues to suppress the itching. In a series of 25 patients, 25% of the patients improved with this treatment; however, in some cases, the response may be temporary. Large quantities of sodium bicarbonate may be purchased economically at bakers' wholesalers.

SECOND LINE THERAPIES

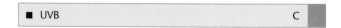

■ UVB	C

Aquagenic pruritus. Steinman HK, Greaves MW. J Am Acad Dermatol 1985;13:91

Because of practical difficulties, treatment with UVB should be considered a second line treatment. Relief usually occurs after 2–4 weeks of treatment but relapse occurs within 3–6 months of cessation of treatment.

THIRD LINE THERAPIES

■ Bath oil	E
■ Emulsifying ointment in the bath water	E
■ PUVA	E
■ Propanolol	E
■ Intramuscular triamcinolone	E
■ Transdermal nitroglycerin	E
■ Naltrexone 50 mg daily	E

The efficacy of psoralen photochemotherapy in the treatment of aquagenic pruritus. Menage HDuP, Norris PG, Hawk JLM, Greaves MW. Br J Dermatol 1993;129:163–5.

Photochemotherapy treatment of pruritus associated with polycythemia vera. Swerlick RA. J Am Acad Dermatol 1985;13:657–75.

PUVA treatment has been effective in the bath itch of polycythemia rubra vera, and has been used successfully in a series of five patients, although maintenance treatment may be necessary.

Aquagenic pruritus responds to propanolol. Thomsen K. J Am Acad Dermatol 1990;22:697.

Aquagenic pruritus: effective treatment with intramuscular triamcinolone. Carson TE. Cutis 1991;48:382.

Sporadic patients are reported to respond to propanolol, intramuscular triamcinolone, and the addition of a bath oil or emulsifying ointment to the bath water.

Aquagenic pruritus response to the exogenous nitric oxide donor, transdermal nitroglycerin. Goihan Yahr M. Int J Dermatol 1994;33:752.

Transdermal nitroglycerin has been used effectively in one patient.

Efficacy and safety of naltrexone, an oral opiate receptor antagonist, in the treatment of pruritus and dermatologi-

Evidence levels A Double-blind study B Clinical trial ≥ 20 subjects C Clinical trial < 20 subjects D Series ≥ 5 subjects E Anecdotal case reports

cal diseases. Metze D, Reinmann S, Beissert S, Luger T. J Am Acad Dermatol 1999;41:533–9.

Naltrexone, at a dose of 50 mg daily, demonstrated a response in the single patient with aquagenic pruritus to whom it was given.

Cholinergic pruritus

Frances Lawlor

Cholinergic pruritus occurs when patients itch, sting, or prickle following a rise in body temperature. The provoking stimuli are exercise (walking, running, dancing, going to the gym), including housework (ironing, vacuuming), heat (hot room, hot food, hot bath, sunny day), and emotion (excitement, stress, fever, embarrassment). A combination of factors may cause a more pronounced itch, for example walking on a sunny day. The intensity, extent, and duration of the itching seem to be directly proportional to the strength of the eliciting stimulus. By definition, no whealing occurs on the skin during an attack. While the prevalence of this condition is not known, it is the author's impression that many people itch when they become warm, although this itching is frequently insufficiently severe or incapacitating to present at a dermatology clinic. Cholinergic pruritus can be regarded as a variant of cholinergic urticaria. There is one case report which describes a patient presenting initially with cholinergic pruritus who progressed to cholinergic urticaria. Since there are no visible skin lesions, it is important to be aware of the condition and to differentiate it from aquagenic pruritus in those who describe itching after a bath or shower.

MANAGEMENT STRATEGY

Explaining the provoking factors and stressing that the condition is not an allergy, related to diet, or related to any underlying disease is helpful. If possible, *minimizing situations in which the itching occurs* can be helpful, and cooling the skin as quickly as possible may lessen the duration of the itching. It is not possible to tell the patient how long the condition will be present before remission takes place. Therapeutic agents typically utilized are *antihistamines*, although *danazol* has been reported to be beneficial.

SPECIFIC INVESTIGATIONS

- Exercise induction
- Warm bath induction (40–41°C)

FIRST LINE THERAPIES

■ Explanation	E
■ Minimally sedating antihistamine: cetirizine 10 mg, fexofenadine 180 mg, loratadine 10 mg	E

An explanation is the most important part of treatment. The patient needs to understand the relationship between the itching and heat and the importance of keeping cool. Treatment with minimally sedating antihistamines generally produces an improvement, although they are unlikely to suppress the condition completely. The standard dose of cetirizine, loratadine, or fexofenadine should be taken either regularly every morning or 2 h before an expected stimulus, in order to assess any response. If the antihistamine proves helpful, the same dose could be repeated 9–12 h later if necessary.

SECOND LINE THERAPIES

■ Danazol	C

Cholinergic pruritus, erythema, and urticaria: a disease spectrum responding to danazol. Berth-Jones J, Graham Brown RAC. Br J Dermatol 1989;121:235–7.

Danazol, which has been used in cholinergic urticaria, may rarely be effective in very severely affected individuals. The recommended dose is 200 mg three times daily. This dose could be continued for approximately 1 month and reduced to the minimum that controls the condition.

Pinta and yaws

Miguel R Sanchez

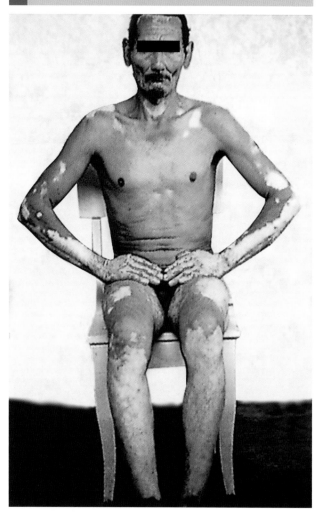

Pinta and yaws are nonvenereal 'endemic' spirochetal infections caused, respectively, by *Treponema carateum* and *Treponema pallidum subspecies pertenue*. Pinta was almost exclusively found in inhabitants of rural, overcrowded, poverty-stricken regions of Mexico, the Caribbean, and the northern part of South America, and has been reported most recently from scattered areas in the Brazilian rain forest. Yaws was prevalent in indigent persons living in tropical, rural, medically underserved areas with high humidity and rainfall within Central Africa, Southeast Asia, Central and northeast South America, and some Pacific Islands, and recently outbreaks have been reported from Papua New Guinea and Guyana. Most patients are children and young adults who acquire the infections by direct contact of abraded skin with another person's exudative infected lesions.

MANAGEMENT STRATEGY

Pinta and yaws are very rare, and familiarity with the types of lesions is essential to differentiate them from syphilis, psoriasis, leprosy, and leukodermas, as well as to establish appropriate treatment. As in syphilis, both infections have three distinct clinical stages.

In pinta signs or symptoms are limited to the skin and lymph nodes, but in yaws the skeletal system and mucous membranes can also be affected. The primary stage of pinta develops after an incubation period of 15 days to months (usually 2–4 weeks) after exposure. One to three erythematous papules erupt, usually on the face or extremities and grow into erythematous scaly plaques, which may become hypochromic or light blue in the center. Nontender regional lymphadenopathy may appear. The secondary stage of pinta usually follows in 2–5 months (sometimes years later) with the appearance of erythematous papules (pintids), which enlarge to form psoriasiform plaques and may remain for years. The plaques, which may be annular or circinate, progress through a range of colors from copper-brown to slate blue or black. Some plaques may be hypochromic. Lymphadenopathy may be present. The tertiary stage is characterized by depigmented patches on the wrists, ankles, elbows, and within old lesions. These develop between 3 months and 10 years after the onset of the secondary stage. At this point patients have a combination of hyperpigmented, hypochromic, achromic, dyschromic, and polychromic patches of different sizes, imparting a mottled appearance to the skin. In 80% of cases, serologic tests become reactive 2–3 months after the onset of the primary lesion and are always reactive in late lesions.

In yaws the primary stage develops after an incubation period of 10 days to 3 months with the appearance usually on a lower extremity of an erythematous, occasionally pruritic papulonodule ('the mother yaw'). This papulonodule enlarges up to 5 cm in circumference and ulcerates with exuberant granulation tissue, which imparts a fraboesiform appearance. The secondary stage usually ensues 10–16 weeks, but as long as 2 years after the onset of the primary stage, with an eruption of reddish, weeping, crust-covered papules ('daughter yaws'), which are similar to but smaller than the primary lesion. In some patients, the clinical findings are similar to secondary syphilis with scaly papules and plaques, hypertrophic condyloma lata resembling lesions on body folds, or lesions resembling mucous patches on mucous membranes. Nodules around the joints are common. Some patients have painful osteoperiostitis of the forearm or leg, and polydactylitis of the hand or foot. In approximately 10% of infected patients, the disease progresses to the tertiary stage with infiltrated plaques and nodules, which ulcerate, leaving deep ulcers with raised granulomatous edges. Skeletal changes include chronic hypertrophic osteoperiostitis, which most commonly affect the tibia (saber shins) or the superior nasal processes of the maxillae. This latter process triggers disfiguring progressive exostosis of new bone (goundou), which in 5–20 years, eventuates in massive destruction and perforation of the nose and the palate (rhinopharyngitis mutilans or gangosa).

The recommended treatment of pinta and yaws is a single intramuscular injection of 1.2 million units of *benzathine penicillin G* in adults, adolescents, and older children, and 0.6 million units in children under 10 years of age. Patients cease to be infectious within 24 h. In pinta primary and secondary lesions heal in 4–12 months, but achromic lesions persist indefinitely. Penicillin-allergic patients older than 8 years of age are treated with a 15-day course of *tetracycline* 250 mg four times daily or *doxycycline* 50 mg twice daily. *Erythromycin* should be reserved for penicillin-allergic children younger than 8 years of age (8 mg/kg four times daily) and for pregnant women (500 mg four times daily).

Evidence levels   **A** Double-blind study   **B** Clinical trial ≥ 20 subjects   **C** Clinical trial < 20 subjects   **D** Series ≥ 5 subjects   **E** Anecdotal case reports

SPECIFIC INVESTIGATIONS

- Serologic tests (cardiolipin flocculation assays, treponemal-specific assays)
- Dark-field microscopy
- Direct fluorescent antibody test
- Histopathology

The endemic treponematoses. Antal GM, Lukehart SA, Meheus AZ. Microbes Infect 2002;4:83–94.

Available serologic tests cannot distinguish yaws or pinta from syphilis. Penicillin treatment often does not lead to seroreversal. Some cases of yaws and pinta may be misdiagnosed as syphilis.

Histopathological aspects of tertiary pinta. Pecher SA, Azevedo EB. Med Cutan Ibero Lat Am 1987;15:239–42.

Treponemes are found on silver impregnation between epidermal cells in primary, secondary, and late-stage hyperpigmented lesions, but not in late hypopigmented patches.

FIRST LINE THERAPIES

■ Penicillin	B

Treponemal infections. WHO Scientific Group. Technical Report Series No. 674. Geneva: World Health Organization; 1982.

Intramuscular benzathine penicillin is the recommended treatment for all patients with pinta or yaws. All household cases and contacts should also be treated in areas where 5% of the population is infected. In areas with 5–10% rates of infection, treatment should be administered to all children under 15 years of age, and in areas with higher infection rates the entire population should be treated with penicillin.

Treatment of pinta with antibiotics. Ketchen DK. Ann N Y Acad Sci 1952;55:1176–85.

This study on Mexican patients with pinta found that, after treatment with penicillin, skin lesions healed completely in all patients with primary lesions, in 69% with secondary lesions, and in 40% with tertiary lesions.

Nonvenereal treponematoses in tropical countries. Engelkens HJ, Vuzevski VD, Stolz E. Clin Dermatol 1999;17:143–52.

This review stresses that penicillin at previously recommended doses remains the treatment of choice.

Failure of penicillin treatment of yaws on Karkar Island, Papua New Guinea. Backhouse JL, Hudson BJ, Hamilton PA, Nesteroff SI. Am J Trop Med Hyg 1998;59:388–92.

Of 39 children 28% developed clinical and/or serologic evidence of relapse after treatment with the recommended dose of intramuscular benzathine penicillin. All but three responded to further penicillin treatment.

Resistance of yaws to penicillin has also been reported from Ecuador.

Efficacy of a targeted, oral penicillin-based yaws control program among children living in rural South America. Scolnik D, Aronson L, Lovinsky R, et al. Clin Infect Dis 2003;36:1232–8.

Clinical cure of yaws lesions was achieved in 94% of 17 children with administration of oral penicillin, 50 mg/kg daily in four divided doses for 7–10 days.

Benzathine penicillin G treatment may not be possible in remote areas because the drug requires refrigeration at a temperature of 2–8°C until 7 days before use, at which time it should be stored at less than 30°C.

Mass treatment programs designed to eradicate endemic treponematosis expose uninfected people to adverse effects and may promote antibiotic resistance. Treatment programs that exclusively target clinically active cases can significantly reduce the prevalence of disease.

Review: endemic treponematoses are not always eradicated. De Schryver A, Meheus A. Med Trop (Mars) 1989;49:237–44.

The infection is highly sensitive to penicillin and resistance has not been reported. Endemic control through treatment of the entire treponemal reservoir with single-dose penicillin is highly successful.

SECOND LINE THERAPIES

■ Tetracycline	E
■ Doxycycline	E
■ Minocycline	E
■ Erythromycin	E

Therapy for nonvenereal treponematosis. Review of the efficacy of penicillin and consideration of alternatives. Brown ST. Rev Infect Dis 1985;7:318–26.

This article reviews studies of the treatment of pinta and yaws. Penicillin is the drug of choice. Tetracycline is also concluded to be effective, but studies were done on patients with yaws. Reports of treatment with erythromycin were scarce. Doxycycline and minocycline appear to be useful alternatives.

Nonvenereal treponematoses: yaws, endemic syphilis, and pinta. Koff AB, Rosen T. J Am Acad Dermatol 1993;29:519–35.

Tetracycline or doxycycline is the treatment of choice in older children and adults who are allergic to penicillin.

Pitted keratolysis

Eunice Tan, John Berth-Jones

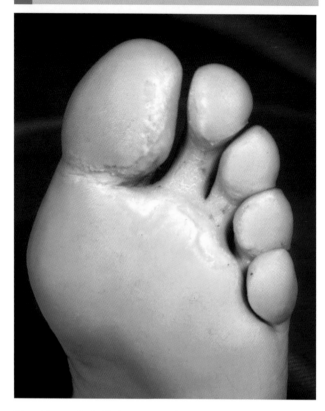

Pitted keratolysis (PK) is a superficial infection of the stratum corneum characterized by shallow, punched-out, circular erosions, primarily on the weightbearing areas of the soles of the feet, and less commonly, on the non-weightbearing areas of the feet and the palms of the hands. Hyperhidrosis, maceration, and a foul odor are usually present. Several species of *Corynebacterium*, *Dermatophilus*, *Actinomyces*, and *Micrococcus* possessing enzymatic keratolytic activity have been isolated.

MANAGEMENT STRATEGY

Most patients experience little or mild irritation. Maceration, foul odor, and soreness are the main reasons for consultation. Sweat retention and immersion are important predisposing factors. Industrial workers wearing rubber shoes and soldiers whose feet are continually wet have a high prevalence of PK. Initial management strategies should include instructions on foot hygiene and avoidance of occlusive footwear.

Treatment of the hyperhidrosis alone will slowly bring the condition under control. However, our usual first line treatment is 2% *fusidic acid cream* applied three to four times daily, sometimes combined with topical *aluminum chloride hexahydrate*. In the USA, where fusidic acid is not available, formulations of *clindamycin*, *erythromycin*, and *tetracycline* designed for the treatment of acne are suitable alternatives. PK has also responded to topical antifungals such as *clotrimazole* and *miconazole*. Clotrimazole 1% cream or miconazole 2% cream or ointment may be applied twice daily. Topical antiseptics can also be effective. Systemic antibiotics are reserved for severe and resistant cases. A 1-week course of *oral erythromycin* at 250 mg four times daily has led to resolution of PK. Penicillins and sulfonamides do not seem to be effective.

Topical 20% aluminum chloride hexahydrate in absolute anhydrous ethyl alcohol may help to reduce the hyperhidrosis. The solution is applied at night and allowed to dry. This should be used daily until the condition is brought under control, and it can then be used less frequently. In palmoplantar hyperhidrosis the response to 20% aluminum chloride hexahydrate is not as complete as in axillary hyperhidrosis.

Formaldehyde 4% solution appears to reduce hyperhidrosis in addition to its antiseptic action. This can be applied with gauze soaks as the patient sits or stands with his or her feet on the gauze in a bowl for 10–15 min once or twice daily.

Iontophoresis has been used in palmar and plantar hyperhidrosis and can be used in the treatment of PK when formaldehyde fails.

Topical 2% buffered glutaraldehyde also reduces hyperhidrosis and has been reported to be effective in PK. Both this and formaldehyde may cause sensitization.

SPECIFIC INVESTIGATIONS

- No investigation is routinely required

Pitted keratolysis. The role of *Micrococcus sedentarius*. Nordstrom KM, McGinley KJ, Cappiello L, et al. Arch Dermatol 1987;123:1320–5.

Isolates of *Micrococcus sedentarius* from PK lesions on the feet of eight patients were tested for antibiotic sensitivities and found to be resistant to penicillin, ampicillin, methicillin, and oxacillin. PK lesions were reproduced in one volunteer inoculated with *M. sedentarius* after 6 weeks of occlusion.

***Kytococcus sedentarius*, the organism associated with pitted keratolysis, produces two keratin-degrading enzymes.** Longshaw CM, Wright JD, Farrell AM, Holland KT. J Appl Microbiol 2002;93:810–6.

This organism (formerly known as *M. sedentarius*), was found to produce two separate keratolytic enzymes, strongly supporting the hypothesis that this organism can cause pitted keratolysis.

FIRST LINE THERAPIES

■ Topical fusidic acid	E
■ Topical aluminum chloride hexahydrate	E
■ Topical formaldehyde	E

Coexistent erythrasma, trichomycosis axillaris, and pitted keratolysis: an overlooked corynebacterial triad? Shelley WB, Shelley ED. J Am Acad Dermatol 1982;7:752–7.

A patient with this triad was treated with oral erythromycin 250 mg four times daily and a solution of 20% aluminum chloride applied nightly to the soles. Three weeks later, the plantar hyperhidrosis and odor were significantly reduced, though the pits remained.

Pitted and ringed keratolysis. A review and update. Zaias N. J Am Acad Dermatol 1982;7:787–91.

Evidence levels A Double-blind study B Clinical trial ≥ 20 subjects C Clinical trial < 20 subjects D Series ≥ 5 subjects E Anecdotal case reports

The author reports personal observations (noncontrolled) that treatment of PK with topical clotrimazole, miconazole, erythromycin, tetracycline, clindamycin, glutaraldehyde, and formaldehyde, and oral erythromycin have been curative. Penicillin has not been useful.

Road rash with a rotten odor. Schissel DJ, Aydelotte J, Keller R. Mil Med 1999;164:65–7.

A soldier was treated with topical clotrimazole cream twice daily, topical clindamycin solution twice daily, and topical ammonium chloride each evening. After 2 weeks he reported resolution of the odor, tenderness, and interdigital pruritus. At 8 weeks there was complete resolution.

SECOND LINE THERAPIES

■ Topical mupirocin	D
■ Topical tetracycline	E
■ Topical clindamycin	E
■ Topical erythromycin	E
■ Topical clotrimazole	E
■ Topical miconazole	E
■ Oral erythromycin	E

Mupirocin ointment for symptomatic pitted keratolysis. Vazquez-Lopez F, Perez-Oliva N. Infection 1996;24:55.

Four patients with symptomatic PK failing to respond to conventional treatments were treated with topical mupirocin ointment with rapid clearance of PK.

Pitted keratolysis: a new form of treatment. Burkhart CG. Arch Dermatol 1980;116:1104.

Three patients with PK were treated with topical 1% clindamycin hydrochloride solution (660 mg dissolved in 55 mL of 70% isopropyl alcohol and 5% propylene glycol). The solution was applied to the plantar surface three times daily, and within 4 weeks there was complete resolution of the clinical lesions.

Pitted keratolysis: a clinicopathologic review. Stanton RL, Schwartz RA, Aly R. J Am Podiatr Med Assoc 1982;72:436–9.

Topical 2% erythromycin applied twice daily resulted in resolution of PK in both feet within 4 weeks of treatment in one case.

Painful, plaque-like, pitted keratolysis occurring in childhood. Shah AS, Kamino H, Prose NS. Pediatr Dermatol 1992;9:251–4.

Two children were reported with these lesions and treatment with topical 2% erythromycin solution twice a day in both patients was curative within 3 weeks of commencing treatment.

Ultrastructure of pitted keratolysis. De Almeida Jr HL, De Castro LAS, Rocha NEM, Abrantes VL. Int J Dermatol 2000;39:698–709.

A patient responded to topical erythromycin.

Pitted keratolysis of the palm arising after herpes zoster. Lee H-J, Roh K-Y, Ha S-J, Kim J-W. Br J Dermatol 1999;140: 974–5.

A report of PK in the palm of a patient who was suffering from postherpetic neuralgia in the same area. This responded within 4 days to oral erythromycin 250 mg twice daily and mupirocin ointment.

THIRD LINE THERAPIES

■ Topical glutaraldehyde	D
■ Topical gentamicin	E
■ Topical Whitfield's ointment	E
■ Topical triamcinolone	E
■ Topical iodochlorhydroxyquin (Vioform®) hydrocortisone	E
■ Topical flexible collodion	E
■ Topical water-repellent ointment	E
■ Formalin ointment	E

Pitted keratolysis: forme fruste old treatments. Gordon HH. Arch Dermatol 1981;117:608.

Buffered glutaraldehyde 2% was used with beneficial results on PK and hyperhidrosis (uncontrolled personal observations). The author also advises that proper instructions on foot hygiene be given and that patients wear sandals as much as possible. He also reports sensitization to glutaraldehyde and advises that when this occurs or when glutaraldehyde treatment has failed, it would be advisable to use antibiotics.

Pitted keratolysis: forme fruste: a review and new therapies. Gordon HH. Cutis 1975;15:54–8.

Buffered glutaraldehyde 2% applied twice daily in five patients resulted in relief of signs and symptoms except in one patient addicted to wearing boots, who continued to have hyperhidrosis. Treatment with gentamicin cream resulted in improvement.

Hyperhidrosis: treatment with glutaraldehyde. Gordon HH. Cutis 1972;9:375–8.

Eight patients with palmar and plantar hyperhidrosis were treated with varying strengths of 2, 2.5, 5, and 10% aqueous glutaraldehyde with good results. Glutaraldehyde 10%, not alkalinized, was rapidly effective but caused brown staining. A starting strength of 5% used three times weekly reduced the staining, and patients were then placed on 2 or 2.5% maintenance treatment as required.

Contact dermatitis has been reported with glutaraldehyde, but none of these patients developed this problem.

Keratolysis plantare sulcatum. Higashi N. Jpn J Clin Dermatol 1972;26:321–5.

Two patients with KP responded to topical gentamicin sulfate cream.

Symptomatic pitted keratolysis. Lamberg SI. Arch Dermatol 1969;100:10–1.

Reports of 12 military personnel with symptomatic PK treated with various topical agents. One foot was used for treatment while the other was used as a control without treatment or as a comparator by application of another topical agent. Treatments included corticosteroid creams, antibiotic creams, iodochlorhydroxyquin-hydrocortisone (Vioform hydrocortisone) cream, flexible collodion, Whitfield's ointment, and formalin in aquaphor (20–40%). Formalin (40%) ointment appeared to be the most effective and was used for the rest of both their asymptomatic and symptomatic patients with PK. All cases returned to full duty with the ointment after a single outpatient visit, and on re-examination PK had resolved.

Pityriasis lichenoides chronica

Alex Milligan, Graham Johnston

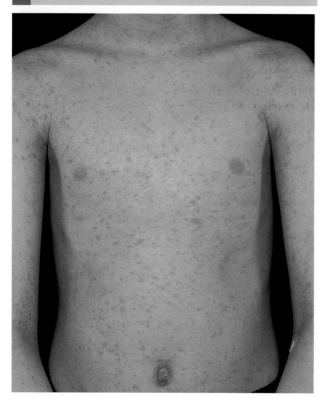

Pityriasis lichenoides chronica (PLC) typically consists of small erythematous papules, which may be purpuric. These develop a characteristic shiny mica scale attached to the center. They occur predominantly over the trunk and proximal limbs. As the name implies, PLC may persist for many years, though spontaneous resolution does occur. Patients should be warned that relapse is common and recurrent courses of therapy may be required.

MANAGEMENT STRATEGY

There are no controlled therapeutic trials for this condition, and case series are only small. In many therapeutic trials PLC has been grouped together with pityriasis lichenoides et varioliformis acuta (see page 498) and management strategies are therefore often similar or interchangeable.

Topical corticosteroids are only reported as effective anecdotally in textbooks rather than in studies. They are often used with *antihistamines* to reduce pruritus, but they are not reported to affect the course of the disease.

The majority of reports describe benefits with *UV therapy*, and therefore either UV alone or with *psoralen plus UVA (PUVA)* therapy is recommended for all patients. The response appears to be unpredictable, however, and the total dose required is extremely variable.

Antibiotics do not appear to be especially helpful, though combination therapy (e.g. *tetracycline* and *topical corticosteroid*) has been suggested.

For severe or refractory cases *methotrexate, cyclosporine,* and *acitretin* have all been described as effective in small numbers of patients.

For most treatment modalities, patients who have been described as improved have usually had fewer new lesions, developing, a shortened disease course and a greater time to relapse compared with untreated patients.

SPECIFIC INVESTIGATIONS

- Consider skin biopsy

Although a skin biopsy is usually unnecessary in clinically obvious cases, it may be useful before commencing aggressive systemic therapy.

An infective etiology is often suggested, but no pathogen has yet been implicated, though an association with toxoplasmosis has been described. These reports tend to come from endemic areas and so investigation for a triggering infection is unnecessary in cases without evidence of specific infections.

The relationship between toxoplasmosis and pityriasis lichenoides chronica. Nassef NE, Hamman MA. J Egypt Soc Parasitol 1997;27:93–9.

Twenty two patients with PLC and 20 healthy controls were examined clinically and serologically for toxoplasmosis. Three (15%) of the controls had toxoplasmosis compared to 8 (36%) of the patients with PLC. Five of the latter had subsidence of skin lesions after pyrimethamine and sulfapyrimidine treatment.

Pityriasis lichenoides and acquired toxoplasmosis. Rongioletti F, Delmonte S, Rebora A. Int J Dermatol 1999;38: 367–76.

A patient with biopsy-proven PLEVA and acute *Toxoplasma* serology is reported. His skin failed to respond to azithromycin but cleared with spiramycin followed by trimethoprim–sulfamethoxazole.

FIRST LINE THERAPIES

■ UVB	D
■ Combined UVA and UVB	D
■ PUVA	D

UV-B Phototherapy for pityriasis lichenoides. Tham SN. Austral J Dermatol 1985;26:9–13.

Seventeen patients with PLC were treated with UVB three to five times per week with a starting dose of 80–90% of the minimal erythema dose. They received an average of 33 treatments, and nine completely cleared while five had 90% clearance. Only half had relapsed at 3-year follow-up.

Phototherapy of pityriasis lichenoides. LeVine MJ. Arch Dermatol 1983;119:378–80.

PLC in 12 patients completely cleared after an average of 30 treatments of minimally erythemogenic doses of UVA/UVB from fluorescent sunlamps. The average UV dose required was 388 mJ/cm².

Comparative studies of treatments for pityriasis lichenoides. Gritiyarangsan P, Pruenglampoo S, Ruangratanarote P. J Dermatol 1987;14:258–61.

In this open study 30 patients with pityriasis lichenoides were recruited, although the authors did not specify how many had PLEVA and how many PLC. The first group of eight were given topical corticosteroid and half had a partial or complete response. The second group were also given oral tetracycline and the majority had a partial response. The third group of eight chronic, refractory cases were given oral methoxsalen 0.6 mg/kg with UVA three times per week for an average of 2 months; five were cleared and two had a partial response.

PUVA therapy of pityriasis lichenoides chronica. Han HK, Kim JK, Kook HL. Korean J Dermatol 1982;20:413–7.

Nine patients with PLC of relatively short duration were treated with oral methoxsalen and UVA and were cleared completely after between eight and 45 treatments.

Experience with UVB phototherapy in children. Tay Y-K, Morelli JG, Weston WL. Pediatr Dermatol 1996;13:406–9.

In an open study of UVB in various dermatoses in younger patients, two children with PLC were given broadband UVB three times a week for an average of 26 treatments (mean total dose 4.2 J/cm²). Both had 90% improvement in lesions and no subsequent relapse.

Long-term follow-up of photochemotherapy in pityriasis lichenoides. Boelen RE, Faber WR, Lambers JCCA, Cormane RH. Acta Dermatol 1982;62:442–4.

Five patients with PLC were treated with PUVA or with a UVB plus UVA light source. All responded and remained clear from 20 to 36 months.

Photochimiotherapie orale du parapsoriasis en gouttes. Thivolet J, Ortonne JP, Gianadda B, Gianadda E. Dermatologica 1981;163:12–8.

Six of eight patients treated with oral methoxsalen PUVA cleared completely.

SECOND LINE THERAPIES

■ Tetracycline	D
■ Erythromycin	E

Tetracycline for the treatment of pityriasis lichenoides. Piamphongsant T. Br J Dermatol 1974;91:319.

Twelve patients in Bangkok were given tetracycline 2 g daily. All responded within 4 weeks. Seven required maintenance therapy of 1 g daily for 6 months.

Pityriasis lichenoides in children: therapeutic response to erythromycin. Truhan AP, Hebert AA, Esterly NB. J Am Acad Dermatol 1986;15:66–70.

Four children aged 4–14 years with biopsy-proven PLC were given oral erythromycin 200–400 mg four times daily. Two improved within a month, and on stopping the drug after 5 and 12 months there was no recurrence. One patient improved on an increased dose and one failed to respond after 6 months of therapy.

THIRD LINE THERAPIES

■ Methotrexate	E
■ Acitretin	E
■ Acitretin plus PUVA	E
■ Cyclosporine	E
■ UVA1	E
■ Topical tacrolimus	E

Methotrexate treatment of pityriasis lichenoides and lymphomatoid papulosis. Lynch PJ, Saied NK. Cutis 1979;23:635–6.

Three patients received methotrexate 25 mg per week intramuscularly or orally. All responded within weeks, but two relapsed on cessation of therapy.

Oral retinoids in the treatment of pityriasis lichenoides. Mastrolonardo M, Cassano N, Coviello C, et al. J Dermatol Treat 1997;8:199–201.

Pityriasis lichenoides in four men treated with 1 mg/kg cleared completely in 6–18 weeks, and on cessation of therapy the men remained disease free for more than 8 months.

Successful treatment of pityriasis lichenoides chronica with acitretin. Hay IC, Omerod AD. J Dermatol Treat 1988;9:53–4.

A further report of a patient with PLC who, having failed to respond to prednisolone, oxytetracycline, dapsone, methotrexate, azathioprine, UVB, and PUVA, responded to 50 mg acitretin daily.

Photochemotherapy for pityriasis lichenoides: 3 cases. Panse I, Bourrat E, Rybojad M, Morel P. Ann Dermatol Venereol 2004;131:201–3.

One patient with pityriasis lichenoides and two patients with PLEVA unresponsive to other therapies including topical corticosteroids, antibiotics, and UVB responded within weeks to acitretin plus PUVA.

Cyclosporine and dermatoses. Gupta AK, Ellis CN, Nickoloff BJ, et al. Arch Dermatol 1990;126:340–1.

In a review of cyclosporine in a wide variety of dermatoses the authors report successful clearance in 8 weeks in a man with a 24-year history of PLC. The dose was 6 mg/kg daily and an improvement in scaling and erythema was noticed after the first week.

Medium-dose ultraviolet A1 therapy for pityriasis lichenoides varioliformis acuta and pityriasis lichenoides chronica. Pinton PC, Capezzera R, Zane C, De Panfilis G. J Am Acad Dermatol 2002;47:410–4.

Eight patients (five with PLC and three with PLEVA) were treated. Three patients with PLC showed complete clinical and histological recovery. Two showed partial improvement.

Refractory pityriasis lichenoides chronica successfully treated with topical tacrolimus. Mallipeddi R, Evans AV. Clin Exp Dermatol 2003;28:456–8.

A 41-year-old woman with an 8-year history of PLC unresponsive to erythromycin, UVB, and PUVA showed almost complete clearance after 4 weeks of treatment with tacrolimus ointment. Subsequent relapses responded to further treatment.

Successful treatment of pityriasis lichenoides with topical tacrolimus. Simon D, Boudny C, Nievergelt H, et al. Br J Dermatol 2004;150:1033–5.

Two children with longlasting refractory PLC were cleared of skin lesions after 14 and 18 weeks of treatment, respectively.

Pityriasis lichenoides et varioliformis acuta

Alex Milligan, Graham Johnston

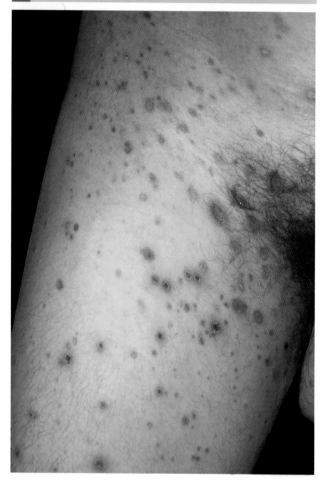

Pityriasis lichenoides et varioliformis acuta (PLEVA, Mucha-Habermann disease) is an eruption of small, erythematous papules, which become vesicular and hemorrhagic. Some ulcerate and necrose, leaving pitted scars. The name refers to the morphology not the duration of the condition because a significant proportion of cases regress with or without treatment, only to recur. Patients should be warned that relapse is common and recurrent courses of therapy may be required. Febrile ulceronecrotic Mucha-Habermann's disease is a rare and severe form of PLEVA characterized by an abrupt onset of an ulceronecrotic eruption associated with a high fever and systemic symptoms.

MANAGEMENT STRATEGY

There are only a handful of controlled trials for this condition and large series are rare. In many therapeutic trials PLEVA is often grouped together with pityriasis lichenoides chronica (see page 496) and management strategies are therefore often similar or interchangeable.

Although a 'wait and see' approach is justifiable in infants, children should be given a 6-week course of *high-dose erythromycin*. Tetracycline should not be given because of its effects on dentition.

Second line therapy in children, and possibly first in adults, is either *UV light* or *psoralen plus UVA (PUVA)* because this has been shown to be more effective in the only comparative study. *Topical corticosteroids* are only reported anecdotally in textbooks rather than in studies. They are used with *antihistamines* to reduce pruritus, but have no reported effect on disease course.

In more extensive or symptomatic disease *low-dose methotrexate* is useful and *systemic corticosteroids* or *cyclosporine* have also been used.

Some authors have suggested that *combination therapy* (e.g. *erythromycin and PUVA* or *methotrexate and PUVA*) is effective, especially in the rare, febrile, ulceronecrotic variant of Mucha-Habermann disease.

SPECIFIC INVESTIGATIONS

- Consider skin biopsy

A diagnostic skin biopsy is unnecessary in clinically obvious cases, but may be useful to exclude lymphomatoid papulosis or before commencing aggressive systemic therapy.

An infective etiology for PLEVA is suggested by reports of clustering of cases, resolution following tonsillectomy, and occurrence in five members of a family. Case reports exist associating PLEVA with parvovirus, adenovirus in the urine, staphylococci from throat cultures, Epstein–Barr virus, toxoplasmosis, and HIV. No organism has been cultured from lesional skin and, unless there are clinical signs of infection, routine investigation for an infective agent does not appear to be useful.

Pityriasis lichenoides: a cytotoxic T-cell-mediated skin disorder. Evidence of human parvovirus B19 DNA in nine cases. Tomasini D, Tomasini CF, Cerri A, et al. J Cutan Pathol 2004;31:531–8.

This study suggests that pityriasis lichenoides is mediated by a cytotoxic T-cell effector population.

The identification of parvovirus B19 DNA in nine cases may be interpreted ambiguously.

Pityriasis lichenoides et varioliformis acuta and group-A beta hemolytic streptococcal infection. English JC III, Collins M, Bryant-Bruce C. Int J Dermatol 1995;34:642–4.

Biopsy-proven PLEVA in association with carriage of Gram-positive cocci cleared with ciprofloxacin in a 35-year-old woman. An identical eruption, in her husband, who was found to have group A β-hemolytic streptococcus from a skin swab, cleared with erythromycin.

Pityriasis lichenoides and acquired toxoplasmosis. Rongioletti F, Delmonte S, Rebora A. Int J Dermatol 1999;38:367–76.

Biopsy-proven PLEVA in a patient with serology indicating acute toxoplasmosis failed to respond to azithromycin, but cleared with spiramycin followed by trimethoprim–sulfamethoxazole.

FIRST LINE THERAPIES

■ Oral erythromycin	D
■ Oral tetracycline	E

Pityriasis lichenoides in children: therapeutic response to erythromycin. Truhan AP, Hebert AA, Esterly NB. J Am Acad Dermatol 1986;15:66–70.

In this retrospective uncontrolled study, 11 children aged 2–11 years with biopsy-proven PLEVA were given oral erythromycin 200 mg three or four times daily. Nine improved within a month, and 2–6 months after stopping the drug, there was only one recurrence. One patient improved on an increased dose and one failed to respond.

Mucha Habermann's disease in children: treatment with erythromycin. Shavin JS, Jones TM, Aton JK, et al. Arch Dermatol 1978;114:1679–80.

Three children responded rapidly to several weeks of erythromycin: 40 mg/kg in the younger patient and 1 g daily in the two adolescents. All subsequently required a second course due to relapse.

Pityriasis lichenoides et varioliformis acuta. Shelley WB, Griffith RF. Arch Dermatol 1969;100:596–7.

A 13-year-old girl who had not responded to oral oxacillin, erythromycin, prednisolone, and intramuscular triamcinolone had complete involution of all lesions on treatment with 2 g of tetracycline daily. Maintenance therapy was required for 1 year.

SECOND LINE THERAPIES

■ UVB	D
■ UVA	D
■ PUVA	D
■ Acitretin and PUVA	D

Pityriasis lichenoides in children: a longterm follow-up of eighty-nine cases. Gelmetti C, Rigoni C, Alessi E, et al. J Am Acad Dermatol 1990;23:473–8.

In a retrospective review of 89 cases the authors did not differentiate between the treatment of PLEVA and pityriasis lichenoides chronica (PLC). However, 77 of the children were treated with 4–8-week courses of UVB phototherapy, which seemed to alleviate symptoms and acute eruptions without modifying the course of the disease. The remaining 12 patients were given oral erythromycin 20–40 mg/kg daily for 1–2 weeks and the response was described as 'moderately effective'.

Medium-dose ultraviolet A1 therapy for pityriasis lichenoides et varioliformis acuta and pityriasis lichenoides chronica. Pinton PC, Capezzera R, Zane C, De Panfilis G. J Am Acad Dermatol 2002;47:410–4.

Three patients received 60 J/cm² UVA1 daily until clinical remission. Lesions inaccessible to UVA1 were used as control lesions. Patients showed complete clinical and histologic recovery and unirradiated control lesions did not improve.

Comparative studies of treatment for pityriasis lichenoides. Gritiyarangsan P, Pruenglampoo S, Ruangratanarote P. J Dermatol 1987;14:258–61.

In this open study 30 patients with pityriasis lichenoides were recruited, although the authors did not specify how many had PLEVA and how many PLC. The first group of eight patients were given topical corticosteroid and half had a partial or complete response. The second group of patients were given corticosteroid plus oral tetracycline and the majority had a partial response. The third group of eight patients with chronic, refractory pityriasis lichenoides were given oral methoxsalen 0.6 mg/kg with UVA three times a week for an average of 2 months; five cleared and two had a partial response.

Erprobung von PUVA bei verscheidenen Dermatosen. Brenner W, Gschnalt F, Honigsmann H, Fritsch P. Hautzart 1978;29:541–4.

Five patients treated with PUVA were symptom free after 2–6 weeks of therapy.

Long-term follow-up of photochemotherapy in pityriasis lichenoides. Boelen RE, Faber WR, Lambers JCCA, Cormane RH. Acta Dermatol 1982;62:442–4.

Three patients required, on average, 30 PUVA exposures to clear their disease. The total energy required was markedly varied. Two patients relapsed and required a further course.

Experience with UVB phototherapy in children. Tay Y-K, Morelli JG, Weston WL. Pediatr Dermatol 1996;13:406–9.

As part of a wider open study of UVB phototherapy, three children with PLEVA were given broadband UVB three times a week for an average of 26 treatments. All had greater than 90% improvement in lesions in this time, though two relapsed after treatment was stopped.

Psoralens and ultraviolet A therapy of pityriasis lichenoides. Powell FC, Muller SA. J Am Acad Dermatol 1984;10:59–64.

Two females were treated with PUVA for longstanding PLEVA. Patient 1 needed 57 treatments over 12 months (total 370.5 J/cm²), and patient 2 required 26 treatments over 3 months (total 189 J/cm²), at which time 80% of lesions had cleared. Patient 2 relapsed after treatment was stopped.

Photochemotherapy for pityriasis lichenoides. Panse I, Bourrat E, Rybojad M, Morel P. Ann Dermatol Venereol 2004;131:201–3.

Two patients, aged 6 and 18 years, presented with a 1-month and 3-month history of PLEVA, respectively. They had received different treatments without significant effect: topical corticosteroids, antibiotic, UVB therapy, and dapsone. A combination of acitretin and PUVA was described as dramatically effective within a few weeks.

THIRD LINE THERAPIES

■ Methotrexate	D
■ Cyclosporine	E
■ Pentoxifylline	D
■ Dapsone	E
■ Systemic corticosteroids	E

Methotrexate for the treatment of Mucha-Habermann disease. Cornelison RL, Knox JM, Everett MA. Arch Dermatol 1972;106:507–8.

Five patients were given oral methotrexate 7.5–20 mg weekly. The authors report rapid clearance of the disease, but swift relapse upon stopping therapy.

Mucha Habermann's disease. Rasmussen JE. Arch Dermatol 1979;115:676–7.

Four adolescents with severe progressive scarring disease unresponsive to erythromycin, tetracycline, and prednisolone all responded to a short course of methotrexate 2.5 mg given every 12 h for three doses.

Zur Behandlung der Pityriasis lichenoides et varioliformis acuta mit Methotrexat. Schleicher H, Waldmann U, Knopf B. Dermatol Monatsschr 1975;161:148–52.

A 60-year-old woman responded to methotrexate 20 mg intravenously initially followed by 15 mg orally per week. She required a maintenance dose of 7.5 mg per week.

Successful long-term use of cyclosporin A in HIV-induced pityriasis lichenoides chronica. Griffiths JK. J Acquir Immune Defic Syndr 1998;18:396.

A 42-year-old woman with AIDS developed biopsy-proven PLC, which then developed into life-threatening, febrile, ulceronecrotic PLEVA. Treatment with cyclosporine 200 mg daily produced a rapid response, though prolonged maintenance treatment was required. Interestingly, the severity of symptoms appeared to parallel viral load.

Pentoxifylline (Trental) therapy for vasculitis of pityriasis lichenoides et varioliformis. Sauer GC. Arch Dermatol 1985;121:1487.

Two females with PLEVA, one extensive, responded to pentoxifylline. This was given at 400 mg twice daily for 2 weeks initially and increased to three times daily thereafter. Efficacy was similar to methotrexate 5 mg a week in one patient.

Febrile ulceronecrotic Mucha-Habermann's disease and its successful therapy with DDS. Nakamura S, Nishihara K, Nakayama K, Hoshi K. J Dermatol 1986;13:381–4.

Oral dapsone 75 mg daily for 20 days, 50 mg daily for 8 days, and 25 mg daily for 6 days produced a dramatic response within 3 days in a 21-year-old man with the ulceronecrotic febrile variant of PLEVA.

Febrile ulceronecrotic Mucha-Habermann's disease managed with methylprednisolone semipulse and subsequent methotrexate therapies. Ito N, Ohshima A, Hashizume H, et al. J Am Acad Dermatol 2003;49:1142–8.

A 12-year-old boy with abdominal pain, hypoprotein-emia, and anemia was successfully treated with methylprednisolone semipulse and subsequent methotrexate therapy.

Evidence levels   **A** Double-blind study   **B** Clinical trial ≥ 20 subjects   **C** Clinical trial < 20 subjects   **D** Series ≥ 5 subjects   **E** Anecdotal case reports

Pityriasis rosea

Anna E Muncaster

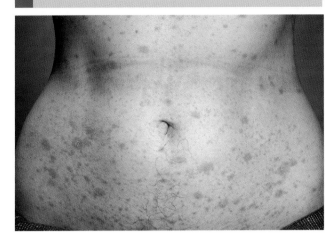

Pityriasis rosea is a common, self-limiting, papulosquamous disorder affecting the trunk and limbs, and usually seen in the 10–35-year age group. It has a classical clinical appearance, is usually asymptomatic, and is associated with little or no constitutional upset.

MANAGEMENT STRATEGY

Pityriasis rosea usually resolves spontaneously after approximately 6 weeks and, because it is commonly asymptomatic, *reassurance* is all that is required. An infectious etiology, most likely viral, is strongly favored, and although some studies have suggested an association with human herpesvirus-6 and -7, this has not been proven; therefore at present investigations are unnecessary. There have been case reports of pityriasis rosea-like eruptions after certain drugs such as captopril and ketotifen, but there is no evidence that pityriasis rosea is drug induced. For patients who do require treatment, usually because of itch or embarrassment over the appearance, *topical corticosteroids* are helpful in suppressing the inflammatory component of the disease, although evidence for these effects is purely anecdotal. *Emollients* and *oral antihistamines* have also been mentioned in the literature as being of some benefit. *UV light* has been mentioned several times in the literature over the past 30 years as being helpful, and studies have shown that UVB light treatment with consecutive daily erythemogenic doses can reduce itch and disease severity. The risk of postinflammatory hyperpigmentation may be increased by phototherapy. For patients with more extensive severe eruptions *oral prednisolone* can be tried because there are reports of improvement with 2–3 weeks of a reducing course of prednisolone. Oral corticosteroids should be used with caution, however, as there are also reports that they exacerbate the condition. More recently, a trial in India of *oral erythromycin* 250 mg four times daily for adults or 25–40 mg/kg in divided doses for children produced complete clearance after 2 weeks in the majority of patients. The best results with all these treatments have been obtained when treatment is started within the first 2 weeks of the appearance of the eruption. Since this trial there has been one case report of vesicular pityriasis rosea responding to 10 days of oral erythromycin at a dose of 250 mg four times daily. There has also been one case report of vesicular pityriasis rosea responding to *dapsone* therapy and a further report of clearance following a short course of oral *acyclovir* (aciclovir).

SPECIFIC INVESTIGATIONS

- In occasional cases mycological examination of scrapings may be helpful to exclude dermatophyte infection or tinea versicolor
- Syphilis serology is sometimes appropriate to exclude secondary syphilis

FIRST LINE THERAPIES

■ Topical corticosteroids	E
■ Emollients	E
■ Oral antihistamines	E

Pityriasis rosea update: 1986. Parsons JM. J Am Acad Dermatol 1986;15:159–67.

The author relates his own experience of using topical corticosteroids, emollients, and oral antihistamines in the treatment of pityriasis rosea. He claims all three treatments to have been of some benefit.

A comprehensive review article.

SECOND LINE THERAPIES

■ UVB	B

Treatment of pityriasis rosea with UV radiation. Arndt KA, Paul BS, Stern RS, Parrish JA. Arch Dermatol 1983;119:381–2.

Twenty patients with symptomatic and extensive pityriasis rosea were treated with UVB phototherapy in a bilateral comparison study using the left side of their body as a control. Five consecutive daily erythemogenic exposures resulted in both clinical and subjective improvement in disease severity and pruritus in 50% of the patients.

UVB phototherapy for pityriasis rosea: a bilateral comparison study. Leenitaphong V, Jiamton S. J Am Acad Dermatol 1995;33:996–9.

Seventeen patients with extensive pityriasis rosea were treated unilaterally with ten daily erythemogenic doses of UVB in a bilateral comparison study using 1 J of UVA to the other half of the body as a control. This resulted in a significant reduction in disease severity in 15 of the 17 patients, but no difference in pruritus.

UVB phototherapy for pityriasis rosea. Valkova S, Trashlieva M, Christova P. J Eur Acad Dermatol Venereol 2004;18:111–2.

In a letter to the editor the authors describe a study of 101 patients (including children) who received broadband UVB either to half the body (24 patients) using UVA on the other half as a control, or to the whole body (77 patients). They showed clearance of the disease in both groups, with those patients having more severe disease requiring significantly more treatments.

THIRD LINE THERAPIES

■ Oral prednisolone	D
■ Oral erythromycin	B
■ Oral acyclovir	E
■ Dapsone	E

One year review of pityriasis rosea at the National Skin Centre, Singapore. Tay YK, Goh CL. Ann Acad Med Singapore 1999;28:829–31.

In this retrospective case note study of 368 patients, 20 with extensive pruritic disease were treated with short reducing courses of prednisolone over 2–3 weeks with improvement.

Pityriasis rosea: exacerbation with corticosteroid treatment. Leonforte JF. Dermatologica 1981;163:480–1.

This was a case series of 18 patients, all of whom had received oral corticosteroids for pityriasis rosea. Five of these patients were observed while they received their corticosteroid course and the other 13 were seen after completing their corticosteroids. In those patients who did report an exacerbation, this was worse the higher the dose of corticosteroid received, the longer the course of treatment, and in those who were treated earlier in their disease.

Erythromycin in pityriasis rosea: a double-blind, placebo-controlled clinical trial. Sharma PK, Yadav TP, Gautam RK, et al. J Am Acad Dermatol 2000;42:241–4.

Ninety patients, including children, were randomly assigned to treatment or control group. Those in the treatment group received 2 weeks of oral erythromycin at doses of 250 mg four times daily for adults or 25–40 mg/kg daily in four divided doses for children. Of patients in the treatment group, 73% had a complete response, compared with none of the controls.

Vesicular pityriasis rosea: response to erythromycin treatment. Miranda SB, Lupi O, Lucas E. J Eur Acad Dermatol Venereol 2004;18:622–5.

A case report of a 32-year-old lady with a 6-week history of biopsy-proven vesicular pityriasis rosea achieved almost complete clearance after 10 days of oral erythromycin at a dose of 250 mg four times daily. No recurrence was observed during a 4-month follow-up period.

Antivirals for pityriasis rosea. Castanedo-Cazares JP, Lepe V, Moncada B. Photodermatol Photoimmunol Photomed 2004; 20:110.

In a letter to the editor the authors relate the successful treatment of a case of pityriasis rosea with a short course of oral acyclovir. Dosage and duration of treatment are not stated.

Dapsone treatment in a case of vesicular pityriasis rosea. Anderson CR. Lancet 1971;2:493.

A case report of a 55-year-old man with histologically proven pityriasis rosea resistant to oral prednisolone that responded to dapsone 100 mg twice daily for 1 month.

Evidence levels A Double-blind study B Clinical trial ≥ 20 subjects C Clinical trial < 20 subjects D Series ≥ 5 subjects E Anecdotal case reports

Pityriasis rubra pilaris

Anne-Marie Tobin, Brian Kirby

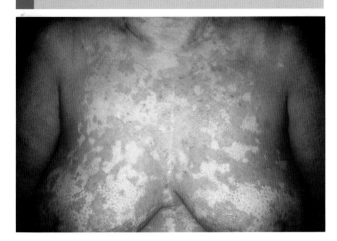

Pityriasis rubra pilaris (PRP) is an uncommon heterogeneous group of papulosquamous disorders. It is classified into six types and the adult classical type (type I) is characterized by the development of circumscribed follicular keratoses, palmoplantar keratoderma, and erythroderma. The onset is abrupt and characterized by the development of erythroderma in a craniocaudal direction within 2–3 months with characteristic islands of sparing of normal skin. It can occur from the first to the eighth decade. The etiology is unknown, but associations with viral infections, notably HIV, and internal malignancies have been reported.

MANAGEMENT STRATEGY

The treatment of PRP is difficult, but 80% of cases resolve spontaneously within 3 years. There are no randomized controlled trials in the literature and retrospective studies suggest that the response to most therapies is variable, reflecting the heterogeneous characteristics of this condition.

Patients with risk factors for the development of HIV infection should be tested for HIV antibodies. There are rare reports of internal malignancies occurring in conjunction with PRP. These reports are for multiple apparently unrelated malignancies and are inconsistent. We recommend that a routine physical examination, routine laboratory investigations, and a chest radiograph are performed at diagnosis, and that further investigations are only necessary if abnormalities are detected on history, physical examination, and the above noninvasive investigations.

In general, patients should be given topical therapy with *bland emollients* to treat the erythroderma. *Retinoids* are probably the most effective treatment for PRP: some series report up to 90% of patients responding. Etretinate (0.75–1.0 mg/ kg daily), isotretinoin (1.0–1.5 mg/kg daily), and acitretin (0.5–1.0 mg/kg daily) have all been reported as effective. Methotrexate (7.5–30 mg weekly) is also effective: one series reported clearance in 17 of 42 patients and another series reported clearance in six of eight patients. In general, the response to methotrexate takes approximately 6–8 weeks and full remission is seen in 3–4 months. The combination of methotrexate and acitretin may be effective in some patients who do not respond to conventional doses of either drug as monotherapy. Azathioprine has only been reported in two case series for PRP, but the response to treatment was excellent, with clearance achieved at doses of 150–200 mg daily. Some patients do not get any response to azathioprine in similar doses (B Kirby, personal communication). The response to cyclosporine appears to be quite variable. HIV-associated PRP may be cleared with antiretroviral therapy.

SPECIFIC INVESTIGATIONS

- Chest radiograph
- Hematology
- Routine biochemistry

FIRST LINE THERAPIES

■ Retinoids	D
■ Methotrexate	D

Pityriasis rubra pilaris: a review of diagnosis and treatment. Cohen PR, Prystowsky JH. J Am Acad Dermatol 1989;20:801–7.

Etretinate was reported as being effective in the majority of patients with PRP in a number of series. The usual dose used is 0.75–1.0 mg/kg daily, with dose tapering according to the response. The usual duration of therapy was 4 months; most studies report a favorable influence on course and prognosis.

Pityriasis rubra pilaris response to 13-cis-retinoic acid (isotretinoin). Goldsmith LA, Weinrich AE, Shupack J. J Am Acad Dermatol 1982;6:710–5.

Isotretinoin treatment of pityriasis rubra pilaris. Dicken CH. J Am Acad Dermatol 1987;16:297–301.

Isotretinoin was reported as effective in treating PRP for 60–95% of patients after 3–6 months of treatment. The combined number of patients treated in these studies was 50. The dosing schedules in these studies varied between 0.48 and 3.19 mg/kg daily, but the usual effective dose seems to be 1.0–1.5 mg/kg daily.

There are few reports in the literature on the use of acitretin in PRP, though this is often used for the condition. In case reports where its success has been reported it was used in combination with photo(chemo)therapy at a dose of 0.5 mg/kg daily.

Pityriasis rubra pilaris. Griffiths WAD. Clin Exp Dermatol 1980;5:105–12.

Methotrexate (7.5–25 mg weekly) was effective in some patients with PRP but, as with retinoids, the response is variable: only 17 of 42 patients in one series showed benefit. However, this retrospective report was based on patients who had received various doses of methotrexate and different dosing schedules.

Adult pityriasis rubra pilaris: a 10 year case series. Clayton BD, Jorizzo MD, Hitchcock MG, et al. J Am Acad Dermatol 1997;36:959–64.

In a case series of 22 patients, 11 received a combination of methotrexate and oral retinoid. Five of these had combination therapy because retinoid monotherapy failed to elicit significant improvement.

This combination may cause significant hepatotoxicity with two case reports of severe hepatitis in patients with psoriasis. Nonetheless, this combination has been used safely in a large number of patients with psoriasis.

SECOND LINE THERAPIES

■ Azathioprine	E
■ Antiretroviral therapy	D
■ Cyclosporine	E

Treatment of pityriasis rubra pilaris with azathioprine. Hunter GA, Forbes IJ. Br J Dermatol 1972;87:42–5.

Azathioprine was reported as effective in seven of eight patients by Griffiths and in four patients by Hunter and Forbes. The doses used were 50 mg three times daily and, in one case, 100 mg daily.

HIV-associated pityriasis rubra pilaris responsive to triple antiretroviral therapy. Gonzalez-Lopez A, Velasco E, Pozo T, Del Villar A. Br J Dermatol 1999;140:931–4.

PRP associated with HIV infection may respond to antiretroviral therapy.

There are case reports of HIV-associated PRP responding to zidovudine (AZT). Results with AZT therapy in non-HIV PRP have been disappointing. Similarly, HIV-associated PRP responds to triple antiretroviral therapy (zidovudine 250 mg 12-hourly, lamivudine 150 mg 12-hourly, and saquinavir 600 mg 8-hourly) and the response corresponds to the fall in HIV viral load.

Three cases of pityriasis rubra pilaris successfully treated with cyclosporin A. Usuki K, Sekiyama M, Shimada T, Kanzaki T. Dermatology 2000;200:324–7.

Cyclosporine at 5 mg/kg daily monotherapy was successful in patients with classical type I PRP. The response was sustained while therapy continued at a dose greater than 1.2 mg/kg daily.

Juvenile pityriasis rubra pilaris: successful treatment with ciclosporin. Wetzig T, Sticherling M. Br J Dermatol 2003;149: 202–3.

A single case report of effective therapy with cyclosporine in classical juvenile PRP.

THIRD LINE THERAPIES

■ Calcipotriol	E
■ Acitretin and narrowband UVB (TL-01)	E
■ Acitretin and UVA1	E
■ Extracorporeal photochemotherapy	E

Topical treatment of pityriasis rubra pilaris with calcipotriol. Van de Kerkhof PC, Steijlen PM. Br J Dermatol 1994;130:675–8.

Calcipotriol was reported as effective in a small series of three patients. Within this study two patients responded and one suffered irritation.

Pityriasis rubra pilaris treated with acitretin and narrow band ultraviolet B (Re-TL-01). Kirby B, Watson R. Br J Dermatol 2000;142:376–7.

Narrowband UVB therapy (TL-01) has been reported as effective when combined with retinoid (Re-TL-01) in a single case of classical juvenile PRP. This patient had not responded to broadband ultraviolet B and it is speculated that TL-01 may have different biological effects than either broadband UVB or photochemotherapy.

One further case of PRP treated with TL-01 has been reported, and this patient developed blisters in lesional skin.

Combined ultraviolet A1 radiation and acitretin therapy as a treatment option for pityriasis rubra pilaris. Herbst RA, Vogelbruch M, Ehnis A, et al. Br J Dermatol 2000;142: 574–5.

This was a single successful case report of long wave UVA (UVA1) in combination with acitretin in the treatment of classical PRP.

Extracorporeal photochemotherapy for the treatment of erythrodermic pityriasis rubra pilaris. Hofer A, Mullegger R, Kerl H, Wolf P. Arch Dermatol 1999;135:475–6.

This was a single report of the successful treatment of PRP with extracorporeal photochemotherapy.

Extracorporeal photochemotherapy for the treatment of exanthematic pityriasis rubra pilaris. Haenssle HA, Bertsch HP, Wolf C, Zutt M. Clin Exp Dermatol 2004;29:244–6.

This is again a single case report of extracorporeal photochemotherapy being effective in recalcitrant type II chronic adult PRP.

Polyarteritis nodosa

Jeffrey P Callen

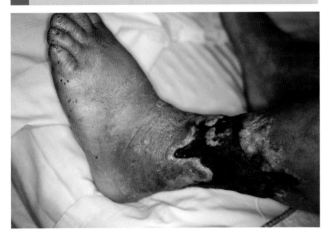

Polyarteritis nodosa (PAN) is a necrotizing vasculitis that involves small or medium-sized arterioles. Classic PAN is characterized by fever, weight loss, cutaneous ulcers, livedo reticularis, myalgias and weakness, arthralgias or arthritis, neuropathy, abdominal pain, ischemic bowel, testicular pain, hypertension, and renal failure. Microscopic polyarteritis (MPA) involves the same-sized vessels as well as smaller vessels and is clinically manifest as a glomerulonephritis and a pulmonary capillaritis with alveolar hemorrhage. Patients with MPA may develop small vessel vasculitis (palpable purpura), livedo reticularis with or without nodules, and/or ulcerations of the skin. Cutaneous PAN (cPAN), sometimes termed benign cutaneous polyarteritis, is characterized by livedo reticularis, nodules and ulceration, usually of the leg; it has been postulated to be a localized necrotizing arteritis that does not affect internal organs and runs a chronic, but benign course. Many reports, however, have linked cPAN to inflammatory bowel disease or hepatitis B or C infection. Occasional reports have linked cPAN to antiphospholipid antibodies, cryoproteins, or antineutrophil cytoplasmic antibodies. cPAN appears to be more prevalent in children. Although it is generally benign, there have been reports of associated neuropathy, as well as visceral involvement.

MANAGEMENT STRATEGY

cPAN causes pain and discomfort and may ulcerate, thus causing disability. These manifestations warrant therapy. Therapy may include local measures, such as *gradient pressure stockings*, or *systemic therapies, including systemic corticosteroids, methotrexate, azathioprine, pentoxifylline* and *intravenous immunoglobulin (IVIG)*. As there are few cases of this disease, most of the reports are anecdotes or small case series. There is no uniformly accepted approach to these patients.

SPECIFIC INVESTIGATIONS

- Skin biopsy
- Serology for hepatitis B and C, antineutrophil cytoplasmic antibody, antiphospholipid antibodies, and cryoproteins
- Assessment for systemic involvement
- Assessment for inflammatory bowel disease
- Assessment for drugs that have been linked to cPAN

Cutaneous periarteritis nodosa: a clinicopathological study of 79 cases. Daoud MS, Hutton KP, Gibson LE. Br J Dermatol 1997;136:706–13.

This retrospective analysis of 79 patients evaluated the clinical and histological features of cPAN and attempted to identify any clinical, pathological, and immunological differences that may distinguish those cases likely to have a prolonged course. Thirty nine patients had ulcers during the course of their illness. Women were affected more than men. Painful nodules on the lower extremities, with edema and swelling, were the most common clinical finding; 22% of patients had some evidence of neuropathy. Most of the laboratory findings were nonspecific. There was no evidence for hepatitis B infection in the 37 patients tested, and hepatitis C infection was present in only one of the 20 patients tested. Five patients had inflammatory bowel disease (four had Crohn's disease and one had ulcerative colitis). Ten patients had rheumatoid arthritis. Most patients (60%) had no associated medical condition. The disease course was prolonged, but benign, and systemic PAN did not develop in any patient. The ulcerative form of disease was more prolonged and frequently associated with neuropathy. Therapy was varied, and the patients with nonulcerative disease responded better than those with ulcers. Observations suggested that agents such as corticosteroids, azathioprine, pentoxifylline, and hydroxychloroquine were effective in individual patients.

This study highlights the associations that might occur in up to 40% of the patients, the fact that neuropathy is relatively common, and that the course and response to treatment are dependent on the presence of ulceration.

Cutaneous polyarteritis nodosa associated with Crohn's disease. Report and review of the literature. Gudbjornsson B, Hallgren R. J Rheumatol 1990;17: 386–90.

A single patient with cPAN developed gastrointestinal symptoms and was found to have Crohn's disease. Resected bowel did not reveal a vasculitis. Prior to the recognition of the bowel disease, her disease was controlled with corticosteroids and cyclophosphamide. Eventually, oral sulfasalazine was effective in controlling the bowel disease and the cPAN.

cPAN has been reported in conjunction with inflammatory bowel disease on numerous occasions. A careful focused history is the preferred method of evaluation. Radiologic or endoscopic studies are not generally necessary.

Cutaneous polyarteritis nodosa in a patient with ulcerative colitis. Volk DM, Owen LG. J Pediatr Gastroenterol Nutr 1986;5:970–2.

A child with cPAN and ulcerative colitis is reported.

Hepatitis C virus infection in cutaneous polyarteritis nodosa: a retrospective study of 16 cases. Soufir N, Descamps V, Crickx B, et al. Arch Dermatol 1999;135:1001–2.

These authors studied 16 patients with cPAN and found antibodies to hepatitis C in five. One patient was coinfected with HIV and one patient had evidence of a prior hepatitis B infection.

Hepatitis C serology should be performed in patients with cPAN. Livedo reticularis with cryoglobulinemia can be seen with hepatitis C infection.

Perinuclear antineutrophilic cytoplasmic antibody-positive cutaneous polyarteritis nodosa associated with minocycline therapy for acne vulgaris. Schaffer JV, Davidson DM, McNiff JM, Bolognia JL. J Am Acad Dermatol 2001;44:198–206

This is the first case linking cPAN to minocycline therapy.

Vasculitic conditions mimicking cPAN have been reported with isotretinoin and amphetamines

FIRST LINE THERAPIES

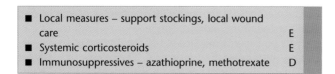

■ Local measures – support stockings, local wound care	E
■ Systemic corticosteroids	E
■ Immunosuppressives – azathioprine, methotrexate	D

Low-dose weekly methotrexate for unusual neutrophilic vascular reactions: cutaneous polyarteritis nodosa and Behçet's disease. Jorizzo JL, White WL, Wise CM, et al. J Am Acad Dermatol 1991;24:973–8.

These authors reported three patients with cPAN who responded dramatically to low-dose weekly methotrexate therapy.

SECOND LINE THERAPIES

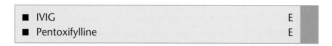

■ IVIG	E
■ Pentoxifylline	E

Intravenous immunoglobulin therapy in a child with cutaneous polyarteritis nodosa. Uziel Y, Silverman ED. Clin Exp Rheumatol 1998;16:187–9.

In this report a 9-year-old boy who developed cPAN was treated with high-dose IVIG, with an immediate favorable response.

Successful treatment of cutaneous PAN with pentoxifylline. Calderon MJ, Landa N, Aguirre A, Diaz-Perez JL. Br J Dermatol 1993;12:706–8.

A patient who failed to respond to aspirin and penicillin was treated with pentoxifylline. Withdrawal of the pentoxifylline resulted in a relapse that again responded to therapy.

THIRD LINE THERAPIES

■ Tamoxifen	E
■ Infliximab	E
■ Tonsillectomy	D

Estrogen-sensitive cutaneous polyarteritis nodosa: response to tamoxifen. Cvancara JL, Meffert JJ, Elston DM. J Am Acad Dermatol 1998;39:643–6.

Tamoxifen, an antiestrogenic agent, at a dose of 10–20 mg daily, led to control of disease in a patient that seemed to worsen with conjugated estrogen therapy. Relapse occurred within 5 days of interruption of the therapy and rapidly responded with re-initiation of the tamoxifen.

Successful response to infliximab in a patient with undifferentiated spondyloarthropathy coexisting with polyarteritis nodosa-like cutaneous vasculitis. Garcia-Porrua C, Gonzalez-Gay MA. Clin Exp Rheumatol 2003;21:S138.

This is a report of an observation in a single patient.

Cutaneous polyarteritis nodosa: therapy and clinical course in four cases. Misago N, Mochizuki Y, Sekiyama-Kodera H, et al. J Dermatol 2001;28:719–27.

In this report of four patients, two treated with tonsillectomy had resolution of their disease. The authors proposed that chronic streptococcal disease might be responsible for cPAN.

Polymorphic light eruption

Warwick L Morison

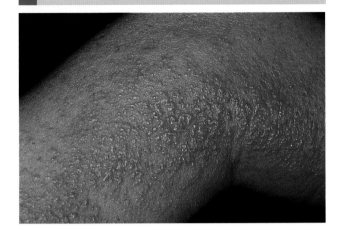

Polymorphic light eruption is the most common photodermatosis and develops hours to a day or more following specific exposure to sunlight. The morphology varies, a papular or papulovesicular form being most common, and plaques, insect-bite type, and erythema multiforme variants much less common. In most patients the tendency to develop polymorphic light eruption diminishes with repeated exposures to sunlight, a phenomenon called hardening.

MANAGEMENT STRATEGY

The treatment of polymorphic light eruption consists of two phases – treatment of established disease after the rash has appeared and second, prevention of the rash in patients known to have the disease. Application of a *mid-potency or high-potency corticosteroid cream or ointment*, two or three times daily, is usually sufficient to reduce symptoms and clear the rash in most patients with established disease. A few patients with extensive disease and marked symptoms require *oral prednisone* in a dose of 60–80 mg for a few days followed by rapid reduction of the dose over a week.

Preventive management is the best choice for patients diagnosed with the disease. The majority of patients with polymorphic light eruption have high-threshold disease so they require prolonged exposure to sunlight or artificial sources of UV radiation to trigger the reaction. Most of these individuals do not seek medical advice, but learn to limit their exposure to levels below their threshold or, in some cases, to prevent the disease by use of *sunscreens*. Patients seeking medical advice usually have low-threshold disease, often triggered by 15–30-minute exposures to sunlight, and this results in marked limitation of outdoor activities.

The initial approach to the prevention of polymorphic light eruption is *avoidance of exposure to sunlight* using a combination of reduction of time spent outdoors, restriction of exposure to early morning and late afternoon hours, wearing of protective clothing, and application of *broadband sunscreens* protecting against both UVA and UVB wavelengths. This strategy is most likely to be effective in patients with high-threshold disease and patients triggered by UVB radiation.

The most effective approach for patients with low-threshold disease is desensitization treatment using a course of *psoralen plus UVA (PUVA)*, *narrowband (311 nm) UVB phototherapy*, or *broadband UVB phototherapy* in spring, followed by regular exposures to sunlight during summer to maintain tolerance. This approach is successful in preventing polymorphic light eruption in up to 90% of patients, but it requires forward planning because treatment lasts for about a month. Patients who develop polymorphic light eruption while on treatment should continue therapy and may require topical or oral corticosteroids to control the rash.

Hydroxychloroquine, beta-carotene, and *nicotinamide* are reported to provide moderate and safe protection in polymorphic light eruption and may be considered in patients unable to undertake or unresponsive to desensitization therapy. Hydroxychloroquine is sometimes a useful preventive measure during a brief winter vacation in a warm climate. It should be started 3 days before the vacation in a dose of 400 mg daily and continued throughout the vacation.

SPECIFIC INVESTIGATIONS

- Skin biopsy
- Phototesting
- Lupus antibodies

Histopathologic findings in papulovesicular light eruption. Hood AF, Elpern DJ, Morison WL. J Cut Path 1986; 13:13–21.

The histologic pattern of this subgroup is characteristic, but not pathognomonic; there is little histologic similarity to lupus erythematosus.

Polymorphous light eruption. Holzle E, Plewig G, von Kries R, Lehmann P. J Invest Dermatol 1987;88:32s–8s.

The histologic patterns in less common subtypes are reviewed. Phototesting reproduced lesions in about 60% of patients and the action spectrum was confined to UVA in 75%, UVB in 10%, and 15% reacted to both wavebands.

Because 100% of patients have developed polymorphic light eruption from exposure to sunlight or an indoor source of UV radiation such as a suntan parlor, the most reliable method of reproducing the eruption is to request the patient to deliberately expose their skin to the source of light that produced their rash and return for inspection and biopsy of the rash.

The prevalence of antinuclear antibodies in patients with apparent polymorphic light eruption. Murphy GM, Hawk JLM. Br J Dermatol 1991;125:448–51.

Of 142 patients with a history consistent with polymorphic light eruption, 6% had a positive Ro antibody test or subsequently developed lupus erythematosus. A lupus package of tests is essential in patients being considered for active desensitization treatment.

FIRST LINE THERAPIES

Restriction of sun exposure	E
Sunscreens	B
Protective clothing	E

New broad-spectrum sunscreen for polymorphic light eruption. Proby M, Baker CS, Morton O, Hawk JLM. Lancet 1993;341:1347–8.

Application of a broad-spectrum sunscreen containing octyl methoxycinnamate, avobenzone and microfined titanium dioxide (SPF 30 for UVA and UVB) applied prior to sun exposure and repeated hourly and after swimming, provided complete protection in 27% of patients and partial protection in another 60% of patients. The sunscreen was cosmetically acceptable and there were no adverse reactions.

Textiles and sun protection. Robson J, Diffey BL. Photodermatol Photoimmunol Photomed 1990;7:32–4.

Transmission of UV radiation through clothing varies greatly, providing an 'SPF' in this study of 2 for a polyester blouse to 1571 for cotton denim jeans. The tightness of the weave is the main variable determining transmission of light. Transmission of UV radiation for all fabrics is increased when a fabric is wet.

Clothing and hats are now available specifically designed to provide protection from sunlight while maintaining a high level of comfort.

SECOND LINE THERAPIES

■ PUVA therapy	C
■ Narrowband (311 nm) phototherapy	C
■ Broadband UVB phototherapy	C

UVB phototherapy and photochemotherapy (PUVA) in the treatment of polymorphic light eruption and solar urticaria. Addo HA, Sharma SC. Br J Dermatol 1987;116: 539–47.

Patients were treated with a regular schedule of oral PUVA or high dose (erythemogenic) broadband UVB phototherapy three times weekly for 5 weeks during the spring and were then instructed to maximize their exposure to sunlight during summer; 90% of PUVA-treated patients and about 70% of UVB-treated patients were free of symptoms of polymorphic light eruption during the summer. Development of the eruption during the active treatment was common, usually mild, and did not interfere with treatment.

A comparison of narrowband (TL-01) and photochemotherapy (PUVA) in the management of polymorphic light eruption. Bilsland D, George SA, Gibbs NK, et al. Br J Dermatol 1993;129:708–12.

A regular schedule of oral PUVA therapy or narrowband (311 nm) phototherapy was given to patients three times a week for 5 weeks in the spring, resulting in about 85% of patients in each treatment group being adequately protected from developing polymorphic light eruption during the summer. The necessity for regular sun exposure every week during the summer may not have been emphasized.

THIRD LINE THERAPIES

■ Prednisolone	A
■ Hydroxychloroquine	A
■ Beta-carotene	C
■ Nicotinamide	B
■ Azathioprine	E
■ Cyclosporine	E

Efficacy of short-course oral prednisolone in polymorphic light eruption: a randomized controlled trial. Patel DC, Bellaney GJ, Seed PT, et al. Br J Dermatol 2000;143:828–31.

A 7-day course of 25 mg prednisolone daily was superior to placebo when started at the onset of the rash. This low dose of corticosteroid is suitable for managing patients who are on brief vacations in a sunny climate. Prednisone would be a suitable alternative medication.

Hydroxychloroquine in polymorphic light eruption: a controlled trial with drug and visual sensitivity monitoring. Murphy GM, Hawk JLM, Magnus IA. Br J Dermatol 1987;116:379–86.

Hydroxychloroquine in a dose of 400 mg, daily for 1 month and 200 mg daily for 2 months was superior to placebo in preventing development of rash, but almost all patients did have rash and irritation during the trial. The degree of protection was judged to be moderate and was related to serum level; the dose of 400 mg daily provided better protection. No visual toxicity was observed.

Comparison of PUVA and beta-carotene in the treatment of polymorphous light eruption. Parrish JA, Le Vine MJ, Morison WL, et al. Br J Dermatol 1979;100:187–91.

Beta-carotene (3.0 mg/kg) in a twice daily divided dose given for the entire summer provided full protection for 30% of patients and partial protection for another 20% of patients. There were no adverse effects.

Treatment of polymorphous light eruption with nicotinamide: a pilot study. Neumann R, Rappold E, Pohl-Markl H. Br J Dermatol 1986;115:77–80.

Nicotinamide given in a dose of 1 g orally three times daily starting 2 days before sun exposure provided complete protection in 60% of patients. The dose was reduced to 2 g daily after 1 week and about half of these patients developed polymorphic light eruption. A few patients had mild fatigue.

Successful treatment of severe polymorphous light eruption with azathioprine. Norris PG, Hawk JLM. Arch Dermatol 1989;125:1377–9.

Two patients with year-round photosensitivity triggered by as little as 1–2 min of sun exposure and unresponsive to all standard treatments were treated with 0.8–2.5 mg/kg of azathioprine daily for 3 months with complete remission of symptoms and normal sun tolerance.

The erythemal responses to UVB radiation were reduced in both patients and to UVA radiation in one patient, which is an unusual finding in typical cases of polymorphic light eruption.

Prophylactic short-term use of cyclosporin in refractory polymorphic light eruption. Lasa O, Trebol I, Gardeazabal J, Diaz-Perez JL. J Eur Acad Dermatol Venereol 2004;18: 747–8.

Cyclosporine in a dose of 3–4 mg/kg daily during 2 or 4 weeks was effective in preventing development of an eruption in three patients during a short vacation in a sunny climate. The patients had not responded to other preventive measures. No adverse effects were observed and this appears to have promise as a prophylactic treatment in patients resistant to other therapies.

Evidence levels **A** Double-blind study **B** Clinical trial ≥ 20 subjects **C** Clinical trial < 20 subjects **D** Series ≥ 5 subjects **E** Anecdotal case reports

Pompholyx

Anne E Burdick, Natalie N Ellis

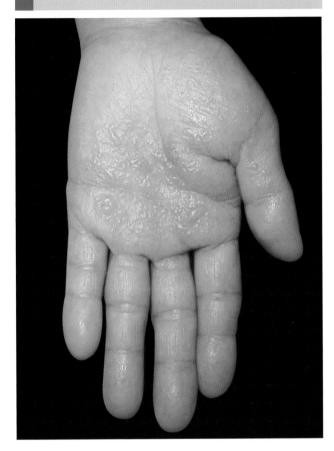

Pompholyx is a recurrent, pruritic, vesicular eruption of the palms, soles, and lateral aspects of the fingers. It is of unknown etiology. This condition is also known as dyshidrosis and dyshidrotic eczema. This cyclical eruption has been associated with atopy, hyperhidrosis, dermatophytosis, emotional stress, contact allergic dermatitis to nickel, and irritant dermatitis.

MANAGEMENT STRATEGY

Although pompholyx may resolve spontaneously, treatment is aimed at control of pruritus and vesicobullous formation. Evaluation is required to exclude dermatophytosis, pustular psoriasis, contact dermatitis, impetigo, herpes simplex, pemphigus vulgaris, and bullous pemphigoid.

For mild localized disease, *topical tacrolimus* once or twice daily alone and/or in combination with *mid- to high-potency corticosteroid creams or ointments* are recommended. *Antipruritic topicals containing pramoxine, camphor, phenol, and menthol* are useful for control of symptoms as are *oral antihistamines*. A course of *oral antibiotics* (cephalosporins or erythromycin) and *emollients* are also beneficial. Vesicles and bullae can be treated with *10% aluminum acetate compresses or soaks in a 1:10 000 solution of potassium permanganate*. Large bullae can be mechanically drained in a sterile manner, leaving the roof intact.

For severe disease, *systemic corticosteroids* are indicated: daily prednisone 0.5–1.0 mg/kg tapered over 2 weeks or intramuscular triamcinolone acetonide (40–60 mg). *Hand*

and foot UVA, with or without oral or topical psoralen, and also *UVA1* are other therapeutic options.

Refractory pompholyx can be treated with *intradermal botulinum toxin* and/or *immunosuppressives such as azathioprine, methotrexate, and cyclosporine*.

SPECIFIC INVESTIGATIONS

- Bacterial culture
- Patch testing for contact allergens
- Potassium hydroxide preparation

Role of contact allergens in pompholyx. Jain V, Passi S, Gupta S. J Dermatol 2004;31:188–93.

Patch testing with the Indian Standard Patch Test Battery was performed on 50 subjects, and 20 (40%) reacted to one or more allergens. Nickel sulfate was the most common offending allergen.

Relation between vesicular eruptions on the hands and tinea pedis, atopic dermatitis and nickel allergy. Bryld L, Agner T, Menne T. Acta Derm Venereol 2003;83:186–8.

A statistically significant risk for vesicular eruptions with tinea pedis was reported in three of 16 patients (19%).

FIRST LINE THERAPIES

■ Topical corticosteroids	A
■ Topical tacrolimus	C
■ Oral antibiotics	D
■ Oral antihistamines	E
■ Oral corticosteroids	D

Therapeutic options for chronic hand dermatitis. Warshaw EM. Dermatol Ther 2004;17:240–50.

A comprehensive review of current therapies.

Pharmacotherapy of pompholyx. Wollina U, Naser MB. Expert Opin Pharmacother 2004;5:1517–22.

A concise review of exacerbating factors, differential diagnosis, and treatments.

Topical tacrolimus (FK 506) and mometasone furoate in treatment of dyshidrotic palmar eczema: a randomized, observer-blinded trial. Schnopp C, Remling R, Mohrenschlager M, et al. J Am Acad Dermatol 2002;46:73–7.

Topical tacrolimus 0.1% ointment was as effective as 0.1% mometasone furoate ointment after 2 weeks, reducing the dyshidrotic and severity index (DASI) to approximately 50% in 16 patients with palmar vesicular pompholyx.

SECOND LINE THERAPIES

■ Psoralen and UVA (PUVA)	C
■ UVA	C
■ UVA1	A
■ Topical PUVA	C
■ Botulinum toxin	C

UVA1 irradiation is effective in chronic vesicular dyshidrotic hand eczema (letter). Schmit T, Abeck D,

Boeck K, et al. Acta Derm Venereol (Stockh) 1998;78: 318–9.

Anecdotal reports of UVA1 efficacy.

A double-blind placebo-controlled trial of UVA-1 in the treatment of dyshidrotic eczema. Polderman M, Govaert J, le Cessie S, Pavel S. Clin Exp Derm 2003;28:584–7.

Twenty-eight patients were randomized to receive UVA1 irradiation (40 J/cm^2) or placebo, five times a week for 3 weeks. The treated patients had significant improvement both subjectively and objectively.

Treatment of recalcitrant dermatosis of the palms and soles with PUVA-bath versus PUVA-cream therapy. Grundmann-Kollmann M, Behrens S, Ru P, Kerscher M. Photodermatol Photoimmunol Photomed 1999;15:87–9.

PUVA-cream therapy was as effective as PUVA-bath therapy in 12 patients.

Treatment of dyshidrotic hand dermatitis with intradermal botulinum toxin. Swartling C, Naver H, Lindberg M, Anveden I. J Am Acad Dermatol 2002;48:667–71.

Ten patients with bilateral vesicular hand dermatitis were injected with 20 µl of Botox® 100 U/mL intradermally on the volar palms and fingers of one hand. Compared to their untreated hand, seven of the 10 patients experienced good or very good results.

THIRD LINE THERAPIES

■ Cyclosporine	E
■ Methotrexate	D
■ Azathioprine	C
■ Mycophenolate mofetil	E
■ Iontophoresis	B

Cyclosporin A responsive chronic severe vesicular hand eczema. Sand Petersen C, Menne T. Acta Derm Venereol (Stockh) 1992;72:436–7.

One patient with refractory pompholyx had marked improvement within 2 weeks on 5 mg/kg cyclosporine daily and maintained good control when tapered to 2.5 mg daily.

Low-dose oral methotrexate treatment for recalcitrant palmoplantar pompholyx. Egan CA, Rallis TM, Meadows KP, Krueger GG. J Am Acad Dermatol 1999;40:612–4.

In five patients with severe pompholyx 12.5–22.5 mg of methotrexate weekly resulted in a decreased dose or discontinuation of prednisone. Superpotent corticosteroids were continued topically.

Azathioprine in dermatological practice. An overview with special emphasis of its use in non-bullous inflammatory dermatoses. Scerri L. Adv Exp Med Biol 1999;455:343–8.

Six patients with severe pompholyx received azathioprine 100–150 mg initially and 50–100 mg daily for maintenance after resolution as monotherapy; three had excellent, one had good, and two had fair responses.

Dyshidrotic eczema treated with mycophenolate mofetil. Pickenacker A, Luger TA, Schwarz T. Arch Dermatol 1998;134:378–9.

Complete clearing occurred in a resistant case after 4 weeks of 1.5 g twice daily and was maintained on 1 g daily.

Successful treatment of dyshidrotic hand eczema using tap water iontophoresis with pulsed direct current. Odia S, Vocks E, Rakoski J, Ring J. Acta Derm Venereol 1996;76: 472–4.

Twenty patients with bilateral mild to moderate palmar pompholyx received 20 high-frequency phase 9 V direct current/9.8 kHz frequency treatments, each for 15 min, within 3 weeks to one hand and a topical nonsteroidal tar and zinc oxide paste to both palms. All patients showed significantly less itching and vesicle formation, with no change in erythema or desquamation.

Evidence levels **A** Double-blind study **B** Clinical trial ≥ 20 subjects **C** Clinical trial < 20 subjects **D** Series ≥ 5 subjects **E** Anecdotal case reports

Porokeratoses

Sandra M Winhoven, Monica Bhushan

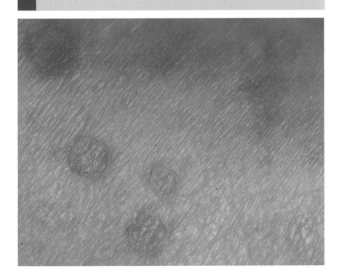

The porokeratoses are disorders of keratinization, histologically characterized by the cornoid lamella. Four clinical variants are recognized: classic porokeratosis of Mibelli (PM); disseminated superficial (actinic) porokeratosis (DSP/DSAP); porokeratosis palmaris et plantaris disseminata (PPPD); and linear porokeratosis (LP). Porokeratoses are believed to be genodermatoses and an autosomal dominant mode of inheritance with reduced penetrance has been established for familial cases. Porokeratotic lesions are usually progressive in nature and there is a risk of malignant transformation, in particular with large, longstanding plaques and the linear variants.

MANAGEMENT STRATEGY

A family history should be obtained. Patients' immune function should be assessed, particularly with the disseminated forms. Discontinuation of immunosuppression has led to resolution of lesions in some patients.

Treatment of porokeratoses may be indicated, not only for cosmetic benefit and symptomatic relief, but also for cancer prevention. It is dependent on the type and extent of porokeratosis. Management should also involve avoidance of irradiation (UV or X-rays) and observation for signs of malignant transformation (squamous cell carcinoma, basal cell carcinoma, Bowen's disease).

The lesions are usually asymptomatic, though pruritus associated with disseminated lesions is often responsive to *topical corticosteroids*. The palmar–plantar variant may cause functional disability due to pain and discomfort.

Localized disease might respond to surgical methods such as *cryotherapy, laser,* or *excision,* but these methods can result in significant scarring. *Topical 5-fluorouracil* may be equally effective and produce less scarring, though a brisk accompanying dermatitis appears to be necessary for efficacy. It might be more efficacious if used under occlusion.

Systemic retinoids have been effective in localized and systemic disease, but there have been reports of exacerbation of pre-existing lesions. Recurrence is common on discontinuation of therapy and a long-term maintenance dose may

be required. This might also reduce the malignant transformation risk.

There are anecdotal reports of the effectiveness of *imiquimod, Vitamin D3 analogues, topical retinoids, dermabrasion, pulsed dye laser, Nd:YAG laser, corticosteroids,* and *Grenz rays.*

Treatment with topical photodynamic therapy in disseminated superficial actinic porokeratosis has been disappointing.

SPECIFIC INVESTIGATIONS

- ■ Skin biopsy
- ■ Dermoscopy
- ■ Assessment for immune function

Porokeratosis of Mibelli. Overview and review of the literature. Schamroth JM, Zlotogorski A, Gilead L. Acta Derm Venereol 1997;77:207–13.

The pathological hallmark of porokeratosis is the cornoid lamella, which is typically found at the border of the lesion. The cornoid lamella forms a column of parakeratosis extending through the orthokeratotic stratum corneum. The granular layer beneath the cornoid lamella is usually absent or markedly reduced in thickness. Dyskeratotic and vacuolated cells are often seen in the spinous layer beneath the cornoid lamella. An inflammatory infiltrate is seen in the dermis.

A good review article.

Gene expression profiling of porokeratosis demonstrates similarities with psoriasis. Hivnor C, Williams N, Singh F, et al. J Cutan Pathol 2004;31:657–64.

The gene expression profile of a cornoid lamella was similar to those found in psoriasis.

This study supports the hypothesis that porokeratosis is a disorder of hyperproliferative keratinocytes exhibiting similarity to psoriasis at a molecular level. Consequently, some therapeutic maneuvers valuable in psoriasis may be beneficial in porokeratotic lesions.

Dermoscopy of disseminated superficial actinic porokeratosis. Zaballos P, Puig S, Malvehy J. Arch Dermatol 2004;140:1410.

Dermoscopy for the diagnosis of porokeratosis. Delfino M, Argenziano G, Nino M. J Eur Acad Dermatol Venereol 2004;18:194–5.

Dermoscopic examination of DSAP showed a characteristic central scar-like area with a single or double 'white track' structure at the margin. The histopathologic correlate of the linear structure was shown to be the cornoid lamella.

FIRST LINE THERAPIES

■ Cryotherapy	D
■ 5-fluorouracil	D

Porokeratosis of Mibelli: successful treatment with cryosurgery. Dereli T, Ozyurt S, Osturk G. J Dermatol 2004;31:223–7.

Eight patients with 20 lesions received treatment with 30-second cycles of cryospray followed by sharp dissection of the lesion border. Most lesions resolved after one treatment; two required one further treatment.

Linear porokeratosis of Mibelli: successful treatment with cryotherapy. Bhushan M, Craven NM, Beck MH, Chalmers RJ. Br J Dermatol 1999;141:389.

A patient with LP was treated on a 6 monthly basis at first and then yearly over a period of 6 years with 20-second freeze–thaw cycles. Treatment resulted in atrophic scarring, but overall a favorable cosmetic improvement, which has been sustained for 2 years.

Cryosurgery of porokeratosis plantaris discreta. Limmer BL. Arch Dermatol 1979;115:582–3.

Twenty one lesions of porokeratosis in 11 patients were treated, resulting in a cure rate of 90.5%. The lesions were pared prior to treatment with cryospray. There was no evidence of recurrence over an average follow-up period of 22 months.

Disseminated superficial porokeratosis: rapid therapeutic response to 5-fluorouracil. Shelley WB, Shelley ED. Cutis 1983;32:139–40.

Resolution of porokeratosis was observed after 3 weeks of daily application of 5% 5-fluorouracil cream. There was no recurrence at 5-month follow-up.

Fluorouracil ointment treatment of porokeratosis of Mibelli. Goncalves JC. Arch Dermatol 1973;108:131–2.

Six patients with facial lesions were treated with 5% fluorouracil ointment three times daily. The treatment was maintained for 8–10 days after a strong inflammatory response occurred. There was no recurrence at 9-month follow-up.

SECOND LINE THERAPIES

■ Systemic retinoids	D
■ CO_2 laser	D

Generalized linear porokeratosis treated with etretinate. Goldman GD, Milstone LM. Arch Dermatol 1995;131:496–7.

A patient with LP on 50–75 mg etretinate daily showed significant improvement within 4 weeks of treatment. Histology at 4 months demonstrated elimination of the cornoid lamella.

Porokeratosis plantaris, palmaris et disseminata. Marschalko M, Somlai B. Arch Dermatol 1986;122:890–1.

A case of familial PPPD was successfully treated with 25–50 mg daily of etretinate. Marked improvement was noted after 3 weeks of treatment.

Etretinate in the treatment of disseminated porokeratosis of Mibelli. Hacham-Zadeh S, Holubar K. Int J Dermatol 1985;24:258–60.

A 30-year-old man with DSP received 50–75 mg of etretinate daily with significant clinical improvement after 2 weeks of treatment.

Etretinate improves localized porokeratosis of Mibelli. Campbell JP, Voorhees JJ. Int J Dermatol 1985;24:261–3.

A patient received etretinate 0.6–1 mg/kg daily for treatment of her psoriasis, resulting in resolution of a single plaque of porokeratosis on her thigh. The lesion continued to resolve after discontinuation of therapy, probably due to the half-life of etretinate. No recurrence was seen at 17 months follow-up.

Disseminated porokeratosis Mibelli treated with RO 10-9359. Bundino S, Zina AM. Dermatologica 1980;160:328–36.

Two patients with DSP were treated with 50–75 mg daily of RO 10-9359 with significant clinical improvement after 5 weeks; 25 mg daily was sufficient to maintain the results. Recurrence was observed 3–4 weeks after cessation of treatment.

Treatment of disseminated superficial actinic porokeratosis with a new aromatic retinoid (Ro 10-9359). Kariniemi A, Stubb S, Lassus A. Br J Dermatol 1980;102:213–4.

Treatment with 50–100 mg daily of Ro 10-9359 led to significant clinical improvement and resolution of pruritus within 40 days of treatment. A dose of 25 mg on alternate days was required to maintain the results. After 6 months of treatment the patient developed follicular hyperkeratosis with tiny keratin horns on the skin of both forearms.

Porokeratosis plantaris, palmaris, et disseminata. Report of a case and treatment with isotretinoin. McCallister RE, Estes SA, Yarbrough CL. J Am Acad Dermatol 1985;13: 598–603.

A patient with familial PPPD received treatment with 1 mg/kg daily of isotretinoin. Significant clinical improvement was noted after 3 months of treatment. Two months after discontinuation of treatment a gradual recurrence was observed.

Treatment of porokeratosis of Mibelli with CO_2 laser vaporization versus surgical excision with split-thickness skin graft. Rabbin PE, Baldwin HE. J Dermatol Surg Oncol 1993;19:199–202.

CO_2 vaporization resulted in better cosmetic and functional improvement compared with split skin graft in one patient.

Reticulate porokeratosis – successful treatment with CO_2-laser vaporization. Merkle T, Hohenleutner U, Braun-Falco O, Landthaler M. Clin Exp Dermatol 1992;17:178–81.

CO_2 laser vaporization of mainly flexural lesions resulted in regression of lesions with slight atrophic scarring and lessening of pruritus. No further treatment was required in a 12-month follow-up period.

Linear porokeratosis: treatment with the carbon dioxide laser. Barnett JH. J Am Acad Dermatol 1986;14:902–4.

First reported case of successful treatment of a patient with LP with CO_2 laser. There was no recurrence at 6-month follow-up.

THIRD LINE THERAPIES

■ Imiquimod	E
■ Vitamin D3 analogues	E
■ Topical retinoids	E
■ Dermabrasion	E
■ Nd:YAG laser	E
■ Corticosteroids	E
■ Grenz ray	E

Evidence levels A Double-blind study **B** Clinical trial ≥ 20 subjects **C** Clinical trial < 20 subjects **D** Series ≥ 5 subjects **E** Anecdotal case reports

Porokeratosis of Mibelli: successful treatment with topical 5% imiquimod cream. Harrison S, Sinclair R. Australas J Dermatol 2003;44:281–3.

Clinical and histological clearance of a large porokeratosis of Mibelli on the shin was achieved with 6 weeks of three times a week application of 5% imiquimod cream without occlusion. A marked inflammatory response was observed. There was no recurrence at 24 months.

Porokeratosis of Mibelli: successful treatment with 5% imiquimod cream. Agarwal S, Berth-Jones J. Br J Dermatol 2002;146:338–9.

A 3-cm lesion of PM on the leg was initially treated with topical imiquimod 5% cream five times a week for 3 months with no improvement. Subsequent treatment with imiquimod 5% cream five times a week under occlusion with an adhesive polythene dressing was successful. There was no recurrence at 1 year.

Disseminated superficial actinic porokeratosis: treatment with topical tacalcitol. Bohm M, Luger TA, Bonsmann G. J Am Acad Dermatol 1999;40:479–80.

DSAP responded to 5 months of topical daily treatment with 0.0004% tacalcitol and remained clear on alternate day maintenance therapy.

Disseminated superficial actinic porokeratosis responding to calcipotriol. Harrison PV, Stollery N. Clin Exp Dermatol 1994;19:95.

Three patients were treated with topical calcipotriol daily for 6–8 weeks. An overall improvement of 50–75% was noted and maintained for up to 6 months in two patients.

Topical tretinoin in Indian male with zosteriform porokeratosis. Agrawal SK, Gandhi V, Madan V, Bhattacharya SN. Int J Dermatol 2003;42:919–20.

Once daily application of topical tretinoin 0.1% gel led to resolution of lesions within 4 months.

Successful treatment of porokeratosis of Mibelli with diamond fraise dermabrasion. Spencer JM, Katz BE. Arch Dermatol 1992;128:1187–8.

No recurrence observed at 15-month follow-up, but the lesion healed with slight hyperpigmentation and mild hypertrophy in a 79-year-old Filipino woman.

Linear porokeratosis: successful treatment with diamond fraise dermabrasion. Cohen PR, Held JL, Katz BE. J Am Acad Dermatol 1990;23:975–7.

Excellent cosmetic result. No recurrence or scarring were observed after 8 months.

Treatment of lichen amyloidosis (LA) and disseminated superficial porokeratosis (DSP) with frequency-doubled Q-switched Nd:YAG laser. Liu HT. Dermatol Surg 2000;26:958–62.

A patient's face and arms were treated four times, 1 month apart, resulting in marked improvement, but not complete clearance of the lesions.

Dexamethasone pulse treatment in disseminated porokeratosis of Mibelli. Verma KK, Singh OP. J Dermatol Sci 1994;7:71–2.

A familial case of progressive porokeratosis received pulses of 100 mg dexamethasone in 5% dextrose intravenously on three consecutive days in a month. No new lesions appeared after the first pulse and clinical improvement was noted after four pulses. There was an 80% improvement after 18 pulses. The patient was then lost to follow-up.

Bullous and pruritic variant of disseminated superficial actinic porokeratosis: successful treatment with grenz rays. Ricci C, Rosset A, Panizzon RG. Dermatology 1999;199:328–31.

Good response to grenz ray treatment, 2 Gy once a day for 5 days. Grenz ray therapy has a low carcinogenic risk, but needs to be used with caution in a condition with a potential for malignant transformation.

Porphyria cutanea tarda

Maureen B Poh-Fitzpatrick

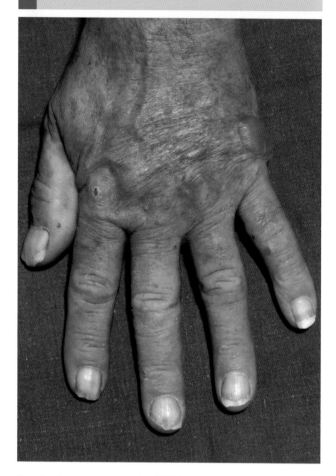

Porphyria cutanea tarda (PCT) is a term encompassing several related inherited or acquired disorders caused by reduced hepatic uroporphyrinogen decarboxylase enzyme activity. The resulting excess porphyrins mediate cutaneous photosensitivity, manifested as fragility, bullae, hypertrichosis, dyspigmentation, sclerodermoid features, and scarring. Multiple factors may contribute to disease expression: mutant uroporphyrinogen decarboxylase or hemochromatosis genes, other predisposing genetic determinants, ethanol, estrogen, iron, hepatitis or human immunodeficiency viruses, hepatotoxic aromatic hydrocarbons and, rarely, hepatic tumors.

MANAGEMENT STRATEGY

Optimal management consists of induction of remissions using strategies that are inappropriate for other porphyrias or pseudoporphyrias, so accurate diagnosis is essential. Associated disorders that may influence management, such as viral infections, hemochromatosis or other causes of excess iron storage, lupus erythematosus, diabetes mellitus, and anemias should be identified.

Eliminating exacerbating factors and pursuing ferrodepletion by *serial phlebotomy, deferoxamine (desferrioxamine) chelation,* or *erythropoietin bone marrow stimulation* can induce biochemical and clinical remissions. Skin should be protected from sunlight exposure and mechanical trauma until full clinical remission is achieved. Porphyrin excretion can be increased using *chloroquine* or *hydroxychloroquine, enteric sorbents,* or *metabolic alkalinization. Interferon-alfa* or *antiretroviral drugs* may benefit PCT associated with hepatitis C or AIDS, respectively. Children can be treated by phlebotomy protocols adjusted for pediatric parameters. Rare reports of chloroquine or hydroxychloroquine treatment of children suggest that cautious low-dose schedules may be safe and effective. *Vitamins E and C, plasmapheresis or plasma exchange, high-flux hemodialysis,* and *cimetidine* have been reported as beneficial alternative or adjunctive therapies. Hepatoerythropoietic porphyria, caused by two mutant genes for uroporphyrinogen decarboxylase in the same individual, resists induction of remission, and requires life-long vigilant skin photoprotection. *Photothermolysis* using selected wavelengths may reduce persistent hypertrichosis.

SPECIFIC INVESTIGATIONS

- Porphyrin concentrations and types in erythrocytes, serum or urine, feces
- Hematological and iron profiles, serum ferritin, hemochromatosis gene analysis
- Liver function profile, liver imaging, liver biopsy if clinically indicated
- Hepatitis A, B, and C viral serology
- HIV serology if risk factors are present
- Fasting blood glucose
- Serum antinuclear antibody

Porphyria cutanea tarda: clinical features and laboratory findings in forty patients. Grossman ME, Bickers DR, Poh-Fitzpatrick MB, et al. Am J Med 1979;67:277–86.

Abnormalities of liver function, glucose tolerance, antinuclear antibody titers, other laboratory parameters, clinical manifestations, skin and liver histopathology, and experience with phlebotomy are surveyed in a large population.

Porphyria cutanea tarda, hepatitis C, and HFE gene mutations in North America. Bonkovsky HL, Poh-Fitzpatrick MB, Pimstone N, et al. Hepatology 1998;27:1661–9.

Of 70 American patients with PCT 53% had evidence of hepatitis C infection, and 43% of 26 patients had HFE gene mutations associated with hereditary hemochromatosis.

Iron overload in porphyria cutanea tarda. Sampietro M, Fiorelli G, Fargion S. Haematologica 1999;84:248–53.

Most patients with PCT have some degree of iron overload, and ferrodepletion leads to remission. Hemochromatosis genes, present in large fractions of various populations, may inhibit uroporphyrinogen decarboxylase directly, or may interact with other genetic or acquired factors that can alter hepatocyte iron homeostasis.

Excess iron may facilitate inhibition of uroporphyrinogen decarboxylase activity and enhanced oxidation of uroporphyrinogen to photoactive uroporphyrin.

FIRST LINE THERAPIES

■ Serial phlebotomies	B
■ Chloroquine, hydroxychloroquine	B

Evidence levels **A** Double-blind study **B** Clinical trial ≥ 20 subjects **C** Clinical trial < 20 subjects **D** Series ≥ 5 subjects **E** Anecdotal case reports

The effect of phlebotomy therapy in porphyria cutanea tarda. Ippen H. Semin Hematol 1977;14:253–9.

Repeated venesection led to reduction of porphyrins and serum iron, improvement of photocutaneous lesions, and normalization of liver function tests in the majority of 351 patients.

Phlebotomy schedules should be adjusted to the tolerance of individual patients, typically ranging from 200 to 500 mL of whole blood at twice-weekly to biweekly or monthly intervals. Keeping hemoglobin over 10–11 g/dL minimizes symptoms of iatrogenic anemia.

Childhood-onset familial porphyria cutanea tarda: effects of therapeutic phlebotomy. Poh-Fitzpatrick MB, Honig PJ, Kim HC, Sassa S. J Am Acad Dermatol 1992;27:896–900.

Phlebotomy guidelines for children are described.

Plasma ferritin levels as a guide to the treatment of porphyria cutanea tarda by venesection. Ratnaike S, Blake D, Campbell D, et al. Australas J Dermatol 1988;29:3–8.

Phlebotomy can be terminated when iron stores, as reflected by plasma ferritin concentration, have fallen to low normal levels.

Reduction of porphyrins in plasma or serum or urine and clinical improvement typically begin during therapy and continue for weeks to months after venesection stops; patients should avoid sunlight and trauma after treatment until photosensitivity remits completely. Clinical improvement precedes full biochemical normalization.

Treatment of porphyria cutanea tarda with chloroquine. Korda V, Semrádová M. Br J Dermatol 1974;90:95–100.

Twenty one adults received oral chloroquine 125 mg twice a week until cutaneous blistering and fragility ceased and urinary uroporphyrins fell below three times the normal limit. Mean duration of treatment was 8.5 months (range 4–11 months) in 19 patients. Serum transaminases and urinary uroporphyrins rose during initial weeks of therapy, then progressively diminished.

Chloroquine risks include irreversible retinopathy after large cumulative doses (>100–300 g), but retinal toxicity is infrequent at dose rates less than 4 mg/kg daily (<6.5 mg/kg daily for hydroxychloroquine). Ophthalmologic examinations at baseline and 6-monthly intervals are recommended. The risk of hemolysis can be minimized by pretreatment testing for glucose-6-phosphate dehydrogenase deficiency and interval monitoring of hematological profiles during therapy.

Childhood-onset porphyria cutanea tarda: successful therapy with low-dose hydroxychloroquine (Plaquenil). Bruce AJ, Ahmed I. J Am Acad Dermatol 1998;38:810–4.

A 4-year-old child given hydroxychloroquine 3 mg/kg twice weekly for 14 months, plus vitamin E 200 U/day, achieved remission without adverse side effects.

Choice of therapy in porphyria cutanea tarda. Adjarov D, Naydenova E, Ivanov E, Ivanova A. Clin Exp Dermatol 1996;21:461–2.

Effectiveness of phlebotomy (500 mL weekly for 4 weeks then monthly) vs oral chloroquine 250 mg twice weekly alone vs combined phlebotomy/chloroquine therapies was retrospectively analyzed in unequal groups totaling 115 patients. Remissions occurred more quickly and reliably with phlebotomy than with chloroquine. Combined therapy shortened the mean total treatment course by approximately 1.5 months only when initial urinary uroporphyrin levels exceeded 3000 nmol/24 h.

Others found that remissions occurred more quickly with chloroquine vs venesection (10.2 months in 24 patients, 12.5 months in 15 patients, respectively), while combination therapy was most rapid (3.5 months in 20 patients) (Seubert et al. Z Hautkr 1990;65:223–5).

Hemochromatosis (HFE) gene mutations and response to chloroquine in porphyria cutanea tarda. Stolzel U, Kostler E, Schuppan D, et al. Arch Dermatol 2003;139:379–80.

Chloroquine was effective in heterozygotes with one, or compound heterozygotes with two, of the major HFE mutations (C282Y, H63D), but C282Y homozygotes failed to improve, and serum iron decreased only in patients with PCT and wild-type HFE. Phlebotomy is the recommended therapy for patients with PCT and HFE gene mutations.

SECOND LINE THERAPIES

■ Deferoxamine (desferrioxamine)	B
■ Erythropoietin	D

Liver iron overload and desferrioxamine treatment of porphyria cutanea tarda. Rocchi E, Cassanelli M, Borghi A, et al. Dermatologica 1991;182:27–31.

Ferrodepletion by desferrioxamine 1.5 g subcutaneous pump infusions 5 days/week (18 patients) or 200 mg/kg infused intravenously once weekly (five patients), or by serial phlebotomies (22 patients) led to clinical remissions after nearly 6 months with all treatments. Normalization of serum ferritin and uroporphyrins occurred at approximately 11 months with chelation, and approximately 13 months with venesection; liver function improved with both modalities.

Chelation is expensive and cumbersome, and thus best reserved for cases in which first line therapies are inadequate or inappropriate.

Haemodialysis-related porphyria cutanea tarda and treatment by recombinant human erythropoietin. Yaqoob M, Smyth J, Ahmad R, et al. Nephron 1992;60:418–31.

A patient receiving erythropoietin 50 U/kg thrice weekly over several months, without adjunctive phlebotomy, exhibited lowered serum ferritin and porphyrin levels and resolution of bullous dermatosis.

Erythropoiesis may be sufficiently stimulated in patients with pre-existing anemias to support serial phlebotomies at judicious volumes and intervals, thus accelerating ferrodepletion. Doses up to 150 U/kg three times weekly may be needed to gain this level of response.

Successful treatment of haemodialysis-related porphyria cutanea tarda with deferoxamine. Pitche P, Corrin E, Wolkenstein P, et al. Ann Dermatol Venereol 2003;130:37–9.

Intravenous deferoxamine 40 mg/kg weekly for 6 weeks led to normalization of clinical and biological signs of PCT in the setting of end-stage renal disease and chronic hemodialysis in one patient that persisted for 12 months.

This rapid and persistent improvement remains to be confirmed in larger trials.

THIRD LINE THERAPIES

■ Antiretroviral therapy	E
■ Interferon-alfa	E
■ Vitamins E and C	D
■ Plasmapheresis, plasma exchange	D
■ High-flux hemodialysis	D
■ Enteric sorbents (cholestyramine, activated charcoal)	D
■ Metabolic alkalinization by oral sodium bicarbonate	D
■ Cimetidine	E
■ Photothermolysis	E

Highly active antiretroviral therapy leading to resolution of porphyria cutanea tarda in a patient with AIDS and hepatitis C. Rich JD, Mylonakis E, Nossa R, Chapnick RM. Dig Dis Sci 1999;44:1034–7.

The association between PCT and HIV infection is less well established than the association of PCT with the hepatitis C virus. It is possible that the hepatitis C virus may trigger PCT in patients with HIV infection.

Dramatic resolution of skin lesions associated with porphyria cutanea tarda – interferon-alpha therapy in a case of chronic hepatitis C. Shiekh MY, Wright RA, Burruss JB. Dig Dis Sci 1998;43:529–33.

The mechanism by which the hepatitis C virus triggers the development of PCT is unknown.

High-dose vitamin E lowers urine porphyrin levels in patients affected by porphyria cutanea tarda. Pinelli A, Trivulzio S, Tomasoni L, et al. Pharmacol Res 2002;45:355–9.

Oral vitamin E (1 g daily) reduced urinary uroporphyrin levels and attenuated skin lesions during a 4-week trial.

Removal of plasma porphyrins with high-flux hemodialysis in porphyria cutanea tarda associated with end stage renal disease. Carson RW, Dunnigan EJ, DuBose TD Jr, et al. J Am Soc Nephrol 1992;2:1445–50.

High-flux hemodialysis may remove porphyrins more effectively than conventional hemodialysis.

Treatment of hemodialysis related porphyria cutanea tarda with plasma exchange. Disler P, Day R, Burman N, et al. Am J Med 1982;72:989–93.

This may aid patients with PCT and chronic renal failure for whom other treatments are unavailable.

The adsorption of porphyrins and porphyria precursors by sorbents: a potential therapy for the porphyrias. Tishler PV, Gordon RJ, O'Connor JA. Methods Find Exp Clin Pharmacol 1982;4:125–31.

Metabolic alkalinization therapy in porphyria cutanea tarda. Perry HO, Mullanax MG, Weigand SE. Arch Dermatol 1970;102:359–67.

Cimetidine in the treatment of porphyria cutanea tarda. Horie Y, Tanaka K, Okano J, et al. Intern Med 1996;35:717–9.

In this report, cimetidine decreased porphyrin levels within 2 weeks. This benign treatment may be of value in patients unwilling or unable to try standard therapeutic approaches.

Management of porphyria cutanea tarda in the setting of chronic renal failure – case report and review. Shieh S, Cohen JL, Lim HW. J Am Acad Dermatol 2000;42:645–52.

This survey of therapies applicable in the context of renal failure includes additional references for several third line agents listed above.

Successful and safe treatment of hypertrichosis by high-intensity pulses of noncoherent light in a patient with hepatoerythropoietic porphyria. Garcia-Bravo M, Lopez-Gomez S, Segurado-Rodriguez MA, et al. Arch Dermatol Res 2004;296:139–40.

Hypertrichosis was almost completely removed after seven sessions without development of skin lesions.

Evidence levels A Double-blind study   **B** Clinical trial ≥ 20 subjects   **C** Clinical trial < 20 subjects   **D** Series ≥ 5 subjects   **E** Anecdotal case reports

Port wine stains

Brandie J Roberts, Lawrence F Eichenfield

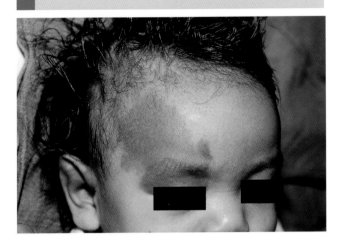

Port wine stains (PWS), are congenital benign capillary malformations of the superficial cutaneous vasculature. They usually present early in life as light pink to red patches that may darken and develop surface irregularities with time. The head and neck are sites of predilection, but any part of the integument can be affected. PWS are not only cosmetically distressing, but may be associated with serious physical, social, and psychological sequelae.

MANAGEMENT STRATEGY

Many therapeutic modalities have been used to treat PWS. Included are surgical excision and grafting, dermabrasion, cryotherapy, radiation therapy, electrotherapy, and tattooing. All have been associated with unfavorable outcomes. Various lasers have been used, including CO_2 laser, Nd:YAG laser, and copper vapor laser, but results have been unsatisfactory. Argon laser was considered at one stage as the best therapeutic method for PWS. However, hypertrophic scarring as a major complication of argon laser limited its use.

Flashlamp-pumped pulsed dye laser is considered by most authorities as the treatment of choice for PWS. Wavelengths of 585–595 nm and pulse durations of 450–1500 µs allow for a deep, safe, and specific action that is confined to the targeted vasculature. Lightening and/or decrease in size of PWS is directly related to the number of laser treatments. Initial treatments usually give the highest percentage of improvement.

Measures to overcome the laser-associated pain and anxiety include topical anesthetics such as a eutectic mixture of lidocaine and prilocaine, liposomal 4% lidocaine, S-Caine Peel®, local lidocaine infiltration, nerve block, and general anesthesia. New generations of flashlamp-pumped pulsed dye lasers with cooling devices markedly decrease the pain of laser procedures.

PWS can either occur as isolated findings or be associated with eye or central nervous system (CNS) structural abnormalities. They may also be associated with limb overgrowth (Klippel–Trenaunay syndrome), or with other vascular malformations (e.g. capillary–venous, capillary–venous–lymphatic, capillary–arteriovenous).

SPECIFIC INVESTIGATIONS

- Ophthalmologic examination
- CT or MRI

Facial port wine stain and Sturge–Weber syndrome. Enjolras O, Riche MC, Merland JJ. Pediatrics 1985;76:48–51.

Sturge–Weber syndrome (SWS) was present in 28.5% of patients with PWS covering the V1 trigeminal sensory area alone or in association with V2 and V3, while 9.5% had glaucoma. None of the patients with PWS located in the V2 and/or the V3 areas had ocular or pial vascular abnormalities.

Location of port wine stains and the likelihood of ophthalmic and/or central nervous system complications. Tallman B, Tan OT, Morelli JG, et al. Pediatrics 1991; 87:323–7.

Among patients with trigeminal PWS, 80% had evidence of eye and/or CNS involvement. PWS of the eyelids, bilateral distribution, and unilateral PWS involving all three branches of the trigeminal nerve were associated with a significantly higher likelihood of having eye and/or CNS complications.

Patients with such presentations should be screened for glaucoma, and the risk of CNS involvement should be discussed with the family and appropriate testing considered.

Sturge–Weber syndrome: age of onset of seizures and glaucoma and the prognosis for affected children. Sujansky E, Conradi S. J Child Neurol 1995;10:49–58.

In this study of 171 patients with SWS, seizures were present in 80% and were almost always associated with PWS in V1 alone or V1 and V2 trigeminal dermatomes. Glaucoma was present in 48% of patients; 92% of the patients with glaucoma had PWS in V1 and V2 areas whereas 8% had only V1 involvement. Glaucoma was diagnosed during the first year of life in 61% and by 5 years of age in 72%.

Children at risk of SWS should have ophthalmologic examination in the neonatal period and require ophthalmologic follow-up because glaucoma may develop subsequent to initial presentation.

Sturge-Weber syndrome. The current neuroradiologic data. Boukobza M, Enjolras O, Cambra M, Merland J. J Radiol 2000;81:765–71.

A neonatal neuroimaging work-up using CT or MRI may not demonstrate the pial anomaly and may be repeated after 6–12 months in an at-risk infant with V1 PWS.

FIRST LINE THERAPIES

■ Pulsed dye laser	B

Anatomic differences of port wine stains in response to treatment with pulsed dye laser. Renfro L, Geronemus RG. Arch Dermatol 1993;129:182–8.

Centrofacial lesions and lesions involving dermatome V2 responded less favorably than lesions located elsewhere on the head and neck.

Port wine stains. An assessment of 5 years of treatment. Orten SS, Waner M, Flock S, et al. Arch Otolaryngol Head Neck Surg 1996;122:1174–9.

Fewer treatments were required for nevus flammeus (NF), forehead and temple, lateral aspect of the face, neck, chest, and shoulder lesions. Lesions involving facial dermatomes, medial and central aspect of face, midline of the face (excluding NF), and the extremities required more treatments. Recurrence rate following completion of treatment was 3.1, 20.8, and 50% at 1, 2, and more than 3 years, respectively.

Facial port wine stains in childhood: prediction of the rate of improvement as a function of the age of the patient, size and location of the port wine stain and the number of treatments with the pulsed dye (585 nm) laser. Nguyen CM, Yohn JJ, Huff C, et al. Br J Dermatol 1998;138:821–5.

Major determinants of treatment response in order of decreasing importance are PWS location, size, and patient age. The most successful responses are seen in young patients (under 1 year of age) with small PWS (less than 20 cm^2) that are located over bony areas of the face such as the central forehead. The greatest percentage of decrease in size occurred after the first five treatments. There was less decrease in size with subsequent treatments.

Treatment of children with port wine stains using the flash lamp pulsed tunable dye laser. Tan OT, Sherwood K, Gilchrest BA. N Engl J Med 1989;320:416–21.

Children less than 7 years of age required fewer sessions than older children.

Flashlamp-pumped pulsed dye laser for port wine stains in infancy: earlier versus later treatment. Ashinoff R, Geronemus RG. J Am Acad Dermatol 1991;24:467–72.

A study of 12 children aged between 6 and 30 weeks that confirmed the safety of pulsed dye laser treatment in infants only a few weeks of age with accelerated response.

Treatment of port wine stains (capillary malformations) with the flash lamp pumped pulsed dye laser. Goldman MP, Fitzpatrick RE, Ruiz-Esparza J. J Pediatr 1993;122:71–7.

Clinical improvement correlated with number of treatments. Initial treatment in children with PWS results in approximately 40% improvement, and each subsequent treatment up to six treatments adds a further increment of 10% improvement. Treatments should be continued as long as there is incremental improvement.

Effect of the timing of treatment of port wine stains with the flash lamp pumped pulsed dye laser. Van der Horst CM, Koster PH, de Borgie CA, et al. N Engl J Med 1998;338:1028–33.

No difference in laser treatment outcome was noticed among different age groups. There were four age groups: 0–5 years, 6–11 years, 12–17 years, and 18–31 years.

Few patients under the age of 12 months were included in this study, making it difficult to compare with others.

High-fluence modified pulsed dye laser photocoagulation with dynamic cooling of port wine stains in infancy. Geronemus RG, Quintana AT, Lou WW, Kauvar AN. Arch Dermatol 2000;136:942–3.

Early intervention during infancy using a modified pulsed dye laser with a longer wavelength (595 nm), broader pulse width (1.5 ms), dynamic cooling spray, and high-energy fluences can result in lightening or clearing of PWS with minimal risk of adverse effects.

Pain relief measures and cooling devices

Effects of percutaneous local anaesthetics on pain reduction during pulse dye laser treatment of port wine stains. McCafferty DF, Woolfson AD, Handley J, Allen G. Br J Anaesth 1997;78:286–9.

Both EMLA® and 4% tetracaine gel were statistically superior to placebo in reducing pain caused by the laser treatment.

The S-Caine peel: a novel topical anesthetic for cutaneous laser surgery. Bryan HA, Alster TS. Dermatol Surg 2002;28:999–1003.

Patients who received S-Caine Peel® experienced significant reduction of pain vs placebo when treated with 595 nm pulsed dye laser. Application for 20 and 30 min were both as effective as 60 min.

Effect of the topical anesthetic EMLA on the efficacy of pulsed dye laser treatment of port wine stains. Ashinoff R, Geronemus RG. J Dermatol Surg Oncol 1990;16:1008–11.

Use of topical anesthetic creams or sedating agents has been shown not to interfere with laser therapy.

Cryogen spray cooling and higher fluence pulsed dye laser treatment improve port wine stain clearance while minimizing epidermal damage. Chang CJ, Nelson JS. Dermatol Surg 1999;25:767–72.

A retrospective study of 196 patients with head and neck PWS indicating the statistically significant advantage of using cryogen spray cooling device with pulsed dye laser by permitting higher light dosages and subsequent higher clearance rate without increasing rate of complications.

General anesthesia for pediatric dermatologic procedures: risks and complications. Cunningham BB, Gigler V, Wang K, et al. Arch Dermatol 2005;141:573–6.

Review of 881 cases performed on 269 pediatric patients, 88% of which were pulsed dye laser treatment of vascular lesions, including PWS. There were no life-threatening events and the mortality rate was zero.

The use of general anesthesia for dermatologic procedures performed in a children's hospital setting is safe with a low rate of complications.

SECOND LINE THERAPIES

■ Intense pulsed light source	B

Treatment of port wine stain with a non-coherent pulsed light source: a retrospective study. Raulin C, Schroeter CA, Weiss RA, et al. Arch Dermatol 1999;125:679–83.

Between 70 and 100% clearing of PWS in 28 of 40 patients treated by intense pulsed light source after an average number of 4.0 treatments for pink PWS (100% clearance), 1.5 for red PWS (100% clearance), and 4.2 for purple PWS (70–99% clearance).

Intense pulsed light source for the treatment of dye laser resistant port-wine stains. Bjerring P, Christiansen K, Troilius A. J Cosmet Laser Ther 2003;5:7–13.

Greater than 50% reduction was achieved after four treatments with intense pulsed light source in 46.7% of 15 patients with PWS previously treated by pulsed dye laser. None of the lesions located in V2 responded.

There are several case reports of successful treatment of resistant PWS with intense pulsed light source. However, controlled studies are needed to confirm this observation.

THIRD LINE THERAPIES

■ Potassium titanyl phosphate (KTP) laser	B

Potassium titanyl phosphate laser treatment of resistant port-wine stains. Chowdhury MU, Harris S, Lanigan SW. Br J Dermatol 2001;144:814–7.

Greater than 50% reduction was seen in 17% of 30 patients with PWS previously treated by pulsed dye laser; 20% of patients experienced side effects, including scarring or hyperpigmentation.

Treatment of PWS with KTP laser is advocated by some, though in studies it has shown limited utility and an increased incidence of scarring.

Pregnancy dermatoses

Wolfgang Jurecka

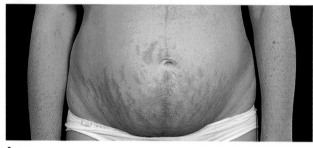

A

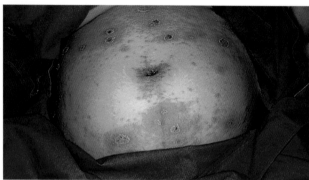

B

Skin changes during pregnancy may range from normal (physiologic) changes that occur with almost all pregnancies through common or pre-existing skin diseases that are not associated with, but influenced by the pregnancy, to eruptions that appear to be specifically associated with pregnancy and the puerperium. In recent years a group of three well-defined dermatoses of pregnancy has been generally accepted. These are: pruritic urticarial papules and plaques of pregnancy (PUPPP) (Figure A), pemphigoid gestationis (Figure B), and pruritus gravidarum (cholestasis of pregnancy).

Pruritic urticarial papules and plaques of pregnancy

Pruritic urticarial papules and plaques of pregnancy (PUPPP) is a common, intensely pruritic dermatosis that usually begins in the third trimester of the first pregnancy, but may be delayed until a few days postpartum (Figure A). It occasionally recurs, less severely, in subsequent pregnancies.

MANAGEMENT STRATEGY

Most women who have PUPPP are relieved to learn that the condition is not serious, that all should be well with them and their baby, and that the rash will disappear at or within a few days after childbirth. However, treatment is usually demanded to provide relief from the intense itching. The skin lesions may closely resemble the very early (urticarial) stage of pemphigoid gestationis. Direct and/or indirect immunofluorescence microscopy of perilesional skin or serum should be performed if pemphigoid gestationis is suspected. All similar eruptions that occur in nonpregnant women may also occur in pregnancy and should not be confused with those dermatoses that are pregnancy specific. Thus erythema multiforme, drug eruptions, contact dermatitis, urticaria, and insect bites should be excluded. In women with localized disease, intense (several times daily) application of *mid-strength or potent topical corticosteroids* provides symptomatic relief after a few days in almost all cases. *Ointments* containing substances such as *betamethasone, mometasone,* or *methylprednisolone* can be regarded as safe during pregnancy. New lesions usually stop appearing within 2 or 3 days and the frequency of applications can be tapered. As the pregnancy continues many patients require therapy only once a day or can even stop treatment before delivery. Topical antipruritic preparations are normally not useful. *Oral H1 antihistamines* may offer some benefit in severely pruritic patients, especially the older sedating antihistamines at bedtime. In more widespread or generalized cases and those which do not respond adequately to topical corticosteroids, a systemic corticosteroid treatment may need to be considered. *Oral methylprednisolone 20–40 mg daily* or its equivalent for 5 days, tapered over the following 2 weeks is very effective. For systemic treatment during pregnancy prednisone, prednisolone, and methylprednisolone are regarded as safer than betamethasone, dexamethasone, cortisone, and hydrocortisone, which may be associated with some risk of malformation.

One striking clinical feature of PUPPP is its onset in the third trimester in association with severe striae. It usually affects first pregnancies in which striae are more common. There have been conflicting reports questioning whether PUPPP is associated with fetal weight and maternal weight gain, resulting in excessive abdominal distention. Some patients have therefore been delivered early with the expectation that this will terminate the PUPPP. This has appeared to be the outcome in some cases, but the resolution of PUPPP is not necessarily related to delivery.

SPECIFIC INVESTIGATIONS

- ■ Biopsy for direct immunofluorescence
- ■ Serum for indirect immunofluorescence

A comparative study of toxic erythema of pregnancy and herpes gestationis. Holmes RC, Black MM, Dann J, et al. Br J Dermatol 1982;106: 499–510.

A comparison of 30 patients with PUPPP and 24 patients with pemphigoid gestationis showed a broad overlap in the morphology of their skin lesions, which may lead to difficulties in the diagnosis of early (urticarial) pemphigoid gestationis. Immunofluorescence is consistently positive in pemphigoid gestationis.

A comparative histopathological study of polymorphic eruption of pregnancy and herpes gestationis. Holmes RC, Jurecka W, Black MM. Clin Exp Dermatol 1983;8:523–9.

There was a broad overlap in the histopathologic changes of skin lesions in patients with PUPPP and pemphigoid gestationis, allowing a clear distinction only when pemphigoid gestationis appears with typical subepidermal blisters.

An immunoelectron microscopy study of the relationship between herpes gestationis and polymorphic eruption of pregnancy. Jurecka W, Holmes RC, Black MM, et al. Br J Dermatol 1983;108:147–51.

This highly sensitive method showed that PUPPP and pemphigoid gestationis are clear separate entities.

Pruritic urticarial papules and plaques of pregnancy: clinical and immunopathologic observations in 57 patients. Aronson IK, Bond S, Fiedler VC, et al. J Am Acad Dermatol 1998;39:933–9.

The clinical features in 57 patients with PUPPP were categorized in three types: (1) mainly urticarial papules and plaques; (2) nonurticarial erythema, papules, or vesicles; (3) a combination of both. Immunofluorescence was consistently negative.

FIRST LINE THERAPIES

■ Topical corticosteroids	B
■ Antihistamines	C

Pruritic urticarial papules and plaques of pregnancy. Clinical experience in twenty-five patients. Yancey KB, Hall RP, Lawley TJ. J Am Acad Dermatol 1984;10:473–80.

Of 25 patients 22 were successfully treated with frequent applications of high-potency topical corticosteroids, providing relief from the pruritus and controlling the eruption.

Pruritic urticarial papules and plaques of pregnancy (PUPPP). A clinicopathologic study. Callen JP, Hanno R. J Am Acad Dermatol 1981;5:401–5.

In 15 cases PUPPP cleared prior to delivery (five cases), within 1 week of delivery (nine cases), and at 6 weeks postpartum (one case). Treatment was performed with various potent topical corticosteroids and antihistamines, namely diphenhydramine in all cases except one. Two cases required additional treatment with hydroxyzine.

Pruritic urticarial papules and plaques of pregnancy. Ahmed AR, Kaplan R. J Am Acad Dermatol 1981;4:679–81.

Two patients were treated with topical corticosteroids and diphenhydramine with good results.

Dermatological therapy during pregnancy and lactation. Sasseville D. In: Harahap M, Wallach R, eds. Skin changes and diseases in pregnancy. New York: Marcel Dekker; 1996: 249–319.

First-generation H1 blockers (antihistamines) are grouped due to their chemical structure in six different classes. Chlorpenamine (chlorpheniramine), diphenhydramine, tripelenamine, cyclizine and meclizine, and cyproheptadine are considered safer for use in pregnancy than the others.

Treating allergic rhinitis in pregnancy. Safety considerations. Mazzotta P, Loebstein R, Koren G. Drug Saf 1999;20:361–75.

First generation (e.g. chlorpheniramine [chlorphenamine]) and second generation (e.g. cetirizine) antihistamines have not been incriminated as human teratogens. However, first generation antihistamines are favored over second generation based on their longevity, leading to more evidence of safety.

Pregnancy outcome after gestational exposure to terfenadine: a multicenter prospective controlled study. Loebstein R, Lalkin A, Addis A, et al. J Allergy Clin Immunol 1999;104:953–6.

One hundred and eighteen women were exposed to terfenadine during pregnancy. Among those exposed during the first trimester (n = 65), only birth weight of the newborns was significantly lower compared with a matched control group. All other parameters were comparable between the groups. On the basis of the limited sample size of this study, it appears that terfenadine is not associated with an increased incidence of malformations. However, further studies will be needed.

SECOND LINE THERAPIES

■ Systemic corticosteroids	D

Pruritic urticarial papules and plaques of pregnancy. Lawley TJ, Hertz KC, Wade TR, et al. JAMA 1979;241:1696–9.

Two of seven patients were treated with oral prednisone (30 mg twice daily and 40 mg daily respectively).

Pruritic urticarial papules and plaques of pregnancy. Clinical experience in twenty-five patients. Yancey KB, Hall RP, Lawley TJ. J Am Acad Dermatol 1984;10:473–80.

Systemic corticosteroids were efficacious in three patients with extensive disease.

Prurigo of late pregnancy. Cooper AJ, Fryer JA. Aust J Dermatol 1980;21:79–84.

Four of five patients were treated successfully with oral prednisone (20 mg daily, tapering by 5 mg every 2 days).

Pruritic urticarial papules and plaques of pregnancy (polymorphic eruption of pregnancy): two unusual cases. Vaughan Jones SA, Dunnill MG, Black MM. Br J Dermatol 1996;135:102–5.

One of two cases required a short course of systemic corticosteroids.

Although only a limited numbers of cases are reported in the literature describing treatment of severe cases of PUPPP with oral corticosteroids, nowadays it is generally accepted that this treatment is effective and safe if prednisone, prednisolone, or methylprednisolone are chosen. However, larger series and prospective studies are missing.

THIRD LINE THERAPIES

■ Early delivery	E

Severe polymorphic eruption of pregnancy occurring in twin pregnancies. Bunker CB, Erskine K, Rustin MHA, Gilkes JJH. Clin Exp Dermatol 1990;15:228–30.

Early delivery to terminate the PUPPP.

Pruritic urticarial papules and plaques of pregnancy: a severe case requiring early delivery for relief of symptoms. Baltrani VP, Baltrani VS. J Am Acad Dermatol 1992;26: 266–7.

Early delivery led to relief of symptoms.

Pruritic urticarial papules and plaques of pregnancy. Carruthers A. J Am Acad Dermatol 1993;29:125.

Resolution of PUPPP is unrelated to delivery, therefore treating of PUPPP by early delivery should not be performed.

Treating an uncomfortable but nonserious dermatosis by such invasive methods with a potential risk for the mother and newborn in the author's view is not indicated and should not be performed anymore, especially as other adequate treatments are available.

Pemphigoid gestationis

Pemphigoid gestationis (herpes gestationis) is a rare, intensely itchy, urticarial or polymorphic or vesiculobullous eruption (Figure B). It affects approximately one in 60 000 pregnancies and usually appears in the second or third trimester, but it may also be associated with hydatiform mole or choriocarcinoma. The term pemphigoid gestationis is preferable because this condition shows many clinical and immunologic similarities with bullous pemphigoid and has no relationship with herpes virus infection.

MANAGEMENT STRATEGY

Although pemphigoid gestationis is a rare disorder, correct diagnosis and optimal management are essential. It occurs only in the presence of paternal tissue (fetus, hydatiform mole, or choriocarcinoma). Once it has manifested, its course may be modulated significantly by changes in estrogen and progesterone levels. Exacerbations may occur postpartum, with oral contraceptives, and during the menstrual cycle, and commonly are more severe in subsequent pregnancies. Circulating autoantibodies are directed against the same target antigens as in bullous pemphigoid, although more commonly against BP 180 antigen than BP 230 antigen. The autoantibodies react with the basement membrane of amnion placenta, resulting in the findings of immune activation in the placenta and evidence of placental insufficiency. Thus skin biopsies for dermatohistopathology, and direct immunofluorescence and indirect immunofluorescence investigations to confirm the diagnosis and to differentiate nonbullous pemphigoid gestationis from PUPPP, are recommended. This is especially important because most patients with pemphigoid gestationis need, at least for a while, treatment with systemic corticosteroids and are therefore at risk of side effects from this treatment. Most cases resolve within a few months postpartum, with just a few urticarial eruptions during the year after delivery. However, some cases have been reported with recurrences more than 10 years postpartum. Even more important is the fetal prognosis. In the older literature an increased risk for fetal morbidity and mortality has been discussed. However, cases with a serious outcome are more likely to be reported. Furthermore, in view of the findings that the placenta is also involved in pemphigoid gestationis, a more severe impact of the disease on the fetus seems reasonable in the precorticosteroid era. More recent studies have recorded a much better fetal prognosis. Patients who have been treated with systemic corticosteroids were no more likely to have children that were small for date compared to those who were not treated with systemic corticosteroids. The current view is that pemphigoid gestationis is associated with premature delivery and a risk of low birth weight. Thus pregnancies of mothers with pemphigoid gestationis should be carefully followed in special units.

The goal of the treatment is to suppress blister formation and to give the patients relief of the intense pruritus. Thus, in mild cases of pemphigoid gestationis, *topical potent or very potent corticosteroids* combined with *a systemic antihistamine* may be sufficient for therapy. First generation antihistamines are favored over second generation antihistamines. Substances such as *chlorpheniramine, diphenhydramine, tripelenamine, cyclizine, meclizine, hydroxyzine,* and *cyproheptadine* may be used (see also discussion on page 520 above about the use of antihistamines in PUPPP). However, most patients require *systemic corticosteroid* treatment during the course of their disease. Initially doses of prednisolone or its equivalent in the range of 20–40 mg daily may be tried, and then adjust the dose depending on the response. In severe cases 1 mg/kg body weight or even higher doses of prednisolone may be necessary to prevent blister formation. If the eruption resolves well the prednisolone can be reduced fairly rapidly in steps, initially twice weekly, later once a week, to a much lower maintenance dose. Some patients then respond to doses of prednisolone of 5–10 mg daily or every second day. Frequently the eruption flares immediately postpartum and then a temporary increase in prednisolone treatment is required.

Newborns of mothers suffering from pemphigoid gestationis may develop bullous lesions similar to those of their mother by passive transfer of the antibasement membrane zone antibody across the placenta. These lesions are transient and require no therapy. If the mother has received high doses of prednisolone for a longer time the infant should be carefully examined by a neonatologist for evidence of adrenal insufficiency.

In severe cases of pemphigoid gestationis that do not respond enough to prednisolone alone or in cases where prolonged treatment with corticosteroids is contraindicated, *plasmapheresis* may be considered. Postpartum treatment may cause difficulties for several reasons as follows.

- If the mother wishes to breastfeed, the drugs pass into the breast milk. Antihistamines may cause drowsiness in the baby and corticosteroids may cause adrenal suppression. The pediatrician should therefore be informed in this situation.
- In general, pemphigoid gestationis tends to improve postpartum: however, it may take weeks, months, or even years until there is complete remission. In those cases *alternative drugs that are contraindicated during pregnancy or while the mother is breastfeeding may be used.* Due to its close relationship to bullous pemphigoid in this situation similar treatment to that of bullous pemphigoid may be tried (see page 99). *Azathioprine, dapsone, sulfapyridine (sulphapyridine),* and *pyridoxine* may be tried as adjunctive therapy with oral corticosteroids or alone. Other drugs that may be used are *goserelin* and *ritodrine. High-dose intravenous immune globulin* alone or in combination with *cyclosporine* or *cyclophosphamide* have been tried with success in rare cases due to their corticosteroid-sparing effect.
- Pemphigoid gestationis tends to exacerbate with menstruation. There may also be dramatic flares with oral contraceptives. Thus, patients should be recommended to *avoid oral contraceptives* as long as the disease is still active.

SPECIFIC INVESTIGATIONS

■ Biopsy for histopathology and direct
immunofluorescence
■ Serum for indirect immunofluorescence and/or
enzyme-linked immunosorbent assay (ELISA)
(immunoblot)

**A comparative study of toxic erythema of pregnancy and
herpes gestationis.** Holmes RC, Black MM, Dann J, et al.
Br J Dermatol 1982;106:499–510.

**A comparative histopathological study of polymorphic
eruption of pregnancy and herpes gestationis.** Holmes RC,
Jurecka W, Black MM. Clin Exp Dermatol 1983;8:523–9.

**An immunoelectron microscopy study of the relationship
between herpes gestationis and polymorphic eruption of
pregnancy.** Jurecka W, Holmes RC, Black MM, et al. Br J
Dermatol 1983;108:147–51.

The disease most often confused with pemphigoid
gestationis is PUPPP. There may be a broad clinical and
histopathologic overlap between these two entities, which
are immunologically distinct with linear C3 deposits
(in 100%) and linear IgG deposits (in approximately 30%)
along the basement membrane zone in pemphigoid
gestationis.

*Clinically pemphigoid gestationis may present either with
prominent annular wheals or target lesions or with grouped vesicles, and then may be confused with either erythema multiforme
or dermatitis herpetiformis. However, these two diseases should be
easily distinguished from pemphigoid gestationis by histopathology and direct immunofluorescence.*

**Herpes gestationis autoantibodies recognize a 180 kD
human epidermal antigen.** Morrison LH, Labib RS, Zone JJ,
et al. J Clin Invest 1988;81:2023–6.

**Immunoblotting and enzyme-linked immunosorbent
assay for the diagnosis of pemphigoid gestationis.** Sitaru C,
Powell J, Messer G, et al. Obstet Gynecol 2004;103:757–
63.

In contrast to bullous pemphigoid, in pemphigoid gestationis the autoantibodies are directed more frequently
against the 180 kD than the 230 kD hemidesmosome target
antigen. By immunoblotting and ELISA, autoantibodies to
bullous pemphigoid antigen 180 were detected in 93 and
86.3% of pemphigoid gestationis patients, respectively, but
in none of the healthy controls. Serum levels of autoantibodies as detected by ELISA paralleled the patients' disease
activity.

*This study shows that immunoblotting and ELISA are
sensitive tools for the detection of autoantibodies to bullous
pemphigoid antigen 180 in patients with pemphigoid gestationis
and that ELISA is useful for monitoring autoantibody serum
levels.*

FIRST LINE THERAPIES

■ Topical corticosteroids	C
■ Systemic corticosteroids	B
■ Antihistamines	C

**Clinical features and management of 87 patients with
pemphigoid gestationis.** Jenkins RE, Hern S, Black MM.
Clin Exp Dermatol 1999;24:255–9.

In this review the clinical data on 142 pregnancies in
87 patients with pemphigoid gestationis are summarized.
Most patients received chlorpheniramine to suppress
the pruritus. Thirteen of 69 (18.8%) patients were treated
with topical corticosteroids alone without systemic treatment. Fifty six of the 69 (81.2%) required systemic corticosteroids with initial doses of prednisolone in the range of 5
to 110 mg daily, resulting in suppression of blistering in
most cases.

*Hitherto this is the largest series of patients ever published,
giving a good overview of the clinical presentation, immunologic
findings, and management strategies. Some patients have also
been treated with azathioprine, dapsone, pyridoxine, sulfapyridine, androgenic steroids, and goserelin. Plasmapheresis was also
used with some temporary relief.*

Fetal and maternal risk factors in herpes gestationis.
Lawley TJ, Stingl G, Katz SI. Arch Dermatol 1979;114:
552–5.

Forty one cases of immunologically proved herpes
gestationis are reviewed. Systemic treatment with corticosteroids is frequently necessary to control maternal signs
and symptoms of herpes gestationis. In eight patients
topical application of corticosteroids was sufficient alone.
Twenty nine patients were treated systemically with
corticosteroids in doses ranging from 20 to 180 mg of prednisone daily. In three of these cases azathioprine was also
used postpartum. Most of the cases responded well to the
treatment.

**Herpes gestationis: clinical and histologic features of
twenty-eight cases.** Shornick JK, Bangert JL, Freemann RG,
Gillian JN. J Am Acad Dermatol 1983;8:214–24.

Prednisone was used during 34 pregnancies, in initial
doses between 20 and 80 mg daily. There was extreme
variability in the need for protracted treatment. Some
women were able to stop prednisone within 5 days of delivery, whereas others needed treatment for up to 18 months.
The typical treatment was for 6–10 weeks postpartum.

*Although topical and systemic corticosteroids alone or together
are regarded as first line treatments in pemphigoid gestationis,
their use has been based only on multiple anecdotal reports and
not on controlled studies.*

SECOND LINE THERAPIES

■ Plasmapheresis	E

Plasma exchange in herpes gestationis. Van de Weil A,
Hart C, Flinkermann J, et al. Br Med J 1980;2:1041–2.

**Herpes gestationis: studies on the binding characteristics,
activity and pathogenetic significance of the complement-
fixing factor.** Carruthers JA, Ewins AR. Clin Exp Immunol
1978;31:38–41.

In single cases it has been shown that if corticosteroid
treatment proves unsuccessful or is contraindicated, then
plasmapheresis should be considered as well during pregnancy as postpartum (see also above).

THIRD LINE THERAPIES

■ High-dose intravenous immunoglobulin	E
■ Azathioprine	E
■ Cyclophosphamide	E
■ Cyclosporine	E
■ Dapsone	E
■ Sulfapyridine	E
■ Pyridoxine	E
■ Ritodrine	E
■ Goserelin	E

High-dose intravenous immune globulin

High dose intravenous immune globulin for the treatment of autoimmune blistering diseases: an evaluation for its use in 14 cases. Harman KE, Black MM. Br J Dermatol 1999;40:865–74.

A retrospective report on the experience of the use of high-dose intravenous immune globulin in several autoimmune blistering disease. The treatment had a corticosteroid-sparing effect with a transient response and repeated courses were required.

Immunosuppressive agents

Fetal and maternal risk factors in herpes gestationis. Lawley TJ, Stingl G, Katz SI. Arch Dermatol 1978;114:552–5.

In three of 41 cases an additional treatment with aza-thioprine besides high doses of corticosteroids was necessary postpartum.

A severe persistent case of pemphigoid gestationis treated with intravenous immunoglobulin and cyclosporin. Hern S, Harman K, Bhogal BS, Black MM. Clin Exp Dermatol 1998;23:185–8.

A patient with severe pemphigoid gestationis in whom the disease persisted for 1.5 years postpartum was treated with immunoglobulin and cyclosporine.

Chronic herpes gestationis and antiphospholipid antibody syndrome successfully treated with cyclophosphamide. Castle SP, Mather-Mondrey M, Bennion S, et al. J Am Acad Dermatol 1996;34:333–6.

Treatment with pulse-dose intravenous cyclophosphamide produced an excellent clinical response.

Immunosuppressive agents for the treatment of pemphigoid gestationis can only be used in the postpartum period while the mother is not breastfeeding.

Other therapies

Clinical features and management of 87 patients with pemphigoid gestationis. Jenkins RE, Hern S, Black MM. Clin Exp Dermatol 1999;24:255–9.

Dapsone, sulfapyridine, and pyridoxine were occasionally used as adjunctive therapy with oral corticosteroids.

The benefit of these drugs on the course of the disease remains questionable.

Herpes gestationis and ritodrine. Dobson RL. J Am Acad Dermatol 1988;18:1145–6.

Ritodrine is a β-adrenergic drug used to prevent premature labor. There has been some support for the suggestion that it may be of benefit in the treatment of pemphigoid gestationis.

Pemphigoid gestationis: response to chemical oophorectomy with goserelin. Garvey MP, Handfield-Jones SE, Black MM. Clin Exp Dermatol 1992;17:443–5.

Goserelin is a gonadotropin releasing hormone (GnRH) analogue and had only initial success in the treatment of continuing disease several years postpartum.

Pruritus gravidarum

Pruritus gravidarum, also known as cholestasis of pregnancy or a mild form of benign recurrent intrahepatic cholestasis, is a hepatic condition that usually occurs in late pregnancy. It first manifests with severe generalized pruritus and may be followed by the clinical appearance of jaundice. Its incidence has been estimated at 0.02–2.4% of pregnancies. It is likely that the irritation results from abnormal hepatic excretion of bile acids induced by endogenous estrogen and progesterone. The itching usually subsides rapidly after childbirth.

MANAGEMENT STRATEGY

The first symptom of pruritus gravidarum is pruritus, followed by secondary excoriations. In mild cases the diagnosis is based on exclusion by differentiating pruritus gravidarum from other itchy conditions that may occur by chance during pregnancy. Thus scabies, eczema, urticaria, drug eruptions, or other conditions, and early cases of PUPPP and pemphigoid gestationis have to be excluded. Liver function tests may occasionally be abnormal with a raised alkaline phosphatase. In fully developed cases numerous excoriations may be seen in conjunction with icterus. The pruritus and the cholestasis usually remit within a few days after delivery. The incidence of prematurity and low birth weight is increased in the offspring of patients with pruritus gravidarum and the pregnancies should be followed carefully. Pruritus gravidarum may recur with subsequent pregnancies and the use of oral contraceptive pills. In mild disease attempts should be made to control pruritus by frequent application of *cooling lotions or creams* and *topical antipruritic agents*. A *1% menthol lotion* or addition of *6–10% polidocanol* may be helpful. In more severe cases *oral antihistamines* are the therapy of choice. First generation antihistamines are preferable to second generation antihistamines (for the use of oral antihistamines during pregnancy see also the discussion of their use in PUPPP above, page 520). From the author's experience *phototherapy with UVB* (290–320 nm) or *UVA* (320–400 nm) may also be of benefit in some cases. *Cholestyramine* and, as shown in numerous recent studies, the administration of *ursodeoxycholic acid* may give adequate relief of symptoms.

SPECIFIC INVESTIGATIONS

■ IgE level
■ Liver function tests

Specific pruritic disease of pregnancy. A prospective study of 3192 pregnant women. Roger D, Vaillant L, Fignon A, et al. Arch Dermatol 1994;130:734–9.

Evidence levels A Double-blind study B Clinical trial ≥ 20 subjects C Clinical trial < 20 subjects D Series ≥ 5 subjects E Anecdotal case reports

Causes of pruritus during pregnancy include not only the specific dermatoses of pregnancy, but also scabies and eczema. The incidence of prematurity and low birth weight is increased in newborns of patients with pruritus gravidarum.

Intrahepatic cholestasis of pregnancy: relationships between bile acid levels and fetal complication rates. Glantz A, Marschall HU, Mattsson LA. Hepatology 2004;40:287–8.

No increase in fetal risk was detected in patients with intrahepatic cholestasis of pregnancy and bile acid levels less than 40 µmol/L.

Clinical outcome in a series of cases of obstetric cholestasis identified via a patient support group. Williamson C, Hems LM, Goulis DG, et al. BJOG 2004;111:676–81.

Intrauterine deaths reported in singleton pregnancies complicated by obstetric cholestasis. Death mainly occurs after 37 weeks. The gestation at which pruritus is first reported may help to predict spontaneous prematurity.

FIRST LINE THERAPIES

■ Emollients and topical antipruritic agents	D
■ Antihistamines	D

Skin changes and diseases in pregnancy. Lawley TJ, Yancey KB. In: Freedberg IM, Eisen AZ, Wolff K, et al., eds. Dermatology in general medicine, 6th edn. New York: McGraw-Hill; 2003:1361–6.

Emollients and topical antipruritic agents should be tried. Antihistamines are of some benefit.

SECOND LINE THERAPIES

■ Phototherapy	E

It is the author's experience that phototherapy with UVB (290–320 nm) or UVA (320–400 nm) is helpful in the treatment of pruritus gravidarum. No studies are available.

THIRD LINE THERAPIES

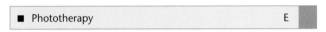

■ Ursodeoxycholic acid	A
■ Cholestyramine	E

Bile acids and progesterone metabolites in intrahepatic cholestasis of pregnancy. Reyes H, Sjovall J. Ann Med 2000;32:94–106.

With the administration of ursodeoxycholic acid to patients with intrahepatic cholestasis of pregnancy, pruritus and liver enzyme values are improved.

Intrahepatic cholestasis of pregnancy: changes in maternal–fetal bile acid balance and improvement by ursodeoxycholic acid. Brites D. Ann Hepatol 2002;1:20–8.

This review focuses on the altered bile acid profiles in maternal and fetal compartments during intrahepatic cholestasis of pregnancy and its recovery by ursodeoxycholic acid administration.

Ursodeoxycholic acid in the treatment of cholestasis of pregnancy: a randomized, double-blind study controlled with placebo. Palma J, Reyes H, Ribalta J, et al. J Hepatol 1997;27:1022–8.

Ursodeoxycholic acid is effective and safe in patients with intrahepatic cholestasis of pregnancy, attenuating pruritus and correcting some biochemical abnormalities in the mother. Relevant aspects of fetal outcome were also improved in patients receiving ursodeoxycholic acid (1 g daily) compared to placebo.

Effect of cholestyramine and phenobarbital on pruritus and serum bile acid levels in cholestasis of pregnancy. Laatikainen M. Am J Obstet Gynecol 1978;132:501–6.

Doses of 4 g cholestyramine two or three times daily have produced a reduction in serum bile acid levels and a relief from pruritus in some patients.

The use of phenobarbital may be contraindicated during pregnancy.

Prescribing in pregnancy

The decision to treat a pregnant woman with a drug should be made by the physician and the pregnant woman together on the best benefit-to-risk ratio, thus the prescription should fulfill each of the following criteria:

■ There should be a strict indication that requires a precise knowledge of the diagnosis and the course of the disease.
■ A drug should be selected with as few active components as possible.
■ The pharmacology of the active component and its safety during pregnancy should be established.
■ A precise knowledge of the duration of the pregnancy (weeks of gestation) is essential.
■ A drug that shows the best benefit-to-risk ratio should be selected.

Pretibial myxedema

Elana T Segal, Warren R Heymann

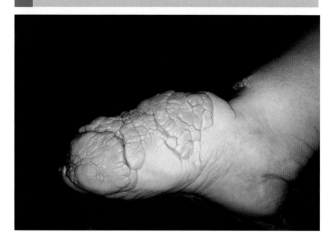

Pretibial myxedema, more accurately termed 'thyroid dermopathy', is characterized by non-pitting edema and flesh colored to violaceous nodules or plaques. These are most commonly distributed pretibially, but sometimes can be seen over the arms, shoulders, head, and neck.

MANAGEMENT STRATEGY

Cases of pretibial myxedema tend to occur following thyroidectomy or radioiodide thyroid ablation in patients with Graves' disease. The condition can, however, develop in hypothyroid and euthyroid patients. It is helpful to look for other clinical evidence of thyroid disease including thyroid acropachy and the presence of a goiter. Pretibial myxedema typically follows the onset of ophthalmopathy. Biopsy may aid in differentiating it from other conditions such as severe stasis dermatitis. Patients usually require therapy, though pretibial myxedema may resolve spontaneously over many years.

Patients with thyroid dermopathy should be started on a trial of *high-potency topical corticosteroids*, alone or under occlusion, for at least 2 months. If symptoms persist, *intralesional corticosteroids* may be effective. A combination of the above in conjunction with *compression bandages* can be beneficial when monotherapy proves inadequate. Both *oral* and *intravenous corticosteroids* have also been shown to improve lesions in several patients. However, their uses have often been limited by systemic side effects.

Pentoxifylline, an analogue of the methylxanthine theobromine, has been shown to reduce the extent of lesions. Although there are conflicting data, the use of *intravenous immunoglobulin (IVIG)* in doses of 400 mg/kg daily given over 3–4 h on five consecutive days for three cycles, followed by maintenance therapy, may improve cases of pretibial myxedema. Subcutaneous or intralesional *octreotide*, a somatostatin analogue, has been an effective strategy in patients unresponsive to other therapies. Plasmapheresis has been reported to be beneficial in improving severe cases.

Temporary improvement with *cytotoxic agents* has been observed. Pretibial myxedema is not a life-threatening condition, and so the use of such agents should be limited to severe, debilitating cases. *Surgical excision* has been shown to be effective in a minority of cases. The high risk of recurrence makes surgical intervention an infrequently used modality. *Complete decongestive physiotherapy* has shown some success in treating the elephantiasic form of pretibial myxedema.

Pretibial ultrasonography to measure skin thickness may be useful in assessing treatment response. Measuring serum hyaluronic acid levels to follow therapeutic response may also be of value.

SPECIFIC INVESTIGATIONS

- Thyroid function tests
- Antithyroglobulin and antithyroid peroxidase antibodies
- Anti-thyroid stimulating hormone (TSH)-receptor antibodies
- Pretibial ultrasound
- Serum hyaluronic acid

Pretibial myxedema as the initial manifestation of Graves' disease. Georgala S, Katoulis AC, Georgala C, et al. J Eur Acad Dermatol Venereol 2002;16:380–3.

A 28-year-old Greek woman presented initially with asymptomatic pretibial myxedema, which ultimately led to a diagnosis of Graves' disease. This patient had elevated anti-TSH-receptor antibodies.

An assessment of thyroid function is warranted because most patients with pretibial myxedema have clinical or laboratory evidence of autoimmune thyroid disease.

Pretibial myxedema associated with Hashimoto's thyroiditis. Cannavo SP, Borgia F, Vaccaro M, et al. J Eur Acad Dermatol Venereol 2002;16:625–7.

A 58-year-old woman with hypothyroid Hashimoto's thyroiditis developed exophthalmos and lesions of pretibial myxedema.

Euthyroid pretibial myxedema. Buljan-Cvijanovic M, Neal JM, Zemtsov A. Endocr Pract 1998;4:375–7.

A 53-year-old man with pretibial myxedema had normal thyroid function and no exophthalmos seen on CT scan of the orbits. He did have an elevated thyroid-stimulating immunoglobulin.

Euthyroid pretibial myxedema. Srebrnik A, Ophir J, Brenner S. Int J Dermatol 1992;31:431–2.

A case of a euthyroid 32-year-old man with pretibial myxedema is presented with no clinical or subclinical evidence of thyroid dysfunction.

FIRST LINE THERAPIES

■ Topical corticosteroids	C
■ Intralesional corticosteroids	D
■ Compression	D

Graves' disease with pretibial myxedema. Roenigk HH, Schermer DR. Arch Dermatol 1969;99:117–9.

Two patients treated with 0.025% fluocinolone acetonide cream twice daily with occlusion at bedtime, and 0.025% flurandrenolone cream with occlusion at bedtime, respectively, had marked improvement in lesions within 3–4 months.

Evidence levels   **A** Double-blind study   **B** Clinical trial ≥ 20 subjects   **C** Clinical trial < 20 subjects   **D** Series ≥ 5 subjects   **E** Anecdotal case reports

Therapy with occlusive dressings of pretibial myxedema with fluocinolone acetonide. Kriss JP, Pleshakov V, Rosenblum A, Sharp G. J Clin Endocrinol Metab 1967;27: 595–604.

All 11 patients treated with topical 0.2% fluocinolone acetonide cream under occlusive dressing at bedtime improved significantly.

Dermopathy of Graves disease (pretibial myxedema): review of 150 cases. Fatourechi V, Pajouhi M, Fransway AF. Medicine 1994;73:1–7.

Treatment with topical 0.05–0.1% triamcinolone acetonide cream under occlusion for 2–10 weeks led to partial remission in 29 of 76 patients in this retrospective study; 1% had complete remission.

Intralesional triamcinolone therapy for pretibial myxedema. Lang PG, Sisson JC, Lynch PJ. Arch Dermatol 1975;111:197–202.

Seven of nine patients treated with monthly injections of 8 mL or less of intralesional triamcinolone acetonide solution (5 mg/mL, 1 mL per injection site) had complete remission of pretibial myxedema after a total of three to seven visits. The other two patients, despite withdrawing from the study prematurely for nonmedical reasons, showed a partial improvement.

Therapy of circumscribed myxedema. James AR. Arch Dermatol 1961;83:161.

Two women in their late forties with pretibial myxedema received intralesional injections of triamcinolone acetonide (10 mg/mL) over two visits separated by 1 week. Both patients showed dramatic improvement when re-examined 1 month after the latter visit.

Pretibial myxedema: a review of the literature and case report. Frisch DR, Roth I. J Am Podiatr Med Assoc 1985; 75:147–52.

A 29-year-old woman with pretibial myxedema was treated with rest, elevation, and topical 0.05% fluocinonide cream under occlusion. Outpatient therapy included weekly intralesional Celestone Soluspan® injections followed by topical 0.05% fluocinonide cream under occlusion. Compression dressings with an Unna boot were applied weekly. After 2 months the lesions were greatly improved.

Compression stockings may also be beneficial. Unless contraindicated, compression should be used in conjunction with any therapeutic approach for this disorder.

Pathogenesis and treatment of pretibial myxedema. Kriss JP. Endocrinol Metab Clin North Am 1987;16:409–15.

Refractory cases of pretibial myxedema, including the elephantiasic form, may benefit from combined therapy with local corticosteroids under occlusion and an Unna boot.

SECOND LINE THERAPIES

■ Pentoxifylline	E

Pentoxifylline inhibits the proliferation and glycosaminoglycan synthesis of cultured fibroblasts derived from patients with Graves' ophthalmopathy and pretibial myxedema. Chang CC, Chang TC, Kao SC, et al. Acta Endocrinol 1993;129:322–7.

Pentoxifylline caused an in vitro dose-dependent decrease in fibroblast proliferation and glycosaminoglycan synthesis in fibroblast cultures taken from pretibial sites. A preliminary trial with a dose of 400 mg intravenously and 800 mg orally daily of pentoxifylline decreased the size of pretibial myxedema lesions within 1 week.

THIRD LINE THERAPIES

■ Intravenous immunoglobulin	D
■ Systemic corticosteroids (including pulse corticosteroid therapy)	D
■ Octreotide	E
■ Plasmapheresis	D
■ Cytotoxic therapy	E
■ Surgery	E
■ Complete decongestive physiotherapy	E

Pretibial myxedema and high-dose intravenous immunoglobulin treatment. Antonelli A, Navarranne A, Palla R, et al. Thyroid 1994;4:399–408.

Improvement of pretibial myxedema began after a few weeks in six patients treated with 400 mg/kg daily of high dose intravenous gamma globulin given over 3–4 h on five consecutive days. The cycle was repeated three times every 21 days. Maintenance therapy of 400 mg/kg for one day was then administered for from 7 to 15 more cycles every 21 days. Total treatment ranged from 7 to 12 months, with maximum response occurring after an average of 6 months.

Lack of response of elephantiasic pretibial myxoedema to treatment with high-dose intravenous immunoglobulins. Terheydem P, Kahaly GJ, Zillikens D, Brocker EB. Clin Exp Dermatol 2003;28:224–6.

IVIG did not significantly improve the lesions of a patient with elephantiasic pretibial myxedema.

Corticoid therapy for pretibial myxedema: observations on the long-acting thyroid stimulator. Benoit FL, Greenspan FS. Ann Intern Med 1967;66:711–20.

Oral prednisolone, begun at 60 mg then tapered, and methylprednisolone starting at 40 mg cleared the pretibial lesions of four patients and improved the lesions of two others. Of the various corticosteroid treatments studied, the best results were obtained with high-dose systemic corticosteroids for 2 weeks.

Localized myxedema, associated with increased serum hyaluronic acid, and response to steroid pulse therapy. Ohtsuka Y, Yamamoto K, Goto Y, et al. Intern Med 1995;34:424–9.

This is a case report of a 66-year-old man with Graves' disease and localized myxedema over the legs, feet, hands, and face. The patient improved with two courses of methylprednisolone pulse therapy (1 g daily) for 3 days each, followed by an oral prednisolone taper begun at 60 mg daily and continued at 10 mg daily for 1.5 years. The patient's serum hyaluronic acid levels decreased as skin lesions improved.

Refractory pretibial myxoedema with response to intralesional insulin-like growth factor 1 antagonist (octreotide): downregulation of hyaluronic acid production by the

lesional fibroblasts. Shinohara M, Hamasaki Y, Katayana I. Br J Dermatol 2000;143:1083–6.

200 mg daily of intralesional octreotide improved the lesions of pretibial myxedema in a male patient with Graves' disease after 4 weeks of therapy.

Octreotide inhibits insulin-like growth factor-1-induced hyaluronic acid secretion by lesional fibroblasts, which may play a role in the pathogenesis of pretibial myxedema.

Octreotide and Graves' ophthalmopathy and pretibial myxoedema. Chang TC, Kao SC, Huang KM. BMJ 1992;304: 158.

Three cases with pretibial myxedema were successfully treated with 100 mg of octreotide tid.

The authors do not comment on the route of administration of the octreotide acetate. According to the Physicians' Desk Reference, the drug may be administered either by subcutaneous injection or intravenously.

Effect of plasmapheresis and steroid treatment on thyrotropin binding inhibitory immunoglobulins in a patient with exophthalmos and a patient with pretibial myxedema. Kuzuya N, DeGroot LJ. J Endocrinol Invest 1982;5:373–8.

Two patients, one with elephantiasis-like lesions, were treated with 16 exchanges over 4–5 months with 1–2 L of the patient's plasma removed and replaced with 1300 mL of purified protein fraction and 700 mL 0.9% saline. Immunoglobulin G fraction was separated out, thereby decreasing total thyrotropin-binding inhibitory immunoglobulin (TBII) activity per unit of serum. The pretibial myxedema was partially and temporarily improved with plasmapheresis and abnormal antibodies were reduced.

Beneficial effects of plasmapheresis followed by immunosuppressive therapy in pretibial myxedema. Noppen M, Velkeniers B, Steenssens L, Vanhaelst L. Acta Clin Belg 1988;43:381–3.

A patient with pretibial myxedema, unresponsive to topical corticosteroids, was cured after 5 days of plasmapheresis followed by 100 mg of azathioprine twice daily for 3 months. Azathioprine was tapered to 50 mg twice daily and continued for a year, at which time no recurrence was noted.

Pretibial myxedema (elephantiasic form): treatment with cytotoxic therapy. Hanke CW, Bergfeld WF, Guirguis MN, Lewis LJ. Cleve Clin Q 1983;50:183–8.

Fibroblasts from pretibial myxedema sites of a 44-year-old male showed decreased DNA content in vitro with the use of cytotoxic agents. Melphalan, which decreased hyaluronic acid levels to the greatest extent, was given orally (8 mg daily) for 4 days, and repeated monthly for 6 months. This regimen provided transient improvement, but the patient's condition then got worse.

Surgical excision of pseudotumorous pretibial myxedema. Pingsmann A, Ockenfels HM, Patsalis T. Foot Ankle Int 1996;17:107–10.

In this case of a 56-year-old woman with Graves' disease, who had undergone subtotal thyroidectomy, surgical excision of the reticular dermis was useful in the elimination of pseudotumorous pretibial myxedema recalcitrant to oral and topical corticosteroids.

Successful combined surgical and octreotide treatment of severe pretibial myxoedema reviewed after 9 years. Felton J, Derrick EK, Price ML. Br J Dermatol 2003;148:825–6.

A 56-year-old man with pretibial myxedema was treated with surgical shave removal followed by daily subcutaneous octreotide injections for 6 months. His lesions did not recur over a 9-year follow-up period.

Pretibial myxedema. Matsuoka LY, Wortsman J, Dietrich JG, Pearson R. Arch Dermatol 1981;117:250–1.

A 47-year-old woman with hypothyroidism had recurrence of pretibial myxedema in a split-thickness skin graft 3 years after placement.

Pretibial myxedema: recurrence after skin grafting. Kucer KA, Herbert A, Luscombe HA, Kauh YC. Arch Dermatol 1980;116:1076–7.

A patient with recurrence of pretibial myxedema in graft sites after wide excision had a good response to topical fluorinated halcinonide cream under occlusion at night and intralesional triamcinolone acetonide every month.

Elephantiasic pretibial myxedema: a novel treatment for an uncommon disorder. Susser WS, Heermans AG, Chapman MS, Baughman RD. J Am Acad Dermatol 2002;46:723–6.

A 67-year-old woman with elephantiasic pretibial myxedema had a 47% reduction of leg edema after 6 weeks of intensive complete decongestive physiotherapy. This response was sustained for 2 years after treatment.

Complete decongestive physiotherapy consists of manual massage of the lower extremities to promote lymphatic drainage followed by compressive bandages, exercise, and skin care.

Prurigo nodularis

*Aleksey Kamenshchikov, Alison Lazinsky,
Mark G Lebwohl*

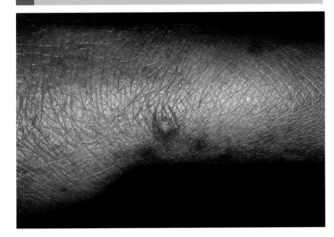

Prurigo nodularis is characterized by extremely pruritic papules, usually concentrated on the scalp and extremities. The papules are caused by repeated scratching and represent a localized form of lichen simplex chronicus.

MANAGEMENT STRATEGY

Underlying causes for the patient's itch must be sought. In patients at risk for HIV infection, HIV serology should be checked. Serum should be sent for liver function tests, BUN, and creatinine to rule out hepatic or renal causes of itching. A history of atopy should be sought and serum IgE measured to look for atopy as a possible etiology. In the elderly, bullous pemphigoid may present with a similar eruption – 'pemphigoid nodularis'. Patients should be advised that repeated scratching can perpetuate the lesions of prurigo nodularis and steps must be taken to minimize itching. Use of *antipruritic agents* containing *menthol* or *phenol*, or *anesthetics* such as *pramocaine*, are helpful. Wearing gloves at night and trimming fingernails short can be beneficial. *Topical corticosteroids* may be used, but even superpotent corticosteroids are often inadequate. Occlusion of corticosteroids with agents such as *flurandrenolide-impregnated tape* (Cordran Tape®, Haelan Tape®) not only treat the lesion but also prevent patients from scratching. When these simple steps are inadequate, *intralesional injection of corticosteroids* is usually beneficial. Triamcinolone acetonide 40 mg/mL can be injected, with less than 0.1 mL per lesion.

For patients refractory to intralesional corticosteroids, *cryotherapy* may be added. When lesions are too numerous to treat topically or by injection, phototherapy with *UVB* or *PUVA* can be administered. In severe cases, oral *thalidomide* is helpful. Sedating *oral antihistamines* are routinely used in patients with prurigo nodularis, despite the lack of evidence that they work.

SPECIFIC INVESTIGATIONS

- Serology for HIV
- Liver function tests
- BUN, creatinine
- Serum IgE
- Histology with immunofluorescence

FIRST LINE THERAPIES

Potent and superpotent corticosteroids	E
Corticosteroids with occlusion	E
Intralesional corticosteroids	E
Occlusion	E
Capsaicin	B

Use of occlusive membrane in prurigo nodularis. Meyers LN. Int J Dermatol 1989;28:275–6.

Four patients with prurigo nodularis responded to weekly application of an occlusive pad (Duoderm®). All lesions resolved, but recurred several weeks later in one patient and several months later in a second. One of these patients responded to application of an occlusive pad and an unspecified tranquilizer, and the second again cleared with application of the occlusive pad.

Apart from possible antipruritic effects of occlusive pads, they physically block scratching, eliminating the cause of prurigo nodularis.

Treatment of prurigo nodularis with topical capsaicin. Stander S, Luger T, Metze D. J Am Acad Dermatol 2001; 44:471–8.

Thirty-three patients with prurigo nodularis were treated with topical capsaicin (0.025% to 0.3%) four to six times daily for periods of between 2 weeks and 10 months. Pruritus resolved in all patients within 12 days, but returned in 16 of 33 patients within 2 months of discontinuation of capsaicin.

SECOND LINE THERAPIES

Cryotherapy	E
UVB phototherapy	E
Narrowband UVB	E

Cryotherapy improves prurigo nodularis. Waldinger TP, Wong RC, Taylor WB, Voorhees JJ. Arch Dermatol 1984;120: 1598–600.

A black female resistant to multiple therapies, including topical corticosteroids, oral hydroxyzine hydrochloride, phototherapy, and tar, was successfully treated with liquid nitrogen. Phototherapy resulted in blistering.

Cryotherapy to the point of blistering can lead to scarring and hypopigmentation, as it did in this patient.

Treatment of prurigo nodularis: use of cryosurgery and intralesional steroids plus lidocaine. Stoll DM, Fields JP, King LE Jr. J Dermatol Surg Oncol 1983;9:922–4.

Two patients were treated with liquid nitrogen applied with a cotton-tipped applicator for a thaw time of 10 s followed by intralesional injection of triamcinolone acetonide 10 mg/mL mixed with lidocaine (lignocaine) 0.75%. All lesions resolved after four to eight injections at 4- to 6-week intervals.

UV treatment of generalised prurigo nodularis. Hans SK, Cho MY, Park YK. J Am Acad Dermatol 1990;29:436–7.

Two patients were treated with UVB administered three times a week for 24 to 30 treatments. Itching resolved and most lesions cleared. Residual large lesions were treated with intralesional injection of corticosteroids and with topical PUVA.

Sequential combined therapy with thalidomide and narrowband (TL01) UVB in the treatment of prurigo nodularis. Ferrandiz C, Carrasocsa JM, Just M, et al. Dermatology 1997;195:359–61.

Four patients with prurigo nodularis were started on thalidomide and subsequently treated with narrowband UVB for up to 37 treatments. One patient who relapsed after 5 months was again controlled with a new course of UVB without thalidomide.

THIRD LINE THERAPIES

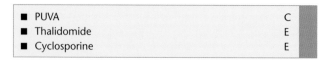

■ PUVA	C
■ Thalidomide	E
■ Cyclosporine	E

Local photochemotherapy in nodular prurigo. Vaatainen N, Hannuksela M, Karvonen J. Acta Derm Venereol 1979;59: 544–7.

Fifteen patients with prurigo nodularis responded to trixosalen baths and UVA. Moderately good results were achieved in 3 weeks. Itching improved dramatically in 4–6 days. Initial doses of 0.1–0.2 J/cm^2 were administered daily and doses increased by approximately 50% every third day.

Oral PUVA has also been used anecdotally in the treatment of prurigo nodularis.

Thalidomide treatment of prurigo nodularis. Winkelmann RK, Connolly SM, Doyle JA, Padilha-Goncalves A. Acta Derm Venereol 1984;64:412–7.

Patients with prurigo nodularis were treated with oral thalidomide, resulting in rapid resolution of itching and subsequent resolution of nodules. Doses of 100–300 mg daily were required. In one patient, lesions recurred after discontinuation of the medication but again responded to restarting the oral thalidomide.

Fatigue, constipation, and neuropathy are potential side effects of this treatment. Thalidomide should not be administered to women of childbearing potential because of the potential for severe birth defects.

Thalidomide treatment for prurigo nodularis in human immunodeficiency virus-infected subjects: efficacy and risk of neuropathy. Maurer T, Poncelet A, Berger T. Arch Dermatol 2004;140:845–9.

Eight HIV-infected patients with prurigo were treated with thalidomide 100 mg daily. After the first month, patients were randomized to receive 100 mg or 200 mg daily and the dose was adjusted if side effects developed. All had more than 50% reduction in itch in an average of 3.4 months, and seven of eight had greater than 50% reduction in skin lesions in an average of 5 months. Thalidomide peripheral neuropathy developed in three patients.

Nodular prurigo responds to cyclosporin. Berth-Jones J, Smith SG, Graham-Brown RAC. Br J Dermatol 1995;132: 795–9.

Two women with prurigo nodularis had marked improvement in lesions on oral cyclosporine at doses of 3–4.5 mg/kg daily, but neither cleared completely.

Prurigo pigmentosa

Yukiko Tsuji-Abe, Hiroshi Shimizu

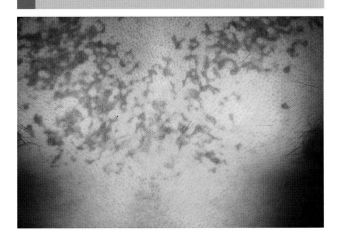

Prurigo pigmentosa has a distinct clinical appearance that starts with pruritic, urticarial papules or papulovesicles followed by a peculiar reticular pigmentation. The majority of reported patients are Japanese with a female predominance, but non-Japanese patients are also described.

MANAGEMENT STRATEGY

The pathogenesis of prurigo pigmentosa is still unknown. Friction from clothing could be one trigger for the disease. In some cases, ketosis caused by diabetes mellitus, sudden weight loss, or anorexia nervosa precedes prurigo pigmentosa, and treatment of these conditions can under some circumstances clear the lesions. There are several case reports of individuals who developed this condition in association with other disorders including contact allergy or *Helicobacter pylori* infection. In these cases, the lesions could also be cleared when the causative agents were removed.

Dapsone (25–100 mg daily) and *minocycline* (100–200 mg daily) are reported as effective against prurigo pigmentosa. The effects are mostly observed within a few days or within a week after treatment, with a reduction in pruritic and papular lesions. Minocycline might be the first choice therapy because it produces less adverse reactions, and remission time is occasionally reported as being longer compared with dapsone. Topical or systemic corticosteroids or antihistamines are usually ineffective.

SPECIFIC INVESTIGATIONS

- Fasting blood sugar and urinary ketones

Ketosis is involved in the origin of prurigo pigmentosa. Teraki Y, Teraki E, Kawashima M, et al. J Am Acad Dermatol 1996;34:509–11.

Prurigo pigmentosa associated with ketosis. Murao K, Urano Y, Uchida N, Arase S. Br J Dermatol 1996;134:379–81.

Prurigo pigmentosa and diabetes. Kubota Y, Koga T, Nakayama J. Eur J Dermatol 1998;8:439–41.

Prurigo pigmentosa (Nagashima) associated with anorexia nervosa. Nakada T, Sueki H, Iijima M. Clin Exp Dermatol 1998;23:25–7.

A young woman with anorexia nervosa developed prurigo pigmentosa. After she gained weight, the lesions cleared completely.

In all these reports, prurigo pigmentosa was associated with ketosis. Disease activity was sometimes correlated with the amount of urinary ketones. In some cases, lesions were cleared simply by treating these conditions.

FIRST LINE THERAPIES

■ Minocycline	C
■ Dapsone	C
■ Treatment for ketosis or any other causative factors	D

Prurigo pigmentosa: a distinctive inflammatory disease of the skin. Boer A, Misago N, Wolter M, et al. Am J Dermatopathol 2003;25:117–29.

Among 25 cases, 16 cases responded well to minocycline (100–200 mg daily) and seven cases responded well to dapsone (25 mg daily).

Prurigo pigmentosa successfully treated with minocycline. Aso M, Miyamoto T, Morimura T, Shimao S. Br J Dermatol 1989;120:705–8.

Five cases of prurigo pigmentosa all responded to minocycline 100–200 mg daily within a week. Two cases previously treated with dapsone had relapsed, but long remission times were observed with minocycline.

Prurigo pigmentosa – clinical observations of our 14 cases. Nagashima M. J Dermatol 1978;5:61–7.

This is the first report of prurigo pigmentosa. The author mentioned friction from clothing could be the trigger of this condition. Dapsone was used in some cases and was highly effective.

Prurigo pigmentosa associated with diabetic ketoacidosis. Ohnishi T, Kita H, Ogata E, Watanabe S. Acta Derm Venereol 2000;80:447–8.

Eighteen cases of prurigo pigmentosa associated with diabetic ketoacidosis. Treatment of ketoacidosis improved eruptions in eight cases, minocycline was effective in five cases, dapsone in three cases, topical corticosteroid in one case, and unknown in one case.

SECOND LINE THERAPIES

■ Roxithromycin	E
■ Clarithromycin	E
■ Doxycycline	E

The successful treatment of prurigo pigmentosa with macrolide antibiotics. Yazawa N, Ihn H, Yamane K, et al. Dermatology 2001;202:67–9.

Two cases of prurigo pigmentosa responded well to 300 mg daily roxithromycin, and another two cases responded well to 400 mg daily clarithromycin. In all cases, the effect appeared quickly and the pruritus and papules disappeared within a week.

Prurigo pigmentosa. Gurses L, Gurbuz O, Demircay Z, Kotiloglu E. Int J Dermatol 1999;38:924–5.

Of two cases, one responded well to doxycycline 200 mg daily, and another case resolved spontaneously.

Prurigo pigmentosa. Gur-Toy G, Gungor E, Artuz F, et al. Int J Dermatol 2002;41:288–91.

Roxithromycin 300 mg daily was effective in two cases of prurigo pigmentosa, and clarithromycin 400 mg daily was effective in another two cases.

Doxycycline and macrolide antibiotics are also effective in prurigo pigmentosa. These therapies are recommended for use in patients who do not or only poorly respond to ordinary therapy, or cannot use first-choice medication because of adverse reactions.

THIRD LINE THERAPIES

■ Potassium iodide	E
■ Sulfamethoxazole	E

Prurigo pigmentosa: 3rd non-Japanese case. Harms M, Mérot Y, Polla L, Saurat JH. Dermatologica 1986;173:202–4.

A 23-year-old woman was first treated with dapsone 50 mg daily, but the disease recurred shortly after stopping therapy. Potassium iodide 500 mg daily was then prescribed and the lesions cleared up.

Prurigo pigmentosa: a possible mechanism of action of sulfonamides. Miyachi Y, Yoshida A, Horio T, et al. Dermatologica 1986;172:82–8.

A 31-year-old woman with a 4-year history of recurrent prurigo pigmentosa responded well to sulfamethoxazole 2.0 g daily.

Most patients with prurigo pigmentosa respond well to first or second line therapies or undergo spontaneous remission, but these alternatives might be useful in exceptional cases.

Evidence levels **A** Double-blind study **B** Clinical trial ≥ 20 subjects **C** Clinical trial < 20 subjects **D** Series ≥ 5 subjects **E** Anecdotal case reports

Pruritus

Jon R Ward, Jeffrey D Bernhard

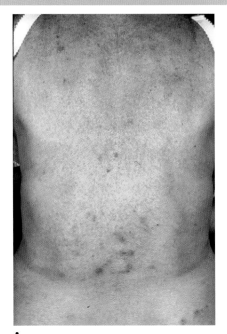

A

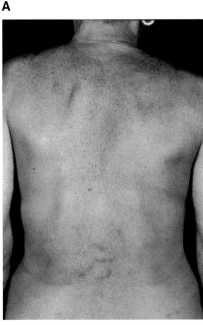

B

Itch can be defined as the urge to scratch. It is a characteristic feature of many diseases of the skin and an unusual sign of some systemic diseases. Generalized itch in the absence of a diagnosable rash can pose both a diagnostic and therapeutic dilemma to even the most seasoned dermatologist. Although there is no magic bullet for pruritus, new understanding of the neurophysiology of itch may lead to specific therapies targeting particular pathways in the central nervous system.

Figure A shows eczematous changes induced by rubbing and scratching on the back of a woman with uremic pruritus. Substantial improvement in itching and in the rash (Figure B) was achieved after treatment with ultraviolet-B phototherapy.

MANAGEMENT STRATEGY

The management of pruritus depends upon the cause, which may not be apparent. Presence of a rash and localization are two clues that can provide important information. Many dermatoses cause itch and it is beyond the scope of this chapter to discuss them all. In the search for a primary dermatosis, one must look for xerosis and scabies, because both can have subtle findings. Generalized pruritus (GP) can be defined as widespread itch without an identifiable primary rash, though nonspecific (and misleading!) secondary changes may be present. In GP, the possibility of systemic disease should be considered and evaluation undertaken. Systemic diseases that may cause GP include hematologic and solid malignancies, HIV, thyroid disease, iron deficiency, renal disease, hepatobiliary disease, connective tissue disease, neurologic disease, parasitosis, and drug hypersensitivity. A complete history and physical examination is mandatory. Interval re-evaluation should be undertaken because pruritus may precede the diagnosis of systemic disease by months to years.

In patients with generalized itching, with or without a rash, one of the more common and embarrassing errors is to miss the diagnosis of scabies; the most serious error is to miss the diagnosis of an underlying systemic disease such as Hodgkin's disease or hyperthyroidism. When it happens, failure to diagnose an underlying systemic illness tends to occur in the setting of a non-diagnostic dermatitis that has been created by rubbing and scratching, but is mistaken for a primary skin disease.

Other causes of GP to consider are psychogenic pruritus and, after all other causes have been excluded, idiopathic pruritus. Idiopathic pruritus is common in the elderly and may be a result of age-related changes of central and/or peripheral neural pathways. It is also important to consider localized forms of pruritus that can go undiagnosed for quite some time. In our experience, it seems that many cases of GP begin as a localized itch. By the time patients fail to respond to various treatments and obtain a dermatology referral, the itch has often been going on for months. The patients can hardly recall where the itch began and secondary changes hide the primary dermatosis. Aggressive treatment of the rash and pruritus may be effective and then reveal a previously localized itch. We have seen this clinical picture in brachioradial pruritus and in stasis dermatitis with autoeczematization.

In the case of most eczematous dermatoses, topical *corticosteroids* or *calcineurin inhibitors* are effective in treating the rash and relieving itch. In the case of xerosis, which may be difficult to recognize, an adequate skin care regimen and *emollients* are indispensable. A good skin care regimen involves the use of unscented bath oils, a humidifier, and the liberal use of emollients, especially after bathing. Irritating soaps, friction from washcloths, and prolonged hot showers should be avoided. In systemic disease, *diagnosis and treatment of the underlying disease* is essential, but symptomatic treatment is often required (e.g. UVB phototherapy for hemodialysis patients with GP). In the management of pruritus that does not respond to simple measures, treatment should be stepwise and individualized based on severity. GP due to hepatic and renal causes is considered separately because they have differing etiology and treatment.

Topical corticosteroid treatment may be tried if there is clinical evidence of inflammation. *Cooling agents* such as menthol may be applied liberally and can provide immediate relief in some cases. *Topical doxepin* is effective for localized itch, but is not recommended for prolonged use or application over a large surface area of skin. *Capsaicin* may be a good option for areas of localized itch, but is not practical for total body application. *Lidocaine patches* and *transcutaneous electrical nerve stimulation* have been effective in patients with localized pruritus as well. Alternative therapies, including *hypnosis* and *acupuncture,* have improved itch according to case reports. *UVB phototherapy* has been reported to relieve itch in patients with idiopathic GP, cholestasis, and renal itch.

Sedating antihistamines are often employed in therapy for patients with itch; it is important to remember that their benefit derives from their soporific side effect. Nonsedating antihistamines may be of benefit, but are not reliably effective unless the disorder is mediated by histamine. The tricyclic antidepressant *doxepin* is a very potent antihistamine; it is unknown if any aspect of its antipruritic effect is independent of sedation. *Amitriptyline* and *mirtazapine* have been effective in brachioradial pruritus and lymphoma-associated pruritus, respectively. *Selective serotonin reuptake inhibitors (SSRIs) paroxetine* and *fluoxetine* have improved pruritus in patients with polycythemia vera. *Gabapentin* has been effective in brachioradial pruritus, but its effect on GP has not yet been reported. Opioid antagonists, *naltrexone* and *naloxone,* have proven effective in randomized and open trials in a number of pruritic conditions.

The pruritus of cholestasis is not completely understood, but may be a consequence of increased levels of endogenous opioids. Treatments for the itch of cholestasis may be targeted at decreasing levels of bile acid or blocking opioid action. *Cholestyramine* and *ursodeoxycholic* acid bind to bile acids in the intestinal tract and interrupt enterohepatic circulation. *Rifampin* and *phenobarbital* are hepatic enzyme inducers that may be effective in suppressing pruritus of cholestasis. *Naltrexone, nalmefene,* and *naloxone* were effective in randomized controlled trials. Opioid antagonists may precipitate a withdrawal syndrome in cholestatic patients due to high levels of endogenous opioids. Paroxetine and mirtazapine have been reported to improve itch in small series of patients with cholestasis. *Ondansetron,* a 5-HT3 receptor antagonist, has shown conflicting results in randomized, controlled trials. A new technique, *extracorporeal albumin dialysis,* led to prolonged remission of intractable pruritus in four patients. Intractable pruritus is an indication for *liver transplantation* in patients with cholestatic pruritus.

Uremic pruritus is a misnomer because blood urea levels do not correlate with itch. Patients with renal itch have increased numbers of dermal mast cells, tend to have dry skin, and may have a variety of unidentified circulating pruritogens, possibly including opioid peptides. UVB phototherapy is a mainstay of treatment and both narrowband and broadband are effective. Emollients improve xerosis and a good skin care regimen can help relieve itch. In patients with elevated calcium and phosphorus, *parathyroidectomy* may lead to improvement of pruritus. *Erythropoietin* was found to improve pruritus and should be considered in any patients not already on this drug. Activated charcoal and thalidomide have been effective in clinical trials. Opioid antagonists were effective in one randomized controlled trial, but subsequent studies have not duplicated these results. Mirtazapine has been effective in a small series of patients. *Renal transplantation* is curative.

SPECIFIC INVESTIGATIONS

Screening
- Careful medication history
- Complete physical exam
- Complete blood count with differential
- Thyroid function testing
- Blood urea nitrogen, creatinine
- Hepatic function testing
- Fasting glucose
- Chest radiograph (posteroanterior and lateral)
- Age-appropriate cancer screening

Additional testing to consider
- HIV testing
- Erythrocyte sedimentation rate
- Serum iron and ferritin
- Serum protein electrophoresis, urine protein electrophoresis
- Stool for ova and parasites

Evaluation of the patient with generalized pruritus. Kantor GR. In: Bernhard, JD ed. Itch: mechanisms and management of pruritus. New York: McGraw-Hill; 1994:337–46.

The diagnostic and therapeutic approach to idiopathic generalized pruritus. Yosipovitch G, David M. Int J Dermatol 1999;38:881–7.

These are two comprehensive reviews relating to the evaluation, work-up, and subsequent treatment of patients without a clear etiology for their itch. The second touches on the new findings in the neural pathways and physiology of itch.

Pruritus in chronic liver disease: mechanisms and treatment. Bergasa NV. Curr Gastroenterol Rep 2004;6:10–6.

This is an excellent and succinct review of cholestatic pruritus. It presents what is known regarding the pathophysiology of itch and cholestasis and then discusses treatments aimed at each step of the process.

FIRST LINE THERAPIES

Localized pruritus	
■ Topical capsaicin	A
■ Lidocaine patch	E
■ Topical doxepin	A
Generalized pruritus (also useful in hepatic or uremic pruritus)	
■ Emollients	E
■ Patient education regarding skin care regimen	E
■ Topical pramoxine	A
■ Antihistamines (for their sedative effect)	A
■ Doxepin	A
Cholestatic pruritus	
■ Cholestyramine	A
■ Naltrexone	A
Uremic pruritus	
■ UVB phototherapy	B
■ Erythropoietin	A

Successful treatment of notalgia paresthetica with topical capsaicin: vehicle-controlled, double-blind, crossover

Evidence levels A Double-blind study B Clinical trial ≥ 20 subjects C Clinical trial < 20 subjects D Series ≥ 5 subjects E Anecdotal case reports

study. Wallengren J, Klinker M. J Am Acad Dermatol 1995; 32:287–9.

In this 10-week study, 20 patients with notalgia paresthetica were treated with capsaicin or placebo five times daily for 1 week and then three times daily for 3 weeks. Treatment was stopped for 2 weeks and then all patients used capsaicin on the same schedule as before; 70% of patients treated with capsaicin improved and 30% on placebo improved. Pruritus did not intensify during the washout period in patients who received capsaicin in the first 4 weeks.

Intractable postherpetic itch and cutaneous deafferentation after facial shingles. Oaklander AL, Cohen SP, Raju SV. Pain 2002;96:9–12.

A case report of a 39-year-old woman with severe itch following zoster unresponsive to multiple treatments that finally responded to a lidocaine patch.

Relief of pruritus in patients with atopic dermatitis after treatment with doxepin cream. Drake LA, Fallon JD, Sober A. J Am Acad Dermatol 1994;31:613–6.

A double-blind, placebo-controlled, multicenter study in 270 patients with atopic dermatitis: 5% doxepin cream was applied to pruritic areas twice on the first day and four times a day for six additional days. Topical doxepin relieved pruritus in 85% of patients compared to relief of pruritus in 57% of vehicle-treated patients. A significant number of patients in the doxepin group experienced drowsiness.

Effect of topical pramoxine on experimentally induced itch in humans. Yosipovitch G, Maibach HI. J Am Acad Dermatol 1997;37:278–80.

A double-blind, placebo-controlled study of 14 patients. Itch induced by intradermal histamine injection was significantly reduced with topical pramoxine.

Suppression of histamine-induced pruritus by three antihistaminic drugs. Rhoades RB, Leifer KN, Cohan R, Wittig HJ. J Allergy Clin Immunol 1975;55:180–5.

Twenty eight normal subjects partook in a double-blind crossover study examining suppression of histamine-induced itch. Hydroxyzine, diphenhydramine, and cyproheptadine were compared to lactose placebo. After ingestion of hydroxyzine, a 750-fold increase in histamine dose was needed to evoke pruritus. A ten-fold increase was needed after diphenhydramine was given. A five-fold increase was needed with both placebo and cyproheptadine.

Pharmacologic modulation of the whealing response to histamine in human skin: identification of doxepin as a potent in vivo inhibitor. Sullivan TJ. J Allergy Clin Immunol 1982;69:260–7.

A randomized, double-blind, placebo-controlled study with five subjects showed that doxepin 5 mg every 12 h led to a 22-fold shift in the histamine dose–response curve.

Double-blind placebo-controlled clinical trial of microporous cholestyramine in the treatment of intra- and extrahepatic cholestasis: relationship between itching and serum bile acids. Di Padova C, Tritapepe R, Rovagnati P, Rossetti S. Methods Find Exp Clin Pharmacol 1984;6:773–6.

A double-blind placebo-controlled study was carried out in ten patients. Microporous cholestyramine 3 g three times daily or placebo were given orally over a 4-week period. The

active drug was superior to placebo in reducing itching intensity and serum bile acids.

Oral naltrexone treatment for cholestatic pruritus: a double-blind, placebo-controlled study. Wolfhagen FH, Sternieri E, Hop WC, et al. Gastroenterology 1997;113: 1264–9.

This study of 16 patients with cholestatic pruritus and five controls showed naltrexone 50 mg daily led to significant improvement in pruritus. Four patients did have an opiate withdrawal syndrome; this was transient in three.

Ultraviolet phototherapy of uremic pruritus. Long-term results and possible mechanism of action. Gilchrest BA, Rowe JW, Brown RS, et al. Ann Intern Med 1979;91:17–21.

This is an open-label study of 38 patients with uremic pruritus treated with UVB phototherapy. A comparison of three schedules varying from one to three treatments weekly showed that the percentage of patients responding was not influenced by frequency of UVB exposure, though patients treated more intensively improved faster. Patients receiving only half-body treatments improved as well, indicating a systemic rather than local effect. Overall 32 of 38 patients improved after a course of six or eight UVB exposures.

Relief of pruritus and decreases in plasma histamine concentrations during erythropoietin therapy in patients with uremia. De Marchi S, Cecchin E, Villalta D, et al. N Engl J Med 1992;326:969–74.

In a double-blind, placebo-controlled, crossover study, eight of ten patients treated with intravenous erythropoietin experienced improvement in pruritus. The pruritus returned within 1 week after the discontinuation of therapy. The improvement was not related to the change in hemoglobin level.

SECOND LINE THERAPIES

Generalized pruritus	
■ UVB phototherapy	B
■ PUVA	C
■ Gabapentin	C
■ Naltrexone	B
■ Mirtazapine	E
Cholestatic pruritus	
■ Rifampin	A
■ Ursodeoxycholic acid	A
■ SSRIs	B
■ S-adenosyl-L-methionine	A
Uremic pruritus	
■ Activated charcoal	A
■ Cholestyramine	A
■ Naltrexone	A

UVB phototherapy is an effective treatment for pruritus in patients infected with HIV. Lim HW, Vallurupalli S, Meola T, Soter NA. J Am Acad Dermatol 1997;37:414–7.

This is a study of 21 HIV-positive patients with pruritus treated three times a week with UVB phototherapy. Significant reductions in pruritus scores were noted. A mean number of 20.7 ± 2.3 treatments resulted in maximal improvement.

Local photochemotherapy in nodular prurigo. Vaatainen N, Hannuksela M, Karvonen J. Acta Derm Venereol 1979; 59:544–7.

Fifteen patients with prurigo nodularis were treated with bath PUVA. All patients had some improvement of symptoms with an average of 3 weeks of treatment.

Brachioradial pruritus: response to treatment with gabapentin. Winhoven SM, Coulson IH, Bottomley WW. Br J Dermatol 2004;150:786–7.

A report of two patients with brachioradial pruritus resistant to other therapies who responded to gabapentin 300 mg three times daily.

Efficacy and safety of naltrexone, an oral opiate receptor antagonist, in the treatment of pruritus in internal and dermatological diseases. Metze D, Reimann S, Beissert S, Luger TA. J Am Acad Dermatol 1999;41:533–9.

Fifty patients with itch of various causes were treated with naltrexone 50 mg daily; 70% of patients achieved a significant therapeutic response as demonstrated by improvement in a visual analogue scale for itch. The authors found naltrexone highly effective in prurigo nodularis.

Mirtazapine for pruritus. Davis MP, Frandsen JL, Walsh D, et al. Pain Symptom Manage 2003;25:288–91.

This case series of four patients with cholestasis, lymphoma, and uremic pruritus showed improvement of pruritus in each patient with mirtazapine 15–30 mg daily.

Treatment of pruritus in primary biliary cirrhosis with rifampin. Results of a double-blind, crossover, randomized trial. Ghent CN, Carruthers SG. Gastroenterology 1988;94:488–93.

Eight of nine patients with primary biliary cirrhosis had significant reduction of pruritus in the first week of treatment. Daily doses of rifampin were 300–450 mg.

Improvement of biliary enzyme levels and itching as a result of long-term administration of ursodeoxycholic acid in primary biliary cirrhosis. Matsuzaki Y, Tanaka N, Osugo T, et al. Am J Gastroenterol 1990;85:15–23.

Six of seven patients treated with ursodeoxycholic acid 600 mg three times a day improved after 1 month of treatment.

Long-term efficacy of sertraline as a treatment for cholestatic pruritus in patients with primary biliary cirrhosis. Browning J, Combes B, Mayo MJ. Am J Gastroenterol 2003;98:2736–41.

A retrospective report of 40 patients enrolled in a prospective study to examine the efficacy of ursodeoxycholic acid in patients with primary biliary cirrhosis. These patients kept itch diaries during the study. Ten patients, seven with itch, were started on sertraline for depression by their primary care providers. Six of seven patients with itch improved significantly on sertraline and were able to discontinue other medications.

Role of S-adenosyl-L-methionine in the treatment of intrahepatic cholestasis. Almasio P, Bortolini M, Pagliaro L, Coltorti M. Drugs 1990;40(suppl 3):111–23.

In four clinical trials involving a total of 639 patients with cholestasis due to acute or chronic liver disease, S-adenosyl-L-methionine in an intravenous dose of 800 mg daily or an oral regimen of 1.6 g daily for 2 weeks was superior to placebo in relieving pruritus.

Relief of idiopathic generalized pruritus in dialysis patients treated with activated oral charcoal. Pederson JA, Matter BJ, Czerwinski AW, Llach F. Ann Intern Med 1980;93:446–8.

Oral charcoal 6 g daily for 8 weeks improved pruritus in ten of 11 hemodialysis patients in this double-blind, placebo-controlled, crossover study.

Cholestyramine in uraemic pruritus. Silverberg DS, Iaina A, Reisin E, et al. Br Med J 1977;1:752–3.

This randomized, placebo-controlled, double-blind study showed cholestyramine 5 g twice daily for 4 weeks improved pruritus in four of five study patients.

Randomised crossover trial of naltrexone in uraemic pruritus. Peer G, Kivity S, Agami O, Fireman E, et al. Lancet 1996;348:1552–4.

Naltrexone 50 mg per day by mouth was given to 15 hemodialysis patients with severe resistant pruritus. The median pruritus scores at the end of the naltrexone treatment were significantly lower than before treatment.

THIRD LINE THERAPIES

Generalized pruritus	
■ Thalidomide	C
Cholestatic pruritus	
■ UVB phototherapy	E
■ Extracorporeal albumin dialysis	D
■ Plasmapheresis	D
■ Dronabinol	E
Uremic pruritus	
■ Thalidomide	A
■ Parathyroidectomy	B

Antipruritic action of thalidomide. Daly BM, Shuster S. Acta Derm Venereol 2000;80:24–5.

The effect of thalidomide on itch was studied in 11 patients with chronic pruritus. Itch was decreased by thalidomide 200 mg on the two nights it was given.

Phototherapy for primary biliary cirrhosis. Perlstein SL. Arch Dermatol 1981;117:608.

A case report of two patients with improvement of pruritus treated with weekly UVB phototherapy.

Extracorporeal albumin dialysis: a procedure for prolonged relief of intractable pruritus in patients with primary biliary cirrhosis. Pares A, Cisneros L, Salmeron JM, et al. Am J Gastroenterol 2004;99:1105–10.

Four patients with primary biliary cirrhosis and severe pruritus were treated with two 7-hour sessions, 1 day apart. Two patients had complete resolution of pruritus and the remaining two patients had a marked decrease in pruritus scores. Long-term remission was obtained in two of the four patients.

Role of plasmapheresis in primary biliary cirrhosis. Cohen LB, Ambinder EP, Wolke AM et al. Gut 1985;26:291–4.

Five patients with intractable pruritus had rapid and sustained improvement while receiving plasmapheresis.

Preliminary observation with dronabinol in patients with intractable pruritus secondary to cholestatic liver disease. Neff GW, O'Brien CB, Reddy KR, et al. Am J Gastroenterol 2002;97:2117–9.

Three patients given dronabinol, a cannabinoid, 5 mg at bedtime reported a decrease in pruritus, marked improvement in sleep, and were able to return to work. The duration of effect was noted to be 4–6 h and more frequent dosing may be needed.

Thalidomide for the treatment of uremic pruritus: a crossover randomized double-blind trial. Silva SR, Viana PC, Lugon NV, et al. Nephron 1994;67:270–3.

Twenty-nine patients in this study were assigned to receive thalidomide or placebo at bedtime for 7 days. After a washout period of 7 days, drugs were crossed over. Over half of the patients had a greater than 50% reduction in pruritus while on thalidomide.

A study on pruritus after parathyroidectomy for secondary hyperparathyroidism. Chou F, Ji-Chen H, Shun-Chen H, Shyr-Ming S. J Am Coll Surg 2000;190:65–70.

Thirty-seven dialysis patients with secondary hyperparathyroidism underwent parathyroidectomy. Twenty-two patients had pruritus prior to parathyroidectomy, and in those patients with itch, pruritus scores improved significantly. This was accompanied by improvement in the calcium–phosphorus product.

Pruritus ani

Gabriele Weichert

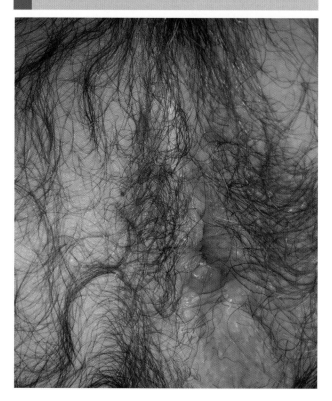

Pruritus ani is a chronic idiopathic intensely pruritic sensation of perianal skin. Longstanding cases are associated with significant discomfort, embarrassment, agitation, and sleep disturbance. Chronic primary pruritus ani is characterized clinically by lichenification and excoriations of the perianal area in the absence of primary skin disorders, infections, or neoplasia.

MANAGEMENT STRATEGY

In evaluating a patient with perianal itch, any contributing primary skin disorders must be identified. These may include atopic dermatitis, psoriasis, or lichen sclerosis. Neoplasia, hemorrhoids, and anal fissures should be ruled out. Infectious etiologies such as genital warts, tinea, candidiasis, infestations (e.g. pinworms, scabies), and bacterial infections (e.g. β-hemolytic streptococcus) must be ruled out with clinical examination and laboratory sampling (potassium hydroxide [KOH], bacterial culture swab, skin scrapings) if necessary. With this approach, most causes of acute or secondary pruritus ani can be identified and treated with directed therapy. It is the patient in whom none of the above factors are identified who has chronic or idiopathic pruritus ani. Patient history may reveal atopy or sensitive skin, leading to an increased itch sensation from all causes. Management history may reveal a sensitizer causing a degree of contact dermatitis. Overcleansing is not uncommon and may be irritating. Many of these patients have low-grade fecal incontinence. This is often evident on examination of the underclothes or of the perianal skin. A history of sleep disturbance may be revealed and can be the most frustrating aspect for many patients.

Management should include *discontinuation of any irritating topical treatments or overzealous cleansing routines*. Potential topical sensitizers should be stopped. A biopsy should be performed if the diagnosis is in doubt. Avoidance of toilet paper to cleanse the area after bowel movements can be helpful because toilet paper may be abrasive. Patients are instructed to *cleanse the perianal* skin twice a day and after bowel movements with cotton balls or cotton squares (such as those sold in pharmacies to remove facial make-up) moistened with warm water or a liquid cleanser. Patients identified with low-grade fecal incontinence should perform this cleansing routine several times a day. A regular cleansing routine has been shown to be as effective as topical corticosteroids. A short few-week course of a *mid-potency corticosteroid* is recommended. Caution must be taken with prolonged high-potency corticosteroid use because the perianal skin is prone to atrophy. Potency should be reduced as the symptoms improve. Corticosteroid *combined with lidocaine* (a rare allergen) have also been reported to be helpful compared to controls. *Topical zinc paste* can limit the degree of irritant dermatitis in patients with fecal incontinence. If a patient fails to improve, anoscopy, proctosigmoidoscopy or colonoscopy should be considered to rule out neoplastic disease. Patch testing should be performed in patients who continue to use potential allergens. Avoidance of caffeine and increased dietary fiber may be helpful.

Second line therapies include a double cycle of *cryotherapy* or *topical capsaicin* 0.006% three times a day for 4 weeks. Capsaicin will cause perianal irritation in most patients during the therapy. Finally, *intralesional corticosteroid injections* to the perianal skin may be considered. *Intradermal methylene blue* injections are reported to damage dermal nerve ending and provide relief. *Injection with phenol in almond oil* has been reported. *Hypnosis* may be helpful if all else fails.

SPECIFIC INVESTIGATIONS

- Mycology
- Bacterial swab
- Fungal culture
- Biopsy
- Skin scrapings for scabies
- Patch testing
- Gastrointestinal investigations

Allergic contact dermatitis in patients with anogenital complaints. Bauer A, Geier J, Elsner P. J Reprod Med 2000; 45:649–54.

A 5-year collection of patients patch tested for consideration of allergic anogenital contact dermatitis demonstrated an increased incidence of benzocaine and (chloro-)-methyl-isothiazolinone allergy. Among 1008 patients, a diagnosis of allergic contact dermatitis was made in 34.8%. The authors recommend using the standard tray plus dibucaine, propolis, bufexamac, and other ingredients gained from the patient's history.

Treatment of persistent pruritus ani in a combined colorectal and dermatological clinic. Dasan S, Neill SM, Donaldson DR, et al. Br J Surg 1999;86:1337–40.

In a series of 40 patients with pruritus ani, 34 had recognizable dermatoses and 18 had a positive patch test result. The authors suggest early assessment by a dermatologist may be appropriate.

Abnormal transient internal sphincter relaxation in idiopathic pruritus ani: physiological evidence from ambulatory monitoring. Forouk R, Duthie GS, Pryde A, et al. Br J Surg 1994;81:603–6.

Abnormal rectal sphincter tone was demonstrated in patients with pruritus ani. This may well be the contributing factor in patients who have occult fecal leakage as a component of their itch.

Pruritus ani. Causes and concerns. Daniel GL, Longo WE, Vernava AM. Dis Colon Rectum 1994;37:670–4.

In this series of 104 patients presenting with pruritus ani as their primary symptom, 52% had anorectal disease (including hemorrhoids, anal fissures, genital warts, and fistulas) and 23% had an existing colorectal or anorectal neoplasm found with investigations. In those without neoplasia, there was a direct correlation between increased caffeine intake and severity of irritation. Patients with primary pruritus ani improved with dietary restrictions (not defined), dietary fiber, corticosteroid creams, and drying agents.

FIRST LINE TREATMENT

■ Hygiene	B
■ Topical corticosteroids	B
■ Topical corticosteroids plus topical anesthetic	A

Idiopathic perianal pruritus: washing compared with topical corticosteroids. Oztas MO, Oztas P, Onder M. Postgrad Med J 2004;80;295–7.

In this study, 28 patients applied topical methylprednisolone cream twice daily for 2 weeks. In a separate group, 32 patients were instructed to cleanse the perianal area twice daily with a liquid cleanser. Effectiveness was similar at 92.3% in the first and 90.6% in the second group (p > 0.05).

Perinal – a new no touch spray to relieve the symptoms of pruritus ani. Allenby CF, Johnstone RS, Chatfield LC, et al. Int J Coloret Dis 1993; 8:184–7.

Twenty-five patients enrolled in a double-blind placebo-controlled crossover study used two to three 0.1 mL sprays of an aqueous solution of 0.2% hydrocortisone and 1% lidocaine for one week. Seventeen of the 23 (p < 0.05) patients who completed the study preferred the active treatment and had a significant decrease in visual analogue pruritus scales.

SECOND LINE TREATMENT

■ Topical capsaicin	A
■ Cryotherapy	C

Topical capsaicin – a novel and effective treatment for idiopathic intractable pruritus ani: a randomised, placebo controlled, crossover study. Lysy J, Sistiery-Ittah M, Israelit Y, et al. Gut 2003;52:1323–6.

In this double-blind placebo-controlled crossover study, capsaicin 0.006% cream was applied three times daily for 1 month followed by 1 month of control treatment using 1% menthol cream; 31 of 44 patients experienced partial relief of symptoms while using the capsaicin cream (p < 0.0001). All patients experienced some degree of perianal burning with capsaicin cream. The menthol cream was not effective.

Note that the strength of the capsaicin cream is lower than that of some of the commercially available preparations.

Cryotherapy for chronic non-specific pruritus ani. Detrano SJ. J Dermatol Surg Oncol 1984;10:483–4.

Eighteen patients were treated with two cycles of cryotherapy lasting 2–3 s; 15 of 18 patients had reduced itch after several months of follow-up. Minor transient itch persisted.

THIRD LINE TREATMENT

■ Intralesional corticosteroid	C
■ Intradermal methylene blue	B
■ Subcutaneous phenol injection	B
■ Hypnotherapy	E

The use of intralesional triamcinolone hexacetonide in the treatment of idiopathic pruritus ani. Minvielle L, Hernandez VL. Dis Colon Rectum 1969;12:340–3.

Nineteen patients were treated weekly for 4 weeks with intralesional triamcinolone at doses of 5–20 mg per week. At the end of the treatment period, 14 of 19 (73.6%) patients had excellent progress, while two reported fair improvement, and three failed to improve. No perianal atrophy was noted at the end of 4 weeks.

Intradermal methylene blue injection for the treatment of intractable idiopathic pruritus ani: results of 30 cases. Mentes BB, Akin M, Leventoglu S, et al. Tech Coloproctol 2004;8:11–4.

In this series, 30 patients were treated with a 15 mL injection of 1% methylene blue to the perianal area. One month later, 24 patients (80%) were symptom free. Four of five partial responders had complete relief with a second injection. After 12 months of follow-up, 23 patients (76.7%) continued to be symptom free.

Methylene blue has been shown by electron microscopy to cause damage to dermal nerve endings. This is the proposed mechanism of action for this modality.

Intra-dermal methylene blue, hydrocortisone and lignocaine for chronic, intractable pruritus ani. Botterill ID, Sagar PM. Colorectal Dis 2002;4:144–6.

Twenty-five patients were treated with perianal injection of 5 mL of 1% methylene blue, 100 mg of hydrocortisone, and 15 mL of lidocaine. After one injection, 16 of 25 (64%) reported symptom relief. Repeat injection in nonresponders led to a total response rate in 22 of the 25 (88%) patients. Three patients failed to respond.

A new concept of the anatomy of the anal sphincter mechanism and the physiology of defecation. XXIII. An injection technique for the treatment of idiopathic pruritus ani. Shafik A. Int Surg 1990;75:43–6.

In this series, 67 patients were treated with an injection of 5% phenol in almond oil; 62 of the 67 (92.5%) experienced complete relief. Five patients relapsed after a period of remission. Repeat injection led to cure.

Hypnosis in a case of long-standing idiopathic itch. Rucklidge JJ, Saunders D. Psychosom Med 1999;61:355–8.

One patient with longstanding vaginal and anal itch unresponsive to standard treatments improved after receiving training in self-hypnosis.

Pruritus vulvae

Ginat Mirowski, Neda Ashourian

Pruritus vulvae is an external sensation of itching that results in a need to scratch or rub the affected vulvar region. Over time the skin becomes lichenified, and occasionally excoriations and pigmentary changes occur. Pruritus vulvae may be primary, or secondary to infections, malignancy, a wide number of dermatoses, and a number of neurologic conditions, or may be multifactorial. Essential pruritus vulvae is the condition in which no primary etiology can be identified.

MANAGEMENT STRATEGY

Pruritus vulvae describes a symptom, not a specific disorder. Pruritus vulvae, in addition to the physical discomfort, may be both psychologically distressing and socially embarrassing. Symptomatic relief is a priority. The tenet of treatment is to break the itch–scratch cycle, restore the damaged barrier layer, and reduce inflammation.

An *underlying etiology should be sought* by obtaining a thorough history and physical exam. The differential diagnosis includes infections, dermatoses, systemic diseases, and malignant and premalignant lesions (Table 1). Appropriate treatment should be instituted when a specific etiology is found, and an adequate course of therapy should be initiated before determining treatment failure.

The mainstay in treatment of pruritus vulvae is to identify and *remove all potential local irritants*. The patient should be instructed to discontinue all local products including soaps, sanitary pads, over-the-counter (OTC) medications, and occlusive/synthetic clothing. The patient should bathe with water only, pad dry, keep the vulva dry, wipe front to back, change underpants daily and rinse them twice after washing. Many patients will be resistant to this because they may believe that they must maintain a 'clean' vulvar region and that natural secretions and odors are offensive and 'unclean'. The patient may have developed elaborate home regimens that contribute to local irritation and contact sensitivity. This may complicate or be the primary cause of a persistent pruritus. Toilet (tissue) paper and commercial wipes should be avoided because their use may contribute to irritation, especially when used to rub or scratch the area. Both may contain allergens such as formaldehyde and fragrances. Urine, stool, and excessive cervical or vaginal secretions may contribute to local irritation. Efforts to treat urinary incontinence and to limit contact with stool (i.e. stool bulking agents and the use of fragrance-free tampons) may be helpful. (Note that bacterial vaginosis must be ruled out by culture prior to initiating the use of tampons.) Cotton washcloths may be used to clean the area. Cool water or Sitz baths are recommended to clean the perineum after urination and defecation. Sitz baths also help restore the normal skin barrier.

The frequent use of *barrier and zinc-based ointments* typically used to prevent diaper rash helps to seal in moisture and protect the affected skin. In low estrogen states, the use of *topical estrogen* may be indicated to restore normal skin.

Systemic or topical corticosteroids are used to reduce inflammation. Topical preparations may contribute to an allergic or irritant contact dermatitis. When topical agents are to be used, ointment-based products, which typically do not contain preservatives, are preferred because they are less likely to contain allergens or irritants. Topical corticosteroid ointment, used sparingly, should be applied once or twice a day. Use of systemic agents to treat infections and for the symptomatic relief of pruritus will limit secondary complications. *Subcutaneous (intralesional) triamcinolone acetonide* injection and systemic corticosteroids are effective for recalcitrant pruritus.

Although corticosteroids decrease pruritus while reducing inflammation, they are often not sufficient to break the itch–scratch cycle. Nightly *antihistamines* such as *hydroxyzine* or *doxepin* are recommended. For daytime pruritus a *low-dose selective serotonin reuptake inhibitor (SSRI)* is more effective than non-drowsy antihistamines.

The use of *intradermal alcohol injection* to treat recalcitrant cases is not advocated. This procedure requires general anesthesia and there is a risk of cellulitis and tissue sloughing. There are no recent data on this procedure and it is no longer recommended. For severe or refractory pruritus vulvae, CO_2 *laser* and the *Mering procedure*, used to partially denervate the area, provide relief of symptoms. *Psychotherapy, acupuncture*, and *hypnosis* are noninvasive methods that have demonstrated efficacy.

Table 1

Type of disorder	Examples
Infections	Candida albicans
	Trichomonas vaginalis
	Group B streptococci
	Enterobius vermicularis
	Phthirius pubis
	Sarcoptes scabiei
	Tinea cruris
	Human papillomavirus
	Herpes simplex virus
	Chlamydia trachomatis
	Gardenella vaginalis
	Neisseria gonorrhoeae
	Corynebacterium minutissimum
	Human immunodeficiency virus
Dermatoses	Allergic contact dermatitis
	Allergic irritant dermatitis
	Atopic dermatitis
	Psoriasis
	Lichen planus
	Seborrheic dermatitis
	Lichen sclerosus et atrophicus
	Fox–Fordyce disease
	Lichen simplex chronicus
	Desquamative inflammatory vaginitis
	Fixed drug eruption
	Estrogen deficiency
	Hypothyroidism
	Sjögren's syndrome
	Syringomas
Systemic diseases	Diabetes mellitus
	Hepatic failure
	Renal failure
	Polycythemia vera
Malignant and premalignant	Squamous cell carcinoma
	Lymphoma
	Vulvar intraepithelial neoplasia
	Bowen's disease
	Extramammary Paget's

Evidence levels **A** Double-blind study **B** Clinical trial ≥ 20 subjects **C** Clinical trial < 20 subjects **D** Series ≥ 5 subjects **E** Anecdotal case reports

SPECIFIC INVESTIGATIONS

- Clinical visual and manual examination of the vulva, vagina, and mucocutaneous integument including scalp and nails
- Direct smear of vaginal secretions (*T. vaginalis*, bacterial vaginosis)
- Whiff test (bacterial vaginosis)
- Potassium hydroxide (fungi, infestation)
- Tape test (*E. vermicularis*)
- Microbiologic cultures (bacteria, fungi, viral)
- Serologic tests (fasting blood glucose, liver/renal/thyroid function)
- Biopsy (hematoxylin and eosin, immunofluorescence)
- Patch testing

Pruritus vulvae: a five-year survey. Pumpianske R, Sheskin J. Dermatologica 1965;131:446–51.

This is an older study that reports the etiology of pruritus vulvae in 1104 gynecologic patients. Nine hundred and forty six (85%) had either candidiasis or *T. vaginalis* infection. Other etiologies, each present in less than 2% of cases, included allergic reactions, kraurosis vulvae, leukoplakia, premenstrual tension, neurodermatitis, and *E. vermicularis* infection.

The prevalence and clinical diagnosis of vaginal candidosis in non-pregnant patients with vaginal discharge and pruritus vulvae. Wright HJ, Palmer A. J R Coll Gen Pract 1978;28:719–23.

Seventeen (45%) of 38 women with pruritus vulvae were diagnosed with *C. albicans* infection. Yeast was not identified in the other patients, and the etiology of their symptoms was not reported.

Pruritus in diabetes mellitus: investigation of prevalence and correlation with diabetes. Neilly JB, Martin A, Simpson N, MacCuish AC. Diabetes Care 1986;9:273–5.

Three hundred diabetic and 100 nondiabetic outpatients were evaluated for the presence of generalized and localized pruritus. Pruritus vulvae, the most common symptom, was noted in 18.4% of diabetic women. This was significant ($p < 0.05$), because only 5.6% of nondiabetic women had pruritus vulvae. Symptoms correlated with glycosylated hemoglobin.

The study suggested that diabetes mellitus should be considered in the differential diagnosis of pruritus vulvae.

Vulvar intraepithelial neoplasia with superficially invasive carcinoma of the vulva. Herod JJ, Shafi MI, Rollason TP, et al. Br J Obstet Gynecol 1996;103:453–6.

In this retrospective study of 26 women with vulvar intraepithelial neoplasia (VIN), pruritus vulvae, the most common symptom, was present in 18 of them (69%).

This study suggested that VIN should be considered in patients with pruritus vulvae.

Contact sensitivity in pruritus vulvae: patch test results and clinical outcomes. Lewis FM, Shah M, Gawkrodger DJ. Am J Contact Dermatitis 1997;8:137–40.

Patch testing was used to evaluate 121 women with pruritus vulvae. Fifty seven (47%) had one or more relevant reactions. Common allergens identified included medica-

tions and components of medications including preservatives, lanolins, quinolone, benzocaine, and fragrances.

Patients with a relevant allergy were significantly ($p < 0.001$) more likely to improve than those without an allergy.

Contact dermatitis of the vulvae. Margesson LJ. Dermatol Ther 2004;17:20–7.

A comprehensive review of common vulvar irritants and their treatments.

FIRST LINE THERAPIES

■ Avoidance of irritants	E
■ Hygiene	E
■ Topical corticosteroids	B
■ Topical estrogen	E

Pruritus vulvae and its treatment with fluocinolone acetonide. Fleckner AN, Anderson C, Yeransian J, et al. J Am Med Womens Assoc 1967;22:460–1.

A series of 65 patients with pruritus vulvae were treated with topical fluocinolone acetonide. Fifty six patients had complete relief of symptoms in 2 days. The six patients who relapsed all responded to a second course of topical corticosteroid.

The treatment of vulvar lichen sclerosus with a very potent topical steroid (clobetasol propionate 0.05%) cream. Dalziel KL, Millard PR, Wojnarowska F. Br J Dermatol 1991;124:461–4.

A series of 13 patients with lichen sclerosus were treated with clobetasol propionate 0.05% cream to determine efficacy. All 13 patients showed marked clinical improvement after 12 weeks of therapy.

Local steroid application for hyperplastic dystrophy of the vulva. Bergman A, Karram M, Bhatia NN. J Reprod Med 1988;33:542–4.

Fifteen patients with pruritus vulvae secondary to hyperplastic dystrophy of the vulva were treated with 0.1% halocidine and crotamiton cream daily. Thirteen (85%) experienced complete relief of symptoms in 6 weeks. The remaining two patients required an additional 3 months of therapy to achieve complete clinical relief.

The common problem of vulvar pruritus. Bornstein J, Pascal B, Abramovici H. Obstet Gynecol Surv 1993;48:111–8.

The authors of this treatment review article recommend stopping use of all soaps, douches, and perfumed deodorants, keeping the vulvar area dry, wearing cotton underpants, and avoiding tight pants as basic principles in the treatment of pruritus vulvae.

Vulvovaginal dryness and itching. Margesson LJ. Skin Therapy Lett 2001;6:3–4.

Author reviews the vulvar signs of estrogen deficiency and offers treatment options.

Pruritus vulvae in prepubertal children. Paek SC, Merritt DF, Mallory SB. J Am Acad Dermatol 2001;44:795–802.

Review of the causes and treatments of vulvar pruritus in prepubertal girls by retrospective evaluation of 44 records; 75% had nonspecific pruritus while lichen sclerosus, bacterial infections, yeast infection, and pinworm infestation were seen in a minority of patients. The authors conclude that in prepubertal girls, poor hygiene and irritants are major contributors to pruritus vulvae.

An approach to the treatment of anogenital pruritus. Weichert GE. Dermatol Ther 2004;17:129–33.

A review of the common causes of acute and chronic anogenital pruritus with a focus on vulvar pruritus. Therapeutic approach to the management of pruritus vulvae in the absence of a clear cause is discussed.

Lichen simplex chronicus (atopic/neurodermatitis) of the anogenital region. Lynch P. Dermatol Ther 2004;17:8–19.

This paper suggests diagnostic tips and differential diagnosis for vulvar lichen simplex chronicus (LSC). The management of LSC is divided into four categories: identification of any underlying disease, repair of the barrier layer function, reduction of inflammation, and break of the itch–scratch cycle. Treatment options for each category are discussed.

SECOND LINE THERAPIES

■ Subcutaneous triamcinolone	B
■ Topical antihistamine	A

Subcutaneous injection of triamcinolone acetonide in the treatment of chronic vulvar pruritus. Kelly RA, Foster DC, Woodruff JD. Am J Obstet Gynecol 1993;169:568–70.

Forty five patients with chronic pruritus vulvae were treated with subcutaneous intralesional injection of triamcinolone acetonide into the vulva. Thirty five experienced relief of vulvar pruritus for more than 1 month (mean 5.8 months).

Efficacy of topical oxatomide in women with pruritus vulvae. Origoni M, Garsia S, Sideri M, et al. Drugs Exp Clin Res 1990;16:591–6.

Double-blind, controlled European study to determine the efficacy of topical oxatomide, an antihistamine not currently available in the USA, in treating pruritus vulvae. The drug was under experimental clinical research. All 29 patients reported improvement in both the intensity and duration of itching. Seven patients experienced complete regression. These results were statistically significant ($p < 0.001$) compared to placebo.

THIRD LINE THERAPIES

■ Intradermal alcohol injection	A
■ Surgery	D
■ CO_2 laser	D
■ Psychotherapy	C
■ Acupuncture	D
■ Hypnosis	E

Treatment of pruritus vulvae by multiple intradermal injections of alcohol. A double-blind study. Sutherst JR. Br J Obstet Gynecol 1979;86:371–3.

A double-blind controlled study reports on the efficacy of intradermal alcohol injections in the treatment of pruritus vulvae. Fourteen of 17 patients reported complete relief of pruritus only on the side treated with alcohol. Pruritus persisted on the placebo-treated side. Treatment with alcohol was significantly better than placebo ($p < 0.05$).

Local alcohol injection in the treatment of vulvar pruritus. Woodruff JD, Thompson B. Obstet Gynecol 1972;40:18–20.

A series of 30 patients with noninfectious longstanding pruritus vulvae were treated with intradermal alcohol injection. All patients had relief of symptoms for at least 4–6 months. Relief persisted beyond 6 months in 80% of patients.

Pruritus vulvae: treatment by multiple intradermal alcohol injections. Ward GD, Sutherst JR. Br J Dermatol 1975;93:201–4.

Twenty five patients with pruritus vulvae were treated with intradermal alcohol injections. Nineteen patients were cured or had marked symptomatic improvement.

A surgical approach to intractable pruritus vulvae. Mering JH. Am J Obstet Gynecol 1952;64:619–27.

A series of 16 women with intractable pruritus vulvae were surgically treated with the Mering procedure (wide undermining of the skin of the vulva, vaginal mucous membranes, and anus). Fifteen patients had immediate relief of symptoms of pruritus. No recurrence was reported at 3 months to 3 years follow-up.

Treatment of pruritus vulvae by means of CO_2 laser. Ovadia J, Levavi H, Edelstein T. Acta Obstet Gynecol Scand 1984;63:265–7.

Four of five women with pruritus vulvae treated with CO_2 laser experienced complete relief of pruritus. The fifth patient had considerable symptomatic improvement.

The diagnosis and treatment of psychosomatic vulvovaginitis. Woodward J. Practitioner 1981;225:1673–7.

Ninety two patients with symptoms of vulvovaginitis and normal physical exam, cytology, and swabs were treated with psychotherapy. Eighty (87%) had complete relief or improvement of symptoms.

56 cases of chronic pruritus vulvae treated with acupuncture. Huang WY, Guo ZR, Yu J, Hu XL. J Tradit Chin Med 1987;7:1–3.

Fifty four of 56 patients with intractable pruritus vulvae experienced symptomatic and clinical improvement with one to seven sessions of acupuncture.

Hypnosis in a case of long-standing idiopathic itch. Rucklidge JJ, Saunders D. Psychosom Med 1999;61:355–8.

This is a case report of a single patient with longstanding pruritus vulvae and ani. She experienced complete relief of symptoms with training in self-hypnosis.

Evidence levels A Double-blind study **B** Clinical trial ≥ 20 subjects **C** Clinical trial < 20 subjects **D** Series ≥ 5 subjects **E** Anecdotal case reports

Pseudofolliculitis barbae

Gary J Brauner

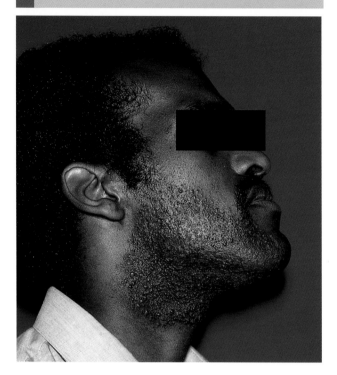

Pseudofolliculitis barbae (PFB) is a chronic inflammatory disease of hair-bearing areas induced by shaving or plucking of curved hairs with resultant transepithelial or transfollicular penetration by the sharpened hair remnant and a foreign body reaction. It is characterized clinically by papules, papulopustules, focal or diffuse postinflammatory hyperpigmentation, growth grooves, and rarely hypertrophic or keloidal scarring.

MANAGEMENT STRATEGY

Because this process is induced by shaving its cure is simple: by not shaving or plucking at all and allowing the hairs to grow to beyond 1 cm in length the disease will spontaneously involute. If a clean shaven appearance is preferred or deemed necessary by occupational or social demands, management involves three elements:

- *Extraction of the foreign body* by lifting of the embedded distal sharpened ends of hairs.
- *Prevention of further embedding* by proper shaving technique or permanent disruption of the follicle's ability to produce new hair.
- *Treatment of postinflammatory hyperpigmentation* or hypertrophic scarring.

Embedded hairs should be *lifted* not plucked just prior to shaving. A safety razor set on its 'gentlest' setting or a preadjusted razor such as the PFB Bumpfighter™ should be used, but with the *opposite hand kept off the face* to prevent skin stretching. Shaving is performed in the direction of hair growth not against the direction, again to prevent too close shaving and transfollicular penetration. A *long presoak* with

a hot wet facecloth will allow hairs to swell and lift; a shaving cream that lathers and holds well will keep those hairs saturated and elevated. Shaving must be performed daily; by 2–3 days of no shaving transepidermal re-entry penetration will occur. If morning shaving is routine, the affected areas should be gently *buffed* or brushed the evening before with a toothbrush, rough dry washcloth, or a Buf Puf™ to loosen hairs about to embed.

Hair clippers will cut hair closely but not so close as to allow transfollicular penetration. Because razor shaving is much closer clippers should be used at least twice daily to avoid a permanent '5 o'clock shadow'.

Powder chemical depilatories are not practical. They are messy to use, hard to mix accurately, difficult to remove rapidly, and, because they are so irritating, can not be used more than every 3 days, which already allows PFB to recur. Lotion depilatories are much easier to apply and remove and, being less irritant, can be used every 2 days to produce a satisfactory cosmetic appearance.

Antibiotics are not necessary topically because this is a sterile foreign body reaction not a pyoderma. Irritants such as *retinoic acid* or *glycolic acid* may enhance lifting of hairs and diminish hyperpigmentation.

Several longer wavelength long pulsed *lasers* (alexandrite, 810 nm diode, and Nd:YAG) in combination with epidermal protective chilling devices can be used to produce dramatic longlasting remission, even in Fitzpatrick types IV, V, and VI patients, and represent a breakthrough treatment for recalcitrant disease.

SPECIFIC INVESTIGATIONS

- Skin biopsy in rare instances
- K6hf gene analysis

No investigations are necessary for usual cases of PFB. Because it is induced by hair manipulation (i.e. shaving or plucking) it is not associated with other diseases. Differentiation of true bacterial folliculitis, requiring systemic antibiotics, must sometimes be considered. Rarely, yeast folliculitis may mimic PFB. Careful clinical inspection and possibly skin biopsy should be performed to rule out granulomatous disease such as sarcoidosis or dental sinusitis in the presence of apparently hypertrophic or keloidal scars. Rarely, cyclosporine (ciclosporin) therapy may induce a pseudofolliculitis-like condition. Recent French literature cites necrotic folliculitis-like lesions and pathergy as common cutaneous presentations of Behçet's syndrome; this 'pseudofolliculitis' is not the PFB of ingrowing hairs.

Scar sarcoidosis in pseudofolliculitis barbae. Norton S, Chesser R, Fitzpatrick J. Mil Med 1991;156:369–71.

A man with hilar adenopathy had smooth firm purplish papules (lupus pernio) on his face and PFB in his beard area. Biopsies of papules of both the lupus pernio and the PFB revealed noncaseating granulomas consistent with sarcoidosis.

Disseminated cryptococcosis presenting as pseudofolliculitis in an AIDS patient. Coker L, Swain R, Morris R, McCall C. Cutis 2000;66:207–10.

A 42-year-old African-American man with AIDS had countless dome-shaped excoriated papules of his trunk, arms and face initially diagnosed as folliculitis (not pseudofolliculitis of ingrowing hairs) with biopsy-proven disseminated cutaneous cryptococcosis.

Hyperplastic pseudofolliculitis barbae associated with cyclosporin. Lear J, Bourke JF, Burns DA. Br J Dermatol 1997;136:132–3.

A condition resembling keloid reactions in PFB is reported as an unusual reaction to cyclosporine.

An unusual Ala12Thr polymorphism in the 1A alpha-helical segment of the companion layer-specific keratin K6hf: evidence for a risk factor in the etiology of the common hair disorder pseudofolliculitis barbae. Winter H, Schissel D, Parry D, et al. J Invest Dermatol 2004;122:652–7. Comment in: J Invest Dermatol 2004;122:xi–xiii.

The authors identify a family with two curly-haired white males with PFB and one straight-haired non-PFB-afflicted female with an unusual dominantly inherited single-nucleotide polymorphism, which gives rise to a disruptive Ala12Thr substitution in the 1A alpha-helical segment of the companion layer-specific keratin K6hf of the hair follicle. In transfected cells this gene seems to be disruptive of filament assembly. A test group of 100 black people, 82% of whom had PFB, and 110 white people (a very high 18% of whom had PFB) showed this unusual gene in 9% of whites, but only 36% of blacks (97% of whom had PFB). The authors somehow conclude that this gene represents a significant genetic risk factor for PFB.

FIRST LINE THERAPIES

■ Beard growth	D
■ Razor shaving technique	D
■ Hair clippers	D
■ Chemical depilatories	D
■ Adjunctive hair extraction	D

Pseudofolliculitis of the beard. Strauss J, Kligman A. Arch Dermatol Syphilol 1956;74:533–42.

The first modern description of the pathogenesis of this disease and the rationale for allowing beard growth and spontaneous involution.

Pseudofolliculitis barbae. Medical consequences of interracial friction in the US Army. Brauner G, Flandermeyer K. Cutis 1979;23:61–6.

PFB is a minor disease affecting only, and almost all, black people who shave. Because of a continued requirement by the US Army of clean shaven faces, significant interracial turmoil and animosity has been aroused. Unclear standards of care of the disease and haphazard policing of shaving habits led to a chaotic process with effective dermatologic care almost paralyzed by the hostile parties. During the Vietnam War era randomly approached lower-ranking enlistees and draftees were much more likely to complain about their disease, even if minor, and were more likely to refuse to shave and be unkempt even without permission to grow a beard (in contravention of Army regulations). Career black enlistees are likely to underreport the severity of their disease and not seek medical help, possibly because of fear of continuous harassment and inability to be promoted by their superiors. Lotion depilatories or hair clippers, combined with routine lifting of ingrown hairs, are the most effective treatments, though complete cessation of shaving is required first.

Pseudofolliculitis barbae. 2. Treatment. Brauner G, Flandermeyer K. Int J Dermatol 1977;16:520–5.

The disease can be cured only by complete cessation of shaving, but it can be adequately controlled in most patients by carefully shaving the hairs neither too close nor too long and by meticulous lifting out of penetrating hairs.

A variety of practical methods of shaving are described in detail.

The causes and treatment of pseudofolliculitis barbae. Crutchfield C. Cutis 1998;61:351–6.

A systematic empiric approach to treatment is given in tabular form.

Pseudofolliculitis barbae and related disorders. Halder R. Dermatol Clin 1988;6:407–12.

Not all regimens will work for each patient. This thorough review discusses beards, triple 'O' electric clippers, chemical depilatories, safety razors including the foil-guarded system to reduce cutting edge, electric razors including the adjustable three-headed rotary razor, manual lifting of hairs, tretinoin lotion, electrolysis, and surgical depilation.

Pathogenesis and treatment of pseudofolliculitis barbae. Brown LA Jr. Cutis 1983;32:373–5.

Specific techniques involving the use of electric clippers, chemical depilatories, manual razors, and complete epilation are discussed. Adjuvant measures such as antibiotics and retinoic acid are presented.

Evaluation of a foil-guarded shaver in the management of pseudofolliculitis barbae. Alexander A. Cutis 1981;27: 534–7,540–2.

Pseudofolliculitis barbae. No 'pseudoproblem'. Conte M, Lawrence J. JAMA 1979;241:53–4.

Ninety six patients with PFB were evaluated and successfully treated by allowing a 30-day period of beard regrowth to eliminate ingrown hairs, twice-daily use of a new polyester skin-cleansing pad, and use of solely electric hair clippers for facial hair removal: 96% of those using this technique could thereafter conform to the Air Force grooming code.

Pseudofolliculitis barbae and acne keloidalis nuchae. Kelly A. Dermatol Clin 2003;21:645–53.

Concise review with good descriptions of various and specific shaving devices.

SECOND LINE THERAPIES

■ Retinoic acid	E
■ Glycolic acid	B
■ Topical clindamycin	A

Pseudofolliculitis of the beard and topically applied tretinoin. Kligman A, Mills O. Arch Dermatol 1973;107: 551–2.

Tretinoin solution is described as a useful adjunctive treatment.

Evidence levels A Double-blind study **B** Clinical trial ≥ 20 subjects **C** Clinical trial < 20 subjects **D** Series ≥ 5 subjects **E** Anecdotal case reports

Pseudofolliculitis – revised concepts of diagnosis and treatment. Report of three cases in women. Hall J, Goetz C, Bartholome C, Livingood C. Cutis 1979;23:798–800.

Three cases of pseudofolliculitis are described in black American women. Topical retinoic acid cream was useful in all three.

Pseudofolliculitis barbae. Chu T. Practitioner 1989;233: 307–9.

In a limited open study, 1% topical clindamycin was found anecdotally effective for pseudofolliculitis and acne keloidalis.

Twice-daily applications of benzoyl peroxide 5%/clindamycin 1% gel versus vehicle in the treatment of pseudofolliculitis barbae. Cook-Bolden F, Barba A, Halder R, Taylor S. Cutis 2004;73(6 suppl):18–24.

Seventy seven men with 16–100 combined papules and pustules on the face and neck were randomized to receive twice-daily benzoyl peroxide 5%/clindamycin 1% (BP/C) gel or vehicle for 10 weeks; 77.3% of the participants were black. All patients were required to shave at least twice a week with a disposable Bumpfighter™ razor and to use a standardized shaving regimen. At weeks 2, 4, and 6, mean percentage reductions from baseline in combined papule and pustule counts were statistically significantly greater with BP/C gel compared with vehicle, but for both were greater than 50% by 10 weeks, particularly in black men. There was a significant change in non-black men, but no difference between test and controls. Although 77% of test patients thought they were much better compared to 47% in the control vehicle group, the authors do not explain the remarkable improvement in the control group nor why nor how they assume their test product alone 'worked'.

Treatment of pseudofolliculitis barbae with topical glycolic acid: a report of two studies. Perricone N. Cutis 1993;52:232–5.

The studies consisted of two placebo-controlled trials in 35 adult men. The results showed that glycolic acid lotion was significantly more effective than placebo in treating PFB. There was a reduction of over 60% in lesions on the treated side, which allowed daily shaving with little irritation.

THIRD LINE THERAPIES

■ Laser depilation	B
■ Surgical depilation	C

Treatment of pseudofolliculitis barbae using the Q-switched Nd:YAG laser with topical carbon suspension. Rogers C, Glaser D. Dermatol Surg 2000;26:737–41.

Nine patients were given two treatments 1 month apart on the neck and mandible. Evaluation as long as 2 months after the last treatment showed a statistically significant decrease in number of papules and pustules compared to the control side.

Pseudofolliculitis of the neck and the shoulder: a new effective treatment with alexandrite laser. Valeriant M, Terracina F, Mezzana P. Plast Reconstr Surg 2002;110:1195–6.

Two Caucasian males with chronic folliculitis and pseudofolliculitis of neck and shoulders were treated with 790 nm alexandrite laser for 30 ms with 10 mm spot size and 16–18 J/cm² for four sessions at 6-week intervals. They had a hair loss of 60–70% and 90% improvement in PFB, which persisted during 1-year follow-up.

Laser treatment of pseudofolliculitis barbae. (Abstract) Kauvar A. Annual Meeting American Society for Dermatologic Surgery; 2 Nov 2000.

Ten subjects of skin types I–IV with PFB of beard, axilla, or bikini areas were treated with an 810 nm diode laser for 15–30 ms at 30–38 J/cm² with three laser treatments at 6–8-week intervals and were followed up 3 months after the last session. There was a hair growth delay of 3–4 weeks and more than 75% improvement of papules. Long pulse alexandrite laser was used in 19 patients with skin types I–IV with 3 ms bursts at 16–18 J/cm² with three laser treatments 6–8 weeks apart. All patients had more than 50% reduction in papules and pustules. There were no pigmentary changes and clinical remission was 6 months.

Treatment of pseudofolliculitis with a pulsed infrared laser. Kauvar A. Arch Dermatol 2000;136:1343–6.

Ten females with Fitzpatrick skin types III–V and a history of pseudofolliculitis on the face, axilla, or groin for at least 1 year had three consecutive treatments at 6–8-week intervals with an 810 nm diode laser and a chill tip at 30–38 J/cm² and 20 ms pulse duration. After their last visit all showed more than 75% improvement in the pseudofolliculitis and had a 50% reduction in hair growth. No blistering occurred.

Laser-assisted hair removal for darker skin types. Battle E, Hobbs L. Dermatol Ther 2004;17:177–83.

The authors carefully review the rationale for use of diode, especially long pulsed diode, and Nd:YAG lasers for highly pigmented patients, as well as testing, dosing, and cooling precautions to improve patient safety

Treatment of pseudofolliculitis barbae in skin types IV, V, and VI with a long-pulsed neodymium:yttrium aluminum garnet laser. Ross E, Cooke L, Timko A, et al. J Am Acad Dermatol 2002;47:263–70.

Thirty seven patients with pseudofolliculitis and Fitzpatrick skin types IV, V, and VI were tested with Nd:YAG laser. There was 33, 43, and 40% hair reduction on the thigh for the 50, 80, and 100 J/cm² fluences, respectively, after 90 days. The highest doses tolerated by the epidermis were 50, 100, and 100 J/cm² for type VI, V, and IV skin, respectively. After testing on the face mean papule counts after 90 days were 6.95 and 1.0 for the control vs treatment sites, respectively.

Treatment of pseudofolliculitis barbae using the long-pulse Nd:YAG laser on skin types V and VI. Weaver S, Sagaral E. Dermatol Surg 2003;29:1187–91.

Twenty subjects with Fitzpatrick type V and VI skin and PFB on the neck or mandible were given two 2 × 2 cm treatments with Nd:YAG laser and 10 mm spot size at 40–50 ms and 24–40 J/cm² 3–4 weeks apart and were assessed by photographic papule/pustule and hair counts at 1, 2, and 3 months after final treatment and compared to a neighboring untreated site. The 76–90% reduction in the number of papules/pustules was statistically significant. Hair reduction of 80% 1 month after testing diminished to 23% by 3 months. Although side effects were noted as transient and

PSEUDOFOLLICULITIS BARBAE

without blistering the two illustrated patients both show scarring.

Long-pulsed Nd:YAG laser-assisted hair removal in pigmented skin: a clinical and histologic evaluation. (Abstract) Alster T, Bryan H. Annual Meeting American Society for Dermatologic Surgery; 2 Nov 2000.

Twenty female patients with skin types IV–VI were treated by 3-monthly applications of long pulse Nd:YAG laser through a cooling disc at 50 ms with 40 J/cm^2 for the face, 45 J/cm^2 for the leg, and 50 J/cm^2 for the axilla. Prolonged hair loss and improvement of PFB held for 6 months after the last treatment, and were best in the axilla and least for the face.

Lasers in the military for cutaneous disease and wound healing. Ross E, Chhieng N. Dermatol Clin 1999;17:135–50, ix.

There are applications for lasers in dermatology in which there is special military relevance. These range from treatment of common diseases such as PFB to noninvasive identification of shrapnel injuries. The authors describe detailed rationale for the types of lasers potentially applicable to removal of deeply situated hair bulbs in medium to darkly pigmented patients.

Recalcitrant scarring follicular disorders treated by laser-assisted hair removal: a preliminary report. Chui C, Berger T, Price V, Zachary C. Dermatol Surg 1999;25:34–7.

Three patients with various scarring follicular disorders (dissecting cellulitis of the scalp, keratosis pilaris spinulosa decalvans, and PFB) were treated with the long pulse non-Q-switched ruby laser and noted improvement of their condition along with decreased hair growth in the treated area.

Surgical depilation for the treatment of pseudofolliculitis or local hirsutism of the face: experience in the first 40 patients. Hage J, Bouman F. Plast Reconstr Surg 1991; 88:446–51.

Forty patients, all but three of whom were Caucasian, were operated on over a 15-year period for local hirsutism in 24, pseudofolliculitis in 11, and beard growth in 12 transgender procedures. The skin of the affected areas was incised and everted in a dermal–subcutaneous plane and the hair bulbs were excised. Marked diminution of hair numbers occurred, but 15 patients required further electrolysis. Side effects were significant, with wound edge necrosis in eight, seroma or hematoma in eight, and significant subcutaneous scar formation in 15, which was later preventable by postoperative long-term (at least 3 months) pressure bandages. See also Comments in Plast Reconstr Surg 1992;90:332–3.

Pseudoxanthoma elasticum

Kenneth H Neldner

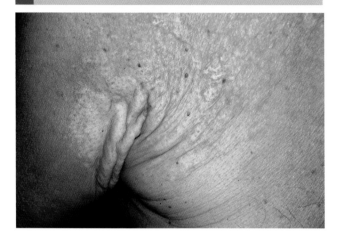

Pseudoxanthoma elasticum (PXE) is a rare, autosomal recessive, hereditary disorder of abnormal calcification of elastic fibers in the skin, retina, and cardiovascular system. Major clinical features include slightly thickened (leather-like) skin lesions in flexural sites, retinal angioid streaks and hemorrhages, with central vision loss. Central cardiac involvement is rare, but intermittent claudication in the peripheral vasculature is more common. Prevalence in the population is approximately one in 70 000. Longevity is usually unaffected. There is an unexplained approximately two to one predominance in females.

MANAGEMENT STRATEGY

Early management ideally begins when the first clinical signs appear as skin lesions on the lateral neck at age 12–15 years, which is also the time when the diagnosis can be made by skin biopsy. Retinal angioid streaks usually appear later, at about age 18–23 years. Retinal hemorrhages become common past the age of 40 years. Intermittent claudication in the legs may appear in the fourth decade, or beyond. Gastric hemorrhages can occur at any age in about 10–15% of the patients and may be severe enough to require blood transfusion.

It is important to recognize that PXE (as well as most hereditary disorders), although basically governed by genetic factors, has a number of controllable environmental factors that influence its natural course. General counseling of the patient and family should include the hereditary nature and general clinical course of PXE, and the nature and average age of onset of the complications. Discuss treatment options for complications and the long- and short-term prognosis.

The early management strategy of PXE is complicated by the fact that the diagnosis is often delayed for many years due to the rarity of the disorder and the fact that very few nondermatologist physicians are familiar with PXE. The effectiveness of most management programs is in direct proportion to the patient's age when they are started. Management includes *dietary calcium restriction*; *avoidance of tobacco*

and platelet inhibitors such as aspirin; *a heart-wise diet and exercise program*; and *limiting activities that traumatize the head*. Any sign of gastrointestinal bleeding requires immediate hospitalization. Threatened retinal hemorrhage (wavy lines on Amsler Grid) requires immediate ophthalmologic consultation.

Overall longevity in PXE is reduced very little, if any. It is important to recognize the nonhereditary forms of PXE in management decisions.

SPECIFIC INVESTIGATIONS

- Skin biopsy (with von Kossa stain)
- Complete lipid profile
- Blood pressure
- Hematology
- Routine liver and kidney laboratory profiles
- Retinal exam and retinal photos. If over age 40 years, get regular eye check and use Amsler grid

Pseudoxanthoma elasticum. Neldner KH. Clin Dermatol 1988;6:1–159.

Epidemiologic studies of 100 patients with PXE showed statistically significant data indicating more adverse long-term effects in those individuals with abnormal lipid profiles, hypertension, high dietary calcium intake during childhood and adolescence, tobacco use, and multiple minor head traumatic episodes, and in women with multiple pregnancies. The diagnosis should be established by skin punch biopsy from an affected skin site. Elastic tissue stains, and particularly the von Kossa stain for calcium salts within the elastic fibers, are the gold standard for diagnosis.

Any hematologic, hepatic, or renal abnormalities should be treated as early as possible. A complete lipid profile should be obtained at the first visit and at 1–2-year intervals thereafter. A dietary history should be obtained for calcium intake and general dietary habits.

FIRST LINE THERAPIES

■ Genetic counseling with patient and family, including discussion of the long-term natural course and complications	B
■ Dietary. Recommend heart-healthy diet, weight control and dietary calcium restriction to approximately 800 mg daily	B
■ Avoid long-term anticoagulants (aspirin, nonsteroidal anti-inflammatory drugs [NSAIDs]), occasional use okay	D
■ Treat hypertension or abnormal lipid profiles vigorously	C
■ Treatment of any apparent complications	E

Pseudoxanthoma elasticum – a connective tissue disease or a metabolic disorder at the genome/environment interface? Uitto J. J Invest Dermatol 2004;122:ix–x.

Mutations of the gene encoding the transmembrane transporter protein ABC-C6 cause pseudoxanthoma elasticum. Struk B, Cai L, Zach S, et al. J Mol Med 2000;78: 282–6.

The chromosome (16p 13.1) and the gene (ABC-C6) have been discovered, but no specific therapy based on genetic information is known at this time.

Pseudoxanthoma elasticum. Neldner KH. Clin Dermatol 1988;6:1–159.

The risk for retinal hemorrhages in the macula and central vision loss to the point of legal blindness increases dramatically beyond the age of 40–45 years. Total blindness does not occur, but central vision loss commonly progresses to a visual acuity of 20/200 bilaterally. Conventional (hot) laser therapy is no longer recommended, due to severe retinal scarring from the procedure. Photodynamic therapy (PDT) is being used in its place. A dye is injected IV, followed by light exposure to the retina with a dye-specific wavelength of light. The most recent addition is so-called Feeder Vessel Therapy. A special camera can photograph deeper retinal vessels that are abnormal and are then exposed to an ultra-narrow laser beam which does relatively little damage to the surrounding macula and fovea. The long term results are still pending adequate follow-up.

Management of upper gastrointestinal hemorrhage in pseudoxanthoma elasticum. McCreedy CH, Zimmermann TJ, Webster SF. Surgery 1989;105:170–4.

Stomach bleeding in PXE is a medical emergency. Of individuals with PXE, 10–15% will have a gastric hemorrhage at some time in their lives; it can occur at any time from adolescence to old age. Blood transfusions are commonly required and gastric surgery is necessary in the most severe cases.

Traumatic retinal hemorrhages with angioid streaks. Levin DB, Dell DK. Arch Ophthalmol 1977;95:1072–3.

Younger individuals in particular (second and third decade) should avoid athletic endeavors involving repeated head trauma, such as boxing, football, soccer, rugby, and heavy weightlifting. Other athletic activities are encouraged.

Pseudoxanthoma elasticum. High dietary calcium intake in early life correlates with severity. Renie WA, Pyrertz RE, Combs J, Fine SL. Am J Med Genet 1984;19:235–44.

Both Renie et al. and Neldner (see above, Clin Dermatol 1988;6:1–159) found that high dietary calcium during childhood and adolescent years aggravated the long-term course of PXE. The daily calcium intake should not exceed 800 mg, particularly during childhood and adolescence. Evidence for a positive benefit for life-long reduced calcium intake is anecdotal, but suggestive. Dietary consultation may be helpful in getting the patient started.

Lipid abnormalities should be controlled with diet and exercise if possible and with medications if necessary. Abnormal lipid values should be followed annually. Tobacco in any form should be avoided.

SECOND LINE THERAPIES

■ Special cardiovascular recommendations	B

Pseudoxanthoma elasticum: a clinical and histologic study. Goodman RM, Smith EW, Paton D. Medicine 1963; 42:297–334.

Cardiovascular symptoms seldom occur before the third or fourth decade of life, and most commonly begin with intermittent claudication in the lower extremities. The ankle/brachial Doppler blood pressure study is a noninvasive procedure that will give a moderately sensitive assessment of lower extremity vascular ischemia and correlates well with the need for therapy if there is intermittent claudication. Pentoxifylline 400 mg three times daily with meals and exercise programs is helpful. Only rarely will vascular surgery be indicated. Direct myocardial involvement is possible, but is very rare.

Pseudoxanthoma elasticum and mitral valve prolapse. Lebwohl MG, Di Stephano D, Prioleau PG, et al. N Engl J Med 1982;307:228–32.

Mitral valve prolapse (MVP) is quite common in PXE, as well as in the general population (exact frequencies are unknown). It is of no clinical significance unless accompanied by a heart murmur over the mitral valve. If this is present, the patient should take antibiotics prior to surgical and dental procedures. An echocardiogram is the best way to diagnose the presence of MVP.

THIRD LINE THERAPIES

■ Plastic surgery	B
■ Complementary and alternative medicine products	E

Pseudoxanthoma elasticum. Neldner KH. Clin Dermatol 1988;6:1–159.

Plastic surgery pre- and postoperative photos are shown with excellent results for the lax skin of the lateral neck if a 'neck lift' procedure is used that leaves no visible scars.

Arch Dermatol 1998;134:1349–1477 and JAMA 1998;280: 1549–1640 (many authors).

Entire issues were devoted to this subject. Free radicals are accepted as causal or aggravating factors in many benign and malignant disorders. Ophthalmologists recommend vitamins A, C, and E, plus zinc, selenium, and copper for patients with retinal diseases, based on their antioxidant properties and known requirements for wound healing.

Antioxidant vitamin and herbal products are widely used, but the beneficial results reported are essentially all anecdotal. Ophthalmologists recommend high doses of vitamins A, C, and E with added selenium, copper, and zinc for patients with macular degeneration (AMD). The long-term results are unknown in AMD and no studies have been done in PXE. Patients with AMD have retinal hemorrhages similar to PXE, but do not have angioid streaks.

OTHER THERAPIES

■ Acquired PXE
■ Provide patients with informational brochures to give to their personal physicians
■ Inform patients of support groups

Localized acquired cutaneous pseudoxanthoma elasticum. Neldner KH, Martinez Hernandez A. J Am Acad Dermatol 1979;1:523–30.

Evidence levels A Double-blind study B Clinical trial ≥ 20 subjects C Clinical trial < 20 subjects D Series ≥ 5 subjects E Anecdotal case reports

An acquired form of PXE occurs predominantly in black, multiparous, obese, hypertensive females. Clinically and histologically typical PXE skin lesions are found on the anterior trunk that mimic hereditary PXE. This condition has also been called periumbilical perforating PXE. The complications of hereditary PXE are lacking, so specific therapeutic recommendations for PXE are not indicated.

Exogenous pseudoxanthoma elasticum: A new case in an old farmer. Neri I, Marzaduris S, Bardazzi F, Patrizi A. Acta Derm Venereol 1998;78:153–4.

Chronic exposure to calcium salts can cause a localized PXE-like reaction in the skin. Treatment consists of avoiding exposure, though the affected skin sites may take many years to clear completely.

National Association for PXE (NAPE) – *www.pxenape.org*, and PXE International.

Encourage patients to join support groups such as the National Association for PXE (NAPE) – *www.pxenape.org* and PXE International.

Psoriasis

Mark G Lebwohl, Peter van de Kerkhof

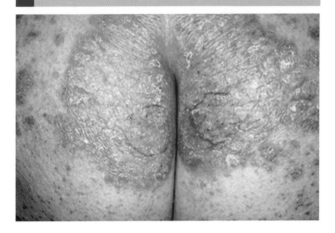

Plaque psoriasis is a common disorder in which environmental factors contribute to the development of sharply demarcated erythematous scaling plaques in genetically predisposed individuals. Because there is an overlap in treatments, guttate psoriasis, inverse psoriasis, and impetigo herpetiformis will be discussed under 'Management Strategy' below. Erythrodermic psoriasis and pustular psoriasis will be discussed at the end of the chapter. Palmoplantar pustulosis is addressed on page 452.

MANAGEMENT STRATEGY

The treatment of psoriasis must take many factors into account, including extent of involvement, areas of involvement, patient's lifestyle, and other health problems and medications. For example, patients who live far from phototherapy centers may not have the option to be treated with psoralen and UVA (PUVA), but a home phototherapy unit can be ordered for patients who can be taught to administer their own UVB therapy. In sunny climates, sun exposure can be added to the therapeutic regimen. If patients are taking medications like lithium that are known to exacerbate psoriasis, alternatives should be sought. In individuals with less than 5% body surface area involvement, topical therapy is usually started unless the patient has previously failed topical therapy or the psoriasis is debilitating because of the site of involvement. In patients with mild localized plaques, *mild, mid-potent or potent topical corticosteroids* can be prescribed, or non-corticosteroids such as *calcipotriol (calcipotriene)* or *tazarotene* can be tried. *Anthralin preparations* have fallen into disfavor because they are messy, but they still offer an effective alternative to corticosteroids and other topical medications. In Europe anthralin preparations are used in day care centers using a care instruction program. Often patients have been using a topical medication that is inadequate as monotherapy. In that case, combination therapy is warranted. The combination of a superpotent corticosteroid and calcipotriol or tazarotene is often effective when monotherapy with either of the agents does not work, and new ointments and creams that combine corticosteroids with vitamin D analogues such as calcipotriol are available or in development.

Some areas may be limited in extent, but require alternative treatments. For example, involvement of the palms and soles can be debilitating, and these areas are notoriously difficult to treat. Pustular psoriasis of the palms and soles, for example, only occasionally responds to topical therapy. Although the palms and soles involve only a small percentage of the body surface area, treatment with oral medications or *phototherapy* may be warranted. The combination of *acitretin* 25 mg daily with 'bath-PUVA' – applied by soaking the hands in a water-filled basin to which *methoxsalen* has been added, followed by UVA irradiation – is a commonly used treatment. *Oral methotrexate, acitretin* and *cyclosporine* are also highly effective for palm and sole psoriasis.

Involvement of the scalp is common and requires gels, solutions, or foams that are not messy rather than ointments and creams. *Shampoos containing tars, salicylic acid, or corticosteroids* are useful adjunctive therapies for the scalp.

The face and intertriginous sites are highly responsive to topical medications, but are particularly sensitive to the side effects of many topical agents. Topical corticosteroids cause cutaneous atrophy, telangiectasia, and striae. Therefore, only milder, safer, corticosteroids should be used on the face and intertriginous sites, and alternating with non-corticosteroids may be optimal if psoriasis recurs. The topical immunomodulators, *tacrolimus 0.1% ointment* and *pimecrolimus 1% cream*, are effective and safe for facial and intertriginous psoriasis, but not as effective on thick plaques on the rest of the body. *Calcipotriol* (50 μg/g) can be irritating on facial or intertriginous psoriasis, and should therefore be alternated with a topical corticosteroid or diluted with petrolatum. Alternative vitamin D analogues such as *calcitriol* (3 μg/g) and *tacalcitol* (2–4 μg/g) (available outside the USA), are less irritating and are therefore particularly suitable for facial and flexural psoriasis. *Tazarotene* may be too irritating to use on genital skin, but it can be used on the face. Preliminary data suggest that tazarotene applied for 1–5 min daily may be highly effective, but less irritating than overnight application of this medication. The irritation of tazarotene can also be minimized by using it in a regimen with topical corticosteroids.

With 5–10% body surface involvement, topical therapy is usually prescribed, but may require the addition of *phototherapy* or *oral medications*. In those with more than 10% body surface involvement, topical therapy may be impractical for all lesions, but may provide a useful adjunct to phototherapy or systemic therapy.

Phototherapy with *UVB* has been in use since the 1920s and has a proven record of safety and efficacy in the treatment of psoriasis. It is particularly useful in patients who have responded well to sun exposure. Patients who have failed UVB or have not done well with sun exposure often respond to *narrowband UVB*. PUVA is one of the most effective treatments for psoriasis and offers long remissions for many patients. Because of its increased risk of cutaneous malignancy, PUVA is usually reserved for those patients who do not achieve adequate remissions with UVB.

In patients who have not achieved satisfactory results with these treatments, *low-dose oral retinoids* can be added. *Acitretin* in doses of 10–25 mg daily dramatically improves the response to UVB and to PUVA. Keeping the dose at 25 mg or less, side effects of acitretin are minimized. For those who are not candidates for UVB phototherapy or PUVA, *oral methotrexate* is highly effective in combination with other treatments or as monotherapy. It is associated with hepatic fibrosis in some patients and regular monitoring of liver function tests in addition to blood counts is necessary. Current guidelines in the USA call for periodic liver biopsies in patients treated with methotrexate. In parts of Europe, the serum level of the amino-terminal propeptide of type III procollagen has been used as a marker for hepatic fibrosis as an alternative to routine use of liver biopsy. *Cyclosporine* is also dramatically effective as monotherapy for psoriasis, but is associated with nephrotoxicity as well as hypertension and a theoretical risk of malignancy with long-term use. Consequently, current guidelines call for limiting use of cyclosporine to 1 or 2 years.

In recent years, the ability to create new drugs that target specific parts of the immune system has led to the development of biologic agents for psoriasis. These drugs are not associated with the nephrotoxicity of cyclosporine or the hepatotoxicity and bone marrow toxicity of methotrexate. The long term side effects of biologics are not known, however, and their cost is often prohibitive. Psoriasis experts are divided on the point at which biologics should be considered. Some consider them first line therapy when the extent of disease is too extensive for topical therapy. Because of their expense, biologics are used by others only after phototherapy or other systemic therapies have been tried.

Because of the toxicities of psoriasis therapy, several concepts have evolved for controlling psoriasis while minimizing side effects. *Rotational therapy*, for example, involves treating psoriasis with a medication such as methotrexate for varying periods of time, followed by switching to PUVA, retinoids, or cyclosporine for limited periods of time. The different treatments used in rotation are determined by patient response. Because biologic therapies have not been associated with major organ toxicity, they are often used long term without the need for rotation.

Combination therapy involves the mixing of two or more treatments. Topical therapies are often used in combination with phototherapy and systemic therapy. Phototherapy with UVB or PUVA is often combined with oral retinoids or methotrexate, thus minimizing the number of treatments and the toxicity of each of the therapies. Low doses of methotrexate and cyclosporine are also commonly used in combination to minimize the nephrotoxicity of cyclosporine and the hepatotoxicity of methotrexate. The latter combination can be effective in patients who have failed monotherapy with either agent.

Sequential therapy refers to the concept of treatment in which potent agents are used to clear the disease and safer, but less effective agents are used to maintain remission. For example, cyclosporine can be used to clear psoriasis and patients can then be switched to oral retinoids in combination with UVB for maintenance. Similarly, sequential therapy can be applied to topical medications. Calcipotriol or tazarotene can be used in combination with superpotent corticosteroids to clear psoriasis and to reduce irritation induced by calcipotriol- or tazarotene monotherapy. The corticosteroid can then be tapered to a regimen where it is used only 2 days per week or eliminated altogether, while the non-corticosteroid agent can be continued.

Guttate psoriasis

Guttate psoriasis is characterized by widespread erythematous, scaling papules. The management of guttate psoriasis is very similar to that of extensive plaque psoriasis. Because streptococcal infection often precedes guttate psoriasis, underlying infection should be sought and treated. Lesions are usually too widespread for topical therapy, so most patients are started on *phototherapy with UVB*. If that is ineffective, *oral retinoids* can be added or patients can be switched to *narrowband UVB or PUVA*. This form of psoriasis frequently responds to phototherapy so it is only occasionally necessary to resort to more aggressive second line or third line therapies listed below; those therapies are also effective for guttate psoriasis.

Inverse psoriasis

Patients with inverse psoriasis develop lesions in the axillae, between the buttocks, on the medial aspects of the thighs, and in the umbilicus. These sites are easily treated with *mild topical corticosteroids,* but are more susceptible to corticosteroid side effects such as atrophy and formation of striae. Consequently, nonsteroidal treatments can be attempted. *Calcipotriol* (50 μg/g) can be irritating on intertriginous sites but is nevertheless effective. Some have advocated diluting *calcipotriol with petrolatum in equal amounts* to minimize irritation. If irritation does not develop, the amount of petrolatum added can be reduced. *Other deltanoids (calcitriol, tacalcitol)* are marketed in lower concentrations and cause less irritation. *Tazarotene* can be used on the face, but is usually too irritating to use in the axillae or groin. *Tars and anthralin* are likewise irritating in intertriginous sites. There are reports of *topical tacrolimus ointment or pimecrolimus cream* being used effectively for psoriasis on the face and in intertriginous sites.

Impetigo herpetiformis

Impetigo herpetiformis is characterized by a generalized pustular eruption with fever and leukocytosis developing during pregnancy. Many consider this to be a variant of pustular psoriasis that occurs during pregnancy. If *bed rest, emollients, compresses,* and *mild topical corticosteroids* are ineffective, *systemic corticosteroids* have been used until recently. Following labor and delivery or termination of the pregnancy, corticosteroids can be replaced by *retinoids* or *methotrexate.*

Most recently, *oral cyclosporine* has proven effective for most variants of psoriasis. This treatment appears to be the least harmful systemic treatment for psoriasis during pregnancy and may therefore be the treatment of choice. Doses of 4–5 mg/kg daily are prescribed. Concerns about cumulative toxicity, such as nephrotoxicity are less worrisome in impetigo herpetiformis because it may resolve at the end of pregnancy, limiting the amount of cyclosporine prescribed.

SPECIFIC INVESTIGATIONS

No investigation is required in the majority of cases. Skin biopsy may be helpful if the diagnosis is in question, but is usually not needed.

As discussed below, a range of investigations are required for screening and monitoring when using systemic therapies.

Routine screening for tuberculosis has been advised for patients treated with infliximab and adalimumab especially in high risk populations. Because methotrexate, cyclosporine, and other biologics are also immunosuppressive, skin testing for tuberculosis and, if positive, chest radiography have been suggested prior to treatment with these agents.

FIRST LINE THERAPIES

■ Anthralin (dithranol)	B
■ Coal tar	A
■ Salicylic acid	C
■ Topical corticosteroids	A
■ Vitamin D analogues (deltanoids)	A
■ Sun exposure	B

Short-duration ('minutes') therapy with dithranol for psoriasis: a new out-patient regimen. Runne U, Kunze J. Br J Dermatol 1982;106:135–9.

High-concentration dithranol (1–3%) applied for only 10–20 min resulted in significantly better clearing than longer application of lower concentrations.

Short-contact anthralin therapy results in less staining and more convenient application of the medication than overnight or day-long applications. Treatment can be started with 1% anthralin for 5 min and increased by 5 min every other day until minimal irritation develops. Triethanolamine can be sprayed on before removal of the anthralin to minimize staining of the skin.

Short- and long-contact therapy using a new dithranol formulation in individually adjusted dosages in the management of psoriasis. Thune P, Brolund L. Acta Derm Venereol Suppl (Stockh) 1992;172:28–9.

Micanol®, a new formulation of anthralin, is effective in short- and long-contact regimens. After 6 weeks of daily treatment, psoriasis severity scores were reduced by 73% in the short-contact group and by 78% in the long-contact group.

The vehicle of Micanol® does not release its anthralin content until it is subjected to skin surface temperatures. This results in less staining of household furniture and laundry and is better accepted by patients.

Efficacy of topical 5% liquor carbonis detergens vs. its emollient base in the treatment of psoriasis. Kanzler MH, Gorsulowsky DC. Br J Dermatol 1993;129:310–14.

5% liquor carbonis detergens resulted in more improvement in psoriasis than its vehicle emollient base in a bilateral-paired comparison study.

Tars are available in gels, creams, emollient creams, and ointments, and are also available in emulsions that are added to the bath. There is a general belief that more cosmetically elegant preparations are better tolerated by patients, but less effective. Crude coal tar is quite effective, but quite messy.

The role of salicylic acid in the treatment of psoriasis. Lebwohl M. Int J Dermatol 1999;38:16–24.

Salicylic acid is a keratolytic agent that removes scale and allows penetration of other topical medications. There is a marked increase in penetration of topical corticosteroids when combined with 2–10% salicylic acid. Combinations of salicylic acid and tar or anthralin have also been used successfully, but salicylic acid inactivates calcipotriol.

Moreover, salicylic acid blocks UVB and should therefore not be applied prior to phototherapy.

Superpotent topical steroid treatment of psoriasis vulgaris – clinical efficacy and adrenal function. Katz HI, Hien NT, Prawer SE, et al. J Am Acad Dermatol 1987;16: 804–11.

Forty patients were treated in a double-blind study with superpotent corticosteroids including betamethasone dipropionate in an optimized vehicle and clobetasol-17-propionate: 75% or greater improvement was achieved in most, but eight of the 40 patients had temporary reversible adrenal suppression as evidenced by low morning plasma cortisols.

Clinically significant adrenal suppression is seldom considered and tests for adrenal function are virtually never performed. Practicing dermatologists are more concerned with side effects of atrophy, telangiectasia, striae, and tachyphylaxis. For all the above reasons, superpotent corticosteroid use should be limited to 2–4 weeks, and less than 50 g per week. Superpotent corticosteroids should not be included and should not be used on the face or intertriginous sites. If at all possible, they should be avoided in children.

Betamethasone dipropionate in optimized vehicle. Intermittent pulse dosing for extended maintenance treatment of psoriasis. Katz HI, Hien NT, Prawer SE, et al. Arch Dermatol 1987;123:1308–11.

Betamethasone dipropionate in optimized vehicle was compared to vehicle in an intermittent pulse dosing regimen where a study medication was applied for three consecutive doses at 12-h intervals once a week, so-called weekend therapy. Improvement in psoriasis was maintained for 12 weeks in 74% of patients with psoriasis treated with betamethasone dipropionate 0.05% in optimized base compared to 21% in the placebo group.

Psoriasis is a chronic recurring disease that can be kept in remission by intermittent dosing regimens such as the weekend therapy regimen described.

Efficacy and safety of calcipotriol (MC 903) ointment in psoriasis vulgaris. A randomized, double-bind, right/left comparative, vehicle-controlled study. Dubertret L, Wallach D, Souteyrand P, et al. J Am Acad Dermatol 1992; 27:983–8.

A double-blind, placebo-controlled, bilateral comparison study of 566 patients with psoriasis demonstrated the efficacy of calcipotriol ointment.

A multicenter trial of calcipotriene ointment and halobetasol ointment compared with either agent alone for the treatment of psoriasis. Lebwohl M, Siskin SB, Epinette W, et al. J Am Acad Dermatol 1996;35:268–9.

In this double-blind study a regimen of calcipotriol ointment applied in the morning and halobetasol propionate ointment applied in the evening proved to be more effective than either agent applied twice daily for 2 weeks.

Calcipotriol ointment and halobetasol ointment in the long-term treatment of psoriasis: effects on the duration of improvement. Lebwohl M, Yoles A, Lombardi K, Lou W. J Am Acad Dermatol 1998;39:447–50.

A regimen of calcipotriol ointment applied twice daily on weekdays and halobetasol ointment applied twice daily on weekends was able to maintain remissions in 76% of patients with psoriasis for 6 months compared to 40% of patients applying halobetasol ointment at weekends only and placebo on weekdays.

Efficacy and safety of topical calcitriol (1,25-dihydroxyvitamin D₃) for the treatment of psoriasis. Perez A, Chen TC, Turner A, et al. Br J Dermatol 1996;134: 238–46.

This double-blind, placebo-controlled, right/left comparison study in 84 patients demonstrated superior efficacy of topical calcitriol ointment over placebo.

Calcitriol ointment is only commercially available in a few countries at present.

Once daily treatment of psoriasis with tacalcitol compared with twice daily treatment with calcipotriol. A double-blind trial. Veien NK, Bjerke JR, Rossmann-Ringdahl I, Jakobsen HB. Br J Dermatol 1997;137:581–6.

Tacalcitol ointment applied once daily was almost as effective as twice daily calcipotriol ointment in this 8-week, double-blind study.

Tacalcitol ointment is available in most European countries and in Japan, but not currently in the USA.

Topical maxacalcitol for the treatment of psoriasis vulgaris: a placebo-controlled, double-blind, dose-finding study with active comparator. Barker JN, Ashton RE, Marks R, et al. Br J Dermatol 1999;141:274–8.

Maxacalcitol 25 mg/g ointment was significantly more effective than vehicle. When applied once daily, marked improvement or clearing occurred in 55% of subjects, which compared favorably with once-daily application of calcipotriol ointment.

Maxacalcitol is not available in the US at this time.

Tazarotene gel, a new retinoid. Weinstein GD, Krueger GG, Lowe NJ, et al. J Am Acad Dermatol 1997;37:85–92.

Tazarotene 0.1% or 0.05% gels were significantly more effective than placebo in this double-blind trial in more than 300 patients. The beneficial effect on psoriasis was sustained for 12 weeks after treatment.

Irritation caused by topical application of tazarotene is the single most limiting side effect. Consequently, this agent is used most frequently in combination with topical corticosteroids.

Tazarotene 0.1% gel plus corticosteroid cream in the treatment of plaque psoriasis. Lebwohl MG, Breneman DL, Goffe BS, et al. J Am Acad Dermatol 1998;39:590–6.

The efficacy of tazarotene 0.1% gel is increased by a combination regimen with mid- or high potency corticosteroids. Most importantly, local cutaneous irritation is reduced in the combination regimen.

Treatment of psoriasis at a Dead Sea dermatology clinic. Abels DJ, Rose T, Bearman JE. Int J Dermatol 1995;34: 134–7.

A retrospective chart review of 1448 consecutive psoriasis patients treated at the Dead Sea revealed improvement in 88%, including 58% with complete clearing. The Dead Sea is the lowest point on earth and has the highest concentration of minerals of any body of water on the earth. The mineral haze in the atmosphere through which sunlight passes results in a unique spectrum of sunlight which accounts for the exceptional therapeutic responses seen there; 2–4 weeks of Dead Sea sun exposure and bathing are required to achieve significant benefit.

SECOND LINE THERAPIES

■ UVB	A
■ Narrowband UVB	A
■ PUVA	A
■ Acitretin	A
■ Adalimumab	A
■ Alefacept	A
■ Efalizumab	A
■ Etanercept	A
■ Infliximab	A
■ Methotrexate	B
■ Cyclosporine	A

Components of the Goeckerman regimen. Le Vine MJ, White HA, Parrish JA. J Invest Dermatol 1979;73:170–3.

The efficacy of UVB phototherapy is improved by the addition of a topical tar preparation or lubricating base; 5% crude coal tar is no more effective than lubricating base when combined with a phototherapy regimen.

The original Goeckerman regimen involved inpatient application of crude coal tar, which was removed prior to daily UVB phototherapy. Most current phototherapy regimens involve outpatient treatment three times per week with topical application of mineral oil or petrolatum.

Narrowband UV-B produces superior clinical and histopathological resolution of moderate-to-severe psoriasis in patients compared with broadband UV-B. Coven TR, Burack LH, Gilleaudeau R, et al. Arch Dermatol 1997; 133:1514–22.

Twenty two patients were treated in a bilateral comparison study with narrowband UVB on one side and broadband UVB on the other. The side treated with narrowband UVB cleared more quickly and more completely than the side treated with broadband.

Narrowband UV-B phototherapy vs photochemotherapy in the treatment of chronic plaque-type psoriasis: a paired comparison study. Tanew A, Radakovic-Fijan S, Schemper M, Honigsmann H. Arch Dermatol 1999;135:519–24.

Twenty five patients were treated in a bilateral paired comparison trial in which one side was treated with narrowband UVB and the other side with PUVA. The Psoriasis Area and Severity Index (PASI) was reduced by a median of 84% on the narrowband treatment side and by 89% on the PUVA-treated side. There was a significantly better response to PUVA in patients with worse psoriasis.

Narrowband UVB is more effective than traditional broadband UVB, but a subset of severely affected patients who do not respond to narrowband UVB may respond to PUVA. Broadband UVB has a long history of safety with very little risk of photocarcinogenicity. Although narrowband UVB has only been in use for a few years, it is probably less carcinogenic than PUVA.

Oral methoxsalen photochemotherapy for the treatment of psoriasis: a cooperative clinical trial. Melski JW, Tanenbaum L, Parrish JA, et al. J Invest Dermatol 1977;68: 328–35.

Fourteen hundred and eight patients were treated two or three times weekly with PUVA. Psoriasis cleared in 88%.

PUVA remains one of the most effective psoriasis therapies available and in many patients provides long periods of remission.

PSORIASIS

553

Side effects of burning, sun sensitivity, and, especially, photo-carcinogenicity are of concern.

PUVA therapy for psoriasis: comparison of oral and bath-water delivery of 8-methoxypsoralen. Lowe NJ, Weingarten D, Bourget T, Moy LS. J Am Acad Dermatol 1986;14:754–60.

Bath-water delivery of methoxsalen (bath-PUVA) is as effective as oral PUVA, but requires less UVA and is not associated with systemic side effects such as nausea. Phototoxicity may be increased.

Topically applied methoxsalen has also been shown to be effective for psoriasis, but is associated with more phototoxicity.

Trioxsalen bath plus UVA effective and safe in the treatment of psoriasis. Hannuksela M, Karvonen J. Br J Dermatol 1978;99:703–7.

Seventy four patients with psoriasis were treated with trioxsalen baths, resulting in good or excellent responses in 92%.

Trioxsalen may be associated with less photosensitivity than methoxsalen.

Baseline and annual eye exams have been suggested for patients treated with PUVA, but initial concerns about the development of cataracts in these patients have not borne out over time. Baseline serologies for lupus were once recommended prior to starting patients on PUVA, but are now only obtained in patients who have other signs or symptoms of the disease.

Acitretin improves psoriasis in a dose-dependent fashion. Goldfarb MT, Ellis CN, Gupta AK, et al. J Am Acad Dermatol 1988;18:655–62.

Thirty eight patients were treated in a double-blind placebo-controlled study comparing varying dosages of acitretin; 10 and 25 mg daily doses were ineffective, but 15–75 mg doses were significantly more effective than placebo. Side effects included hair loss, cheilitis, hyperlipidemia, and elevated liver function tests.

When used in combination with UVB or PUVA, daily doses of 10–25 mg acitretin are highly effective with very few side effects. Monotherapy for plaque psoriasis requires higher doses. With any dose, teratogenicity must be considered.

Treatment with oral retinoids requires baseline liver function tests and lipids, which are then repeated at intervals during therapy.

Methotrexate in psoriasis: consensus conference. Roenigk HH Jr, Auerbach R, Maibach H, et al. J Am Acad Dermatol 1998;38:478–85.

Methotrexate remains one of the most effective systemic agents for psoriasis. Following an initial test dose of 2.5–7.5 mg, weekly doses ranging from 15 to 30 mg can be used to clear psoriasis in most patients. The most worrisome side effects are hepatotoxicity and bone marrow suppression.

This article reviews many of the publications on methotrexate and covers laboratory monitoring guidelines including blood work and liver biopsy, dosage guidelines, drug interactions, and side effects.

Patients treated with methotrexate should have baseline blood and platelet counts as well as liver function tests and creatinine. If baseline liver function tests are elevated, serological studies for hepatitis B and hepatitis C are warranted. Assays for the amino terminal propeptide of type III procollagen are obtained in Europe.

In the USA, baseline liver biopsies are no longer obtained in patients without a history of liver disease. Many dermatologists in the USA and Europe still obtain periodic liver biopsies to monitor hepatic fibrosis.

Isotretinoin–PUVA in women with psoriasis. Anstey A, Hawk JL. Br J Dermatol 1997;136:798–9.

A report of four young adult female patients demonstrating a good response to isotretinoin combined with PUVA.

Isotretinoin appears generally to be less effective than acitretin or etretinate in the treatment of psoriasis, but in combination with PUVA it seems to effectively reduce the PUVA exposure required. This may be particularly useful for fertile female patients for whom acitretin is contraindicated. Women must still be advised to avoid pregnancy for at least 31 days after stopping isotretinoin.

Cyclosporine consensus conference: with emphasis on the treatment of psoriasis. Lebwohl M, Ellis C, Gottlieb A, et al. J Am Acad Dermatol 1998;39:464–75.

Oral cyclosporine in doses up to 5 mg/kg daily is dramatically effective for psoriasis, but is limited by the development of nephrotoxicity.

This article presents guidelines regarding dosage and monitoring, drug interactions, and complications of cyclosporine.

In patients treated with cyclosporine, blood and platelet count as well as comprehensive serum chemistries are warranted including blood urea nitrogen, creatinine, potassium, magnesium, uric acid, liver function tests, and lipids. Two baseline serum creatinines and two baseline blood pressure measurements should be obtained prior to starting cyclosporine therapy.

An international, randomized, double-blind, placebo-controlled phase 3 trial of intramuscular alefacept in patients with chronic plaque psoriasis. Lebwohl M, Christophers E, Langley R, et al; Alefacept Clinical Study Group. Arch Dermatol 2003;139:719–27.

Five hundred and seven patients with psoriasis were treated with placebo, alefacept 10 mg, or alefacept 15 mg, administered weekly for 12 weeks; 33% of patients treated with 15 mg achieved 75% improvement in PASI scores at some point during the course of therapy or 12 weeks of follow-up. Of patients who achieved 75% improvement in PASI scores (PASI 75), 50% reduction in PASI (PASI 50) was maintained throughout the 12-week follow-up in 71%. Reductions in CD4 counts were noted in some patients.

Long remissions are the primary advantage of this agent, which does not achieve PASI 75 in the majority of treated patients, and improvement is slow, with maximal benefit usually occurring several weeks after the last injection. More patients improve with additional therapy, and longer remissions are achieved following two courses of treatment. Baseline total lymphocyte and CD4 counts must be obtained prior to starting patients on alefacept, and current guidelines recommend that these be repeated weekly during therapy, although some are obtaining these every other week.

Etanercept as monotherapy in patients with psoriasis. Leonardi CL, Powers JL, Matheson RT, et al; Etanercept Psoriasis Study Group. N Engl J Med 2003;349:2014–22.

Six hundred and seventy two patients were treated in this double-blind multiple dose trial. Of patients treated with etanercept 50 mg twice weekly, 49% achieved PASI 75 after

Evidence levels **A** Double-blind study   **B** Clinical trial ≥ 20 subjects   **C** Clinical trial < 20 subjects   **D** Series ≥ 5 subjects   **E** Anecdotal case reports

12 weeks and 59% achieved PASI 75 after 24 weeks. In those patients treated with 25 mg subcutaneously twice a week, 34 and 44% achieved PASI 75 after 12 weeks and 24 weeks, respectively.

To achieve an initial rapid response, etanercept has been approved by the FDA in the USA and the European EMEA at a dose of 50 mg twice a week for 12 weeks. At that point, it has been recommended that etanercept doses are reduced to 25 mg subcutaneously twice a week. Some patients, however, require the 50 mg dose to maintain their benefit.

Efalizumab for patients with moderate to severe plaque psoriasis: a randomized controlled trial. Gordon KB, Papp KA, Hamilton TK, et al; Efalizumab Study Group. JAMA 2003;290:3073–80.

Five hundred and fifty six patients with psoriasis were treated in a double-blind controlled trial in which they received either efalizumab 1 mg/kg weekly for 12 weeks or placebo; 27% of the efalizumab treated patients achieved PASI 75 after 12 weeks.

Open-label studies in which efalizumab is administered for periods exceeding 1 year have resulted in much higher response rates. Efalizumab should not be discontinued abruptly because discontinuation has been associated with rebound of psoriasis. Patients must therefore be transitioned to other therapies if discontinuation is necessary. Efalizumab for psoriasis has been approved by the FDA in the USA and the European EMEA.

For patients treated with efalizumab, baseline platelet counts have been recommended and these are repeated monthly for the first 3 months.

Infliximab induction therapy for patients with severe plaque-type psoriasis: a randomized, double-blind, placebo-controlled trial. Gottlieb AB, Evans R, Li S, et al. J Am Acad Dermatol 2004;51:534–42.

Two hundred and forty nine patients were treated with three intravenous infusions of infliximab 3 mg/kg or 5 mg/kg, or placebo, at baseline, week 2, and week 6; 88% of patients treated with infliximab 5 mg/kg achieved PASI 75. Improvement was seen as early as 2 weeks after the first infusion.

Infliximab infusions must be administered over at least 2 h and require frequent monitoring. When used for other conditions such as Crohn's disease, approximately 5% of infusions are complicated by reactions. Fortunately, most infusion reactions are mild and can be prevented by treatment with acetaminophen and antihistamines.

Adalimumab: efficacy and safety in psoriasis and rheumatoid arthritis. Patel T, Gordon KB. Dermatol Ther 2004;17: 427–31.

Adalimumab administered in doses of 40 mg subcutaneously once a week or every other week results in substantial improvement of psoriasis.

Data reveal as many as 80% of patients achieve PASI 75 with 12 weekly 40 mg subcutaneous injections of adalimumab. Over 50% of patients treated with adalimumab subcutaneously every other week achieve PASI 75.

Routine screening for tuberculosis has been advised for patients treated with infliximab and adalimumab.

THIRD LINE THERAPIES

■ Topical 5-fluorouracil	C
■ Topical propylthiouracil	C
■ Intralesional 5-fluorouracil	C
■ Combination therapy	A
■ Sulfasalazine (sulphasalazine)	A
■ Mycophenolate mofetil	B
■ Hydroxyurea	B
■ 6-Thioguanine	C
■ Azathioprine	C
■ FK-506	A
■ Fumaric acid esters	B
■ Antibiotics	C
■ Colchicine	C
■ Propylthiouracil	B
■ Excimer laser	C
■ Cryotherapy	C
■ Grenz rays	B
■ Photodynamic therapy	C
■ CTLA4Ig	A

Weekly pulse dosing schedule of fluorouracil: a new topical therapy for psoriasis. Pearlman DL, Youngberg B, Engelhard C. J Am Acad Dermatol 1986;15:1247–52.

Fourteen patients were treated with topical 5-fluorouracil with occlusion 2–3 days per week for a mean of 15.7 weeks. Eleven patients achieved 90% clearing of treated lesions compared to 6% for placebo.

Because of concern about absorption, topical 5-fluorouracil should only be used on isolated plaques. Irritation is the main side effect.

A controlled trial of topical propylthiouracil in the treatment of patients with psoriasis. Elias AN, Dangaran X, Barr RJ, et al. J Am Acad Dermatol 1994;31:455–8.

Nine patients with psoriasis were treated in a double-blind study in which some lesions were treated with topical propylthiouracil and others with placebo. Study medications were applied three times daily for 4–8 weeks. There was greater clearing of lesions treated with propylthiouracil, including near complete clearing in two patients. Systemic side effects did not occur.

Weekly psoriasis therapy using intralesional fluorouracil. Pearlman DL, Youngberg B, Engelhard C. J Am Acad Dermatol 1987;17:78–82.

Eleven patients were treated with intralesional injection of 1 mL of fluorouracil (50 mg/mL). Injections were repeated at 1- to 2-week intervals with each patient receiving an average of two injections. Nine of 11 patients improved, with maximal clearing occurring 4 weeks after the first injection. There were no systemic side effects but local irritation and hyperpigmentation occurred.

Proceedings of the psoriasis combination and rotation therapy conference. Deer Valley, Utah, Oct. 7–9, 1994. Menter MA, See JA, Amend WJ, et al. J Am Acad Dermatol 1996;34:315–21.

Side effects of psoriasis treatments can be minimized and efficacy enhanced by combining low doses of different psoriasis therapies. Rotational therapy refers to a method in which patients cleared with one psoriasis therapy are subsequently treated with different therapies to minimize the cumulative toxicity of any given psoriasis treatment. Thus, the hepatotoxicity of cumulative doses of methotrexate, the nephrotoxicity of cyclosporine, and the carcinogenicity of PUVA can be minimized.

The most commonly used combinations involve retinoids and UVB, and retinoids and PUVA. UVB and PUVA have been used in combination with one another as well as with methotrexate. Retinoids are among the safest systemic agents for psoriasis and have been combined with methotrexate and cyclosporine, though liver function tests should be watched carefully when methotrexate and acitretin are used together. The combination of methotrexate and cyclosporine is a dramatically effective therapy, as is the combination of cyclosporine and hydroxyurea. Methotrexate has also been used with hydroxyurea, but blood counts must be watched very carefully. Etanercept has been used with methotrexate and cyclosporine for the treatment of rheumatoid arthritis, so we will undoubtedly be seeing more combination therapy for psoriasis as well.

Sulfasalazine improves psoriasis. A double-blind analysis. Gupta AK, Ellis CN, Siegel MT, et al. Arch Dermatol 1990;126:487–93.

Fifty patients participated in this double-blind, placebo-controlled trial. Marked improvement was reported in 41% of the sulfasalazine treated patients and moderate improvement in another 41%. Over one-quarter of the sulfasalazine treated patients discontinued the study because of side effects of rash or nausea.

Mycophenolate mofetil (CellCept) for psoriasis: a two-center, prospective, open-label clinical trial. Zhou Y, Rosenthal D, Dutz J, Ho V. J Cutan Med Surg 2003;7:193–7.

Twenty-three patients were treated in an open-label study of mycophenolate mofetil 2–3 g daily for 12 weeks. At the end of 12 weeks PASI scores improved by 47%. Only 22% of patients did not have a significant response. Five patients developed nausea and one patient developed transient leukopenia.

Mycophenolate mofetil is highly effective in a subset of psoriasis patients. Gastrointestinal side effects can be limited by administering the drug in four divided daily doses instead of the twice-daily dosing recommended in the package insert.

Hydroxyurea in the management of therapy resistant psoriasis. Layton AM, Sheehan-Dare RA, Goodfield MJ, Cotterill JA. Br J Dermatol 1989;121:647–53.

Eighty five patients with psoriasis were treated with long-term hydroxyurea in doses of 0.5–1.5 g daily. Remissions occurred in 61%. Reversible bone marrow suppression occurred in 35% of patients. Four patients developed cutaneous side effects.

6-Thioguanine treatment of psoriasis: experience in 81 patients. Zackheim HS, Glogau RG, Fisher DA, Maibach HI. J Am Acad Dermatol 1994;30:452–8.

This was a retrospective study of 81 patients treated with 6-thioguanine for psoriasis. Improvement was maintained in nearly 50% of patients for a median of 33 months. Treatment with 6-thioguanine had to be discontinued most commonly because of reversible bone marrow suppression.

Pulse dosing of thioguanine in recalcitrant psoriasis. Silvis NG, Levine N. Arch Dermatol 1999;135:433–7.

Bone marrow suppression can be avoided by treating patients with oral thioguanine two to three times per week with maintenance doses ranging from 120 mg twice per week to 160 mg three times per week. In this open study, marked improvement was noted in ten of 14 patients.

Azathioprine in psoriasis. Greaves MW, Dawber R. Br Med J 1970;2:237–8.

Azathioprine can be effective monotherapy for psoriasis, but its use is limited by bone marrow toxicity.

As with 6-thioguanine and hydroxyurea, the therapeutic effective dose of azathioprine is close to doses that are toxic to the bone marrow. With all three of these drugs, frequent blood counts are essential.

Systemic tacrolimus (FK 506) is effective for the treatment of psoriasis in a double-blind, placebo-controlled study. The European FK 506 Multicentre Psoriasis Study Group. Arch Dermatol 1996;132:419–23.

Fifty patients with psoriasis were treated in this double-blind, placebo-controlled study for 9 weeks. Starting doses were 0.05 mg/kg daily and could be increased up to 0.15 mg/kg daily. Tacrolimus treated patients had significantly greater improvements in PASI scores than those receiving placebo. Diarrhea, paresthesias, and insomnia were the most commonly reported side effects.

Treatment of psoriasis with fumaric acid esters: results of a prospective multicentre study: German Multicentre Study. Mrowietz U, Christophers E, Altmeyer P. Br J Dermatol 1998;138:456–60.

Of 101 patients who started this prospective study, 70 completed 4 months of treatment. There was an 80% reduction in PASI scores. Side effects consisted of lymphocytopenia, gastrointestinal complaints, and flushing.

Although not noted in this study, nephrotoxicity has been a recognized side effect of fumaric acid therapy.

Use of rifampin with penicillin and erythromycin in the treatment of psoriasis. Preliminary report. Rosenberg EW, Noah PW, Zanolli MD, et al. J Am Acad Dermatol 1986;14:761–4.

All nine patients with streptococcal-associated psoriasis responded to a 5-day course of rifampin (rifampicin) in combination with 10–14 days of oral penicillin or erythromycin.

The use of oral antibiotics has been championed by Rosenberg and colleagues. Although supported by sound theories and numerous anecdotes, the use of antibiotics for psoriasis has not been supported by controlled clinical trials. Other agents that have been used include oral nystatin and oral fluconazole; even tonsillectomy has been advocated.

Therapeutic trials with oral colchicine in psoriasis. Wahba A, Cohen H. Acta Derm Venereol 1980;60:515–20.

Twenty two patients were treated in an open trial of colchicine 0.02 mg/kg daily for 2–4 months. Of the nine patients with thin papules and plaques, eight noted marked improvement or clearing, but there was little improvement in patients with thick plaques.

Propylthiouracil in psoriasis: results of an open trial. Elias AN, Goodman MM, Liem WH, Barr RJ. J Am Acad Dermatol 1993;29:78–81.

Propylthiouracil at a dose of 100 mg was administered orally every 8 h for 8 weeks to ten patients with psoriasis. Seven had marked improvement in their psoriasis and the others showed moderate improvement. Thyroid function

Evidence levels **A** Double-blind study **B** Clinical trial ≥ 20 subjects **C** Clinical trial < 20 subjects **D** Series ≥ 5 subjects **E** Anecdotal case reports

tests were unaffected except for mild increase in serum thyroid stimulating hormone after 6 weeks of therapy in a single patient.

308-nm excimer laser for the treatment of psoriasis: a dose–response study. Asawanonda P, Anderson RR, Chang Y, Taylor CR. Arch Dermatol 2000;136:619–24.

Target lesions in 13 patients were treated with eight doses in a dose escalation study that ranged from 0.5 to 16 multiples of the minimal erythema dose. High fluences were significantly more effective than low fluences.

The excimer laser has been approved for the treatment of psoriasis in the USA and is proven to be one of the fastest modalities for treating plaques. It is useful for plaques of limited size, but is impractical to use when large parts of the body surface area are affected.

Cryotherapy for psoriasis. Nouri K, Chartier TK, Eaglstein WH, Taylor JR. Arch Dermatol 1997;133:1608–9.

Target plaques of psoriasis were treated with cryotherapy resulting in improvement. Local reactions including pain and vesiculation were the only side effects other than discoloration.

As with lasers, cryotherapy is only practical for isolated, localized plaques. Despite the Koebner phenomenon, psoriasis does not commonly occur in frozen plaques, but scarring or discoloration can occur.

Psoriasis of the scalp treated with Grenz rays or topical corticosteroid combined with Grenz rays. A comparative randomized trial. Lindelof B, Johannesson A. Br J Dermatol 1988;119:241–4.

Forty patients were treated with either Grenz rays or Grenz rays plus topical corticosteroids for scalp psoriasis. Grenz rays were administered at a dosage of 4 Gy at weekly intervals for six treatments; 84% of the Grenz ray treated patients and 72% of the Grenz ray plus corticosteroid group healed. The addition of topical corticosteroids offered little benefit.

The association between X-ray therapy and squamous cell carcinomas, particularly in patients subsequently treated with PUVA, has led to a reduction in experience with this useful modality.

Improved response of plaque psoriasis after multiple treatments with topical 5-aminolaevulinic acid photodynamic therapy. Robinson DJ, Collins P, Stringer MR, et al. Acta Derm Venereol 1999;79:451–5.

Topical application of 5-aminolevulinic acid was followed by exposure to broad-band visible radiation. Treatment was performed up to three times per week, with a maximum of 12 treatments, using a light dose of 8 J/cm^2 delivered at a dose rate of 15 mW/cm^2. Eight of ten patients showed a clinical response, though only four of 19 treated sites cleared, ten improved, and five failed to improve. The authors concluded that the unpredictability of the response and the discomfort associated with the treatment made this approach unsuitable for the treatment of psoriasis.

Much more work needs to be done before 5-aminolevulinic acid photodynamic therapy is used for psoriasis. However, research continues and it seems possible that better results may be obtainable.

Administration of DAB389IL-2 to patients with recalcitrant psoriasis: a double-blind, phase II multicenter trial. Bagel J, Garland WT, Breneman D, et al. J Am Acad Dermatol 1998;38:938–44.

A double-blind, placebo-controlled study of DAB389IL-2 was conducted to examine the safety and efficacy of this medication in psoriasis. Patients received either placebo, or 5, 10, or 15 mg/kg intravenously for three consecutive days each week. At least 50% improvement was achieved in 41% of patients during the course of this regimen compared to 25% of controls. Ten patients discontinued treatment because of adverse effects including flu-like symptoms and, in one patient, vasospasm and coagulopathy.

Diphtheria fusion toxin has been demonstrated to be effective for psoriasis, but is limited by its side effects. Because it is already approved for the treatment of cutaneous T cell lymphoma, efforts are underway to see if it can be made tolerable for psoriasis.

CTLA4Ig-mediated blockade of T-cell costimulation in patients with psoriasis vulgaris. Abrams JR, Lebwohl MG, Guzzo CA, et al. J Clin Invest 1999;103:1243–52.

Forty three patients were treated in this 26-week, open-label, dose-escalation study in which patients received four intravenous infusions of this fusion protein; 46% of patients achieved 50% or greater improvement with significantly greater responses in patients treated with higher doses.

Erythrodermic psoriasis

Erythrodermic psoriasis is characterized by angry erythema and scaling affecting the entire cutaneous surface. All the protective functions of the skin are lost including protection against infection, temperature control, and prevention of fluid loss. Loss of nutrients through the skin leads to anemia and electrolyte imbalance. The most common precipitating cause of erythrodermic psoriasis is the withdrawal of systemic corticosteroids, and these should therefore be avoided in patients with psoriasis. Excessive use of topical superpotent corticosteroids, phototherapy burns, and infection have also been implicated as causes of erythrodermic psoriasis.

Patients may require *hospitalization with bed rest, emollients,* and *application of mild topical corticosteroids.* Because sepsis and shock are complications of erythrodermic psoriasis, *monitoring of temperature, blood pressure, urine output,* and *weight* may be important depending on the severity of the condition. In males and in females not of childbearing potential, *oral retinoids* are among the safest treatments for erythrodermic psoriasis, but are not as reliably effective as *infliximab, cyclosporine,* or *methotrexate.* Acitretin can be started in doses of 25 mg daily and can be increased to 50 mg or higher. Cyclosporine in doses of 4–5 mg/kg daily results in rapid improvement. Oral methotrexate starting at 15 mg per week and gradually increasing up to 30 mg/week is effective within a few weeks. Once erythema has cleared with topical or systemic agents, patients can be switched to *phototherapy* or *PUVA.* Infliximab is rapidly effective for erythrodermic psoriasis, and is emerging as an important treatment option. Because antichimeric antibodies are more likely to develop against this agent if treatments are not maintained, long-term therapy with infliximab infusions must be considered if this treatment is chosen.

When the above agents either do not work or cannot be used, many of the third line therapies listed for psoriasis are effective. For example, there are anecdotal reports of

6-thioguanine, mycophenolate mofetil, azathioprine, and *hydroxyurea* working for erythrodermic psoriasis. *Combination therapy* such as the combination of methotrexate and cyclosporine in low doses or the combination of methotrexate and infliximab can also be effective. There are also anecdotal reports of *carbamazepine* clearing erythrodermic psoriasis.

FIRST LINE THERAPIES

■ Emollients	D
■ Topical corticosteroids	D

SECOND LINE THERAPIES

■ Retinoids	B
■ Cyclosporine	B
■ Infliximab	E
■ Methotrexate	B

THIRD LINE THERAPIES

■ Combination therapy	D
■ 6-Thioguanine	E
■ Mycophenolate mofetil	E
■ Hydroxyurea	E
■ Azathioprine	E
■ Carbamazepine	E

Pustular and erythrodermic psoriasis. Prystowsky JH, Cohen PR. Dermatol Clin 1995;13:757–70.

The treatments used for pustular and erythrodermic psoriasis are reviewed and a general approach to the management of these difficult conditions is presented.

Use of short-course class 1 topical glucocorticoid under occlusion for the rapid control of erythrodermic psoriasis. Arbiser JL, Grossman K, Kaye E, Arndt KA. Arch Dermatol 1994;130:704–6.

Erythrodermic psoriasis will respond rapidly to oral corticosteroids or to superpotent corticosteroids with occlusion, but withdrawal of these agents often results in a more severe flare. Consequently, those treatments are avoided in patients with erythrodermic psoriasis.

Management of erythrodermic psoriasis with low-dose cyclosporine. Studio Italiano Muticentrico nella Psoriasi (SIMPSO). Dermatology 1993;187(suppl 1):30–7.

Thirty three patients with erythrodermic psoriasis were treated with cyclosporine starting with up to 5 mg/kg daily; 67% achieved complete remission in a median of 2–4 months and another 27% noted substantial improvement.

Erythrodermic, recalcitrant psoriasis: clinical resolution with infliximab. Rongioletti F, Borenstein M, Kirsner R, Kerdel F. J Dermatolog Treat 2003;14:222–5.

A patient with a 12-year history of erythrodermic psoriasis responded dramatically to infliximab infusion.

Treatment of pustulous and erythrodermic psoriasis with PUVA therapy and methotrexate. (German) Lekovic B, Dostanic I, Konstantinovic K, Kneitner I. Hautarzt 1982;33: 284–5.

The combination of PUVA and methotrexate successfully treated five patients with erythrodermic psoriasis and two patients with pustular psoriasis. According to the authors, annual methotrexate doses could be reduced by 50% by adding PUVA to the regimen.

It is difficult to distinguish a PUVA burn from erythrodermic psoriasis. Nevertheless, some patients with erythrodermic psoriasis are successfully controlled with PUVA. Monotherapy with methotrexate is used more typically.

The treatment of psoriasis with etretinate and acitretin: a follow up of actual use. Magis NL, Blummel JJ, Kerkhof PC, Gerritsen RM. Eur J Dermatol 2000;10:517–21.

In a retrospective review of 94 patients treated with retinoids, there were no serious side effects after 10 years of follow-up. The efficacy of retinoids for pustular and erythrodermic psoriasis was stressed.

Accidental success with carbamazepine for psoriatic erythroderma. Smith KJ, Skelton HG. N Engl J Med 1996;335: 1999–2000.

An patient with HIV infection and erythrodermic psoriasis was inadvertently treated with carbamazepine instead of etretinate. The patient's erythroderma cleared.

Carbamazepine in doses of 200–400 mg daily has been reported to clear erythrodermic psoriasis in some but not all patients. Further controlled clinical studies are warranted.

Pustular psoriasis

Management of pustular psoriasis begins with *removal of precipitating causes.* Lithium, antimalarials, diltiazem, propranolol and irritating topical therapy with tar have all been implicated, but the most common cause is the withdrawal of systemic corticosteroids. As in erythrodermic psoriasis, all the protective functions of skin are compromised and patients are susceptible to infection, fluid loss, electrolyte imbalance, loss of nutrients through the skin, and loss of temperature control. Supportive care and treatment of infection are mandatory. *Oral acitretin* results in rapid improvement. In women of childbearing potential, *isotretinoin* may be preferred because the period of teratogenicity of this drug is shorter than with acitretin. *Cyclosporine, infliximab* and *methotrexate* are also highly effective for this life-threatening condition. *Hydroxyurea, 6-thioguanine, mycophenolate mofetil, azathioprine, dapsone,* and *colchicine* have also been used in isolated patients.

FIRST LINE THERAPIES

■ Topical corticosteroids	E
■ Retinoids	B
■ Cyclosporine	E
■ Infliximab	E
■ Methotrexate	B

Evidence levels A Double-blind study B Clinical trial ≥ 20 subjects C Clinical trial < 20 subjects D Series ≥ 5 subjects E Anecdotal case reports

SECOND LINE THERAPIES

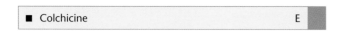

■ Topical calcipotriol	E
■ Etanercept	E
■ 6-Thioguanine	E
■ Hydroxyurea	E
■ Mycophenolate mofetil	E
■ Azathioprine	E

THIRD LINE THERAPIES

■ Colchicine	E

Isotretinoin vs etretinate therapy in generalized pustular and chronic psoriasis. Moy RL, Kingston TP, Lowe NJ. Arch Dermatol 1985;121:1297–301.

Although isotretinoin was less effective than etretinate for plaque psoriasis, ten of 11 patients with pustular psoriasis responded.

Many consider acitretin or isotretinoin to be the treatment of choice for patients with pustular psoriasis. Apart from the shorter period of teratogenicity of isotretinoin, it also causes less hair loss than acitretin.

Generalized pustular psoriasis (von Zumbusch) responding to cyclosporine A. Meinardi MM, Westerhof W, Bos JD. Br J Dermatol 1987;116:269–70.

This is one of numerous case reports documenting the dramatic response of pustular psoriasis to cyclosporine.

Cyclosporine in doses of 4–5 mg/kg daily is usually effective in the treatment of pustular psoriasis.

Rapid response to infliximab in severe pustular psoriasis, von Zumbusch type. Newland MR, Weinstein A, Kerdel F. Int J Dermatol 2002;41:449–52.

This case report describes the rapid improvement seen in generalized pustular psoriasis following treatment with infliximab.

Pustular psoriasis induced by infliximab. Thurber M, Feasel A, Stroehlein J, Hymes SR. J Drugs Dermatol 2004; 3:439–40.

Despite several reports describing the efficacy of infliximab in pustular psoriasis, there are a small number of reports of pustular psoriasis developing in patients treated with infliximab for other indications.

Generalised pustular psoriasis: response to topical calcipotriol. Berth-Jones J, Bourke J, Bailey K, et al. BMJ 1992; 305:868–9.

Three cases of pustular psoriasis responded to topical application of calcipotriol and the treatment was well tolerated.

It is important to monitor serum calcium when using calcipotriol in this way. Although irritation was not a problem in the reported cases, some care is required in case this develops.

Generalised pustular psoriasis induced by cyclosporin A withdrawal responding to the tumour necrosis factor alpha inhibitor etanercept. Kamarashev J, Lor P, Forster A, et al. Dermatology 2002;205:213–6.

This case report describes the use of etanercept 25 mg subcutaneously twice per week to improve psoriatic arthritis and pustular psoriasis induced by withdrawal of cyclosporine.

Systemic corticosteroids and folic acid antagonists in the treatment of generalized pustular psoriasis. Evaluation and prognosis based on the study of 104 cases. Ryan TJ, Baker H. Br J Dermatol 1969;81:134–45.

Despite short-term benefit of systemic corticosteroids for pustular psoriasis, once the dose is reduced rebound flares occur. In this study a significant proportion of patients treated with systemic corticosteroids died.

Methotrexate remains a highly effective modality for the treatment of pustular psoriasis. Doses beginning at 15 mg per week (following an initial test dose) are used.

Pustular psoriasis. Farber EM, Nall L. Cutis 1993;51:29–32.

The diagnosis and treatment of pustular psoriasis are discussed.

This review presents many of the usual and unusual treatments for pustular psoriasis including methotrexate, hydroxyurea, retinoids, dapsone, and cyclosporine. Even systemic corticosteroids are discussed, though most experts believe these should be avoided.

Colchicine in generalized pustular psoriasis: clinical response and antibody-dependent cytotoxicity by monocytes and neutrophils. Zachariae H, Kragballe K, Herlin T. Arch Dermatol Res 1982;274:327–33.

Three of four patients with pustular psoriasis cleared within 2 weeks of starting oral colchicine.

Colchicine 0.6 mg twice daily can be effective for pustular psoriasis. The dose can be increased by one pill daily, but side effects of diarrhea frequently intervene.

Pyoderma gangrenosum

John Berth-Jones

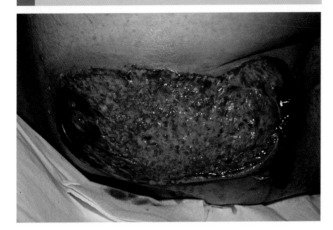

Pyoderma gangrenosum (PG) is a clinically diagnosed entity presenting as pustules that enlarge, forming ulcers with a dark, necrotic, undermined margin. Any skin site may be affected. Although PG is usually self-limiting there is a danger of disfiguring scarring.

MANAGEMENT STRATEGY

There are no controlled trials of treatment for PG, perhaps due to the relatively rare and sporadic occurrence of this disease. The pathogenesis is not well understood so treatment has developed largely on an empirical basis, and the mechanisms of action of the treatments employed are highly speculative.

No treatment is always effective. The most consistent results are reported with *systemic corticosteroids* and *cyclosporine (ciclosporin)* and these effective, but potentially toxic modalities can be employed when the severity of the disease justifies the risks (e.g. when there is facial involvement or rapid progression). The evidence regarding other modalities is less conclusive. PG tends to resolve spontaneously so some of the reports of therapeutic success may simply be the result of the disease following its natural course.

In cases where scarring is not a major concern, consideration should be given to *conservative treatment with wound dressing* only, because most lesions resolve spontaneously. When required, relatively nontoxic first line treatments should be tried first and second line modalities should be employed if there is no response. *Topical tacrolimus* offers an interesting novel approach to first line therapy. A wide variety of potentially hazardous and expensive treatments are employed occasionally, and these third line modalities should be considered only when others are ineffective.

The many recognized associations with PG include rheumatoid disease, inflammatory bowel disease, plasma cell dyscrasias, and other myeloproliferative disease. These may warrant investigation and may also influence the choice of treatment. *Effective management of an underlying pathology* such as ulcerative colitis often seems to result in improvement of the PG.

PG may demonstrate the Köbner phenomenon (pathergy); care should be taken to avoid trauma to the skin. When surgery is unavoidable in patients with a history of PG, the surgeon should be made aware of this risk. Surgical incisions should be kept as short as possible. Careful wound closure may be helpful. Prophylactic systemic corticosteroids or cyclosporine may be indicated perioperatively.

SPECIFIC INVESTIGATIONS

- Hematology
- Plasma protein electrophoresis
- Rheumatoid factor
- Antineutrophil cytoplasmic antibodies

In selected patients where clinically indicated
- Gastrointestinal workup for inflammatory bowel disease

Pyoderma gangrenosum associated with Wegener's granulomatosis: partial response to mycophenolate mofetil. Le Hello C, Bonte I, Mora JJ, et al. Rheumatology (Oxford) 2002;41:236–7.

In addition to more familiar associations, there are now many reports of PG lesions developing as a feature of Wegener's granulomatosis.

FIRST LINE THERAPIES

Topical tacrolimus	C
Topical corticosteroids	D
Clofazimine	D
Dapsone	D
Intralesional corticosteroids	D
Minocycline	D
Nicotine chewing gum	E
Sodium cromoglycate	D
Sulfasalazine (sulphasalazine)	D

Topical tacrolimus for pyoderma gangrenosum. Reich K, Vente C, Neumann C. Br J Dermatol 1998;139:755–7.

Tacrolimus ointment, 0.1%, proved effective when used in combination with systemic cyclosporine and also when used alone. The formula comprised 100 mg FK506 powder obtained from tablets of Prograf®, mixed into 100 g of hydrophilic petrolatum (white petrolatum with 8% bleached beeswax, 3% stearyl alcohol, and 3% cholesterol).

Topical tacrolimus in the management of peristomal pyoderma gangrenosum. Lyon CC, Stapleton M, Smith AJ, et al. J Dermatol Treat 2001;12:13–7.

Seven of eleven cases of peristomal PG healed completely after 2–10 weeks of applying tacrolimus 0.3% in carmellose sodium paste (Orabase®). Serum levels of tacrolimus were undetectable in all cases. In this open study, results were at least as good as those for clobetasol propionate.

Topical tacrolimus would seem to be safe enough to use as a first line treatment, though experience remains limited.

Pyoderma gangrenosum of the scalp. Peachey RDG. Br J Dermatol 1974;90:106.

A case of PG involving the scalp showed slow but steady improvement on treatment with 0.1% betamethasone valerate lotion applied under polythene occlusion at night.

Evidence levels A Double-blind study **B** Clinical trial ≥ 20 subjects **C** Clinical trial < 20 subjects **D** Series ≥ 5 subjects **E** Anecdotal case reports

The efficacy of systemic corticosteroids would suggest that topical application might also be beneficial. However, there are only sparse anecdotal reports to support their efficacy. Potent compounds are generally used (e.g. betamethasone dipropionate 0.05% cream or clobetasol propionate 0.05% cream) applied once daily to the lesion under an occlusive dressing of paraffin gauze or hydrocolloid.

Clofazimine. A new agent for treatment of pyoderma gangrenosum. Michaelsson G, Molin L, Ohman S, et al. Arch Dermatol 1976;112:344–9.

These authors employed clofazimine with the rationale that the ability of this drug to enhance neutrophil phagocytosis would be beneficial in PG. A good response was observed in eight cases and was often apparent within a few days. The dose used was 300–400 mg daily.

Clofazimine in the treatment of pyoderma gangrenosum. Thomsen K, Rothenborg HW. Arch Dermatol 1979;115: 851–2.

A good response was reported in seven of ten cases which healed within 2–5 months on 100 mg three times daily.

Sulfapyridine and sulphone-type drugs in dermatology. Lorincz AL, Pearson RW. Arch Dermatol 1962;85:42–56.

Dapsone was successfully employed in the treatment of PG at doses of up to 400 mg daily. Low cost and the familiarity of dermatologists with this drug probably contribute to its popularity.

Dapsone has often been used in combination with other modalities, especially systemic corticosteroids. There are also many published cases in which this drug has proved ineffective. Dapsone has been successfully used in children with PG. The mechanism of action is believed to be inhibition of neutrophil migration and the myeloperoxidase system.

Triamcinolone and pyoderma gangrenosum. Gardner LW, Acker DW. Arch Dermatol 1972;106:599–600.

A case of multifocal PG responded to intralesional triamcinolone acetonide 10 mg/mL. Doses ranging from 40 to 200 mg were injected at any one time.

Intralesional or perilesional injection of corticosteroids appears to be very helpful in some cases.

The corticosteroid is usually injected into the skin around the active margins of lesions. The risk of inducing cutaneous atrophy is small using these concentrations and is not unacceptable in view of the scarring that will develop without treatment.

The successful use of minocycline in pyoderma gangrenosum – a report of seven cases and review of the literature. Berth-Jones J, Tan SV, Graham-Brown RAC, Pembroke AC. J Dermatol Treat 1989;1:23–5.

Seven cases responded to minocycline used at doses of 100 mg twice daily or 200 mg twice daily. Improvement was often observed within a few days.

Nicotine for pyoderma gangrenosum. Kanekura T, Usuki K, Kanzaki T. Lancet 1995;345:1058.

This is an isolated report of PG responding to nicotine chewing gum three tablets daily, each tablet containing 2 mg nicotine.

Pyoderma gangrenosum. A study of nineteen cases. Perry HO, Brunsting LA. Arch Dermatol 1957;75:380–6.

Six of seven patients with PG associated with colitis demonstrated a good response to sulfasalazine using 0.5 g every 3 h. A good response was also seen in three of four cases of PG when colitis was not present. This drug may be particularly useful in cases of PG associated with inflammatory bowel disease and it can also be effective in those that are not. The initial dose ranges from 0.5 to 2 g four times daily. Doses at the upper end of this range are usually reduced for maintenance therapy.

The treatment of pyoderma gangrenosum with sodium cromoglycate. De Cock KM, Thorne MG. Br J Dermatol 1980;102:231–3.

Two cases responded to sodium cromoglycate aqueous solution (2% w/v, Rynacrom® nasal spray). In one patient, healing occurred within 3 weeks.

This is a remarkably safe treatment. Solutions of this drug have been applied to lesions of PG in concentrations ranging from 1 to 4%. Various nasal sprays and nebulizer solutions have proved suitable for direct application to PG lesions. The solution can be sprayed on to the ulcer or applied on gauze or under occlusion with a hydrocolloid dressing. This drug may act by inhibiting neutrophil migration or cytotoxicity.

SECOND LINE THERAPIES

■ Cyclosporine	C
■ Systemic corticosteroids	C

Treatment of pyoderma gangrenosum with cyclosporine: results in seven patients. Elgart G, Stover P, Larson K, et al. J Am Acad Dermatol 1991;24:83–6.

Six of seven patients, including cases associated with rheumatoid disease and cryoglobulinemia improved on cyclosporine, four healing completely.

The response to cyclosporine seems to be fairly consistent. Because the toxicity of cyclosporine is largely related to prolonged use it can be a reasonably safe approach for gaining control of PG, which is often a brief self-limiting illness. High doses have been used (5–10 mg/kg daily), and are probably safe for a few days in an urgent situation. However, it is likely that lower doses of 5 mg/kg daily will often be adequate.

Pyoderma gangrenosum. Clinical and laboratory findings in 15 patients with special reference to polyarthritis. Holt PJA, Davies MG, Saunders KC, Nuki G. Medicine 1980; 59:114–33.

Twelve of these patients received, and responded to, corticosteroid treatment. Doses of up to 100 mg daily were required to induce remission.

Systemic corticosteroids (prednisone/prednisolone) have been one of the most frequently used treatments for PG and extensive published experience indicates that they are generally considered to be highly effective. High doses of 40–100 mg daily may be required and the morbidity may be considerable. Lower doses of 7.5–20 mg daily are sometimes adequate for maintenance. Other systemic and topical agents are usually employed simultaneously to minimize the dose.

Pulse therapy. Therapeutic efficacy in the treatment of pyoderma gangrenosum. Johnson RB, Lazarus GS. Arch Dermatol 1982;118:76–84.

Intravenous doses of methylprednisolone 1 g daily for 5 days induced prompt responses in three cases.

THIRD LINE THERAPIES

■ Alkylating agents (cyclophosphamide, chlorambucil)	D
■ Plasmapheresis (plasma exchange)	E
■ Leukocytapheresis	D
■ Human immunoglobulin	D
■ Intralesional cyclosporine	E
■ Tacrolimus	D
■ Azathioprine and mercaptopurine	D
■ Colchicine	D
■ Thalidomide	D
■ Topical nitrogen mustard (mechlorethamine)	E
■ Mycophenolate mofetil	D
■ Granulocyte macrophage-colony stimulating factor (GM-CSF)	E
■ Methotrexate	E
■ Infliximab	D
■ Etanercept	E
■ Topical platelet-derived growth factor	E
■ Hyperbaric oxygen	D
■ Surgical repair by graft or flap	E

Pyoderma gangrenosum. Response to cyclophosphamide therapy. Newell LM, Malkinson FD. Arch Dermatol 1983;119:495–7.

A very refractory case of PG responded to cyclophosphamide 150 mg daily. Healing was evident after 14 days and almost complete after 109 days.

Intravenous cyclophosphamide pulses in the treatment of pyoderma gangrenosum associated with rheumatoid arthritis: report of 2 cases and review of the literature. Zonana-Nacach A, Jimenez-Balderas FJ, Martinez-Osuna P, Mintz G. J Rheumatol 1994;21:1352–6.

Two cases improved on pulsed intravenous cyclophosphamide at doses of 500 mg/m², combined with oral corticosteroid. The first received three pulses over 5 weeks and the second seven pulses over 14 weeks. In both cases, remission was subsequently maintained using oral cyclophosphamide 100 mg daily.

Chlorambucil is an effective corticosteroid-sparing agent for recalcitrant pyoderma gangrenosum. Burruss JB, Farmer ER, Callen JP. J Am Acad Dermatol 1996;35:720–4.

Chlorambucil was successfully used in six cases, both alone and in combination with systemic corticosteroids. The doses used ranged from 2 to 4 mg daily.

Pyoderma gangrenosum – response to topical nitrogen mustard. Tsele E, Yu RCH, Chu AC. Clin Exp Dermatol 1992;17:437–40.

The application of nitrogen mustard 20 mg/100 mL in aqueous solution on gauze swabs proved helpful in a single case associated with IgA paraprotein, which had not responded to many other treatment modalities. Patients can prepare this solution at home using tap water. Plasmapheresis was also helpful in this case. This was performed weekly for 2 years, successfully controlling the PG during this time.

Plasmapheresis is a relatively safe treatment involving removal of plasma while returning the blood cells to the circulation. Exchanges have generally been performed one to three times weekly and prompt responses have been reported.

Leukocytapheresis treatment for pyoderma gangrenosum. Fujimoto E, Fujimoto N, Kuroda K, Tajima S. Br J Dermatol 2004;151:1090–2.

Granulocyte and monocyte adsorption apheresis for pyoderma gangrenosum. Kanekura T, Maruyama I, Kanzaki T. J Am Acad Dermatol 2002;47:320–1.

These treatments, which involve extracorporeal removal of leukocytes, are now reported to have been effective in several cases of PG occurring in isolation and in association with ulcerative colitis and rheumatoid disease. Treatment was performed once weekly for 4–5 weeks.

Efficacy of human intravenous immune globulin in pyoderma gangrenosum. Gupta AK, Shear NH, Sauder DN. J Am Acad Dermatol 1995;32:140–2.

This case was treated for 5 days at 0.4 g/kg daily followed by a course of 1 g/kg daily for 2 days while cyclosporine and prednisone were continued.

Successful treatment of pyoderma gangrenosum with intravenous human immunoglobulin. Dirschka T, Kastner U, Behrens S, Altmeyer P. J Am Acad Dermatol 1998;39:789–90.

This case received 2-day courses of 1 g/kg daily repeated every month until complete healing was achieved after 4 months while also receiving prednisone, which was gradually reduced from 60 mg to 10 mg daily.

Superficial granulomatous pyoderma treated with intravenous immunoglobulin. Dobson CM, Parslew RA, Evans S. J Am Acad Dermatol 2003;48:456–60.

Superficial granulomatous pyoderma has been described as a distinct variant of PG. This case had proved refractory to many treatments over a 5-year period, but improved rapidly after a 5-day course of intravenous immunoglobulin (IVIG) 400 mg/kg body weight daily, healing completely during the ensuing 3 months.

Human IVIG has proved effective in cases that had previously failed to respond to high doses of systemic corticosteroids and cyclosporine. However, this treatment is somewhat costly and because IVIG is derived from pooled plasma carries a theoretical risk of transmitting infection.

Clearing of pyoderma gangrenosum by intralesional cyclosporin A. Mrowietz U, Christophers E. Br J Dermatol 1991;125:498–9.

A lesion on the shoulder improved after two injections in one week of 35 mg cyclosporine into the active edges and beneath the lesion. The injection was formulated by diluting Sandimmun® with normal saline in a 1:3 ratio.

Resolution of severe pyoderma gangrenosum in a patient with streaking leukocyte factor disease after treatment with tacrolimus (FK506). Abu-Elmagd K, Van Thiel DH, Jegasothy BV, et al. Ann Intern Med 1993;119:595–8.

These authors used an initial dose of 0.15 mg/kg twice daily and reduced this gradually to the lowest effective dose.

Recalcitrant pyoderma gangrenosum treated with systemic tacrolimus. Lyon CC, Kirby B, Griffiths CE. Br J Dermatol 1999;140:562–4.

A refractory case of peristomal PG responded to oral tacrolimus 0.15 mg/kg daily.

Successful therapy of refractory pyoderma gangrenosum and periorbital phlegmona with tacrolimus (FK506) in ulcerative colitis. Baumgart DC, Wiedenmann B, Dignass AU. Inflamm Bowel Dis 2004;10:421–4.

Two cases of PG associated with ulcerative colitis responded to oral tacrolimus 0.1 mg/kg daily.

Combination oral and topical tacrolimus in therapy-resistant pyoderma gangrenosum. Jolles S, Niclasse S, Benson E. Br J Dermatol 1999;140:564–5.

Tacrolimus ointment, 0.1%, was used concomitantly with systemic administration of this drug at the dose of 0.3 mg/kg daily after higher systemic doses had proved too nephrotoxic. The addition of the topical application was followed by healing over 3 months.

Pyoderma gangrenosum treated with 6-mercaptopurine and followed by acute leukemia. Maldonado N, Torres VM, Mendez-Cashion D, et al. J Pediatr 1968;72:409–14.

These authors reported a response to mercaptopurine used alone, at the relatively high dose of 2.5 mg/kg daily, though the patient, a 7-year-old boy, subsequently developed leukemia.

Crohn's disease with cutaneous involvement. Parks AG, Morson BC, Pegum JS. Proc Roy Soc Med 1965;58:241.

Mercaptopurine was used at the lower dose of 75 mg daily in combination with prednisone 20 mg daily.

Azathioprine has often been employed for treatment of PG, both alone and as a corticosteroid-sparing agent. Doses have generally ranged from 100 to 150 mg daily. Less often, higher doses of up to 2.5 mg/kg daily are used. This drug seems to be useful in some cases, but results are not consistent. Mercaptopurine is the active metabolite of azathioprine.

Treatment of pyoderma gangrenosum with colchicine. Paolini O, Hebuterne X, Flory P, et al. Lancet 1995;345:1057–8.

Colchicine was effective and well tolerated in PG associated with Crohn's colitis. The dose used was 1 mg daily.

Colchicine in pyoderma gangrenosum. Rampal P, Benzaken S, Schneider S, Hebuterne X. Lancet 1998;351:1134–5.

Response was maintained using 1 mg daily for 3 years and the drug was well tolerated.

Case report: severe pyoderma associated with familial Mediterranean fever – favorable response to colchicine in three patients. Lugassy G, Ronnen M. Am J Med Sci 1992;304:29–31.

Colchicine was effective in three cases of PG associated with familial Mediterranean fever. Treatment was commenced at 2 mg daily and reduced to 1 mg daily for maintenance.

Pyoderma gangrenosum with severe pharyngeal involvement. Buckley C, Bayoumi AHM, Sarkany I. J Roy Soc Med 1990;83:590–1.

An adult case refractory to several other modalities responded to thalidomide 100 mg daily.

Pyoderma gangrenosum chez un enfant: traitement par la thalidomide. Venencie PY, Saurat J-H. Ann Pediatr 1982;1:67–9.

A 3-year-old child refractory to other treatments responded well to thalidomide 150 mg daily.

Pyoderma gangrenosum associated with Behçet's syndrome – response to thalidomide. Munro CS, Cox NH. Clin Exp Dermatol 1988;13:408–10.

A case refractory to prednisolone 100 mg daily combined with dapsone 100 mg daily responded within 48 hours to thalidomide 400 mg daily.

Thalidomide may be of particular value in cases associated with Behçet's disease because it is also reportedly effective in severe aphthous ulceration.

Mycophenolate mofetil and cyclosporin treatment for recalcitrant pyoderma gangrenosum. Hohenleutner U, Mohr VD, Michel S, Landthaler M. Lancet 1997;350:1748.

Mycophenolate mofetil proved useful for a severe case of PG in combination with cyclosporine, intravenous corticosteroids, and topical application of platelet-derived wound-healing factors. The effective dose was 2 g daily.

Treatment of recalcitrant ulcers in pyoderma gangrenosum with mycophenolate mofetil and autologous keratinocyte transplantation on a hyaluronic acid matrix. Wollina U, Karamfilov T. J Eur Acad Dermatol Venereol 2000;14:187–90.

This case improved when mycophenolate 2 g daily was used in combination with an intravenous infusion of prednisolone 100 mg daily.

Mycophenolate mofetil in pyoderma gangrenosum. Lee MR, Cooper AJ. J Dermatol Treat 2004;15:303–7.

Mycophenolate 1–2.5 g daily was used in combination with prednisolone in three cases and as monotherapy (with 500 mg twice daily) in one.

Mycophenolate has most often been used in combination with other agents such as cyclosporine and corticosteroids.

Pyoderma gangrenosum in myelodysplasia responding to granulocyte macrophage-colony stimulating factor (GM-CSF). Bulvic S, Jacobs P. Br J Dermatol 1997;136:637–8.

This case responded to GM-CSF in a dose of 400 µg daily injected subcutaneously.

Pyoderma gangrenosum successfully treated with perilesional granulocyte-macrophage colony stimulating factor. Shpiro D, Gilat D, Fisher-Feld L, et al. Br J Dermatol 1998;138:368–9.

In this case the GM-CSF was injected perilesionally at a weekly dose of 400 mg for 4 weeks.

The use of GM-CSF has also been reported to aggravate PG. A variety of hypersensitivity reactions, including anaphylaxis, have occasionally occurred.

Treatment of pyoderma gangrenosum with methotrexate. Teitel AD. Cutis 1996;57:326–8.

A case of PG failing to respond to prednisone 60 mg daily improved within 2 weeks of adding in methotrexate 15 mg weekly.

Improvement of pyoderma gangrenosum and psoriasis associated with Crohn disease with anti-tumor necrosis factor alpha monoclonal antibody. Tan MH, Gordon M, Lebwohl O, et al. Arch Dermatol 2001;137:930–3.

Treatment of pyoderma gangrenosum with infliximab in Crohn's disease. Sapienza MS, Cohen S, Dimarino AJ. Dig Dis Sci 2004;49:1454–7.

Several cases of PG associated with inflammatory bowel disease have now been reported to respond within 4 weeks to infusion of infliximab. In some cases a single infusion of 5 mg/kg has been adequate.

Treatment of pyoderma gangrenosum with etanercept. McGowan JW 4th, Johnson CA, Lynn A. J Drugs Dermatol 2004;3:441–4.

A single case responding to etanercept.

Topical platelet-derived growth factor accelerates healing of myelodysplastic syndrome-associated pyoderma gangrenosum. Braun-Falco M, Stock K, Ring J, Hein R. Br J Dermatol 2002;147:829–31.

Complete healing occurred over 9 weeks in this case after platelet-derived growth factor (Becalpermin®) was added to the treatment regimen.

Pyoderma gangrenosum treated with hyperbaric oxygen therapy. Wasserteil V, Bruce S, Sessoms SL, Guntupalli KK. Int J Dermatol 1992;31:594–6.

Hyperbaric oxygen has been reported as beneficial in several cases of PG. However, as with all other treatments, it is not effective in all cases. This treatment may be worth trying when facilities are available.

Split skin grafts in the treatment of pyoderma gangrenosum: a report of four cases. Cliff S. Dermatol Surg 1999; 25:299–302.

Free flap coverage of pyoderma gangrenosum leg ulcers. Classen DA, Thomson C. J Cutan Med Surg 2002;6:327–31.

Surgical approaches are generally best avoided in PG, at least while the disease is active, because the disease is likely to develop in sites of trauma. Although the use of split skin grafts and microvascular free flaps have been reported to successfully accelerate healing, surgery is probably best reserved for use once the disease is inactive.

Evidence levels A Double-blind study B Clinical trial ≥ 20 subjects C Clinical trial < 20 subjects D Series ≥ 5 subjects E Anecdotal case reports

Radiation dermatitis

Joshua A Zeichner, Jack F Dalton

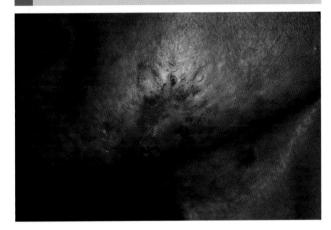

Radiation dermatitis refers to skin changes that occur after cutaneous radiation exposure, as during interventional radiologic procedures or treatment of malignancies. The dermatitis may be categorized as either acute or chronic. Appendageal structures and basal layer cells are the most sensitive to radiation exposure, and their damage leads to the acute skin changes. These include pruritus, dry and moist desquamation, erythema, epilation, edema, and blistering. Atrophy, hyper- or hypopigmentation, telangiectasia, fibrosis, ulceration, and necrosis are later effects that depend more on dermal and vascular damage. Certain chemotherapeutic drugs such as doxorubicin and dactinomycin may induce similar skin changes at sites of previous radiation exposure, referred to as radiation recall dermatitis.

MANAGEMENT STRATEGY

Treatment of radiation dermatitis begins with prevention, and the severity of skin changes correlates with the cumulative dose of ionizing radiation the patient receives. Radiation therapy is an integral part of many cancer treatment regimens, however, and cannot always be avoided. Therefore, much of the management of radiation dermatitis consists of supportive care, pain control, and prevention of infection.

Topical therapies are the mainstay of treatment for acute radiation dermatitis. *Cornstarch and emollient creams* help dry desquamation (painless peeling of the skin). Management of moist desquamation (painful, full-thickness loss of the epidermis) is similar to that of burns, with *occlusive dressings and care to prevent infections*. *Topical corticosteroids* control pruritus and decrease inflammation, particularly in sundamaged areas. Patients should also avoid friction on the skin from tight-fitting clothing. *Topical antifungal ointments* treat and may provide prophylaxis against fungal infections of the skin, especially in the intertriginous areas. Patients may gently wash skin with water and mild soaps.

Similar to acute changes, chronic radiation dermatitis is treated symptomatically. Topical emollient creams and corticosteroids can be employed as needed. Skin necrosis or ulceration must be carefully monitored for signs of infection.

Some recommend physical massage of the skin to improve fibrosis.

SPECIFIC INVESTIGATIONS

- History of previous radiation exposure and chemotherapeutic drugs
- Evaluation of affected skin for development of malignancy

Radio-induced malignancies of the scalp about 98 patients with 150 lesions and literature review. Maalej M, Frikha H, Kochbati L, et al. Cancer Radiother 2004;8:81–7.

Basal cell carcinomas are the most common malignancies to develop in the skin at sites of previous radiation exposure, especially on the head and the neck.

FIRST LINE THERAPIES

Prevention	
■ Avoidance of excessive ionizing radiation exposure	
Acute radiation dermatitis	
■ Emollient creams	E
■ Topical corticosteroids	A
■ Topical calendula	A
■ Dexpanthenol	A
Chronic radiation dermatitis	
■ Emollient creams	E

Prevention and treatment of acute radiation dermatitis: a literature review. Wickline MM. Oncol Nurs Forum 2004;31:237–47.

This review discusses the current therapies available for prevention and treatment of acute radiation dermatitis. Many products on the market have not been proven to be effective. These include trolamine (Biafine®), some herbal creams and ointments, and topical vitamin C. The benefit of aloe vera gel is still unclear. Certain skin dressings, sucralfate cream, and corticosteroids have been shown to improve radiation dermatitis.

Potent corticosteroid cream (mometasone furoate) significantly reduces acute radiation dermatitis: results from a double blind, randomized study. Bostrom A, Lindman H, Swartling C, et al. Radiother Oncol 2001;59:257–65.

Topical corticosteroid treatment is effective in improving skin outcome after radiation treatment.

Topical corticosteroid therapy for acute radiation dermatitis: a prospective, randomized, double-blind study. Schmuth M, Wimmer MA, Hofer S, et al. Br J Dermatol 2002;146:983–91.

The authors of this article found that neither topical corticosteroids nor topical dexpanthenol prevented the onset of radiation dermatitis. However, both decreased the severity of the skin changes compared to the control group, and the members of the topical corticosteroid group showed less severe skin reactions than the dexpanthenol group.

Phase III randomized trial of *Calendula officinalis* compared with trolamine for the prevention of acute dermatitis during irradiation for breast cancer. Pommier P, Gomez F, Sunyach MP, et al. J Clin Oncol 2004;22:1447–53.

This randomized trial compared the use of topical calendula to topical trolamine (Biafine®) at sites of irradiation in patients receiving radiation treatment for breast cancer. Acute radiation dermatitis developed in a significantly higher percentage of patients using trolamine compared to calendula.

Skin treatment with Bepanthen cream versus no cream during radiotherapy – a randomized control trial. Lokkevik E, Skovlund E, Reitan JB, et al. Acta Oncol 1996;35: 1021–6.

This study demonstrated the efficacy of dexpanthenol-containing cream in treating radiation dermatitis.

SECOND LINE THERAPIES

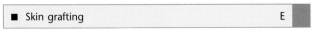

■ Amifostine	B
■ Pentoxifylline (under investigation)	A
■ Celecoxib (under investigation)	E

The cytoprotective effect of amifostine in acute radiation dermatitis: a retrospective analysis. Kouvaris J, Kouloulias V, Kokakis J, et al. Eur J Dermatol 2002;12:458–62.

Amifostine is a cytoprotective drug used to reduce toxicities from cancer chemotherapy and radiation therapy. In this retrospective analysis, the authors found a significant protective effect in the skin in patients receiving radiation therapy.

Prophylactic effect of pentoxifylline on radiotherapy complications: a clinical study. Aygenc E, Celikkanat S, Kaymakci M, et al. Otolaryngol Head Neck Surg 2004;130:351–6.

Many late changes in radiation dermatitis are thought to be due to vascular insufficiency. In this trial, the group taking pentoxifylline had less severe fibrosis and necrosis than the placebo group. This report is the only case series of its kind in the literature. Pentoxifylline is still under investigation for this application. Confirmatory studies have not yet been published.

Celecoxib reduces skin damage after radiation: selective reduction of chemokine and receptor mRNA expression in irradiated skin but not irradiated mammary tumor. Liang L, Hu D, Liu W, et al. Am J Clin Oncol 2003; 26:S114–21.

In a mouse model, celecoxib was shown to decrease necrosis, inflammatory infiltrate, and chemokine expression in irradiated skin. This effect was selective for the skin, without affecting the irradiated tissue of the tumor in question. Cyclooxygenase-2 (COX-2) inhibitors are currently not a standard part of treatment for radiation dermatitis, but this discovery warrants further investigation.

THIRD LINE THERAPIES

■ Skin grafting	E

Chronic radiodermatitis injury after cardiac catheterization. Barnea Y, Amir A, Shafir R, et al. Ann Plast Surg 2002;49:668–72.

The authors present two cases of patients with painful, nonhealing wounds at the site of chronic radiation dermatitis. The patients underwent wound excision with skin grafting. The skin healed completely, but pain was only partially relieved. In practice, skin grafting is extremely rare.

Evidence levels   A Double-blind study   **B** Clinical trial ≥ 20 subjects   **C** Clinical trial < 20 subjects   **D** Series ≥ 5 subjects   **E** Anecdotal case reports

Raynaud's disease and phenomenon

Brian S Fuchs, Marsha L Gordon

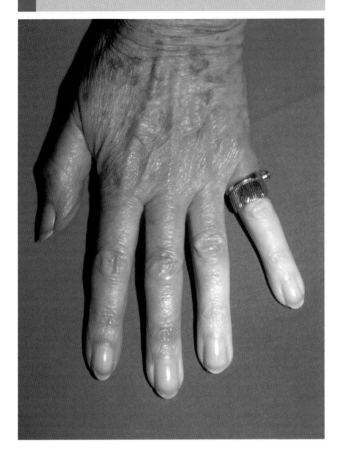

Both Raynaud's disease and Raynaud's phenomenon (RP) are characterized by intermittent peripheral vasoconstriction leading to pallor, cyanosis, and reactive vasodilation of the arterioles of the fingers and toes. They are caused by vasospasm in response to cold, emotion, hormones, and certain vasospastic drugs. Primary Raynaud's disease is a milder, idiopathic form while secondary Raynaud's phenomenon coexists with autoimmune connective tissue disorders such as systemic lupus erythematosus and systemic sclerosis or other conditions that reduce blood flow.

MANAGEMENT STRATEGY

For prognostic and therapeutic reasons, it is important to determine if Raynaud's phenomenon (RP) is associated with a connective tissue disorder such as systemic lupus erythematosus, CREST syndrome, scleroderma or, less frequently, rheumatoid arthritis, Sjögren's syndrome, mixed connective tissue disease, cryoglobulinemia, or dermatomyositis. Treatment of the underlying condition, if present, is essential.

Avoidance of triggers such as cold (especially sudden drops in temperature) and vibration (in cases where vibration is the precipitant) should be stressed. Drugs that may exacerbate the condition include β-blockers, bleomycin, caffeine, cisplatin, ergot preparations, interferon, methysergide, nicotine, oral contraceptives, reboxetine, tegaserod, and vinblastine.

Use of *warming devices* such as 'toe warmers' (Grabber Performance Group, Grand Rapids, MI 49512, USA) is beneficial.

First line medications include *calcium channel blockers* such as nifedipine (10–20 mg three or four times daily) or diltiazem (60 mg three or four times daily). *Vasodilators* (e.g. glyceryl trinitrate paste 2%), and the serotonin receptor blocker, *ketanserin*, have been employed with benefit, as have the *angiotensin converting enzyme (ACE) inhibitors*. *Low-dose acetylsalicylic acid and dipyridamole* can be used in combination to treat patients with RP who have digital ulcers.

For severe cases, *prostacyclin* or *prostaglandin E1* may work well. *Calcitonin gene-related peptide*, a potent vasodilator, has been used with success as have *plasma exchange, L-arginine, triiodothyronine (T3)*, and *Helicobacter pylori eradication*. *Sympathectomy* is the option of last resort.

Digital ulcers resulting from severe RP are to be treated with *aggressive local therapy* including *topical or oral antibiotics*, if necessary, and *occlusive dressings*. Severe ischemic attacks in older patients with comorbidities such as atherosclerosis or heart disease may necessitate *hospitalization*. Other therapies such as *acupuncture, biofeedback, and dietary supplementation with fish oil and evening primrose oil* have proved beneficial as well.

SPECIFIC INVESTIGATIONS

- Occupational history – vibration-associated 'white finger'
- Drug history
- Nailfold capillaroscopy
- Hematology
- Erythrocyte sedimentation rate
- Lupus serology
- Scl-70 antibody
- Anticentromere antibody
- Rheumatoid factor
- Cryoglobulins

Nailfold digital capillaroscopy in 447 patients with connective tissue disease and Raynaud's disease. Nagy Z, Czirjak L. J Eur Acad Dermatol Venereol 2004;18:62–8.

This article concludes that the scleroderma capillary pattern is often present in systemic sclerosis and dermato/polymyositis. Evidence from this study suggests that capillarmicroscopy is useful for early selection of patients who are candidates for developing scleroderma spectrum disorders.

Raynaud's phenomenon: a proposal for classification. LeRoy EC, Medsger TA Jr. Clin Exp Rheumatol 1992;10:485–8.

The authors have proposed a classification system in which patients with RP are considered to have secondary RP if they have any of the following: antinuclear antibodies, abnormal nailfold capillaries, digital pitting or gangrene, and certain organ abnormalities.

Anticardiolipin, anticentromere, and anti-Scl-70 antibodies in patients with systemic sclerosis and severe digital ischaemia. Herrick AL, Heaney M, Hollis S, Jayson MI. Ann Rheum Dis 1994;53:540–2.

The findings of this study suggest that patients who are positive for either anticentromere or anti-Scl-70 antibodies may be at risk of digital loss and should be treated accordingly.

Raynaud's phenomenon induced by drugs acting on neuro-transmission: two cases under reboxetine and one under tegaserod. Bertoli R, Girardin F, Russmann S, Lauterburg B. Eur J Clin Pharmacol 2003;58:717.

The authors suggest that the temporal relationship to tegaserod or reboxetine and the improvement upon de-challenge provides convincing evidence of drug-induced RP in the three cases examined.

Interferon-α induced Raynaud's syndrome. Kruit WH, Eggermont AMM, Stoter G. Ann Oncol 2000;11:1501–2.

During treatment with interferon-α, as adjuvant therapy for melanoma, two patients developed Raynaud's syndrome.

Microvascular abnormalities in patients with vibration white finger. Littleford RC, Khan F, Hindley MO, et al. QJM 1997;90:525–9.

Abnormal nailfold capillary patterns exist in patients with vibration white finger (VWF) and can be used to diagnose or confirm VWF.

FIRST LINE THERAPIES

■ Calcium channel blockers (nifedipine, diltiazem)	A
■ Vasodilators (inositol nicotinate [Hexopal®], glyceryl trinitrate 2% transdermal patch)	A
■ Dipyridamole and low-dose acetylsalicylic acid	A

Objective benefit of nifedipine in the treatment of Raynaud's phenomenon. White CJ, Phillips WA, Abrahams LA, et al. Am J Med 1986;80:623–5.

Nine of 11 patients with moderate to severe RP experienced improvement of their symptoms after treatment with nifedipine. Digital skin recovery time measurements after immersing the hand in cold water confirmed that nifedipine is an effective treatment for RP.

Acute effects of nifedipine on digital blood flow in human subjects with Raynaud's phenomenon: a double-blind placebo controlled trial. Wise RA, Malamet R, Wigley FM. J Rheumatol 1987;14:278–83.

The authors caution against the use of nifedipine in patients with severe RP because nifedipine can reduce blood flow by reducing perfusion pressure.

A double-blind placebo controlled crossover randomized trial of diltiazem in Raynaud's phenomenon. Rhedda A, McCans J, Willan AR, Ford PM. J Rheumatol 1985;12:724–7.

Reduction in severity, duration, and frequency of attacks was significant in patients with either primary or secondary RP.

A double-blind randomized placebo controlled trial of Hexopal in primary Raynaud's disease. Sunderland GT, Belch JJ, Sturrock RD, Forbes CD, McKay AJ. Clin Rheumatol 1988;7:46–9.

Hexopal 4 g daily is an effective treatment for patients with primary Raynaud's disease, especially during the winter months.

Hexopal® is inositol nicotinate or inositol hexanicotinate. It is not available in the USA.

Sustained-release transdermal glyceryl trinitrate patches as a treatment for primary and secondary Raynaud's phenomenon. Teh LS, Manning J, Moore T, et al. Br J Rheumatol 1995;34:636–41.

Glyceryl trinitrate patches (0.2 mg/h) were shown to be effective in reducing the number and severity of Raynaud's attacks in this study of 42 patients with primary and secondary RP. Headache was a frequent side effect.

These patches contain nitroglycerine paste 2%.

A double-blind controlled trial of low dose acetylsalicylic acid and dipyridamole in the treatment of Raynaud's phenomenon. van der Meer J, Wouda AA, Kallenberg CG, Wesseling H. Vasa Suppl 1987;18:71–5.

This analgesic and antithrombotic combination is safe and helpful in treating patients with RP who have severe digital ulceration.

SECOND LINE THERAPIES

■ Selective serotonin reuptake inhibitors (fluoxetine)	B
■ Captopril	A
■ Losartan	B
■ Serotonin antagonists (ketanserin)	A

Treatment of Raynaud's phenomenon with the selective serotonin reuptake inhibitor fluoxetine. Coleiro B, Marshall SE, Denton CP, et al. Rheumatology 2001;40:1038–43.

This study of 26 patients with primary and 27 patients with secondary RP demonstrates the tolerability of fluoxetine and suggests it would be an effective treatment.

The effect of captopril on cutaneous blood flow in patients with primary Raynaud's phenomenon. Rustin MH, Almond NE, Beacham JA, et al. Br J Dermatol 1987;117:751–8.

Captopril (25 mg three times daily) improved blood flow, but did not decrease the frequency or severity of attacks.

Losartan therapy for Raynaud's phenomenon and scleroderma: clinical and biochemical findings in a fifteen-week, randomized, parallel-group, controlled trial. Dziadzio M, Denton CP, Smith R, et al. Arthritis Rheum 1999;42:2646–55.

Treatment with losartan (50 mg daily) was shown to reduce the severity and frequency of Raynaud's attacks in patients with scleroderma-associated RP.

The effectiveness of ketanserin in patients with primary Raynaud's phenomenon. A randomized, double-blind, placebo controlled study. van de Wal HJ, Wijn PF, van Lier HJ, Skotnicki SH. Int Angiol 1987;6:313–22.

This serotonin antagonist showed no side effects and proved effective in minimizing subjective complaints in patients with primary RP.

Evidence levels A Double-blind study B Clinical trial ≥ 20 subjects C Clinical trial < 20 subjects D Series ≥ 5 subjects E Anecdotal case reports

THIRD LINE THERAPIES

■ Prostaglandin E1 (alprostadil)	A
■ Prostacyclin	A
■ Calcitonin gene-related peptide	C
■ L-arginine	D
■ H-O-U therapy	C
■ T3	C
■ *Helicobacter pylori* treatment	B
■ Sympathectomy	C
■ Low level laser therapy	A
■ Acupuncture	A
■ Evening primrose oil supplementation	A
■ Fish oil supplementation	A
■ Biofeedback	C
■ Botulinum toxin	D
■ Sildenafil	E
■ Spinal cord stimulation	E

Efficacy evaluation of prostaglandin E1 against placebo in patients with progressive systemic sclerosis and significant Raynaud's phenomenon. Bartolone S, Trifiletti A, De Nuzzo G, et al. Minerva Cardioangiol 1999;47:137–43.

Alprostadil infusions at 60 μg in 250 mL for 6 days reduced the frequency and severity of attacks of RP in patients with secondary RP.

Intravenous iloprost infusion in patients with Raynaud phenomenon secondary to systemic sclerosis. Wigley FM, Wise RA, Seibold JR, et al. Ann Intern Med 1994;120:199–206.

In this study, 131 patients with systemic sclerosis were treated with 6-h infusions of iloprost (0.5–2.0 ng/kg per min). The number of attacks was reduced in patients receiving iloprost (39.1%) compared with placebo (22.2%). Improvement during the 9-week follow-up was greater in patients given iloprost.

In a published study of another prostacyclin, epoprostenol, it was reported that the vasodilatory effect is not sustained after 1 week.

Oral iloprost in Raynaud's phenomenon secondary to systemic sclerosis: a multicentre, placebo-controlled, dose-comparison study. Black CM, Halkier-Sorensen L, Belch JJ, et al. Br J Rheumatol 1998;37:952–60.

Oral iloprost 50 μg or 100 μg twice a day was effective in reducing the duration of attacks, but not the severity or frequency. In this study of 103 patients, the 50 μg dose was better tolerated.

Negative reports about beraprost (another oral prostacyclin analogue) and oral iloprost exist as well.

Calcitonin gene-related peptide in treatment of severe peripheral vascular insufficiency in Raynaud's phenomenon. Bunker CB, Reavley C, O'Shaugnessy DJ, Dowd PM. Lancet 1993;342:80–3.

Calcitonin gene-related peptide, a potent vasodilator, given intravenously (0.6 μg/min for 3 h per day for 5 days) resulted in an increase in blood flow, ulcer healing, and effective vascular dilation in patients with severe RP.

Oral L-arginine can reverse digital necrosis in Raynaud's phenomenon. Rembold CM, Ayers CR. Mol Cell Biochem 2003;244:139–41.

The authors demonstrate a beneficial response to oral L-arginine therapy. L-arginine reversed digital necrosis and improved the symptoms of severe RP. This evidence suggests that a defect in nitric oxide synthesis or metabolism is associated with RP and demonstrates the potential effectiveness of L-arginine therapy.

Treatment of severe Raynaud's syndrome by injection of autologous blood pretreated by heating, ozonation, and exposure to ultraviolet light (H-O-U) therapy. Cooke ED, Pockley AG, Tucker AT, et al. Int Angiol 1997;16:250–4.

Treatment was successful for patients with severe RP. Results included reduction of attacks for at least 3 months and for some, no attacks at all.

Triiodothyronine treatment for Raynaud's phenomenon: a controlled trial. Dessein PH, Morrison RC, Lamparelli RD, van der Merwe CA. J Rheumatol 1990;17:1025–8.

T3, 80 μg, given daily in this trial increased finger skin temperature and reduced recovery times after cold exposure. Treatment is recommended for patients with severe RP and digital ulcers.

Helicobacter pylori **eradication ameliorates primary Raynaud's phenomenon.** Gasbarrini A, Massari I, Serrichio M, et al. Dig Dis Sci 1998;43:1641–5.

Of 46 RP patients, 36 were infected with *H. pylori*. After treatment for *H. pylori*, RP disappeared in 17% of patients; 72% of the remaining patients noticed a reduction in frequency and duration of their vasospastic attacks.

The use of digital artery sympathectomy as a salvage procedure for severe ischemia of Raynaud's disease and phenomenon. McCall TE, Petersen DP, Wong LB. J Hand Surg [Am] 1999;24:173–7.

In six of seven patients, the use of digital artery sympathectomy was effective; the patients' digital ulcers healed and amputation was avoided.

Double-blind, randomised, placebo controlled low laser therapy study in patients with primary Raynaud's phenomenon. Hirschl M, Katzenschlager R, Ammer K, et al. Vasa 2002;31:91–4.

This study examined 15 patients with primary RP and demonstrated that low-level laser therapy reduced the intensity of attacks during laser irradiation without significantly affecting the frequency of attacks. Additionally, after laser irradiation the temperature gradient following cold exposure was reduced, but there was no effect on the number of fingers showing prolonged rewarming.

Treatment of primary Raynaud's syndrome with traditional Chinese acupuncture. Appiah R, Hiller S, Caspary L, et al. J Intern Med 1997;241:119–24.

Thirty three patients with primary Raynaud's disease (16 control, 17 treatment) were studied. Overall, attacks were reduced by 63%.

Evening primrose oil (Efamol) in the treatment of Raynaud's phenomenon: a double-blind study. Belch JJ, Shaw B, O'Dowd A, et al. Thromb Haemost 1985;54:490–4.

Twenty one patients were studied. Evening primrose oil (12 capsules daily) provided symptomatic improvement.

Fish-oil dietary supplementation in patients with Raynaud's phenomenon: a double-blind controlled, prospective study. DiGiacomo RA, Kremer JM, Shah DM. Am J Med 1989;86:158–64.

Supplementation with omega-3 fatty acids was shown to be of benefit in patients with primary, but not secondary, RP in this trial involving 32 patients.

Use of biofeedback training in treatment of Raynaud's disease and phenomenon. Yocum DE, Hodes R, Sundstrom WR, Cleeland CS. J Rheumatol 1985;12:90–3.

Biofeedback training elevates baseline temperatures. *Reserved for the well-motivated patient.*

***Botulinum* toxin in the treatment of Raynaud's phenomenon: a pilot study.** Sycha T, Graninger M, Auff E, Schnider P. Eur J Clin Invest 2003;34:312–3.

Based on clinical evaluation in addition to laser Doppler interferometry measurements, data from this study demonstrate a beneficial effect of *Botulinum* toxin A in two patients with primary and secondary RP. Additionally, both patients seemed to experience mild systemic effects on fingers that were not injected.

Sildenafil improved pulmonary hypertension and peripheral blood flow in a patient with scleroderma-associated lung fibrosis and the Raynaud phenomenon. Rosenkranz S, Diet F, Karasch T, et al. Ann Int Med 2003;139:871–3.

An examination of a 65-year-old woman suggests that sildenafil improved RP because the severity and frequency of acrocyanosis decreased with treatment.

Clinical and objective data on spinal cord stimulation for the treatment of severe Raynaud's phenomenon. Neuhauser B, Perkmann R, Klingler PJ, et al. Am Surg 2001;67:1096–7.

Spinal cord stimulation was shown to effectively improve red blood cell velocity, capillary density, and capillary permeability in a 77-year-old woman with severe RP.

Evidence levels **A** Double-blind study   **B** Clinical trial ≥ 20 subjects   **C** Clinical trial < 20 subjects   **D** Series ≥ 5 subjects   **E** Anecdotal case reports

Reactive arthritis (formerly Reiter's syndrome)

Karen S McGinnis, Sam Kim, Abby S Van Voorhees

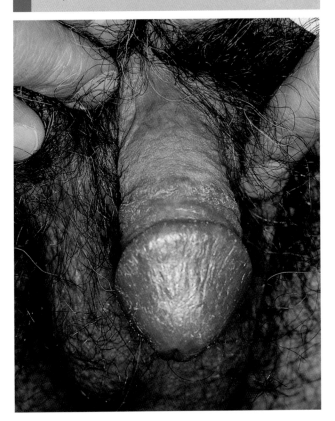

Reactive arthritis is a genetically determined and immune-mediated disease primarily affecting the skin and joints after an antecedent infection of the gastrointestinal or urinary tract. It is characterized by a triad of urethritis, conjunctivitis, and arthritis. The classic skin manifestations of reactive arthritis include keratoderma blennorrhagica and circinate balanitis. Recent controversy regarding the naming of this syndrome after a Nazi war criminal, Hans Reiter, has led to it being renamed 'Reactive Arthritis'.

MANAGEMENT STRATEGY

The mucocutaneous lesions of uncomplicated reactive arthritis are self-limited and clear within a few months. Severe, extensive, and chronic cutaneous presentations, which are more common in the setting of HIV infection, are generally treated in the same manner as pustular psoriasis. Initial therapy for limited skin disease includes *topical corticosteroids, calcipotriene (calcipotriol),* and *tazarotene.* Second line agents include *UVB* and *systemic retinoids.* Extremely severe skin disease can be treated with *psoralen plus UVA (PUVA)* and *immunosuppressive agents* such as *methotrexate* and *cyclosporine.* A case report of treatment with *infliximab* has also been described. The potential efficacy of these agents has to be balanced against the possibility of inducing further immune suppression when HIV disease is also present.

Antibiotic therapy remains a controversial topic. In the absence of controlled studies and practical methods to monitor persistence of infection, the decision to use antibiotics varies with each individual case and ultimately rests on physician judgment. If a specific inciting organism is documented by culture or molecular diagnostics (e.g. following chlamydial urethritis), antibiotics are indicated. The most beneficial antibiotic as well as the optimal dose and duration of therapy remain to be clarified. In our experience, the incidence of severe psoriasis and reactive arthritis in the setting of advanced HIV disease has dramatically decreased since the advent of highly active antiretroviral therapy (HAART). HIV-positive individuals with reactive arthritis should be referred for initiation of effective antiviral agents and monitoring of viral load. Conversely, new onset of reactive arthritis has been reported as part of the immune reconstitution syndrome seen with the commencement of HAART. In this particular case a rapid and sustained response occurred after a 2-week course of doxycycline.

The symptoms of arthritis and enthesopathy usually dictate the focus of treatment in most patients with reactive arthritis. *Nonsteroidal anti-inflammatory drugs (NSAIDs)* are the first line of therapy. *Sulfasalazine* has been shown in a prospective trial to be well tolerated and effective in cases unresponsive to NSAIDs. *Methotrexate* and *azathioprine* are reserved for severe, intractable disease. Exercise and physical therapy are important adjuncts to therapy.

Transient and mild conjunctivitis does not require specific therapeutic intervention. Symptoms of uveitis, on the other hand, should prompt immediate referral to an ophthalmologist. Treatment includes topical and often systemic corticosteroids as well as other immunosuppressive agents such as methotrexate and cyclosporine.

SPECIFIC INVESTIGATIONS

- Recent history of gastrointestinal or genitourinary infection or symptoms
- Skin biopsy
- Urethral smear and urinalysis
- Urethral, cervical, and stool cultures for bacteria
- Serum antibody titers to *Chlamydia* spp. or specific enteric organisms
- Erythrocyte sedimentation rate (ESR) and C-reactive protein
- Rheumatoid factor and antinuclear antibody
- Radiographic imaging
- Joint fluid analysis and synovial biopsy
- Molecular diagnostics to detect microbial components in synovial biopsies and synovial fluid
- HLA-B27 typing
- HIV testing
- Ophthalmological evaluation with slit lamp exam

European guideline for the management of sexually acquired reactive arthritis. Int J STD AIDS 2001;12 (suppl 3):94–102.

A recent history of urethral discharge and/or dysuria is present in approximately 80% of men with sexually acquired reactive arthritis (SARA). Conjunctivitis occurs in 20–50% of patients with SARA and iritis is seen in 2–11%. Slit-lamp examination is necessary to differentiate between them. Posterior uveitis and optic neuritis have also been described.

Reiter's syndrome. Amor B. Rheum Dis Clin North Am 1998;24:677–95.

Laboratory tests such as the ESR and C-reactive protein can help confirm the inflammatory nature of the disease. However, a normal ESR is not incompatible with the diagnosis. Radiographs of affected joints are typically normal. Enthesopathic lesions can be visualized by MRI. Synovial fluid analysis typically shows an inflammatory process with a majority of polymorphonuclear leukocytes. Synovial biopsy shows vascular congestion and a perivascular neutrophilic infiltrate. Synovial fluid and tissue cultures are negative. HLA-B27 is present in 50–80% of cases.

Although HLA typing is probably unnecessary from a diagnostic standpoint, HLA-B27 positivity is associated with more severe and protracted disease. Thus, testing may be useful in more difficult cases for prognostic reasons.

HIV-related psoriasis and Reiter's syndrome. Weitzul S, Duvic M. Semin Cutan Med Surg 1997;16:213–8.

Assessment of HIV status is important because the use of conventionally effective immunosuppressive agents may be counterproductive and even harmful in patients with HIV infection.

FIRST LINE THERAPIES

Cutaneous disease	
■ Topical corticosteroids	D
■ Calcipotriene (calcipotriol)	E
■ Tazarotene	E

Reiter syndrome. Rothe MJ, Kerdel FA. Int J Dermatol 1991; 30:173–80.

Mucocutaneous lesions may necessitate only local care for mucosal erosions and topical corticosteroids for psoriasiform lesions.

As treatment in Reiter's syndrome is typically directed towards the musculoskeletal component and urethritis, there is a paucity of studies in the literature designed specifically for the treatment of cutaneous disease. However, despite the lack of controlled studies, topical corticosteroids are accepted in practice as first line therapy for mild cutaneous lesions.

Successful treatment of chronic skin diseases with clobetasol propionate and a hydrocolloid occlusive dressing. Volden G. Acta Derm Venereol 1992;72:69–71.

Two patients described as having skin lesions of Reiter's syndrome and 19 patients with palmoplantar pustulosis responded to clobetasol propionate lotion once a week under an occlusive patch. The mean interval to complete remission was 3 weeks for skin lesions of Reiter's syndrome and 2.2 weeks for palmoplantar pustulosis.

Reiter's disease in a homosexual HIV-positive male. Vaughan Jones SA, McGibbon DH. Clin Exp Dermatol 1994; 19:430–3.

A case report of a 32-year-old man with AIDS whose widespread psoriasiform lesions improved following 2 weeks of topical corticosteroids and a course of flucloxacillin.

The use of topical calcipotriene/calcipotriol in conditions other than plaque-type psoriasis. Thiers BH. J Am Acad Dermatol 1997;37:S69–71.

A 47-year-old man with relapsing Reiter's syndrome, who had pustules and hyperkeratotic plaques on his palms and soles, as well as circinate balanitis, responded to a 14-day regimen of oral doxycycline (100 mg twice daily) and topical calcipotriene.

Treatment of keratoderma blennorrhagicum with tazarotene gel 0.1%. Lewis A, Nigro M, Rosen T. J Am Acad Dermatol 2000;43:400–2.

A case report of a 64-year-old man with Reiter's syndrome who responded to once-daily application of tazarotene gel 0.1% to his sole.

SECOND LINE THERAPIES

Cutaneous disease	
■ Systemic retinoids	C
■ UVB/PUVA	E
■ Zidovudine	D

Acitretin and AIDS-related Reiter's disease. Blanche P. Clin Exp Rheum 1999;17:105–6.

A case report of a 46-year-old patient with AIDS and Reiter's syndrome whose arthritis and skin lesions responded dramatically after 2 weeks of acitretin (25 mg daily). The acitretin was continued for 5 months; however, there was recurrence several months after the acitretin was stopped and while the patient was maintained on highly active antiretroviral therapy. Acitretin was resumed at the same dosage, resulting in prompt resolution of disease, and continued for 6 months. No recurrence was observed after 13 months.

Reiter's syndrome-like pattern in AIDS-associated psoriasiform dermatitis. Romani J, Puig L, Baselga E, De Moragas JM. Int J Dermatol 1996;35:484–8.

A retrospective review of seven HIV-positive patients with Reiter's-like psoriasiform dermatitis. Etretinate alone and RePUVA (etretinate 1 mg/kg daily, 8-methoxypsoralen 0.6 mg/kg followed by UVA) were safe and effective in controlling skin disease. Methotrexate (15 mg weekly in three divided doses) was effective, but was complicated by hematologic toxicity in two patients. Cyclosporine (2.5 mg/kg daily) was moderately effective and was not associated with progression of AIDS.

Successful treatment of severe Reiter's syndrome associated with human immunodeficiency virus infection with etretinate. Report of 2 cases. Louthrenoo W. J Rheumatol 1993;20:1243–6.

A report of two cases of HIV-related Reiter's syndrome responding dramatically to etretinate (0.5–1.0 mg/kg daily) after 4 weeks of treatment.

Zidovudine improves psoriasis in human immunodeficiency virus-positive males. Duvic M, Crane MM, Conant M, et al. Arch Dermatol 1994;130:447–51.

Nineteen of 20 HIV-positive patients with psoriasis and Reiter's syndrome had either a partial (58%) or complete (32%) improvement of skin disease with zidovudine therapy (1200 mg daily).

Evidence levels **A** Double-blind study **B** Clinical trial ≥ 20 subjects **C** Clinical trial < 20 subjects **D** Series ≥ 5 subjects **E** Anecdotal case reports

THIRD LINE THERAPIES

Cutaneous disease	
■ Methotrexate	C
■ Cyclosporine	E
■ Infliximab	E

A review of methotrexate therapy in Reiter syndrome. Lally EV, Ho G Jr. Semin Arthritis Rheum 1985;15:139–45.

A case report and review of the literature. Eighteen of 20 patients (90%) noted dramatic improvement in skin lesions within 2 weeks of receiving methotrexate. There was also significant improvement in arthritis in 15 of 20 patients (75%), although the response was generally slower than that of skin lesions. Methotrexate was generally well tolerated, but the drug had to be discontinued in three cases (15%) due to adverse effects. The majority of patients who received methotrexate were treated for exacerbations and were discontinued successfully from the drug after clinical improvement. The usual dosage was 10–50 mg/week administered either orally or parenterally.

Successful treatment of Reiter's syndrome in a patient with AIDS with methotrexate and corticosteroids. Berenbaum F, Duvivier C, Prier A, Kaplan G. Br J Rheumatol 1996;35:295–301.

A case report of a 37-year-old man with AIDS and severe Reiter's syndrome who responded to prednisone 20 mg daily and methotrexate 20 mg/week. This was combined with antiviral therapy, chemoprophylaxis of infection, and aggressive therapy of Kaposi's sarcoma without exacerbations of his AIDS.

Successful treatment of severe recurrent Reiter's syndrome with cyclosporine. Kiyohara A, Takamori K, Niizuma N, Ogawa H. J Am Acad Dermatol 1997;36:482–3.

A case report of a 48-year-old man who had a recurrence of Reiter's syndrome while on etretinate that responded dramatically to cyclosporine (3–5 mg/kg daily). No recurrence was seen 18 months after discontinuation of therapy.

Infliximab in the treatment of an HIV positive patient with Reiter's syndrome. Gaylis N. J Rheumatol 2003;30:2.

A case report of a 41-year-old man with Reiter's syndrome who responded to infliximab added to a regimen of methotrexate and systemic corticosteroids. During therapy his arthritis resolved as did the severe onycholysis and keratoderma blennorrhagica of the soles. The patient was able to discontinue systemic corticosteroids and was maintained on intravenous infliximab at a dose of 300 mg (3 mg/kg) every 6–7 weeks and intramuscular methotrexate at a dose of 15 mg/week for 18 months, without a decrease in his CD4 cells or a rise in his viral load.

Relapsing polychondritis

Paul H Bowman, Donald Rudikoff

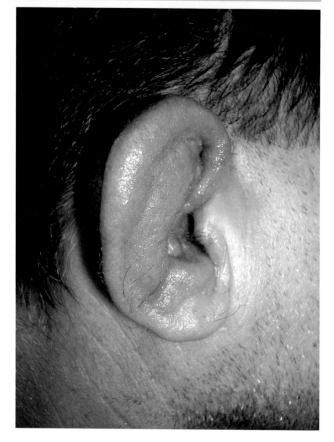

Relapsing polychondritis is a rare, multisystemic disease of unknown etiology, characterized by recurrent inflammation of cartilage and connective tissue. Patients with the **MAGIC** syndrome (**M**outh **A**nd **G**enital ulcers with **I**nflamed **C**artilage), a combination of Behçet's disease (Ch. 24) and relapsing polychondritis, may also benefit from the treatment strategy outlined in this chapter.

MANAGEMENT STRATEGY

Treatment of relapsing polychondritis is aimed at decreasing inflammation, which often progressively destroys affected structures in the ears, nose, eyes, joints, respiratory tract, and cardiovascular system. A multidisciplinary approach is crucial to evaluate and treat the multiple organ systems which can be affected.

Systemic corticosteroids are the cornerstone of therapy, and doses of 80 to 100 mg daily can reliably abate acute attacks in most patients. Maintenance use (10 to 25 mg daily) can decrease the frequency and severity of recurrences, but does not stop disease progression in the more aggressive cases. In addition, long-term side effects necessitate the use of steroid-sparing agents. *Nonsteroidal anti-inflammatory agents* (NSAIDs) such as aspirin and indometacin are safer first line agents, but as monotherapy often do not fully control the disease. *Dapsone* should also be tried, as some patients show excellent improvement when it is used either as mono-

therapy or in combination with steroids. When present, the response to dapsone usually occurs within 1 to 2 weeks, although higher doses (200 mg daily) are often required.

Azathioprine (50–150 mg daily) and *cyclophosphamide* (100–150 mg daily) have both traditionally been used as steroid-sparing agents. More recently, *cyclosporine* has shown good response in several cases at doses of 5–15 mg/kg daily, and has been effectively used at lower doses in combination with steroids. Medium-dose *methotrexate* (10–15 mg per week) has been effectively used to lower steroid requirements, and at higher doses (20–25 mg per week) has been successful as monotherapy.

A trial of *colchicine* (0.6 mg twice daily) may be worthwhile as it is a comparatively benign drug, although it has been reported to be successful only in a minority of patients. For relapsing polychondritis unresponsive to other therapies, *salazosulfapyridine* and *plasmapheresis* have each been effective when combined with first and second line agents. In late-stage disease with significant functional pulmonary involvement, interventions such as *tracheostomy* and/or *tracheobronchial stent placement* may improve respiratory function.

SPECIFIC INVESTIGATIONS

- ■ Pulmonary evaluation
  - – Chest radiograph and/or computed tomography/ magnetic resonance imaging (CT/MRI)
  - – Pulmonary function tests (especially flow volume loops)
  - – Endobronchial ultrasonography
- ■ Cardiovascular examination
  - – Electrocardiogram and/or echocardiogram
- ■ Ophthalmologic examination
  - – Audiometry
- ■ Complete blood count
- ■ Erythrocyte sedimentation rate

Pulmonary function in patients with relapsing polychondritis. Mohsenifar Z, Tashkin DP, Carson SA, Bellamy PE. Chest 1982;81:711–7.

The authors describe detailed physiologic and radiographic studies of the respiratory tract in five patients with pulmonary involvement with relapsing polychondritis.

Airway manifestations are ultimately present in over 50% of patients with relapsing polychondritis and are the leading cause of death in patients with this disease. Airway obstruction may be asymptomatic in the earlier stages, detected only on pulmonary function testing. Other sources stress the importance of plain radiography, CT, and MRI for early detection of tracheal narrowing and upper airway disease.

Cardiovascular involvement in relapsing polychondritis. Del Rosso A, Rosa Petrix N, Pratesi M, Bini A. Semin Arthritis Rheum 1997;26:840–4.

Cardiovascular complications eventually occur in half of all patients with relapsing polychondritis, and are the second most frequent cause of mortality. Aortic valve inflammation, the most common cardiac manifestation of relapsing polychondritis (10% of patients), has been reported in asymptomatic patients, and can silently progress during seemingly effective systemic corticosteroid therapy.

Evidence levels **A** Double-blind study **B** Clinical trial ≥ 20 subjects **C** Clinical trial < 20 subjects **D** Series ≥ 5 subjects **E** Anecdotal case reports

Progressive aortic valve inflammation occurring despite apparent remission of relapsing polychondritis. Buckley LM, Ades PA. Arthritis Rheum 1992;35:812–4.

Subclinical aortic valve inflammation requiring valve replacement was discovered in a 37-year-old patient whose relapsing polychondritis had been asymptomatic (and thus not treated) for 7 months. The authors suggest baseline echocardiography and regular follow-up with cardiac auscultation, electrocardiography, and chest radiography in every patient with relapsing polychondritis.

Scleritis in relapsing polychondritis. Hoang-xuan T, Foster CS, Rice BA. Ophthalmology 1990;97:892–8.

Ocular inflammation is one of the most constant features of relapsing polychondritis (developing in up to 63% of patients), can affect almost any part of the eye, and can reduce vision. The authors stress the importance of early detection of this serious consequence of the disease.

Otolaryngological aspects of relapsing polychondritis: course and outcome. Yettser S, Inal A, Taser M, Ozkaptan Y. Rev Laryngol Otol Retinol 2001;122:195–200.

Analysis of the otolaryngologic manifestations of relapsing polychondritis in seven patients.

Several of the reviews referenced below (McAdam et al. 1976, Trentham et al. 1998) also discuss the importance of screening audiometry in patients with relapsing polychondritis: up to 46% of patients suffer from impaired hearing, and inadequately treated cases can suffer permanent hearing loss.

Association of myelodysplastic syndrome and relapsing polychondritis: further evidence. Hebbar M, Brouillard M, Wattel E, et al. Leukemia 1995;9:731–3.

Twenty-eight percent of all patients (5 of 18 cases) diagnosed with relapsing polychondritis at the authors' institution over a period of 13 years were also found to have myelodysplastic syndromes. Multiple other such cases have been reported elsewhere in the literature.

Anemia is a poor prognostic sign in patients with relapsing polychondritis; those with concurrent myelodysplasia often develop refractory anemia requiring transfusions, and several have progressed to leukemia.

McAdam et al. (1976, below) and others suggest that since the erythrocyte sedimentation rate is generally increased during periods of disease activity, it may be useful in monitoring response to therapy.

Relapsing polychondritis: a clinical review. Letko E, Zafrakis P, Baltatzis S, et al. Semin Arthritis Rheum 2002; 31:384–95.

A nice review article.

Endobronchial ultrasonography in the diagnosis and treatment of relapsing polychondritis with tracheo-bronchial malacia. Miyazu Y, Miyazawa T, Kurimoto N, et al. Chest 2003;124:2393–5.

In two cases of relapsing polychondritis, endobroncheal ultrasonography revealed a poorly defined bronchial wall structure with two patterns of cartilaginous damage: fragmentation and edema. Successful treatment was achieved by the implantation of nitinol stents, the sizes of which were determined by endobroncheal ultrasonography.

FIRST LINE THERAPIES

■ Systemic corticosteroids	C
■ NSAIDs	D
■ Dapsone	C

Relapsing polychondritis: prospective study of 23 patients and review of the literature. McAdam LP, O'Hanlan MA, Bluestone R, Pearson CM. Medicine (Baltimore) 1976;55: 193–215.

In this report, 18 of 23 patients were treated with prolonged systemic corticosteroid therapy (average prednisone maintenance dose of 25 mg daily) while 6 of 23 were well controlled using NSAIDs (aspirin, indometacin, phenylbutazone).

Although the use of systemic corticosteroids for relapsing polychondritis has not been evaluated with controlled clinical trials, multiple small series in the literature report corticosteroids as being the most uniformly reliable therapy in abating acute exacerbations and decreasing the frequency and severity of recurrences. Unfortunately, they do not always halt disease progression.

Relapsing polychondritis: excellent response to naproxen and aspirin. Kremer J, Gates SA, Parhami N. J Rheumatol 1979;6:719–20.

A case report of a 59-year-old man with an acute flare of relapsing polychondritis which responded well to a combination of naproxen (250 mg twice daily) and salicylate (975 mg four times daily) therapy. The authors discuss that mild cases of relapsing polychondritis (and even some acute flares) usually respond to NSAIDs.

Treatment of relapsing polychondritis with dapsone. Barranco VP, Monor DB, Solomon H. Arch Dermatol 1976; 112:1268–88.

Three patients were successfully treated with dapsone (100 to 200 mg daily), each showing complete resolution of an acute attack of relapsing polychondritis within 2 weeks of starting therapy.

While not all patients respond to dapsone, those that do are usually reported as having a dramatic improvement within 1–2 weeks of initiating therapy. Effectiveness of dapsone seems to be dose-dependent, with 200 mg daily being the most commonly reported effective dose.

Relapsing polychondritis – report of ten cases. Damiani JM, Levine HL. Laryngoscope 1979;89:929–44.

In this report of 10 cases of relapsing polychondritis seen at the Cleveland Clinic over a 20-year period, systemic steroids and dapsone were each reliable in abating episodes of disease activity and in decreasing recurrences. Based on their review of the 211 case reports of relapsing polychondritis existing at the time, the authors proposed that response to steroids and/or dapsone be a diagnostic criterion for the disease.

Although one might expect a synergistic anti-inflammatory effect from a combination regimen of steroids and dapsone, this has not been conclusively shown to be advantageous over either agent alone.

Relapsing polychondritis in HIV-infected patients: a report of two cases. Dolev JC, Maurer TA, Reddy SG, et al. J Am Acad Dermatol 2004;51:1023–5.

Two cases of relapsing polychondritis as a possible manifestation of immune reconstitution following highly active antiretroviral therapy (HAART) are presented. In one case, dapsone plus prednisone, and in the other, dapsone alone, were effective treatments.

SECOND LINE THERAPIES

■ Azathioprine	D
■ Cyclosporine	D
■ Methotrexate	D
■ Cyclophosphamide	E

Relapsing polychondritis in a Latin American man. Waller ES, Raebel MA. Am J Hosp Pharm 1979;36;806–10.

In this case report of a 33-year-old man with severe relapsing polychondritis, including respiratory tract chondritis requiring tracheostomy, addition of azathioprine (150 mg daily) allowed reduction in prednisone dosage from 60 mg daily to 25 mg daily.

Cyclosporin A in the treatment of relapsing polychondritis with severe recurrent eye involvement. Priori R, Paroli MP, Luan FL, et al. Br J Rheumatol 1993;32:352.

A 54-year-old female with relapsing polychondritis and severe recurrent necrotizing nodular scleritis was refractory to steroids and azathioprine but achieved complete remission with cyclosporine 5 mg/kg daily.

This and other case reports suggest that cyclosporine may be especially useful for ocular manifestations of relapsing polychondritis when they are refractory to other therapies.

Relapsing polychondritis. Trentham DE, Le CH. Ann Intern Med 1998;129:114–22.

In this review of the authors' experience with 36 patients with relapsing polychondritis, 23 of 31 patients were able to decrease their prednisone dose from an average of 19 mg daily to 5 mg daily by adding methotrexate (average weekly methotrexate dose 15.5 mg).

A good review article.

Steroid sparing effect of methotrexate in relapsing polychondritis. Park J, Gowin KM, Schumacher HR. J Rheumatol 1996;23:937–8.

Two patients with auricular conduits were able to decrease or discontinue their dose of prednisone by taking methotrexate 15–20 mg per week, while a third patient responded to monotherapy with methotrexate 22.5 mg per week.

Relapsing polychondritis with glomerulonephritis: improvement with prednisone and cyclophosphamide. Ruhlen JL, Huston KA, Wood WG. JAMA 1981;245:847–8.

A 32-year-old man with relapsing polychondritis and life-threatening upper airway obstruction responded to high-dose corticosteroid therapy but subsequently developed progressive renal insufficiency despite continued treatment. The addition of oral cyclophosphamide, 150 mg daily, led to substantial improvement in renal function and sustained improvement for 21 months of follow-up, despite subsequent reduction of prednisone dose. The authors suggest monitoring renal function in relapsing polychondritis and suggest a regimen of prednisone and cyclophosphamide in cases with glomerulonephritis.

THIRD LINE THERAPIES

■ Colchicine	E
■ Minocycline	E
■ Pentoxifylline	E
■ Salazosulfapyridine	E
■ Anti-CD4 monoclonal antibody	E
■ Plasmapheresis	E
■ Tracheostomy/tracheobronchial stent placement	D
■ Infliximab	D

Colchicine for treatment of relapsing polychondritis. Askari AD. J Am Acad Dermatol 1984;10:507–10.

Oral colchicine, 0.6 mg twice daily, abated three attacks of chondritis in two patients with relapsing polychondritis. Marked improvement was noted within several days of starting the drug.

Colchicine and indomethacin for the treatment of relapsing polychondritis. Mark KA, Franks AG. J Am Acad Dermatol 2002;46(2 Suppl Case Reports):S22–4.

One patient with steroid-dependent disease had marked improvement and decreased steroid doses after adding colchicine, 0.6 mg two to four times daily, and indometacin, 25 mg three times daily.

Antibiotic therapy for rheumatoid arthritis: scientific and anecdotal appraisals. Trentham DE, Dynesius-Trentham RA. Rheum Dis Clin North Am 1995;21:817–34.

Oral minocycline, as used for rheumatoid arthritis, was associated with improvement in a patient who had developed methotrexate toxicity.

Mouth and genital ulcers with inflamed cartilage (MAGIC syndrome): a case report and literature review. Imai H, Motegi M, Mizuki N, et al. Am J Med Sci 1997;314:330–2.

A 39-year-old woman with relapsing polychondritis and Behçet's disease (MAGIC syndrome) had improvement in oral ulcers, erythema nodosum, and arthritis when treated with a combination of methotrexate (5 mg weekly) and pentoxifylline (300 mg daily).

[A refractory case of relapsing polychondritis]. Nosaka Y, Nishio J, Nanki T, et al. Nihon Rinsho Meneki Gakkai Kaishi 1998;21:80–6. In Japanese.

A 15-year-old girl with severe relapsing polychondritis was initially partially responsive to separate courses of oral corticosteroids and cyclosporine, but later had a complete remission when both these agents were used in combination with salazosulfapyridine.

Anti-CD4 monoclonal antibody for relapsing polychondritis. Van der Lubbe PA, Miltenburg AM, Breedveld FC. Lancet 1991;337:1349.

[Auricular chondritis, malignant glomerulonephritis and pulmonary hemorrhage]. Dracon M, Noel C, Ramon P, et al. Nephrologie 1991;12;139–41. In French.

A 41-year-old man with auricular chondritis, subacute renal failure, and pulmonary involvement had rapid improvement with plasmapheresis and prednisone treatment.

Evidence levels A Double-blind study **B** Clinical trial ≥ 20 subjects **C** Clinical trial < 20 subjects **D** Series ≥ 5 subjects **E** Anecdotal case reports

Since antibodies to type II collagen seem to be important in the pathogenesis of relapsing polychondritis, plasmapheresis may have a role in the management of these patients.

Management of airway manifestations of relapsing polychondritis: case reports and review of the literature. Sarodia SD, Dasgupta A, Mehta AC. Chest 1999;116:1669–75.

Five patients with severe respiratory involvement from relapsing polychondritis (three of whom required continuous mechanical ventilation due to airway collapse) benefited from placement of self-expandable metallic tracheobronchial stents. A total of 17 stents of varying sizes were placed in these patients over a period of 3 years, with favorable overall outcome in four patients.

When severe, progressive disease leads to extensive destruction of the tracheobronchial tree despite maximal medical therapy, tracheostomy or tracheobronchial stent placement may preserve or improve respiratory function and decrease patients' reliance on mechanical ventilation.

Successful treatment of relapsing polychondritis with infliximab. Richez C, Dumoulin C, Coutoly X, Schaeverbeke T. Clin Exp Rheumatol 2004;22:629–31.

One patient had marked improvement in symptoms 4 days after an infusion of infliximab 4 mg/kg. Control was maintained with repeat treatments every 6–8 weeks.

Infliximab seems to be an effective therapy for relapsing polychondritis unresponsive to conventional therapy, as well as a steroid-sparing agent.

Severe septicemia in a patient with polychondritis and Sweet's syndrome after initiation of treatment with infliximab. Matzkies FG, Manger B, Schmitt-Haendle M, et al. Ann Rheum Dis 2003;62:81–2.

A 51-year-old diabetic man with relapsing polychondritis had an excellent clinical response to infliximab 3 mg/kg, but then developed a parasternal abscess 11 days later, caused by penicillin-resistant *Staphylococcus aureus*, and expired from subsequent septicemia.

This report underscores the importance of monitoring at-risk patients closely for infection.

Rhinophyma

John Berth-Jones, Sheila M Clark, Catriona A Henderson

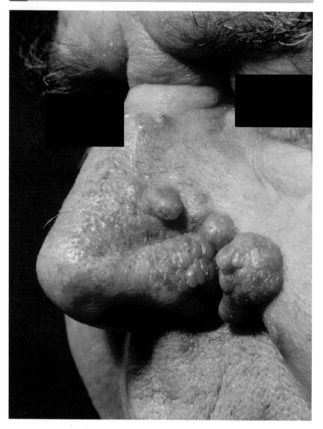

Phymas, of which rhinophyma is much the most common, are localized swellings of facial soft tissues due to a variable combination of fibrosis, sebaceous hyperplasia, and lymphedema. These occur on the nose (rhinophyma) and, less often, the ears (otophyma), forehead (metophyma), or chin (gnathophyma). They are seen much more frequently in males than in females. Rhinophyma may develop in patients with a long history of rosacea, when it is often regarded as a complication or 'end stage' of the disease. However, rhinophyma is also seen in patients who do not have any history of rosacea. Occasionally, rhinophyma is complicated by the development of a malignancy.

MANAGEMENT STRATEGY

Phymas require physical ablation or removal – usually by surgery. Remodeling is most often achieved simply by paring off the excess tissue with a scalpel. Other techniques which can be useful in the hands of those with the necessary expertise include electrosurgery, excision/vaporization with argon, CO_2, Nd:YAG, or erbium:YAG lasers, and cryotherapy. Ionizing radiation has been used in cases with coexisting malignancy. Systemic isotretinoin can significantly reduce the bulk of rhinophyma, although it does not restore normal skin contours. It is possible, but not established, that treatment of rosacea may inhibit the development of rhinophyma.

SPECIFIC INVESTIGATIONS

- Biopsy is occasionally indicated to exclude malignancy

Rhinophyma and coexisting occult skin cancers. Lutz ME, Otley CC. Dermatol Surg 2001;27:201–2.

Rhinophyma can be complicated by the development of a malignancy which can be difficult to recognize.

FIRST LINE THERAPIES

■ Surgical paring	C

Triple approach to rhinophyma. Curnier A, Choudhary S. Ann Plast Surg 2002;49:211–4.

The authors report pleasing results in six patients treated by tangential excision for debulking, the use of scissors for sculpting, and mild dermabrasion for final contouring.

SECOND LINE THERAPIES

■ Electrosurgery	C
■ Argon laser	C
■ CO_2 laser	C
■ Nd:YAG laser	E
■ Erbium:YAG laser	D
■ Cryotherapy	D
■ Isotretinoin	C
■ Microdebrider	E
■ Shaw scalpel	E
■ Radiotherapy	E

Electrosurgical treatment of rhinophyma. Clark DP, Hanke CW. J Am Acad Dermatol 1990;22:831–7.

This treatment was inexpensive and associated with few complications and gave good or excellent cosmetic results in 13 cases.

Surgical management of rhinophyma: report of eight patients treated with electrosection. Rex J, Ribera M, Bielsa I, et al. Dermatol Surg 2002;28:347–9.

Eight male patients were treated using radiofrequency electrosurgery to remove thin layers of tissue until the nose shape was recreated. All patients achieved acceptable cosmetic results.

Rhinophyma treated by argon laser. Halsbergen-Henning JP, van Gemert MJ. Lasers Surg Med 1983;2:211–5.

Thirteen cases were treated. This laser is believed to work by selectively coagulating capillaries causing redness of the nose and which feed the hypertrophic regions, as well as by direct coagulation shrinkage of the hypertrophic connective tissue. The result was a smooth and more natural appearance of the nose, without redness. Pustulosis was also reduced.

Comparison of CO_2 laser and electrosurgery in the treatment of rhinophyma. Greenbaum SS, Krull EA, Watnick K. J Am Acad Dermatol 1988;18:363–8.

The results from the CO_2 laser and electrosurgery were compared in three patients by treating one side of the nose by each method. There was little to choose between them in terms of results, but electrosurgery was more cost effective.

Evidence levels A Double-blind study B Clinical trial ≥ 20 subjects C Clinical trial < 20 subjects D Series ≥ 5 subjects E Anecdotal case reports

Spectrum of results after treatment of rhinophyma with the carbon dioxide laser. El Azhary RA, Roenigk RK, Wang TD. Mayo Clin Proc 1991;66:899–905.

A review of 30 patients treated with the CO_2 laser and followed up for 1 to 4 years. Milder cases were treated with laser vaporization, more severe cases with CO_2 laser excision and then vaporization. Dilated pores developed in many patients. Leukoderma, unilateral alar lift, and mild hypertrophic scarring developed in single cases.

Excision of rhinophyma with Nd:YAG laser: a new technique. Wenig BL, Weingarten RT. Laryngoscope 1993;103: 101–6.

Treatment of rhinophyma with Er:YAG laser. Orenstein A, Haik J, Tamir J, et al. Lasers Surg Med 2001;29:230–5.

Use of a dual-mode erbium:YAG laser for the surgical correction of rhinophyma. Fincher EF, Gladstone HB. Arch Facial Plast Surg 2004;6:267–71.

In each of these reports, six cases of rhinophyma were treated with satisfactory outcome. The erbium:YAG laser provides both controlled ablation of tissue and hemostasis.

Rhinophyma treated by liquid nitrogen spray cryosurgery. Sonnex TS, Dawber RPR. Clin Exp Dermatol 1986;11:284–8.

Five cases were treated using two freeze–thaw cycles, each freeze lasting 30 s after the ice field was established, with a 4-min intervening thaw. A pethidine and diazepam premedication was used. In three cases, small residual prominent areas responded to further treatment after 2 months. The final result was satisfactory in each case, with no scarring.

Isotretinoin in the treatment of rosacea and rhinophyma. Irvine C, Kumar P, Marks R. In: Marks R, Plewig G, eds. Acne and Related Disorders. London: Martin Dunitz; 1989: 311–5.

A study in which nine men with rhinophyma were treated with isotretinoin 1 mg/kg daily for up to 18 weeks. Isotretinoin reduced the volume of rhinophyma (assessed objectively using molds of the noses) by 9–23%. However, it did not restore normal skin contours in advanced cases.

The authors report good results in five cases and consider this their treatment of choice.

New surgical adjuncts in the treatment of rhinophyma: the microdebrider and FloSeal®. Kaushik V, Tahery J, Malik TH, Jones PH. J Laryngol Otol 2003;117:551–2.

This is a report of a single case treated using this approach. The microdebrider is a powered rotary shaving device. FloSeal® is a hemostatic mixture of thrombin and gelatin, applied topically after the surgery. The use of these adjuncts allowed precise sculpting and immediate hemostasis.

Surgical treatment of rhinophyma with the Shaw scalpel. Eisen RF, Katz AE, Bohigian RK, Grande DJ. Arch Dermatol 1986;122:307–9.

The Shaw scalpel is a device in which a scalpel blade can be heated. A rhinophyma was treated using a temperature of 150°C to achieve hemostasis while paring. Contours were then refined using a CO_2 laser and light dermabrasion.

Rhinophyma, associated with carcinoma, treated successfully with radiation. Plenk HP. Plast Reconstr Surg 1995; 95:559–62.

Two patients with basal cell carcinoma complicating rhinophyma had complete control of both conditions by radiotherapy with orthovoltage X-radiation. The authors suggest that this modality might be useful for rhinophyma alone.

Rickettsial infections

Philippe Berbis

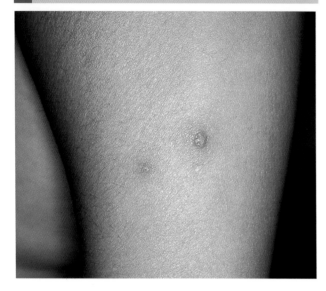

The family Rickettsiaceae is a group of obligate intracellular bacteria that includes the agents of spotted fevers, typhus, rickettsialpox, Q fever, and ehrlichiosis.

Spotted Fevers

These comprise African tick bite fever (*R. africae*), Astrakhan fever (*R. conorii*), Flinders island spotted fever (*R. honei*), Indian tick typhus (*R. conorii*), Israeli spotted fever (*R. conorii*), Japanese spotted fever (*R. japonica*), Mediterranean spotted fever (*R. conorii*), Queensland tick typhus (*R. australis*), Rocky Mountain spotted fever (*R. rickettsii*), and Siberian tick typhus (*R. sibirica*).

MANAGEMENT STRATEGY

Treatment should be initiated whenever there is clinical suspicion of the disease, before confirmation by serology. *Doxycycline* is the treatment of choice, 100 mg twice daily in adults. Children over 8 years should receive 4 mg/kg daily.

Patients are treated orally until they have been afebrile for at least 2 days and for a total treatment duration of no less than 7 days. Significant improvement is observed within 36 to 48 h after initiation of treatment. Apyrexia is commonly obtained by 72 h. *Tetracycline* (500 mg 6-hourly) is efficacious but is contraindicated in patients with renal failure. Tetracyclines are contraindicated during pregnancy and in children under the age of 8 years. *Chloramphenicol* (50–75 mg/kg daily, divided into four doses) is the recommended treatment during pregnancy and of pediatric cases. However, few data are available and relapses have been noted. The intravenous route is recommended for severe cases which should be hospitalized. Oxygen supplementation, intravenous hydration, fluid maintenance, and nutritional support are necessary in more severe cases. Oliguria, anuria, or renal failure may necessitate hemodialysis.

Prompt recognition and early initiation of effective treatment are the most important factors affecting prognosis. Prevention reposes on avoidance of tick-infested areas and avoidance of physical contact with dogs in endemic areas. Topical insect repellents should be applied on any exposed skin. Unfortunately, most skin repellents have short-lasting efficacy. Frequent and careful examination of the skin (at least twice a day in endemic areas) with special attention to the scalp, pubic, and axillary hair, and prompt and careful tick removal are important preventive measures. Long protective clothing diminishes the risk of exposure to skin. Clothing can be impregnated with acaricidal compounds. No vaccine is currently available, but immunogenic surface protein antigens have been cloned and sequenced.

SPECIFIC INVESTIGATIONS

- Serology: indirect immunofluorescence
- Polymerase chain reaction (PCR)

Polymerase chain reaction-based diagnosis of Mediterranean spotted fever in serum and tissue samples. Leitner M, Yitzhaki S, Rzotkiewicz S, Keysary A. Am J Trop Med Hyg 2002;67:166–9.

A nested PCR has been developed in the diagnosis of Mediterranean spotted fever. Specific primers were derived from a *Rickettsia conorii* 17-kD protein gene. Sera and tissue samples are suitable for this test.

Spotless rickettsiosis caused by *Rickettsia slovaca* and associated with *Dermacentor* ticks. Raoult D, Lakos A, Fenollar F, et al. Clin Infect Dis 2002;34:1331–6.

Rickettsia slovaca infections were confirmed by PCR in 17 of 67 patients with lesions of the scalp and enlarged cervical lymph nodes after receiving a bite from a *Dermacentor* tick.

FIRST LINE THERAPIES

- Tetracycline or doxycycline   A

Erythromycin versus tetracycline for treatment of Mediterranean spotted fever. Munoz-Espin T, Lopez-Pares P, Espejo-Arenas E, et al. Arch Dis Child 1986;6:1027–9.

A randomized trial assessed tetracycline hydrochloride versus erythromycin stearate in 81 children with Mediterranean spotted fever. Clinical symptoms and fever disappeared significantly more quickly in patients treated with tetracycline.

Relapse of rickettsial Mediterranean spotted fever and murine typhus after treatment with chloramphenicol. Shaked Y, Samra Y, Maier MK, Rubinstein E. J Infect 1989;18:35–7.

Relapse occurred in 10 of 24 patients treated with chloramphenicol, compared with none of 108 patients treated with tetracycline.

Analysis of risk factors for fatal Rocky Mountain spotted fever: evidence for superiority of tetracyclines for therapy. Holman RC, Paddock CD, Curns AT, et al. J Infect Dis 2001;184:1437–44.

US national surveillance 1981–1998 noted 6388 patients with Rocky Mountain spotted fever. Older patients, patients treated with chloramphenicol only, and patients for whom treatment was delayed by 5 or more days after onset of symptoms were at higher risk for death.

SECOND LINE THERAPIES

■ Azithromycin	B
■ Clarithromycin	B
■ Ciprofloxacin	B
■ Chloramphenicol	D

Clarithromycin versus azithromycin in the treatment of Mediterranean spotted fever in children: a randomized controlled trial. Cascio A, Colomba C, Antinori S, et al. Clin Infect Dis 2002;34:154–8.

This open-label randomized trial compared clarithromycin (15 mg/kg daily in two divided doses for 7 days) with azithromycin (10 mg/kg daily in one dose for 3 days) in the treatment of children with Mediterranean spotted fever. These two agents could be acceptable treatments for children aged ≤8 years.

Typhus group

MANAGEMENT STRATEGY

Epidemic typhus

Epidemic typhus is due to *R. prowazekii*, transmitted from the body louse. *Doxycycline* is effective orally (200 mg daily for 5 days) or intravenously in more severe cases. *Chloramphenicol* is also effective. Prevention is essential by bathing, washing clothes, and use of insecticides.

Murine typhus

Murine typhus (or endemic typhus) is due to *R. typhi*, transmitted from the rat flea and the rat louse. Recommended treatment in adults is *doxycycline* 200 mg daily for 7 to 15 days (or until 3 days after defervescence). *Chloramphenicol* may also be used but relapses have been reported. Prevention reposes on control of rat population and insecticides.

Scrub typhus

Scrub typhus is caused by *R. tsutsugamushi*, transmitted from larval mites. *Tetracyclines* are the agents recommended for the treatment of scrub typhus in adults: *doxycycline* (200 mg daily) or *tetracycline* (2 g daily) for 2 to 14 days. *Chloramphenicol* is also effective but acts more slowly than tetracyclines.

SPECIFIC INVESTIGATIONS

Epidemic typhus
■ Serology: microimmunofluorescent and plate microagglutination tests
Murine typhus
■ Serology: indirect fluorescent antibody, latex agglutination, solid phase immunoassay
Scrub typhus
■ Serology: indirect fluorescent antibody test

FIRST LINE THERAPIES

Epidemic typhus	
■ Doxycycline	A
Murine typhus	
■ Doxycycline	A
Scrub typhus	
■ Doxycycline	A
■ Rifampicin	A

Comparison of the effectiveness of five different antibiotic regimens on infection with Rickettsia typhi: therapeutic data from 87 cases. Gikas A, Doukakis S, Pediaditis J, et al. Am J Trop Med Hyg 2004;70:576–9.

In 87 patients with endemic typhus, the mean time to defervescence was 2.9 days for doxycycline, 4 days for chloramphenicol, and 4.2 days for ciprofloxacin (retrospective study).

Paediatric scrub typhus in Thailand: a study of 73 confirmed cases. Silpapojakul K, Varachit B, Silpapojakul K. Trans R Soc Trop Med Hyg 2004;98:354–9.

In 73 children with scrub typhus (median age, 9 years), defervescence occurred a median of 1 day after initiation of doxycycline and 3 days after initiation of chloramphenicol, compared with 5 days for those who received none or other antibiotics.

Doxycycline and rifampicin for mild scrub-typhus infections in northern Thailand: a randomised trial. Watt G, Kantipong P, Jongsakul K, et al. Lancet 2000;356:1057–61.

Adult patients with mild scrub typhus were randomly assigned to 1 week of daily oral treatment with 200 mg doxycycline (n = 28), 600 mg rifampicin (n = 26), or 900 mg rifampicin (n = 24). The median duration of pyrexia was significantly shorter in the patients treated with rifampicin at either dose level than in the patients treated with doxycycline.

SECOND LINE THERAPIES

Epidemic typhus	
■ Chloramphenicol	D
Murine typhus	
■ Chloramphenicol	D
Scrub typhus	
■ Chloramphenicol	D

Rickettsialpox

MANAGEMENT STRATEGY

Rickettsialpox is caused by *R. akari*. This self-limited illness is transmitted from the reservoir (house mouse) by mites. The treatment in adults is *doxycycline* (200 mg daily) for 2 to 5 days.

SPECIFIC INVESTIGATIONS

■ Serology: complement fixation	

FIRST LINE THERAPIES

■ Doxycycline	A

Rickettsialpox: report of an outbreak and a contemporary review. Brettman LR, Lewin S, Holzman RS, et al. Medicine 1981;60:363–72.

Antibiotics serve to shorten the duration of symptoms to 24–48 h.

Q fever

Q fever is due to *Coxiella burnetii*, transmitted to human from urine, feces, or birth products of ungulates (hoofed mammals) by aerosolization.

MANAGEMENT STRATEGY

Acute Q fever

Doxycycline (200 mg daily for 2 or 3 weeks) is the treatment of choice of acute Q fever in adults. *C. burnetii* is also susceptible in vitro to *quinolones, chloramphenicol, rifampin,* and *trimethoprim–sulfamethoxazole.*

Chronic Q fever

Endocarditis (chronic Q fever) is difficult to treat because all antibiotics are bacteriostatic and not bactericidal against *C. burnetii*. A combination of a *quinolone* and *doxycycline* for a minimum of 3 years is proposed. The combination of *hydroxychloroquine and* doxycycline should increase bactericidal activity.

SPECIFIC INVESTIGATIONS

Acute Q fever	
■ Serology: complement fixation, immunofluorescent antibody	
Chronic Q fever	
■ Echocardiography	
■ Serology	

FIRST LINE THERAPIES

Acute Q fever	
■ β-lactams	B
■ Doxycycline	B
■ Macrolides	B
■ Quinolones	B
Chronic Q fever	
■ Quinolone and doxycycline	B
■ Doxycycline and hydroxychloroquine	B

Q fever: epidemiology, clinical features and prognosis. A study from 1983 to 1999 in the South of Spain. Alarcon A, Villanueva JL, Viciana P, et al. J Infect 2003;47:110–6.

A retrospective study of 231 cases of acute Q fever. No difference in the duration of fever was observed with the treatment received (β-lactams, macrolides, doxycycline, or quinolones). Antimicrobial treatment was more effective if it was administered in the first 2 weeks.

Q fever in the Greek island of Crete: epidemiologic, clinical, and therapeutic data from 98 cases. Tselentis Y, Gikas A, Kofteridis D, et al. Clin Infect Dis 1995;20:1311–6.

A retrospective study including 98 cases of Q fever in Crete showed that there was no difference in the duration of fever whether the patient received therapy with tetracycline or erythromycin, but this finding may be explained by the delay in initiating tetracycline therapy.

Comparison of different antibiotic regimens for therapy of 32 cases of Q fever endocarditis. Levy PY, Drancourt M, Etienne J, et al. Antimicrob Agents Chemother 1991;35:533–7.

Thirty-two cases of Q fever endocarditis diagnosed in France between 1985 and 1989 were studied. In terms of effect on mortality, the combination of doxycycline and quinolone was statistically more beneficial than doxycycline alone. The authors advise a minimum duration of treatment of 3 years.

Treatment of Q fever endocarditis: comparison of 2 regimens containing doxycycline and ofloxacin or hydroxychloroquine. Raoult D, Houpikian P, Tissot Dupont H, et al. Arch Intern Med 1999;159:167–73.

Thirty-five patients with Q fever endocarditis were treated with doxycycline and quinolone or with doxycycline and hydroxychloroquine. The combination of doxycycline and hydroxychloroquine for at least 18 months allows shortening of the duration of therapy and reduction in the number of relapses.

Ehrlichiosis

MANAGEMENT STRATEGY

Human ehrlichiosis includes two tick-borne zoonoses: human monocytic (due to *E. chaffeensis*) and human granulocytic (due to *E. equi*). Ehrlichioses are transmitted from mammalian reservoirs (deer, dogs, horses) by ticks. *Doxycycline* (100 mg twice daily for adults or 4 mg/kg daily in children over 8 years) is recommended. The treatment has to be continued for 3 days after defervescence, for a minimal total duration of 7 days.

SPECIFIC INVESTIGATIONS

■ Serology: immunofluorescent antibody	

Evidence levels **A** Double-blind study **B** Clinical trial ≥ 20 subjects **C** Clinical trial < 20 subjects **D** Series ≥ 5 subjects **E** Anecdotal case reports

FIRST LINE THERAPIES

■ Doxycycline	A

Human granulocytic ehrlichiosis: a case series from a medical center in New York State. Aguero-Rosenfeld ME, Horowitz HW, Wormser GP, et al. Ann Intern Med 1996;125:904–8.

All 18 patients were successfully treated with doxycycline.

SECOND LINE THERAPIES

■ Rifampin	D

Successful treatment of human granulocytic ehrlichiosis in children using rifampin. Krause PJ, Corrow CL, Bakken JS. Pediatrics 2003;112:252–3.

The authors report two cases of children with human granulocytic ehrlichiosis successfully treated with rifampin.

Rocky Mountain spotted fever

Rachel Nazarian, Mark G Lebwohl

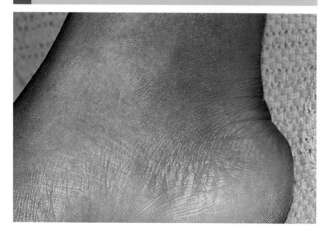

Rocky Mountain spotted fever has become a misnomer because it is endemic to almost all areas of the USA and rash is not always a reliable diagnostic sign. Diagnosis is difficult to make and is often delayed because the critical early stages frequently fail to present with the classic triad of tick bite, characteristic rash, and fever. The infection runs a rapid course and requires immediate treatment initiated in the first 3–4 days of illness. Beyond 5 days of illness onset, untreated RMSF has a higher incidence of death. Response to treatment is apparent within 24 h and it should be noted that early discontinuation of therapy may result in relapse. In its classic presentation, pink macules start on the wrists and ankles and become petechial and purpuric, quickly spreading to the palms, soles, extremities, trunk, and face. The diagnostic sign of skin rash is absent in nearly 10% of patients, and usually does not present until the third day of illness. Occasional atypical presentation of rash, limited to one area of the body, has also been noted.

Nearly half of patients have gastrointestinal symptoms such as nausea, vomiting, diarrhea, and abdominal pains, noted most often within the onset of illness, and commonly lead to misdiagnosis or delay in therapy. Cases have been reported of vascular injury to the small intestine, appendix, and gallbladder, and even the mimicking of acute cholecystitis. Nearly all patients with RMSF have fever, severe headache, and myalgias, most commonly presenting as bilateral calf pain.

MANAGEMENT STRATEGY

The use of *tetracycline* as the best first line agent for treating RMSF has been supported by immense amounts of experimental data as well as clinical experience. It should be noted that when dealing with pregnant patients, alternative treatment to tetracycline, *chloramphenicol*, is the therapy of choice. In addition to antibiotic therapy, supportive care plays a significant role in recovery. It remains important to uphold a high-protein diet and maintain adequate fluid intake, continuously monitoring blood volume. Specialized therapy may be necessary for cases of RMSF with complications of renal, pulmonary, and cardiac dysfunction.

SPECIFIC INVESTIGATIONS

- Skin biopsy, direct immunofluorescence/immunoperoxidase
- Liver function tests
- Complete blood count
- Serologic testing for antirickettsial antibodies

Diagnosis is most often based on clinical features in a patient who has been to an endemic area, particularly if a history of tick bite can be elicited. Because mortality increases if treatment is delayed, initiate therapy as soon as the diagnosis is suspected. Direct immunofluorescence or immunoperoxidase staining of skin biopsy specimens is a fast way of making this diagnosis. Serologic tests are available for detection of antirickettsial antibodies and include indirect immunofluorescence, latex agglutination, and enzyme immunoassay. Because antibodies are not detectable until 7–10 days after illness onset, these tests usually appear negative in the critical first days of the disease. Testing of acute and convalescent phase serum samples can be used to confirm the diagnosis. The most useful of the serologic tests remains the indirect hemagglutination antibody and immunofluorescent antibody tests. Both have exceptional sensitivity and specificity and are often employed, especially the immunofluorescent test due to its ability to measure IgG and IgM.

It may be judicious to obtain a complete blood count because most patients will have varying degrees of anemia or decreased white blood cell count, though the white blood count can be elevated. Thrombocytopenia can occur in severe cases. However, most of the laboratory studies are nonspecific and a complication or death associated with RMSF can be avoided with early diagnosis of RMSF and the early employment of empiric therapy.

Cultures of blood or skin biopsy can retrospectively confirm the diagnosis, but take too long to help establish the diagnosis early in the course of RMSF.

Although it is a Gram-negative bacterial parasite, *Rickettsia rickettsii* does not stain well with Gram stain, and instead may be stained with Giemsa, Machiavello's or Castaneda's stains.

Laboratory diagnosis of Rocky Mountain spotted fever. Walker DH, Burday MS, Folds JD. South Med J 1980;73: 1143–6.

Skin biopsies from 16 patients showed immunofluorescence staining of skin biopsies as the best procedure for early diagnosis of RMSF. Sensitivity rates were recorded at 70% with overall specificity rates of 100%. Immunofluorescence staining for *R. rickettsii* is successful as a diagnostic tool, but must be initiated within 48 h after beginning antirickettsial therapy.

Immunoperoxidase and immunofluorescent staining of *Rickettsia rickettsii* in skin biopsies: a comparative study. Procop GW, Burchette JL, Howell DN, Sexton DJ. Arch Pathol Lab Med 1997;121:894–9.

Results of immunofluorescent staining for *R. rickettsii* were compared with results of immunoperoxidase staining for *R. rickettsii* on formalin-fixed, paraffin-embedded skin biopsies in 26 patients. Although sensitivity and specificity for both stains were identical, results found the immunofluorescent technique to be quicker, which is of high

Evidence levels A Double-blind study B Clinical trial ≥ 20 subjects C Clinical trial < 20 subjects D Series ≥ 5 subjects E Anecdotal case reports

importance with patients with RMSF, but found immunoperoxidase staining to have easier antigen localization and the convenient ability to view the histopathology simultaneously.

FIRST LINE THERAPIES

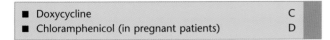

■ Doxycycline	C
■ Chloramphenicol (in pregnant patients)	D

Rickettsia rickettsii is sensitive to chloramphenicol, tetracycline, and rifampin. Doxycycline is the therapy of choice and should be administered early in illness onset. Adults and children weighing 45 kg or more should take 100 mg doses of doxycycline at 12-h intervals orally or intravenously. Children weighing less than 45 kg should be given 0.9 mg/kg, divided into two doses.

Should tetracycline be contraindicated for therapy of presumed RMSF in children less than 9 years of age? Abramson JS, Givner LB. Pediatrics 1990;86:123–4.

Staining of teeth related to administration of tetracycline appears to be dose related and children younger than 5 years of age who were treated with less than six courses (6 days per course) of tetracycline had negligible tooth discoloration. Treatment with chloramphenicol is not advised due to serious complications such as aplastic anemia.

The benefits of tetracycline in patients less than 9 years old who have RMSF outweigh the risks according to these authors.

Rocky Mountain spotted fever: a clinician's dilemma. Masters EJ, Olson GS, Weiner SJ, et al. Arch Intern Med 2003;163:769–74.

The success of treatment of RMSF is dependent upon the expediency of its deliverance. The most common factors associated with a failure to diagnose and adequately treat upon initial clinical evaluation are (1) absence of a skin rash, (2) absence of a tick bite by history, (3) inappropriate geographic and seasonal exclusion, (4) misdiagnosis due to nonspecific symptoms, and (5) failure to treat with appropriate doses of doxycycline.

The reported mortality rate was 6.5% for those treated within 5 days of onset and 22.9% for those treated 5 days or more after onset (Therapeutic delay and mortality in cases of Rocky Mountain spotted fever. Kirkland KB, Wilkinson WE, Sexton DJ. Clin Infect Dis 1995;20:1118–21).

SECOND LINE THERAPIES

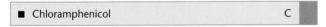

■ Chloramphenicol	C

Analysis of risk factors for fatal Rocky Mountain spotted fever: evidence for superiority of tetracyclines for therapy. Holman RC, Paddock CD, Curns AT, et al. J Infect Dis 2001;184:1437–44.

Study of 5600 confirmed and probable cases of RMSF using reports submitted to the Center for Disease Control and Prevention by state health departments and private physicians from 1981 to 1998. Patients were stratified using criteria including age, race, and time of treatment with

respect to onset of illness. Patients were studied based on four treatments for therapy divided into tetracycline without chloramphenicol, chloramphenicol without tetracycline, chloramphenicol with tetracycline, and neither chloramphenicol nor tetracycline. Risk for death was significantly greater for RMSF patients who did not receive tetracycline-only treatment, for those treated with chloramphenicol only, and for those who did not receive treatment with either a tetracycline or chloramphenicol. These findings were consistent with all varying groups of patients.

Although a range of risk factors and medical conditions that may predispose patients to a greater severity of illness were not taken into consideration, it remains that tetracycline-class antibiotics administered early in illness onset significantly reduce the risk of death in patients with RMSF.

THIRD LINE THERAPIES

■ Quinolones	E

Evaluation of the antirickettsial activities of fluoroquinolones. Keren G, Hzhaki A, Oron C, Keysarg A. Drugs 1995;49(suppl 2):208–10.

In-vitro tissue culture testing showed inhibition of *Rickettsia conorii* and other *Rickettsia* spp. with the use of fluoroquinolones at concentrations less than 1 mg/mL. Although this would suggest the use of fluoroquinolones for treatment of RMSF, in-vivo studies on humans are not available, and thus further studies are required.

COMPLICATIONS

Complications of RMSF include edema of the periorbital areas or lower extremity, which was reported in half of children studied with RMSF. Edema appears to be more common in children, and mirrors a similar level of intensity of the rash. Further, conjunctivitis is often present, involving the palpebral and bulbar conjunctivae. Due to vascular involvement of the optic nerve, papilledema is also sometimes seen. During the acute stages of RMSF, temporary deafness can occur; permanent deafness is seldom, if ever, noted.

Long-term sequelae of Rocky Mountain spotted fever. Archibald LK, Sexton DJ. Clin Infect Dis 1995;20:1122–5.

Twenty five patients were followed in this study, which found cases of long-term sequelae including paraparesis, peripheral neuropathy, hearing loss, and language disorders. Data were conclusive in finding long-term sequelae common with severe cases of RMSF.

Rocky Mountain spotted fever complicated by gangrene: report of six cases and review. Kirkland KB, Marcom PK, Sexton DJ, et al. Clin Infect Dis 1993;16:629–34.

Cutaneous necrosis and gangrene are complications of RMSF. The authors report six patients who developed gangrene. Four patients required multiple amputations; one died.

Although most patients with RMSF recover without long-term complications, gangrene and loss of digits can occur.

Rosacea

John Berth-Jones, Sheila M Clark, Catriona A Henderson

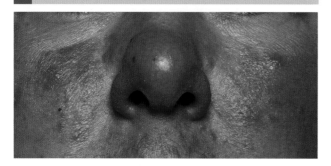

Rosacea is a common inflammatory skin disease. The eruption is generally confined to the face, principally the cheeks, forehead, nose, and chin. In some cases, lesions may extend onto the scalp and occasionally also onto the neck and the upper part of the body. A common early feature is flushing, often accompanied by a burning sensation. Papulation and pustulation develop to some degree in most cases and may become florid. Telangiectasia and erythema are frequently observed. These are initially mild but may later become very conspicuous. Other later features are the development of lymphedema, thickening, and induration. On the nose and, less often, the ears, forehead, or chin, hypertrophy and lymphedema of subcutaneous tissue may develop into distinct swellings known as phymas, of which rhinophyma is most familiar. The etiology and pathogenesis of rosacea remain poorly understood. Improvements in our understanding of the etiology would probably facilitate a more rational approach to treatment, which has, of necessity, developed along largely empiric lines. Treatments for rhinophyma and perioral dermatitis are described in separate chapters.

MANAGEMENT STRATEGY

Patients may find it beneficial to avoid alcohol, spicy food, hot drinks, etc., which may induce flushing and promote the development of telangiectasia. Cosmetic camouflage of the erythema and telangiectasia can be helpful for female patients. Facial massage may promote lymphatic drainage and reduce the development of lymphedema. Papulation, pustulation, and erythema can be effectively suppressed using a variety of topical and systemic antibiotics, retinoids, and other agents described below. Unfortunately, these modalities are usually not very effective for suppressing flushing and have little effect on established telangiectasia. Flushing is usually the most difficult feature to treat. Telangiectasia can be effectively treated by physical measures to ablate the vessels, such as vascular lasers or intense pulsed light. Rosacea is often complicated by ocular changes, conjunctivitis, keratitis, iritis, etc. These often seem to improve during treatment in parallel with the inflammatory changes in the skin but will not be specifically addressed in this chapter.

SPECIFIC INVESTIGATIONS

In selected cases:	
■ Urine 5HIAA to exclude carcinoid syndrome	A
■ Serology to help exclude lupus	A

FIRST LINE TREATMENTS

■ Topical metronidazole	A
■ Topical azelaic acid	A
■ Oral tetracyclines	A
■ Oral erythromycin	C

Treatment of rosacea with 1% metronidazole cream. A double-blind study. Nielson PG. Br J Dermatol 1983;108: 327–32.

Eighty-one patients were treated with 1% metronidazole cream or vehicle for 2 months. Metronidazole cream was significantly more effective than placebo in suppression of inflammatory lesions and erythema.

The efficacy of metronidazole 1% cream once daily compared with metronidazole cream twice daily and their vehicles in rosacea: a double-blind clinical trial. Jorizzo JL, Lebwohl M, Tobey RE. J Am Acad Dermatol 1998;39:502–4.

This study also demonstrated improvements in counts of inflammatory lesions and in erythema relative to placebo. However, there was no apparent difference between once-daily and twice-daily application.

Topical metronidazole maintains remissions of rosacea. Dahl MV, Katz HI, Krueger GG, et al. Arch Dermatol 1998; 134:679–83.

Eighty-eight patients who had responded to treatment with systemic tetracycline and topical metronidazole were randomized to receive 0.75% metronidazole gel or placebo gel for 6 months. Among those applying the metronidazole gel, 23% developed a relapse of papulopustular lesions, and 55% a worsening of erythema, compared with 42% and 74% of patients, respectively, in the placebo gel group.

Topical azelaic acid in the treatment of rosacea. Carmichael AJ, Marks R, Graupe KA, Zaumseil RP. J Derm Treat 1993;4 (suppl 1):19–22.

Topical azelaic acid 20% cream was shown to be more effective than the base alone in a double-blind, controlled, split-face study with 33 patients. Treatment was given for 9 weeks and improvement was seen in papules, pustules, and erythema, but not telangiectasia.

Double-blind comparison of azelaic acid 20% cream and its vehicle in treatment of papulo-pustular rosacea. Bjerke R, Fyrand O, Graupe K. Acta Derm Venereol 1999;79:456–9.

A 3-month, randomized, double-blind study compared the efficacy and safety of azelaic acid 20% cream, applied twice daily, with its vehicle in 116 patients. Azelaic acid cream produced significantly greater mean reductions in total inflammatory lesions than vehicle; 73.4% vs 50.6%, respectively. Erythema also responded.

A comparison of topical azelaic acid 20% cream and topical metronidazole 0.75% cream in the treatment of patients with papulopustular rosacea. Maddin S. J Am Acad Dermatol 1999;40:961–5.

A double-blind, randomized, split-face study in 40 patients comparing topical azelaic acid 20% cream with metronidazole 0.75% cream, each applied twice daily for 15 weeks. The treatments were similarly effective.

A comparison of 15% azelaic acid gel and 0.75% metronidazole gel in the topical treatment of papulopustular rosacea. Elewski BE, Fleischer AB, Pariser DM. Arch Dermatol 2003;139:1444–50.

A double-blind study in 251 patients with papulopustular rosacea. In these formulations, azelaic acid proved superior to metronidazole for reducing inflammatory lesions and erythema. Metronidazole was somewhat better tolerated.

A clinical trial of tetracycline in rosacea. Sneddon IB. Br J Dermatol 1966;78:649–52.

A double-blind trial with 78 evaluable patients, comparing tetracycline 250 mg twice daily with placebo after 4 weeks' treatment. There was a significantly superior response to active treatment even though a pronounced placebo effect was observed. During subsequent follow-up it was found that some patients could be completely controlled using only 100 mg daily.

Safety of long-term tetracycline therapy for acne. Sauer GC. Arch Dermatol 1976;112:1603–5.

A study of 325 patients treated with oral tetracycline for 3 years or more showed the drug was generally well tolerated. However, elevated bilirubin and alkaline phosphatase levels were found in approximately 5% of cases (the majority being minimally so or returning to normal on repeat testing), suggesting that liver function should be monitored in patients on long-term therapy. One patient developed mild jaundice while taking 500 mg of tetracycline daily.

A double-blind study of 1% metronidazole cream versus systemic oxytetracycline therapy for rosacea. Nielsen PG. Br J Dermatol 1983;109:63–5.

In this randomized, double-blind trial, 51 patients were treated for 2 months with 1% metronidazole cream and placebo tablets or with oxytetracycline 250 mg twice daily and placebo cream. Improvement occurred in 90% of the patients. There was no significant difference between the treatments.

Steroid rosacea in prepubertal children. Weston WL, Morelli JG. Arch Pediatr Adolesc Med 2000;154:62–4.

A retrospective evaluation of 106 children younger than 13 years with steroid rosacea. Abrupt cessation of topical corticosteroid use and initiation of treatment with oral erythromycin stearate for 4 weeks produced complete clearing in 86% of children within 4 weeks and 100% by 8 weeks.

The efficacy of oral tetracyclines seems to be well established, although most of the trials on the use of these antibiotics have been against active comparators rather than placebo. Both tetracycline and oxytetracycline are generally used at the dose of 250–500 mg twice daily in rosacea. Other systemic tetracyclines, such as minocycline 100 mg daily, doxycycline 100 mg daily, and lymecycline 408 mg daily, are also often prescribed. These offer the advantage of once-daily administration and their absorption is less influenced by dietary calcium, so they can be taken with food. Erythromycin 250–500 mg twice daily is also often

prescribed and widely held to be effective and can be useful when rosacea occurs in children, for whom tetracyclines are contraindicated.

SECOND LINE TREATMENTS

■ Topical erythromycin	C
■ Topical clindamycin	C
■ Oral metronidazole	A
■ Topical benzoyl peroxide	A
■ Ampicillin	A
■ Azithromycin	C

Topically applied erythromycin in rosacea. Mills OH, Kligman AM. Arch Dermatol 1976;112:553–4.

A 2% solution applied twice daily to 15 patients produced a 50–100% improvement in 87% of cases and treatment was effective by 4 weeks. Once-daily application was sufficient after the disease had been controlled.

Treatment of rosacea: topical clindamycin versus oral tetracycline. Wilkin JK, DeWitt S. Int J Dermatol 1993;32:65–7.

A randomized, blinded trial comparing topical clindamycin lotion twice daily with oral tetracycline in 43 patients evaluated over 12 weeks. Similar improvements were found in both groups, though clindamycin was superior in eradication of pustules.

Treatment of rosacea by metronidazole. Pye RJ, Burton JL. Lancet 1976;1:1211–2.

A double-blind, placebo-controlled, parallel-group trial demonstrating the efficacy of oral metronidazole 200 mg twice daily after 6 weeks of treatment. Ten of 14 patients treated with metronidazole showed a good response.

A double-blinded trial of metronidazole versus oxytetracycline therapy for rosacea. Saihan EM, Burton JL. Br J Dermatol 1980;102:443–5.

Forty patients were treated for 12 weeks with oxytetracycline 250 mg twice daily or metronidazole 200 mg twice daily. For both drugs, the degree of improvement was greater after 12 weeks than after 6 weeks. There was no significant difference between the two therapies.

Although metronidazole is generally well tolerated and it has been used long term, there is a risk of peripheral neuropathy if it is used for longer than 3 months.

Topical treatment of acne rosacea with benzyl peroxide acetone gel. Montes LF, Cordero AA, Kriner J. Cutis 1983;32:185–90.

Benzoyl peroxide gel (5% increasing to 10%) was significantly superior to vehicle, although it was poorly tolerated and there was a high dropout rate.

Comparative effectiveness of tetracycline and ampicillin in rosacea. A controlled trial. Marks R, Ellis J. Lancet 1971;2:1049–52.

A double-blind, placebo-controlled trial lasting 6 weeks and completed by 56 patients. Both antibiotics were significantly more effective than placebo. Tetracycline was apparently (but not significantly) more effective than ampicillin.

A novel treatment for acne vulgaris and rosacea. Elewski BE. J Eur Acad Dermatol Venereol 2000;14:423–4.

Ten patients were treated in an open study of azithromycin: 500 mg on day 1, followed by 250 mg daily on days 2–5, beginning on the 1st and 15th day of each month, for 3 months. All patients improved and nine were clear by 3 months.

Therapeutic potential of azithromycin in rosacea. Bakar O, Demircay Z, Gurbuz O. Int J Dermatol 2004;43:151–4.

In a 12-week open study in 18 patients, azithromycin was used at the dose of 500 mg daily for three consecutive days each week for the first 4 weeks, 250 mg daily on 3 days for the next 4 weeks, and 500 mg once weekly for the last 4 weeks. Both inflammatory lesions and erythema improved markedly in the 14 evaluable subjects.

Oral use of azithromycin for the treatment of acne rosacea. Fernandez-Obregon A. Arch Dermatol 2004;140:489–90.

Ten patients responded well to azithromycin 250 mg daily, for 3 days each week (Monday, Wednesday, and Friday), within 4 weeks. Ocular symptoms also improved.

Azithromycin has a relatively long half life and is therefore suited to this sort of regimen.

THIRD LINE TREATMENTS

■ Systemic isotretinoin	B
■ Topical tretinoin	C
■ Topical sulfur	B
■ Topical corticosteroids	D
■ Topical ketoconazole	D
■ Systemic ketoconazole	D
■ Topical bifonazole	D
■ Ondansetron	E
■ Spironolactone	D
■ *Demodex* eradication	B
■ *Helicobacter pylori* eradication	D
■ Sunscreens	E
■ Topical tacrolimus	C
■ Octreotide	C
■ Inhibition of ovulation	C
■ Topical NADH	C

Treatment of rosacea with isotretinoin. Hoting E, Paul E, Plewig G. Int J Dermatol 1986;25:660–3.

This open study involving 92 patients is the largest on the use of isotretinoin in rosacea. Results were beneficial, although seven patients were intolerant of the drug.

Continuous microdose isotretinoin in adult recalcitrant rosacea. Hofer T. Clin Exp Dermatol 2004;29:204–5.

In this report on 12 patients, isotretinoin was commenced at 10 or 20 mg daily for a period of 4–6 months, then reduced individually to lower doses. The treatment was well tolerated and quality of life, assessed using the Dermatology Life Quality Index (DLQI), was improved relative to a control group.

There have been several reports of the use of isotretinoin at doses ranging from 10 to 60 mg daily or 0.5 to 1 mg/kg daily for 6–28 weeks. Variable relapse rates have been reported after discontinuing the drug, there being a trend toward more frequent relapse in those given lower total doses. However, doses often need to be kept low to avoid aggravating ocular symptoms. Partly for this reason, other investigators have advocated the use of continuous low-dose therapy with isotretinoin.

Topical tretinoin for rosacea; a preliminary report. Kligman AM. J Dermatol Treat 1993;4:71–3.

Topical tretinoin 0.025% for 6–12 months improved rosacea in about 70% of cases in this open study with 19 patients. Improvement was seen in telangiectasia as well as in erythematous and papulosquamous lesions.

A comparison of the efficacy of topical tretinoin and low-dose oral isotretinoin in rosacea. Ertl GA, Levine N, Kligman AM. Arch Dermatol 1994;130:319–24.

In this study involving 22 patients, topical tretinoin (0.025% cream), low-dose isotretinoin (10 mg daily), and a combination of both these treatments appeared equally effective after 16 weeks.

Topical treatment with sulfur 10% for rosacea. Blom I, Hornmark A-M. Acta Derm Venereol 1984;64:358–9.

A randomized study with 40 patients. Treatment duration was 4 weeks. Topical sulfur 10% in a cream base (Diprobase®) was as effective as oral lymecycline 150 mg daily. A greater reduction in inflammatory lesions was observed in the group treated with sulfur, although there were a greater number of lesions at baseline in this group.

The treatment of rosacea: the safety and efficacy of sodium sulfacetamide 10% and sulfur 5% lotion (Novacet) is demonstrated in a double-blind study. Saunder DN, Miller R, Gratton D, et al. J Dermatol Treat 1997;8:79–85.

The efficacy of a lotion of 10% sodium sulfacetamide and 5% sulfur was demonstrated in an 8-week, double-blind, randomized, vehicle-controlled, parallel-group, multicenter study of 103 patients.

Comparative study of triamcinolone acetonide and hydrocortisone 17-butyrate in rosacea with special regard to the rebound phenomenon. Go MJ, Wuite J. Dermatologica 1976;152(suppl 1):239–46.

The place of steroids in rosacea is ill defined and probably very limited, although their use has been reported in conjunction with standard treatments. In this study with 19 patients, topical steroids given in conjunction with tetracycline did not cause a rebound phenomenon when the steroids were discontinued.

Treatment of rosacea with ketoconazole. Utas S, Unver U. J Eur Acad Dermatol Venereol 1997;8:69–70.

A double-blind, placebo-controlled study of oral ketoconazole 400 mg daily, ketoconazole 2% cream, and both treatments combined in 53 patients. Improvement was reported in all three actively treated groups after 2 weeks.

Treatment of rosacea with bifonazole cream: a preliminary report. Veraldi S, Schianchi-Veraldi R. Ann Ital Derm Clin Sper 1990;44:169–71.

Topical bifonazole 1% cream was used successfully in eight cases of rosacea, with no recurrence at 3 months.

The response of erythematous rosacea to ondansetron. Wollina U. Br J Dermatol 1999;140:561–2.

Two cases of resistant rosacea responded to the serotonin receptor antagonist ondansetron. This drug, which is used mainly as an antiemetic, was given intravenously at a dose of 12 mg daily and later orally at doses of 4–8 mg twice daily.

Evidence levels A Double-blind study B Clinical trial ≥ 20 subjects C Clinical trial < 20 subjects D Series ≥ 5 subjects E Anecdotal case reports

Oral spironolactone therapy in male patients with rosacea. Aizawa H, Niimura M. J Dermatol 1992;19:293–7.

Spironolactone at a dose of 50 mg daily for 4 weeks was reported to benefit seven of 13 male patients with rosacea. Two of the patients did not tolerate the drug.

***Demodex folliculorum* and topical treatment: action evaluated by standardized skin surface biopsy.** Forton F, Seys B, Marchal JL, Song AM. Br J Dermatol 1998;138:461–6.

There have been several reports of increased numbers of *Demodex* mites in rosacea – circumstantial evidence to suggest they might be implicated in the pathogenesis in some cases. This has provided a rationale for the use of a range of therapies aimed at eradication of the mites. This study of 34 patients with high *Demodex* carriage compared the miticidal effect of topical metronidazole, permethrin, sulfur, lindane, crotamiton, and benzyl benzoate. Benzyl benzoate and crotamiton had particular effects on the mite population, suggesting that they may be appropriate treatment for some cases of rosacea and 'rosacea-like demodecosis'.

A pilot study of 5% permethrin cream versus 0.75% metronidazole gel in acne rosacea. Signore RJ. Cutis 1995; 56:177–9.

Six patients who applied 5% permethrin cream to one side of the face and 0.75% metronidazole gel to the other showed similar responses to the two topical agents.

Permethrin 5% cream versus metronidazole 0.75% gel for the treatment of papulopustular rosacea. A randomized double-blind placebo-controlled study. Koçak M, Yagli S, Vahapoglu G, Eksioglu M. Dermatology 2002;205:265–70.

Permethrin 5% cream was compared with metronidazole 0.75% gel and placebo, applied twice daily for 2 months, in a randomized parallel-group study of 63 patients. Permethrin was more effective than placebo in improving erythema and papules and as effective as metronidazole 0.75% gel, but it had no effect on telangiectasia, rhinophyma, or pustules. The reduction in *Demodex* counts was significantly greater with permethrin than with the other treatments.

Treatment of rosacea-like demodicidosis with oral ivermectin and topical permethrin cream. Forstinger C, Kittler H, Binder M. J Am Acad Dermatol 1999;41:775–7.

A patient suffering from a follicular, papulopustular, facial eruption with a long history of unsuccessful treatment responded to ivermectin 200 µg/kg. This was followed by once-weekly application of 5% permethrin cream to prevent reinfestation.

***Helicobacter pylori* eradication treatment reduces the severity of rosacea.** Utas S, Ozbakir O, Turasan A, Utas C. J Am Acad Dermatol 1999;40:433–5.

Thirteen cases of rosacea with evidence of *H. pylori* infection received a course of amoxicillin 500 mg three times daily for 2 weeks, metronidazole 500 mg three times daily for 2 weeks, and bismuth subcitrate 300 mg four times daily for 4 weeks. There was a significant decrease in severity of the rosacea at the end of treatment.

The response of rosacea to eradication of *Helicobacter pylori*. Son SW, Kim IH, Oh CH, Kim JG. Br J Dermatol 1999;140:984–5.

Twenty cases of rosacea were treated with amoxicillin 2.25 g daily for 2 weeks, clarithromycin 1.5 g daily for 2

weeks, and nizatidine 300 mg daily for 6 weeks. The 13 who had evidence of *H. pylori* infection demonstrated significantly greater improvement in erythema than the seven who did not.

Effect of treatment of *Helicobacter pylori* infection on rosacea. Bamford JL, Tilden RL, Blankush JL, Gangeness DE. Arch Dermatol 1999;135:659–63.

A randomized, double-blind, controlled trial of *H. pylori* eradication with clarithromycin and omeprazole, or placebo. There was no difference in the rosacea between the two groups at 60 days.

Several investigators have proposed an association between H. pylori and rosacea, although this remains highly controversial.

Effective sunscreen ingredients and cutaneous irritation in patients with rosacea. Nichols K, Desai N, Lebwohl MG. Cutis 1998;61:344–6.

Patients with rosacea are particularly susceptible to the irritation caused by sunscreen ingredients. Formulations with protective constituents, such as dimethicone and cyclomethicone, may be preferable.

Epidemiological studies of the influence of sunlight on the skin. Berg M. Photodermatology 1989;6:80–4.

Individuals with rosacea experienced improvement more often than impairment from exposure to sunlight.

Tacrolimus ointment for the treatment of steroid-induced rosacea: a preliminary report. Goldman D. J Am Acad Dermatol 2001;44:995–8.

Corticosteroid-induced rosacea resolved in three patients after 7 to 10 days of treatment with topical tacrolimus 0.075% ointment in conjunction with avoidance of topical corticosteroids and other possible exacerbating factors.

Tacrolimus effect on rosacea. Bamford JTM, Elliott BA, Haller IV. J Am Acad Dermatol 2004;50:107–8.

Topical tacrolimus 0.1% reduced erythema but not papulopustular lesions in this open study with 24 patients.

Induction of rosaceiform dermatitis during treatment of facial inflammatory dermatoses with tacrolimus ointment. Antille C, Saurat JH, Lübbe J. Arch Dermatol 2004;140:457–60.

Rosacea-like eruptions developed or worsened in six patients with facial dermatoses treated with tacrolimus.

If there is a role for topical tacrolimus and pimecrolimus in the management of rosacea, it remains to be clarified.

Incidental control of rosacea by somatostatin. Piérard-Franchimont C, Quatresooz P, Piérard GE. Dermatology 2003;206:249–51.

A report of four cases of rosacea which improved during incidental treatment of diabetic retinopathy with a long-acting octreotide injection (Sandostatine®) 20 mg monthly.

Octreotide is a somatotstatin analogue known to be highly active in suppressing the secretion of vasoactive hormones by carcinoid tumours and reduces the flushing associated with the carcinoid syndrome.

It is also worth observing that carcinoid syndrome has occasionally been misdiagnosed as rosacea in the past.

Effect of oral inhibitors of ovulation in treatment of rosacea and dermatitis perioralis in women. Spirov G, Berova N, Vassilev D. Aust J Derm 1971;12:149–54.

Inhibition of ovulation with an oral contraceptive was associated with improvement of rosacea in 90% of 30 women. An open, uncontrolled study.

Topical application of NADH for the treatment of rosacea and contact dermatitis. Wozniacka A, Sysa-Jedrzejowska A, Adamus J, Gebicki J. Clin Exp Dermatol 2003;28:61–3.

Ten cases of rosacea were treated in an open study with 1% NADH in an ointment base. Nine showed some degree of improvement. The response is proposed to be due to the antioxidant properties of NADH.

ROSACEA TELANGIECTASIA

■ Cosmetic camouflage	C
■ Vascular lasers	C
■ Intense pulsed light	B

Decorative cosmetics improve the quality of life in patients with disfiguring skin diseases. Boehncke WH, Ochsendorf F, Paeslack I, et al. Eur J Dermatol 2002;12: 577–80.

Twenty female patients with a range of dermatoses, including nine with rosacea, completed the DLQI questionnaire before and after instruction by a cosmetician. The mean score dropped significantly from 9.2 to 5.5.

Selective destruction of facial telangiectasia using a copper vapor laser. Key JM, Waner M. Arch Otololaryngol Head Neck Surg 1992;118:509–13.

Twenty patients with facial telangiectasia were treated with the 578-nm option of a copper vapor laser in an office setting. Eighteen experienced satisfactory clearance.

Argon laser treatment of the red nose. Dicken CH. J Dermatol Surg Oncol 1990;16:33–6.

A good result was reported in seven patients with telangiectasia due to rosacea.

Flash lamp pumped dye laser for rosacea-associated telangiectasia and erythema. Lowe NJ, Behr KL, Fitzpatrick R, et al. J Dermatol Surg Oncol 1991;17:522–5.

This laser gave good or excellent reduction of telangiectasia and erythema in 24 of 27 patients after one to three treatments. Papulation and pustulation were also improved.

Pulsed dye laser therapy for rosacea. Tan ST, Bialostocki A, Armstrong JR. Br J Plast Surg 2004;57:303–10.

Forty patients were treated and all considered that the treatment was worthwhile. When improvement in erythema and telangiectasis was assessed on a five-point scale by an independent panel of 10 members, there was a mean score of 3.7, i.e. between slight (3) and moderate (4) improvement.

How laser surgery can help your rosacea patients. West T. Skin Aging 1998;March:43–6.

A review of the use of lasers and intense pulsed light (IPL) for rosacea telangiectasia. IPL is considered to require more operator skill than the potassium titanyl phosphate (KTP) or pulsed dye lasers. This article includes recommended parameters for the use of lasers and IPL.

Objective and quantitative improvement of rosacea-associated erythema after intense pulsed light treatment.

Mark KA, Sparacio RM, Voigt A, et al. Dermatol Surg 2003; 29:600–4.

Objective assessments were performed on four patients before and after IPL therapy for rosacea. Five treatments at 3-week intervals were undertaken using the Photoderm VL® machine, with a 515-nm filter, a single pulse of 3 ms duration, and various fluences. Facial blood flow was decreased by 30%, the area of the cheek occupied by telangiectasia was reduced by 29%, and erythema intensity was reduced by 21%.

Treatment of rosacea with intense pulsed light. Taub AF. J Drugs Dermatol 2003;2:254–9.

Thirty-two patients underwent one to seven treatments: 83% had reduced redness, 75% noted reduced flushing, and 64% noted fewer acneiform breakouts. The treatment was well tolerated.

Treatment of facial vascular lesions with intense pulsed light. Angermeier MC. J Cutan Laser Ther 1999;1:95–100.

Two hundred patients with facial pathologies were treated with an IPL source (PhotoDerm VL®) using various treatment parameters. Indications included telangiectasia, hemangiomas, rosacea, and port wine stains. Of the 188 patients who returned for follow-up at 2 months, 174 achieved 75% to 100% clearance after one to four treatment sessions. Side effects were minimal, with no instances of scarring, and were considered less frequent than with laser treatment.

IPL seems likely to emerge as the treatment of choice for rosacea telangiectasia. It can improve not only telangiectasia but also erythema and flushing. IPL is also generally better tolerated than lasers. However, considerable expertise is required for optimal results.

ROSACEA FLUSHING

■ Clonidine	D
■ Beta blockers	D
■ Naloxone	D
■ Rilmenidine	D
■ Cosmesis	C
■ Pulsed dye laser	D
■ Intense pulsed light	D
■ Hypnosis	E

Clonidine and facial flushing in rosacea. Cunliffe WJ, Dodman B, Binner JG. Br Med J 1977;1:105.

Clonidine 0.05 mg twice daily was compared with placebo in a crossover trial involving 17 patients. Five of these reported an improvement in severity and frequency of flushing while on clonidine.

Flushing in rosacea: a possible mechanism. Guarrera M, Parodi A, Cipriani C, et al. Arch Dermatol Res 1982;272: 311–16.

A study of possible pharmacologic inhibitors of rosacea flushing. A single 0.15 mg dose of clonidine inhibited the flushing induced by ingestion of 100 ml of beer in all five patients tested. The testing was undertaken 1 h after the oral dose so that the blood level of clonidine was at its peak during the investigation.

Evidence levels **A** Double-blind study **B** Clinical trial ≥ 20 subjects **C** Clinical trial < 20 subjects **D** Series ≥ 5 subjects **E** Anecdotal case reports

Effect of subdepressor clonidine on flushing reactions in rosacea. Change in malar thermal circulation index during provoked flushing reactions. Wilkin JK. Arch Dermatol 1983;119:211–14.

Clonidine can reduce menopausal flushing. In this study, clonidine 0.05 mg given orally twice daily did not suppress flushing reactions provoked by water at 60°C, red wine, and chocolate. Clonidine did reduce the temperature of malar skin, suggesting a vasoconstrictor effect.

Rilmenidine in rosacea: a double-blind study versus placebo. Grosshans E, Michel C, Arcade B, Cribier B. Ann Dermatol Venereol 1997;124:687–91.

Rilmenidine is a centrally acting hypotensive drug similar in action to clonidine but with less tendency to cause sedation. In this trial with 34 evaluable patients, the reduction in flushing was higher on rilmetidine 1 mg daily than on placebo, but the difference was not quite significant (p = 0.076).

Effect of nadolol on flushing reactions in rosacea. Wilkin JK. J Am Acad Dermatol 1989;20:202–5.

A placebo-controlled trial of nadolol 40 mg daily. Spontaneous flushing and flushing provoked in the laboratory by challenges with hot drinks, alcohol, and nicotinic acid were evaluated in 15 patients. Nadolol had no effect on objective measurements of provoked flushing. There was a trend toward improvement in patient-reported spontaneous flushing.

Alcohol-induced rosacea flushing blocked by naloxone. Bernstein JE, Soltani K. Br J Dermatol 1982;107:59–61.

In an experimental setting, five subjects with rosacea were investigated to determine whether alcohol-induced rosacea flushing could be inhibited by naloxone 0.8 mg subcutaneously, placebo injection, or chlorphenamine (chlorpheniramine) 12 mg orally. Naloxone effectively prevented alcohol-induced rosacea flushing. Chlorphenamine (chlorpheniramine) and placebo had no consistent effect. This suggests that there may be a role for opioid antagonists in inhibition of this reaction.

Pulsed dye laser treatment of rosacea improves erythema, symptomatology, and quality of life. Tan SR, Tope WD. J Am Acad Dermatol 2004;51:592–9.

Sixteen patients with erythematotelangiectatic rosacea were treated with the pulsed dye laser, 15 of them on two occasions. Not only telangiectasia and erythema but also symptoms including flushing, burning, and stinging were improved.

The use of IPL is discussed above under treatment of telangiectasia. It would seem plausible that the pulsed dye laser and IPL may reduce flushing as a secondary effect by reducing the number of dilated capillaries.

Hypnosis in dermatology. Shenefelt PD. Arch Dermatol 2000;136:393–9.

Hypnosis has been reported to improve the blushing associated with rosacea.

This is a comprehensive review of the many potential applications for hypnosis in dermatology.

ROSACEA FULMINANS

Rosacea fulminans (pyoderma faciale) is a very severe facial eruption of sudden onset with prominent pustulation and abscess formation. In addition to conventional treatment modalities for rosacea, a short course of systemic corticosteroids is often indicated to reduce the acute inflammation. Isotretinoin seems to be useful in this condition.

■ Systemic corticosteroids	C
■ Topical corticosteroids	D
■ Isotretinoin	C
■ Systemic antibiotics	C
■ Dapsone	E

Pyoderma faciale: a review and report of 20 additional cases: is it rosacea? Plewig G, Jansen T, Kligman AM. Arch Dermatol 1992;128:1611–17.

Ten of these 20 cases were hospitalized to commence treatment. Prednisolone was commenced at 1 mg/kg daily for 1–2 weeks before adding isotretinoin 0.2–0.5 mg/kg daily. The corticosteroid was then tapered off over 2–3 weeks and the isotretinoin continued for 3–4 months.

Treatment of rosacea fulminans with isotretinoin and topical alclometasone dipropionate. Veraldi S, Scarabelli G, Rizzitelli G, Caputo R. Eur J Dermatol 1996;6:94–6.

Five cases were treated successfully with this combination. Alclometasone dipropionate cream (a moderate potency corticosteroid) was applied twice daily for 10 days, then daily for 10 days. The initial dose of isotretinoin was 0.5 mg/kg daily for 1 month, followed by 0.7 mg/kg daily for 3 months. Combined cyproterone acetate/ethinylestradiol was used as a contraceptive. Marked improvement was observed after 1 month and complete resolution after 4 months.

Pyoderma faciale – a clinical study of 29 patients. Massa MC, Su WP. J Am Acad Dermatol 1982;6:84–91.

Thirteen of these patients were hospitalized. All were treated with antibiotics, most frequently tetracycline, minocycline, or erythromycin. Vleminckx packs (containing sulfur, calcium polysulfide, and calcium thiosulfate) were used for 21 cases and were considered the most effective topical treatment. Other modalities employed included benzoyl peroxide and UVB.

Dapsone in rosacea fulminans. Bormann G, Gaber G, Fischer M, Marsch WC. J Eur Acad Dermatol Venereol 2001;15:385.

Dapsone resulted in complete clearance of rosacea fulminans after 5 weeks in a 56-year-old woman whose condition had not previously responded to standard therapy.

Sarcoidosis

Erum N Ilyas, Warren R Heymann

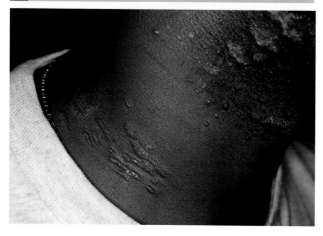

Sarcoidosis is a multisystem disease of unknown etiology characterized histologically by noncaseating granulomas. It is considered to be immune-mediated with a Th1-predominant cytokine profile. Skin manifestations are observed in approximately 25% of cases. Therapy for erythema nodosum associated with sarcoidosis is addressed on page 204.

MANAGEMENT STRATEGY

The treatment of cutaneous sarcoidosis is dependent upon the type and extent of lesions present. Therapy is directed at suppressing the formation of granulomas. Guidelines for treating extracutaneous involvement can be found elsewhere, but it should be recognized that therapy for internal involvement may take precedence over skin disease and that response to treatment may be variable depending on the type of tissue involved.

In small papular or extremely localized sarcoidosis, treatment with *potent topical corticosteroids* or *intralesional triamcinolone acetonide* (3.3–10 mg/mL) is reasonable. If this is ineffective or involvement is more diffuse, *oral chloroquine* (initial dose 250 mg twice daily) or *hydroxychloroquine* (initial dose 200 mg twice daily) may be effective. If no response is seen with antimalarials or disfiguring lesions are present, *oral prednisone* can be used at a dose of 1 mg/kg daily (maximum 60 mg) for up to 3 months and then tapered if improvement or a stable level is reached, to a maintenance dose of 5–10 mg on alternate days for several months. Periodic escalations in dose are necessary with flares.

Methotrexate may be used as a corticosteroid-sparing agent or as monotherapy in those patients with lupus pernio, ulcerative sarcoidosis, or severe disease that has not responded to prednisone. Initial doses of 15–20 mg weekly are favored. *Thalidomide, azathioprine, chlorambucil, isotretinoin,* or *allopurinol* could be considered if methotrexate fails in this subset of patients. Azathioprine and chlorambucil are better studied in patients with pulmonary sarcoidosis. Thalidomide seems to be more effective than isotretinoin and allopurinol in cutaneous disease. Reported failures are described with etretinate and allopurinol.

Localized disease that does not respond to topical or intralesional corticosteroids, and where the use of systemic antimalarials or corticosteroids is undesirable, may represent a niche for alternative therapy such as *excision, laser, intralesional chloroquine,* or *phonophoresis.*

SPECIFIC INVESTIGATIONS

- Special stains, cultures, and polarization of biopsy specimens
- Electrolytes, blood urea nitrogen, creatinine, serum calcium, liver function tests, complete blood count, 24-hour urine calcium, and serum angiotensin-converting enzyme (ACE)
- Ophthalmologic evaluation, including slit-lamp examination
- Chest radiograph, pulmonary function tests
- Electrocardiogram

Sarcoidosis: etiology, immunology, and therapeutics. Vourlekis JS, Sawyer RT, Newman LS. Adv Intern Med 2000; 45:209–57.

A review on the appropriate history, physical examination, referrals, and laboratory tests.

Sarcoidosis: an updated review. Kerdel FA, Moschella SL. J Am Acad Dermatol 1984;11:1–19.

The histopathologic presence of granulomas is nonspecific and may be seen in a variety of clinical situations, including tuberculosis, deep fungal infections, berylliosis, zirconiosis, leishmaniasis, and tuberculoid leprosy.

Serum angiotensin-converting enzyme activity in evaluating the clinical course of sarcoidosis. De Remee RA, Rohrbach MS. Ann Intern Med 1980;92:361–5.

Thirty five patients with sarcoidosis were monitored for ACE activity. The ACE level was regarded as a sensitive index for evaluating the course of sarcoidosis. Cutaneous lesions were a variable in assessing clinical change.

FIRST LINE THERAPIES

■ Topical corticosteroids	C
■ Intralesional corticosteroids	C
■ Oral corticosteroids	C
■ Chloroquine	B
■ Hydroxychloroquine	C

Successful treatment of chronic skin diseases with clobetasol propionate and a hydrocolloid occlusive dressing. Volden G. Acta Derm Venereol 1992;72:69–71.

Three patients with sarcoidosis were treated with clobetasol propionate lotion under occlusion. Complete remissions were observed in a mean of 4 weeks.

Potent topical corticosteroid use is reported to be of some value in anecdotal reports. Most authors feel that intralesional corticosteroids are more effective, yet this too is anecdotal. Small lesions would be optimal candidates, but lupus pernio has also been reported to respond.

Intralesional triamcinolone for cutaneous palpebral sarcoidosis. Bersani TA, Nichols CW. Am J Ophthalmol 1985;99:561–2.

A case report of a 32-year-old woman responding to intralesional triamcinolone, 10 mg/mL, administered three times over a 4-week period.

Evidence levels A Double-blind study **B** Clinical trial ≥ 20 subjects **C** Clinical trial < 20 subjects **D** Series ≥ 5 subjects **E** Anecdotal case reports

Anecdotal reports suggest small, papular sarcoid responds best. Strength of the triamcinolone acetonide varies from 2 to 10 mg/mL, and frequency varies from weekly to monthly.

Cutaneous sarcoidosis: prognosis and treatment. Veien NK. Clin Dermatol 1986;4:75–87.

When dermatologic manifestations are the main indication for systemic treatment, the author suggests prednisone 30 mg on alternate days until the granulomas fade. The dose is then tapered over several months to 15 mg on alternate days. Recurrences are managed by increasing back to the initial dose.

Another suggested regimen of prednisone in cutaneous sarcoidosis is 20–40 mg daily for 8–12 weeks, then tapered to 5–10 mg daily. Pulmonary sarcoidosis therapy is better studied, and has been supported by a few randomized, controlled, long-term trials. However, the pulmonary literature has no consensus on initial starting dose or whether oral corticosteroids affect long-term morbidity and mortality. Some protocols suggest prednisone 30–40 mg daily with a gradual taper to 10–20 mg on alternate days for 1 year, or prednisone 1 mg/kg daily (maximum 60 mg) for 8–12 weeks with a taper to 0.25 mg/kg daily and continued for 6 months.

Treatment of cutaneous sarcoidosis with chloroquine: review of the literature. Zic JA, Horowitz DH, Arzubiaga C, King LE. Arch Dermatol 1991;127:1034–40.

A review of the efficacy and safety of chloroquine in the treatment of cutaneous sarcoidosis. The article cites four studies – three open clinical trials and one case series – that support the use of chloroquine. The authors recommend an initial dose of 250 mg twice daily for 14 days then 250 mg daily for long-term suppression, though most studies have used 500 mg daily for several months. Relapses after discontinuation of treatment are frequent.

Hydroxychloroquine is effective therapy for control of cutaneous sarcoidal granulomas. Jones EJ, Callen JP. J Am Acad Dermatol 1990;23:487–9.

Seventeen patients were treated with 200 mg daily or 400 mg daily of hydroxychloroquine. Cutaneous lesions regressed in 12 patients within 4–12 weeks, and three patients had a partial response. In the 12 patients with the best response, six had a recurrence after a dosage reduction or discontinuation.

Hydroxychloroquine may have a better safety profile than chloroquine; however, chloroquine has been better studied in sarcoidosis. Furthermore, a case series of 15 patients has documented a poor response to hydroxychloroquine at 500–1000 mg daily.

SECOND LINE THERAPIES

■ Methotrexate	C

Weekly low-dose methotrexate therapy for cutaneous sarcoidosis. Webster GF, Razsi LK, Sanchez M, Shupack JL. J Am Acad Dermatol 1991;24:451–4.

Three patients with severe, treatment-resistant cutaneous sarcoidosis were initially treated with methotrexate 15–22.5 mg weekly (in three 12-hour interval doses). A favorable response was seen after several weeks, and after 4–6 months the dose was tapered to 10 mg weekly.

Methotrexate may be particularly useful for those with ulcerative sarcoidosis.

Prolonged use of methotrexate for sarcoidosis. Lower EE, Baughman RP. Arch Intern Med 1995;155:846–51.

Fifty patients were treated with methotrexate, 10 mg weekly, for a minimum of 2 years. Most patients did not have cutaneous involvement, but in those who did, a good response was seen. In many patients methotrexate was used in conjunction with prednisone with favorable results.

THIRD LINE THERAPIES

■ Thalidomide	D
■ Allopurinol	D
■ Isotretinoin	E
■ Azathioprine	E
■ Chlorambucil	E
■ Quinacrine	D
■ Minocycline, doxycycline	D
■ Clofazimine	E
■ Etanercept	E
■ Fumaric acid esters	E
■ Topical tacrolimus	E
■ Intralesional chloroquine	E
■ Excision	D
■ Laser	E

Treatment of cutaneous sarcoidosis with thalidomide. Nguyen YT, Dupuy A, Cordoliani F, et al. J Am Acad Dermatol 2004;50:235–41.

A retrospective evaluation of 12 patients with cutaneous sarcoidosis, two patients with systemic involvement, ten of whom were treated successfully with a treatment duration of two to more than 16 months with a daily dose of thalidomide ranging from 50–200 mg daily. Two patients received combined therapy with oral corticosteroids (dose ranging from 7.5 to 30 mg daily), one patient used potent topical corticosteroids, and one received combined therapy with methotrexate (dose 25 mg weekly). The average response time was 2–3 months. The main adverse effect noted in this series of patients was deep venous thrombosis in one patient.

Allopurinol: a therapeutic alternative for disseminated cutaneous sarcoidosis. Brechtel B, Haas N, Henz BM, Kolde G. Br J Dermatol 1996;135:307–9.

A 57-year-old woman with truncal and extremity plaque sarcoidosis achieved a complete response after 12 weeks of allopurinol (increased to 300 mg daily after the first 3 weeks).

A few case reports demonstrate efficacy of allopurinol with doses from 100 to 300 mg daily, alone and in conjunction with oral corticosteroids.

Cutaneous sarcoidosis: complete remission after oral isotretinoin therapy. Georgiou S, Monastirli A, Pasmatzi E, Tsambaos D. Acta Derm Venereol 1998;78:457–9.

A 31-year-old woman with nodules and plaques on the trunk and extremities showed a complete remission with 8 months of isotretinoin at 1 mg/kg daily; 15-month follow-up revealed continuing remission.

Two other cases report improvement with a 30-week course (0.67–1.34 mg/kg daily) and a 6-month course (0.4–1 mg/kg daily) of isotretinoin.

Long-term use of azathioprine as a steroid-sparing treatment. Hof DG, Hof PC, Godfrey WA. Am J Resp Crit Care Med 1996;153:870A.

Of the 21 patients in this study, eight had 'multisystem' involvement and one had skin-only involvement. All patients with extrapulmonary disease achieved a complete remission with azathioprine and a tapering dose of prednisone.

Chlorambucil in sarcoidosis. Kataria YP. Chest 1980;78: 36–43.

Three patients were treated for cutaneous sarcoidosis: two underwent complete remission, and one had an incomplete response. The initial dose of chlorambucil was 4–6 mg daily and two patients received concomitant prednisone.

Two cases of sarcoidosis treated with mepacrine. Soderstrom N. Lancet 1960;2:947–8.

Quinacrine (mepacrine) 100 mg three times daily resulted in dramatic improvement within 2–3 weeks in two patients.

The yellow discoloration of the skin and sclera observed with quinacrine (one-third of patients), make chloroquine and hydroxychloroquine better alternatives.

The use of tetracyclines for the treatment of sarcoidosis. Bachelez H, Senet P, Cadranel J, et al. Arch Dermatol 2001; 137:69–73.

Twelve patients with cutaneous sarcoidosis, three of whom had systemic involvement, were treated with minocycline at a daily dose of 200 mg for a median duration of 12 months. Ten patients showed a response, eight complete and two partial, while one patient's symptoms remained stable and one patient's disease progressed. For patients experiencing relapse after discontinuation of minocycline, doxycycline was used, resulting in remission.

Disseminated small-node cutaneous sarcoidosis. Schwarzenbach R, Djawari D. Dtsch Med Wochenschr 2000; 125:560–2.

An 83-year-old woman with cutaneous sarcoidosis without systemic involvement was treated with clofazimine 300 mg daily tapered over 4 months with resolution of cutaneous findings.

Etanercept ameliorates sarcoidosis, arthritis and skin disease. Khanna D, Liebling MR, Louie JS. J Rheumatol 2003;30:1864–7.

Case report of a patient with therapy-resistant sarcoidosis responding to etanercept.

Successful treatment of recalcitrant cutaneous sarcoidosis with fumaric acid esters. Nowack U, Gambichler T, Hanefeld C, et al. BMC Dermatol 2002;24:215.

Report of three patients with cutaneous sarcoidosis treated with fumaric acid esters for 4–12 months resulting in complete clearance of cutaneous lesions.

Successful topical treatment of cutaneous sarcoidosis with tacrolimus. Gutzmer R, Volker B, Kapp A, Werfel T. Hautarzt 2003;54:1193–7.

Topical tacrolimus was used for cutaneous sarcoidosis of the face for 3 months with nearly complete remission lasting for at least 4 months.

Intralesional chloroquine for the treatment of cutaneous sarcoidosis. Liedtka JE. Int J Dermatol 1996;35:682–3.

Multiple injections of intralesional chloroquine hydrochloride (50 mg/mL) were effective in treating five lesions in a single patient with minimal side effects.

Cutaneous nasal sarcoidosis – treatment by excision and split-skin grafting. Goldin JH, Jawad SMA, Reis AP. J Laryngol Otol 1983;97:1053–6.

Split-thickness and full-thickness skin grafts, dermabrasion, and primary closure have been attempted with mixed results. Surgery has been used in ulcerative and nonulcerative sarcoidosis.

CO_2 laser vaporization for disfiguring lupus pernio. Young HS, Chalmers RJ, Griffiths CE, August PJ. J Cosmet Laser Ther 2002;4: 87–90.

CO_2 laser resurfacing was used in two patients with lupus pernio with a favorable cosmetic result.

Flashlamp pulsed dye laser and Q-switched ruby laser have been beneficial in one case report of lupus pernio. However, exacerbations of lupus pernio, namely generalized ulceration in treated and untreated lesions, have been reported following this therapy.

Evidence levels   **A** Double-blind study   **B** Clinical trial ≥ 20 subjects   **C** Clinical trial < 20 subjects   **D** Series ≥ 5 subjects   **E** Anecdotal case reports

Scabies

William F G Tucker

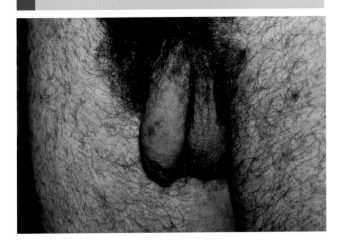

Scabies is a characteristically pruritic skin condition due to infestation by the itch mite, *Sarcoptes scabiei*. Patients can be of any age or social strata, and personal hygiene is no guarantor of freedom from infection. Heavy parasitization results in crusted or 'Norwegian scabies', and tends to occur in the elderly, and people who are mentally deficient or immunocompromised.

MANAGEMENT STRATEGY

Infection with the scabies mite results from close personal contact with an infected individual, and generally requires prolonged skin-to-skin contact, such as handholding, sexual intercourse, and/or sharing a bed. Where an infected person is heavily colonized, as in crusted scabies, their clothing and surroundings can become sufficiently contaminated with live mites as to cause a significant hazard to their attendants and companions.

Because newly infected patients do not begin to itch until 4–8 weeks after being colonized, and may have little or no visible rash, infection is passed on easily. Once sensitized to the mite, reinfestation results in immediate symptoms. Itching at night and when warm is a hallmark feature.

Suspicion is the prerequisite for disease control because many patients are assumed by family physicians and other medical attendants to have eczema or other skin disorders.

Total isolation from other people is clearly unnecessary with a causative organism that cannot jump or fly, and can survive for only approximately 72 hours away from the skin.

Topical application of antiscabetic agents is standard practice. *Sulfur* was the first effective agent, and is still used in many countries, and when nothing else is suitable, as in very young infants. *Benzoyl benzoate* has been the mainstay of therapy, and is cheap and effective if used properly. It has an unfortunate tendency to cause eczematous rashes after repeat applications, and has fallen from favor in most western countries. *Lindane (gamma benzene hexachloride)* was in very widespread use until recently, and is very effective. Unfortunately it accumulates in body fat stores and has been implicated in causing neurologic damage in infants; it has been withdrawn in the UK. Where lindane is used, the risk of toxicity is reduced by not bathing before treatment, showering 12 hours later, and not having more than two treat-

ments per month. *Malathion* is well tolerated, and has the theoretic advantage of prolonged retention in the epidermis, so that reinfection may be reduced. *Permethrin* has been the latest agent to be used and seems to be well tolerated and effective. *Crotamiton* is favored in primary care because it is also antipruritic. *Monosulfiram soap* was reported effective, but has been withdrawn from the UK market.

With all topical agents the key to success is to ensure that adequate concentrations of the scabicide are in contact with the skin for long periods. It is generally accepted that the face and scalp do not need treatment except in infants and the immunocompromised, although some may argue this is a source of treatment failure. Other reservoirs of infection include the subungual areas. What is essential is that *all intimates of the patient, whether apparently infected or not, are treated* at about the same time. Many clinicians find a simple explanatory leaflet, which can also emphasize the need to *launder clothes and bedding*, helpful.

However, what should be done if this doesn't work, there is severe eczematization, and/or compliance is doubtful? Oral therapy would seem to be the answer, and *ivermectin* in single doses of 200 µg/kg has been shown to be very effective in a number of studies. It is unlicensed for this use in humans, but is widely and safely used in onchocerciasis.

SPECIFIC INVESTIGATIONS

- Visualization of mites and burrows

The one specific investigation for scabies is to isolate the mite; nothing is more guaranteed to ensure compliance than to show a patient their co-dweller under the bench microscope. Dermatologists take a great delight in capturing their quarry, and each will be an advocate of one particular method. With standard scabies, burrows are generally easiest to find around the hands, and the mite can often be seen as a dark dot at one end. With the aid of a blunt needle or sewing pin, the mite is then winkled out and placed on a glass slide. It should be noted that hypodermic needles are useless for this purpose because they slice and shred the mite! Alternatively, the burrow is carefully scraped or shaved with a 15 Bard-Parker blade and the slice of stratum corneum placed on a glass slide with some immersion oil. As the slide warms up the mite can be seen moving, and her eggs may also be seen. Both methods require practice and skill. Scraping/shaving is the test of choice in crusted scabies. If you have neither the time, equipment, or expertise for this, mite presence can be proven in a number of other ways. Skin biopsy is often illuminating, particularly because the mite may be a surprise finding! A dermatoscope can actually enable you to visualize the mite in situ, and is a useful aid in visiting elderly persons in residential homes.

The single most useful piece of diagnostic equipment is a fountain pen, however. A blob of ink is carefully applied to a suspected burrow, left for a minute or so, and wiped off with an isopropyl alcohol swab. If a burrow is present, then capillary action will have led to tracking of the ink into the burrow, leaving a wiggly line. Less traditional doctors substitute felt-tip pens with apparent success. Tetracycline solution has been used for the same purpose, along with a UV lamp, but why complicate matters?

Laboratory testing will frequently show a mild eosinophilia in peripheral blood.

FIRST LINE THERAPIES

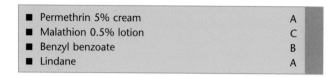

■ Permethrin 5% cream	A
■ Malathion 0.5% lotion	C
■ Benzyl benzoate	B
■ Lindane	A

Permethrin 5% dermal cream: a new treatment for scabies. Taplin D, Meinking TL, Porcelain SL, et al. J Am Acad Dermatol 1986;15:995–1001.

Fifty two patients in a rural Panama community with a high endemic scabies infection rate, were randomly selected, with microscopic confirmation of mite presence in all but five. They were given a single head-to-toe application of either lindane 1% lotion or permethrin 5% cream. Microscopic confirmation of cure was sought at 2 and 4 weeks, with permethrin coming out ahead curing 21 of 23 patients compared with a cure rate of 15 of the 24 patients treated with lindane.

Sarcoptes scabiei infestation treated with malathion liquid. Hanna NF, Clay JC, Harris JRW. Br J Vener Dis 1978; 54:354.

A noncontrolled study using 0.5% malathion liquid in 30 patients, yielding an 83% cure rate at 4 weeks. Surprisingly, since this has become the recommended first line treatment for scabies in the *British National Formulary*, there has been a dearth of randomized controlled trials showing its efficacy.

A family based study on the treatment of scabies with benzyl benzoate and sulphur ointment. Gulati PV, Singh KP. Ind J Dermatol Venereol Leprol 1978;44:269–73.

One hundred and fifty eight clinically diagnosed patients were randomly allocated to use either 25% benzyl benzoate emulsion or 5% sulfur ointment. Treatment was applied at least three times over 24 hours. The sulfur seems to have been marginally more effective.

Interventions for treating scabies. Walker GJA, Johnstone PW. (Cochrane Review) in The Cochrane Library, Issue 4, 2001. Oxford: Update Software.

A very comprehensive review of all published work, but with strict exclusion criteria. Overall permethrin comes out best.

SECOND LINE THERAPIES

■ Sulfur	B
■ Crotamiton	B
■ Ivermectin	A

Therapeutic efficacy, secondary effects, and patient acceptability of 10% sulfur in either pork fat or cold cream for the treatment of scabies. Avila-Romay A, Alvarez-Franco M, Ruiz-Maldonada R. Pediatr Dermatol 1991;8:64–6.

Readers will be pleased to learn that cold cream came out best, with no clinical failures at day 10 in the 26 patients (of 51) assigned to this arm of the trial. Interestingly, there were more side effects, such as pruritus and burning sensations, in the pork-fat group. However sulfur was effective and of course cheap.

Permethrin versus crotamiton and lindane in the treatment of scabies. Amer M, El-Gharib I. Int J Dermatol 1992;31:357–8.

Comparison of crotamiton 10% cream (Eurax) and permethrin 5% cream (Elimite) for the treatment of scabies in children. Taplin D, Meinking TL, Chen JA, Sanchez R. Pediatr Dermatol 1990;7:67–73.

Both these studies show superior efficacy for permethrin, with clinical cures of 91 of 97 vs 72 of 97 patients. The Taplin et al. study also measured parasitic cure, and by this outcome permethrin was much more effective curing 42 of 47 vs 28 of 47.

Tratamiento de la escabiasis con ivermectina por via oral. Macotela-Ruiz E, Pena-Gonzalez G. Gac Med Mex 1993;129:201–5.

This randomized trial compared the treatment of 55 patients with a clinical diagnosis of scabies by either a single dose of ivermectin 200 µg/kg or placebo. After 7 days the code was broken because there was such a significant improvement in the treated group: 23 of 29 vs 4 of 26.

Comparison of ivermectin and benzyl benzoate for treatment of scabies. Glaziou P, Cartel JL, Alzieu P, et al. Trop Med Parasitol 1993;44:331–2.

A randomized study in French Polynesia comparing a single dose of 100 µg/kg ivermectin with 10% benzyl benzoate lotion applied below the neck and repeated 12 hours later. Both were equally effective.

Treatment of scabies with ivermectin. Offidani A, Cellini A, Simonetti O, Fumelli C. Eur J Dermatol 1999;9:100–1.

Six patients with heavy mite infestation received a single dose of 200 µg/kg ivermectin. All were clinically cured.

Deaths associated with ivermectin treatment of scabies. Barkwell R, Shields S. Lancet 1997;349:1144–5.

This is the only 'fly in the ointment' with ivermectin; the authors report on the treatment of a large cohort of 47 elderly, mentally disadvantaged residents of an institution with a single dose of ivermectin at 150–200 µg/kg body weight. All had failed to respond to multiple earlier courses of lindane and crotamiton. All were cured, but over the next 6 months 15 died, of a number of causes, whereas five died in an equivalent, matched population within the same unit.

With a mean age of 73.4 years, and no excess fatalities reported in other studies, you can draw your own conclusions.

THIRD LINE THERAPIES

■ Monosulfiram soap	C
■ Topical thiabendazole solution	B
■ Cotrimoxazole	D

Control of scabies by use of soap impregnated with tetra-ethylthiuram monosulphide ('tetmosol'). Gordon FM, Davey TH, Unsworth K, et al. Br Med J 1944;2:803–6.

A bath a day for 6 days using 20% tetmosol soap cured all six patients; three baths on alternate days cured 88 of 110 patients.

Presumably the limiting factor in wartime Britain was the availability of hot bathwater!

Evidence levels **A** Double-blind study **B** Clinical trial ≥ 20 subjects **C** Clinical trial < 20 subjects **D** Series ≥ 5 subjects **E** Anecdotal case reports

Scabies prophylaxis using 'tetmosol' soap. Mellanby K. Br Med J 1945;1:38–9.

A nonrandomized open study carried out in a large mental hospital showed significant reductions in infection rates.

Where has this soap gone?

Topically applied thiabendazole in the treatment of scabies. Hernandez-Perez E. Arch Dermatol 1976;112:1400–1.

Forty patients with scabies were treated with a single external application of a 10% suspension of thiabendazole.

Thirty two (80%) seemed to be cleared, while six needed a second course.

Perhaps worth trying when patients have had adverse reactions to other topical agents.

A trial of cotrimoxazole in scabies. Shashindran CH, Gandhi IS, Lal S. Br J Dermatol 1979;100:483.

Whereas some clinicians use oral cotrimoxazole as a concomitant treatment for secondarily infected scabies, these authors chose to leave out the scabicide. It didn't work.

Scleredema

Lori M DiRusso, Stephen E Helms,
Robert T Brodell

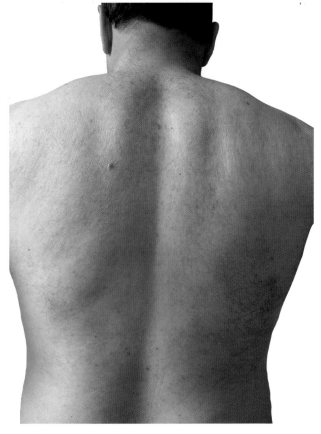

Scleredema (scleredema adultorum or scleredema of Buschke) is a connective tissue disorder characterized by progressive, symmetric induration and thickening of the skin, principally over the posterior neck and upper back. The three clinical forms are: scleredema following acute viral or bacterial infection, which usually resolves spontaneously in 6 months to 2 years; scleredema associated with diabetes mellitus, which persists indefinitely; and scleredema associated with monoclonal gammopathy.

MANAGEMENT STRATEGY

Treatment of scleredema is difficult. There are case-based data to support the effectiveness of several therapies. In many cases, a frank discussion with the patient regarding limitations of treatment, cost, and side effects will lead to a decision to withhold treatment. This is particularly appropriate in patients with the postinfectious form, which can resolve spontaneously without any specific skin treatment. Of course, identification of a specific etiology, such as streptococcal pharyngitis, should lead to appropriate antibiotic treatment even in the absence of evidence that this would alter the rate of clearing in this self-limited form of scleredema. In the forms associated with diabetes mellitus and monoclonal gammopathy, however, progressive involvement can lead to discomfort, unsightly thickening, and even systemic complications such as restrictive pulmonary func-

tion, dysphagia secondary to tongue swelling, and cardiac arrhythmias. In these cases, patients will demand treatment.

Bath or cream psoralen PUVA is recommended as initial therapy in moderately severe disease. *Electron beam therapy* would be the primary recommendation for patients with severe disease, especially cases with restrictive pulmonary function. Alternative therapies would include *cyclosporine* and *high-dose penicillin*. Antidiabetic therapy has no effect on the evolution of scleredema in diabetics, as the progression of scleredema has been found to be unrelated to control of serum glucose levels.

SPECIFIC INVESTIGATIONS

- Fasting blood sugar, glucose tolerance test, hemoglobin A1c (glycosylated hemoglobin)
- Serum protein electrophoresis, immunoelectrophoresis
- Antistreptolysin O, bacterial culture, other efforts to identify an acute infectious agent, erythrocyte sedimentation rate

Scleredema adultorum due to streptococcal infection. Alp H, Orbak Z, Aktas A. Pediatr Int 2003;45:101–3.

Scleredema occurs within a few days to 6 weeks following an acute febrile illness in 65–95% of cases. Of these, 58% of the infections are streptococcal. These infections may present as tonsillitis, pharyngitis, scarlet fever, erysipelas, cervical adenitis, pneumonia, otitis media, pyoderma, impetigo, or rheumatic fever, and appropriate studies will rapidly help determine if one of these is the cause of scleredema.

Since 50% of cases of scleredema occur in childhood, the term adultorum is a misnomer.

Monoclonal gammopathy in scleredema: observations in three cases. Kovary PM, Vakilzadeh F, Macher E, et al. Arch Dermatol 1981;117:536–9.

Immunoelectrophoresis studies in six patients with severe persistent scleredema revealed that three of the patients also had monoclonal gammopathy, and many subsequent reports have also discussed this association. The skin manifestations often precede the development of the gammopathy and thus it is recommended that immunoelectrophoresis be performed at regular intervals in all cases of widespread scleredema.

Scleredema and diabetes mellitus. Fleischmajer R. Arch Dermatol 1970;101:21–6.

Scleredema in patients with diabetes mellitus generally follows a progressive course that is unrelated to control of serum glucose levels.

FIRST LINE THERAPIES

- Identify and treat any underlying disease (diabetes mellitus, monoclonal gammopathy, acute infection)   D
- Conservative management using the principle 'Do no harm'   D

Scleredema: a review of thirty-three cases. Venencie PY, Powell FC, Su D, Perry HO. J Am Acad Dermatol 1984;11: 128–34.

Evidence levels A Double-blind study   B Clinical trial ≥ 20 subjects   C Clinical trial < 20 subjects   D Series ≥ 5 subjects   E Anecdotal case reports

A review of 33 cases of scleredema in which systemic corticosteroids, methotrexate, and D-penicillamine had no effect on the disease course. Both diabetic and nondiabetic patients were studied, and although some patients in both groups had mild complications such as dysphagia and ECG changes, the authors emphasize that, for the most part, scleredema is a mild disease that does not pose a threat to overall health.

Scleredema adultorum. Not always a benign self-limited disease. Curtis AC, Shulak BM. Arch Dermatol 1965;92: 526–41.

A review of 223 scleredema patients revealed that 25% had had symptoms for more than 2 years. The following were found to have no therapeutic benefit: calcium gluconate, estradiol, fever, hot baths, hyaluronidase, nicotinic acid, ovarian extract, para-amino benzoate, penicillin, pituitary extract, corticosteroids, thyroid hormone, and vitamin D.

Due to the expense and potential side effects of the second line therapies discussed below, as well as the recognition that many patients with mild scleredema either improve without treatment or do not respond to the therapy, a policy of 'do no harm' and withholding of treatment is recommended in patients with mild disease.

SECOND LINE THERAPIES

■ Electron beam therapy	E
■ Bath PUVA and cream PUVA	E
■ High-dose penicillin	E
■ Cyclosporine	E
■ Extracorporeal photophoresis	E

Scleredema of Buschke successfully treated with electron beam therapy. Tamburin LM, Pena JR, Meredith R. Arch Dermatol 1998;134:419–22.

A patient with scleredema and insulin-dependent diabetes mellitus experienced complete resolution of skin induration after receiving electron beam therapy twice weekly for 36 days. Prior treatment with topical, intralesional, and systemic corticosteroids had failed. This patient also suffered significant restrictive pulmonary disease thought to be secondary to scleredema, and pulmonary function tests following electron beam therapy revealed marked improvement in lung function. This treatment should be considered in patients with severe persistent disease and systemic complications.

Electron-beam therapy in scleredema adultorum with associated monoclonal hypergammaglobulinaemia. Angeli-Besson C, Koeppel M, Jacquet P, et al. Br J Dermatol 1994;130:394–7.

Ten sessions of electron beam therapy produced significant clinical improvement in the skin lesions of a patient with scleredema associated with IgA κ monoclonal gammopathy. A trial of factor XIII and cyclofenil had proved unsuccessful in this patient. Although the patient had initially responded to systemic corticosteroids, she subsequently became resistant and the condition progressed. At that point, electron beam therapy was begun.

Bath-PUVA therapy in three patients with scleredema adultorum. Hager CM, Sobhi HA, Hunzelmann N, et al. J Am Acad Dermatol 1998;38:240–2.

Bath PUVA therapy (median of 59 treatments) produced substantial clinical improvement in three patients with scleredema. Although one patient did not have a history of diabetes mellitus or preceding infection, the remaining two patients had diabetes. The successful use of bath PUVA in these cases may be significant, since diabetic patients with scleredema tend to have a long unremitting course without treatment.

Cream PUVA therapy for scleredema adultorum. Grundmann-Kollmann M, Ochsendorf F, Zollner TM, et al. Br J Dermatol 2000;142:1058–9.

Cream PUVA therapy (35 irradiations) produced marked clinical improvement and softening of the skin in a patient with a 10-year history of scleredema who also suffered non-insulin-dependent diabetes mellitus. Bath PUVA was contraindicated in this patient due to coronary artery disease, and prior treatment with intravenous penicillin was unsuccessful. Cream PUVA therapy is easier to administer than bath PUVA and may become an important treatment option for scleredema.

Persistent scleredema of Buschke in a diabetic: improvement with high-dose penicillin. Krasagakis K, Hettmannsperger U, Trautmann C, et al. Br J Dermatol 1996; 134:597–8.

High-dose (3×10^6 IU daily) intravenous penicillin for 7 days led to a reduction in the degree of scleredema in a patient with comorbid severe diabetes mellitus. The antifibrotic action of penicillin, causing a decreased dermal thickness, is postulated to be the mechanism of action in this case. The observation that treatment with erythromycin was not effective in this patient and that antibiotics in general have not been successful in treating scleredema supports the role of an antifibrotic rather than antibiotic action of penicillin at work in this case.

Cyclosporine in scleredema. Mattheou-Vakali G, Ioannides D, Thomas T, et al. J Am Acad Dermatol 1996; 35:990–1.

Cyclosporine at a dose of 5 mg/kg daily for 5 weeks was effective in completely clearing scleredema in two patients, neither of whom had coexistent monoclonal gammopathy or diabetes mellitus. Both patients presented with the postinfectious form of scleredema and thus would have likely experienced resolution of their symptoms even without treatment.

Scleredema associated with paraproteinemia treated by extracorporeal photophoresis. Stables GI, Taylor PC, Highet AS. Br J Dermatol 2000;142:781–3.

A patient with scleredema associated with paraproteinemia demonstrated a significant improvement in skin lesions following treatment with extracorporeal photophoresis. When the treatment sessions were reduced from two per month to one, the patient's condition deteriorated, suggesting that the improvement was due to therapy rather than spontaneous resolution. Since scleredema associated with paraproteinemia usually has a progressive course, this treatment should be considered in patients with a similar presentation.

Beneficial effect of aggressive low-density lipoprotein apheresis in a familial hypercholesterolemic patient with severe diabetic scleredema. Koga N. Ther Apher 2001;5: 506–12.

A 59-year-old woman with diabetic scleredema and familial hypercholesterolemia, treated with weekly LDL apheresis over a period of 3 years, had significant improvement in her scleredema when her lipid levels were reduced to normal. Histopathologic as well as clinical improvement was noted. The author concluded that LDL apheresis therapy is an effective second line treatment for resistant diabetic scleredema.

Treatment with chemotherapy of scleredema associated with IgA myeloma. Santos-Juanes J, Osuna CG, Iglesias JR, et al. Int J Dermatol 2001;40:720–1.

A 70-year-old woman with IgA myeloma and scleredema was treated with oral melphalan and prednisone over a 6-month period. During the 18 months she was followed, clinical evidence of softening of the indurated and taut skin was observed. Similar cases were cited in which chemotherapy for myeloma resulted in significant improvement of associated scleredema.

Evidence levels **A** Double-blind study **B** Clinical trial ≥ 20 subjects **C** Clinical trial < 20 subjects **D** Series ≥ 5 subjects **E** Anecdotal case reports

Scleroderma

Timothy H Clayton, Stephanie Ogden, Mark J D Goodfield

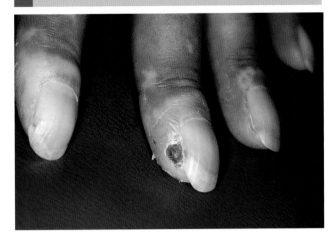

Systemic sclerosis (SSc) is a rare multiorgan connective tissue disorder. It can affect any organ system, particularly skin, gastrointestinal tract, kidney, heart, and lungs. Patients typically present with cutaneous sclerosis or Raynaud's phenomenon (RP). The degree of skin involvement defines the clinical subset of the disease. Diffuse cutaneous SSc (dcSSc) involves the skin proximal to the neck, elbows, or knees, whereas involvement remaining distal to these sites is known as limited cutaneous SSc (lcSSc); some authors include an intermediate group.

MANAGEMENT STRATEGY

Being a multisystem disorder, SSc requires a multidisciplinary approach with careful follow-up. In most cases cutaneous lesions and RP precede systemic involvement. The face and hands are typically involved, with patients displaying a characteristic shiny appearance of the skin and complaining of increased skin tightness or firmness.

There is no specific therapy for the skin although *topical emollients* have a role in prevention of skin breakdown. Topical 0.025–0.05% tretinoin may improve the perioral radial furrows and facial tightening. *UVA phototherapy* – psoralen and UVA (PUVA) and UVA1 – has been reported to be effective in reducing skin thickness.

Vasodilators such as nifedipine reduce vasospasm and improve peripheral blood flow. More recently, *losartan*, an antagonist of angiotensin II receptor type I, has been found to be effective in reducing severity and frequency of attacks of RP. *Parenteral prostacyclin analogues* such as iloprost also improve both the severity and frequency of RP.

A number of immunosuppressant drugs have been used to treat SSc. Both *low-dose prednisolone* 20 mg daily, and *methotrexate (MTX)* 15–25 mg/week have been shown to reduce skin thickness scores. *Cyclosporine* 3–4 mg/kg daily may improve skin induration, but has no effect on internal organ involvement. It should be used with caution because renal involvement with SSc is not uncommon. *Cyclophosphamide* 1–2 mg/kg daily is of proven value in reducing skin scores and preventing the development of lung fibrosis and other complications. Respiratory complications of SSc develop in roughly 30% of patients. Pulmonary hyper-

tension may occur and should be confirmed by right heart catheterization. *Iloprost infusions* have also been shown to reduce PAH. *Angiotensin-converting enzyme (ACE) inhibitors* are particularly effective in reducing the renal complications of the disease, and early treatment may prevent the onset of renal failure. *Proton pump inhibitors* treat esophageal disease effectively. Recent randomized controlled trials have suggested that oral minocycline and D-penicillamine are not effective in SSc. Although SSc carries a high case-specific mortality, there have been significant advances in the management of skin, renal, and pulmonary complications. The introduction of targeted, cytokine-directed therapies is likely to have a significant impact on the treatment of SSc.

SPECIFIC INVESTIGATIONS

- Skin biopsy
- Renal function tests
- Anticentromere and anti-Scl-70 antibodies
- Chest radiograph
- Pulmonary function tests
- Echocardiography

Evidence-based guidelines for the use of immunologic tests: anticentromere, Scl-70, and nucleolar antibodies. Reveille JD, Solomon DH. Arthritis Care Res 2003;49: 399–412.

This excellent, thorough review by the American College of Rheumatology found anticentromere antibodies (ACA) detected by immunofluorescence and anti-Scl-70 antibodies to be particularly useful in the diagnosis of SSc.

Determination of ACA early in the course of disease is useful in predicting whether skin involvement will remain limited. Anti-Scl-70 is also useful in predicting a greater likelihood for developing diffuse cutaneous disease and lung involvement. Once a patient is determined as being anti-Scl-70 or ACA positive or negative, there is little justification for serial determinations.

Scleroderma – clinical and pathological advances. Denton CP, Black CM. Best Pract Res Clin Rheumatol 2004;18:271–90.

This review focuses on the current assessment and treatment of patients with SSc. It recommends that all patients with SSc should be regularly screened for pulmonary disease. Regular monitoring of blood pressure improves outcome.

FIRST LINE THERAPIES

■ Nifedipine	A
■ Iloprost	A
■ ACE inhibitors	B

Iloprost and cisaprost for Raynaud's phenomenon in progressive systemic sclerosis. Pope J, Fenlon D, Thompson A, et al. Cochrane Database Syst Rev 2000(2):CD000953.

This Cochrane review confirms the view that intravenous iloprost is effective in the treatment of RP secondary to scleroderma by decreasing the frequency and severity of attacks and preventing or healing digital ulcers. However, cisaprost has minimal or no efficacy when given orally for the treatment of RP secondary to scleroderma.

It also suggests that oral iloprost may have less efficacy than intravenous iloprost.

Controlled double-blind trial of nifedipine in the treatment of Raynaud's phenomenon. Rodeheffer RJ, Rommer JA, Wigley F, Smith CRN. N Engl J Med 1983;308:880–3.

Calcium channel blockers inhibit smooth muscle cell contraction by reducing the uptake of calcium. Nifedipine was effective in reducing severity of RP.

The efficacy of nifedipine in RP was confirmed by additional studies.

Outcome of renal crisis in systemic sclerosis: relation to availability of angiotensin converting enzyme (ACE) inhibitors. Steen VD, Costantino JP, Shapiro AP, Medsger TA Jr. Ann Intern Med 1990;113:352–7.

Patients with SSc who develop hypertension should be treated with an ACE inhibitor. Improved survival and successful discontinuation of dialysis are possible when ACE inhibitors are used to treat scleroderma renal crisis.

A multicenter randomized control trial involving the use of quinapril in SSc is currently underway.

SECOND LINE THERAPIES

■ Methotrexate	A
■ Cyclophosphamide	B
■ Prednisolone	B
■ Losartan	B
■ Acitretin	C
■ Colchicine	C
■ UVA	C

Comparison of methotrexate with placebo in the treatment of systemic sclerosis: a 24-week randomized double-blind trial, followed by a 24-week observational trial. Van den Hoogen FH, Boerbooms AM, Swaak AJ, et al. Br J Rheumatol 1996;35:364–72.

Twenty nine patients with SSc received 15–25 mg weekly injections of MTX or placebo, for a 24-week period in a randomized, double-blind trial. Improvement in skin severity score and hand grip was noted in the treated group.

However, a more recent randomized, controlled trial failed to reproduce these findings (see below).

A randomized, controlled trial of methotrexate versus placebo in early diffuse scleroderma. Pope JE, Bellamy N, Seibold JR, et al. Arthritis Rheum 2001;44:1351–8.

In this trial 35 patients received between 7.5 mg and 50 mg weekly doses of MTX vs 36 patients who received placebo, and no significant differences were found between each group. However there was a significant improvement on severity of skin involvement in the first few months in the arm treated with MTX.

The efficacy of oral cyclophosphamide plus prednisolone in early diffuse systemic sclerosis. Calguneri M, Apras S, Ozbalkan Z, et al. Clin Rheumatol 2003;22:289–94.

In this study 27 patients with early diffuse SSc were treated with oral cyclophosphamide (1–2 mg/kg daily) plus oral prednisolone (40 mg every other day) between the years 1995 and 1998. The results regarding the efficacy and toxicity of cyclophosphamide were compared with those of 22 patients with early SSc who had been treated with oral D-penicillamine between 1992 and 1995. There was a significant improvement on the skin score, maximal oral opening, flexion index, predicted forced vital capacity and

carbon monoxide diffusing capacity in the cyclophosphamide group. The decrease in skin score in the cyclophosphamide group started earlier than in the D-penicillamine group.

Treatment of early diffuse cutaneous systemic sclerosis patients in Japan by low-dose corticosteroids for skin involvement. Takehara K. Clin Exp Rheumatol 2004;22(3 suppl 33):S87–9.

Twenty three patients with early dcSSc were treated with low-dose 20 mg/kg of prednisolone, with significant reduction in skin scores.

The vitamin A derivative etretinate improves skin sclerosis in patients with systemic sclerosis. Ikeda T, Uede K, Hashizume H, Furukawa F. J Dermatol Sci 2004;34:62–6.

This small study of 31 patients showed that patients taking oral etretinate had significant improvements in skin thickness compared to patients not taking etretinate.

Losartan therapy for Raynaud's phenomenon and scleroderma: clinical and biochemical findings in a fifteen-week, randomized, parallel-group, controlled trial. Dziadzio M, Denton CP, Smith R, et al. Arthritis Rheum 1999;42:2646–55.

Losartan is an antagonist of angiotensin II receptor type I. In this randomized, controlled trial, 25 patients with primary RP and 27 patients with RP secondary to SSc were treated with either losartan (50 mg daily) or nifedipine (40 mg daily). Losartan reduced the frequency and severity of RP.

Long-term evaluation of colchicine in the treatment of scleroderma. Alarcon-Segovia D, Ramos-Niembro F, Ibanez de Kasep G, et al. J Rheumatol 1979;6:705–12.

In this early uncontrolled study, 19 patients with SSc of varying clinical types were treated with colchicine, 10.1 mg per week with a follow up of 19–57 months. They reported improvement in skin elasticity, mouth opening, finger mobility, and a reduction in dysphagia.

Different low doses of broad-band UVA in the treatment of morphea and systemic sclerosis. El-Mofty M, Mostafa W, El-Darouty M, et al. Photodermatol Photoimmunol Photomed 2004;20:148–56.

Fifteen patients with SS received 20 sessions of UVA (320–400 nm), and all patients improved clinically.

UVA is well tolerated. There is experimental evidence that UVA1 may be beneficial. Further trials are required to confirm efficacy.

THIRD LINE THERAPIES

■ Extracorporeal photochemotherapy	B
■ Cyclosporine	C
■ Thalidomide	D
■ Etanercept	D
■ Minocycline	F

Treatment of systemic sclerosis with extracorporeal photochemotherapy. Results of a multicenter trial. Rook AH, Freundlich B, Jegasothy BV, et al. Arch Dermatol 1992;128:337–46.

This multicenter trial showed a reduction in skin induration, but no effect on pulmonary function.

Additional studies were not able to corroborate the above data. Furthermore, extracorporeal photopheresis is not approved by the Food and Drug Administration (FDA) for the treatment of SSc.

Ciclosporin in systemic sclerosis. Clements PJ, Lachenbruch PA, Sterz M, et al. Arthritis Rheum 1993;36:75–83.

Cyclosporine is an immunosuppressive drug that selectively inhibits the release of interleukin (IL)-2, which has been shown to be increased in SSc serum. This study showed that cyclosporine may improve skin induration, but had no effect on internal organ involvement.

The high incidence of nephrotoxicity with cyclosporine therapy reduces its use in SSc where renal crisis and hypertension may occur.

Reduced fibrosis and normalisation of skin structure in scleroderma patients treated with thalidomide. (Abstract) Oliver SJ, Moreira A, Kaplan G. Arthritis Rheum 1999; 42(suppl):s187.

Open trial on ten patients, with improvement noted in skin repigmentation, and healing of digital ulcers.

Etanercept as treatment for diffuse scleroderma: a pilot study. (Abstract) Ellman MH, McDonald PA, Hayes FA. Arthritis Rheum 2000;43(suppl):s392.

This targeted fusion protein blocks tumor necrosis factor (TNF)-α. Four of ten patients treated with etanercept 25 mg subcutaneously, twice weekly had improvements of skin scores and healing of digital ulcers.

Minocycline in early diffuse scleroderma. Le CH, Morales A, Trentham DE. Lancet 1998;352:1755–6.

Eleven patients with early SSc were treated with minocycline (100 mg daily for 4 weeks; 200 mg daily for 11 months). Four patients showed complete resolution of skin involvement following 9 and 12 months of therapy.

A more recent study reported that minocycline is not an effective therapy for SSc (see below).

Minocycline is not effective in systemic sclerosis: results of an open-label multicenter trial. Mayes MD, O'Donnell D, Rothfield NF, Csuka ME. Arthritis Rheum 2004;50:553–7.

This open label trial recruited 36 patients, and no significant change in skin score was found.

OTHER THERAPIES – INTERNAL ORGAN INVOLVEMENT

Prostacyclin for pulmonary hypertension in adults. Paramothayan NS, Lasseron TJ, Wells AU, Walters EH. Cochrane Database Syst Rev 2002(4), CD002994.

This meta-analysis of seven randomized trials assessed the benefit of prostacyclin or one of its analogues in primary pulmonary hypertension or pulmonary hypertension secondary to connective tissue disease such as SSc. The authors concluded that prostacyclin can increase exercise capacity, New York Heart Association functional class, and symptoms in patients with primary or secondary pulmonary hypertension.

Bosentan therapy for pulmonary arterial hypertension. Rubin LJ, Badesch DB, Barst RJ, et al. N Engl J Med 2002;346:896–903.

In this randomized control trial of patients with pulmonary arterial hypertension, the dual endothelin receptor antagonist bosentan improved exercise capacity. SSc patients with pulmonary arterial hypertension were shown to have improved exercise capacity on subgroup analysis.

Cyclophosphamide is associated with pulmonary function and survival benefit in patients with scleroderma and alveolitis. White B, Moore WC, Wigley FM, et al. Ann Intern Med 2000;132:947–54.

This retrospective cohort study involving 103 patients with SSc showed that lung inflammation (alveolitis) treated with cyclophosphamide improves lung function outcome and survival.

Renal transplantation in scleroderma. Chang YJ, Spiera H. Medicine 1999;78:382–5.

Retrospective study from data collected by the United Network for Organ Sharing (UNOS) Scientific Renal Transplant Registry. From 1987 to 1997, 86 patients with SSc had renal transplantation. At 5-year follow-up, 47% of the patients were alive. Patients whose renal function does not improve with ACE inhibitors should be considered for renal transplantation.

Autologous stem cell transplantation in the treatment of systemic sclerosis: report from the EBMT/EULAR Registry. Farge D, Passweg J, van Laar JM, et al. Ann Rheum Dis 2004;63:974–81.

The use of stem cell transplantation to treat severe SSc is currently being studied. Prospective randomized controlled trials are awaited.

Omeprazole in the long-term treatment of severe gastro-oesophageal reflux disease in patients with systemic sclerosis. Hendel L. Aliment Pharmacol Ther 1992;6:565–77.

Twenty-five patients treated with omeprazole showed significant improvement of gastrointestinal symptoms.

Sebaceous gland hyperplasia

Agustin Martin-Clavijo, John Berth-Jones

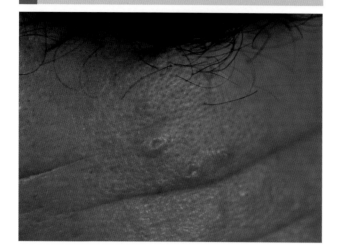

Sebaceous gland hyperplasia is a common benign condition. It affects adults of middle age and older and its incidence increases with age. It presents as single or multiple soft yellowish papules, often with central umbilication, mainly on the face (commonly nose, cheeks, and forehead), but it can present in other areas such as chest, areola, mouth, and genitalia. Its frequency is increased in immunocompromised patients, especially after transplantation in patients on cyclosporine and corticosteroids.

Alta prevalencia de hiperplasias sebaceas en transplantados renales. Perez-Espana L, Prats I, Sanz A, Mayor M, Nefrologia 2003;23:179–80.

The authors looked at 163 renal transplant patients; 25.9% had sebaceous hyperplasia. This was highest in patients on cyclosporine. However, there was no significant increase in the incidence of sebaceous gland hyperplasia with other immunosuppressants (azathioprine, mycophenolate mofetil, and tacrolimus).

MANAGEMENT STRATEGY

Sebaceous gland hyperplasia is a benign condition, with no potential for malignant transformation. Usually it is asymptomatic and therefore needs to be treated only for cosmetic reasons. *Cautery (electrodesiccation)* or *cryotherapy* are usually used as first line therapies. Other treatments include *surgical excision, laser, isotretinoin,* and *chemical peels.* It is important to stress to the patient the risk of scarring with many of these techniques.

SPECIFIC INVESTIGATIONS

No specific investigations are usually needed because this is a clinical diagnosis. The differential diagnosis includes rhinophyma, nevus sebaceus, basal cell carcinoma, dermal nevus, plane warts, molluscum, lupus milia disseminatus faciei, and syringoma. If the diagnosis is uncertain, a biopsy will show enlargement of individual glands with increase in the number of fully mature lobules with no atypia or dysplasia.

FIRST LINE THERAPIES

■ Conservative management/cosmetic camouflage	E
■ Electrodesiccation/cautery	C
■ Cryotherapy	E

Guidelines of care for cryosurgery. American Academy of Dermatology Committee on Guidelines of Care. J Am Acad Dermatol 1994;31:648–53.

The authors include sebaceous hyperplasia as a condition treatable with cryotherapy.

Surgical pearl: intralesional electrodesiccation of sebaceous hyperplasia. Bader RS, Scarborough DA. J Am Acad Dermatol 2000;42:127–8.

The authors describe the technique for intralesional electrodesiccation. They have used it on more than 30 patients with no recurrences after 7 months.

SECOND LINE THERAPIES

■ Isotretinoin	C
■ Diode laser	D
■ Pulsed dye laser	D
■ Argon laser	E
■ CO_2 laser	E
■ Erbium:YAG laser	E

Premature familial sebaceous hyperplasia: successful response to oral isotretinoin in three patients. Grimalt R, Ferrando J, Mascaro JM. J Am Acad Dermatol 1997;37:996–8.

Three closely related patients with premature familial sebaceous hyperplasia were treated with isotretinoin 1 mg/kg daily for 6 weeks. Response was maintained with isotretinoin 20 mg orally on alternate days in one case and isotretinoin gel 0.05%. Follow-up was 5 months.

Isotretinoin for the treatment of sebaceous hyperplasia. Grekin RC, Ellis CN. Cutis 1987;34:90–2.

Two patients were treated with isotretinoin. Both had a good response, but relapsed after the treatment was withdrawn, needing maintenance treatment. The first patient had 20 mg daily with a maintenance dose of 10 mg orally on alternate days. The second had 40 mg on alternate days with a maintenance dose of 40 mg twice a week.

Although the mucocutaneous side effects of short-term oral isotretinoin are manageable, the benefits of long-term isotretinoin therapy must be weighed against the potential for bony side effects and calcification of ligaments and tendons.

Sebaceous hyperplasia treated with a 1450-nm diode laser. No D, McLaren M, Chotzen V, Kilmer SL. Dermatol Surg 2004;30:382–4.

The authors treated ten patients. Both objective and subjective improvement were noted in the majority of the patients with very few side effects.

Elucidating the pulsed-dye laser treatment of sebaceous hyperplasia in vivo with real-time confocal scanning laser microscopy. Aghassi D, Gonzalez E, Anderson RR, et al. J Am Acad Dermatol 2000;43:49–53.

Evidence levels A Double-blind study **B** Clinical trial ≥ 20 subjects **C** Clinical trial < 20 subjects **D** Series ≥ 5 subjects **E** Anecdotal case reports

The authors treated 29 lesions on seven different patients with pulsed dye laser. There was improvement in 93% of lesions with complete clearance in 28%. No scarring or hyperpigmentation was noted. However, 28% of the lesions reappeared and 7% returned to the original size.

A three year experience with the argon laser in dermatotherapy. Landthaler M, Haina D, Waidelich W, Braun-Falco O. J Dermatol Surg Oncol 1984;10:456–61.

The authors report on 477 patients with different cutaneous lesions treated with argon laser, including sebaceous hyperplasia.

Sebaceous gland hyperplasia as a side effect of cyclosporin A. Treatment with the CO$_2$ laser. Walther T, Hohenleutner U, Landthaler M. Dtsch Med Wochenschr 1998;123:798–800.

This article reports the treatment of a patient with CO$_2$ laser. The lesions cleared without scarring.

[Controlled cosmetic dermal ablation in the facial region with the erbium:YAG laser.] (German) Riedel F, Bergler W, Baker-Schreyer A, et al. HNO 1999;47:101–6.

This article looks at 216 patients with different facial lesions. The authors report good-to-excellent results with sebaceous hyperplasia.

THIRD LINE THERAPIES

■ Photodynamic therapy	E
■ Topical aminolevulinic acid and pulsed dye laser	D
■ Bichloroacetic acid	C
■ Surgery/curettage	E

Photodynamic therapy of sebaceous hyperplasia with topical 5-aminolaevulinic acid and slide projector. Horio T, Horio O, Miyaichi-Hashimoto H, et al. Br J Dermatol 2003;148:1270–90.

The authors treated one patient with photodynamic therapy who had a good response and no scarring or hyperpigmentation at 12-month follow-up.

Photodynamic therapy with topical aminolevulinic acid and pulsed dye laser irradiation for sebaceous hyperplasia. Alster TS, Tanzi EL. J Drugs Dermatol 2003;2:501–4.

Ten patients were treated with topical aminolevulinic acid followed 1 h later with pulsed dye laser. They were compared with untreated lesions and laser-only treated lesions; 70% of lesions had total clearing after one treatment, the remaining 30% after two treatments.

The treatment of benign sebaceous hyperplasia with the topical application of bichloracetic acid. Rosian R, Goslen JB, Brodell RT. J Dermatol Surg Oncol 1991;17:876–9.

The authors treated 67 lesions on 20 patients; 66 cleared after one application of 100% bichloroacetic acid with minimal scarring.

Surgical removal

Occasionally, sebaceous hyperplasia is treated surgically. This has the advantage of providing tissue for histology when there is any doubt about the diagnosis.

Seborrheic eczema

Corinna Mendonca, Ian Coulson

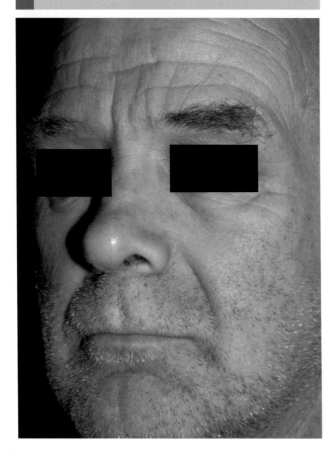

Seborrheic eczema is a chronic dermatitis affecting between 3 and 10% of adults. The signs and symptoms comprise erythema, greasy scaling, pruritus, burning, and dryness in a typical distribution pattern affecting the scalp, the face, particularly the nasolabial folds, eyebrows, ears, upper trunk, and flexures. Seborrheic eczema can also affect infants up to the age of 3–4 months in the napkin area (see page 166). It is more common in patients with Parkinson's disease, particularly those with neuroleptic-induced disease and is particularly severe and recalcitrant in HIV infection.

MANAGEMENT STRATEGY

Seborrheic eczema is a chronic relapsing dermatitis. It responds to a variety of immunosuppressive therapies, but there are no cures.

Seborrheic eczema of the face is dry and flaky so soap avoidance and substitution with a *light emollient cleanser* will help. Facial and flexural disease responds to *mild topical corticosteroids* alone or in combination with a variety of *topical antipityrosporal agents such as miconazole, clotrimazole, ketoconazole, itraconazole, ciclopiroxolamine,* or *sulfur*. An ointment containing *lithium gluconate/lithium succinate* may also be helpful. Recent studies have demonstrated short-term efficacy with the topical calcineurin inhibitors *tacrolimus* and *pimecrolimus*. Resistant cases may respond to short course of *oral itraconazole*. Scalp seborrheic dermatitis can be helped with *topical azoles, zinc pyrithione, selenium sulfide,* and *tar* shampoos, or a *propylene glycol* preparation formulated for scalp use. Severe cases with marked hyperkeratosis or pityriasis amiantacea may require topical keratolytics such as *salicylic acid ointment* or *coconut compound ointment*.

SPECIFIC INVESTIGATIONS

- Tests for HIV infection
- Zinc

Cutaneous findings in HIV-1 positive patients: a 42-month prospective study. Smith KJ, Skelton HG, Yeager J, et al. J Am Acad Dermatol 1994;31:746–54.

In this study of 912 HIV-positive patients, seborrheic dermatitis was the third commonest skin disorder diagnosed (53% of cases).

Seborrheic dermatitis in neuroleptic-induced parkinsonism. Binder RL, Jonelis FJ. Arch Dermatol 1983;119:473–5.

Comparison of 42 hospitalized patients with drug-induced parkinsonism with psychiatric patients as controls showed an incidence of seborrheic dermatitis of 59.5% in the patients with parkinsonism compared with 15% in the control group.

In neonates and children consider acrodermatitis enteropathica or transient neonatal zinc deficiency, which can mimic recalcitrant seborrheic dermatitis. A similar eruption in parenterally fed adults can occur due to zinc deficiency.

Non-scalp disease

FIRST LINE THERAPIES

■ Topical ketoconazole	A
■ Topical hydrocortisone	A

Double-blind treatment of seborrhoeic dermatitis with 2% ketoconazole cream. Skinner RB, Noah PW, Taylor RM, et al. J Am Acad Dermatol 1985;12:852–6.

This paper reports a controlled double-blind trial in 37 patients, reporting a 75–95% improvement, in 18 of 20 patients treated with the ketoconazole cream compared with a vehicle control for a 4-week treatment period.

Ketoconazole 2% cream versus hydrocortisone 1% cream in the treatment of seborrhoeic dermatitis. A double-blind comparative study. Stratigos JD, Antoniou C, Katsambas A, et al. J Am Acad Dermatol 1988;19:850–3.

In a double blind study 72 patients were treated daily for 4 weeks with either 2% ketoconazole cream or 1% hydrocortisone cream; 80.5% of the ketoconazole group compared to 94.4% of the hydrocortisone group showed significant improvement in all symptoms. There was no significant difference between the two treatment groups in relapse rates at 2 and 4 weeks following treatment.

SECOND LINE THERAPIES

■ Lithium succinate/lithium gluconate	A
■ Topical ciclopiroxolamine cream	A
■ Tacrolimus 0.1% ointment	C
■ Pimecrolimus ointment	B

Evidence levels **A** Double-blind study **B** Clinical trial ≥ 20 subjects **C** Clinical trial < 20 subjects **D** Series ≥ 5 subjects **E** Anecdotal case reports

A double-blind, placebo-controlled, multicenter trial of lithium succinate ointment in the treatment of seborrhoeic dermatitis. Multicenter trial group. The Efalith Multicenter Trial Group. J Am Acad Dermatol 1992;26:452–7.

A multicenter, placebo-controlled, double-blind study in 227 patients showed that lithium succinate ointment was significantly more effective than placebo in treating all symptoms of non-scalp seborrheic dermatitis.

Lithium gluconate 8% vs ketoconazole 2% in the treatment of seborrhoeic dermatitis: a multicentre, randomized study. Dreno B, Chosidow O, Revuz J, Moyse D. Br J Dermatol 2003;148:1230–6.

A randomized, non-inferiority study comparing 8% lithium gluconate and ketoconazole 2% in moderate to severe seborrheic dermatitis for 2 months – 269 patients were treated. Lithium was 22% more effective than ketoconazole in giving complete remission of seborrheic dermatitis.

Randomized, placebo-controlled, double-blind study on clinical efficacy of ciclopiroxolamine 1% cream in facial seborrhoeic dermatitis. Dupuy P, Maurette C, Amoric JC, Chosidow O. Br J Dermatol 2001;144:1033–7.

One hundred and twenty seven patients were randomized to receive either twice daily 1% ciclopiroxolamine cream for 28 days followed by once daily application for a further 28 days or placebo. At the end of the treatment, 63% (43 patients) responded in the ciclopiroxolamine group.

An open pilot study using tacrolimus ointment in the treatment of seborrheic dermatitis. Meshkinpour A, Sun J, Weinstein G. J Am Acad Dermatol 2003;49:145–7.

In this study, 18 patients used 0.1% tacrolimus twice a day for 28 days or until complete clearance was achieved – 61% showed 100% clearance of their seborrheic dermatitis and 39% showed 70–90% clearance.

Pimecrolimus cream 1% vs. betamethasone 17-valerate 0.1% cream in the treatment of seborrheic dermatitis. A randomized open-label clinical trial. Rigopoulos D, Ioannides D, Kalogeromitros D, et al. Br J Dermatol 2004;151:1071–5.

Twenty patients with seborrheic dermatitis were included in this study, 11 patients in the pimecrolimus 1% cream group and nine patients in the betamethasone 17-valerate 0.1% cream group. Similar efficacy was seen in both groups, but pruritus returned more slowly on treatment discontinuation in the pimecrolimus group.

The authors point out that betamethasone is potent and not to be recommended for long-term facial use.

THIRD LINE THERAPIES

■ Oral itraconazole	B
■ Phototherapy	E
■ Benzoyl peroxide	C
■ Oral terbinafine	B

Itraconazole in the treatment of seborrhoeic dermatitis: a new treatment modality. Baysal V, Yildirim M, Ozcanli C, Ceyhan M. Int J Dermatol 2004;43:63–6.

Twenty eight patients took 200 mg daily itraconazole for 1 month followed by 200 mg daily for 2 days of the following 11 months. Nineteen patients showed complete improvement (more than 71% clear), six showed moderate improvement and three slight improvement.

Narrow-band ultraviolet B (TL-01) phototherapy is an effective and safe treatment option for patients with severe seborrhoeic dermatitis. Pirkhammer D, Seeber A, Honigsmann H, Tanew A. Br J Dermatol 2000;143:964–8.

In this study 18 patients were treated three times weekly until complete clearing or to a maximum of 8 weeks. Six showed complete clearance and 12 marked improvement.

Benzoyl peroxide in seborrheic dermatitis. Bonnetblanc JM, Bernard P. Arch Dermatol 1986;122:752.

Twenty eight of 30 patients showed improvement with 1 week of use of 2.5% benzoyl peroxide preparation. Patients relapsed within 2–12 weeks of stopping treatment.

Evaluation of the efficacy and tolerability of oral terbinafine in patients with seborrhoeic dermatitis. A multicentre, randomized, investigator-blinded, placebo-controlled trial. Scaparro E, Quadri G, Virno G, et al. Br J Dermatol 2001;144:854–7.

Sixty patients with moderate to severe seborrheic dermatitis were treated with terbinafine 250 mg daily for 4 weeks or a moisturizing cream twice daily. Terbinafine statistically reduced severity scores compared to baseline and placebo.

For the scalp

FIRST LINE THERAPIES

■ Ketoconazole shampoo	A
■ Ciclopirox shampoo	A
■ Zinc pyrithione shampoo	B

Successful treatment and prophylaxis of scalp seborrhoeic dermatitis and dandruff with 2% ketoconazole shampoo: results of a multicentre, double-blind, placebo-controlled trial. Peter RU, Richarz-Barthauer U. Br J Dermatol 1995;132:441–5.

Five hundred and seventy-five patients with moderate to severe scalp seborrheic dermatitis and dandruff were treated with 2% ketoconazole shampoo twice weekly for 2 months, producing clearance in 88%. Responders were then randomized to active treatment or placebo once weekly. There were fewer relapses in the ketoconazole prophylactic treatment group after 6 months.

Safety and efficacy of ciclopirox 1% shampoo for the treatment of seborrheic dermatitis of the scalp in the US population: results of a double-blind, vehicle-controlled trial. Lebwohl M, Plott T. Int J Dermatol 2004;43(suppl 1):17–20.

Ciclopirox was found to be significantly better than vehicle in effectively treating scalp seborrheic dermatitis when 499 patients with seborrheic dermatitis of the scalp were randomized to apply either ciclopirox shampoo 1% or vehicle twice weekly for 4 weeks.

The effects of a shampoo containing zinc pyrithione on the control of dandruff. Marks R, Pearse AD, Walker AP. Br J Dermatol 1985;112:415–22.

Thirty two patients with dandruff were treated with a shampoo containing 1% zinc pyrithione to half the scalp, the other half being washed in a shampoo with base alone. Each scalp was washed one, three, six, or nine times. The actively treated group showed a progressive reduction in dandruff on the actively treated side. The difference was statistically significant after three, six, and nine washes.

SECOND LINE THERAPIES

■ Propylene glycol lotion	A
■ Miconazole	C
■ Selenium sulfide	C

Propylene glycol in the treatment of seborrhoeic dermatitis of the scalp: a double-blind study. Faergemann J. Cutis 1988;42:69–71.

Thirty nine patients with scalp seborrheic dermatitis were treated in a double-blind controlled study with 15% propylene glycol in a base of 50% ethanol and 35% water or vehicle alone – 89% in the group treated with propylene glycol showed healing compared to 32% in the control group.

A randomized, double-blind, placebo-controlled trial of ketoconazole 2% shampoo versus selenium sulfide 2.5% shampoo in the treatment of moderate to severe dandruff. Danby FW, Maddin WS, Margeson LJ, Rosenthal D. J Am Acad Derm 1993;29:1008–12.

A total of 236 patients were included in the study. Both medicated shampoos were statistically better than placebo in treating scaling and itching. However, ketoconazole was superior to selenium shampoo.

Seborrhoeic dermatitis and *Pityrosporum orbiculare*: treatment of seborrhoeic dermatitis of the scalp with miconazole-hydrocortisone (Daktacort), miconazole and hydrocortisone. Faergemann J. Br J Dermatol 1986;114: 695–700.

Sixty seven patients were treated twice daily for 6 weeks and those cured received prophylactic treatment twice monthly for 3 months. Nineteen of 21 patients were cured in the Daktacort group, 15 of 22 in the miconazole group, and 17 of 24 in the hydrocortisone group. Daktacort and miconazole were significantly better than hydrocortisone as prophylaxis.

Evidence levels **A** Double-blind study **B** Clinical trial ≥ 20 subjects **C** Clinical trial < 20 subjects **D** Series ≥ 5 subjects **E** Anecdotal case reports

Seborrheic keratosis

Richard J Motley

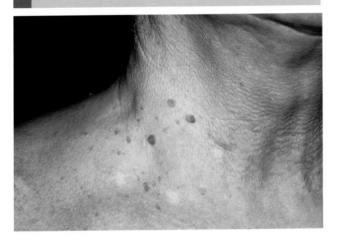

Seborrheic keratosis is a benign, exophytic, warty, lightly pigmented growth of the skin surface that becomes increasingly common with age. Mainly found on the trunk, often at sites of pressure, it is a cosmetic nuisance and rarely a cause for diagnostic confusion. Several variants exist and are described below.

MANAGEMENT STRATEGY

Many patients present with seborrheic keratoses because of concern about possible melanoma and reassurance may be all that is required. Occasionally the lesion can become 'irritated' and show erythema, crusting, and itching. In this case the appearance may resemble a pyogenic granuloma or squamous cell carcinoma.

Where treatment is requested there are several options and the choice will depend on patient and physician preference. *Surgical excision*, although effective, is never the treatment of choice and usually indicates that the surgeon failed to make the correct clinical diagnosis or is unfamiliar with alternative treatments. When the diagnosis is in doubt then material should be taken for histologic examination, preferably by a *'shave'* or *tangential biopsy* technique or by *sharp curettage*. Blunt curettage provides poor material for histologic assessment. *Cautery* is very effective at softening the lesion and often allows it to be removed with minimal effort, the heat separating the lesion at the dermal–epidermal junction. The 'melting' of the lesion observed after the application of heat is almost diagnostic. Smaller lesions can be 'flicked off' the skin using a traditional curette, often without local anesthesia. Heat can be applied to the surface of the lesion followed by curettage and, for superficial lesions, 'curettage' can be achieved using a cotton gauze swab to wipe away the softened lesion. Cautery can also be used after shave excision to treat any tissue remnants. With all these treatments the aim is to remove the lesion, but little of the underlying skin surface.

Cryotherapy using a liquid nitrogen spray is an alternative method of treatment. Liquid nitrogen is sprayed onto the lesion until frozen and then continued for 5–10 s. It can be undertaken without local anesthesia because freezing reduces sensations of pain and this can be an advantage when treating multiple lesions. After a day or two the treated lesion blisters and crumbles away. The underlying wound heals over after several days and is often quite exudative, requiring daily cleansing by the patient. Overall the recovery period is longer and the wound slower to heal than following curettage and cautery. Whereas following cautery hyperpigmentation is common, following cryotherapy, hypopigmentation occurs. For this reason it is not recommended in black people.

Seborrheic keratosis variants

Senile or 'solar' lentigines can be considered to be flat versions of the seborrheic keratosis. Sometimes referred to as 'age' or 'liver' spots, these small pigmented papules and plaques are more commonly seen on areas of frequent sun exposure such as the face and dorsa of the hands. Their true nature can be recognized by the slight velvety texture to the lesional surface, which is best seen with tangential lighting. This indicates that the lesion is not a true lentigo, but a superficial keratosis. These lesions are amenable to very minor treatments. Topical *tretinoin* cream can be effective. Other treatments include light abrasion with an *exfoliating cream, light dermabrasion* or *laser resurfacing, cryotherapy,* or *chemical peels* using trichloracetic acid or phenol. A favorite treatment is minimal cautery followed by 'curettage' with a cotton gauze swab. This leaves an erythematous superficial wound that heals rapidly.

Dermatosis papulosa nigra is commonly seen on the cheeks of black adults. These small seborrheic warts are easily treated by light cautery or diathermy, followed by cotton gauze curettage, but patients should be warned about the possibility of hyperpigmentation.

Stucco keratoses are small grayish-white seborrheic keratoses, which are typically found on the forearms and lower legs and are easily removed with curettage without bleeding. The edge of these lesions is often curled up away from the skin surface.

Giant seborrheic keratoses are large lesions, usually found on the scalp, and are often several centimeters in diameter.

Multiple seborrheic keratoses

Seborrheic keratoses may have a familial tendency, especially in patients with multiple lesions. It is these patients who are often the most challenging to treat – and also the most affected by their condition. Many middle-aged to elderly patients will not undress for sporting activities such as swimming because they are embarrassed by the appearance of their skin. Patients not infrequently present with multiple lesions and requesting their complete removal. In these circumstances it is reasonable to offer several different types of treatment so that the patient can determine their preference.

The sudden onset of multiple seborrheic keratoses may be associated with underlying malignancy – the sign of Leser-Trelat – and should prompt a full clinical examination for underlying malignancy.

SPECIFIC INVESTIGATIONS

> ■ Consider the sign of Leser-Trelat and investigate for underlying malignancy

Sign of Leser-Trelat. Schwartz RA. J Am Acad Dermatol 1996;35:88–95.

The sign of Leser-Trelat is rare. The sudden eruption of multiple seborrheic keratoses or their rapid increase in size is caused by a malignancy. Its association with malignant acanthosis nigricans, seen in 35% of patients, is one of several of its features that support its legitimacy as a true paraneoplastic disorder.

FIRST LINE THERAPIES

■ Reassurance	E
■ Curettage and cautery	B
■ Cryotherapy	B

Curettage of small basal cell papillomas with the disposable ring curette is superior to conventional treatment. Long CC, Motley RJ, Holt PJ. Br J Dermatol 1994;131:732–3.

Ring curettage followed by aluminum chloride 25% in 70% isopropyl alcohol gave a superior cosmetic result compared to using a traditional curette and light cautery.

Skin tumours: seborrhoeic warts. Motley R. Dermatol Pract 1997;5:6–7.

A practical review of treatment options.

Cutaneous cryotherapy: principles and practice. Dawber R, Colver G, Jackson A, eds. London: Martin Dunitz; 1997.

A well-illustrated practical guide to all that is cutaneous cryosurgery, including seborrheic warts!

SECOND LINE THERAPY

■ Chemical peels for smaller, superficial lesions and dermatosis papulosa nigrans	C
■ Lasers (pulsed CO$_2$, erbium:YAG)	C

Focal trichloroacetic acid peel method for benign pigmented lesions in dark-skinned patients. Chun EY, Lee JB, Lee KH. Dermatol Surg 2004;30;512–6.

After cleansing the skin with alcohol, 65% trichloroacetic acid was focally applied to seborrheic keratoses, using a sharpened wooden applicator, to create evenly frosted spots on each lesion. Crusts separated from the skin with gentle washing after 4–7 days and healing was completed 10–14 days later. Twenty three patients required a mean of 1.5 treatments and in 57% of these the results were rated as excellent.

Use of the Alexandrite laser for treatment of seborrhoeic keratoses. Mehrabi D, Brodell RT. Dermatol Surg 2002; 28:437–9.

A patient with multiple seborrheic keratoses was treated in four sessions with a normal-mode Alexandrite laser (755 nm wavelength) spot size 8 mm, fluence 100 J/cm^2. The entire surface of each lesion was treated in a checkerboard fashion. Twelve-day follow-up revealed excellent cosmetic resolution of the lesions with minimal scarring and hypopigmentation, especially when compared to areas previously treated with liquid nitrogen cryotherapy.

Treatment of verruca vulgaris, seborrheic keratoses, lentigines, and actinic cheilitis. Clinical advantage of the CO$_2$ laser superpulsed mode. Fitzpatrick RE, Goldman MP, Ruiz-Esparza J. J Dermatol Surg Oncol 1994;20;449–56.

Continuous and superpulsed CO$_2$ lasers were compared in their effect on a variety of lesions including seborrheic keratoses. Ideal parameters prevent unwanted thermal damage.

Ablation of cutaneous lesions using an erbium:YAG laser. Khatri KA. J Cosmet Laser Ther 2003;5;150–3.

Erbium:YAG laser was used to remove multiple benign skin lesions and found to safe and effective for this purpose.

THIRD LINE THERAPIES

■ 5-Fluorouracil	E

Giant seborrhoeic keratosis on the frontal scalp treated with topical fluorouracil. Tsuji T, Morita A. J Dermatol 1995;22:74–5.

An unusual giant scalp seborrheic keratosis was successfully treated with topical fluorouracil.

Evidence levels **A** Double-blind study **B** Clinical trial ≥ 20 subjects **C** Clinical trial < 20 subjects **D** Series ≥ 5 subjects **E** Anecdotal case reports

Spitz nevus

Ronald P Rapini

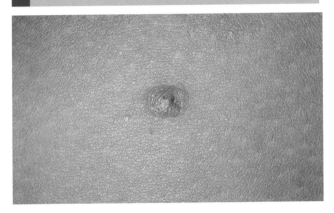

Spitz nevus is a benign 'mole' of children and young adults that can be difficult to distinguish histologically from malignant melanoma (see page 387). Because melanoma can metastasize and kill the patient, the treatment of Spitz nevus depends upon the relative certainty of the diagnosis.

MANAGEMENT STRATEGY

Spitz nevi are benign, and *no treatment is needed if the clinician and pathologist are both certain of the diagnosis*. Unfortunately, this 'certainty' can be elusive in up to 10% of cases. Some expert dermatologists, especially pediatric dermatologists, may feel confident enough to monitor a classic Spitz nevus without a biopsy or any other treatment, but it is usually wise to perform a biopsy or excision for histologic confirmation. Spitz nevus can resemble juvenile xanthogranuloma, mastocytoma, pyogenic granuloma, hemangioma, and other lesions, besides the very rare childhood melanoma.

Most Spitz nevi are less than 10 mm in diameter; it is therefore usually best to *excise the entire lesion with margins of 2 mm* and suture. The smallest lesions can often be quickly removed by the use of a *punch biopsy* instrument. Punch biopsy of just a portion of a lesion is not recommended because the overall architecture of the entire lesion is then not apparent to the pathologist. Because many children are moving targets unless sedated, some clinicians prefer a *quick shave biopsy*. This has the disadvantage of providing the pathologist with a smaller, more superficial specimen, and Spitz nevi are prone to recur when incompletely excised. Regrowth of the lesion may cause more concern, and then a second procedure may have to be performed. Biopsies may be easier to obtain after sedation, or with topical anesthetics such as EMLA (Eutectic Mixture of Local Anesthetics).

SPECIFIC INVESTIGATIONS

- ■ Skin biopsy and evaluation of specimen by dermatopathologist

Clinical review of 247 case records of Spitz nevus. Dal Pozzo V, Benelli C, Restano L, et al. Dermatology 1997;194: 20–5.

Spitz nevi are pigmented in 72% of cases, and they may be exceptionally black like a melanoma. They are usually asymptomatic smooth papules or nodules. Textbooks often emphasize that some Spitz nevi are red and amelanotic, but erythematous lesions account for only a fourth of cases, and these are more common on the head or neck.

Although these authors found the lower extremities to be the most common site, other reviews have found Spitz nevi of the head or neck to be more common. The trunk is also a common site, so overall they may be found almost anywhere on the body. Most patients are Caucasians.

Spitz nevus or melanoma? Rapini RP. Semin Cutan Med Surg 1999;18:56–63.

This review article discusses the clinical and histologic criteria for Spitz nevus as compared with melanoma. The biopsy is best reviewed by an expert dermatopathologist because the literature is replete with documentation of the difficulty in excluding a melanoma. Because Spitz nevus is most common in children and young adults, a diagnosis of Spitz nevus should be viewed very suspiciously in middle-aged or older adults. The diagnosis of melanoma should be viewed suspiciously in children. About 73% of Spitz nevi are less than 6 mm in diameter, whereas most melanomas are greater than 6 mm. Ulceration is uncommon in Spitz nevi, unlike melanoma. No single histologic criterion is 100% reliable, so a variety of features must be considered together. Compared with melanomas, Spitz nevi are more likely to have 1. sharp demarcation, 2. symmetry, 3. maturation of smaller, less atypical melanocytes in the deeper portion, 4. epithelial hyperplasia that often clutches melanocytic nests, 5. clefts around the junctional nests, 6. a predominance of spindle or epithelioid melanocytes, with uniform nest size and shape, less tendency to be confluent in the dermis, and 7. Kamino bodies. Mitoses, inflammation, and pagetoid cells can be seen in both Spitz nevus and melanoma. A more detailed discussion of histologic minutiae is beyond the scope of this book.

'Atypical' Spitz's nevus, 'malignant' Spitz's nevus, and 'metastasizing' Spitz's nevus: a critique in historical perspective of three concepts flawed fatally. Mones JM, Ackerman AB. Am J Dermatopathol 2004;26:310–33.

Some authorities have used the term 'atypical Spitz tumor' to describe cases where the distinction from melanoma was uncertain. 'Malignant Spitz nevus' is a controversial diagnosis that was used by one set of authors to describe cases of 'Spitz nevi' that metastasized to regional lymph nodes, but did not spread further, and the patients did well (perhaps these were really childhood melanomas that had a better than average outcome).

'Safe' Spitz and its alternatives. LeBoit PE. Pediatr Dermatol 2002;19:163–5.

Lesions with larger diameters, ulceration, abnormal mitoses, necrosis, and other worrisome features ought to be excised with clear surgical margins.

Other sophisticated investigations have been used to help to distinguish Spitz nevi from melanomas, but their use is controversial and sometimes not readily available. Spitz nevi are more likely to have MIB-1 (Ki-67) positive staining in less than 2% of the cells, whereas more than 10% of the cells are positive in melanoma. HMB-45 staining tends to be positive diffusely in many melanomas, but mainly stains the superficial portion rather than the deep dermal portion of Spitz nevi (so-called 'stratification of staining'), which is also seen with MIB-1. Comparative genomic hybridization (CGH) may show a gain or loss of chromosome 9 or 9p in melanoma, but may show a gain of chromosome 11p in Spitz nevus. BRAF mutations may occur in melanoma, but generally not in Spitz nevi.

FIRST LINE THERAPIES

■ Complete excision to adipose with closure by sutures	B

The surgical management of Spitz nevi. Murphy ME, Boyer JD, Stashower ME, Zitelli JA. Dermatol Surg 2002;28: 1065–9.

Management of Spitz nevi: a survey of dermatologists in the United States. Gelbard SN, Tripp JM, Marghoob AA, et al. J Am Acad Dermatol 2002;47:224–30.

Most authorities recommend complete excision with conservative margins (2–5 mm margins) for the average Spitz nevus. Wider margins may be needed for equivocal cases, but seldom is wide excision with margins of 10–20 mm needed except in those cases in which the possibility of melanoma is a real concern.

SECOND LINE THERAPIES

■ Biopsy with no further treatment	C
■ No treatment with no biopsy	C
■ Electrodesiccation	D
■ Sentinel lymph node biopsy for equivocal cases	D
■ Cryotherapy	E
■ Laser ablation	E

Spindle and epithelioid cell nevus (Spitz nevus). Natural history following biopsy. Kaye VN, Dehner LP. Arch Dermatol 1990;126:1581–3.

Only 39% of 49 Spitz nevi in this study were initially completely excised. Six were re-excised, and no evidence of residual nevus was found in five of those six cases. None of the 49 patients had a recurrence during an average follow-up period of 5 years. Clinical follow-up alone is recommended after a subtotal excision when the pathologic diagnosis is unequivocal.

The literature does not clearly document the natural history of untreated Spitz nevi. They may have rapid growth for the first 3–12 months, and then they often remain static. It is uncertain whether they generally eventually regress or persist. The rate of spontaneous resolution is not documented. At least some incompletely excised Spitz nevi will recur (average 7–16% in the literature) within an average time of 1 year.

Sentinel lymph node biopsy in patients with diagnostically controversial spitzoid melanocytic tumors. Lohmann CM, Coit DG, Brady MS, et al. Am J Surg Pathol 2002;26:47–55.
Sentinel lymph node biopsy for patients with problematic spitzoid melanocytic lesions: a report on 18 patients. Su LD, Fullen DR, Sondak VK, et al. Cancer 2003;97:499–507.

In both these studies, sentinel lymph nodes were used to evaluate problematic spitzoid lesions. Some patients with positive regional nodes had regional lymphadenectomy. All patients in these two studies, even those with positive nodes, remained alive and well.

What do these cells prove? LeBoit PE. Am J Dermatopathol 2003;25:355–6.

Even though some reports tell us of cases in which diagnostic uncertainty was settled by means of a sentinel node biopsy, the presence of small clusters of melanocytes within nodes do not prove malignancy. Small nests of melanocytes can be found within nodes draining ordinary benign nevi and apparently benign Spitz nevi.

Evidence levels **A** Double-blind study **B** Clinical trial ≥ 20 subjects **C** Clinical trial < 20 subjects **D** Series ≥ 5 subjects **E** Anecdotal case reports

Sporotrichosis

Wanda Sonia Robles

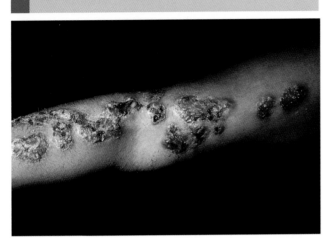

Sporotrichosis is a chronic infection usually limited to the skin and subcutaneous tissues, although occasionally it may become widely disseminated. The causative organism is a dimorphic fungal pathogen known as *Sporothrix schenckii*, which infects humans and animals. The lesions develop following inoculation or traumatic implantation of *S. schenckii*. The initial lesion appears at the site of a skin injury as an erythematous, ulcerated, or verrucous nodule, commonly followed by nodular lymphangitic spread. Localized skin lesions without lymphangitis, fixed-type sporotrichosis, also occur. Primary systemic involvement may occur following inhalation and, rarely, can follow cutaneous inoculation with subsequent hematogenous dissemination.

MANAGEMENT STRATEGY

While cases of sporotrichosis have been described as having spontaneous remissions, it is common practice to give patients some form of treatment. Historically, uncomplicated lymphangitic and fixed forms of sporotrichosis have been treated with *oral potassium iodide* in high doses and it is advisable to continue this treatment for 3–4 weeks after clinical cure. This is known to be a cheap and effective form of treatment but with well-recognized gastrointestinal side effects. In some cases, the application of *topical heat* has also been effective. If either of these forms of treatment fails, or if the patient is seriously ill, one may consider systemic chemotherapy with one of the antifungal drugs. *Itraconazole* in doses of 100–200 mg daily is known to be effective. *Terbinafine* has also been successfully used in the treatment of cutaneous sporotrichosis. Intravenous *amphotericin B* or *miconazole* may be used in complicated cases of sporotrichosis, including those with involvement of one or more joints, or in those with disseminated disease. These may also be used in patients who have failed to respond to treatment with itraconazole or terbinafine.

Recently, a case of disseminated sporotrichosis associated with treatment with tumor necrosis factor-α antagonists has been reported. This certainly illustrates the potential for infectious disease in patients on these forms of treatment.

SPECIFIC INVESTIGATIONS

- Culture
- Histology
- Serology for HIV infection (where relevant)

Direct microscopy of infected material is usually a futile exercise in view of the scarcity of the infective organisms in tissue. Culture is usually very rewarding and this is considered the most sensitive means of diagnosis. Infected material, which consists of pus or biopsy tissue from a lesion, is inoculated onto fungal culture media. The colonies are initially white or creamy with a wrinkled surface, and, as the colony ages, they become progressively darker until they are dark brown or black. To confirm the identification, it is important to convert the dimorphic fungus to the yeast phase, which is best achieved on brain–heart infusion agar and incubated at 37°C. The yeasts are either oval or cigar shaped.

Histologic examination of biopsies from patients reveals an area of central necrosis with an inflammatory infiltrate that consists of neutrophils, mixed granulomatous reaction with macrophages, and giant cells. The fungus is usually evident in the form of a small, cigar-shaped or oval yeast. Fungi may be surrounded by structures known as asteroid bodies, which consist of a yeast surrounded by a thick radiating eosinophilic material.

Successful treatment of AIDS-related disseminated cutaneous sporotrichosis with itraconazole. Bonifaz A, Peniche A, Mercadillo P, Saul A. AIDS Patient Care STDS 2001;15:603–6.

Case report of a 28-year-old male patient who developed disseminated cutaneous sporotrichosis and was successfully treated with itraconazole 300 mg daily.

Disseminated *Sporothrix schenckii* infection with arthritis in a patient with acquired immunodeficiency syndrome. Lipstein-Kresch E, Isenberg HD, Singer C, et al. J Rheumatol 1985;12:805–8.

A patient with a previous history of drug abuse is reported as the first case of sporotrichosis in AIDS. It presented as a disseminated infection with skin lesions and arthritis.

Disseminated sporotrichosis in a patient with HIV infection after treatment for acquired factor VIII inhibitor. Bibler MR, Luber HJ, Glueck HI, Estes SA. J Am Med Assoc 1986;256:3125–6.

Case report of a 71-year-old female patient with HIV infection due to transfusion therapy for an acquired factor VIII inhibitor who developed sporotrichosis 3 years later.

Acquired immunodeficiency syndrome presenting as disseminated cutaneous sporotrichosis. Fitzpatrick JE, Eubanks S. Int J Dermatol 1988;27:406–7.

Report of a 43-year-old homosexual patient in whom sporotrichosis was a presenting clinical feature of AIDS. The condition responded partially to treatment with amphotericin B.

Sporotrichosis in the acquired immunodeficiency syndrome. Shaw JC, Levinson W, Montanaro A. J Am Acad Dermatol 1989;21:1145–7.

A case report of a homosexual male with antibodies to HIV who presented with Kaposi's sarcoma and disseminated sporotrichosis of the skin and joints simultaneously. The patient failed to respond to treatment with amphotericin B alone and in combination with ketoconazole, followed by a trial of flucytosine.

Sporotrichosis may be a presenting opportunistic infection in patients with HIV infection or AIDS, in whom it tends to be disseminated at the time of diagnosis.

FIRST LINE THERAPIES

■ Potassium iodide	D
■ Itraconazole	C
■ Terbinafine	B

Practice guidelines for the management of patients with sporotrichosis. For the Mycoses Study Group, Infectious Diseases Society of America. Kauffman CA, Hajjeh R, Chapman SW. Clin Infect Dis 2000;30:684–7.

Derived from multicenter, nonrandomized clinical trials, small retrospective studies, and case reports. There are no randomized comparative studies reported to date. For fixed cutaneous or lymphocutaneous sporotrichosis: itraconazole for 36 months. For osteoarticular sporotrichosis: itraconazole for 48 months. For pulmonary disease that responds poorly to treatment: amphotericin B. Mild to moderate infection can be treated with itraconazole. For meningeal and disseminated disease (rare): amphotericin B. For AIDS patients with disseminated infection: amphotericin B followed by life-long treatment with itraconazole.

Potassium iodide remains the most effective therapy for cutaneous sporotrichosis. Sandhu K, Gupta S. J Dermatolog Treat 2003;14:200–2.

Case report of a patient with cutaneous sporotrichosis who failed to respond to treatment with itraconazole and went on to be successfully treated with potassium iodide.

Treatment of the superficial and subcutaneous mycoses. Roberts SOB. In: Speller DCE, ed. Antifungal Chemotherapy. Chichester: John Wiley; 1980:225–83.

Potassium iodide is recommended, with a schedule of five drops initially, increasing to 4–6 mL of saturated potassium iodide, three times daily. A lower maximum dose may be required for patients with poor tolerance to this medication.

Sporotrichosis: case report and successful treatment with itraconazole. Tay YK, Goh CL, Ong BH. Cutis 1997;60:87–90.

Report of a 51-year-old male patient who presented with a 6-month history of lymphocutaneous sporotrichosis on the right arm. Treatment was carried out with itraconazole 100 mg daily, with complete remission of the lesions after 5 months of treatment.

Verrucous sporotrichosis in an infant treated with itraconazole. Qwon KS, Yim CS, Jang HS, et al. J Am Acad Dermatol 1998;38:112–4.

Report of a 16-month-old Korean girl who developed a verrucous plaque on the dorsum of the left hand. She was successfully treated with itraconazole 3 mg/kg daily for 14 weeks. No recurrence was observed after 15 months of therapy.

Itraconazole therapy in lymphocutaneous sporotrichosis: a case report and review of the literature. Karakayali G, Lenk N, Alli N, et al. Cutis 1998;61:106–7.

This describes a 24-year-old male with 6-month history of asymptomatic nodules on the right hand. Improvement of the lesions was recorded after 2 months of treatment with itraconazole.

Case report. Sporotrichosis successfully treated with itraconazole in Japan. Noguchi H, Hiruma M, Kawada A. Mycoses 1999;42:571–6.

This describes a 65-year-old female patient with lymphocutaneous sporotrichosis that had developed from the dorsum of the nose to the left buccal area. The patient was treated with itraconazole 100 mg daily, with clearance of the lesion after 10 weeks. Treatment was continued for a total of 16 weeks. Fourteen months after completion of treatment, there was no evidence of recurrence. According to this report, the response to itraconazole in a series of 43 cases has been an 88% success rate. The mean dose of itraconazole used was 100 mg daily and the mean duration of treatment was 11 weeks.

This is a good review.

Disseminated cutaneous sporotrichosis treated with itraconazole. Stalkup JR, Bell K, Rosen T. Cutis 2002;69:371–4.

A 72-year-old male patient with diabetes who was receiving immunosuppressive treatment with prednisone and methotrexate was diagnosed with disseminated cutaneous sporotrichosis. Use of prednisone was discontinued, the dose of methotrexate was decreased, and treatment with oral itraconazole 400 mg daily was instituted. The patient's lesions cleared within 5 months, and no recurrence was noted during a 3-month follow-up.

Comparative evaluation of the efficacy and safety of two doses of terbinafine (500 and 1000 mg day⁻¹) in the treatment of cutaneous or lymphocutaneous sporotrichosis. Chapman SW, Pappas P, Kauffmann C, et al. Mycoses 2004;47:62–8.

This was a multicenter, randomized, controlled trial to evaluate the safety and efficacy of oral terbinafine (500 and 1000 mg daily) in the treatment of cutaneous or lymphocutaneous sporotrichosis. Sixty-three patients were involved in the study. The cure rate was significantly higher in patients treated with terbinafine 1000 mg daily than in those treated with only 500 mg daily (87% vs 52%). Tolerance to the drug was very good in both treatment groups.

SECOND LINE THERAPIES

■ Fluconazole	B

Treatment of lymphocutaneous and visceral sporotrichosis with fluconazole. Kauffman CA, Pappas PG, McKinsey DS, et al. Clin Infect Dis 1996;22:46–50.

This is a clinical trial involving 30 patients with sporotrichosis who were treated with fluconazole 200–800 mg daily. Of these, 14 patients had lymphocutaneous infection and 16 had osteoarticular or visceral sporotrichosis. Eleven of the 30 patients had previously been treated with other forms of

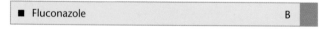

Evidence levels **A** Double-blind study **B** Clinical trial ≥ 20 subjects **C** Clinical trial < 20 subjects **D** Series ≥ 5 subjects **E** Anecdotal case reports

antifungal therapy without success. Most patients were treated with fluconazole 400 mg daily. Four patients received fluconazole 200 mg daily and another four received 800 mg daily. This form of treatment is reported to have cured 10 (71%) of 14 patients with lymphocutaneous sporotrichosis. However, only five (31%) of the 16 patients with osteoarticular or visceral sporotrichosis responded to treatment. The conclusion is that fluconazole is only modestly effective for treatment of sporotrichosis and should be considered second line therapy in patients who are unable to take itraconazole.

Case report. An unusual case of cutaneous sporotrichosis and its response to weekly fluconazole. Ghodsi SZ, Shams S, Naraghi Z, et al. Mycoses 2000;43:75–7.

Case report of a patient with both lymphocutaneous and fixed clinical forms of sporotrichosis treated with fluconazole 150 mg weekly. The fixed lesions responded well, healing after 4 months. However, the lymphocutaneous lesions did not resolve even after 6 months of treatment.

Sporotrichosis. Morris-Jones R. Clin Exp Dermatol 2002;27: 427–31.

A good review article about this infection. It highlights the importance of potassium iodide as the treatment of choice in endemic areas, as it is an effective and inexpensive therapy, but also stresses the effectiveness of itraconazole treatment.

THIRD LINE THERAPIES

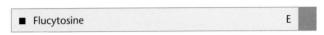

■ Flucytosine	E

Disseminated sporotrichosis of the skin and bone cured with 5-fluorocytosine: photosensitivity as a complication. Shelley WB, Sica PA Jr. J Am Acad Dermatol 1983;8:229–35.

Report of a disseminated form of cutaneous and osteoarticular sporotrichosis in a patient who failed to respond to treatment with potassium iodide for a period of 6 months. Following failure of iodide therapy, the patient showed some improvement after a 2-month course of intravenous amphotericin B. However, relapse was experienced 12 days after the amphotericin B was stopped. Cure was only achieved after 6 months of treatment with flucytosine (8 g daily) in combination with amphotericin B (total dose, 4.8 g). Photosensitivity is reported as a rare complication of treatment with flucytosine.

Squamous cell carcinoma

Stephanie A Diamantis, Heidi A Waldorf

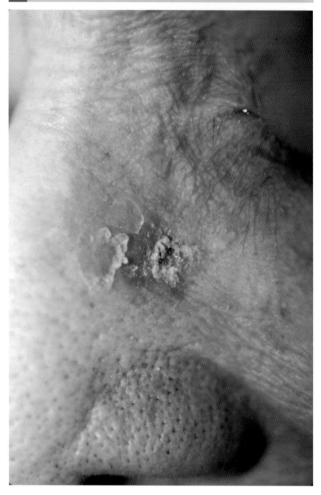

Squamous cell carcinoma is a malignant neoplasm arising from epithelial keratinocytes of the skin and mucous membranes that generally appears as an erythematous, keratotic papule or nodule, which may become ulcerated. Although it is most commonly associated with chronic sun exposure in light-skinned individuals, squamous cell carcinoma can arise secondary to scarring processes (burns, chronic ulcers, hidradenitis suppurativa), chemical carcinogens (arsenic, tobacco tar, hydrocarbons), human papillomavirus (types 16, 18, 30, 33, 35), and ionizing radiation exposure (X-rays, gamma rays, radium). Immunosuppression due to disease or drug therapy is an instigating factor.

MANAGEMENT STRATEGY

Management of squamous cell carcinoma is dependent upon the histopathologic classification and clinical setting. Risk of local recurrence and of metastasis are correlated with poor histologic differentiation, perineural invasion, tumor size (>2 cm), tumor depth (>4 mm), tumor location (lip, ear, temple, genitalia), treatment modality, history of recurrence, host immunosuppression, and precipitating factors other than UV light. Regional lymphadenopathy is a poor prognostic sign.

Accurate histopathologic diagnosis is the most critical investigation. Differential diagnosis may include verruca vulgaris, actinic keratosis, squamous cell carcinoma in situ (Bowen's disease), and keratoacanthoma (these conditions are described in separate chapters). Specimens for histopathologic diagnosis should include epidermis and dermis. A deep curette or scoop shave biopsy is generally sufficient, but an incisional or excisional biopsy is useful if there is concern regarding obtaining adequate tissue.

Regional lymph node palpation is performed when an aggressive tumor is suspected, based upon the criteria specified above. In the absence of palpable lymphadenopathy, additional radiologic and surgical studies are performed if deep invasion (bone, cartilage, parotid) or perineural spread is suspected.

Small, superficial squamous cell carcinoma may be effectively treated utilizing a destructive modality. *Cryosurgery* destroys tumor if it is frozen to −40 to −70°C – generally two cycles of at least 60-s thaw time. *Curettage and electrodesiccation* involves a sequence of three curette scrapings and electrodesiccations. A treatment margin of 3 or 4 mm around the tumor should be treated with cryosurgery and with curettage and desiccation. Adequately treated lesions often require several weeks to heal and may leave hypopigmented, atrophic, or hypertrophic scars. Cosmetically sensitive areas, concave surfaces, and skin prone to keloid formation should be avoided. Cure rates are highly technique dependent.

Standard surgical excision, utilizing 3–4 mm margins beyond the clinically apparent tumor, is a reasonable option for well-demarcated squamous cell carcinoma, particularly of the trunk and extremities. Recent studies have suggested that light curettage of the lesion prior to excision, traditionally used to better define tumor margins, may not be efficacious. Extensive tumors of the limbs involving bone may require amputation.

The gold standard for treatment of squamous cell carcinoma is *Mohs' micrographic surgery*, a technique in which the surgeon also acts as pathologist. The tumor is extirpated in a series of thin layers, which are precisely oriented, horizontally sectioned, and immediately processed for evaluation. The process is continued until all margins are clear to maximize tumor extirpation and tissue conservation. Indications for Mohs' micrographic surgery include tumor size, location (cosmetically or functionally sensitive, high recurrence rate), indistinct margins, history of recurrence, aggressive histopathology, and young patient age. *Adjuvant radiation therapy* following Mohs' micrographic surgery should be considered for facial squamous cell carcinoma greater than 2 cm in diameter and those with perineural spread.

Although use of radiation therapy as a primary modality has decreased, it remains a good treatment option for selected patients, particularly those of advanced age or poor surgical risk, with uncomplicated tumors of the head and neck. A total of 4000–7000 cGy is given sequentially over several weeks. One standard schedule is administration of 500 cGy three to five times per week over 2–6 weeks. Complications include hypopigmentation, telangiectasia, loss of adnexa, radiation dermatitis, and late (10–20 years) tumor recurrence.

For patients with squamous cell carcinoma not amenable to surgical extirpation or radiation due to advanced stage

Evidence levels A Double-blind study B Clinical trial ≥ 20 subjects C Clinical trial < 20 subjects D Series ≥ 5 subjects E Anecdotal case reports

of disease or large number of lesions, *topical therapy with imiquimod or 5-fluorouracil, intralesional therapy with bleomycin, 5-fluorouracil, or interferon, or systemic therapy with retinoids or interferon* may be effective. *Photodynamic therapy*, most commonly using topical porphyrins followed by selective irradiation with visible light, is another alternative.

SPECIFIC INVESTIGATIONS

- Histopathology
- Physical examination for lymphadenopathy
- Radiologic examination (MRI, CT scan)
- Sentinel lymphadenectomy

Demonstration of additional pathological findings in biopsy samples initially diagnosed as actinic keratosis. Carag HR, Priento VG, Yballe LS, Shea CR. Arch Dermatol 2000;136:471–5.

One-third of 69 skin biopsy specimens showing features of actinic keratoses on the initial section revealed additional pathology on step sections, 3% of which were invasive squamous cell carcinoma. These findings correlated with the presence of ulceration on the first level, clinical suspicion of skin cancer, and prior history of biopsy-proven skin cancer in the source individual.

Keratoacanthoma: when to observe and when to operate and the importance of accurate diagnosis. Netscher DT, Wigoda P, Green LK, Spira M. South Med J 1994;87:1272–6.

Case reports of two biopsy-diagnosed keratoacanthomas, one of which regressed without therapy after a rapid growth phase; the other rapidly recurred after medical treatment. Histology of the recurrent lesion revealed an invasive squamous cell carcinoma, suggesting that the initial diagnosis of keratoacanthoma was inaccurate.

Regional lymph node metastasis from cutaneous squamous cell carcinoma. Kraus DH, Carew JF, Harrison LB. Arch Otolaryngol Head Neck Surg 1998;124:582–7.

Despite a variable combination of neck dissection, parotidectomy, and radiation therapy, 45 patients with cutaneous squamous cell carcinoma of the head and neck metastatic to regional lymph nodes had 2- and 5-year survival rates of only 33 and 22%, respectively. Clinical stage of the neck was the only factor that predicted outcome in this series.

Nonmelanoma cutaneous malignancy with regional metastasis. Chu A, Osguthorpe JD. Otolaryngol Head Neck Surg 2003;128:663–73.

This is a retrospective study of 28 patients who underwent a variable combination of parotidectomy, neck dissection, and postoperative radiation for management of regional metastasis from non-melanoma cutaneous malignancies of the head and neck. Only 39% of these patients were disease-free at follow-up (mean follow-up 34 months), indicating that patients with regional metastasis have a poor prognosis even with aggressive treatment.

Sentinal node biopsy for high-risk nonmelanoma cutaneous malignancy. Wagner JD, Evdokimow DZ, Weisberger E, et al. Arch Dermatol 2004;140:75–9.

A study population of 24 patients with high-risk non-melanoma cutaneous malignancies, the majority squamous cell carcinoma (n = 17), underwent preoperative dermato-lymphoscintigraphy and sentinal lymphadenectomy. Although these patients had non-palpable lymph nodes at presentation, 29.2% had tumor-positive sentinal nodes. The sensitivity of the sentinal node procedure was 88%, and the specificity was 100%.

FIRST LINE THERAPIES

Curettage and electrodesiccation	C
Cryosurgery	C
Standard excision	B
Mohs' micrographic surgery	B
Radiation therapy	C

Cryosurgery for cutaneous malignancy. An update. Kuflik EG. Dermatol Surg 1997;23:1081–7.

A review article outlining the techniques and advantages of cryotherapy, including low cost and speed.

Surgical margins for excision of primary squamous cell carcinoma. Brodland DG, Zitelli JA. J Am Acad Dermatol 1992;27:241–8.

Based upon prospective study of subclinical microscopic tumor extension, it was recommended that minimal margins of 4 mm be taken around clinical borders of squamous cell carcinoma. Margins of at least 6 mm were proposed for tumors 2 cm or larger, histologic grade 2 or higher, with invasion of subcutaneous tissue, and/or location in high-risk areas.

Efficacy of curettage before excision in clearing surgical margins of nonmelanoma skin cancer. Chiller K, Passaro D, McCalmont T, Vin-Christian MD. Arch Dermatol 2000; 136:1327–32.

A retrospective, nonrandomized case–control series of 1983 basal cell carcinomas and 849 squamous cell carcinomas treated with pre-excisional curettage followed by simple excision. Pre-excisional curettage decreased the frequency of tumor margin involvement compared to non-curetted lesions for basal cell carcinomas, but not squamous cell carcinomas.

An assessment of the suitability of Mohs' micrographic surgery in patients aged 90 years and older. MacFarlane DF, Pustelny BL, Goldberg LH. Dermatol Surg 1997;23: 389–92.

A retrospective analysis of 115 patients over 90 years old (average age 92.4 years) who underwent Mohs' micrographic surgery from 1988 to 1996 for tumors, including 33 squamous cell carcinomas, revealed only one complication.

Prognostic factors for local recurrence, metastasis, and survival rates in squamous cell carcinoma of the skin, ear, and lip, implications for treatment modality selection. Rowe DE, Carroll RJ, Day CL. J Am Acad Dermatol 1992;26:976–90.

A review of all studies since 1940 revealed lower recurrence rates for Mohs' micrographic surgery than with other modalities including standard excision for primary squamous cell carcinoma of the skin and lip (3.1 vs 10.9%), of the ear (5.3 vs 18.7%), with diameter greater than 2 cm (25.2 vs 41.7%), with perineural involvement (0 vs 47%), poorly differentiated (32.6 vs 53.6%), and squamous cell carcinoma locally recurrent after previous treatment (10 vs 23.3%).

Squamous cell carcinoma of skin with perineural invasion. Lawrence N, Cottel WI. J Am Acad Dermatol 1994;31: 30–3.

Recurrences occurred in three of 44 squamous cell carcinomas with perineural invasion treated with Mohs' micrographic surgery. Follow-up reached 3 years or more in 33 cases.

Adjuvant radiotherapy after excision of cutaneous squamous cell carcinoma. Geohas J, Roholt NS, Robinson JK. J Am Acad Dermatol 1994;30:633–6.

A case report and review of the literature suggesting adjuvant radiotherapy following Mohs' micrographic surgery of high-risk cutaneous squamous cell carcinoma.

Ionizing radiation therapy in dermatology. Goldschmidt H, Breneman JC, Breneman DL. J Am Acad Dermatol 1994; 30:157–82.

Five-year cure rate following radiotherapy for primary squamous cell carcinoma is estimated to be between 91.3 and 92.3%.

A review article.

SECOND LINE THERAPIES

■ Topical imiquimod	D
■ Topical 5-fluorouracil	D
■ Intralesional 5-fluorouracil	B
■ Electrochemotherapy with bleomycin	B
■ Intralesional interferon-alfa	C

Successful treatment with topical 0.5% fluorouracil and imiquimod 5% cream in the treatment of a patient with actinic keratoses and a squamous cell carcinoma. Torok HM. J Am Acad Dermatol 2004;50:129.

A case report of clinical clearance of multiple actinic keratoses and a 1.2 × 1.2 cm squamous cell carcinoma of the scalp using concomitant application of 0.5% 5-fluorouracil cream at night and 5% imiquimod cream in the morning for 2 weeks for a patient who had previously failed treatment with imiquimod alone. There was no recurrence at 1 year.

Successful treatment of invasive squamous cell carcinoma using topical imiquimod. Hengge UR, Schaller J. Arch Dermatol 2004;140:404–6.

Case report of a biopsy-proven invasive squamous cell carcinoma of the scalp in an immunosuppressed renal transplant patient treated to histologic clearance with thrice weekly overnight application of imiquimod cream for 12 weeks.

Intratumoral chemotherapy with fluorouracil/epinephrine injectable gel: a nonsurgical treatment of cutaneous squamous cell carcinoma. Kraus S, Miller BH, Swinehart JM, et al. J Am Acad Dermatol 1998;38:438–42.

One biopsy-proven squamous cell carcinoma on each of 25 patients was treated weekly over 6 weeks with up to 1 mL of a 5-fluorouracil/epinephrine (adrenaline)/bovine collagen gel. Histology of tumor site and margins at 4 months

revealed clearance in 96% of the 23 patients available for follow-up with good to excellent cosmetic results.

A prior study done by this group resulted in 91% cure.

Treatment of cutaneous and subcutaneous tumors with electrochemotherapy using intralesional bleomycin. Heller R, Jaroszeski MJ, Reintgen DS, et al. Cancer 1998; 83:148–57.

In 34 patients, 130 of 143 (91%) tumor nodules had a complete response, defined clinically and by random biopsies, to intralesional injection of bleomycin followed by the direct application of electric pulses.

Effective treatment of cutaneous and subcutaneous malignant tumours by electrochemotherapy. Mir LM, Glass LF, Sersa G, et al. Br J Cancer 1998;77:2336–42.

A prospective clinical trial of 291 tumors including 87 squamous cell carcinomas of the head and neck in 50 patients revealed clinical complete responses in 154 (56.4%) and partial responses in 79 (28.9%) of all tumors using electrochemotherapy with intralesional bleomycin. Follow-up was limited to 1 month after treatment.

Treatment of cutaneous squamous cell carcinomas by intralesional interferon alpha-2b therapy. Edwards L, Berman B, Rapini RP, et al. Arch Dermatol 1992;128:1486–9.

In an open-label study, complete histologic response rate of 88.2% was achieved for 36 actinically-induced primary squamous cell carcinomas under 2.0 cm diameter (28 invasive, eight in situ), 18 weeks after completing a 3-week course of intralesional injection of 1.5 million units of interferon-alfa-2b three times a week.

THIRD LINE THERAPIES

■ Amputation	D
■ Photodynamic therapy	C
■ Systemic retinoids	B
■ Systemic interferon-alfa	C

Squamous cell carcinoma arising in osteomyelitis and chronic wounds. Treatment with Mohs' micrographic surgery vs. amputation. Kirsner RS, Spencer J, Falanga V, et al. Dermatol Surg 1996;22:1015–8.

Patients with extensive local or metastatic squamous cell carcinoma of the leg involving bone may require amputation if Mohs' micrographic surgery would render the remaining limb unstable.

A review of laser and photodynamic therapy for the treatment of nonmelanoma skin cancer. Marmur ES, Schmults CD, Goldberg DJ. Dermatol Surg 2004;30:264–71.

Photodynamic therapy involves administration of a photosensitizer preferentially absorbed in tumor tissue followed by selective irradiation with visible light. The most common treatment protocol involves application of topical 20% aminolevulinic acid followed by exposure to an incoherent light source. When used to treat squamous cell carcinoma, photodynamic therapy achieves only an 8% clearance rate and has a recurrence rate of 82%. Although useful in certain populations, this modality remains inferior to standard surgical excision.

A good review article.

Evidence levels A Double-blind study B Clinical trial ≥ 20 subjects C Clinical trial < 20 subjects D Series ≥ 5 subjects E Anecdotal case reports

13-cis-retinoic acid and interferon alpha-2a: effective combination therapy for advanced squamous cell carcinoma of the skin. Lippman SM, Parkinson DR, Itri LM, et al. J Natl Cancer Inst 1992;84:235–41.

Of 28 patients with inoperable cutaneous squamous cell carcinoma, 19 (68%) had a partial response and seven (25%) had a complete response to a regimen of oral isotretinoin, 1 mg/kg daily, and subcutaneous interferon-alfa-2a, 3 million units daily. The major dose-limiting side effect was fatigue.

Beneficial effect of low-dose systemic retinoid in combination with topical tretinoin for the treatment and prophylaxis of premalignant and malignant skin lesions in renal transplant recipients. Rook AH, Jaworsky C, Nguyen T. Transplantation 1995;59:714–9.

In a study of 11 renal allograft patients a combination of topical tretinoin cream and oral etretinate, 10 mg daily, significantly reduced the number of existing lesions and decreased the recurrence rate of new squamous cell carcinomas.

Acitretin suppression of squamous cell carcinoma: case report and literature review. Lebwohl M, Tannis C, Carrasco D. J Dermatolog Treat 2003;14(suppl 2);3–6.

A 40-year-old man with a history of severe psoriasis began developing numerous cutaneous squamous cell carcinomas after treatment with psoralen and ultraviolet A (PUVA) for 4.5 years. Because of a flare in his psoriasis, he was started on 25 mg daily of acitretin, which resulted in a dramatic decrease in the number of squamous cell carcinomas. This report reviews the mechanism by which retinoids are thought to act and describes how oral retinoids may be an important therapy in patients at risk for developing multiple cutaneous malignancies.

Oral retinoid use reduces cutaneous squamous cell carcinoma risk in patients with psoriasis treated with psoralen-UVA: a nested cohort study. Nijsten TEC, Stern RS. J Am Acad Dermatol 2003;49:644–50.

To assess whether oral retinoids reduce the risk of developing cutaneous squamous cell carcinoma, a nested cohort of 135 patients participating in the PUVA follow-up study with at least 1 year of substantial retinoid use was identified. Each patient's tumor incidence during retinoid therapy was compared to the incidence of squamous cell carcinoma development in periods of no use. Overall, a 30% reduction in squamous cell carcinoma incidence was noted when patients were on oral retinoid therapy.

Retinoids (isotretinoin, acitretin) may play a role in the treatment of patients with squamous cell carcinoma not amenable to surgical extirpation due to advanced stage of disease or large number of lesions. Several studies have shown an overall response rate of about 70%. Systemic retinoids may play a greater role in chemoprevention of new and recurrent malignancy in susceptible individuals, such as organ transplant recipients and those with xeroderma pigmentosa, than in treatment.

Staphylococcal scalded skin syndrome

Anna Martinez, John Harper

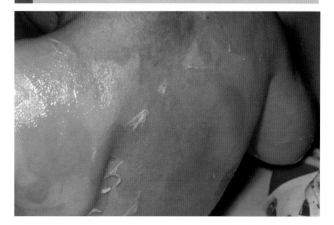

Staphylococcal scalded skin syndrome (SSSS) is the term used to describe a blistering skin disease caused by exfoliative toxins (ETs) of certain strains of *Staphylococcus aureus*. SSSS was first described in 1878 by Ritter von Rittershain and the term Ritter's disease is still used to describe generalized SSSS in neonates. This condition primarily affects neonates and young children; it is rare in adults. Outbreaks of SSSS infection tend to occur in clusters as a consequence of cross-infection. Typically neonatal and maternity staff infected or colonized with ET-producing *S. aureus* are the source of these outbreaks. Although most toxigenic strains of *S. aureus* belong to phage group II (types 71 and 55), toxin producers have also been identified among phage groups I and III.

Histopathology of the skin shows superficial intraepidermal splitting without epidermal necrosis and with very few inflammatory cells. The cleavage is in the granular layer of the dermis, while in toxic epidermal necrolysis (TEN), the cleavage is at the dermal–epidermal junction.

Severity varies from localized bullous impetigo to generalized SSSS involving the entire skin surface. Infections leading to SSSS typically originate in the nasopharynx, and frequently are unrecognized. Other primary foci of infection include the umbilicus, urinary tract, conjunctivae, and blood. Sudden onset of fever, irritability, cutaneous tenderness, and erythema are hallmarks of the syndrome. The erythema is often accentuated in flexural and periorificial areas. Flaccid blisters and erosions develop within 24–48 h. The blisters and erosions yield no organisms. Easy disruption of the skin with pressure (Nikolsky's sign) is present. Complications of sepsis and serious fluid and electrolyte disturbances increase the morbidity and mortality rates of this condition.

MANAGEMENT STRATEGY

Therapy for SSSS should be directed toward eradication of *S. aureus*, which generally requires *intravenous antistaphylococcal antibiotics*. Topical agents are ineffective.

Usually, oral antibiotic therapy can be substituted within several days. The use of suitable antibiotics combined with *supportive skin care* and *appropriate attention to fluid and electrolyte management* in the face of disrupted barrier function will usually ensure rapid recovery. Neonates are nursed in incubators to *maintain body temperature*, and *analgesia* should be used as required. Intravenous fluids may be required if clinical dehydration develops, otherwise we encourage oral fluids and carefully monitor the intake and urinary output. *Nonadherent dressings*, such as petrolatum-impregnated gauze can be applied to the skin. Nonadherent dressings should also be used where topical anesthetic is applied before intravenous cannulation.

Within 2–3 days the fever subsides and the erythema resolves with cessation of blister formation. The superficial nature of the erosions in SSSS makes rapid re-epithelialization with minimal or no scarring a predictable result following appropriate therapy. The prognosis of SSSS in children with appropriate treatment is usually very good, with complete resolution within 2–3 weeks and no permanent sequelae. The mortality risk is low, but has been quoted as up to 5%.

It is vital to recognize the potential for epidemic SSSS in newborn nurseries, and *identification of healthcare workers colonized or infected with toxigenic strains* of *S. aureus* is an integral part of managing the problem. *Control measures should be applied*, including strict enforcement of *chlorhexidine handwashing*, *oral antibiotic therapy for infected workers*, and *mupirocin ointment for eradication of persistent nasal carriage*.

In adults, SSSS carries a less favorable prognosis, partly because it tends to occur in debilitated and immunocompromised patients.

Skin biopsy can be helpful, but this is usually not necessary because the clinical diagnosis is straightforward in most cases. The most common problem in differential diagnosis, particularly in adults, is TEN. This can be rapidly differentiated by histological examination of a frozen section of blister roof because the full thickness necrosis of the epidermis and a subepidermal split in TEN contrast to the very superficial blister formation within the granular layer in SSSS (see TEN, page 657).

SPECIFIC INVESTIGATIONS

- Nose and throat swabs
- Other swabs dependent on the suspected site of primary infection
- Full blood count
- Serum biochemistry
- Blood culture
- Histological examination of frozen section of blister roof
- Skin biopsy (not generally required)

Early hospital discharge and cross-infection. Bell FG, Fenton PA. Lancet 1993;342:120.

An outbreak of mild SSSS due to carriage of an exfoliative toxin-producing strain of *Staphylococcus* by pediatrician. This was not initially recognized because many cases developed after discharge from hospital.

Very careful hygiene is required in the presence of toxigenic strains of S. aureus. *In the event of outbreaks occurring, thorough screening of healthcare personnel is essential to exclude asymptomatic carriage.*

Isolating *Staphylococcus aureus* from children with suspected staphylococcal scalded skin syndrome is not clinically useful. Ladhani S, Robbie S, Chapple DS, et al. Pediatr Infect Dis J 2003;22:284–6.

Fifty-four *Staph. aureus* isolates were obtained from skin lesions of children clinically suspected of having generalized SSSS during a 4-year period and subjected to polymerase chain reaction (PCR) that identifies the presence of the *eta* and *etb* genes and Western blot analysis. Only 17 of 54 (31%) samples produced exfoliative toxin and in the remaining 37 isolates (69%), there was no evidence of exfoliative toxin production.

Failure to detect S. aureus *from skin lesions of children with suspected SSSS does not exclude the diagnosis because more than two-thirds of the isolates do not produce exfoliative toxins.*

FIRST LINE THERAPIES

■ Intravenous penicillinase-resistant penicillin (e.g. flucloxacillin)	D

Outbreak of staphylococcal scalded skin syndrome among neonates. Dancer SJ, Simmons NA, Poston SM, Noble WC. J Infect 1988;16:87–103.

Twelve cases were successfully treated with short courses of intravenous flucloxacillin (50 mg/kg body weight total daily dose for patients up to 7 days of age and 75 mg/kg for those older).

This report from Guy's Hospital further demonstrates the tendency for SSSS to occur in outbreaks that seem to be the result of carriage of the organism by hospital staff.

Treatment of staphylococcal toxic epidermal necrolysis. Rudolph RI, Schwartz W, Leyden JJ. Arch Dermatol 1974; 110:559–62.

These authors describe their treatment of 18 cases of SSSS. A good outcome was observed with the use of penicillinase-resistant penicillins – nafcillin sodium 50 mg/kg intravenously for 3–8 days followed by dicloxacillin sodium monohydrate orally 50 mg/kg for 5–10 more days. The use of systemic corticosteroids was associated with a less favorable outcome, especially when these were used without antibiotics.

The title of this citation reflects the past variation in terminology. The term toxic epidermal necrolysis is no longer taken to include SSSS. However, these results all relate to true SSSS.

SECOND LINE THERAPIES

■ Intravenous macrolide (erythromycin or clarithromycin)	E

Staphylococcal scalded skin syndrome in an adult and a child. Sturman SW, Malkinson FD. Arch Dermatol 1976;112: 1275–9.

Two cases of SSSS caused by penicillin-resistant organisms. Oral erythromycin 250 mg four times daily for 2 days and increased to 1.5 g daily for the next 5 days, combined with an ointment containing flurandrenolide and neomycin sulphate, was used in the adult's case. The child, aged 14 months, was treated orally with cloxacillin sodium 250 mg orally every 6 h and topically with an ointment containing polymyxin B sulphate and zinc bacitracin. Both recovered rapidly.

THIRD LINE THERAPIES

■ Cephalosporins	E
■ Vancomycin	E

Microbiology characteristics of exfoliative toxin-producing *Staphylococcus aureus*. Murono K, Fujita H. Pediatr Infect Dis J 1988;7:313–5.

A Japanese study of 74 strains of *S. aureus* including 61 producing exfoliating toxins. No toxigenic strains were resistant to penicillin G, methicillin, cephalosporins, lincomycin, or vancomycin; 5% were resistant to gentamicin, 2% to chloramphenicol, 7% to tetracycline, and 18% to erythromycin.

Other reports have found penicillin G resistance in toxigenic strains.

Staphylococcal scalded skin syndrome in a liver transplant patient. Strauss G, Mogensen AM, Rasmussen A, Kirkegaard P. Liver Transpl Surg 1997;3:435–6.

A case successfully treated with vancomycin.

Steatocystoma multiplex

Roy A Palmer, Martin Keefe

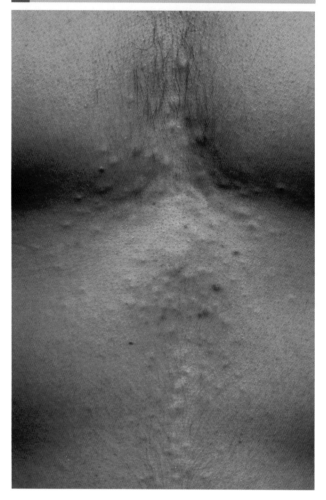

Although probably genetically heterogeneous, steatocystoma multiplex often demonstrates an autosomal dominant pattern of inheritance. It is characterized by the development in adolescence or early adulthood of cysts on the trunk and proximal limbs, or in some patients on the face and scalp. The cysts are true 'sebaceous cysts' because sebaceous gland lobules are present in the walls. Overlap with eruptive vellus hair cysts and association with pachyonychia congenita type II have been reported.

MANAGEMENT STRATEGY

The cysts persist indefinitely. Although usually a minor cosmetic problem, they can be highly disfiguring. Paradoxically, those patients who would benefit most from treatment are sometimes regarded as being unsuitable for surgery because they have too many cysts to excise. The *surgical* technique described below is quick, so it can be used on large numbers of lesions in one session. The procedure produces good cosmetic results.

Lesions can become inflamed, due to rupture of the cyst wall with leakage of the contents into the dermis, or due to

bacterial infection. Suppuration and scarring may follow. The clinical picture then resembles cystic acne and is called steatocystoma multiplex suppurativum. Oral *isotretinoin* is an effective treatment of inflammatory lesions, but not noninflamed cysts. This suggests it operates by a direct anti-inflammatory effect rather than by reducing the sebum excretion rate. Alternatively, inflamed cysts can be treated with *incision and drainage, intralesional triamcinolone, tetracycline* 1 g daily, or *minocycline* 100–200 mg daily.

Topical treatment is largely ineffective because it does not penetrate to reach the cyst wall.

SPECIFIC INVESTIGATIONS

- Skin biopsy if diagnosis is in doubt

FIRST LINE THERAPIES

Lesions inflamed:	
■ Isotretinoin	D
■ Antibiotics	E
■ Incision and drainage	E
Lesions not inflamed	
■ Surgical incision and extraction of cyst wall	D

Steatocystoma multiplex suppurativum: treatment with isotretinoin. Schwartz JL, Goldsmith LA. Cutis 1984;34: 149–53.

The treatment of steatocystoma multiplex suppurativum with isotretinoin. Statham BN, Cunliffe WJ. Br J Dermatol 1984;111:246.

Isotretinoin in the treatment of steatocystoma multiplex: a possible adverse reaction. Rosen BL, Broadkin RH. Cutis 1986;115:115–20.

Steatocystoma multiplex treated with isotretinoin: a delayed response. Mortiz DL, Silverman RA. Cutis 1988;42: 437–9.

Treatment of steatocystoma multiplex and pseudofolliculitis barbae with isotretinoin. Friedman SJ. Cutis 1987;39: 506–7.

These five papers report a total of seven patients treated with oral isotretinoin, at a dose of approximately 1 mg/kg daily for about 20 weeks. Inflammation of cysts was greatly reduced. Noninflammatory lesions were unaffected, and in one patient appeared to increase in size and number. One successfully treated patient relapsed 10 weeks after ceasing therapy, but other patients did not relapse during a follow-up period of up to 8 months.

Successful treatment of steatocystoma multiplex by simple surgery. Keefe M, Leppard BJ, Royle G. Br J Dermatol 1992;127:41–4.

Five generations with steatocystoma multiplex congenita: a treatment regimen. Pamoukian VN, Westreich M. Plast Reconstr Surg 1997;99:1142–6.

Surgical pearl: mini-incisions for the extraction of steatocystoma multiplex. Schmook T, Burg G, Hafner J. J Am Acad Dermatol 2001;44:1041–2.

Evidence levels **A** Double-blind study **B** Clinical trial ≥ 20 subjects **C** Clinical trial < 20 subjects **D** Series ≥ 5 subjects **E** Anecdotal case reports

A simple surgical technique for the treatment of steatocystoma multiplex. Kaya TI, Ikizoglu G, Kokturk A, Tursen U. Int J Dermatol 2001;40:785–8.

Suggestion for the treatment of steatocystoma multiplex located exclusively on the face. Duzova AN, Senturk GB. Int J Dermatol 2004;43:60–2.

These five reports describe variants of a simple surgical technique for noninflamed cysts. Local, regional, general, or no anesthesia is used depending on the exact technique and the number of cysts being treated. In most cases a 1–10 mm incision is made with a surgical blade, the contents of the cyst are expressed, then fine artery forceps are passed through the opening to grasp the base of the cyst, which is pulled out. The incisions heal by secondary intention. Good cosmetic results and a very low recurrence rate are reported.

Excision of cysts and aspiration have also been described.

SECOND LINE THERAPIES

■ CO₂ laser therapy	E

CO₂ laser therapy for steatocystoma multiplex. Krahenbuhl A, Eichmann A, Pfaltz M. Dermatologica 1991;183:294–6.

'Fairly good' results were reported.

THIRD LINE THERAPIES

■ Cryotherapy	E

Treatment of lesions of steatocystoma multiplex and other epidermal cysts by cryosurgery. Notowicz A. J Dermatol Surg Oncol 1980;6:98–9.

Three or 4 days after cryotherapy, the necrotic skin overlying the cyst was removed and the intact cyst expressed through the opening.

Stoma care

Eric Berkowitz, Mark G Lebwohl

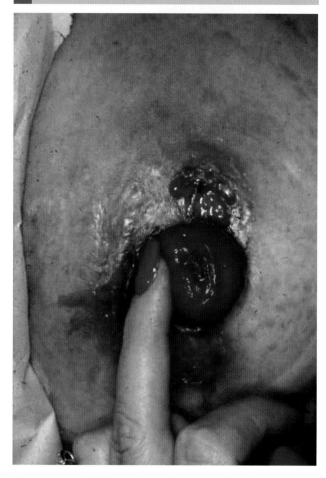

Stomas are artificial openings that are produced to maintain proper drainage from internal structures. The most commonly formed stomas are colostomies, ileostomies, and urostomies. They may be formed either under emergency conditions or electively, and may be permanent or temporary. There is a high prevalence of peristomal cutaneous complications, ranging from 37% in patients with colostomies to over 80% in ileostomy patients.

MANAGEMENT STRATEGY

Even with the best of preventative measures dermatologic problems often arise. The pathophysiology leading to cutaneous peristomal dermatitis can be caused by external irritants, body fluid irritants, infections, and pre-existing skin disorders.

The typical peristomal dermatitis is caused by enzyme degradation from leakage of fluid from the stoma. The content of the fluid varies depending on the type of stoma, but is usually rich in lipases, peptidases, and polysaccharidases. When the fluid comes into contact with skin it can cause inflammation and hypergranulation. Ideally, the ostomy appliance should fit snugly around the opening of the stoma covering as much skin as possible without blocking the opening. If the margin of the device is too small, the disc may rub and irritate protruding mucosa; if the opening is too large, excess skin may be exposed to the content of the fluid. The key to treating peristomal irritation is to *correct the cause*. Primary treatments for inflammation are to change an ill-fitting device and treat with anti-inflammatory creams such as *topical corticosteroid creams, tacrolimus ointment,* or *pimecrolimus cream. Flurandrenolide tape,* an occlusive corticosteroid therapy, is particularly useful because the stoma device can be applied over the tape. Hypergranulation can be treated with *silver nitrate* or by *curettage and electrodessication.* Mechanical stress and pressure necrosis also occur, though are less common, and are usually caused by an ill fitting device.

Allergic contact dermatitis, while rare, is another problem. The allergen is most often a component of the cementing material, the pouch, or the barrier. Patch testing may be required to identify the offending agent. Treatment includes substituting the offending agent and resolution of the inflammation with *topical or systemic corticosteroids* and *antipruritic agents.*

Infection, specifically intertrigo, is another potential problem. The closed, moist, and warm environment can lead to maceration, folliculitis, and other types of infection. Proper treatment leading to resolution consists of careful drying after washing, powders, and the use of *antifungals and/or antibacterials* if infection is demonstrated.

Other difficulties occur with less frequency. Inflammatory processes cause the skin to adhere to adjacent structures, and degeneration of the common wall results in fistula formation. Inflammatory conditions that commonly cause fistulae are radiation damage, tumor-induced inflammation and adhesions, infection, Crohn's disease, and diverticular disease. Other causes of fistula formation are trauma and surgical injury. Chronic papillomatous dermatitis is characterized by 2–10 mm high, domed red-brown hyperplastic, papulonodules that usually occur with urostomies. Treatment measures usually consist of changing the appliance and acidifying the urine.

Pre-existing skin disorders may occur in the skin surrounding the stoma mimicking inflammation caused by other pathologies. Some of the common pre-existing dermatologic disorders that particularly affect stomas are psoriasis, seborrheic dermatitis, cutaneous Crohn's disease, pyoderma gangrenosum, and eczema.

SPECIFIC INVESTIGATIONS

- Skin biopsy
- Wound culture
- Patch testing
- Radiographic studies to look for fistulae

The spectrum of skin disorders in abdominal stoma patients. Lyon CC, Smith AJ, Griffiths CEM, Beck MH. Br J Dermatol 2000;143:1248–60.

This large cohort study documented the many different types of skin disorders that can occur around a stoma. Initial evaluations for patients presenting with inflammation include a bacterial swab because infections are relatively common and easy to treat. Allergic contact hypersensitivity should be suspected in any patient

Evidence levels **A** Double-blind study **B** Clinical trial ≥ 20 subjects **C** Clinical trial < 20 subjects **D** Series ≥ 5 subjects **E** Anecdotal case reports

with persistent disease that is unresponsive to treatment. And finally, in any peristomal skin disorder with ulceration or a papular component a biopsy should be performed.

A comprehensive review discussing the various different pathologies that can occur with a stoma and how to evaluate them.

FIRST LINE THERAPIES

■ Change appliance	D
■ Absorbent powders	D
■ Antibiotics	D
■ Topical corticosteroids	B

Dermatologic considerations of stoma care. Rothstein MS. J Am Acad Dermatol 1986;15;411–32.

Ill-fitting devices can cause stomal irritation and skin irritation. The chemical irritation caused from the stomal effluent, mechanical irritation, and contact dermatitis can all be alleviated by replacing the stoma device at the earliest sign of irritation. Additionally, careful drying of the skin after washing and the use of absorbent powders will alleviate irritation caused by intertrigo and ill-fitting devices. Infection is another cause of complications and treatment is dependent on the causative organism.

Peristomal dermatoses; a novel indication for topical steroid lotions. Lyon CC, Smith AJ, Griffiths CEM, Beck MH. J Am Acad Dermatol 2000:43;679–82.

This large clinical study demonstrated the benefits of treating inflammatory peristomal skin diseases with topical corticosteroids formulated in an aqueous alcohol lotion. This formulation was found advantageous because it did not interfere with ostomy bag adhesion to the skin, allowing treatment of the skin disease as well as proper ostomy bag application.

SECOND LINE THERAPIES

■ Intralesional corticosteroids	E
■ Tacrolimus ointment or pimecrolimus cream	E
■ Amikacin gel	C
■ Sucralfate	C

Topical sucralfate in the management of peristomal skin disease: an open study. Lyon CC, Stapelton M, Smith AJ, et al. Clin Exp Dermatol 2000:25;584–8.

The authors demonstrated the ability of sucralfate to help treat peristomal erosions. Sucralfate is a basic aluminum salt of sucrose octasulfate that polymerizes in acidic environments and provides a viscous barrier on mucosal surfaces. Sucralfate was effective for erosions and irritation caused by either feces or urine. However, it was ineffective for peristomal pyoderma gangrenosum.

Peristomal pyoderma gangrenosum. Keltz M, Lebwohl M, Bishop S. J Am Acad Dermatol 1992;27:360–4.

A patient with peristomal pyoderma gangrenosum is described who responded well to intralesional corticosteroids.

This article also discusses the difficulties in diagnosing peristomal pyoderma gangrenosum.

Topical tacrolimus in the management of peristomal pyoderma gangrenosum. Lyon CC, Stapelton M, Smith AJ, et al. J Dermatol Treat 2001;12:13–7.

Topical tacrolimus in conjunction with other treatments was found to rapidly heal pyoderma gangrenosum.

Amikacin gel administration in the treatment of peristomal dermatitis. La Torre F, Nicolai AP. Drugs Exp Clin Res 1998;24:153–7.

Local daily application of amikacin sulfate 5% gel was a successful treatment for patients with moderate to severe peristomal dermatitis.

THIRD LINE THERAPIES

■ Topical cromolyn sodium	E
■ Oral dapsone	E
■ Cyclosporine	D
■ Tumor necrosis factor (TNF)-blocking drugs	E
■ Collagen injections	E
■ Lipectomy	E
■ Embolization	E
■ Surgery	
■ Cholestyramine	E

Clinical features and treatment of peristomal pyoderma gangrenosum. Hughes AP, Jackson JM, Callen JP. JAMA 2000;284:1546–8.

Peristomal pyoderma gangrenosum is a difficult and frequently misdiagnosed condition. It was observed in this study that six of seven patients required either dapsone, topical cromolyn sodium, cyclosporine, mycophenolate mofetil, or infliximab and that these treatments are beneficial in treating peristomal pyoderma gangrenosum rather than other peristomal ulcers.

Infliximab for peristomal pyoderma gangrenosum. Mimouni D, Anhalt GJ, Kouba DJ, Nousari HC. Br J Dermatol 2003;148:813–6.

The authors report three cases of patients with peristomal pyoderma gangrenosum that was unresponsive to various immunomodulating therapies. Infliximab resulted in rapid and complete resolution of the peristomal pyoderma gangrenosum in two patients and significant improvement in the third patient.

Stomal varices: treatment by percutaneous transhepatic embolization. Kaneyuki T, Matsunaga N. Cardiovasc Intervent Radiol 1999;22:523–5.

In a patient with portal hypertension who had uncontrolled stomal variceal bleeding, the bleeding was treated and controlled with percutaneous transhepatic embolization.

Correction of dermal contour defect with collagen injection: a simple management technique for difficult stomal care. Arai Y, Okubo K. J Urol 1999;161:601–2.

Peristomal dermal deformity such as skin creasing and scarring makes appliance placement troublesome. The authors report a case of a dermal contour defect that was successfully treated with intradermal injections of collagen.

Troublesome colostomies and urinary stomas treated with suction assisted lipectomy. Samdal F, Amlamd PF, Bakka A, Aasen AO. Eur J Surg 1995;161:361–4.

This study demonstrated the usefulness of syringe-assisted lipectomy for stomas with significant leakage. The ability to reduce the amount of leakage and irritation led to significant patient satisfaction.

Complications of colostomies. Porter JA, Salvati EP, Rubin RJ, Eisenstat TE. Dis Colon Rectum 1989;32:299–303.

This cohort study related the many different complications associated with stomas and reported that occasionally stomas must be surgically corrected.

Treatment of skin irritation around enterostomies with cholestyramine ointment. Rodriguez JT, Huang TL, Ferry GD, et al. J Pediatr 1976;88:659–61.

This study found that the irritation caused by stomas can be treated with cholestyramine ointment.

Evidence levels A Double-blind study B Clinical trial ≥ 20 subjects C Clinical trial < 20 subjects D Series ≥ 5 subjects E Anecdotal case reports

Striae

Jonathan E Blume

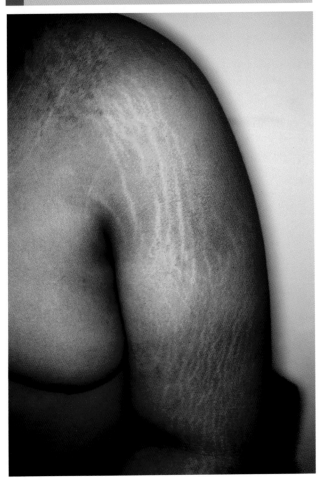

Striae distensae are common lesions that are of significant cosmetic concern to many patients. Striae are initially slightly elevated and have a pink to violaceous color. Over time, these striae rubra evolve into striae alba, which are white, atrophic, linear bands of skin. They are considered by most to be atrophic dermal scars and are probably the result of a combination of factors including genetics, mechanical stress, and hormones (e.g. cortisol and estrogen).

MANAGEMENT STRATEGIES

The goal of treatment is gradual, incremental improvement. In general, 'older' striae alba respond more slowly and less dramatically to therapy than 'newer' striae rubra. The best results are achieved by combining multiple treatment modalities.

Several studies have shown that *topical tretinoin* improves the appearance of striae. Based on these reports, striae rubra respond better to this therapy. Although not formally investigated, it is expected that *other topical retinoids (e.g. tazarotene, adapalene)* may also provide some improvement.

Nonablative lasers likely produce improvement by stimulating an increase in dermal collagen and elastin. The *pulsed dye laser* is the laser that has been most studied. Early reports suggest that this laser is helpful for both striae rubra and alba. However, more recent studies suggest that improve-

ment is more common in early striae that are pink to red in color.

The *excimer laser, intense pulsed light,* and *glycolic acid products* appear to be the most promising treatments for mature striae.

SPECIFIC INVESTIGATIONS

- Thorough history and physical examination
- Skin biopsy (not generally necessary)
- Serum adrenocorticotropin (ACTH) levels, 24-hour urine free cortisol level, plasma cortisol levels

The diagnosis and cause of striae are usually straightforward. When the lesions are particularly severe and the cause is unknown, laboratory testing to exclude Cushing's syndrome is advised. Occasionally, striae may be confused with linear focal elastosis, which are stria-like, slightly palpable, yellow bands commonly found on the lower back of older adults. Histological evaluation, with specific attention given to the elastic fiber content, will clearly differentiate these two entities.

FIRST LINE THERAPIES

■ Observation	D

Adolescent striae. Ammar NM, Roa B, Schwartz RA, Janniger CK. Cutis 2000;65:69–70.

Striae cutis distensae. Nigam PK. Int J Dermatol 1989;28: 426–7.

It is well known that striae tend to become less conspicuous with time. Thus, reassurance may be all that is required for the patient who is not overly concerned about his or her striae.

SECOND LINE THERAPIES

■ Topical tretinoin	B
■ Pulsed dye laser (585 nm)	C

Topical tretinoin 0.1% for pregnancy-related abdominal striae: an open-label, multicenter, prospective study. Rangel O, Aries I, García E, Lopez-Padilla S. Adv Ther 2001;18:181–6.

Twenty patients who were 1-week post-delivery applied tretinoin cream 0.1% once a day for 3 months to half of the abdomen: 80% of patients noted a marked or moderate improvement. Measured striae decreased by 20% in length and by 23% in width.

Topical tretinoin for management of early striae. Kang S. J Am Acad Dermatol 1998;38:S90–2.

Twenty six patients with early erythematous striae were randomized to either tretinoin cream 0.1% or placebo for 24 weeks: 80% of the patients in the treatment arm experienced improvement or marked improvement with decreased length and width of striae.

Topical tretinoin (retinoic acid) improves early stretch marks. Kang S, Kim KJ, Griffiths CEM, et al. Arch Dermatol 1996;132:519–26.

In this double-blind study, 22 patients with early striae applied either tretinoin cream 0.1% or placebo cream daily for 6 months: 80% of the patients who used tretinoin showed improvement or marked improvement.

Low-dose tretinoin does not improve striae distensae: a double-blind, placebo-controlled study. Pribanich S, Simpson FG, Held B, Yarbrough CL, White SN. Cutis 1994; 54:121–4.

No difference was noted in the treatment group compared with the control group.

It should be noted that this study was very small (only 11 subjects) and low-dose tretinoin (0.025% cream) was used.

Treatment of striae distensae with topical tretinoin. Elson ML. J Dermatol Surg Oncol 1990;16:267–70.

All patients applied Retin-A® cream 0.1 % once a day for 12 weeks: 15 of 16 patients experienced significant improvement, while some patients had total resolution. Although not specifically quantified, some of the patients who showed improvement had striae alba.

Treatment of striae rubra and striae alba with the 585-nm pulsed-dye laser. Jiménez G, Flores F, Berman B, Gunja-Smith Z. Dermatol Surg 2003;29:362–5.

Nine patients with striae rubra and 11 patients with striae alba were treated at baseline and again at 6 weeks. The treatment was moderately effective in decreasing the erythema of striae rubra, but no improvement was noted in late stage striae. The authors warn against using the pulsed dye laser in patients with skin types V and VI.

Comparison of the 585 nm pulsed dye laser and the short pulsed CO_2 laser in the treatment of striae distensae in skin types IV and VI. Nouri K, Romagosa R, Chartier T, et al. Dermatol Surg 1999;25:368–70.

This study confirmed that laser treatment for patients with skin types IV, V, or VI should be avoided or used only with extreme caution.

Treatment of mature striae with the pulsed dye laser. Nehal KS, Lichtenstein DA, Kamino H, et al. J Cutan Laser Ther 1999;1:41–4.

Five patients with late-stage striae were treated with multiple sessions of the pulsed dye laser. All five patients felt that their striae had improved. However, physician, photographic, textural, and histologic assessments could not confirm this improvement.

Treatment of stretch marks with the 585-nm flashlamp-pumped pulsed dye laser. McDaniel DH, Ash K, Zukowski M. Dermatol Surg 1996;22:332–7.

Thirty nine striae were treated once with the pulsed dye laser. Except for one stria, all were of the alba type. All of the striae showed at least minimal improvement that continued for six or more months after the treatment.

THIRD LINE THERAPIES

■ Excimer laser (308 nm)	C
■ Intense pulsed light	C
■ Copper bromide laser (577–511 nm)	C
■ 20% glycolic acid/0.05% tretinoin	C
■ 20% glycolic acid/10% L-ascorbic acid	C
■ 70% glycolic acid gel/40% trichloroacetic acid (TCA) chemical peel	D
■ *Centella asiatica* extract	A
■ Microdermabrasion	E

The safety and efficacy of the 308-nm excimer laser for pigment correction of hypopigmented scars and striae alba. Alexiades-Armenakas MR, Bernstein LJ, Friedman PM, Geronemus RG. Arch Dermatol 2004;104:955–60.

In this randomized controlled trial, nine patients with striae alba experienced repigmentation after treatment with the excimer laser. The pigment normalization is temporary and requires maintenance treatment every 1–4 months.

Intense pulsed light in the treatment of striae distensae. Hernández-Pérez E, Colombo-Charrier E, Valencia-Ibiett E. Dermatol Surg 2002;28:1124–30.

In this prospective study, 15 women with late-stage striae of the abdomen were treated with five sessions of intense pulsed light. All patients showed clinical and microscopic improvement in their striae

Two-year follow-up results of copper bromide laser treatment of striae. Longo L, Postiglione MG, Marangoni O, Melato M. J Clin Laser Med Surg 2003;21:157–60.

Thirteen of 15 patients experienced improvement in their striae that remained after 1–2 years. One-third of the patients had total disappearance of selected striae.

Comparison of topical therapy for striae alba (20% glycolic acid/0.05% tretinoin versus 20% glycolic acid/10% L-ascorbic acid). Ash K, Lord J, Zukowski M, McDaniel DH. Dermatol Surg 1998;24:849–56.

Ten patients with skin types I through V and abdominal and thigh striae associated with childbirth applied glycolic acid in the morning and either tretinoin or L-ascorbic acid in the evening for a total of 12 weeks. All patients in the study felt that they had improvement of their striae.

Chemical peel of nonfacial skin using glycolic acid gel augmented with TCA and neutralized based on visual staging. Cook KK, Cook WR. Dermatol Surg 2000;26:994–9.

The authors comment about their experience treating over 3100 patients with nonfacial peels using a combination of 70% glycolic acid gel combined with 40% TCA. It is reported that striae, including atrophic hypopigmented striae, can be improved with this treatment.

Prophylaxis of striae gravidarum with a topical formulation: a double blind trial. Mallol J, Belda MA, Costa D, et al. Int J Cosmetic Sci 1991;3:51–7.

One hundred pregnant women applied either Trofolastin cream (contains *C. asiatica*, α-tocopherol, and collagen–elastin hydrolysates) or placebo daily from 12 weeks' gestation until labor. The product, which is only available in Europe, helped women who already had striae from developing additional striae in pregnancy.

Extracts of C. asiatica, a medicinal plant, are widely used outside the USA for many dermatologic conditions including striae, keloids, hypertrophic scars, chronic venous insufficiency, leprosy sores, slow-healing wounds, and cellulitis.

Laser therapy of stretch marks. McDaniel DH. Dermatol Clin 2002;20:67–76.

The author states that microdermabrasion has become part of the adjunctive armamentarium for striae, often combined with laser, topical agents, and chemical peels.

Subacute cutaneous lupus erythematosus

Jeffrey P Callen

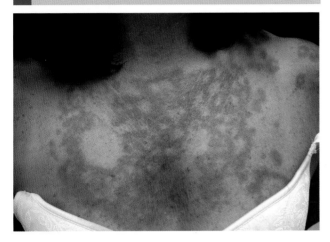

Subacute cutaneous lupus erythematosus (SCLE) is a non-scarring, non-atrophy-producing variant of lupus erythematosus that was first distinguished from other cutaneous variants in 1979. In the original article Sontheimer et al. (1979) described two subsets: patients with annular disease, and patients with papulosquamous disease. It might be debated whether tumid LE belongs to the SCLE subset of LE, because these patients have nonscarring lesions; however, they have chronic disease and rarely manifest a positive serology, in contrast to the patient with SCLE in whom ANA positivity is frequent and anti-Ro (SS-A) is common. At least half of the patients with SCLE have or develop four or more of the features that allow classification as systemic LE. In general, however, their prognosis is better than unselected patients with systemic LE.

MANAGEMENT STRATEGY

Therapy of cutaneous lesions in patients with LE involves both an empiric as well as a scientific approach. Unfortunately, there are few double-blind, placebo-controlled trials of drugs used in the treatment of cutaneous LE.

The goals of management of the patient with discoid lupus erythematosus (DLE) or SCLE are to improve the patient's appearance and prevent the development of deforming scars, atrophy, or dyspigmentation. In addition, the majority of patients with SCLE have disease that primarily affects their skin and may be reassured that their prognosis is relatively benign. Cosmetic problems are often of major importance to the patient with cutaneous LE. Dyspigmentation may follow both DLE and SCLE and may be effectively hidden by agents such as Covermark® or Dermablend®.

Once a diagnosis of subcutaneous LE has been made, management must involve *sun avoidance* and *sun protection* and *elimination of medications that might be responsible for the skin lesions*. Treatment with the most benign drugs possible should be stressed. *Topical corticosteroids* and *oral anti-*

malarials are the most commonly prescribed medications. Although *systemic corticosteroids* may be highly effective, attempts should be made to reduce their dosage and use other medications in their place to avoid corticosteroid side effects.

SPECIFIC INVESTIGATIONS

- Thorough evaluation to exclude systemic disease
- History of drug ingestion that might be responsible for the disease
- History of smoking

The cornerstone of the management of DLE and SCLE is correct diagnosis and thorough evaluation. The patient should have a careful history, physical examination, and laboratory studies directed at uncovering systemic manifestations that might occur in patients with LE. The risk of serious systemic involvement in patients with SCLE is probably around 10%, though many patients, roughly 50%, with SCLE have sufficient criteria to classify them as systemic lupus erythematosus (SLE).

Subacute cutaneous lupus erythematosus associated with hydrochlorothiazide therapy. Reed BR, Huff JC, Jones SK, et al. Ann Intern Med 1985;103:49–51.

This was the first report that linked a drug ingestion to SCLE. These authors linked hydrochlorothiazide to SCLE. Discontinuation of the drug led to a clearing of the disease.

Subacute cutaneous lupus erythematosus induced or exacerbated by terbinafine: a report of five cases. Callen JP, Hughes AP, Kulp-Shorten CL. Arch Dermatol 2001;137:1196–8.

This report links terbinafine to SCLE. Four of the five patients did not have documented onychomycosis. Also, this report suggests that patients with a prior history of LE or photosensitivity may be predisposed to the development of this eruption.

Drug-induced, Ro/SSA-positive cutaneous lupus erythematosus. Srivastava M, Rencic A, Diglio G, et al. Arch Dermatol 2003;139:45–9.

This study detailed only patients with cutaneous disease who were anti-Ro/SS-A positive. However, they found that among 70 such patients, 15 had a link to a new drug within 6 months of the diagnosis of SCLE. Most of these instances were linked to antihypertensive agents, but two patients with statin-induced disease were reported.

A complete list of the patient's medications will assist in the exclusion of drug-induced cutaneous LE. Drugs that have been linked as causes of SCLE primarily include antihypertensive agents such as hydrochlorothiazide, calcium channel blockers, and angiotensin converting enzyme inhibitors. In addition, there are multiple reports of terbinafine and tumor necrosis factor-alpha (TNF-α) inhibitors that have been linked to the development of SCLE.

Report of an association between discoid lupus erythematosus and smoking. Gallego H, Crutchfield CE III, Lewis EJ, Gallego HJ. Cutis 1999;63:231–4.

These authors suggest that cutaneous LE is more severe in patients who smoke.

Patients with cutaneous lupus erythematosus who smoke are less responsive to antimalarial treatment. Jewell ML, McCauliffe DP. J Am Acad Dermatol 2000;42:983–7.

These authors compared antimalarial-responsive patients to those who did not respond. Their results indicate that patients with cutaneous LE who smoke are significantly less likely to respond to antimalarial therapy.

Patients who smoke should be encouraged to stop for the benefit of their skin disease. In personal observations, I have noted marked improvement in some patients who take this advice.

FIRST LINE THERAPIES

■ Cosmetics	E
■ Sunscreens and protective clothing	C
■ Topical corticosteroids	E
■ Antimalarials	D
■ Topical retinoids	E

Experimental reproduction of skin lesions in lupus erythematosus by UVA and UVB radiation. Lehmann P, Holze E, Kind P, Goerz G, Plewig G. J Am Acad Dermatol 1990;22:181–7.

The action spectrum was defined by photoprovocation testing and includes UVA, UVB and occasionally visible light.

Broad-spectrum sunscreens, protective clothing, and sun avoidance are important parts of an input therapy regimen.

Evaluation of the capacity of sunscreens to photoprotect lupus erythematosus patients by employing the photoprovocation test. Stege H, Budde MA, Grether S, Krutmann J. Photodermatol Photoimmunol Photomed 2000;16:256–9.

These authors examined the capacity of three sunscreens to prevent the development of skin lesions by provocative phototesting. Although each of the three sunscreens tested prevented lesions, the extent to which they did so varied greatly. The sunscreen that was most effective contained Octocrylene® as the UVB protectant, Mexoryl SX®, Mexoryl XL® and Parsol 1789® as UVA protectants, and titanium oxide. This sunscreen's SPF was 60. Their study was of only 11 patients (nine men and two women), of whom eight had SCLE and three had DLE.

Intralesional triamcinolone is effective for discoid lupus erythematosus of the palms and soles. Callen JP. J Rheumatol 1985;12:630–3.

Intralesional injections of corticosteroids are often effective in patients with lesions that are refractory to topical corticosteroids. Small amounts of triamcinolone acetonide may be injected with a 30-gauge needle into multiple areas. These injections are often very effective in control of the lesions, but do not prevent the development of new lesions.

The potential for cutaneous atrophy and/or dyspigmentation similar to that seen with the disease should be discussed with the patient; however, in most cases an experienced dermatologist is able to inject without a great risk. Alternative agents for intralesional injection have not been well tested.

The association of the two antimalarials chloroquine and quinacrine for treatment-resistent chronic and subacute cutaneous lupus erythematosus. Feldmann R, Salomon D, Saurat JH. Dermatology 1994;189:425–7.

The first line therapy is the use of an antimalarial drug. The antimalarial preferred by the author is hydroxychloroquine sulfate

(Plaquenil®). This drug is used in doses of 200 mg orally once or twice daily, or in a dose of less than 6.5 mg/kg daily. The onset of action of the antimalarial agents is roughly 4–8 weeks and for this reason some physicians have advocated higher initial loading doses. Hydroxychloroquine is also of benefit for the joint symptoms and malaise that may accompany SCLE. Hydroxychloroquine is less toxic, but also less effective than chloroquine phosphate (Aralen®), which is used in doses of 250–500 mg daily. Thus patients who fail to fully respond to hydroxychloroquine may be switched to chloroquine, but the two should not be used together because of the concern that ophthalmologic toxicity may be enhanced. Another antimalarial, quinacrine hydrochloride (Atabrine®), may add benefit to either hydroxychloroquine or chloroquine and is not associated with ophthalmologic toxicity. This agent is not readily available, but several compounding pharmacies in the USA have it.

Cutaneous lupus treated with topical tretinoin: a case report. Seiger E, Roland S, Goldman S. Cutis 1991;47:351–5.

This is a case report of hypertrophic lupus erythematosus treated with topical tretinoin.

Treatment of localized discoid lupus erythematosus with tazarotene. Edwards KR, Burke WA. J Am Acad Dermatol 1999;41:1049–50.

Several other topical agents might be of use in individual patients with SCLE. None of these agents has been tested in any systematic manner. It appears that they are more likely to be effective in chronic cutaneous LE. Other topical nonsteroidal agents that might be considered in the future would be tacrolimus and imiquimod.

Topical tacrolimus therapy of resistant cutaneous lesions in lupus erythematosus: a possible alternative. Lampropoulos CE, Sangle S, Harrison P, et al. Rheumatology 2004;43:1383–5.

This is an open-label study of 12 patients with various types of cutaneous lesions who had disease that was recalcitrant to previous therapies including systemic therapies. The patients with a malar photosensitive eruption responded best and those with discoid LE lesions responded less well. Two of the four patients with SCLE included in this study responded to therapy with topical tacrolimus.

Pimecrolimus 1% cream for cutaneous lupus erythematosus. Kreuter A, Gambichler T, Breuckmann F, et al. J Am Acad Dermatol 2004;51:407–10.

This is an open-label study of 11 patients with various forms of cutaneous LE. The two patients with SCLE within this study had excellent responses. These patients differ from those in the tacrolimus study in that they were not selected for recalcitrant disease and therefore this method of selection may have been associated with an improved response rate.

SECOND LINE THERAPIES

■ Dapsone	E
■ Gold	B
■ Antibiotics	E
■ Thalidomide	B
■ Retinoids	C
■ Immunosuppressive agents – methotrexate, azathioprine, mycophenolate mofetil	C

Evidence levels **A** Double-blind study **B** Clinical trial ≥ 20 subjects **C** Clinical trial < 20 subjects **D** Series ≥ 5 subjects **E** Anecdotal case reports

Dapsone is an effective therapy for the skin lesions of subacute cutaneous lupus erythematosus and urticarial vasculitis in a patient with C2 deficiency. Holtman J, Neustadt D, Callen JP. J Rheumatol 1990;17:122–5.

A case of SLE with acute, subacute and chronic cutaneous lesions successfully treated with dapsone. Neri R, Mosca M, Bernacchi E, Bombardieri S. Lupus 1999;8:240–3.

Low-dose dapsone in the treatment of subacute cutaneous lupus erythematosus. Fenton DA, Black MM. Clin Exp Dermatol 1986;11:102–3.

Dapsone, given in doses of 25–200 mg daily, has been useful for SCLE lesions and for the vasculitic lesions that may accompany SCLE, as well as for patients with bullous LE.

Auranofin in the treatment of discoid lupus erythematosus. Stenjker B. J Dermatol Treat 1991;2:27–9.

Auranofin (Ridura®), an oral form of gold, has been used for cutaneous LE. Complete remission occurs in a minority of patients, about 15%, while a partial response has been noted in about two-thirds of those treated.

Treatment of chronic discoid lupus erythematosus with an oral gold compound (auranofin). Dalziel K, Going G, Cartwright PH, et al. Br J Dermatol 1986;115:211–6.

Nineteen of 23 patients responded to oral gold in this open study, with complete resolution of lesions in four of the patients.

The author's personal experience has been encouraging in a small number of patients. Auranofin is begun at a dose of 3 mg daily and after 1 week the dose may be raised to twice daily if the patient experiences no problem with nausea, diarrhea, or headache. Monitoring with regular complete blood counts and urinalysis is suggested. The author has seen one patient with a lichenoid drug eruption presumed to be due to the auranofin.

Long-term cefuroxime axetil in subacute cutaneous lupus erythematosus. A report of three cases. Rudnicka L, Szymanska E, Walecka I, Stowinska M. Dermatology 2000;200:129–31.

A variety of antibiotics have been used for the treatment of SCLE. Rudnicka et al. reported that the antibiotic cefuroxime axetil resulted in the clearing of skin lesions in three patients with SCLE at a dose of 500 mg daily. Cefuroxime axetil is a second generation β-lactamase oral cephalosporin. Others must replicate this observation before it can be recommended for widespread use, but it is a relatively benign form of treatment.

Traitment du lupus erythemateux chronique par la sulfasalazine: 11 observations. Delaporte E, Catteau B, Sabbagh N, et al. Ann Dermatol Venereol 1997;124:151–6.

Another group has reported the successful use of sulfasalazine in eight of 11 patients. Sulfasalazine is a combination drug used for inflammatory bowel disease and various arthritides. These authors administered 2 g daily, but noted that the minimal effective daily dose was 1.5 g. The eight patients who responded were all rapid acetylators, while the three who failed to respond were all slow acetylators. No serious toxicity was noted in this small open-label case series.

Sulfasalazine in the treatment of cutaneous lupus erythematosus: open trial in six cases. (Abstract) LaGrange S, Piette J-C, Becherel P-A, et al. Lupus 1998;7:21.

LaGrange et al. noted a drug eruption in five of six patients treated with sulfasalazine and in only two patients did they feel that there was a beneficial effect.

Treatment of cutaneous lesions of systemic lupus erythematosus with thalidomide. Atra E, Sato EI. Clin Exp Rheumatol 1993;11:487–93.

Of 23 patients with SLE treated with thalidomide 300 mg daily, 18 had complete remission of cutaneous lesions, two had partial improvement, and three discontinued treatment because of side effects. Drowsiness and abdominal distention were the most common adverse effects and were dose related.

American experience with low-dose thalidomide therapy for severe cutaneous lupus erythematosus. Duong JD, Spigel T, Moxley RT III, Gaspari AA. Arch Dermatol 1999; 135:1079–87.

Thalidomide in the treatment of cutaneous lupus erythematosus refractory to conventional therapy. Ordi-Ros J, Cortes F, Cucurull E, et al. J Rheumatol 2000;27:1429–33.

Six of seven patients treated with low-dose, long-term thalidomide experienced marked resolution or complete clearing of cutaneous lesions in an average of 2.2 months. Sedation, constipation, weight gain, intermittent shaking, and paresthesias occurred.

Low-dose thalidomide therapy for refractory cutaneous lesions of lupus erythematosus. Housman TS, Jorizzo JL, McCarty MA, et al. Arch Dermatol 2003;139:50–4.

This is a retrospective analysis of 23 patients treated with thalidomide for at least 1 month for various skin lesions of LE including three patients with SCLE; 74% of the patients had complete resolution of their disease, but with discontinuation of thalidomide relapse was frequent. Neurological toxicity was common, occurring in five patients as documented by nerve conduction studies.

Thalidomide in cutaneous lupus erythematosus. Pelle MT, Werth VP. Am J Clin Dermatol 2003;4:379–87.

This is an excellent compilation of reports of the use of thalidomide for cutaneous lupus erythematosus.

Thalidomide inhibits UVB-induced mouse keratinocyte apoptosis by both TNF-α-dependent and TNF-α-independent pathways. Lu KQ, Brenneman S, Burns R, et al. Photodermatol Photoimmunol Photomed 2003;19:272–80.

These authors used a mouse model to ascertain the mechanism by which thalidomide may exert its effects.

Thalidomide has recently become more available and is being used for patients with cutaneous LE with some regularity. Its mechanism of action is believed to involve a decrease in inflammatory mediators, particularly TNF-α and Fas ligand. Open-label trials suggest that it is highly effective, and may result in an increase in the lymphocyte count and a decrease in the C-reactive protein level. Induction with 100–300 mg daily at bedtime results in improvement in 90% of the patients who are able to tolerate the drug. Toxicity commonly associated with thalidomide use includes drowsiness, headache, weight gain, amenorrhea, and dizziness. Drowsiness and dizziness may persist during the following day. Neuropathy, usually sensory, may limit the ability of patients to continue thalidomide on a long-term basis. Neuropathy may be reversible, but there are patients whose neuropathy has progressed despite stopping the drug. Whether nerve conduction studies should be performed at the onset of therapy and periodically is not known, but in their recent summary paper, Pelle and Werth suggest this study at baseline and every 6 months while on therapy. I choose not to perform nerve conduction studies unless symptoms develop. Thalidomide is a potent teratogen and accordingly the company has developed a program to prevent the chance of pregnancy in patients exposed to the drug. The program requires that the prescribing physician and the pharmacy be registered with the company and that the patient use extra precautions in taking the drug. No more than a 1-month supply may be written for at any one time. Unfortunately the response to thalidomide is not durable in most patients, therefore long-term, low-dose maintenance therapy may be necessary.

Mechanism-oriented assessment of isotretinoin in chronic or subacute cutaneous lupus erythematosus. Newton RC, Jorizzo JL, Solomon AR, et al. Arch Dermatol 1986;122: 180–6.

Eight of ten patients with cutaneous LE had an excellent response to oral isotretinoin 80 mg daily for 16 weeks.

Treatment of cutaneous lupus erythematosus with etretinate. Ruzicka T, Meurer M, Brown-Falco O. Acta Derm Venereol 1985;65:324–9.

Eleven of 19 patients with cutaneous lupus erythematosus had excellent results after 2–6 weeks of treatment with etretinate.

Oral retinoids are effective in many patients who have failed to respond to previous less toxic therapies. Isotretinoin and acitretin (formerly etretinate was used) have both been used in doses similar to those used for acne vulgaris or psoriasis, respectively. The response is not durable and after short courses the patient will still need further suppressive therapy. These agents are particularly helpful in patients with hypertrophic lesions of chronic cutaneous LE. Experience in SCLE is limited.

Azathioprine: an effective, corticosteroid-sparing therapy for patients with recalcitrant cutaneous lupus erythematosus or with recalcitrant cutaneous leukocytoclastic vasculitis. Callen JP, Spencer LV, Burruss JB, Holtman J. Arch Dermatol 1991;127:515–22.

Three of six patients with chronic cutaneous LE had an excellent response to azathioprine, permitting prednisone doses to be reduced.

Management of cutaneous lupus erythematosus with low-dose methotrexate: indication for modulation of inflammatory mechanisms. Boehm IB, Boehm GA, Bauer R. Rheumatol Int 1998;18:59–62.

Ten of 12 patients with cutaneous LE responded to weekly low-dose methotrexate (10–25 mg). Five of the patients had long remissions (5–24 months) after stopping the methotrexate.

Successful treatment of subacute cutaneous lupus erythematosus with mycophenolate mofetil. Schanz S, Ulmer A, Rassner G, Fierlbeck G. Br J Dermatol 2002;147:174–8.

Two patients with SCLE were treated with mycophenolate mofetil.

Treatment of resistent discoid lupus erythematosus of the palms and soles with mycophenolate mofetil. Goyal S, Nousari HC. J Am Acad Dermatol 2001;45:142–4.

Mycophenolate mofetil has been used successfully to treat cutaneous disease.

Treatment of discoid and subacute cutaneous lupus erythematosus with cyclophosphamide. Schulz EJ, Menter MA. Br J Dermatol 1971;85:60–5.

Several cytotoxic agents have been reported to be beneficial for the control of cutaneous LE lesions. Azathioprine has perhaps had the greatest number of reports, but methotrexate and mycophenolate mofetil have also been reported to benefit patients with 'recalcitrant' disease. Individual reports have suggested that cyclophosphamide may be effective.

THIRD LINE THERAPIES

■ Clofazimine	E
■ Phenytoin	B
■ High-dose intravenous immune globulin	C
■ Cytokine therapy	D

Clofazimine (Lamprene) in the treatment of discoid lupus erythematosus. Krivanek JFC, Paver WKA, Kossard S, Cains G. Australas J Dermatol 1976;17:108–10.

Clofazimine failed to demonstrate efficacy in all but one report.

Phenytoin in the treatment of discoid lupus erythematosus. Rodriquez-Castellanos MA, Rubio JB, Gomez JFB, Mendoza AG. Arch Dermatol 1995;131:620–1.

This group studied 93 patients with cutaneous LE and observed excellent results in 90%. They administered oral phenytoin 300 mg daily to their patients for up to 6 months. Relapse occurred in at least one-third of patients for whom follow-up data were available, but prolonged remission of 6–12 months was noted in 33 patients. Toxicity was minimal in prevalence and severity.

The author has not tried this agent in patients with cutaneous LE.

Intravenous immunoglobulin (IVIg) for therapy-resistant cutaneous lupus erythematosus. Goodfield M, Davison K, Bowden K. J Dermatolog Treat 2004;15:46–50.

This is an open-label study of 12 patients with various forms of cutaneous LE, all of whom had SLE. Three of the patients had SCLE. Of the ten evaluable patients, five had excellent responses, two had partial responses and three had limited or no responses. One patient develop an acute cutaneous vasculitis otherwise there were no significant adverse reactions.

High-dose intravenous immune globulin has been used successfully – 1 g/kg daily for two consecutive days monthly was administered to these patients who had failed to respond to multiple previous therapies. Although there might be an excellent response in some patients, the response is often short-lived. Toxicity is minimal, but this therapy is extremely expensive.

Response of discoid and subacute cutaneous lupus erythematosus to recombinant interferon alpha-2a. Nicolas J-F, Thivolet J, Kanitkis J, Lyonnet S. J Invest Dermatol 1990; 95:142S–5S.

Interferon-alfa has been used successfully; however, all patients on this regimen develop toxicity and long-term remission is rarely achieved.

Treatment of severe cutaneous lupus erythematosus with a chimeric CD4 monoclonal antibody, cM-T412. Prinz JC,

Meurer M, Reiter C, et al. J Am Acad Dermatol 1996;34: 244–52.

Prinz and colleagues have used chimeric CD4 monoclonal antibody infusions in five patients with severe, refractory cutaneous LE. Longlasting improvement was noted, with a restoration of responsiveness to conventional treatments.

If other cytokines can be administered and result in the restoration of response to less toxic therapy, then perhaps we will be able to induce remission with one agent and maintain it with another.

Regression of subacute cutaneous lupus erythematosus in a patient with rheumatoid arthritis treated with a biologic tumor necrosis factor alpha-blocking agent: comment on the article by Pisetsky and the letter from Aringer et al. Fautrel B, Foltz V, Frances C, et al. Arthritis Rheum 2002; 46:1408–9.

This is a single case report. There have been multiple reports linking TNF-α antagonists to the development of cutaneous as well as systemic LE.

There are many new biologic agents that might prove to be useful for cutaneous LE. Caution should be used with the TNF antagonists because although an individual case of benefit has been reported, there are many patients in whom these drugs have resulted in development of the disease. Properly conducted observational studies followed by placebo-controlled trials will be helpful.

Subcorneal pustular dermatosis

Rebecca C C Brooke, Robert J G Chalmers

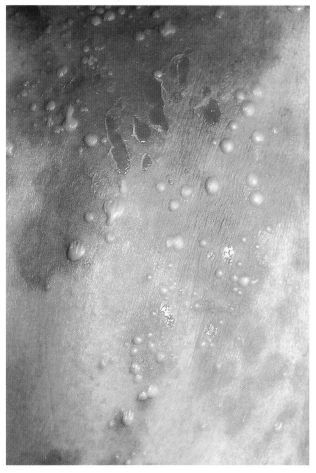

Subcorneal pustular dermatosis is a rare, chronic, neutrophilic dermatosis of unknown etiology, in which flaccid pustules and vesicopustules, classically forming a hypopyon, arise in crops on truncal and flexural skin. The condition occurs in any age, more commonly in females, and usually follows a relapsing and remitting course, but generally the patient remains systemically well. Long-term follow-up is required because monoclonal IgA paraproteinemia or myeloma may occur many years after presentation. The condition may be difficult to differentiate from other vesicopustular dermatoses and some cases may eventuate into pustular psoriasis.

MANAGEMENT STRATEGY

Dapsone is the treatment of choice (25–200 mg daily) and normally results in resolution of the rash within 4 weeks; the drug usually needs to be continued long term because relapse is common on withdrawal of therapy. After control is gained, the dose should be tapered to the lowest dose required to maintain remission. Other sulfones (*sulfapyri-dine, salazosulfapyridine*) have also been reported to be beneficial in isolated reports.

In a proportion of cases the response to dapsone is poor; *retinoids* (formerly etretinate, now replaced by acitretin) have been substituted with success, using an initial dose of 0.5–1.0 mg/kg daily and then reducing to the lowest dose that will maintain control. Alternatively, for those unable to tolerate dapsone in the dose required, retinoids have been added to dapsone; this has enabled lower doses of each to be used. There are a few case reports detailing good response to *phototherapy – psoralen and UVA (PUVA), narrowband UVB, or broadband UVB* – in combination with dapsone or retinoids.

Both *topical* and *systemic corticosteroids* have been reported to provide some degree of control in isolated cases. Unacceptably high doses of systemic corticosteroids may be required, but combination with *dapsone, cyclosporine, vitamin E, or antibiotics (minocycline, tetracycline)* may allow control with lower doses.

Subcorneal pustular dermatosis tends to run a chronic course. Maintenance of a continuing beneficial response may be difficult, as may be inferred from the extensive range of treatment options described. Although dapsone appears to offer the best chance of a good therapeutic response, treatment regimens for this condition have not been formally evaluated.

Immunofluorescence studies have shown that a subset of patients have intraepidermal deposits of IgA. These have been given various alternative designations including IgA pemphigus, intraepidermal IgA pustulosis, or intercellular IgA dermatosis and in a number of them desmocollin 1 has been identified as the target antigen.

SPECIFIC INVESTIGATIONS

- Full blood count
- Immunoglobulin levels
- Immunoelectrophoresis
- Bence–Jones protein
- Autoantibodies
- Biopsy with immunofluorescence

Subcorneal pustular dermatosis: a clinical study of ten patients. Lutz ME, Daoud MS, McEvoy MT, Gibson LE. Cutis 1998;61:203–8.

Four of seven patients tested had paraproteinemia, three of IgA and one of IgG type. A further three had subcorneal deposits of IgA on direct immunofluorescence.

Subcorneal pustular dermatosis (Sneddon–Wilkinson disease) in association with a monoclonal IgA gammopathy: a report and review of the literature. Kasha EE, Epinette WW. J Am Acad Dermatol 1988;19:854–8.

Subcorneal pustular dermatosis and IgA λ myeloma: an uncommon association but probably not coincidental. Vaccaro M, Cannavò SP, Guarneri F. Eur J Dermatol 1999;9:644–6.

A case report of IgA λ myeloma. Treatment of the underlying myeloma had no effect on the skin disease.

Sneddon–Wilkinson disease in association with rheumatoid arthritis. Butt A, Burge SM. Br J Dermatol 1995;132:313–5.

Useful overview of all reported cases associated with either seronegative or seropositive arthritis.

Subcorneal pustular dermatosis. Reed J, Wilkinson J. Clin Dermatol 2000;18:301–13.

Review, with detailed tables of associations and differential diagnoses.

Intraepidermal IgA pustulosis. Wallach D. J Am Acad Dermatol 1992;27:993–1000.

Overview of all reported cases.

Subcorneal pustular dermatosis has also been reported in association with pyoderma gangrenosum, Crohn's disease, ulcerative colitis, systemic lupus erythematosus, morphea, myeloproliferative disorders, hyperthyroidism, multiple sclerosis, solid tumors, and infections, particularly mycoplasma. Isolated reports detail resolution with treatment of the associated disorder. Two drugs have been implicated: diltiazem and thiols (bucillamine or gold sodium thiomalate). In one case the condition arose at the site of injection of recombinant human granulocyte-macrophage colony stimulating factor.

FIRST LINE THERAPIES

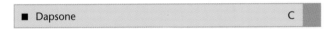

■ Dapsone	C

Subcorneal pustular dermatosis. Sneddon IB, Wilkinson DS. Br J Dermatol 1956;68:385–93.

Three of six patients responded to dapsone 50–100 mg daily.

Sneddon–Wilkinson disease in association with rheumatoid arthritis. Butt A, Burge SM. Br J Dermatol 1995;132: 313–5.

A further five patients who responded to dapsone.

Dapsone is the treatment of choice with over 20 reports of successful control. Combination with other drugs has been reported to be helpful.

Subcorneal pustular dermatosis and IgA gammopathy. Burrows D, Bingham EA. Br J Dermatol 1984;111(suppl 26): 91–3.

Addition of etretinate enabled control in a patient intolerant of higher dose dapsone.

Subcorneal pustular dermatosis treated with PUVA therapy. Bauwens M, De Coninck A, Roseeuw D. Dermatology 1999;198:203–5.

A patient resistant to dapsone alone responded well to combination with PUVA.

Sneddon-Wilkinson disease. Four cases report. Launay F, Albes B, Bayle P, Carriere M, et al. Rev Med Interne 2004; 25:154–9.

Three responded to dapsone, one to etretinate.

Subcorneal pustular dermatosis in a young boy. Garg BR, Sait MA, Baruah MC. Indian J Dermatol 1985;30:21–3.

Report of dapsone use in a child.

SECOND LINE THERAPIES

■ Sulfones	D
■ Corticosteroids	D
■ Etretinate (no longer marketed)	D
■ Acitretin	E
■ PUVA	D
■ Narrowband UVB	E
■ Broadband UVB	E

Subcorneal pustular dermatosis. Sneddon IB, Wilkinson DS. Br J Dermatol 1956;68:385–93.

Two patients were controlled on sulfapyridine 1 g twice daily.

Pyoderma gangrenosum followed by subcorneal pustular dermatosis in a patient with IgA paraproteinemia. Kohl PK, Hartschuh W, Tilgen W, Frosch PJ. J Am Acad Dermatol 1991;24:325–8.

Sulfasalazine (salazosulfapyridine) 3 g daily provided control in this patient.

Subcorneal pustular dermatosis in children. Johnson SAM, Cripps DJ. Arch Dermatol 1974;109:73–7.

Two children were controlled but not cleared with topical and systemic corticosteroids.

Role of tumour necrosis factor-α in Sneddon–Wilkinson subcorneal pustular dermatosis. Grob JJ, Mege JL, Capo C, et al. J Am Acad Dermatol 1991;25:944–7.

Methylprednisolone induced remission in this patient who failed to respond to dapsone, etretinate, or plasma exchange. A maintenance dose of 12 mg daily was required.

An unusual severe case of subcorneal pustular dermatosis treated with cyclosporine and prednisolone. Zachariae CO, Rossen K, Weismann K. Acta Derm Venereol 2000;80:386–7.

After failure with dapsone and prednisolone (because of abnormal liver enzymes), cyclosporine (400 mg daily) was substituted for dapsone; onset of resolution was swift, and cyclosporine was stopped after 3 weeks; prednisolone was slowly tailed off over a 2-month period with no recurrence.

Treatment of subcorneal pustulosis by etretinate. Iandoli R, Monfrecola G. Dermatologica 1987;175:235–8.

A patient who failed to respond to dapsone 300 mg daily and topical corticosteroids responded well to etretinate 1 mg/kg daily. A maintenance dose of 0.75 mg/kg daily was required.

Successful treatment of subcorneal pustular dermatosis (Sneddon–Wilkinson disease) by acitretin: report of a case. Marlière V, Beylot-Barry M, Beylot C, Doutre M-S. Dermatology 1999;199:153–5.

This paper reviews the use of retinoids for subcorneal pustular dermatosis.

Subcorneal pustular dermatosis treated with PUVA therapy. Bauwens M, De Coninck A, Roseeuw D. Dermatology 1999;198:203–5.

This paper contains a useful overview of PUVA therapy.

Subcorneal pustular dermatosis (Sneddon–Wilkinson disease) treated with narrowband (TL-01) UVB phototherapy. Cameron H, Dawe RS. Br J Dermatol 1997;137:150–1.

This patient was initially controlled with minocycline 200 mg daily and topical corticosteroids, but suffered a flare that was poorly responsive. Narrowband UVB phototherapy enabled corticosteroids to be withdrawn and control maintained with minocycline alone.

Subcorneal pustular dermatosis responsive to narrowband (TL-01) UVB phototherapy. Orton DI, George SA. Br J Dermatol 1997;137:149–50.

After long-term PUVA treatment this patient achieved a satisfactory response with narrowband UVB phototherapy.

Subcorneal pustular dermatosis treated with phototherapy. Park YK, Park HY, Bang DS, Cho CK. Int J Dermatol 1986;25:124–6.

After failure of dapsone, prednisolone, and topical fluocinolone acetonide, lasting remission was achieved with broadband UVB.

THIRD LINE THERAPIES

■ Infliximab	E
■ Tacalcitol (1α,24-dihydroxyvitamin D₃)	E
■ Mizoribine	E
■ Ketoconazole	E
■ Tetracycline, minocycline	E
■ Benzylpenicillin	E
■ Vitamin E	E
■ Mebhydrolin	E

Infliximab (anti-tumor necrosis factor alpha antibody): a novel, highly effective treatment of recalcitrant subcorneal pustular dermatosis (Sneddon–Wilkinson disease). Voigtlander C, Luftl M, Schuler G, Hertl M. Arch Dermatol 2001;137:1571–4.

Intravenous infliximab, after suitable work-up, at a dose of 5 mg/kg over 2 h was given after therapeutic trials of multiple agents failed, enabling oral methylprednisolone to be withdrawn and the dose of acitretin to be stabilized at 0.4 mg/kg daily. After 14 days the patient developed new pustules and a second dose of infliximab was given, again with excellent results. Over a 3-month period complete remission was achieved with oral methylprednisolone and acitretin.

Recalcitrant subcorneal pustular dermatosis and bullous pemphigoid treated with mizoribine, an immunosuppressive, purine biosynthesis inhibitor. Kono T, Terashima T, Oura H, et al. Br J Dermatol 2000;143:1328–30.

Two patients responded to mizoribine (Bredinin®) 150 mg daily, one to mizoribine alone, the other with combined prednisolone 50 mg and mizoribine 150 mg daily.

A case of subcorneal pustular dermatosis treated with tacalcitol (1alpha,24-dihydroxyvitamin D₃). Kawaguchi M, Mitsuhashi Y, Kondo S. J Dermatol. 2000;27:669–72.

Topical vitamin D3 led to sustained resolution of lesions.

Ketoconazole as a therapeutic modality in subcorneal pustular dermatosis. Verma KK, Pasricha JS. Acta Derm Venereol 1977;77:407–8.

After failing to respond to dapsone a patient achieved remission using ketoconazole 200 mg daily. Although initially started in conjunction with dapsone, on withdrawal she flared and was controlled subsequently on ketoconazole alone.

Subcorneal pustular dermatosis (Sneddon–Wilkinson). Mandel EH, Gonzales V. Arch Dermatol 1969;99:246–7.

Tetracycline 250 mg four times daily controlled new pustule formation.

Cutaneous manifestations of neutrophilic disease. Vignon-Pennamen MD, Wallach D. Dermatologica 1991;183:255–64.

An overview of seven cases with various neutrophilic dermatoses.

Subcorneal pustular dermatosis with polyarthritis. Lin RY, Schwartz RA, Lambert WC. Cutis 1986;37:123–6.

Intravenous benzylpenicillin (20 million units daily), plus topical triamcinolone resolved both the arthritis and rash over a period of 8 days. No follow-up information given.

Subcorneal pustular dermatosis controlled by vitamin E. Ayres S, Mihan R. Arch Dermatol 1974;109:74.

Vitamin E (400 IU D-α-tocopheryl acetate), when added to prednisolone 40 mg daily, enabled the dosage of prednisolone to be reduced to 5 mg daily.

Subcorneale pustulose Sneddon Wilkinson, therapie mit Mebhydrolin. Dorittke P, Wassilew SW. Z Hautkrankheiten 1988;63:1025–7.

Mebhydrolin, 50 mg three times daily, was successful.

Subcutaneous fat necrosis of the newborn

Bernice R Krafchik

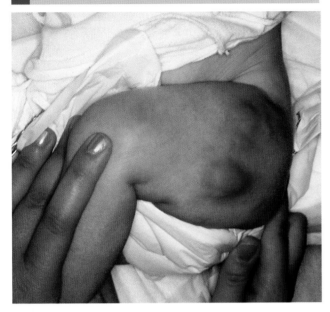

Subcutaneous fat necrosis (SFN) is a rare, self-limiting, skin disease occurring in neonates and affecting areas where fat tissue is found. The condition is thought to arise from perinatal stress; it usually resolves spontaneously within 3–6 months with no scarring, although occasionally small pits are left. Treatment is seldom necessary, except in the rare instances when liquefaction of the fat tissue occurs or when persistent hypercalcemia develops.

MANAGEMENT STRATEGY

Biopsy is usually not warranted because the clinical picture is typical. MRI scans may demonstrate characteristic features. The lesions of SFN heal over a few months leaving normal skin or small pitted scars, and very occasionally absence of fat tissue in the affected areas. The rare occurrence of liquefaction in the lesions is treated by *removal of the liquid with a large-bore needle*.

Hypercalcemia and hypercalciuria may develop (in about one-third of patients in one series, who were admitted to the hospital). Hypercalcemia is diagnosed by the blood sampling that is performed routinely in patients with SFN or more rarely if symptoms supervene. The symptoms are nonspecific and consist of fever, vomiting, lethargy, constipation, feeding difficulties, failure to thrive, and seizures. In normal infants or those with perinatal stress the calcium levels may be low in the first 2 weeks. It is important to monitor those with SFN with repeated serum calcium levels weekly or biweekly for up to 5 months to ensure that hypercalcemia does not occur. Very occasionally thrombocytopenia and hypoglycemia may occur.

Treatment regimens are determined by the levels of hypercalcemia and hypercalcuria. If serum levels are marginally raised, monitoring the serum and urine calcium may suffice and a spontaneous return to normal levels usually occurs. If the higher levels persist or rise further, treatment should be instigated. Mild hypercalcemia is treated by the *withdrawal of vitamin D and using a low calcium diet*. This is best accomplished with *breastfeeding* because breast milk is low in both vitamin D and calcium. If this is not possible or helpful a formula low in calcium with no vitamin D should be used. If a reduction in calcium does not occur or the levels rise, *intravenous saline at 1.5 times the maintenance requirement* is given to promote the renal excretion of calcium. This is augmented with furosemide, which further promotes excretion. Other options for nonresponders include calcitonin (4–8 IU/kg every 6–12 h), bisphosphonates (pamidronate), and oral corticosteroids (hydrocortisone or prednisone). The latter treatments should be instituted with the help of a pediatric endocrinologist.

SPECIFIC INVESTIGATIONS

- Follow serum and urine calcium for 5 months
- If hypercalcemia occurs, calcium should be monitored biweekly
- Monitor calcium/creatinine ratio in the urine
- Ultrasound of kidneys for nephrocalcinosis and nephrolithiasis; other organs may be involved and should be checked radiologically

Subcutaneous fat necrosis of the newborn. Anderson DR, Narla LD, Dunn NL. Pediatr Radiol 1999;29:794–6.

MRI findings in a case of SFN of the newborn are presented for the first time.

Radiological case of the month. Subcutaneous fat necrosis of the newborn. Bellini C, Oddone M, Biscaldi E, Serra G. Arch Pediatr Adolesc Med 2001;155:1381–2.

A report of the diagnosis of SFN made from an MRI examination. The characteristics on MRI are typical. This procedure circumvents the necessity of performing a biopsy.

Asymptomatic hypercalcemia in subcutaneous fat necrosis. Lum CK, Solomon IL, Bachrach LK. Clin Pediatr (Phila) 1999;38:547–50.

Patients with high levels of calcium associated with SFN may remain asymptomatic. It is therefore imperative that patients with SFN continue to be monitored for serum calcium levels even after the SFN has resolved for up to 5 months.

FIRST LINE THERAPIES

No treatment for the majority of patients	C
If mild hypercalcemia develops with or without symptoms, treatment should be instigated	C
Low calcium diet and low vitamin D (either breast milk or formula)	D

Subcutaneous fat necrosis of the newborn: a review of 11 cases. Burden AD, Krafchik BR. Pediatr Dermatol 1999;16:384–7.

A review of SFN in patients admitted to the hospital. Ten of eleven patients had been delivered by caesarean section for fetal distress, and four of eleven developed hypercalcemia. Patients should be monitored for 5 months, even after the lesions of SFN have disappeared.

SECOND LINE THERAPIES

■ Intravenous saline	E
■ Furosemide 1 mg/kg two to three times daily	E

Subcutaneous fat necrosis of the newborn following hypothermia and complicated by pain and hypercalcaemia. Wiadrowski TP, Marshman G. Australas J Dermatol 2001;42:207–10.

A female infant was delivered with complications of severe meconium aspiration and birth asphyxia. She was diagnosed with SFN, which was complicated by pain resistant to treatment with opiates. Asymptomatic hypercalcemia was noted at 7 weeks on periodic testing, and treated by rehydration, diuretics, prednisolone, etidronate and a low-calcium and -vitamin D diet. Treatment of hypercalcemia in SFN is reviewed.

Subcutaneous fat necrosis of the newborn: hypercalcaemia with hepatic and atrial myocardial calcification. Dudink J, Walther FJ, Beekman RP. Arch Dis Child Fetal Neonatal Ed 2003;88:F343–5.

This case report discusses the various treatments of SFN and the calcification of organs that may result from severe involvement. The need to monitor serum levels of calcium is stressed.

THIRD LINE THERAPIES

■ Oral prednisone 1–3 mg/kg daily in divided doses for 48 h to three weeks	E
■ Subcutaneous calcitonin 4–8 IU/kg every 6–12 h	E
■ Pamidronate 0.5 mg/kg infused intravenously over 4 h	E

Intravenous bisphosphonate for hypercalcemia accompanying subcutaneous fat necrosis: a novel treatment approach. Khan N, Licata A, Rogers D. Clin Pediatr (Phila) 2001;40:217–9.

Oral bisphosphonates are poorly absorbed. This is the first report of intravenous administration of a bisphosphonate that resulted in fast normalization of the hypercalcemia from SFN. The drug acts by slowing the calcium turnover from bone.

Etidronate therapy for hypercalcemia in subcutaneous fat necrosis of the newborn. Rice AM, Rivkees SA. J Pediatr 1999;134:349–51.

SFN may occasionally be associated with hypercalcemia and even more rarely this may become life-threatening. Etidronate, a bisphosphonate may be used to control hypercalcemia in infants with SFN.

Expanding role of bisphosphonate therapy in children. Shoemaker LR. J Pediatr 1999;134:264–7.

The initial report of improvement with bisphosphonates appeared over 30 years ago, but pediatric experience has been limited. Although the first adverse effects on the growing skeleton have been exaggerated, physicians should warn parents that careful monitoring is important.

Sweet's syndrome

*Sarah E Dick, Joel M Gelfand,
William D James*

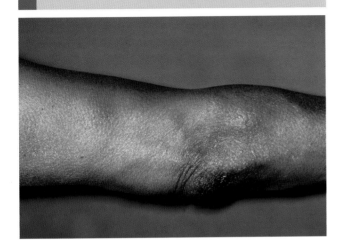

Sweet's syndrome is a neutrophilic dermatosis with characteristic clinical and histopathologic features.

MANAGEMENT STRATEGY

Sweet's syndrome is characterized clinically by multiple, painful, well-demarcated, nonscarring, erythematous plaques or pustules on the face, neck, upper trunk, and extremities. There can be a pseudovesicular appearance. Fever, leukocytosis, arthralgias, myalgias, headaches, and general malaise may occur. Oral, ocular, and internal organ involvement is rarely present. Neutrophilic dermatosis of the dorsal hands (NDDH) is a recently identified entity and is classified as an anatomically limited subset of Sweet's syndrome. Histologically, there is a diffuse neutrophilic infiltrate in the upper dermis without evidence of primary leukocytoclastic vasculitis.

Sweet's syndrome often affects adult women. It is usually idiopathic, but may be associated with malignancy (most commonly acute myelogenous leukemia, but also lymphomas, dysproteinemias, and carcinomas), inflammatory bowel disease, infection (commonly *Streptococcus* or *Yersinia*), medication (usually to granulocyte colony stimulating factor [G-CSF]), and pregnancy. A work-up including skin biopsy, complete physical examination, and laboratory studies is indicated. Treatment of the underlying associated condition or discontinuation of the causative medication may lead to resolution of skin lesions.

The standard treatment for Sweet's syndrome is *oral corticosteroids*. Pulse *intravenous corticosteroid* therapy has been successful for refractory and recurrent disease. High-potency *topical corticosteroids or intralesional corticosteroids* are beneficial for mild or localized disease. For patients with contraindications to corticosteroids, or in cases where a corticosteroid-sparing agent is desired, therapies such as *potassium iodide, colchicine, indomethacin, dapsone*, and *clofazimine* may be used. Antibiotics including *doxycycline* and *metronidazole* have been reported to be beneficial in some patients with and without dermatosis-associated infections. In recalcitrant cases, *cyclosporine, interferon-α, cyclophosphamide, chlorambucil*, or *oral retinoids* may be utilized.

SPECIFIC INVESTIGATIONS

- History and physical examination
- Complete blood count with differential and erythrocyte sedimentation rate
- Medical work-up as indicated by history and physical examination
- Cultures as indicated by history and physical examination
- Pregnancy test (in women of childbearing potential)
- Rule out medication etiology

Sweet's syndrome revisited: a review of disease concepts. Cohen PR, Kurzrock R. Int J Dermatol 2003;42:761–78.
Excellent review of the literature.

Neutrophilic dermatosis of the dorsal hands: pustular vasculitis revisited. Galaria NA, Junkins-Hopkins JM, Kligman D, et al. J Am Acad Dermatol 2000;43:870–4.

Review of three cases of neutrophilic dermatosis limited to the dorsal hands. The term NDDH is proposed for this entity. Given the lack of primary leukocytoclastic vasculitis on biopsy findings, it is categorized as a subset of Sweet's syndrome rather than a type of vasculitis.

FIRST LINE THERAPIES

■ Oral corticosteroids	C
■ Topical and intralesional corticosteroids	C

Sweet's syndrome: a review of current treatment options. Cohen PR, Kurzrock R. Am J Clin Dermatol 2002;3:117–31.

Excellent review of the literature and treatment options.

Corticosteroid therapy (oral prednisone 0.5–1.5 mg/kg daily tapered over 4–6 weeks) results in rapid relief of systemic symptoms (e.g. within 1–2 days) and skin lesions within 3–9 days. Up to one-third of patients will relapse.

High-potency topical corticosteroids and intralesional corticosteroids may be useful as monotherapy for patients with limited or mild disease, or as adjuvant treatment.

SECOND LINE THERAPIES

■ Potassium iodide	C
■ Colchicine	C
■ Indomethacin	C
■ Pulse intravenous corticosteroids	D
■ Dapsone	D
■ Clofazimine	D
■ Doxycycline	E
■ Metronidazole	E

Potassium iodide in dermatology: a 19th century drug for the 21st century – uses, pharmacology, adverse effects, and contraindications. Sterling JB, Heymann WR. J Am Acad Dermatol 2000;43:691–7.

Review of potassium iodide use in dermatology with review of the literature.

Usual dosage is 40–60 mg orally three times a day up to 300 mg three times a day. A supersaturated solution of potassium iodide (SSKI) may also be used. Start at three drops orally three times daily and increase one drop per dose up to ten drops (500 mg) three times daily until clear, then taper.

Long-term suppression of chronic Sweet's syndrome with colchicine. Ritter S, George R, Serwatka LM, et al. J Am Acad Dermatol 2002;47:323–4.

Case report of successful long-term treatment using colchicine with review of the literature.

Indomethacin treatment of eighteen patients with Sweet's syndrome. Jeanfils S, Joly P, Young P, et al. J Am Acad Dermatol 1997;36:436–9.

Prospective open-label noncontrolled study of 18 patients treated with indomethacin 150 mg daily for 7 days followed by 100 mg daily from days 7 to 21. Seventeen of 18 patients responded within 48 h and no relapses occurred.

Association of acute neutrophilic dermatosis and myelo-dysplastic syndrome with (6;9) chromosome translocation: a case report and review of the literature. Megarbane B, Bodemer C, Valensi F, et al. Br J Dermatol 2000;143: 1322–4.

Case report of Sweet's syndrome associated with a myelodysplastic syndrome treated successfully with pulse intravenous methylprednisolone followed by oral pred-nisone.

Pulse corticosteroid therapy has been successful for refractory and/or recurrent Sweet's syndrome. Intravenous doses of methyl-prednisolone up to 1000 mg daily for 3–5 days have been used, followed by a low-dose tapering schedule of an oral corticosteroid with or without another immunosuppressant agent.

Sweet's syndrome and malignancy in the UK. Bourke JF, Keohane S, Long CC, et al. Br J Dermatol 1997;137:609–13.

Review of 87 cases with Sweet's syndrome. Dapsone was used successfully as first line therapy in five of six cases.

Dapsone may be used as monotherapy or in combination therapy. Initial oral doses range from 100 mg daily to 200 mg daily. Sulfapyridine might also be efficacious.

Sweet's syndrome in association with generalized granu-loma annulare in a patient with previous breast cancer. Anthony F, Holden CA. Clin Exp Dermatol 2001;26:668–70.

Case report of Sweet's syndrome successfully treated with clofazimine.

Clofazimine 200 mg daily for 4 weeks followed by 100 mg daily for 4 weeks has been reported to be an effective dosage regimen in six patients.

Sweet's syndrome. Amichai B, Lazarov A, Halevy S. J Am Acad Dermatol 1995;33:144–5.

Case report of a patient with Sweet's syndrome as-sociated with a chlamydial infection who responded to tetracycline.

Tetracycline, doxycycline, and minocycline have been effective in cases of Sweet's syndrome with and without associated Chlamydia or Yersinia spp. infections.

Sweet's syndrome in association with Crohn's disease: report of a case and review of the literature. Rappaport A, Shaked M, Landau M, et al. Dis Colon Rectum 2001;44: 1526–9.

Case report of a patient with Sweet's syndrome and Crohn's disease treated successfully with metronidazole and prednisone.

THIRD LINE THERAPIES

■ Cyclosporine	E
■ Interferon	E
■ Cyclophosphamide	E
■ Chlorambucil	E
■ Etretinate	E

Peripheral ulcerative keratitis – an extracutaneous neu-trophilic disorder: report of a patient with rheumatoid arthritis, pustular vasculitis, pyoderma gangrenosum, and Sweet's syndrome with an excellent response to cyclosporine therapy. Wilson DM, John GR, Callen JP. J Am Acad Dermatol 1999;40:331–4.

Case report of a patient with Sweet's syndrome who responded to cyclosporine.

Initial doses of 2–10 mg/kg daily have been used successfully. Cyclosporine should generally be limited to short-term use given its potential renal toxicity when used chronically.

Systemic interferon-alpha treatment for idiopathic Sweet's syndrome. Bianchi L, Masi M, Hagman JH, et al. Clin Exp Dermatol 1999;24:443–5.

Case report of one patient who responded to interferon-α 3 million units intramuscularly three times weekly plus hydroxycarbamide (hydroxyurea) 500 mg twice daily for 30 days tapered to 500 mg daily for 30 days. The patient then maintained remission for 2 years with intramuscular inter-feron-α as monotherapy.

Lymphocytic infiltrates as a presenting feature of Sweet's syndrome with myelodysplasia and response to cyclo-phosphamide. Evans AV, Sabroe RA, Liddell K, et al. Br J Dermatol 2002;146:1087–90.

Case report of one patient who responded to oral cyclophosphamide 50 mg daily, with an occasional need for oral prednisolone to alleviate exacerbations.

The use of pulse methylprednisolone and chlorambucil in the treatment of Sweet's syndrome. Case JD, Smith SZ, Callen JP. Cutis 1989;44:125–9.

Case report of chronic and relapsing Sweet's syndrome successfully treated with pulse intravenous methylpred-nisolone. Remission was maintained with oral chlorambu-cil 4 mg daily.

Sweet's syndrome in a patient with idiopathic myelofibro-sis and thymoma–myasthenia gravis-immunodeficiency complex: efficacy of treatment with etretinate. Altomare G, Capella GL, Frigerio E. Haematologica 1996;81:54–8.

Case report of one patient who responded to etretinate 50 mg orally daily.

Etretinate has been withdrawn from some countries and replaced by acitretin, but as yet there are no reports about the use of acitretin in Sweet's syndrome.

640

Syphilis (Lues)

Miguel R Sanchez

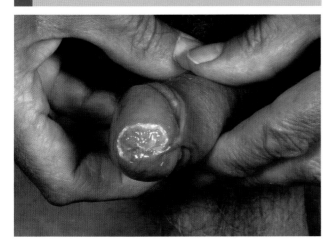

Syphilis is a chronic systemic infection with a variable clinical course, caused by the motile, corkscrew-shaped human spirochete, *Treponema pallidum* (ssp. *pallidum*). In adults, the infection is transmitted almost exclusively through sexual contact with infectious mucocutaneous lesions, and only rarely through transfusion or accidental inoculation. About one-third of persons become infected after a single episode of unprotected sexual intercourse with a partner with infectious syphilis.

MANAGEMENT STRATEGY

Accurate staging of syphilis is required before choosing the correct treatment regimen. The course of the infection is divided into three clinically distinct stages and two asymptomatic epidemiologic stages. The primary stage begins with the appearance of a chancre at the site of treponemal penetration, usually after an incubation period of approximately 3 weeks (range 10–90 days). The secondary stage usually presents with an eruption that appears 2–10 weeks after the onset of the chancre. The clinical manifestations of secondary syphilis heal in 4–12 weeks, at which point the patient is asymptomatic and the infection is only diagnosable through a positive serologic test (latent syphilis). Latent syphilis is classified as early (less than 1 year in duration) or late (greater than 1–2 years in duration). Latent cases in whom the onset of infection cannot be determined are diagnosed as having syphilis of indeterminate duration. Although patients are not infectious during the latent stage, approximately 25% of patients will develop one or more relapses of highly infectious secondary syphilis lesions, usually during the first year. Nearly 60% of these patients cannot recall the presence of an eruption and about 25% fail to remember having had a chancre. Without treatment about one-third of untreated patients with latent syphilis progress to tertiary syphilis (cardiovascular disease, neurosyphilis, or gummata).

Parenteral penicillin G is the treatment of choice for all stages, but the selected preparation, dose, and duration of treatment depend on the clinical stage and disease manifestations. The recommended treatment for patients with primary, secondary, or early latent syphilis is a single dose of *benzathine penicillin G*, 2.4 million IU, intramuscularly. For patients with syphilis of indeterminate duration, late latent syphilis, or tertiary syphilis, this regimen should be repeated weekly for three doses. Patients who are pregnant or HIV seropositive should be treated only with penicillin and should be desensitized to penicillin if there is a history of previous allergy. Other patients who are allergic to penicillin may be treated orally with *tetracycline* (500 mg four times daily), *doxycycline* (100 mg twice daily), or *erythromycin* (500 mg four times daily) for 14 days for early syphilis or 28 days for late latent syphilis. Treatment efficacy should be evaluated by serologic and clinical examinations at 6 and 12 months and, if needed, at 24 months in healthy patients, and at 3-month intervals for the first year and annually thereafter in HIV-seropositive patients. Serologic serum titers should decline fourfold within 6 months after treatment for primary or secondary syphilis, but may decrease more slowly in late syphilis. Patients whose nontreponemal test titers increase fourfold from baseline or a preceding test, or do not decrease fourfold within 12 months of treatment are considered to have failed treatment and should be evaluated with CNS examination and re-treated accordingly with regimens for late latent syphilis or for neurosyphilis.

Penicillin is the only proven effective drug for neurosyphilis and these patients should be treated with *intravenous aqueous crystalline penicillin G* 18–24 million IU daily administered as 3–4 million IU every 4 h. An alternative regimen is a 10-day course of *procaine benzylpenicillin (procaine penicillin)*, 2–4 million IU, administered as a single daily intramuscular injection *in addition to oral probenecid*, 500 mg four times daily.

SPECIFIC INVESTIGATIONS

- Dark-field microscopy
- Direct fluorescence antibody test
- Serologic tests
- Cerebrospinal fluid (CSF) examination

Comparison of methods for the detection of *Treponema pallidum* in lesions of early syphilis. Cummings MC, Lukehart SA, Marra C, et al. Sex Transm Dis 1996;23:366–9.

Definitive diagnosis of syphilis rests on the demonstration of spirochetes in the exudate of a chancre by dark-field examination or direct fluorescence antibody staining or in biopsied skin treated with silver stains.

Laboratory methods of diagnosis of syphilis for the beginning of the third millennium. Wicher K, Horowitz HW, Wicher V. Microbes Infect 1999;1:1035–49.

The diagnosis of syphilis is confirmed with serologic tests. The less costly, easier to perform, highly sensitive but less specific nontreponemal tests, such as the Venereal Disease Research Laboratory (VDRL) and the rapid plasma reagin (RPR) tests, are widely used for screening. These assays use cardiolipin antigens to detect antibodies to *T. pallidum*, and may be falsely reactive (2% of tests) in patients with narcotic abuse, connective tissue disease, viral and spirochetal infections, and malignancy, as well as other acute infections and systemic illnesses. Therefore, a reactive VDRL or RPR result should be confirmed with a treponemal test, such as the fluorescent treponemal antibody absorbed (FTA-ABS) assay and the microhemagglutination assay for antibody to *T. pallidum* (MHA-TP). Treponemal tests are highly specific as well as sensitive, but are rarely reactive in some connective tissue diseases and other treponemal infections. However, the presence of reactive nontreponemal and treponemal serologic tests in a patient provides compelling evidence for a presumptive diagnosis of syphilis.

Because enzyme-linked immunosorbent assays (ELISA) are as easy to perform as nontreponemal tests and as sensitive and more specific than nontreponemal tests, they are becoming the standard test for syphilis screening; however, nontreponemal tests will continue to be used to monitor treatment response.

Sexually transmitted diseases treatment guidelines 2002. Centers for Disease Control. MMWR Recomm Rep 2002;51: 18–29

CSF examination is indicated to exclude neurosyphilis in patients with neurologic signs, cardiovascular syphilis, gummata, iritis, auditory symptoms, HIV infection (late latent syphilis and syphilis of unknown duration), treatment failure, or slow decline in serologic titers after treatment with a medication other than penicillin.

Syphilis and HIV: a dangerous combination. Lynn WA, Lightman S. Lancet Infect Dis 2004;4:456–66.

Patients with syphilis should be tested for HIV antibodies and patients with HIV infection should be regularly screened for syphilis. Contact with the primary chancre of a person coinfected with HIV and *T. pallidum* enhances the transmission of HIV infection. There is an increased rate of early neurological and ophthalmic involvement. HIV infection can exacerbate the progression of syphilis and increase the risk of developing neurosyphilis.

In most patients with HIV infection, serologic tests are accurate and reliable for following the response to treatment. Unusually high or low serologic titers may be seen in some coinfected patients. Delayed seroconversion is rare. In the absence of reactive serology, the diagnosis of syphilis requires confirmation of the clinical presentation by biopsy and direct microscopy.

Invasion of the central nervous system by *Treponema pallidum*: implications for diagnosis and treatment. Lukehart SA, Hook EW, Baker-Zander SA, et al. Ann Intern Med 1988;109:855–62.

Treponema pallidum was isolated from the CSF of 30% of 40 patients with untreated primary and secondary syphilis. Concurrent HIV infection did not predispose to the presence of *T. pallidum* in the CSF, but appears to prevent clearance after appropriate treatment.

FIRST LINE THERAPIES

■ Benzathine penicillin	A
■ Procaine penicillin plus probenecid	A

Penicillin in the treatment of syphilis. The experience of three decades. Idsøe O, Guthe T, Willcox RR. Bull WHO 1972;47:1–68.

In studies totaling 1381 patients with seronegative primary syphilis, 97% of treated patients were clinically well and serologically negative. Treatment failures were attributed to reinfection.

Relapse of secondary syphilis after benzathine penicillin G: molecular analysis. Myint M, Bashiri H, Harrington RD, Marra CM. Sex Transm Dis 2004;31:196–9.

Relapse of infectious syphilis after treatment with the recommended doses of penicillin is rare, but does occur. For this reason, it is important to follow treated patients clinically and serologically. These patients respond to higher and more prolonged doses of penicillin

Efficacy of treatment for syphilis in pregnancy. Alexander JM, Sheffield JS, Sanchez PJ, et al. Obstet Gynecol 1999;93:5–8.

Centers for Disease Control recommended regimens for the treatment of maternal syphilis infection were found to prevent congenital syphilis in 98.2% of cases (27/27 with primary syphilis, 71/75 with secondary syphilis, 100/102 with early latent syphilis, and 136/136 with late latent syphilis).

A randomized trial of enhanced therapy for early syphilis in patients with and without human immunodeficiency virus infection. Rolfs RT, Joesoef MR, Hendershot EF, et al. N Engl J Med 1997;337:307–14.

In a multicenter, randomized, double blind trial of 501 syphilis patients, which included 101 patients with HIV infection, treatment with 2 g of amoxicillin and 500 mg of probenecid three times a day for 10 days in addition to benzathine penicillin was not superior to treatment with benzathine penicillin alone.

Acceptability and compliance with daily injections of procaine penicillin in the outpatient treatment of syphilis-treponemal infection. Crowe G, Theodore C, Forster GE, Goh BT. Sex Transm Dis 1997;24:127–30.

In some European countries, such as England, the recommended treatment is daily procaine benzylpenicillin (procaine penicillin) injections with or without oral probenecid for 8–21 days depending on the stage of the disease.

SECOND LINE THERAPIES

■ Tetracycline	B
■ Doxycycline	B
■ Amoxicillin plus probenecid	B

National guideline for the management of early syphilis. Clinical Effectiveness Group (Association of Genitourinary Medicine and the Medical Society for the Study of Venereal Diseases). Sex Trans Infect 1999;75:S29–33.

The recommended treatment of primary, secondary, or early latent syphilis in immunocompetent persons who are allergic to penicillin is orally administered doxycycline, 100 mg twice daily, or tetracycline, 500 mg four times daily for 14 days. Amoxicillin, 500 mg four times daily plus probenecid 500 mg four times daily for 14 days is not as effective as parenteral penicillin due to poorer compliance with this regimen.

National guideline for the management of early syphilis. Clinical Effectiveness Group (Association of Genitourinary Medicine and the Medical Society for the Study of Venereal Diseases). Sex Trans Infect 1999;75:S34–7.

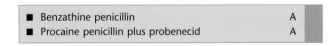

Evidence levels   **A** Double-blind study   **B** Clinical trial ≥ 20 subjects   **C** Clinical trial < 20 subjects   **D** Series ≥ 5 subjects   **E** Anecdotal case reports

Doxycycline 100 mg by mouth twice daily for 28 days is recommended for immunocompetent patients with uncomplicated late latent syphilis or syphilis of unknown duration. *Some experts prefer a dose of 200 mg twice daily.*

Therapeutic effect of oral doxycycline on syphilis. Onoda Y. Jpn J Antibiot 1980;33:18–28.

The response of 100 mg twice daily of doxycycline for 28 days in 81 patients with syphilis was 100% for primary, 91.7% for early, 63.0% for late, and 61.8% for congenital disease in adults.

THIRD LINE THERAPIES

■ Erythromycin	C
■ Azithromycin	B
■ Ceftriaxone	B

Ceftriaxone therapy for syphilis: report from the emerging infections network. Augenbraun M, Workowski K. Clin Infect Dis 1999;29:1337–8.

A single injection of 1 g of ceftriaxone is not effective for treating infectious syphilis. Daily or every other day injections for 8–10 days appear to be efficacious, but more data are needed to evaluate late failures.

Response of HIV-infected patients with asymptomatic syphilis to intensive intramuscular therapy with ceftriaxone or procaine penicillin. Smith NH, Musher DM, Huang DB, et al. Int J STD AIDS. 2004;15:328–32.

In this prospective pilot study of 31 patients with HIV infection and latent syphilis or syphilis of unknown duration, a fourfold or greater decline in serologic titers occurred in 71% (ten of 14) of patients treated with a daily 1 g intramuscular injection of ceftriaxone for 15 days and 70% (seven of ten) of those treated with a daily 2.4 million IU intramuscular injection of procaine penicillin (plus probenecid 500 mg orally four times daily) for 15 days. Two penicillin treated and one ceftriaxone treated patients relapsed and two patients failed ceftriaxone therapy. Three penicillin treated, and two ceftriaxone treated patients remained serofast.

A pilot study evaluating ceftriaxone and penicillin G as treatment agents for neurosyphilis in human immunodeficiency virus-infected individuals. Marra CM, Boutin P, McArthur JC, et al. Clin Infect Dis 2000;30:540–4.

There was no difference in CSF abnormalities after treatment with intravenous ceftriaxone or intravenous penicillin in HIV-seropositive patients with neurosyphilis.

A randomized, comparative pilot study of azithromycin versus benzathine penicillin G for treatment of early syphilis. Hook EW 3rd, Martin DH, Stephens J, et al. Sex Transm Dis 2002;29:486–90.

In a randomized pilot study comparing intramuscular injections of benzathine penicillin G and azithromycin in early syphilis, the response rate of a single 2.0 g dose of azithromycin was comparable (94% – 16 of 17 persons) to that of a single injection of benzathine penicillin G (86% – 12 of 14 persons). An additional dose of azithromycin 1 week after the initial treatment did not improve the response of a single dose (83% – 24 of 29 persons).

Macrolide resistance in *Treponema pallidum* in the United States and Ireland. Lukehart SA, Godornes C, Molini BJ, et al. N Engl J Med 2004;351:154–8.

Azithromycin treatment failures in syphilis infections – San Francisco, California, 2002–2003. Centers for Disease Control and Prevention. MMWR Morb Mortal Wkly Rep 2004;53:197–8.

Treatment of eight patients with either primary syphilis or seronegative contacts of partners with syphilis with a single 2 g dose of azithromycin failed to prevent progression to symptomatic or serologic infection or to heal the chancres. Five of the patients had HIV infection. A 2 g dose of azithromycin is an alternative to doxycycline for penicillin-allergic patients with early syphilis, but only when close follow-up can be assured because treatment efficacy is not well documented and has not been studied in persons with HIV infection.

Syringomata

James A A Langtry

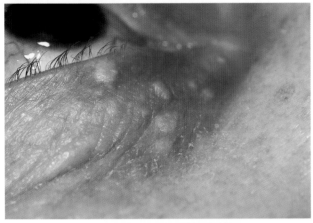

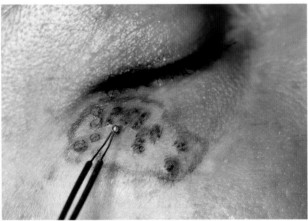

Syringomata are benign appendageal tumors of the intraepidermal eccrine sweat duct which have a characteristic histologic appearance. The typical clinical presentation is of individual skin- or tan-colored papules, with a rounded or flat surface, 1–5 mm in diameter. Single tumors can occur, but more commonly they are multiple and symmetric, more common in females and from adolescence onwards. Linear distribution and familial occurrence have been described. Syringomata are usually limited to the lower eyelids, although they may occur at other sites, including the cheeks, axillae, abdomen, and vulva.

MANAGEMENT STRATEGY

Syringomata of the eyelids and cheeks are in a prominent site, may appear conspicuous, and treatment may be sought to improve appearance. The syringomata are situated in the upper to mid dermis. Available treatments aim to remove or flatten the papule produced by each syringoma. All are ablative modalities and include surgical excision with primary suturing (some patients are troubled by a few individual lesions and in this situation simple excision is an option; large numbers preclude use of this technique for most cases). The modalities are: scissor excision with secondary intention healing; surgical excision of the entire cosmetic unit of the lower eyelids in patients who would in addition benefit from lower eyelid blepharoplasty; electrocautery;

electrodesiccation; intralesional electrodesiccation; dermabrasion; cryotherapy; and ablation with CO_2 or erbium:YAG laser.

Local anesthesia is needed prior to treatment and this may be topical, or by local injections with or without nerve blocks. Local anesthetic injections producing a field block are most commonly employed, as good anesthesia is helpful when using ablative treatments near the eye. Patients should be warned about the possibility of postoperative bruising. Eye protection is of paramount importance and specific precautions relevant to the use of lasers must be taken if laser treatment is used.

Ablative treatments will produce scarring to some degree and the aim is to make this imperceptible and produce an excellent cosmetic result. Possible noticeable sequelae, including scarring and hypo- or hyperpigmentation (especially with increasing skin pigmentation), should always be discussed prior to treatment.

There are no studies comparing different treatment modalities for syringomata and there is very little long-term follow-up data on which to base recommendations for treatment. On the basis of experience and the limited evidence available, it is not necessary to have the latest and most expensive technology to achieve good results. Expertise and good outcomes with simple, 'low-tech' methods are as important as expertise and good outcomes with 'high-tech' modalities. Each have benefits as well as pitfalls for the novice or unwary. It is more important to be expert in the use and application of one particular modality.

SPECIFIC INVESTIGATIONS

The clinical features of periorbital syringomata are usually typical and a skin biopsy is only necessary if there is diagnostic doubt.

FIRST LINE THERAPIES

■ Surgical excision	E
■ Snip excision and secondary intention healing	E
■ Electrocautery	E
■ Intralesional electrodesiccation	D
■ CO_2 laser	D

Cosmetic Dermatologic Surgery, 2nd edn. Stegman SS, Tromovitch TA, Glogau RG, eds. Chicago: Year Book Medical; 1992:32.

A commonsense approach to treatment of syringomata, advocating the use of surgical excision, electrosurgery, or laser.

An easy method for removal of syringoma. Maloney ME. J Dermatol Surg Oncol 1982;8:973–5.

A single case is reported with a good outcome following removal of four to six lesions per session, in 12 sessions over 5 months.

A good photographic demonstration of the removal of periorbital syringomata with fine ophthalmic spring action scissors.

True electrocautery in the treatment of syringomas and other benign cutaneous lesions. Langtry JAA, Carruthers JA. J Cutan Med Surg 1997;2:60–3.

The technique of electrocautery is described, and good results reported in a number of benign skin lesions, including syringomata.

Intralesional electrodesiccation of syringomas. Karma P, Benedetto AV. Dermatol Surg 1997;23:921–4.

Electrodesiccation via a fine electrode into the center of the syringoma with the aim of localizing the effect and minimizing scarring. Twelve patients were treated, all with reported excellent results and no recurrence after a follow-up of 18–48 months. Two patients with Fitzpatrick skin type IV had focal hyperpigmentation which cleared in 2–3 months.

Treatment of multiple facial syringomas with the carbon dioxide (CO_2) laser. Wang JI, Roenigk HH Jr. Dermatol Surg 1999;25:136–9.

A description of 10 patients treated with CO_2 laser reporting excellent results. Patients with larger numbers needed more treatment sessions. The median follow-up was 16 months and one patient had new syringomata at other periorbital sites 18 months after treatment. Erythema lasted 6–12 weeks in all patients. One patient with Fitzpatrick type IV skin had minimal focal areas of hyperpigmentation clearing after 2–3 months.

SECOND LINE THERAPIES

■ Electrodesiccation and curettage	E
■ Cryotherapy	E
■ Combination of CO_2 laser and trichloroacetic acid	D

Syringoma: removal by electrodesiccation and curettage. Stevenson TR, Swanson SA. Am Plast Surg 1985;15:151–4.

The technique is described and well illustrated. Good results are reported, but there is no description of numbers of patients treated, clinical details, or follow-up data using this technique.

Cryosurgery. Dawber RPR. In: Lask GP, Moy RL, eds. Principles and Techniques of Cutaneous Surgery. New York: McGraw-Hill; 1996:154.

Syringoma is listed as a condition treatable by cryotherapy.

Details are not given and periorbital syringomata are not specifically mentioned.

A new treatment for syringoma. Combination of carbon dioxide laser and trichloroacetic acid. Kang H, Kim NS, Kim YB, Shim WC. Dermatol Surg 1998;24:1370–4.

This study evaluates the histopathology and efficacy of combined CO_2 laser and 50% trichloroacetic acid treatment of 20 Korean patients with periorbital syringomata. Results were reported as excellent (11 patients), good (6 patients), and fair (3 patients), without complications such as scarring, infection, or textural change, using the technique detailed.

THIRD LINE THERAPIES

■ Dermabrasion	E
■ Trichloroacetic acid	E

Dermabrasion by diamond fraises revolving at 85 000 revolutions per minute. Fulton JE. J Dermatol Surg Oncol 1978;4:777–9.

High-speed dermabrasion is described and good results are reported in 65 patients with acne scarring, actinic damage, adenoma sebaceum, and syringomata.

The treatment of eruptive syringomas in an African American patient with a combination of trichlororoacetic acid and CO_2 laser destruction. Frazier CC, Camacho AP, Cockerell CJ. Dermatol Surg 2001;27:489–92.

Single case report of eruptive facial syringomata in an African-American woman treated by 35% trichloroacetic acid peel, followed 2 weeks later by CO_2 laser, with acceptable cosmetic results and without significant side effects.

Tinea capitis

David T Roberts, David J Bilsland

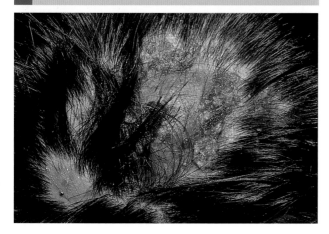

Tinea capitis is the term used to describe a scalp infection caused by dermatophyte species of fungi. A number of different species of dermatophytes are responsible and produce either ectothrix or endothrix type of infection. Ectothrix infection involves both the inside and outside of the hair shaft whereas endothrix infection only involves the inside of the hair shaft. Infections of both types may be anthropophilic, where man is the primary host, or zoophilic, where infection is contracted from an animal host.

MANAGEMENT STRATEGY

Treatment is aimed at eradicating the organism to prevent spread of infection and to prevent scarring, which results in permanent alopecia. Established tinea capitis cannot be treated topically, and systemic therapy is always necessary. *Griseofulvin*, although only a weakly fungistatic drug, is very effective in the management of all varieties of tinea capitis although treatment periods are often lengthy. In most countries, griseofulvin remains the only systemic antifungal agent licensed for use in children, in whom the disease is most prevalent, and the drug must be given in adequate doses for long periods. The aim must be to eradicate the infection, and each case should be individually monitored using a Wood's light (for those infections that fluoresce) and by sending specimens to the laboratory for mycological examination.

Recently the azoles – *ketoconazole, fluconazole,* and *itraconazole* – and the allylamine *terbinafine* have become available for systemic use. Numerous open, placebo-controlled and comparative therapeutic trials have been carried out with these agents in various types of tinea capitis. These studies have demonstrated at least equal efficacy to griseofulvin, often over shorter treatment durations. Cure rates in such studies are never 100%, but the aim must be to cure 100% of cases in the clinical setting.

Very recently, the use of intermittent or pulsed treatment regimens has been investigated using both fluconazole and itraconazole. This therapeutic strategy is based on the long half-life of these drugs in keratin; this is likely to be a property of the target organ rather than the drug. Such regimens are not likely to produce any advantages in cure rates, but may reduce the total acquisition cost of drugs.

Ectothrix infections are generally caused by zoophilic *Microsporum canis* or the anthropophilic *Microsporum audouinii* and nearly always occur in children. Griseofulvin remains the treatment of choice in a dose of 15–20 mg/kg, continued for as long as is necessary, which is often 3–4 months. Endothrix infections, most commonly *Trichophyton tonsurans* or *Trichophyton violaceum*, should be treated similarly in children, but 2 months or so of treatment is much more likely to be effective. *Topical azoles and allylamines* are sometimes used in conjunction with systemic therapy, which may shorten the time during which the patient is infectious.

SPECIFIC INVESTIGATIONS

- ■ Examination of hair and skin scales by direct microscopy and culture
- ■ Direct observation using a Wood's light

Essentials of medical mycology. Evans EGV, Gentles JC. Edinburgh: Churchill Livingstone; 1985:60.

Hairs infected with *M. adouinii, M. canis,* and *Trichophyton schoenleinii* fluoresce bright green under Wood's light.

Fungal infection: diagnosis and management. Richardson MD, Warnock DW. Oxford: Blackwell; 1993:45–8.

Direct microscopic examination of hairs reveals arthrospores of the fungus located outside (ectothrix) or inside (endothrix) the infected hair. Each species can be identified by specific appearances in culture.

Treatment of tinea capitis often needs to be started before laboratory confirmation is available. However, appropriate specimens should always be taken prior to treatment.

FIRST LINE THERAPIES

■ Griseofulvin	A
■ Terbinafine	A
■ Itraconazole	A

Comparison of terbinafine and griseofulvin in the treatment of tinea capitis. Caceres-Rios H, Rueada M, Ballona R, Bustamante B. J Am Acad Dermatol 2000;42:80–4.

A double-blind, randomized study involving 50 pediatric patients with clinical and mycological diagnosis of tinea capitis. One group received 4 weeks of terbinafine followed by 4 weeks of placebo. The doses used were 250 mg once daily for those with body weight over 40 kg, half this dose for those weighing 20–40 kg, and a quarter of the dose for those weighing less than 20 kg. The other group had 8 weeks of griseofulvin 500 mg once daily, reduced in the same proportions for patients weighing less than 40 kg. The majority had *T. tonsurans* infection (74%) and a minority *M. canis* (26%). At week 8, griseofulvin cure rates were 76% and terbinafine 72%. At week 12, recurrences were noted in the griseofulvin group (efficacy reduced to 44%). Efficacy was unchanged in the terbinafine group.

This study established that terbinafine given for 4 weeks was as effective as griseofulvin for 8 weeks and there were more recurrences in the griseofulvin group during the ensuing 4 weeks. This study suggests that terbinafine may well become the treatment of choice when licensed for use in children.

Evidence levels A Double-blind study   B Clinical trial ≥ 20 subjects   C Clinical trial < 20 subjects   D Series ≥ 5 subjects   E Anecdotal case reports

A randomized comparison of 4 weeks of terbinafine vs. 8 weeks of griseofulvin for the treatment of tinea capitis. Fuller LC, Smith CH, Cerio R, et al. Br J Dermatol 2001; 144:321–7.

A prospective open randomized multicenter study of children aged 2–16 years; 210 patients enrolled to either 4 weeks of treatment with oral terbinafine or 8 weeks in the same doses as quoted in the above study (Caceres-Rios H, et al. J Am Acad Dermatol 2000;42:80–4) and oral griseofulvin in a dose of 10 mg/kg body weight. Selenium sulfide shampoo was additionally used twice weekly for the first 2 weeks of treatment.

The majority of the 147 patients evaluated were infected with *Trichophyton* spp. (83 and 84%, in each group); 77 patients were treated with terbinafine and 70 with griseofulvin. At weeks 4, 8, 12, and 24 the percentage of patients rated as cured (clinical plus mycological clearance) was 26, 55, 57, and 64% (terbinafine) and 17, 49, 57, and 67% (griseofulvin). No statistically significant differences between the two drugs were observed with regard to treatment efficacy or tolerability. There appeared to be a better response to griseofulvin than terbinafine in patients with *M. audouinii*.

A randomized double-blind parallel-group duration-finding study of oral terbinafine and open-label high-dose griseofulvin in children with tinea capitis due to *Microsporum* species. Lipozencic J, Skerley M, Orofino-Costa R, et al. Br J Dermatol 2002:146:816–23.

A multicenter study comparing shorter courses of terbinafine (6 and 8 weeks) with 12 weeks of griseofulvin in a mainly pediatric population with *Microsporum* sp. infection (*M. canis* in 98%). Higher mycological cure rates were observed in the patients treated with griseofulvin (84%) as opposed to terbinafine (60%).

These studies indicate that, in countries where terbinafine is not licensed in children, griseofulvin is still an effective treatment. This is particularly so if doses of 20 mg/kg daily are used and if the infection is caused by Microsporum *spp.*

A double-blind randomized comparative trial of itraconazole versus terbinafine for 2 weeks in tinea capitis. Jahangir M, Hussain I, Ul Hasan M, Harron TS. Br J Dermatol 1998;139:672–4.

A randomized, double-blind study comparing itraconazole (n = 28) and terbinafine (n = 27). Daily doses were 200 mg and 250 mg, respectively, for patients weighing more than 40 kg and the doses were halved for those weighing 20–40 kg, and halved again for those weighing less than 20 kg. *Trichophyton violaceum* was the major pathogen in both groups. Final evaluation at week 12 showed cure rates of 85.7 and 77.8%, respectively (difference not significant).

This study showed terbinafine and itraconazole to be equally effective over a short treatment duration of only 2 weeks.

Itraconazole versus griseofulvin in the treatment of tinea capitis: a double-blind randomized study in children. Lopez-Gomez S, Del Palacio A, Van Cutsem J, et al. Int J Dermatol 1994;33:743–7.

Itraconazole 100 mg daily versus griseofulvin 500 mg daily, were both given for six consecutive weeks, with final evaluation at 8 weeks. Fifteen of 17 patients treated with itraconazole and 14 of 15 patients treated with griseofulvin had *M. canis* infection. Cure rates were similar: 15 of the 17 patients treated with itraconazole and 15 of 17 patients

treated with griseofulvin were cured at the end of the treatment period. This small study of mainly ectothrix infections reveals remarkably high cure rates without follow-up data and requires confirmation in a larger, better designed study.

SECOND LINE THERAPIES

■ Terbinafine	B
■ Fluconazole	B

Once weekly fluconazole is effective in children in the treatment of tinea capitis: a prospective multicentre study. Gupta AK, Dlova N, Taborda P, et al. Br J Dermatol 2000; 142:965–8.

An open, multicenter evaluation of 61 children enrolled and treated once weekly with fluconazole (8 mg/kg for 8 weeks), with an extra 4 weeks of the drug if clinically indicated. Organisms involved in tinea capitis were dominated by *T. violaceum* (33 cases), *T. tonsurans* (11), and a smaller group of *M. canis* (17). Clinical and mycological cure appear to be similar in both groups. A majority of patients (47) received the drug for 8 weeks, while ten required 12 weeks, and three 16 weeks.

Short duration treatment with terbinafine for tinea capitis caused by *Trichophyton* or *Microsporum* species. Hamm H, Schwinn A, Brautigam M, Weidinger G. Br J Dermatol 1999;140:480–2.

A double-blind comparison of either 1 or 2 weeks of terbinafine in 35 patients (mean age 9 years). Doses were 250, 125, or 62.5 mg according to body weight as described above. Patients were observed for 12 weeks. Nonresponders were offered an additional 4 weeks of treatment. Causative organisms included *M. canis* (12 cases), *T. tonsurans* (12), and other *Trichophyton* species (11). Cure rate after 1 week of therapy was 56%, and after 2 weeks of treatment 86%. In the *Microsporum* group, one of seven responded after 1 week of treatment and none of the five treated for 2 weeks responded. However, treatment was effective in four of these six nonresponders after an additional 4 weeks of therapy.

A randomized double-blind comparative study of terbinafine for 1, 2 and 4 weeks in tinea capitis. Haroon TS, Hussain I, Aman S, et al. Br J Dermatol 1996;135:86–8.

Of 161 patients aged 3–13 years, 53 were treated for 1 week, 51 for 2 weeks, and 57 for 4 weeks. Doses of terbinafine were the same as those described above (Caceres-Rios H, et al. J Am Acad Dermatol 2000;42:80–4). *Trichophyton violaceum* was the predominant fungus (71.5%). Cure rates (final evaluation at 12 weeks) were 73.6, 80.4, and 85.9, in the 1-, 2-, and 4-week treatment groups, respectively.

These studies are all relatively small or consist of infections with mainly a single species. They suggest, but certainly do not confirm, that both short-term treatment and intermittent treatment may be effective and also that ectothrix infections are likely to be more recalcitrant.

THIRD LINE THERAPIES

■ Prednisolone	B
■ Ketoconazole shampoo	B
■ Selenium sulfide shampoo	B

A randomized, comparative trial of treatment of kerion celsi with griseofulvin plus oral prednisolone vs. griseofulvin alone. Hussain I, Muzaffar F, Rashid T, et al. Med Mycol 1999;37:97–9.

Thirty patients were randomized to treatment with either griseofulvin and oral prednisolone in combination or oral griseofulvin alone in the treatment of scalp kerion. Final evaluation at week 12 showed similar cure rates, but apparently no additional benefit of oral prednisolone.

The use of systemic corticosteroids in inflammatory tinea capitis to reduce inflammation and thus alopecia, is controversial. There are those, the authors included, who always use them in combination with antifungal therapy, whereas other authorities claim little benefit. This study tends to support the latter view, but is by no means conclusive.

Comparison of 1% and 2.5% selenium sulphide in treatment of tinea capitis. Gibbens TG, Murray MM, Baker RC. Arch Pediatr Adolesc Med 1995;149:808–11.

Fifty four pediatric patients received either 2.5% selenium sulfide lotion or 1% selenium sulfide shampoo or an unmedicated shampoo as a control in addition to griseofulvin 15 mg/kg daily. Survival data indicated that selenium sulfide lotion and shampoo both reduced surface counts of the organism.

Successful treatment of tinea capitis with 2% ketoconazole shampoo. Greer DL. Int J Dermatol 2000;39: 302–4.

Sixteen pediatric patients were treated daily for 8 weeks with 2% ketoconazole shampoo. A marked clinical improvement was noted in all patients. Five of 15 patients were cured after 8 weeks. There was no recurrence in these five patients. Patients with positive cultures after 8 weeks were placed on oral griseofulvin.

Both these studies indicate a reduction in colony count following the use of antifungal shampoos, which may reduce the period during which these patients are infectious during the initial phase of systemic treatment.

Evidence levels A Double-blind study   **B** Clinical trial ≥ 20 subjects   **C** Clinical trial < 20 subjects   **D** Series ≥ 5 subjects   **E** Anecdotal case reports

Tinea pedis and skin dermatophytosis

David T Roberts, David J Bilsland

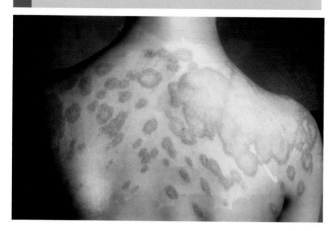

Tinea pedis (athlete's foot) is among the commonest dermatologic diseases. It usually produces maceration and fissures in the toe clefts, but can spread onto the soles, where it appears as dry, hyperkeratotic scale. Tinea cruris is caused by the same fungi and affects the groin area, nearly always in males. Tinea corporis (ringworm) appears as annular lesions on the trunk and may be the result of spread from the feet or sometimes from infected animals.

MANAGEMENT STRATEGY

Relapse is common in tinea pedis and may be the result of recurrence following inadequate treatment or reinfection. The fungi involved – *Trichophyton rubrum, Trichophyton interdigitale,* and occasionally *Epidermophyton floccosum* – are endemic in communal bathing places. Topical therapy is usually sufficient for toe cleft infection, and *terbinafine* is the most potent agent, eradicating the fungus more quickly than *topical azoles. Antifungal foot powders are only of value prophylactically.* Small areas of tinea cruris and tinea corporis can be treated topically, but many cases require systemic therapy. *Griseofulvin* (15 mg/kg body weight) works well in glabrous skin infection, but must be given for at least 4 weeks. *Terbinafine and itraconazole* work equally well in doses of 250 mg daily and 200 mg daily, respectively, over 2 weeks' duration. Infections of the palms (tinea manum) and soles (moccasin tinea pedis) require treatment systemically in similar doses and duration.

The choice of topical or systemic treatment of tinea pedis and dermatophytoses of glabrous skin therefore depends upon both the site and extent of the lesions.

SPECIFIC INVESTIGATIONS

- Examination of skin scrapings by direct microscopy and culture
- Direct observation using Wood's light

Essentials of medical mycology. Evans EGV, Gentles JC. Edinburgh: Churchill Livingstone; 1985:56–60.

Skin scrapings should be taken outwards from the edge of the lesion, cleared in 20% potassium hydroxide (KOH) and examined directly. The remainder of the material submitted should be cultured at 25–30.8°C in 4% malt extract or Sabouraud's dextrose agar. Many annular lesions are misdiagnosed, and exclusion of a fungal infection is always worthwhile. Topical therapy for athlete's foot is now so efficient that the condition has generally cleared before the laboratory result is available.

FIRST LINE THERAPIES

Topical	
■ Terbinafine	A
■ Clotrimazole	A

Comparison of terbinafine and clotrimazole in treating tinea pedis. Evans EGV, Dodman B, Williamson DM, et al. Br Med J 1993;307:645–7.

This is a study of 256 patients with proven tinea pedis randomized to receive either terbinafine 1% cream applied twice daily for a week plus placebo cream for a further 3 weeks vs clotrimazole 1% cream twice daily for 4 weeks. At week 4, mycological cure rates were 97.2% and 83.7% for terbinafine and clotrimazole, respectively.

Topical terbinafine and clotrimazole in interdigital tinea pedis; a multicenter comparison of cure and relapse rates with 1 and 4 week treatment regimens. Bergstresser PR, Elewski B, Hanifin J, et al. J Am Acad Dermatol 1993; 28:648–51.

This study showed 1 week of treatment with terbinafine (76% cure) to be as effective as 4 weeks of terbinafine (86% cure) assessed at week 12. These values are similar to those seen with 4 weeks of clotrimazole (70% cure), but superior to 1 week of clotrimazole (35% cure).

Terbinafine versus miconazole in patients with tinea pedis. Vermeer BJ, Staats CC, van Houwelingen JC. Ned Tijdschr Geneeskd 1996;140:1605–8.

Cure rates following 1 week of 1% terbinafine cream were 95%, as opposed to 87% following 4 weeks of miconazole 1% cream.

These important studies reveal terbinafine to be effective over a much shorter treatment duration than clotrimazole and miconazole. Compliance over a 1-week treatment duration is clearly likely to be better than 4 weeks, thus reducing relapse rates. Terbinafine 1% cream should therefore be considered the topical treatment of choice for tinea pedis.

Treatment of dermatomycoses with topically applied allylamines: naftifine and terbinafine. Jones TC. J Dermatol Treat 1990;1(suppl 2):29–32.

This paper summarizes five studies of terbinafine cream in tinea cruris and tinea corporis and reports an overall mycological cure rate of 93%.

Treatment of tinea cruris with topical terbinafine. Greer DL, Jolly HW Jr. J Am Acad Dermatol 1998;23(suppl):800–4.

This study was a double blind comparison of terbinafine 1% cream and its vehicle given for 2 weeks and followed for a further 2 weeks. At the end of week 4, the cure rates for the terbinafine group were over 80% as opposed to just over 20% for the placebo.

There are no published comparisons of topical terbinafine vs a topical azole in tinea corporis and tinea cruris. It can be assumed, however, that the comparative efficacy would be similar to that seen in tinea pedis, and terbinafine would be equally effective over a shorter treatment period. Currently published studies suggest that topical treatment using terbinafine 1% cream in tinea corporis and tinea cruris should be continued for 2 weeks.

SECOND LINE THERAPIES

Systemic agents	
■ Griseofulvin	A
■ Terbinafine	A
■ Itraconazole	A
■ Fluconazole	A

Oral terbinafine versus griseofulvin in the treatment of moccasin-type tinea pedis. Savin RC. J Am Acad Dermatol 1990;23:807–9.

This small study compared 16 patients receiving terbinafine 250 mg daily and 12 receiving griseofulvin 500 mg daily over a 6-week treatment period. Follow-up 2 weeks after cessation of therapy revealed clinical and mycological cure of 88% in the terbinafine group and 45% in the griseofulvin group.

Although small, this study reveals terbinafine to be significantly superior to griseofulvin over 6 weeks of treatment and superior at follow-up. The treatment duration for griseofulvin is probably too short for this notably recalcitrant disease.

A double-blind study of itraconazole versus griseofulvin in patients with tinea pedis and tinea manus. Wishart JM. N Z Med J 1994;107:126–8.

Patients were randomized to receive itraconazole 100 mg or griseofulvin 500 mg once daily for 4 weeks. After 6 weeks of therapy 70% of the itraconazole group and 50% of the griseofulvin group had negative microscopy. The clinical score comparison was in favor of itraconazole, and this study suggested it to be superior to griseofulvin in this indication.

This study shows itraconazole to be superior to griseofulvin.

Two week oral treatment of tinea pedis, comparing terbinafine (250 mg/day) with itraconazole (100 mg/day): a double-blind multicentre study. De Keyser P, De Backer M, Massart DL, Westelink KJ. Br J Dermatol 1994;130(suppl 43):22–5.

This study involved 366 patients with both interdigital and moccasin tinea pedis. Four weeks after cessation of therapy, 86.3% of the terbinafine group were negative mycologically as opposed to 54.5% of the itraconazole group.

A comparison of two weeks of terbinafine 250 mg per day with four weeks of itraconazole 100 mg per day in plantar type tinea pedis. Hay RJ, MacGregor JM, Wuite J, Ryatt KS, et al. Br J Dermatol 1995;132:604–8.

One hundred and twenty nine evaluable patients were treated and randomized to one of the two groups. At the end of week 16, 71% of the terbinafine group and 55% of the itraconazole group were negative mycologically with minimal or absent clinical signs. Cure rates were closer at other follow-up periods and the authors concluded that the two drugs were of similar efficacy over the treatment durations examined.

These two studies show terbinafine to be effective in recalcitrant forms of tinea pedis over a 2-week treatment period. The comparison with itraconazole is less valid because it is now recognized that 100 mg daily is a suboptimal dose of itraconazole.

Itraconazole for the treatment of tinea pedis: a dosage of 400 mg/day given for one week is similar in efficacy to 100 or 200 mg/day given for 2–4 weeks. Gupta AK, de Donker P, Heremans A, et al. J Am Acad Dermatol 1997;36:789–92.

This study reveals cure rates similar to those seen with terbinafine 250 mg daily over 2 weeks in the itraconazole 400 mg daily for 1 week treatment group.

It would appear that itraconazole in this significantly increased dose is effective over a 1-week treatment period in tinea pedis.

One week therapy with oral terbinafine in cases of tinea cruris/corporis. Farag A, Taha M, Halim S. Br J Dermatol 1994;131:684–6.

This open study of 22 patients revealed 100% cure rates at the end of the 6-week follow-up.

A comparison of itraconazole and griseofulvin in the treatment of tinea corporis and tinea cruris: a double-blind study. Panagiotidou D, Kousidou T, Chaidemenos G, et al. J Int Med Res 1992;20:392–400.

Forty patients were treated with either itraconazole 100 mg daily or griseofulvin 500 mg daily for 15 days. Mycological cure rates at the 15-day follow-up were 77.8% of the itraconazole group as opposed to 66.7% of the griseofulvin group; this was just significant.

Once weekly oral doses of fluconazole 150 mg daily in the treatment of tinea corporis/cruris and cutaneous candidiasis. Suchil P, Gei FM, Robles M, et al. Clin Exp Dermatol 1992;17:397–401.

Ninety five patients with tinea corporis/cruris were given a mean 2.6 doses of fluconazole. Clinical cure was achieved in 92% of patients and mycology was negative in 85 of 86 patients at 30 days following the last dose.

Studies in tinea corporis and tinea cruris tend to be smaller and of rather lower quality than those found for tinea pedis. This perhaps reflects the lower prevalence of the disease. However, all studies reveal satisfactory cure rates with all of the newer agents – terbinafine, itraconazole, and fluconazole. The latter drug, however, has not been extensively studied and is not licensed in very many countries for dermatophytosis. Terbinafine and itraconazole are therefore likely to be the treatments of choice in doses of 250 mg and 200 mg daily respectively, both for 2 weeks in tinea corporis and tinea cruris.

Tinea unguium

David T Roberts, David J Bilsland

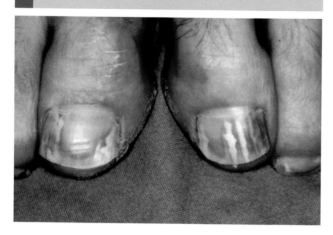

Tinea unguium is defined as dermatophyte infection of the nail, and dermatophytes are the offending pathogens in over 90% of cases. Onychomycosis covers both tinea unguium and those remaining cases caused by yeasts, mainly of the *Candida* species, and various nondermatophyte molds. The disease begins at the hyponychium, usually laterally, and progresses proximally resulting in onycholysis, discoloration, and subungual hyperkeratosis. Ultimately the nail becomes grossly dystrophic and friable.

MANAGEMENT STRATEGY

Tinea unguium is a disease of insidious onset and relentless progression and does not resolve spontaneously. The fungus enters the nail from an infected foot and the great toenail is usually, but not invariably, affected first. Ultimately, the disease spreads to involve other toenails and, in about 20% of cases, the fingernails as well. Various studies of prevalence suggest that 5–10% of the population of Western societies are affected, and treatment of all of these involves considerable cost.

Although a number of topical preparations are available it is likely that systemic treatment will always provide optimal cure rates. *Griseofulvin* was, for a considerable period, the only oral agent available for the treatment of this disease and cure rates were disappointing (around 30%) especially in toenails. The drug requires to be given in a dose of at least 1 g daily for 12–18 months for toenail infection and 6–12 months for fingernail infection.

The recent advent of newer, more potent systemic antifungal drugs for oral use has much improved cure rates. *Terbinafine* and *itraconazole* are the major players in the treatment of tinea unguium, and both drugs are more effective than griseofulvin.

Terbinafine is the most potent antidermatophyte agent in vitro, having a minimum fungicidal concentration (MFC) around 100 times greater than itraconazole. Terbinafine is given in a dose of 250 mg daily for 3 months for toenail infection and for 6 weeks for fingernail infection, and cure rates of around 80% can be confidently expected.

Itraconazole is now mostly used in a pulsed or intermittent fashion where the drug is given in a dose of 400 mg daily for 1 week per month for 3 or 4 months for toenail infection tind for 2 months for fingernail infection. Cure rates vary across a number of studies, but are not likely to be as good as those achieved with terbinafine.

Terbinafine is therefore the drug of choice in tinea unguium, followed by itraconazole if there are any contraindications to the use of terbinafine.

SPECIFIC INVESTIGATIONS

- Microscopy and culture of specimens submitted for mycological examination

Essentials of medical mycology. Evans EGV, Gentles JC. Edinburgh: Churchill Livingstone; 1985.

Nail clippings or preferably subungual debris are cleared in 20% potassium hydroxide and examined microscopically for the presence of fungal hyphae. Part of a sample is cultured on 4% malt extract agar or Sabouraud's dextrose agar at 25–30°C for at least 3 weeks. *Trichophyton rubrum* is the predominant pathogen and is found in excess of 80% of cases, followed by *Trichophyton interdigitale*. *Epidermophyton floccosum* is a rare pathogen of nails, as are some other dermatophytes.

It is essential to confirm the diagnosis of tinea unguium prior to the commencement of therapy. Treatment is both lengthy and costly, and other diseases, notably psoriasis, can produce nail dystrophy that closely mimics tinea unguium. Fungal infection of the nail is, however, the cause of about 50% of all nail dystrophies at presentation and is always worth excluding.

FIRST LINE THERAPIES

■ Terbinafine	A
■ Itraconazole	A

Double-blind randomised study of continuous terbinafine compared with intermittent itraconazole in treatment of toenail onychomycosis. The L.I.O.N. study group. Evans EG, Sigurgeirsson B. Br Med J 1999;318:1031–5.

This study compared terbinafine 250 mg daily for 3 and 4 months with itraconazole 400 mg daily for 1 week per month for 3 and 4 months in tinea unguium. More than 120 patients were entered into each of the four treatment groups and final follow-up was at 72 weeks. At this time mycological cure rates were 75.7% in the 3-month terbinafine group and 80.8% in the 4-month terbinafine group. This contrasted with 38.3% and 49.1% in the 3-month and 4-month itraconazole pulsed groups respectively. Secondary clinical outcome measures were significantly in favor of terbinafine at week 72. The number of adverse events in this study was similar for all four treatment groups.

This study is the largest double-blind comparison of terbinafine and pulsed itraconazole and has the longest follow-up period. It is therefore considered to be the most definitive comparison thus far and the results are heavily in favor of terbinafine.

Twelve weeks of continuous oral therapy for toenail onychomycosis caused by dermatophytes: a double-blind comparative trial of terbinafine 250 mg/day versus itraconazole 200 mg/day. De Backer M, De Vroey C, Lesaffre E, et al. J Am Acad Dermatol 1998;38:S57–63.

A total of 186 patients in each treatment group with confirmed dermatophyte infection were entered and final assessment was at week 48. Mycological cure rates were 73% in the terbinafine group vs 45.8% in the itraconazole group.

A randomized double-blind multicentre comparison of terbinafine and itraconazole for the treatment of toenail tinea infection. Brautigam M, Nolting S, Schopf RE, Weidinger G. Br J Dermatol 1996;134(suppl 46):18–21.

One hundred and ninety five patients were randomized into two groups and given terbinafine 250 mg daily or itraconazole 200 mg daily for 12 weeks with follow-up at a further 40 weeks. At that time mycological cure rates were 81% for the terbinafine group and 63% for the itraconazole group.

These two studies compared terbinafine with continuous itraconazole in a dose of 200 mg daily. Both revealed terbinafine to be superior, and continuous itraconazole is now rarely recommended, having been supplanted by the pulsed regimen discussed above.

Terbinafine in fungal infections of the nails; a meta-analysis of randomized clinical trials. Haugh M, Helou S, Boissel JP, Cribier BJ. Br J Dermatol 2002;147:118–21.

This meta-analysis includes comparison of terbinafine (n = 622) with itraconazole (n = 642) in four studies. A statistically significant advantage in favor of terbinafine was observed at the end of these trials. Studies comparing terbinafine with both continuous and pulse itraconazole were included.

This meta-analysis confirms the superiority of terbinafine as suggested in single studies.

SECOND LINE THERAPIES

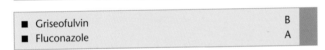

■ Griseofulvin	B
■ Fluconazole	A

Mycological and clinical evaluation of griseofulvin for chronic onychomycosis. Davies RR, Everall JD, Hamilton E. Br Med J 1957;3:464–8.

In this original study of griseofulvin in tinea unguium, the drug was given for 12 months for toenail infection; cure rates were about 30%.

A double-blind, randomized study to compare the efficacy and safety of terbinafine (Lamisil) with fluconazole (Diflucan) in the treatment of onychomycosis. Havu V, Heikkila H, Kuokkanen K, et al. Br J Dermatol 2000;142:97–102.

This study compared terbinafine 250 mg daily for 12 weeks with fluconazole 150 mg once weekly for 12 or 24 weeks. A total of 137 patients were divided into three groups and at week 60 the mycological cure rate for terbinafine was 89% vs 51% and 49%, respectively, for the 12- and 24-week fluconazole groups.

The original griseofulvin study reveals relatively poor cure rates in toenails and subsequent studies have shown sometimes poorer and sometimes better cure rates. However, clinical experience over many years suggested that the original cure rates of 30% are accurate and, furthermore, relapse rates are high. The comparison of terbinafine with fluconazole revealed terbinafine to be superior, although results with higher dosage regimens of fluconazole may be better. Such regimens are likely to be much more costly than terbinafine even if they are clinically comparable.

In terms of mycological cure rate, therefore, all these studies confirm terbinafine as the drug of choice.

How often does oral treatment of toenail onychomycosis produce a disease-free nail? An analysis of published data. Epstein E. Arch Dermatol 1998;134:1551–4.

An analysis of 26 articles found that standard courses of terbinafine achieved a disease-free nail in approximately 35–50% of patients whereas itraconazole produced a disease-free nail in 25–40% of cases.

This paper analyzes published data in a meta-analytical fashion to try to establish which is the superior drug. Again, terbinafine appears to be better than itraconazole, but it may appear that the percentage of disease-free nails produced is still disappointing. However, the criteria used to assess normality, usually a scoring system involving thickening, discoloration, and onycholysis, are very strict and a large percentage of toenails would not be considered 'normal' prior to infection. Patients' assessment of their own disease reveals satisfaction in approximately the same percentage of cases as demonstrated by mycological cure and this may be a more accurate assessment than a strict scoring system.

The latter point is important for fear that healthcare providers do not consider the disease to be worth treating because the production of a disease-free target organ is, on the face of it, disappointing.

THIRD LINE THERAPIES

■ Topical amorolfine	B
■ Topical ciclopirox	B
■ Topical tioconazole	D

Amorolfine in the treatment of onychomycoses and dermatomycoses (an overview). Zaug M, Bergstrausser M. Clin Exp Dermatol 1992;17(suppl 1):61–70.

A total of 727 patients were treated for 6 months (range 1–14 months) with 2% and 5% amorolfine lacquer. At follow-up visit 3 months after the end of treatment 45–50% of the patients treated once weekly were cured. The paper recommends that 5% amorolfine nail lacquer be applied once or twice weekly until clinical cure is achieved.

Topical therapy of onychomycoses with nail varnish containing 8% ciclopirox. Effendy I, Kolczak H, Ossowski B, Hohler T. Fortschr Med 1993;111:39–42.

Forty seven patients were treated with a nail varnish containing ciclopirox once daily for 6 months. At the end of the 6-month follow-up period mycological and clinical cure was seen in 59.5%, mycological cure in an additional 12.8%, and complete failure in 27.7%.

An open, noncomparative study.

Tioconazole. A review of its antimicrobial activity and therapeutic use in superficial mycoses. Clissold SP, Heel RC. Drugs 1986;31:29–51.

This review article reports tioconazole to be effective in superficial fungal infections of the skin.

Topical treatments for fungal infections of the skin and nails of the foot. Crawford F, Hart R, Bell-Syer S, et al. Cochrane Database Syst Rev 2000;(2):CD001434.

Evidence levels   A Double-blind study   B Clinical trial ≥ 20 subjects   C Clinical trial < 20 subjects   D Series ≥ 5 subjects   E Anecdotal case reports

This review concentrated mainly on skin infection but the authors commented that, in two trials of nail infections that fulfilled the strict criteria for consideration, there was no evidence of any benefit of topical treatments compared with placebo.

The first three references above detail open studies of the use of three nail lacquers for tinea unguium. The numbers in the amorolfine paper are large and cure rates do not appear to be too bad. Apart from the review there is no specific study of the efficacy of tioconazole, and clinical experience does not suggest that it is effective. Ciclopirox does appear to be effective in some cases, but again there are no comparative data with systemic treatments, and the last reference, which is a critical review of published data, suggests that there is no evidence that topical treatment works at all.

However, topical treatment is available for those patients who do not wish to take, or in whom there is a contraindication to, systemic therapy.

A randomized trial of 5% amorolfine solution nail lacquer combined with oral terbinafine compared with terbinafine alone in the treatment of dermatophytic toenail onychomycosis affecting the matrix region. Baran R, Feuilhade M, Datry A, et al. Br J Dermatol 2000;142:1177–83.

This study examined potential synergy between topical and oral treatment, and the mycological and clinical cure rate at 18 months was 44.0% in the group given terbinafine for 6 weeks together with a weekly application of nail lacquer. Of those given terbinafine for 12 weeks together with lacquer 73.2% were cured, whereas only 37.5% of patients who took terbinafine alone were cured.

The results obtained in this study were unusual in that the group that received only terbinafine produced cure rates that are approximately half as good as those one would expect. Indeed, the cure rates for the combination of 12 weeks plus the nail lacquer were about the same as seen in many other studies with terbinafine alone and there does not seem to be evidence that the hard core of 20% failures are responding here. However, this work requires to be repeated because the results are not what one would expect.

Tinea versicolor (pityriasis versicolor)

Jan Faergemann, Rachel Nazarian

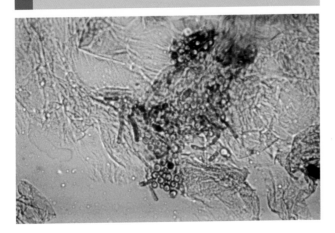

Tinea versicolor, also known as pityriasis versicolor, is a chronic superficial fungal infection and one of the more commonly found pigmentary disorders with a worldwide distribution. It is caused by the lipophilic yeast *Malassezia* (previously called *Pityrosporum*), an agent that is part of the normal human skin flora and carried by 90–100% of the population. It consists of both a yeast form and a mycelial form, which is a lipophilic fungus that requires exogenous fatty acids for growth, leading to its affinity for mature sebaceous glands. Subsequent to this attribute, tinea versicolor is frequently seen after puberty on the back, trunk, upper arms, and scalp: areas with a high density of sebaceous glands. Hair shafts or mucosae are not involved, though occasionally hair follicles may be due to the available environment of free fatty acids and triglycerides, causing *Pityrosporum* folliculitis.

Clinically, tinea versicolor presents with hypo- or hyperpigmented lesions that are slightly scaling and papular or nummular. High temperatures and a high relative humidity increase susceptibility to tinea versicolor, which correlates with findings that the disease has a higher incidence in hot tropical zones with humid climates. Additional factors that play a role include immunodeficiency or immunosuppression, elevated corticosteroids, hyperhidrosis, pregnancy, greasy skin, and a possible hereditary influence. The high rate of recurrence with tinea versicolor, reaching 60% after 1 year and 80% after 2 years, is due to the difficulty in eradicating predisposing factors. Consequently, a prophylactic treatment regimen is necessary to avoid recurrence.

MANAGEMENT STRATEGY

This superficial fungus can be cleared by targeting the outer stratum corneum. *Synthetic antifungal creams or shampoos* are often the most effective choice of treatment. Studies have found ketoconazole 2% shampoo, zinc pyrithione shampoo, and sulfur–salicylic acid shampoo work well. Selenium sulfide 2.5% may be used, but the patient sometimes com-plains about the offensive odor and stinging sensation on the skin after application. Due to the presence of the fungus even on unaffected skin, topical lotions are applied from the neck down to the knees and left on for 10–15 min once a day for 2 weeks. *Topical application of bifonazole, clotrimazole, econazole, or miconazole* once or twice daily for 2 weeks is also effective, with bifonazole 1% shown to be effective for infants as well. These topical antifungals are effective, but cost may be a limiting factor. A topical application of *terbinafine 1%* as a solution, cream, gel, or even spray has also been found effective. *Propylene glycol 50% in water* presents an ideal solution because it is cheap, effective, and cosmetically elegant.

Systemic therapy is primarily indicated for extensive lesions, for lesions resistant to topical treatment, and for frequent relapse. *Fluconazole, itraconazole,* and *ketoconazole* are all effective oral treatments for tinea versicolor. It is judicious to note that oral treatments taken for longer than 4 weeks increase the risk for hepatotoxicity. However, the risk of side effects with systemic therapy may be minimized with short-term treatment and therefore oral antifungals may be used, even for other indications.

Additional successful methods of management include *Whitfield's ointment* and *ciclopirox gel*. Recently topical applications of equal part mixtures of *honey, olive oil, and beeswax* have been shown to be efficacious in treating tinea versicolor when applied three times daily for 4 weeks.

Regardless of method of treatment, recurrence is common with tinea versicolor, and *applications should be repeated every 1 or 2 weeks to keep the cutaneous fungal infection in remission.*

Patients are often left with hypopigmentation even with successful treatment, which may lead them to believe the fungus is still present. Tanning is advised to restore even-toned skin.

SPECIFIC INVESTIGATIONS

- Wood's light
- Parker ink/potassium hydroxide (KOH) preparation of scale
- Albert's ink/KOH preparation of scale

Although the diagnosis of tinea versicolor is relatively easy to make clinically, it may often look similar to other dermatoses such as pityriasis alba, epidermodysplasia verruciformis, hypopigmented mycosis fungoides, seborrheic dermatitis, and leprosy. A few simple investigations can be done to confirm the diagnosis. The long-wave UV radiation from a Wood's lamp can highlight the lesions with a pale yellow fluorescence. Skin scrapings may be taken from the suspected lesion, though often skin strippings can be taken using a strip of Scotch tape. The strippings are placed on a slide in KOH 20% or 1% methylene blue. Results may be easier and faster to read when using Albert's solution or Parker ink. Both methods will stain fungal elements, and under microscopic examination will reveal the characteristic spores and hyphae that have been nicknamed 'meatballs and spaghetti'.

Evidence levels **A** Double-blind study **B** Clinical trial ≥ 20 subjects **C** Clinical trial < 20 subjects **D** Series ≥ 5 subjects **E** Anecdotal case reports

FIRST LINE THERAPIES

Topical antifungals	
■ Ketoconazole	A
■ Terbinafine	A
■ Clotrimazole	A
■ Selenium sulfide	A
■ Tioconazole	B
■ Sulfur salicylic acid shampoo	B
■ Zinc pyrithione shampoo	A
■ Bifonazole 1% shampoo/gel	B

Ketoconazole 2% shampoo in the treatment of tinea versicolor: a multicenter, randomized, double-blind, placebo-controlled trial. Lange DS, Richards HM, Guarnieri J, et al. J Am Acad Dermatol 1998;39:944–50.

A 31-day comparison of the efficacy of once-a-day applications of ketoconazole 2% shampoo versus three-a-day applications vs placebo on 312 patients with mycologically confirmed tinea versicolor. Both treatments with ketoconazole were significantly more successful than placebo, with the clinical responses of three-a-day and one-a-day ketoconazole being 73 and 69%, respectively. Either treatment was considered safe and effective. No serious side effects were noted.

Terbinafine. An update of its use in superficial mycoses. McClellan KJ, Wiseman LR, Markham A. Drugs 1999;58:179–202.

Topical terbinafine 1% is shown to be effective for tinea versicolor when applied twice daily for 2 weeks. Mycological cure was seen in 80% or more of patients.

Comparative study of tioconazole and clotrimazole in the treatment of tinea versicolor. Alchorne MM, Paschoalick RC, Forjaz MH. Clin Ther 1987;9:360–7.

Thirty two patients with tinea versicolor were treated with either 1% tioconazole lotion or 1% clotrimazole solution, applied twice daily for 28 days. All patients were clinically and mycologically cured by the end of treatment. It was noted that there was a substantial diminution of rash in those patients treated with 1% tioconazole during the second week of treatment. No side effects were noted in either patient population.

A double-blind comparative study of sodium sulfacetamide lotion 10% versus selenium sulfide lotion 2.5% in the treatment of pityriasis (tinea) versicolor. Hull CA, Johnson SM. Cutis 2004;73:425–9.

A double-blind study comparing sodium sulfacetamide lotion 10% and selenium sulfide lotion 2.5% when used once a day to treat patients with tinea versicolor for a maximum of 28 days. Selenium sulfide had a cure rate of 76.2% compared to 47.8% for sodium sulfacetamide. No side effects were noted.

Treatment of tinea versicolor with sulfur–salicylic shampoo. Bamford JT. J Am Acad Dermatol. 1983;8:211–3.

Patients with tinea versicolor were treated with sulfur–salicylic acid shampoo applied as a lotion nightly for 1 week. Half of the patients were placebo tested. After 3 months of treatment, 19 of 22 patients were negative by KOH examination. Only one of 16 controls was negative. Skin irritation was the only side effect and it did not diminish the effectiveness.

Double-blind comparison of a zinc pyrithione shampoo and its shampoo base in the treatment of tinea versicolor. Fredriksson T, Faergemann J. Cutis 1983;31:436–7.

Twenty patients with tinea versicolor were treated with 1% zinc pyrithione shampoo every night for 2 weeks; 20 additional patients with tinea versicolor were treated with placebo. The 20 patients treated with zinc pyrithione shampoo cleared without side effects, while the 20 patients treated with placebo did not clear.

Butenafine: an update of its use in superficial mycoses. Gupta AK. Skin Therapy Lett 2002;7:1–2, 5.

Butenafine is a safe and effective synthetic benzylamine antifungal agent, applied once daily for 2 weeks. The effectiveness lasted 4 weeks after the termination of therapy, which suggests retention of the drug in the skin.

Evaluation of in vitro activity of ciclopirox olamine, butenafine HCl and econazole nitrate against dermatophytes, yeasts and bacteria. Kokjohn K, Bradley M, Griffiths B, Ghannoum M. Int J Dermatol 2003;42(Suppl 1):11–7.

The three antifungals were compared against various cutaneous fungal infections; butenafine was found to have no activity against *M. furfur*.

Treatment of pityriasis versicolor with a shampoo containing 1% bifonazole (Agispor® shampoo) in children. Amichai B. Clin Exp Dermatol 2000;25:660.

An evaluation of the clinical efficacy of a shampoo with 1% bifonazole on 22 children aged 9–14 years. The children had been diagnosed with tinea versicolor, ranging from mild to severe. Shampoo was applied once a day for 3 weeks, with all children achieving a clinical cure.

SECOND LINE THERAPIES

Oral antifungals	
■ Itraconazole	A
■ Ketoconazole	A
■ Fluconazole	A

Single-dose fluconazole versus itraconazole in pityriasis versicolor. Partap R, Kaur I, Chakrabarti A, Kumar B. Dermatology 2004;208:55–9.

A comparison of the efficacy in curing tinea versicolor of single oral doses of fluconazole compared to itraconazole in 40 patients. After 8 weeks, 65% of patients taking fluconazole tested KOH negative and culture negative for *M. furfur*, and 20% taking itraconazole were culture and KOH negative. Relapse was 25% higher in the itraconazole group than in the fluconazole group. Both drugs were found to be equally safe.

Efficacy of itraconazole in the prophylactic treatment of pityriasis (tinea) versicolor. Faergemann J, Gupta AK, Mofadi AA, et al. Arch Dermatol 2002;138:69–73.

Patients were given itraconazole 200 mg twice daily one day per month prophylactically for six months. 88% were still free of lesions compared with 57% in the placebo group (p < .001).

Two years of follow-up of oral ketoconazole therapy in 60 cases of pityriasis versicolor. Alteras I, Sandbank M, Segal R. Dermatologica 1987;175:142–4.

Sixty patients with pityriasis versicolor were given 200 mg of oral ketoconazole daily for 24 days; 95% of patients had a clinical cure after 3 months. After 2 years, 60% of patients showed a relapse of tinea versicolor.

Long-term ketoconazole would raise concerns about liver toxicity, making single, weekly dosage for 2 weeks the preferred treatment.

Fluconazole versus ketoconazole in the treatment of tinea versicolor. Farschian M, Yaghoobi R, Samadi K. J Dermatolog Treat 2003;13:73–6.

A randomized, double-blind study in 128 patients with tinea versicolor, diagnosed through KOH preparation and examination with Wood's light fluorescence. Half received two 150 mg fluconazole capsules as a single weekly dosage for 2 weeks; half received two 200 mg ketoconazole tablets as a single weekly dosage for 2 weeks. The results showed no significant difference between either therapy with regards to efficacy, safety, or tolerability. Side effects were not noted, and the maximum cure rate was noted 8 weeks after commencement of therapy.

THIRD LINE THERAPIES

■ Whitfield's ointment	B
■ Propylene glycol	B
■ Ciclopirox	A
■ Honey, olive oil, beeswax	B

Comparison of clotrimazole cream, Whitfield's ointment and nystatin ointment for the topical treatment of ringworm infections, pityriasis versicolor, erythrasma and candidiasis. Clayton YM, Connor BL. Br J Dermatol 1973;89:297–303.

Thirty one patients with tinea versicolor were treated with either Whitfield's ointment or clotrimazole cream,

twice daily for 4 weeks. Clotrimazole had a cure rate of 88% and Whitfield's ointment had a cure rate of 86%.

The difficulty in applying ointments or creams over large body surface areas render these less practical than shampoos, lotions, or sprays, and hence, they are listed as third line therapies.

Propylene glycol in the treatment of tinea versicolor. Faergemann J, Fredriksson T. Acta Derm Venereol 1980;60:92–3.

Propylene glycol 50% in water was used to treat 20 patients with tinea versicolor using an application of twice daily for 2 weeks. Two weeks following the cessation of therapy all patients were reported as cured. Two patients experienced a slight burning of their skin after applying the solution.

Ciclopirox for the treatment of superficial fungal infections: a review. Gupta AK, Skinner AR. Int J Dermatol. 2003;42(Suppl 1):3–9.

Ninety patients with diagnosed pityriasis/tinea versicolor were treated with 0.1% ciclopirox olamine for 4 weeks. Clinical cure was achieved in 75% of patients; 86% cure was achieved after an additional 4 weeks of therapy.

An alternative treatment for pityriasis versicolor, tinea cruris, tinea corporis and tinea faciei with topical application of honey, olive oil and beeswax mixture: an open pilot study. Al-Waili NS. Complement Ther Med 2004;12:45–7.

A mixture of equal parts (1:1:1) of honey, olive oil, and beeswax was applied to the lesions of 37 patients with tinea versicolor, three times a day for 4 weeks. A clinical response was noted in 86% of patients, while mycological cure was noted in 75%.

Honey is known to have an inhibitory effect on fungi, but three applications daily for 4 weeks is a daunting schedule.

Toxic epidermal necrolysis and Stevens–Johnson syndrome

Nicholas M Craven

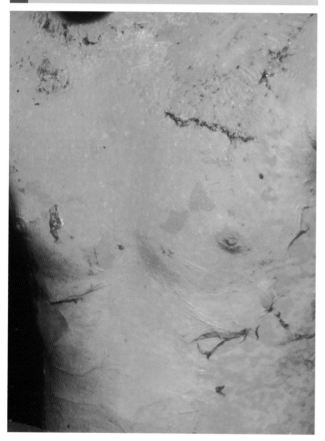

Toxic epidermal necrolysis (TEN) and Stevens–Johnson syndrome (SJS) form a spectrum of rare, potentially life-threatening conditions manifesting widespread erythematous macules or atypical target lesions and severe erosions of mucous membranes. Confluence of cutaneous lesions leads to epidermal loss, which by definition involves less than 10% of total body surface area (BSA) in SJS, 10–30% in overlap cases, and greater than 30% in TEN. Complications develop similar to those seen after burns. In most cases, TEN and SJS can be attributed to a drug reaction.

MANAGEMENT STRATEGY

The causative drug should be identified and discontinued. In general, drugs introduced in the 4 weeks before the onset of symptoms are usually responsible. If in doubt, all drugs should be stopped if possible.

The patient should be *managed in a burns unit* or appropriate *high-dependency unit.* Supportive therapy is directed at *fluid replacement*, maintaining a warm environment to *reduce heat loss*, topical *antiseptic preparations, hydrocolloid dressings or skin substitutes* to reduce colonization of the skin, and

regular monitoring for sepsis. Fluid replacement requirements depend upon the extent of involvement of the skin and mucous membranes, and may be 5–7 L in the first 24 h. Peripheral lines are preferable to central lines, which increase the risk of sepsis. *Nutritional support* requires fine-bore nasogastric tube feeding until the oral mucosa has healed. All lines should be checked daily for signs of infection, should be changed at least every 3 days, and the tips of all discarded lines and catheters should be sent for culture. Antibiotics should not be given routinely because this promotes resistance. If signs of sepsis develop (rising or falling temperature, rigors, hypotension, fall in urine output, deterioration of respiratory status, diabetic control, or level of consciousness), initial *antibiotic therapy* can be guided by the results of swabs taken from the skin and mucous membranes. Necrolytic epidermis should be removed gently once it starts to fold over to reduce the risk of infection.

Ophthalmological review should be obtained as soon as possible after diagnosis to minimize the risk of conjunctival scarring and blindness. Regular instillation of *antiseptic eye drops* and *separation of newly forming synechiae* are required. *Oral and nasal debris should be cleaned regularly* and an *antiseptic mouthwash* used several times a day.

Analgesia with opiates is often required, and care should be taken to monitor for respiratory depression. Respiratory failure may develop, requiring *ventilation* in an intensive care facility.

The use of *systemic corticosteroids* in the management of TEN and SJS remains controversial (see below). Several reports suggest that the use of corticosteroids increases morbidity and mortality, usually through increasing the risk of sepsis. Conversely, a number of case reports and short studies advocate the use of high-dose corticosteroids in the early part of the evolution of these conditions. It is possible, therefore, that high-dose corticosteroids may prove beneficial in aborting further epithelial loss in patients with evolving TEN/SJS, but this has not yet been tested in a randomized, controlled trial. Nevertheless, it is generally accepted that continuing administration of corticosteroids is counterproductive once extensive skin loss has occurred.

Several other potential disease-modifying treatments (*intravenous immunoglobulin (IVIG), cyclosporine, pentoxifylline, plasmapheresis, cyclophosphamide*) have been reported in small numbers of patients, but at the present time there is no strong evidence base for recommending any specific intervention other than supportive care.

Survivors of TEN and SJS, and their close relatives should avoid exposure to the culprit drug and related compounds.

SPECIFIC INVESTIGATIONS

- Histology
- Biochemical and hematological monitoring

Diagnosis of established TEN can usually be made clinically. Biopsy and immunofluorescence of an affected area of skin can exclude conditions such as staphylococcal scalded skin syndrome and paraneoplastic pemphigus. Histological examination of the roof of a fresh blister (even on frozen section specimens) may be adequate to distinguish TEN from staphylococcal scalded skin syndrome.

Supportive care of the patient involves regular monitoring of full blood count, urea, creatinine, electrolytes (including calcium and phosphate), transaminases, glucose, blood gases, swabs from infected areas and flexures, blood and urine cultures, and urine output.

Pulmonary complications in toxic epidermal necrolysis: a prospective clinical study. Lebargy F, Wolkenstein P, Gisselbrecht M, et al. Intensive Care Med 1997;23:1237–44.

Dyspnea, bronchial hypersecretion, and marked hypoxemia in the presence of a normal chest radiograph suggests bronchial injury from TEN, indicating a likely need for ventilation and a poor prognosis.

Incidence of Stevens–Johnson syndrome and toxic epidermal necrolysis in patients with the acquired immunodeficiency syndrome in Germany. Rzany B, Mockenhaupt M, Stocker U, et al. Arch Dermatol 1993;129:1059.

Patients with AIDS have an incidence of TEN/SJS of around one case per 1000 per year, compared with an incidence in the total population of 1.2–1.4 per 10^6 per annum.

HIV testing should be considered for high-risk patients presenting with TEN/SJS.

Medication use and the risk of Stevens–Johnson syndrome or toxic epidermal necrolysis. Roujeau J-C, Kelly JP, Naldi L, et al. N Engl J Med 1995;333:1600–7.

The main culprit drugs are sulfonamides, anticonvulsants, oxicam nonsteroidal anti-inflammatory drugs (NSAIDs), allopurinol, chlormezanone, and corticosteroids, but the excess risk associated with the use of these drugs is less than five cases per million users per week.

SCORTEN: a severity-of-illness score for toxic epidermal necrolysis. Bastuji-Garin S, Fouchard N, Bertocchi M, et al. J Invest Dermatol 2000;115:149–153.

Assessment of seven clinical parameters within the first 24 h of admission (age over 40 years; history of malignancy; tachycardia > 120 bpm; skin loss > 10%; urea > 10 mmol/L; glucose > 14 mmol/L; bicarbonate < 20 mmol/L) can be used to predict risk of mortality (score 0 or 1 – 3% risk of death; 2 – 12%; 3 – 35%; 4 – 58%; 5+ – 90%).

FIRST LINE THERAPIES

■ Supportive measures	E
■ Analgesia	E

Toxic epidermal necrolysis (Lyell syndrome). Roujeau J-C, Chosidow O, Saiag P, Guillaume J-C. J Am Acad Dermatol 1990;23:1039–58.

Useful review article covering all aspects of TEN. Practical guidance is given on therapy including fluid replacement, nutritional support, antimicrobial measures, topical treatments, and other aspects of supportive care.

Skin coverage with Biobrane® biomaterial for the treatment of patients with toxic epidermal necrolysis. Arévalo JM, Lorente JA. J Burn Care Rehabil 1999;20:406–10.

The authors describe their experience in treating eight consecutive TEN patients on a burn care unit with extensive early debridement of necrotic skin areas followed by wound coverage with a temporary semisynthetic skin substitute.

These patients also received cyclosporine (see below). Reported benefits of Biobrane® include decreased pain and fluid loss, facilitation of re-epithelialization, and decreased risk of sepsis.

SECOND LINE THERAPIES

■ Cyclosporine	C
■ Systemic corticosteroids	C
■ Intravenous immunoglobulin	C

Treatment of toxic epidermal necrolysis with cyclosporin A. Arévalo JM, Lorente JA, González-Herrada C, Jiménez-Reyes J. J Trauma 2000;48:473–8.

An improved outcome is reported in 11 consecutive patients with TEN treated with cyclosporine 3 mg/kg daily compared to six historical controls treated with cyclophosphamide and corticosteroids. Both groups were of comparable age, with similar extent of skin loss and delay between onset of TEN and admission. Patients treated with cyclosporine had more rapid re-epithelialization, were less likely to suffer multiorgan failure, and had a lower mortality (0 of 11 vs 3 of 6).

Toxic epidermal necrolysis associated with severe hypocalcaemia, and treated with cyclosporin. Zaki I, Patel S, Reed R, Dalziel KL. Br J Dermatol 1995;133:337–8.

A case induced by amoxicillin. This case had not responded to prednisolone 60 mg daily. Improvement occurred within 48 h of starting cyclosporine 4 mg/kg daily (route not stated). After 10 days, when the dose of cyclosporine was reduced to 2 mg/kg daily, the disease flared again, but improved on restoration of the original cyclosporine dose.

Toxic epidermal necrolysis treated with cyclosporin. Hewitt J, Ormerod AD. Clin Exp Dermatol 1992;17:264–5.

Two cases of TEN improving on cyclosporine. One followed an upper respiratory tract infection treated with Dequacaine® lozenges and pholcodeine linctus and was treated with 3.6 mg/kg daily (route not stated). The other followed amoxicillin treatment for an upper respiratory tract infection (treated with 3 mg/kg daily orally), and recurred following ciprofloxacin treatment for a urinary infection, again resolving on cyclosporine 5 mg/kg.

There are now several reports of the successful use of cyclosporine in TEN. Because most of the hazards of this drug are associated with long-term use it seems logical to use high doses in TEN as treatment will only be needed for a few days.

High-dose systemic corticosteroids can arrest recurrences of severe mucocutaneous erythema multiforme. Martinez AE, Atherton DJ. Pediatr Dermatol 2000;17:87–90.

Two children, one with SJS and one with bullous erythema multiforme (typical target lesions), were subject to recurrent attacks, which appeared to be abated by intravenous methylprednisolone (20 mg/kg daily for 3 days), commenced within 24–48 h of the onset of skin signs.

Toxic epidermal necrolysis and systemic corticosteroids. Stables GL, Lever RS. Br J Dermatol 1993;128:357.

Case report of a patient with TEN whose skin showed reduction in erythema 12 h after commencing prednisolone 60 mg daily.

Corticosteroid therapy in an additional 13 cases of Stevens–Johnson syndrome: a total series of 67 cases. Tripathi A, Ditto AM, Grammer LC, et al. Allergy Asthma Proc 2000;21:101–5.

Latest in a series of reports from this group. Thirteen patients with SJS were treated with intravenous methyl-prednisolone 160–240 mg daily on admission to the unit (1–14 days after onset of symptoms). One patient died from unrelated causes; all others survived. This extends to 67 the authors' series of patients with SJS treated with corticosteroids.

Clinical descriptions are incomplete, but surprisingly few of the patients had bullous lesions. It is possible that a significant number of these 67 patients would be classified by dermatologists as having hypersensitivity syndrome rather than SJS.

Erythema multiforme in children. Response to treatment with systemic corticosteroids. Rasmussen JE. Br J Dermatol 1976;95:181–6.

A retrospective study comparing the progress of 17 children with SJS treated with prednisolone 40–80 mg/m² with 15 treated with supportive care only. Both groups were similar in terms of age, sex, and extent of cutaneous and mucosal involvement. The corticosteroid group had more complications (mostly infections) and a longer mean duration of hospitalization (21 vs 13 days) than the noncorticosteroid group. No patients died.

It is likely that a number of these cases recorded as having iris lesions would now be classified as bullous erythema multiforme rather than SJS.

Characteristics of toxic epidermal necrolysis in patients undergoing long-term glucocorticoid therapy. Guibal F, Bastuji-Garin S, Chosidow O, et al. Arch Dermatol 1995;131:669–72.

TEN can occur in patients already taking high-dose corticosteroids. The onset of TEN is delayed following exposure to the culprit drug, but its progression is not halted.

Improved burn center survival of patients with toxic epidermal necrolysis managed without corticosteroids. Halebian PH, Corder VJ, Madden MR, et al. Ann Surg 1986;204:503–12.

Fifteen consecutive TEN patients treated in a burns unit with supportive measures only had an overall mortality rate of 33%, compared with a 66% mortality rate in the historical control group treated with corticosteroids. Eleven of the 'noncorticosteroid' group had nevertheless been commenced on corticosteroids by the referring institutions prior to arrival at the burns unit.

Inhibition of toxic epidermal necrolysis by blockade of CD95 with human intravenous immunoglobulin. Viard I, Wehrli P, Bullani R, et al. Science 1998;282:490–3.

Series of ten consecutive patients with TEN treated with IVIG at 0.2–0.75 g/kg daily for 4 days. Progression of skin disease stopped within 24–48 h, and all patients survived.

Intravenous immunoglobulin treatment for Stevens–Johnson syndrome and toxic epidermal necrolysis: a prospective noncomparative study showing no benefit on mortality or progression. Bachot N, Revuz J, Roujeau JC. Arch Dermatol 2003;139:33–6.

Prospective open trial of 34 patients with SJS, TEN, or overlap treated with IVIG 2 g/kg over 2 days; 11 deaths occurred (32% – mostly elderly patients with impaired renal function), compared to a predicted mortality of 8.2 deaths based on SCORTEN data. No measurable effect was observed on the progression of epidermal detachment or on the speed of re-epithelialization.

Treatment of toxic epidermal necrolysis with high-dose intravenous immunoglobulins: multicenter retrospective analysis of 48 consecutive cases. Prins C, Kerdel FA, Padilla RS, et al. Arch Dermatol 2003;139:26–32.

Multicenter retrospective analysis of 48 consecutive TEN patients treated with IVIG, mean dose 2.7 g/kg. Treatment was associated with a rapid cessation of skin and mucosal detachment in 43 patients (90%) and survival in 42 (88%). It was noted that patients who responded to IVIG had received treatment earlier in the course of disease and had higher doses of IVIG. The authors therefore recommend early treatment with IVIG at a total dose of 3 g/kg over three consecutive days (1 g/kg daily for 3 days).

Intravenous immunoglobulin does not improve outcome in toxic epidermal necrolysis. Shortt R, Gomez M, Mittman N, Cartotto R. J Burn Care Rehabil 2004;25:246–55.

Outcome data for 16 patients with TEN treated with IVIG was compared with that of 16 historical controls treated without IVIG. The mortality rate of the IVIG group was 25%, compared to 38% in the control group (not statistically significant). There were no significant differences between the groups with respect to the duration of stay, duration of ventilation, the incidence of sepsis, or time to healing. There was a trend towards less severe wound progression in patients who received IVIG.

As with all data on treatment of TEN, interpretation of the available literature is limited by lack of uniformity in the treatment regimens used, by the lack of adequate control data, and by the relatively small size of the studies.

THIRD LINE THERAPIES

■ Plasmapheresis	C
■ Cyclophosphamide	D
■ Pentoxifylline	E

Plasmapheresis as an adjunct treatment in toxic epidermal necrolysis. Egan CA, Grant WJ, Morris SE, et al. J Am Acad Dermatol 1999;40:458–61.

Retrospective study of 16 patients, six of whom were selected for plasmapheresis (one to four treatments) based on rapid progression of disease in the 24 h after admission. None of the patients treated with plasmapheresis died, whereas four of the other ten patients died.

Lack of significant treatment effect of plasma exchange in the treatment of drug-induced toxic epidermal necrolysis? Furubacke A, Berlin G, Anderson C, Sjoberg F. Intensive Care Med 1999;25:1307–10.

Comparison of outcome of eight patients with TEN affecting 12–100% BSA who received one to eight plasma exchange treatments with the results in two other centers that used almost identical treatment protocols but without plasma exchange showed no benefit in terms of mortality

(12.5%), time to re-epithelialization, or duration of stay in the burns intensive care unit. The authors concluded that the results did not support the use of plasma exchange in the treatment of TEN.

Plasma exchange in patients with toxic epidermal necrolysis. Bamichas G, Natse T, Christidou F, et al. Ther Apher 2002;6:225–8.

Retrospective study of 13 patients with TEN with involvement of 17–100% BSA treated with two to five sessions of plasmapheresis carried out daily or on alternate days. Three patients died (mortality rate 23%).

Efficacy of cyclophosphamide in toxic epidermal necrolysis. Heng MCY, Allen SG. J Am Acad Dermatol 1991;25:778–86.

Series of five patients with TEN; four survived following treatment with cyclophosphamide 100–300 mg daily and corticosteroid (prednisolone 60–120 mg or methylprednisolone 1 g daily). The fifth died having had supportive treatment only.

Pentoxifylline in toxic epidermal necrolysis and Stevens–Johnson syndrome. Sanclemente G, De La Roche CA, Escobar CE, Falabella R. Int J Dermatol 1999;38:878–9.

Two children with SJS and SJS/TEN overlap were treated with intravenous pentoxifylline 12 mg/kg daily. In both cases skin loss stopped on commencement of treatment, and in one of the children the skin deteriorated when pentoxifylline was temporarily discontinued.

Randomised comparison of thalidomide versus placebo in toxic epidermal necrolysis. Wolkenstein P, Latarjet J, Roujeau J-C, et al. Lancet 1998;352:1586–9.

Patients with TEN were randomized to either a 5-day course of thalidomide 400 mg daily (12 patients) or placebo (ten patients). The study was stopped early due to excess mortality in the treatment arm.

Evidence levels   **A** Double-blind study   **B** Clinical trial ≥ 20 subjects   **C** Clinical trial < 20 subjects   **D** Series ≥ 5 subjects   **E** Anecdotal case reports

Transient acantholytic dermatosis (Grover's disease)

Stuart C Murray, Susan M Burge

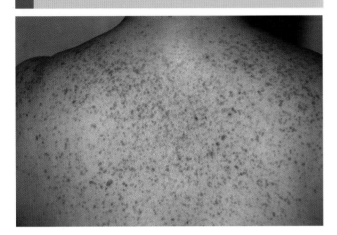

Grover's disease is an acquired, pruritic, papulovesicular eruption characterized histologically by focal acantholytic dyskeratosis. It is predominantly self-limiting. It is more common in middle-aged and elderly people, especially males, and involves mainly the trunk. The evolution is acute or chronic. The etiology is unknown, but excessive UV exposure, heat, sweating, and ionizing radiation are linked to the disease.

MANAGEMENT STRATEGY

Grover's disease is a common disorder characterized by discrete erythematous, edematous, papulovesicles or keratotic papules. The duration of the eruption may be weeks to months and it may be persistent or recurrent. Pruritus of variable intensity is experienced by most patients and may be out of proportion to the clinical signs. Constitutional symptoms are usually absent.

Treatment is difficult. There have been no large clinical trials and reports are based on small numbers.

Patients should be advised to *avoid excessive sun exposure, strenuous exercise, heat and occlusive fabrics*. In mild cases, simple antipruritic measures such as *avoidance of soap* and *aqueous cream and soothing baths with emollient bath oils or colloidal oatmeal* may be of benefit. *Wet compresses with zinc oxide, calamine, or topical corticosteroids* may help to relieve the itching. *Antihistamines* may aid in the control of pruritus, but do not prevent the development of new lesions.

Topical calcipotriol (ointment) twice daily 50 μg/g may be helpful after 3–4 weeks of treatment. *Topical vitamin A acid (retinoic acid)* is of limited use due to skin irritation.

Systemic therapy may be indicated in more extensive and persistent disease. *Oral vitamin A* has been recommended in the past. The aromatic retinoid, *etretinate*, has been used successfully in doses of 25–50 mg daily or *acitretin* 0.5 mg/kg daily. Isotretinoin 40 mg daily has been used for periods ranging from 2 to 12 weeks. It may be administered on a reducing regimen if the initial response is rapid, with a maintenance dose of 10 mg daily. Side effects include dry skin, cheilitis, teratogenicity, and cholesterol and triglyceride elevation.

Systemic corticosteroids have been used to suppress inflammation and pruritus, but relapses frequently occur on withdrawing the drug.

Psoralen with UVA (PUVA) may be useful, but an initial exacerbation may occur. There are anecdotal reports of the success of narrow-band UVB and of medium-dose ultraviolet A1 phototherapy.

Topical 5-fluorouracil, dapsone, antibiotics, and cryotherapy are ineffective.

SPECIFIC INVESTIGATIONS

- Skin biopsy

Acantholysis is the characteristic epidermal change. The histologic changes may mimic Darier's disease, pemphigus, and Hailey-Hailey disease. Hyperkeratosis, parakeratosis, and spongiosis are other common epidermal changes.

FIRST LINE THERAPIES

■ Emollients	E
■ Avoid heat/sweating	D
■ Topical corticosteroids	D
■ Antihistamines	D

Transient acantholytic dermatosis. Heenan PJ, Quirk CJ. Br J Dermatol 1980;102:515–20.

This study looked at a series of 24 cases of transient acantholytic dermatosis. Most of them required topical fluorinated corticosteroids to control the pruritus, and two patients required intermittent courses of oral corticosteroids. Antihistamines were of limited value in controlling pruritus.

Incidence of transient acantholytic dermatosis (Grover's disease) in a hospital setting. French LE, Piletta PA, Etienne A, et al. Dermatology 1999;198:410–1.

A prospective study of 28 hospital inpatients diagnosed with Grover's disease. In over 80% of cases, the duration of hospitalization exceeded 2 weeks and was associated with strict bed rest. The authors suggested a sweat-related pathogenesis.

Transient acantholytic dermatosis (Grover's disease). Hu H, Michel B, Farber EM. Arch Dermatol 1985;121:1439–41.

Seven cases of Grover's disease are presented in this article, which demonstrated a causal association with heat and sweating. Five of the cases are reported to have responded to topical corticosteroids.

SECOND LINE THERAPIES

■ Isotretinoin/acitretin	D
■ Systemic corticosteroids	D
■ PUVA	E
■ Vitamin A	D

Persistent acantholytic dermatosis. Dodd HJ, Sarkany I. Clin Exp Dermatol 1984;9:431–4.

A case report of a 41-year-old male with a 5-year history of an itchy truncal and lower limb rash consistent with persistent acantholytic dermatosis. Bath emollients and aqueous cream BP afforded minor relief. Etretinate (50 mg daily) cleared the skin lesions and reduced the itching.

Etretinate has been replaced by its active metabolite, acitretin. Lower doses of the latter drug may be effective.

Grover's disease treated with isotretinoin. Helfman RJ, Gables C. J Am Acad Dermatol 1985;12:981–4.

Four patients with biopsy-proven Grover's disease responded to 40 mg daily of isotretinoin. They completed a 2–4-month course of treatment. In two patients most lesions had cleared after 3–4 weeks of treatment. Their dose was reduced 10 mg daily for a further 8 weeks. One patient required 40 mg daily for 8 weeks. These patients remained in remission up to 10 months after treatment. The final case obtained partial relief and then discontinued treatment due to elevated triglycerides.

Transient acantholytic dermatosis treated with isotretinoin. Mancuso A, Cohen EH. Int J Dermatol 1989;28:58–9.

A 48-year-old man with severe pruritus had a 2-month history of Grover's disease. Systemic corticosteroids initially relieved his symptoms. On discontinuation of prednisone he relapsed. Isotretinoin was commenced at an initial dose of 1 mg/kg daily (40 mg twice daily) and then reduced to 40 mg daily due to adverse effects. He had improved by 6 weeks. Lesions and pruritus resolved after 3 months of therapy.

Response of transient acantholytic dermatosis to photochemotherapy. Paul BS, Arndt KA. Arch Dermatol 1984;120:121–2.

A 59-year-old male with persistent Grover's disease was unresponsive to oral prednisone and vitamin A (300 000 units daily). PUVA was initiated with 50 mg (0.6 mg/kg) methoxsalen and 2 J/cm² of UVA. Treatment was twice weekly and the UVA dosage was increased by 0.5 J/cm² with each treatment. The patient experienced a flare after four treatments, but improved by week 6 with maximal improvement by week 8. Therapy was then tapered off over the following 4 weeks with complete clearing. No recurrence had occurred 25 months after therapy.

Photochemotherapy beyond psoriasis. Honig B, Morison WL, Karp D. J Am Acad Dermatol 1994;31:775–90.

The authors comment that Grover's disease may occur in patients receiving PUVA for other skin conditions. Contin-

uation of PUVA clears the rash, with the pruritus resolving within ten treatments and the eruption clearing within 20–30 treatments. No numbers are supplied.

Reports show that approximately ten treatments are required for resolution of pruritus and 20–30 treatments may be needed for clearing of the eruption. Paradoxically, Grover's disease may complicate PUVA prescribed for other conditions.

Treatment of transient acantholytic dermatosis. Rohr JR, Quirk CJ. Arch Dermatol 1979;115:1033–4.

Eight patients were treated with vitamin A 50 000 units three times a day for up to 2 weeks, with all patients responding. Once initial improvement was noted the dose was reduced to 50 000 units daily as maintenance for several weeks. No signs of toxicity were noted. One patient required reinstitution of the drug due to recurrence on ceasing vitamin A.

THIRD LINE THERAPIES

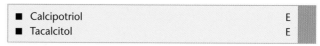

■ Calcipotriol	E
■ Tacalcitol	E

Treatment of Grover's disease with calcipotriol (Dovonex). Keohane SG, Cork MJ. Br J Dermatol 1995;132:832–3.

A 50-year-old man had a 13-month history of Grover's disease. He responded poorly to oxytetracycline, topical corticosteroids, dapsone, and etretinate. Lesions cleared following hospitalization and prednisone 100 mg daily, but he relapsed with any decrease in dose. Oral corticosteroids were stopped and he was commenced on an alternating regimen of calcipotriol ointment and betamethasone valerate 1:4. There was complete clearance of lesions following 1 month of treatment. The disease relapsed when treatment was stopped.

Successful treatment of Grover's disease with calcipotriol. Mota AV, Correia TM, Lopes JM, Guimaraes JM. Eur J Dermatol 1998;8:33–5.

Case report of an 84-year-old man with a 2-year history of Grover's disease. He improved significantly, despite initial moderate irritation, following a 3-week course of calcipotriol 50 µg/g applied twice daily. Lesions did not recur during a 6-month follow-up.

Treatment of Grover's disease with tacalcitol. Hayashi H. Clin Exp Dermatol 2002;27:160.

A 31-year-old man with a 2-month history of Grover's disease that failed to respond to topical corticosteroid was commenced on tacalcitol ointment twice daily. He improved dramatically within 1 week and was in remission after 1 month of therapy.

Evidence levels A Double-blind study **B** Clinical trial ≥ 20 subjects **C** Clinical trial < 20 subjects **D** Series ≥ 5 subjects **E** Anecdotal case reports

Trichotillomania

Ian Coulson, Leslie G Millard

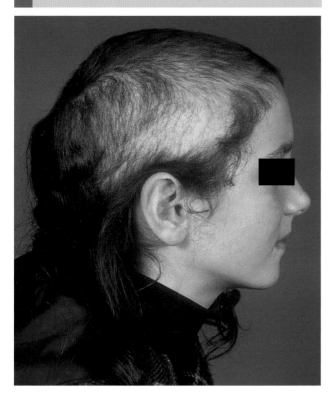

Trichotillomania is defined as the irresistible urge to pull out the hair, accompanied by the sense of relief after the hair has been plucked. The term was originally used by Hallopeau in 1889 and its literal meaning is that of a morbid craving to pull out the hair. Its definition includes trichotillomania as an impulse control disorder and it is co-classified with compulsive gambling and kleptomania. In children and adolescents it is more likely to be a stress-induced habit response, whereas in adults chronic disease is associated with significant psychopathology.

MANAGEMENT STRATEGY

The most important management strategy is to establish the diagnosis. This may be more difficult than it first appears. The textbook descriptions of trichotillomania emphasize the appearance of chronic hair loss with broken-off hairs and localized patches of hair loss more often in areas of handed dominance. The differential diagnosis includes alopecia areata, where the exclamation mark hairs may be confused with the stubby, broken, plucked hairs evident in localized and diffuse forms. Habitual hair shaving or cutting will produce subtly different clinical signs.

In children the problem is usually seen on the scalp and is usually asymmetrical, though with chronicity it may involve both sides of the scalp and, in time, involve the eyebrows and lashes. In adults, in whom the condition is invariably chronic, there is almost always a stubbly hair loss showing multiple broken-off hairs. Chronic trichotillomania usually involves the scalp, face, and also secondary sexual hair.

A very small proportion of patients may have weight loss, anorexia, and vomiting because of the formation of a hair ball (trichobezoar). When the ingested hair extends further into the small intestine (Rapunzel syndrome), signs of intestinal obstruction become evident with pain, vomiting, and dehydration. Barium meal examination or CT scan will show this. The treatment is surgical.

Patients with acute trichotillomania are usually children or adolescents. This physical response needs to be linked to some contemporary stressful episode within the child's environment, often school-linked stresses such as bullying, or home-linked events such as physical and sexual abuse by parents and fellow siblings. In older children, associations with anorexia/bulimia and substance abuse are well recorded.

In adults, this destructive behavior pattern quite commonly has persisted since the teens.

Chronic trichotillomania is a destructive impulse disorder with features of an obsessive–compulsive disorder, and an explanation of this to the patient will usually be empathically received. Hair loss may be disguised using wigs and hats, and hair colorants make the most of the remaining hair.

A significant proportion of patients with chronic trichotillomania have a depressive illness. Management of these associated conditions is essential. A combined approach using *behavioral modification, habit reversal, and hypnotherapy* techniques can be used with selective serotonin reuptake inhibitors (SSRI) such as *venlafaxine, fluvoxamine,* and *citalopram. Risperidone* in addition to a SSRI may be advantageous in recalcitrant disease. *Olanzapine* has shown efficacy in recent studies. Chronicity in children and continuing destructive behavior in adults may respond to *behavioral cognitive techniques* that mean intervention by the clinical psychologist or psychiatrist. *www.tric.org* is a trichotillomania learning resource that patients and carers alike may find useful.

SPECIFIC INVESTIGATIONS

- Hair microscopy
- Scalp biopsy
- Full blood count and ferritin
- Consider investigations for trichobezoar

Trichotillomania: a histopathological study in 66 patients. Miller S. J Am Acad Dermatol 1990;23:56–62.

Description of the definitive signs on scalp biopsy and differentiation from alopecia areata.

Hair microscopy may help to show the broken-off and fractured hairs. Scalp biopsy is helpful in differentiating between trichotillomania and alopecia areata.

There is a relationship to iron deficiency and full blood count, and ferritin levels are useful indicators of associated aggravating factors such as anorexia/bulimia and pica.

Trichotemnomania: obsessive–compulsive habit of cutting or shaving the hair. Happle R. J Am Acad Dermatol 2005;52:157–9.

Compulsive shaving or cutting of the hair can mimic both trichotillomania and alopecia areata.

Gastric trichobezoar. Phillips MR, Zaheer S, Drugas GT. Mayo Clinic Proc 1998;73:653–6.

Description of symptoms and treatment options.

Laparoscopic removal of large gastric trichobezoar. Nirasawa Y, Mari T, Ito Y, Tanaka H. J Pediatr Surg 1998;33: 663–5.

The presence of a trichobezoar needs surgical intervention. This can be performed either by open removal or laparoscopy.

FIRST LINE THERAPIES

■ Supportive psychotherapy	A
■ Directive and autogenic training	B
■ SSRI antidepressants	C

For children with acute trichotillomania, reassurance and explanation about the impulsive reactive nature of the condition is all that is required. Elucidation of the stress and corrective counseling usually relieve the problem.

Trichotillomania and related disorders in children and adolescents. Hanna GL. Child Psychiatry Hum Dev 1997;27: 255–68.

Common psychological factors to consider in counseling.

The characterization and treatment of trichotillomania. Christenson GA, Crow SJ. J Clin Psychiatry 1996;57(suppl 8):42–8.

Discussion of current treatment options. For chronic trichotillomania and multisite involvement, particularly in adults, explanation of the problem and recognition of the obsessional impulsive nature of the disease establishes an empathic response.

Trichotillomania treatment. Van Hasselt VB. Sourcebook of psychological treatment manual for adult disorders. New York: Plenum Press; 1996:657–87.

Treatment with pharmacological agents such as SSRIs produces a favorable response in up to 60% of patients.

Controlled trial of venlafaxine in trichotillomania. Ninan PT, Knight B, Kirk L, et al. Psychopharmacol Bull 1998;34:221–4.

Venlafaxine was effective in significantly reducing the symptoms of trichotillomania; eight of 12 patients were considered responders. The implications of the efficacy of venlafaxine in trichotillomania are discussed, including its important advantages over other available antidepressant and anxiolytic medications.

Fluvoxamine treatment of trichotillomania. Stanley MA, Breckenridge KA, Swann AC, et al. J Clin Pharmacol 1997;17:278–83.

Fluvoxamine was helpful in a subset of patients with trichotillomania; in some patients it did not reduce hair pulling, but did improve associated anxiety and depressive symptoms.

Use of the selective serotonin reuptake inhibitor citalopram in treatment of trichotillomania. Stein DJ, Bouwer C, Maud CM. Eur Arch Psychiatry 1997;247:234–6.

Citalopram was used in doses of up to 60 mg daily over 12 weeks in 14 patients; one-third were responders. Citalopram appears to be safe in trichotillomania, and it may be effective in a subset of patients.

SECOND LINE THERAPIES

■ Behavior therapy/habit retraining	B
■ Atypical neuroleptics (risperidone, olanzapine)	C
■ Hypnotherapy	C

Simplified habit reversal treatment for chronic hair pulling. Rapp JT, Miltenberger RG, Long ES, et al. J Appl Behav Anal 1998;31:299–302.

Three adolescents with chronic hair pulling were treated with a simplified habit reversal procedure consisting of awareness training, competing response training, and social support. Treatment resulted in an immediate reduction to near-zero levels of hair pulling, with one to three booster sessions required to maintain these levels. The results were maintained from 18 to 27 weeks after treatment.

Retrospective review of treatment outcome for 63 patients with trichotillomania. Keuthen NJ, O'Sullivan RL, Goodchild P. Am J Psychiatry 1998;155:560–7.

Recent behavioral and pharmacological therapy in a specific trichotillomania clinic offered significant clinical benefit.

Treatment of trichotillomania with behavioral therapy or fluoxetine: a randomized, waiting-list controlled study. van Minnen A, Hoogduin KA, Keijsers GP, et al. Arch Gen Psychiatry 2003;60:517–22.

Behavioral therapy was found to be superior to 60 mg of fluoxetine daily.

Risperidone augmentation of SSRI in obsessive–compulsive and related disorders. Stein DJ, Bouwer C, Hawkridge S, Emsley RA. J Clin Psychiatry 1997;58:119–22.

The addition of risperidone to SSRI antidepressants proved valuable in five patients with refractory trichotillomania.

An open-label, flexible-dose study of olanzapine in the treatment of trichotillomania. Stewart RS, Nejtek VA. J Clin Psychiatry 2003;64:49–52

Eighteen patients were enrolled in a 3-month open-label study of olanzapine for trichotillomania (diagnosis based on modified DSM-IV criteria). Patients with comorbid psychiatric disorders or on treatment with psychoactive medication were excluded. Olanzapine was titrated gradually in 2.5 mg/week increments up to a maximum dose of 10 mg daily. Hair pulling was reduced by 66%.

Hypnotherapeutic management of pediatric and adolescent trichotillomania. Kohen DP. J Dev Behav Pediatr 1996;17:328–34.

This report presents five cases of trichotillomania in which self-monitoring, dissociative hypnotic techniques, and self-hypnosis (relaxation/mental imagery) practices were used in teaching children successful management of chronic trichotillomania.

Evidence levels A Double-blind study B Clinical trial ≥ 20 subjects C Clinical trial < 20 subjects D Series ≥ 5 subjects E Anecdotal case reports

Hypnosis as a vehicle for choice and self-agency in the treatment of children with trichotillomania. Iglesias A. Am J Clin Hypn 2003;46:129–37.

Three cases of hypnosis helping childhood trichotillomania.

THIRD LINE THERAPIES

■ Psychiatric referral	A

Comorbid self-injurious behaviour in 71 female hair pullers. Simeon D, Cohen LJ, Stein DJ, Schmeidler J. J Nerv Ment Dis 1997;185:117–19.

Treatment of continuing depression and obsessive–compulsive disorder needs specialist psychiatric referral.

Tuberculosis and tuberculids

Anita Takwale, John Berth-Jones

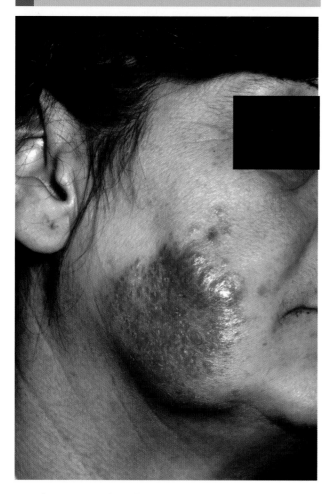

Mycobacterium tuberculosis is the predominant etiologic agent in cutaneous tuberculosis. Occasionally *Mycobacterium bovis* and bacille Calmette-Guérin (BCG) may produce skin lesions. True cutaneous tuberculosis has a wide variety of clinical presentations: inoculation tuberculosis, from an exogenous source (e.g. tuberculous chancre, warty tuberculosis, lupus vulgaris); secondary cutaneous tuberculosis, from an endogenous source (e.g. scrofuloderma, via contiguous spread; orificial tuberculosis, via autoinoculation); hematogenous tuberculosis (e.g. acute miliary tuberculosis, lupus vulgaris, tuberculous gumma). Tuberculids are considered to be immune reactions within the skin due to *M. tuberculosis* or mycobacterial antigen in an individual with strong antituberculosis cell-mediated immunity. This group includes lichen scrofulosorum, papular/papulonecrotic tuberculid, and erythema induratum (Bazin's disease).

MANAGEMENT STRATEGY

Diagnosis of cutaneous tuberculosis requires the correlation of clinical findings with diagnostic testing. Acid-fast bacilli (AFB) are almost never seen microscopically because the majority of cases are paucibacillary. Intradermal tests based on tuberculin reactivity cannot distinguish between an active and previous infection or vaccination. The only absolute criteria are a positive culture of *M. tuberculosis* from the lesion or identification of mycobacterial DNA by polymerase chain reaction (PCR). Because of the rising emergence of drug-resistant tuberculosis, wherever possible drug susceptibilities should be obtained.

In the UK, all patients with tuberculosis must be *notified*. This initiates *contact tracing* where appropriate. A careful search for an underlying focus of disease and coexistent infections is necessary. *HIV testing*, with informed consent and counseling should be considered if there are widespread lesions and in multidrug-resistant cases.

The aim of treatment is to cure the disease as rapidly as possible. The Joint Tuberculosis Committee (JTC) 1998 recommends treatment of all patients should be supervised by physicians (in most cases respiratory) with full training in the management of such cases. Directly observed therapy (DOT) is recommended for patients who are unlikely to comply.

The standard treatment regimens recommended are based on extensive controlled trials carried out for pulmonary tuberculosis. There have been few controlled trials for treatment of extrapulmonary tuberculosis and the use of such short-course regimens is based on analogy. The practice in the past of treating lupus vulgaris with *isoniazid (INH)* alone and treatment regimens shorter than 6 months for tuberculids are not recommended. The standard 6-month regimen for adults comprises *rifampin (rifampicin) 10 mg/kg, INH 5 mg/kg, pyrazinamide 35 mg/kg*, and *ethambutol 15 mg/kg* for the initial 2 months followed by rifampin and INH for a further 4 months in the continuation phase. Ethambutol can be omitted in patients with a low risk of resistance to INH. In countries where resources to provide rifampin are not available, ethambutol and INH are the drugs recommended by the World Health Organization (WHO) for the continuation phase. Occasionally longer treatment regimens may be necessary to achieve a complete cure.

In patients with HIV infection the continuation phase may need to be extended for seven or more months. Cases of multidrug-resistant tuberculosis should be managed at specialist centers whenever possible. Other measures may also be used. *Excision* may be effective for small early lesions of lupus vulgaris or warty tuberculosis. Local destruction of small residual nodules of lupus vulgaris may have a place in the management. *Surgery* may be useful in scrofuloderma. *Plastic surgery* may help the disfigurement left by treated lupus vulgaris.

The latest advances in management of pulmonary tuberculosis include *newer rifampin derivatives*, and *quinolones, interferon-α, tuberculous vaccine*, and *recombinant human interleukin-2* as an immunomodulator in tuberculosis. There are no trials of these in cutaneous tuberculosis, but they may influence the treatment of cutaneous infection in future.

SPECIFIC INVESTIGATIONS

- Skin biopsy for histopathology, and tissue or pus for mycobacterial culture
- Polymerase chain reaction (PCR) for *Mycobacterium tuberculosis* DNA in skin
- Tuberculin test
- Screening for extracutaneous tuberculosis: chest radiography is essential; consider also culture of sputum, bronchoscopy, early morning urine for AFB, and lymph node biopsy.

Detection of *Mycobacterium tuberculosis* complex DNA by the polymerase chain reaction for rapid diagnosis of cutaneous tuberculosis. Margall N, Baselga E, Coll P, et al. Br J Dermatol 1996;135:231–6.

Thirty seven of 48 (77.1%) of paraffin-embedded specimens from 32 patients with different variants of cutaneous tuberculosis were positive by PCR. The assay consisted of amplification of the 123 bp fragment of the IS6110 insertion sequence specific for *M. tuberculosis* complex. No false-positive results were obtained from the negative controls. Of the 20 biopsy specimens tested by PCR and conventional culture (Ziehl-Neelsen method, Lowenstein-Jensen medium, and BACTEC 12B liquid medium), 90% (18 samples) were positive on PCR and 65% (13 samples) on culture.

Cutaneous tuberculosis in Indian children: the importance of screening for involvement of internal organs. Pandhi D, Reddy BS, Chowdhary S, Khurana N. J Eur Acad Dermatol Venereol 2004;18:546–51.

Of 142 patients with cutaneous tuberculosis, 68 were children aged from 9 months to 14 years. Scrofuloderma was the most common presentation encountered in 30 (44.1%) patients, Fifteen (22.1%) patients had lupus vulgaris, 16 had lichen scrofulosorum, three had tuberculosis verrucosa cutis, and four had more than one type of tuberculosis. Involvement of the lung, involvement of the bone, and involvement of both the lung and bone was found in 14 (20.6%), seven (10.2%), and four (5.9%) patients, respectively.

FIRST LINE THERAPIES

- Antituberculous drugs   A

Chemotherapy and management of tuberculosis in the United Kingdom: recommendations 1998. Joint Tuberculosis Committee of the British Thoracic Society. Thorax 1998;53:536–48.

The Joint Tuberculosis Committee of the British Thoracic Society recommend an initial phase of 2 months of treatment with four drugs: INH 5 mg/kg, rifampin 10 mg/kg, pyrazinamide 35 mg/kg, and ethambutol 15 mg/kg. This is followed by a continuation phase of 4 months using INH and rifampin for pulmonary and extrapulmonary tuberculosis. The fourth drug (ethambutol) can be omitted in patients with a low risk of resistance to INH.

Treatment of tuberculosis: guidelines for National Programmes. Maher D, Chaulet P, Spinaci S, Harries A. Geneva: WHO; 1997.

The antituberculosis drugs recommended are INH (H) 5 mg/kg, rifampin (R) 10 mg/kg, pyrazinamide (Z) 25 mg/kg, streptomycin (S) 15 mg/kg, ethambutol (E) 15 mg/kg, and thiacetazone (T) 2.5 mg/kg. A common regimen employed is 2 months HRZE/6 months HE.

Cutaneous tuberculosis in Blackburn district (U.K): a 15-year prospective series, 1981–95. Yates VM, Ormerod LP. Br J Dermatol 1997;136:483–9.

Of the 1065 cases of tuberculosis in the Blackburn district, UK, 47 (4.4%) had forms of cutaneous tuberculosis. Scrofuloderma was the commonest form with 23 cases (55.3%). Ten cases were diagnosed as tuberculids, with erythema induratum being the commonest. All patients received antituberculosis drugs. A 6-month regimen was used from 1989 onwards. Shared management with the drug therapy decided, supervised, and monitored by the respiratory physicians had been practiced throughout the 15-year series. No patients had significant drug-related toxicity, all had good clinical response, and none relapsed.

Comparative efficacy of drug regimens in skin tuberculosis. Ramesh V, Misra RS, Saxena U, Mukherjee A. Clin Exp Dermatol 1991;16:106–9.

Three antituberculosis drug regimens were employed to study the response in 90 patients with cutaneous tuberculosis. The first two regimens contained rifampin (adults 450 mg, children 15 mg/kg), INH (adults 300 mg, children 5 mg/kg), and either pyrazinamide (adults 1500 mg, children 30 mg/kg) or thiacetazone (adults 150 mg, children 4 mg/kg), and the third regimen had rifampin and INH only. The patients with lupus vulgaris and warty tuberculosis cleared with all three regimens in 4 and 5 months for localized and generalized disease, respectively. Patients with scrofuloderma responded well to both triple drug regimens, with the skin lesions subsiding completely within 5 months in the localized and 6 months in the widespread forms of the disease. However 9–10 months of treatment was necessary in the group receiving INH and rifampin.

Lupus vulgaris. Clinical, histopathologic, and bacteriologic study of 10 cases. Marcoval J, Servitje O, Moreno A, et al. J Am Acad Dermatol 1992;26:404–7.

All but one of the ten patients responded satisfactorily to a 9-month course of combined antituberculosis chemotherapy using INH 5–10 mg/kg, and rifampin 10–20 mg/kg supplemented with ethambutol 15–25 mg/kg in the initial 3-month phase. The patient on INH alone relapsed twice after two courses of 9 months of treatment each time.

Erythema induratum (Bazin's disease). Rademaker M, Lowe DG, Munro DD. J Am Acad Dermatol 1989;21:740–5.

A series of 26 patients with erythema induratum is reviewed. Of four patients receiving INH alone two relapsed, and of 13 patients on INH and rifampin or INH and para-aminosalicylic acid, six relapsed. The duration of treatment for these was between 1 and 12 months. Of the eight patients who had a relapse, five cleared on triple therapy. All nine patients receiving triple therapy for 9 months (combinations of INH, pyrazinamide, rifampin, and ethambutol) achieved remission.

SECOND LINE THERAPIES

■ Local excision	D

Scrofuloderma of the lower extremity treated with wide resection: a case report and review of the literature. Connolly B, Pitcher JD Jr, Roth B, et al. Am J Orthop 1999;28:417–20.

A report on an immunocompromised patient who presented with scrofuloderma of the lower extremity. This failed to resolve with the standard antituberculosis regimen consisting of four drugs – INH, rifampin, pyrazinamide, ethambutol for 2 months followed by INH and rifampin for 3 months – but was then successfully treated with wide resection under spinal anesthesia.

Lupus vulgaris of the ear lobe. Okazaki M, Sakurai A. Ann Plast Surg 1997;39:643–6.

A 59-year-old woman with an initial diagnosis of hemangioma had surgical treatment, followed by antituberculosis therapy (INH, rifampin, and pyridoxine for 9 months) for lupus vulgaris of the ear lobe.

Primary inoculation tuberculosis. Hooker RP, Eberts TJ, Strickland JA. J Hand Surg 1979;4:270–3.

A case of primary inoculation tuberculosis of the finger is reported in which Mantoux test conversion reverted after prompt surgical and medical treatment with INH 300 mg daily for 1 year and ethambutol 200 mg daily for the initial 3 months.

Urticaria and angioedema

Frances Humphreys

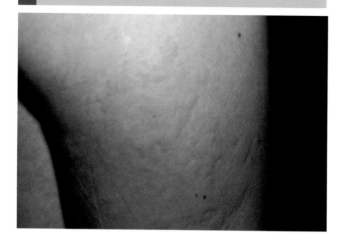

Urticaria is the result of plasma leakage and is characterized by short-lived, itchy, raised wheals due to dermal edema. In angioedema the swelling is deeper, resulting in more diffuse and prolonged edema, particularly affecting the face. These conditions are defined as chronic if symptoms have lasted longer than 6 weeks.

Hereditary angioedema (HAO) and the physical urticarias are covered on pages 267 and 486, respectively.

MANAGEMENT STRATEGY

Explanation of the nature of the disorder and prognosis is important. Most patients with chronic urticaria become asymptomatic within 2 years. Patients with a longer history and those with physical urticarias are less likely to remit. It is important to exclude causative and exacerbating factors, particularly drugs (i.e. aspirin, nonsteroidal anti-inflammatory drugs [NSAIDs], angiotensin-converting enzyme [ACE] inhibitors). IgE-mediated allergy is rarely a cause of chronic symptoms and does not need to be tested for routinely. Blood tests and chest radiography should only be performed if history or examination dictate. There is an increased incidence of positive thyroid autoantibodies. Of patients with chronic disease, 30–40% have a positive autologous serum skin test providing evidence of autoimmunity. This test does not need to be performed in routine practice. HAO should be excluded in those with angioedema without urticaria. Individual urticarial lesions lasting over 24 h may indicate urticarial vasculitis, necessitating skin biopsy and appropriate investigation if confirmed.

Potent nonsedating antihistamines are the mainstay of treatment and are usually given regularly, but occasionally as required for intermittent symptoms. Many patients show a diurnal variation in symptoms, and timing of once-daily treatment should be adjusted accordingly. In practice *acrivastine, cetirizine/levocetirizine, fexofenadine, loratadine/desloratadine* and *mizolastine* are all effective. Individual responses to different antihistamines vary and tachyphylaxis is frequently reported so changing H1 antagonists is warranted. Increasing the dose, combining two different long-acting ones 12 h apart, or adding a short-acting anti-histamine for breakthrough symptoms can all be useful maneuvers.

There is some evidence that *exclusion diets* may help in urticaria. It seems logical to try a low-salicylate diet for a 4-week assessment period in patients who report exacerbation of symptoms with aspirin or NSAIDs. *Systemic corticosteroids* do not help all patients with urticaria and, if introduced and effective, can be very difficult to withdraw. A short course of prednisolone 20–30 mg daily for 3 days can reduce the severity and time course of attacks of angioedema and acute urticaria. *Intramuscular epinephrine (adrenaline)* is not routinely used, but may be necessary for severe angioedema affecting the upper respiratory tract.

H2 antagonists have been used in combination with H1 antagonists, but their benefit in practice is disappointing. There is increasing evidence for a beneficial effect of *leukotriene antagonists, montelukast* being used most commonly. Limited evidence exists for *doxepin* (a tricyclic with H1 antagonist properties), *nifedipine, psoralen and UVA (PUVA)*, and *warfarin*. Some authors have used *thyroxine* with variable results. Conflicting evidence exists for *Helicobacter pylori eradication therapy. Rofecoxib* was used in a very small number of patients in open studies prior to its withdrawal; it is not known whether other cyclooxygenase-2 (COX-2) inhibitors have any effect. Like leukotriene antagonists these drugs can also cause urticaria.

There is now good evidence for an autoimmune etiology in chronic urticaria. Because most patients have a self-limiting and non-life-threatening condition, *immunosuppressive therapy* is not indicated for the majority. In those with severe and unremitting problems who are experiencing considerable morbidity associated with the condition, *cyclosporine, plasmapheresis* and *intravenous immunoglobulin* have all now been shown to be effective. The benefit of such treatment may be short-lived. A recent open study has shown that 4 weeks of cyclosporine gives the same degree of benefit as 12 weeks of treatment.

SPECIFIC INVESTIGATIONS

- None; or
- Screening tests based on history and physical examination

Recurrent urticaria: clinical investigation of 330 patients. Juhlin L. Br J Dermatol 1981;104:369–81.

Laboratory investigation in chronic urticaria was of little value in the absence of history or signs of other disease.

The autologous serum skin test: a screening test for autoantibodies in chronic idiopathic urticaria. Sabroe RA, Grattan CEH, Francis DM, et al. Br J Dermatol 1999;140:446–52.

In the hands of two experienced investigators 65–70% sensitivity and 80% specificity were obtained for this test. It is time consuming and best performed regularly by an experienced observer. In-vitro validation is useful.

FIRST LINE THERAPIES

■ Nonsedating H1 antagonists	A

Appraisal of the validity of histamine-induced wheal and flare to predict the clinical efficacy of antihistamines. Monroe EW, Daly AF, Shalhoub RF. J Allergy Clin Immunol 1997;99:S798–806.

This paper presents data from a number of open and placebo-controlled studies of antihistamines in chronic idiopathic urticaria (CIU). A therapeutic effect of these drugs has been shown, but no individual antihistamine is superior clinically despite some differences in effect on histamine wheal and flare reactions.

SECOND LINE THERAPIES

■ Leukotriene antagonists	A
■ Diet	B
■ Corticosteroids	B
■ H2 antagonists	B
■ Doxepin	B
■ Nifedipine	C
■ PUVA	C
■ Warfarin	C
■ Thyroid hormone	E

The addition of zafirlukast to cetirizine improves the treatment of chronic urticaria in patients with positive autologous skin tests. Bagenstose SE, Leven L, Bernstein JA. J Allergy Clin Immunol 2004;113:134–40.

This double-blind study showed a small but significant improvement by the addition of zafirlukast 20 mg twice daily, particularly in those who were autologous skin test positive. A previous study had failed to show an effect.

Urticaria is also reported as a side effect of these drugs.

Randomized placebo-controlled trial comparing desloratadine and montelukast in monotherapy and desloratadine plus montelukast in combined therapy for chronic idiopathic urticaria. Di Lorenzo G, Pacor ML, Mansueto P, et al. J Allergy Clin Immunol 2004;114:619–25.

One hundred sixty patients were treated with 5 mg of desloratadine once daily (n = 40), 10 mg of montelukast once daily (n = 40), 5 mg of desloratadine in the morning plus montelukast 10 mg in the evening (n = 40), or matched placebo (n = 40). The study demonstrated that desloratadine is highly effective for the treatment of patients with CIU, but the regular combined therapy of desloratadine plus montelukast did not seem to offer a substantial advantage with respect to desloratadine alone.

Pseudoallergen-free diet in the treatment of chronic urticaria. Zuberbier T, Chantraine-Hess S, Hartmann K, Czarnetski BM. Acta Derm Venereol 1995;75:484–7.

Seventy three per cent of 64 patients with CIU improved on a 2-week pseudoallergen-avoidance diet in an open study. Only 19% reacted to pseudoallergens on provocation testing. An additive-free, stringently controlled diet may provide a means of treating some patients with chronic urticaria.

Acute urticaria: clinical aspects and therapeutic responsiveness. Zuberbier T, Ifflander J, Semmler C, Henz BM. Acta Derm Venereol 1996;76:295–8.

Prednisolone 50 mg daily for 3 days was significantly better than loratadine in inducing remission of acute urticaria.

Cimetidine and chlorpheniramine in the treatment of chronic idiopathic urticaria: a multi-centre randomized double-blind study. Bleehan SS, Thomas SE, Greaves MW, et al. Br J Dermatol 1987;117:81–8.

Forty patients whose symptoms were not abolished by treatment with chlorpheniramine (chlorphenamine) alone were treated with either chlorpheniramine and placebo or chlorpheniramine and cimetidine 400 mg four times daily. A significant improvement in wheals and pruritus was shown for the active treatment.

Double-blind crossover study comparing doxepin with diphenhydramine for the treatment of chronic urticaria. Green SL, Reed CE, Schroeter AL. J Am Acad Dermatol 1985;12:669–75.

Fifty patients with CIU were treated with doxepin 10 mg three times daily compared with diphenhydramine 25 mg three times daily, with control of symptoms in 74 and 10%, respectively.

In practice, sedation can limit the usefulness of this drug.

Therapy of chronic idiopathic urticaria with nifedipine: demonstration of beneficial effect in a double-blinded, placebo-controlled, crossover trial. Bressler RB, Sowell K, Huston DP. J Allergy Clin Immunol 1989;83:756–63.

Ten patients with refractory urticaria had nifedipine (up to 20 mg three times daily) or placebo added to their treatment for 4 weeks. A beneficial effect was shown for seven patients who completed the study.

Treatment of chronic urticaria with PUVA or UVA plus placebo: a double-blind study. Olafsson JH, Larko O, Roupe G, et al. Arch Dermatol Res 1986;278:228–31.

This study showed improvement with PUVA and UVA plus placebo, suggesting either a therapeutic effect of UVA or a placebo effect.

Warfarin treatment of chronic idiopathic urticaria and angio-oedema. Parslew R, Pryce D, Ashworth J, Friedmann PS. Clin Exp Allergy 2000;30:1161–5.

Six of eight treatment-resistant patients showed a therapeutic effect of warfarin in an open study. Three responders then took part in a double-blind study, which confirmed an improvement in pruritus and angioedema scores.

Chronic urticaria and angioedema associated with thyroid autoimmunity: review and therapeutic implications. Heymann WR. J Am Acad Dermatol 1999;40:229–32.

In patients with chronic idiopathic urticaria who have documented antithyroid autoantibodies, the administration of thyroid hormone may suppress urticaria in selected cases.

THIRD LINE THERAPIES

■ Cyclosporine	A
■ Plasmapheresis	D
■ Intravenous immunoglobulin	D

Randomized double-blind study of cyclosporin in chronic 'idiopathic' urticaria. Grattan CEH, O'Donnell BF, Francis DM, et al. Br J Dermatol 2000;143:365–72.

Thirty patients with severe CIU who were autologous skin test positive were treated with 4 mg/kg daily cyclosporine or placebo for 4 weeks double blind, and nonresponders were then offered 4 weeks of treatment with cyclosporine on an open basis. In all, 19/30 responded to cyclosporine, but 14 relapsed by 20 weeks after treatment.

Plasmapheresis for severe, unremitting, chronic urticaria. Grattan CEH, Francis DM, Slater NP, et al. Lancet 1992;339: 1078–80.

Eight patients with severe disease and serum histamine-releasing activity underwent plasmapheresis with beneficial effect in six.

Intravenous immunoglobulin in autoimmune chronic urticaria. O'Donnell BF, Barr RM, Kobza Black A, et al. Br J Dermatol 1998;138:101–6.

An open, uncontrolled study showed benefit in nine of ten patients with severe CIU and evidence of autoimmunity –0.4 g/kg was used daily for 5 days.

Varicella

*Christine Soon, Malobi Ogboli,
John Berth-Jones*

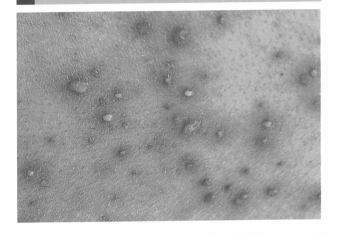

Varicella, or chickenpox, is the exanthematic illness caused by infection with the herpes virus, varicella zoster (VZV). It is common and highly contagious. Varicella spreads by direct person-to-person contact or by airborne droplets. It has a typical incubation period of 10–14 days. Fever and malaise can precede the development of erythema, papules, and vesicles, which have been likened to 'dew drops on rose petals'. The vesicles tend to appear in crops over 2–4 days in a centripetal distribution and crust over before healing. The mucosae are often involved. Pruritus is commonly a prominent feature. The disease is contagious from 48 h before the rash appears until after the vesicles crust. It occurs most commonly in young children and systemic symptoms are usually mild, though complications may occur. In patients with atopic dermatitis, varicella may closely resemble eczema herpeticum. In adolescents, adults, and immunocompromised individuals it is a more severe disease with a higher complication rate. Treatment is most commonly recommended for this group of individuals. Potential complications include secondary bacterial infection of the skin, bacterial pneumonia, and varicella pneumonitis. Rare complications of varicella include aseptic meningitis, encephalitis, cerebellar ataxia, myocarditis, corneal lesions, nephritis, arthritis, acute glomerulonephritis, Reye's syndrome, bleeding diathesis, and hepatitis. Herpes zoster (shingles), a delayed consequence of infection with VZV is discussed on page 277.

MANAGEMENT STRATEGY

Routine *vaccination* of healthy persons 12 months of age or older who have not had varicella is now recommended in the United States. In the UK vaccination is recommended for nonimmune individuals (principally healthcare workers) who are in frequent contact with patients who would be especially vulnerable to the infection (the purpose being primarily to protect those patients from infection). A live, attenuated vaccine is used. Postexposure immunization may also be effective for household contacts if given within 3 days of the appearance of the rash in the index case.

In healthy children below the age of 12 years, symptomatic treatment is all that is generally required. *Aceta-*minophen (paracetamol) is suitable. Aspirin should be avoided because of the risk of Reye's syndrome. If a child is the second affected case in a family, the illness can run a more severe course and antiviral therapy should be considered. *Oral acyclovir* is the antiviral of choice and should be started within 24 h of the rash developing.

In healthy adolescents and adults, oral acyclovir commenced within 24 h of development of the rash has been shown to be beneficial. Heavy smokers and people with chronic lung disease are at greater risk of developing complications, particularly varicella pneumonitis. Treatment with acyclovir should be given if they are seen within 24 h of the rash developing. There is no evidence to indicate significant benefit if treatment is started after 24 h in cases where infection is following the normal course and there are no complications. Treatment should be symptomatic and patients should be advised to return promptly if they deteriorate. All patients with complications require hospital assessment.

Immunocompromised patients with varicella, including patients on oral corticosteroids or with a history of oral corticosteroid intake for more than 3 weeks in the preceding 3 months, should be admitted to hospital and treated with *intravenous acyclovir* because they are most at risk of severe disease and complications. Newer anti-VZV drugs that have been developed include *valacyclovir, famciclovir,* and *brivudin.* These are currently licensed for treatment of herpes zoster, but not varicella. Resistance to acyclovir can occur in immunocompromised individuals following long-term acyclovir therapy. In patients with proven acyclovir-resistant VZV strains, *intravenous foscarnet* is currently the antiviral agent of choice.

Pregnant women are at a higher risk of severe and complicated disease, and careful consideration should be given to treating these patients. Nonimmune pregnant women who have had contact with a person with varicella should receive specific *varicella zoster immunoglobulin* (VZIG). VZIG is effective up to 10 days after contact. This has been shown to prevent varicella or modify disease severity. It also reduces the risk of fetal transmission if disease develops. The potential benefit is greatest when exposure to varicella occurs during the first 20 weeks of pregnancy or near term (within 21 days of the estimated date of delivery).

Maternal varicella during the first 20 weeks of pregnancy is associated with a 1–2% risk of fetal varicella syndrome, and this risk needs to be weighed against the theoretical possibility of a teratogenic effect of treatment. Acyclovir is not a recognized teratogen. Oral acyclovir is recommended if the patient is beyond 20 weeks of gestation and is seen within 24 h of the onset of the rash. Pregnant women who are smokers, have chronic lung disease, are taking corticosteroids, or are in the latter half of pregnancy are at greater risk of developing systemic symptoms. *Hospitalization* should be considered in late pregnancy and in women with chest or neurological symptoms, a hemorrhagic rash, bleeding, or very severe disease with a dense rash and mucosal lesions.

Neonates with varicella whose mothers developed varicella within 7 days prior to delivery may develop severe disease and should be treated with intravenous acyclovir. Treatment should also be considered within 48 h of development of the rash in other infants with congenital varicella (rash within 16 days of delivery) and severe clinical disease.

Oral acyclovir has been effective in postexposure prophylaxis. It is given approximately 9 days after exposure for

Evidence levels   **A** Double-blind study   **B** Clinical trial ≥ 20 subjects   **C** Clinical trial < 20 subjects   **D** Series ≥ 5 subjects   **E** Anecdotal case reports

1 week. This aborts disease or reduces its severity. Post-exposure prophylaxis with VZIG is also given to neonates whose mothers had varicella 7 days before to 7 days after delivery, and immunocompromised individuals. It is most effective if given within 72 h, but may still modify disease if given up to 10 days after exposure.

SPECIFIC INVESTIGATIONS

- Virology on vesicle fluid
- Tzanck smear
- Immunostaining
- Polymerase chain reaction (PCR)
- Serology on acute and convalescent sera

The diagnosis of viral infections. Kangro HO. In: Parker MT, Collier LH, eds. Topley and Wilson's principles of bacteriology, virology and immunity. London: Edward Arnold; 1999: 227–42.

This is a general review of diagnostic virology, including VZV. The virus can be identified by electron microscopy, immune electron microscopy, tissue culture or shell viral culture, immunofluorescence, immunostaining, or detection of viral DNA by PCR.

FIRST LINE THERAPIES

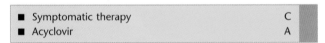

■ Symptomatic therapy	C
■ Acyclovir	A

Acyclovir for treating varicella in otherwise healthy children and adolescents. Klassen TP, Belseck EM, Wiebe N, Hartling L. Cochrane Database Syst Rev 2004;(2):CD002980.

This systematic review concluded that acyclovir initiated within 24 h after onset of the rash shows a therapeutic benefit in reducing the duration of fever and the maximum number of lesions in immunocompetent children. There were no clinically important differences in the number of complications and adverse effects among acyclovir and placebo groups.

The use of oral acyclovir in otherwise healthy children with varicella. Hall CB, Granoff DM, Gromisch DS, et al. Pediatrics 1993;91:674–6.

A helpful review article with treatment recommendations. Oral acyclovir therapy is safe but the cost–benefit ratio of treatment in otherwise healthy children remains to be established. Treatment initiated within 24 h of onset will typically reduce fever duration by 1 day and also reduce the severity of the eruption.

Symptomatic treatment with analgesics and topical agents such as calamine lotion or crotamiton cream and daily baths are all that is required in most children.

When required, acyclovir is the antiviral of choice for varicella infection. It is usually given orally. In children up to 12 years of age it is given at a dose of 20 mg/kg 6-hourly (to a maximum of 800 mg/dose) for 5 days. In adolescents and adults the dose is 800 mg five times daily for 7 days. Acyclovir is given intravenously in severe disease and in immunocompromised individuals.

Acyclovir treatment of varicella in otherwise healthy adolescents. Balfour Jr HH, Rotbart HA, Feldman S, et al. J Pediatr 1992;120:627–33.

A double blind, placebo-controlled trial with 62 evaluable subjects. Acyclovir, 800 mg orally four times daily for 5 days, significantly reduced the severity and duration of the illness.

Treatment of adult varicella with oral aciclovir: a randomized, placebo-controlled trial. Wallace MR, Bowler WA, Murray NB, et al. Ann Intern Med 1992;117:358–63.

A study on 148 evaluable military personnel hospitalized for varicella treated with acyclovir, 800 mg orally five times daily for 7 days, or placebo. Patients treated within 24 h of onset of the rash had fewer lesions and shorter time to crusting. Treatment after 24 h had no effect on the disease.

SECOND LINE THERAPIES

■ Foscarnet	D
■ Valacyclovir	D

Foscarnet therapy in five patients with AIDS and aciclovir resistant varicella zoster virus infection. Safrin S, Berger TG, Wolfe PR, et al. Ann Intern Med 1991;115:19–21.

Five patients with AIDS and acyclovir-resistant VZV were treated with foscarnet. Four had healing of the lesions and negative cultures during foscarnet therapy. Fluorescent antigen testing remained positive in two patients – one healed completely, but the other had clinical failure of therapy.

Foscarnet is used in patients who have developed resistance to acyclovir. The dose is 40 mg/kg 8-hourly in 1-hour infusions for 10 days.

Varicella in a pediatric heart transplant population on nonsteroid maintenance immunosuppression. Dodd DA, Burger J, Edwards KM, Dummer JS. Pediatrics 2001;108:E80

Six of 14 pediatric heart transplant patients with varicella were treated with oral valacyclovir, dose range from 61 to 88 mg/kg daily, for 7 days, one with oral acyclovir for 10 days and seven with intravenous acyclovir for 3 days followed by oral acyclovir for 7 days. All treatment regimens were well tolerated without complications.

PROPHYLAXIS

■ Vaccines	A
■ VZIG	B
■ Intravenous immunoglobulin	C
■ Acyclovir	A

Oka/Merck varicella vaccine in healthy children: final report of a 2-year efficacy study and 7-year follow-up studies. Kuter BJ, Weibel RE, Guess HA, et al. Vaccine 1991;9:643–7.

A large, placebo-controlled trial in children aged 1–14 years demonstrating the varicella vaccine to be 70–90% effective for preventing varicella and more than 95% effective for preventing severe varicella.

Evaluation of varicella zoster immune globulin: protection of immunosuppressed children after household exposure to varicella. Zaia JA, Levin MJ, Preblud SR, et al. J Infect Dis 1983;147:737–43.

VZIG is effective for prophylaxis.

Intravenous immunoglobulin prophylaxis in children with acute leukaemia following exposure to varicella. Chen SH, Liang DC. Pediatr Hematol Oncol 1992;9:347–51.

Five children with leukemia received a single dose (200 mg/kg) of intravenous immunoglobulin within 3 days of exposure to varicella. None developed the infection. Intravenous immunoglobulin appears to be an effective and safe alternative when hyperimmune zoster immunoglobulin or VZIG is unavailable.

Postexposure prophylaxis of varicella in family contact by oral acyclovir. Asano Y, Yoshikawa T, Suga S, et al. Pediatrics 1993;92:219–22.

Twenty five children were treated with oral acyclovir 40 or 80 mg/kg daily in four divided doses, 7–9 days after household exposure to varicella. Twenty five age-matched control subjects who had been exposed, but did not receive treatment were also followed. Twenty of the 25 treated subjects were protected from disease, but four of these failed to seroconvert. All 25 control subjects developed varicella.

Antiviral prophylaxis and treatment in chickenpox. A review prepared for the UK Advisory Group on Chickenpox on behalf of the British Society for the Study of Infection. Ogilvie MM. J Infect 1998;36(suppl 1):31–8.

A review of the use of VZIG, live attenuated varicella vaccine, and acyclovir. Oral acyclovir is only considered effective if begun within 24 h of onset of rash. It is recommended for treatment of varicella in otherwise healthy adults and adolescents, but not for routine use in children under 13 years of age unless they are sibling contacts or have other medical conditions. Acyclovir has a high therapeutic index and good safety profile, but caution is advised with use in pregnancy.

Chickenpox in pregnancy. Guideline No.13. Royal College of Obstetricians and Gynaecologists. http://www.rcog.org.uk/resources/Public/Chickenpox_No13.pdf.

Current UK guidelines for the treatment of pregnant women with varicella and advice on postexposure prophylaxis. VZIG is recommended for postexposure prophylaxis. Oral acyclovir is recommended if patients present within 24 h of the rash and they are more than 20 weeks of gestation. If delivery occurs within 5 days of maternal infection, or if the mother develops chickenpox within 2 days of giving birth, the neonate should be given VZIG. The infant should be monitored for signs of infection for 14–16 days. If neonatal infection occurs, the neonate should be treated with acyclovir.

Viral exanthems: rubella, roseola, rubeola

Karen Wiss

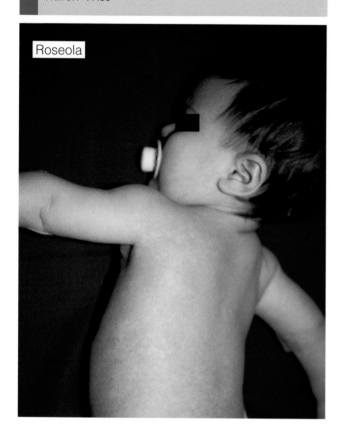

Roseola

Rubella

Rubella (German measles, 3-day measles) is usually a mild disease of low-grade fever, generalized erythematous macules and papules, and generalized lymphadenopathy. It is caused by an enveloped RNA virus in the Togaviridae family. Maternal rubella during pregnancy can cause fetal death or the congenital rubella syndrome.

MANAGEMENT STRATEGY

In children, there is typically no prodrome. In adolescents and adults, a prodrome of fever, malaise, sore throat, nausea, anorexia, and generalized lymphadenopathy is often seen. The pink erythematous macules and papules start on the face and neck and spread from the neck down and out in a centrifugal fashion in 1–2 days. The lesions disappear from the face and neck and down in 2–3 days. An enanthem, called Forchheimer spots, consisting of petechiae on the hard palate, may accompany the rash.

Rubella is a self-limiting illness that resolves spontaneously. The treatment is *supportive* in most cases. Some individuals, especially teenagers and adults, may have tran-

sient polyarthralgia and polyarthritis. Thrombocytopenia and encephalitis are extremely rare. Maternal rubella during the first trimester of pregnancy can result in fetal death or the congenital rubella syndrome. The main fetal anomalies include eye findings (cataracts, glaucoma, microphthalmia, and chorioretinitis), sensorineural deafness, cardiac abnormalities (patent ductus arteriosus, atrial septal defects, ventricular septal defects), pulmonic stenosis, and blueberry muffin lesions (extramedullary hematopoiesis).

It can be difficult to distinguish rubella from other viral exanthems, in particular enteroviruses. Rubella may also mimic measles, and infection by parvovirus B19, human herpesvirus-6 (HHV-6), and arboviruses. It is essential that the correct diagnosis is confirmed during pregnancy and with suspected congenital infection.

Rubella virus can be isolated from the nose and throat in postnatal infection and from blood, urine, cerebrospinal fluid, and throat in congenitally infected infants. Antibody testing for rubella-specific IgM will suggest recent infection. A fourfold or greater increase in antibody titer between acute and convalescent IgG titers over several months also suggests infection.

Children with rubella should be *excluded from school for 7 days after onset of the rash*. *Rubella vaccine* is recommended in combination with the measles and mumps vaccine (MMR) at 12–15 months of age, with a second dose at school entry between 4 and 6 years of age. Postpubertal females can be tested for rubella IgG antibody and vaccinated. Because the vaccine contains live virus, it should not be given to pregnant women.

SPECIFIC INVESTIGATIONS

- Viral culture
- Acute IgM antibody titers
- Acute and convalescent IgG antibody titers

Rubella virus replication and links to teratogenicity. Lee JY, Bowden DS. Clin Microbiol Rev 2000;13:571–87.

The virus has been readily grown in tissue culture and has some unusual features of replication that likely play a role in the teratogenesis.

Comparison of five different methods of rubella IgM antibody testing. Cubie H, Edmond E. J Clin Pathol 1985;38:203–7.

The radioimmunoassay and enzyme-linked assays were more sensitive than the traditional hemagglutination inhibition method for detecting rubella-specific IgM antibody.

FIRST LINE THERAPIES

■ Antipyretics – acetaminophen (paracetamol), ibuprofen	E
■ Analgesics – nonsteroidal anti-inflammatory drugs (NSAIDs)	E
■ School avoidance for 7 days	A
■ Immunization	A

The changing epidemiology of rubella in the 1990s: on the verge of elimination and new challenges for control and prevention. Reef SE, Frey TK, Theall K, et al. JAMA 2002;287:464–72.

Rubella and congenital rubella syndrome are on the verge of elimination in the United States due to effective immunization programs.

Safety of combination vaccines: perception versus reality. Halsey NA. Pediatr Infect Dis J 2001;20:S40–4.

Combination vaccines have been used safely and effectively for over 50 years. New combination vaccines will reduce the number of injections and prevent additional diseases.

Roseola

Roseola infantum (exanthem subitum, sixth disease) is an exanthem of young childhood caused by primary infection with HHV-6 or -7. The clinical findings include high fever in a well-appearing child and a rash with defervescence. The exanthem consists of pink macules and papules that spread from neck down to the trunk and proximal extremities.

MANAGEMENT STRATEGY

Roseola is an illness of children aged between 6 and 36 months. The first sign of illness is high fever (>39.5°C) that persists for 3–7 days. Fever is followed by pink macules and papules on the trunk that last hours to days. *Typically, no treatment is necessary* and the illness resolves spontaneously in a few days. Febrile seizures are commonly seen in infants during the febrile phase of the illness. These infants usually require emergency room care.

Identification of virus, either HHV-6 or HHV-7, by culture from the peripheral blood is presently available only in specialized research laboratories. Amplification of the viruses by polymerase chain reaction (PCR) is available. However, it can be difficult to distinguish active from latent infection or from chronic persistence. PCR of plasma has been shown to be sensitive and specific for diagnosing primary HHV-6 infection in immunocompetent children. HHV-6 IgM serology is available, but is not very reliable by itself. Seroconversion of IgG antibody in sera collected 2–3-weeks apart with a fourfold increase in titer can be more reliable. There is considerable cross-reactivity between HHV-6, HHV-7, and cytomegaloviruses.

Most individuals harbor HHV-6 and HHV-7 in their saliva throughout their lives. Reactivation of the virus may cause more severe disease especially in immunocompromised hosts. Reactivation may manifest as fever, bone marrow suppression, hepatitis, pneumonia, lymphoproliferative disorders, and encephalitis. In these patients, *ganciclovir* and *foscarnet* have been recommended by some. Ganciclovir and foscarnet are inhibitors of HHV-6 replication in vitro. Individual case reports have suggested benefit from these agents in ill patients.

SPECIFIC INVESTIGATIONS

- None
- HHV-6 IgM
- HHV-6 IgG – acute and convalescent titers
- PCR for HHV-6

Early diagnosis of primary human herpesvirus 6 infection in childhood: serology, polymerase chain reaction, and virus load. Chiu SS, Cheung CY, Tse CY, Peiris M. J Infect Dis 1998;178:1250–6.

Using a combination of these methods improves the sensitivity of diagnosing primary HHV-6 infection.

FIRST LINE THERAPIES

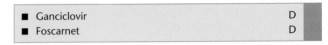

■ Antipyretics – acetaminophen, ibuprofen	E

SECOND LINE THERAPIES

■ Ganciclovir	D
■ Foscarnet	D

Determination of antiviral efficacy against lymphotropic herpesviruses utilizing flow cytometry. Long MC, Bidanset DJ, Williams SL, et al. Antiviral Res 2003;58:149–57.

Flow cytometry was used successfully to evaluate HHV-6 and showed inhibition by foscarnet and ganciclovir.

Human herpesvirus type 6 and human herpesvirus type 7 infections of the central nervous system. Dewhurst S. Herpes 2004;11:105A–11A.

Ganciclovir and foscarnet may be used for managing HHV-6-related disease. Ganciclovir but not foscarnet may be useful for HHV-7-related illness.

Antiviral prophylaxis may prevent human herpesvirus-6 reactivation in bone marrow transplant recipients. Rapaport D, Engelhard D, Tagger G, et al. Transpl Infect Dis 2002;4:10–16.

In six bone marrow transplant recipients, ganciclovir prevented HHV-6 reactivation.

Rubeola

Rubeola (measles) is a systemic illness caused by a paramyxovirus. The clinical signs and symptoms consist of fever, cough, coryza, conjunctivitis, morbilliform rash, and Koplik spots. Complications include pneumonia, croup, diarrhea, acute encephalitis, brain damage, and death from respiratory and neurologic complications. Subacute sclerosing panencephalitis (SSPE) due to persistent measles infection is a rare degenerative neurologic disease that can occur years after the original infection.

MANAGEMENT STRATEGY

The measles rash consists of erythematous macules and papules that begin along the hairline and behind the ears and spread down the body. A pathognomonic enanthem called Koplik spots occurs before the onset of the rash. It is important to distinguish the measles rash from other viral infections, in particular enterovirus infections. Drug eruptions and Kawasaki disease are frequently considered in the differential diagnosis.

Perhaps most clinically useful is a rapid diagnostic technique with immunofluorescence obtained by collecting

Evidence levels A Double-blind study B Clinical trial ≥ 20 subjects C Clinical trial < 20 subjects D Series ≥ 5 subjects E Anecdotal case reports

desquamated nasal mucosa cells. Measles-specific IgM antibody tests from sera collected at the onset of the eruption can be quite useful. Although diagnosis will be delayed, acute and convalescent IgG antibody can be obtained. Measles virus can also be isolated from nasopharyngeal secretions during the febrile phase of the illness.

Children with measles need to be *isolated for 4 days after the onset of the rash*. In the United States and in the UK, suspected cases of measles should be *notified* to the appropriate monitoring authorities.

Measles *vaccine* contains live attenuated virus and is recommended as part of the MMR vaccine at 12–15 months of age and again at 4–6 years of age. It can also be given as a measles-only formulation. The vaccine is very effective. Two doses are usually recommended for maximum immunity.

Individuals with poor nutritional states are at greatest risk for complications from measles. *Dietary supplementation with vitamin A* may reduce the morbidity and mortality of the disease. Vitamin A should be given to children aged 6 months to 2 years who are hospitalized for complications of measles. Any children with measles who are immunocompromised, have vitamin A deficiency or malnutrition, or recently immigrated from areas with high mortality rates for measles are candidates for treatment. Vitamin A supplementation is recommended by the World Health Organization in all communities in which vitamin A deficiency is a problem. The dose suggested is 100 000–200 000 IU as a single oral dose. The dose is given the next day and at 4 weeks if there is clinical evidence or great risk for vitamin A deficiency.

Immunoglobulin prophylaxis can prevent or modify measles in a susceptible person within 6 days of exposure. It is recommended for susceptible household contacts, especially if those contacts are younger than 1 year of age or are pregnant or immunocompromised.

Measles virus is susceptible to *ribavirin* in vitro. It has been given intravenously and nasally to treat children with severe illness and immunocompromise.

SPECIFIC INVESTIGATIONS

- Immunofluorescence
- IgM antibody
- IgG antibody – acute and convalescent
- Viral culture

Use of immunofluorescence to identify measles virus infections. Minnich LL, Goodenough F, Ray CG. J Clin Microbiol 1991;29:1148–50.

Nasopharyngeal throat swabs had a high yield with indirect immunofluorescence in identification of measles virus infection.

Difficulties in clinical diagnosis of measles: proposal for modified clinical case definition. Ferson MJ, Young LC, Robertson PW, Whybin LR. Med J Aust 1995;163:364–6.

Clinical diagnosis of measles is unreliable. Cases must be confirmed by serological tests.

FIRST LINE THERAPIES

■ Antipyretics – acetaminophen, ibuprofen	E
■ Report to local or state health department	A
■ Measles vaccine	A

Measles surveillance in the United States: an overview. Guris D, Harpaz R, Redd SB, et al. J Infect Dis 2004; 189:S177–84.

The elimination of measles is facilitated by reporting and investigation of all suspected measles cases.

Worldwide measles prevention. Orenstein WA, Markowitz LE, Atkinson WL, Hinman AR. Isr J Med Sci 1994;30:469–81.

Measles immunization has dramatically reduced measles rates in the world. One million deaths still occur each year. Two-dose schedules are needed to eliminate the disease.

SECOND LINE THERAPIES

■ Oral vitamin A	A
■ Immunoglobulin prophylaxis	A

Vitamin A for the treatment of children with measles – a systematic review. D'Souza RM, D'Souza R. J Trop Pediatr 2002;48:323–7.

Meta-analysis of randomized controlled trials comparing vitamin A with placebo concluded that 200 000 IU repeated on 2 days should be used for measles treatment in areas where case fatality is high.

Vitamin A supplementation and child mortality. A meta-analysis. Fawzi WW, Chalmers TC, Herrera MG, Mosteller F. JAMA 1993;269:898–903.

Meta-analysis of studies examining vitamin A supplementation and child mortality showed a significant reduction in mortality.

THIRD LINE THERAPIES

■ Ribavirin	D

Severe measles in immunocompromised patients. Kaplan LJ, Daum RS, Smaron M, McCarthy CA. JAMA 1992;267: 1237–41.

Ribavirin resulted in rapid defervescence in measles among these immunocompromised patients.

Viral warts

Imtiaz Ahmed

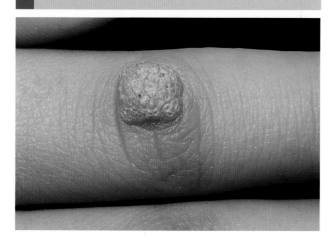

This common disease is caused by infection with various strains of the human papillomavirus. Children present most commonly with warts on the hands and feet. Presentation is often as verruca vulgaris (common wart). Plane warts are frequently seen on the dorsum of hands or on the face. Genital warts are considered in another chapter.

MANAGEMENT STRATEGY

Most warts will resolve spontaneously with time. Treatment is, however, demanded by patients and, in the case of children, by their parents, for various reasons. Warts may be painful, an object of ridicule, lead to loss of confidence and distorted self image, worry of loss of employment, a cosmetic concern, or a public health and safety issue. Immunosuppressed patients may have extensive and resistant warts. Before presenting to the physician, patients have usually treated themselves with over-the-counter preparations containing keratolytics or caustics. *Salicylic acid (SA)* in various concentrations and different bases is the most commonly used application. This can be applied with or without occlusion. It may cause irritation of the surrounding skin. *Formaldehyde soaks, glutaraldehyde solution,* or *silver nitrate pencils* are also available.

When seen by a physician, the diagnosis and the possibility of spontaneous resolution should be explained. The patient should be educated on how to accurately apply the topical preparations. Keeping the warts well pared down with the use of a *file or pumice stone* after soaking is important. *Liquid nitrogen cryotherapy* is one of the commonest treatments used when patients are referred to a dermatologist. Cryotherapy can be applied with a cotton bud or a cryospray. The wart is frozen from the center to include a 2-mm rim and the freeze maintained for 5 s. Cryotherapy is usually repeated at 1–3-weekly intervals. Hyperkeratotic warts should be pared before cryotherapy and plantar warts treated by two freeze–thaw cycles. This treatment is painful and not tolerated well by young children. The warts can be sore or occasionally blister afterwards. In pigmented skin, post-treatment hypo- and hyperpigmentation can be a problem. Liquid nitrogen cryotherapy can be combined with topical preparations. Cryotherapy with CO_2 snow or

dimethylether applicators does not produce temperatures as low as liquid nitrogen and is considered less effective.

If cryotherapy is not successful then various other options are available. *Immunotherapy* with topical application of *diphencyprone or squaric acid* and *intralesional mumps/candida antigen* can be effective. Treatment may need to be done repeatedly before a response is obtained. *Intralesional bleomycin* using a solution containing 1 mg/mL of bleomycin can be injected into the wart or the solution applied to the wart and then repeatedly pricked through with a lancet. This treatment is quite painful and should only be done by someone with experience. *Surgical excision, CO_2 laser ablation,* or *curettage and cautery* of troublesome and resistant single warts can be attempted, but the risk of scarring and recurrence in the scar can be a problem. *Pulsed dye laser treatment,* by theoretically targeting the rich capillary network in the wart, is sometimes effective.

Other treatments such as *oral high-dose cimetidine, oral retinoids, topical retinoids for plane warts, topical 5-fluorouracil (5-FU),* and *oral levamisole* can be tried. In some published series of patients, cimetidine has been shown to be effective, particularly in children; however, controlled trials have not shown an advantage over placebo. *Localized heat therapy* by means of various devices has been effective in some cases. *Photodynamic therapy using 5-aminolevulinic acid (ALA)* or other photosensitizers may find a place in the treatment of resistant warts. *Topical imiquimod* may also emerge as a useful treatment in the future after its success in genital warts. *Hypnotherapy* and suggestion has been described to work and may be tried as a first or last resort depending, perhaps, on the suggestibility of the physician. *Duct tape occlusion* may work on the same principle or by some other unknown mechanism.

FIRST LINE THERAPIES

■ Salicylic acid preparations	B
■ Glutaraldehyde	B
■ Silver nitrate stick	B

An assessment of methods of treating viral warts by comparative treatment trials based on a standard design. Bunney MH, Nolan MW, Williams DA. Br J Dermatol 1976;94:667–79.

This is the seminal work on the treatment of warts, describing a series of 11 trials on 1802 patients. In a randomized blind trial involving 389 patients with hand warts, SA with lactic acid (SAL) paint was as effective as liquid nitrogen cryotherapy done by the physician. Patients having both treatments concurrently had a better cure rate (78%). The SAL paint comprised one part (17%) SA, one part (17%) lactic acid, and four parts (66%) of flexible collodion. In another study of 382 plantar warts, 84% of patients with simple plantar warts (n = 296) were cured after 12 weeks of regular SAL paint application. In a separate study (n = 94), 45% of patients with mosaic warts were cured with SAL paint compared to 47% of patients applying 10% glutaraldehyde.

Monochloroacetic acid and 60% salicylic acid as a treatment for simple plantar warts: effectiveness and mode of action. Steele K, Shirodaria P, O'Hare M, et al. Br J Dermatol 1988;118:537–44.

In this double blind study of 57 patients with plantar warts, a preparation of monochloroacetic acid and 60% SA ointment was applied to the wart and left on for 1 week. After this single application, 19 (66%) were cured at week 6 assessment, compared to five (18%) in the placebo group. In view of the severe irritant effect of this preparation, it had to be applied very carefully. In the active group a significant number of patients complained of pain, and one patient developed cellulitis.

Local treatment for cutaneous warts. Gibbs S, Harvey I, Sterling JC, Stark R. Cochrane Database Syst Rev 2003;(3): CD001781.

Fifty two trials fulfilled the criteria for inclusion in this review. The best evidence was for the use of preparations containing SA. Data pooled from six placebo-controlled trials showed a cure rate of 75% in the SA group compared to 48% in the placebo group.

Efficacy of silver nitrate pencils in the treatment of common warts. Yazar S, Basaran E. J Dermatol 1994;21: 329–33.

A randomized, placebo-controlled study with 35 patients in each group, showed that 1 month after treatment, 15 (43%) patients were cleared of warts by three applications of a silver nitrate pencil at 3-day intervals. Only four (11%) of the placebo group responded.

SECOND LINE THERAPIES

■ Liquid nitrogen cryotherapy	B

An assessment of methods of treating viral warts by comparative treatment trials based on a standard design. Bunney MH, Nolan MW, Williams DA. Br J Dermatol 1976; 94:667–79.

This series of trials described a standardized method of cryotherapy using liquid nitrogen applied to the wart with a cotton wool bud. Liquid nitrogen was applied with a cotton wool bud just smaller than the wart, using slight vertical pressure, until a frozen halo appeared around its base (5–30 s depending on the thickness of the wart). After 3 months of cryotherapy at 3-week intervals the cure rate in hand warts was 68.6% with liquid nitrogen alone and 78% when combined with nightly applications of SAL (number of patients in each group around 100). In a separate trial comparing cure rates for hand warts treated when cryotherapy was performed at 2-, 3-, or 4-week intervals for 3 months, the authors conclude that the cure rate for 4-weekly treatments (40%) was significantly less than that for the 2- or 3-weekly treatment groups (78%, 75%).

Value of a second freeze–thaw cycle in cryotherapy of common warts. Berth-Jones J, Bourke J, Eglitis H, et al. Br J Dermatol 1994;131: 883–6.

This randomized parallel group study of 300 patients suggests that a double freeze–thaw cycle in the cryotherapy of plantar warts (n = 121) may be considerably more effective than a single freeze.

Cryotherapy of common viral warts at intervals of 1, 2 and 3 weeks. Bourke JF, Berth-Jones J, Hutchinson PE. Br J Dermatol 1995;132:433–6.

This study carried out on 225 patients showed that the cure rate (45%) with liquid nitrogen cryotherapy of hand and foot warts is related to the number of treatments received and independent of the interval between treatments.

Liquid nitrogen cryotherapy of common warts: cryo-spray versus cotton wool bud. Ahmed I, Agarwal S, Ilchyshyn A, et al. Br J Dermatol 2001;144:1006–9.

This prospective study of 363 patients compared cotton wool bud application with cryospray. The authors conclude that cryotherapy with liquid nitrogen for hand and foot warts is equally effective when applied with a cotton wool bud or by means of a cryospray (47 and 44%, respectively) after 3 months of treatment.

THIRD LINE THERAPIES

Local	
■ Immunotherapy with diphencyprone	C
■ Immunotherapy with squaric acid dibutylester (SADBE)	C
■ Immunotherapy with mumps or candida antigen	D
■ Intralesional bleomycin	A
■ Surgery, curettage and cautery, and laser treatment	C
■ Topical imiquimod	C
■ Topical 5-FU	A
■ Photodynamic therapy	A
■ Topical tretinoin	B
■ Intralesional interferon (IFN)	C
■ Formaldehyde soaks	C
■ Localized heat therapy	C
■ Intralesional formic acid	B
■ Topical α-lactalbumin-oleic acid	A
■ Duct tape application	B
■ Sodium salicylate iontophoresis	D
Systemic and others	
■ Oral cimetidine	C
■ Oral levamisole	A
■ Oral zinc sulphate	B
■ Oral retinoids	C
■ Hypnotherapy	C
Anecdotal reports	
■ Cidofovir	E
■ Vitamin D3 derivatives	E
■ Imiquimod and SA	E

Local

Recalcitrant viral warts treated by diphencyprone immunotherapy. Buckley DA, Keane FM, Munn SE, et al. Br J Dermatol 1999;141:292–6.

This is a retrospective case series of 60 patients with resistant hand and foot warts. Forty-two of 48 (88%) patients who attended regularly were cleared of warts after a mean of five (range 1–22) treatments. A concentration of 0.01–6% diphencyprone was used after initial sensitization and treatments done at an interval of 1–4 weeks. Painful local blistering (n = 11), blistering at site of sensitization (n = 9), and a pompholyx-like or more generalized eczematous eruption (n = 11) were significant adverse events. Six patients withdrew due to side effects.

In another retrospective series 211 patients were sensitized for treatment of recalcitrant palmoplantar and periungual warts. Of 154 evaluable patients, 135 (87.7%) were cleared of warts completely with an average of five treatments over a 6-month period (Upitis JA, Krol A. J Cutan Med Surg 2002;6:214–7).

A further case series of resistant warts in 111 patients treated at weekly intervals for up to 8 weeks revealed a 60% response rate, with 49 complete and 18 partial remissions (Rampen FH, Steijlen PM. Dermatology 1996;193:236–8).

Squaric acid immunotherapy for warts in children.
Silverberg NB, Lim JK, Paller AS, Mancini AJ. J Am Acad Dermatol 2000;42:803–8.

This is a retrospective series of 61 children with warts, treated by home application with SADBE after initial sensitization. The treatment was done for between three and seven nights a week for at least 3 months at a starting concentration of 0.2%. Eleven patients had concomitant therapies. Thirty-four (56%) patients completely cleared and 11 (18%) improved with the treatment. Only two patients had to discontinue treatment due to side effects.

Another retrospective case series of 29 patients showed a 69% clearance with SADBE contact immunotherapy when treated at 2-weekly intervals by a physician (Lee AN, Mallory SB. J Am Acad Dermatol 1999;41:595–9).

Immunotherapy for recalcitrant warts in children using intralesional mumps or candida antigens.
Clifton MM, Johnson SM, Roberson PK, et al. Pediatr Dermatol 2003;20: 268–71.

In this study 47 patients with recalcitrant warts were treated intralesionally with mumps or candida antigen at 3-week intervals with an average of 3.8 treatments to the largest wart. Complete response of treated wart was seen in 22 patients (47%); 14 of these patients experienced resolution of all distant warts as well.

Another study comparing standard treatment with intralesional Candida albicans *allergenic extract showed complete clearing of warts in 44 of 87 patients (51%) after an average of 2.3 treatments. In the standard treatment group 46 of 95 patients (48%) were cleared of warts after an average of 1.6 treatments (Signore RJ. Cutis 2002;70:185–92).*

A further study showed that 146 of 206 (70.9%) patients treated with a combined candida, mumps and trichophyton antigen cleared after an average of 4.7 treatments (Johnson SM, Horn TD. J Drugs Dermatol 2004;3:263–5).

Bleomycin in the treatment of recalcitrant warts.
Shumer SM, O'Keefe EJ. J Am Acad Dermatol 1983;9:91–6.

In this double blind, placebo-controlled, crossover trial, intralesional injections of bleomycin (1 IU/mL) or saline placebo were performed on two occasions, 2 weeks apart. The warts persisting after two treatments were then treated with the other agent. Twenty-nine of the 40 patients treated with bleomycin were cleared of their warts compared to none in the placebo group. Large plantar warts and periungual warts were significantly painful and tender after bleomycin injection.

Curettage and cautery

Curettage can be an effective treatment for single or few warts particularly filiform warts. Destruction with electrocautery can be tried, but is painful and can result in scarring.

Long-term follow-up evaluation of patients with electrosurgically treated warts.
Gibbs RC, Scheiner AM. Cutis 1978;21:383–4.

A questionnaire study looked at response of warts on extremities following electrocautery and curettage under local anaesthesia. 100 questionnaires were sent. In 22 of 23 patients who replied, the warts had responded to treatment and not recurred.

Pulsed-dye laser versus conventional therapy in the treatment of warts: a prospective randomized trial.
Robson KJ, Cunningham NM, Kruzan KL, et al. J Am Acad Dermatol 2000;43:275–80.

In this trial of 40 patients pulsed dye laser or cryotherapy treatment was performed at 1-month intervals. The response rates after four treatments were similar (66 vs 70%, respectively) in the two groups.

Pulsed-dye laser therapy for viral warts.
Kenton-Smith J, Tan ST. Br J Plast Surg 1999;52:554–8.

In this series of 28 patients, 95 of 103 recalcitrant warts (> 2 years' duration, and failed to respond to at least one conventional treatment) cleared after a mean of 2.1 treatments. They used a power setting of 6–9 J/cm^2, spot size 5–7 mm, spots overlapped by 1 mm, treatment extending 5 mm beyond the clinical margin of the wart, and gave three passes over each area.

Successful treatment of recalcitrant warts in pediatric patients with carbon dioxide laser.
Serour F, Somekh E. Eur J Pediatr Surg 2003; 13:219–23.

In this case series of 40 children (mean age 12.7 years), 54 warts were treated with CO_2 laser ablation under local anesthesia or ring block. Healing time was 4–5 weeks. There was no recurrence at 12 months. No significant or disabling scarring was noticed, but hypopigmentation was noticed in 11 (27.5%) cases.

Er:YAG laser followed by topical podophyllotoxin for hard-to-treat palmoplantar warts.
Wollina U. J Cosmet Laser Ther 2003;5:35–7.

Recalcitrant warts in 35 patients were ablated once with Er:YAG laser and then treated with topical podophyllotoxin for up to six cycles (one cycle = 3 days on, 4 days off topical application). Complete resolution was observed in 31 (88.6%) patients. Mild burning and prickling was noted during podophyllotoxin treatment.

5-Fluorouracil in the treatment of common warts of the hands: a double-blind study.
Almeida Goncalves JC. Br J Dermatol 1975;92:89–91.

In this trial of 27 women working in a fowl slaughter house in Lisbon, a combination of 5-FU and 10% SA varnish was compared with 10% SA varnish alone in the treatment of hand warts. After daily treatment for up to 9 weeks, 50% of the warts treated with the combination of 5-FU and SA cleared, compared to 4% treated with SA alone.

Topical treatment of warts and mollusca with imiquimod.
Hengge UR, Goos M. Ann Intern Med 2000;132:95.

In this open trial, 28/50 (56%) patients were cleared of their recalcitrant warts after a mean treatment of 9.5 weeks. Some of these patients were immunosuppressed.

In another uncontrolled study of resistant warts, ten of 37 patients were cleared of their warts after a mean treatment of 19 weeks with imiquimod applied twice daily (Grussendorf-Conen

EI, Jacobs S, Rubben A, Dethlefsen U. Topical 5% imiquimod long-term treatment of cutaneous warts resistant to standard therapy modalities. Dermatology 2002;205:139–45).

A controlled trial on the use of topical 5-fluorouracil on viral warts. Hursthouse MW. Br J Dermatol 1975;92:93–5.

This is a placebo-controlled, double blind, right-left comparison of 5-FU applied daily under occlusion for 4 weeks in 60 patients including 40 children. In 48 assessable patients, 29 (60%) in the active group cleared compared to eight (17%) in the placebo group. Onycholysis occurred in 11 patients with fingertip or periungual warts treated with 5-FU.

Photodynamic therapy with 5-aminolaevulinic acid or placebo for recalcitrant foot and hand warts: randomised double-blind trial. Stender I-M, Na R, Fogh H, et al. Lancet 2000;355:963–6.

In this study 5-ALA photodynamic therapy (PDT) was compared with placebo in a blinded, randomized fashion in the treatment of resistant warts. Three treatments were done at weekly intervals and repeated if the warts persisted 4 weeks after the last treatment. Sixty-four of 104 (61%) warts cleared in the active group whereas 47 of 102 (46%) warts cleared in the group who were exposed to placebo and light. The pain associated with the treatment was significant and classified as unbearable in some cases. The authors conclude that ALA PDT is superior to placebo PDT.

Evaluation of the efficacy and safety of 0.05% tretinoin cream in the treatment of plane warts in Arab children. Kubeyinje EP. J Dermatol Treat 1996;7:21–2.

In a randomized controlled study of 25 children, 85% of warts cleared compared to 32% in controls.

Treatment of verrucae with alpha-2 interferon. Berman B, Davis-Reed L, Silverstein L, et al. J Infect Dis 1986;154:328–30.

In this study of recalcitrant warts, patients were given a 0.1 mL injection containing either 100 000 units of IFN or placebo injection into the wart. Single warts were treated in eight patients. Three of the four patients treated with IFN were cured after a course of nine injections given over a period of 3 weeks compared to one of four patients in the placebo group.

Treatment of plantar warts in children. Vickers CFH. Br Med J 1961;2:743–5.

A survey of 646 children with plantar warts showed that 3% formalin foot-soaks 15–20 min each night for 6–8 weeks cured 80% of all plantar warts up to 1 cm in diameter.

Controlled localized heat therapy in cutaneous warts. Stern P, Levine N. Arch Dermatol 1992;128:945–8.

In this controlled, randomized trial, 13 patients with 29 warts were treated by a handheld radiofrequency heat generator device. They were treated on between one and four occasions for 30 s so that a temperature of 50°C was achieved in the warts. Twenty-five of the 29 (86%) treated warts cleared, compared to 7 of 17 (41%) control warts.

Nd:YAG laser hyperthermia in the treatment of recalcitrant verrucae vulgares (Regensburg's technique). Pfau A, Abd el Raheem TA, Baumler W, et al. Acta Derm Venereol 1994;74:212–14.

Hyperthermia of the warts achieved by this method was effective in a 54-year-old woman with recalcitrant verrucae vulgares on the little finger of her right hand and on her left sole. Laser energy was applied twice with an interval of 6 weeks. Laser output power was 10 W, spot size 8 mm, and irradiation time up to 20 s.

Topical formic acid puncture technique for the treatment of common warts. Bhat RM, Vidya K, Kamath G. Int J Dermatol 2001;40:415–19.

This was a nonrandomized, placebo-controlled trial of 100 patients with common warts comparing 85% formic acid puncture technique with saline placebo. A maximum number of 12 treatments were done on alternate days: 46 (92%) of the patients in the active group showed clearance of warts after a mean of 4.6 treatments; in the placebo group only three (6%) cleared after a mean of 11.6 treatments. A mild sensation of burning was felt by all patients with formic acid and six patients in this group developed secondary infection requiring systemic antibiotics.

Treatment of skin papillomas with topical alpha-lactalbumin-oleic acid. Gustafsson L, Leijonhufvud I, Aronsson A, Mossberg A-K, Svanborg C. N Engl J Med 2004;350:2663–72.

In this randomized, placebo-controlled, double-blind study of 40 patients with warts, 20 patients were randomized to have topical application of α-lactalbumin-oleic acid under occlusion for 3 weeks. The active agent is a complex produced by binding of α-lactalbumin (from human milk) and oleic acid, which can induce apoptosis in transformed cell lines. Wart volume was reduced by over 75% in all 20 patients in the active group compared to only three of 20 in the placebo group.

The efficacy of duct tape vs cryotherapy in the treatment of verruca vulgaris (the common wart). Focht DR 3rd, Spicer C, Fairchok MP. Arch Pediatr Adolesc Med 2002;156:971–4.

Fifty one patients were randomized to either cryotherapy or duct tape occlusion of one target wart. Cryotherapy was done with a 10 s freeze for a maximum of six treatments every 2–3 weeks. Duct tape was applied every 6 days, the wart being debrided upon removal of tape, for a maximum of 2 months. Twenty two (85%) of 26 in the duct tape arm had complete resolution of their warts compared to 15 (60%) of 25 in the cryotherapy group.

Treatment of plantar verrucae using 2% sodium salicylate iontophoresis. Soroko YT, Repking MC, Clemment JA, et al. Phys Ther 2002;82:1184–91.

Twenty patients with plantar warts were treated using 2% sodium salicylate solution with iontophoresis on three occasions a week apart and assessed 3 months after treatment. One patient had complete clearance of warts, three patients demonstrated a large reduction in wart area and 12 patients exhibited a measurable reduction in wart area.

Systemic and other

Cimetidine therapy for recalcitrant warts in adults. Glass AT, Solomon BA. Arch Dermatol 1996;132:680–2.

An open, uncontrolled, prospective study of cimetidine, 30–40 mg/kg daily, in 20 adult patients with recalcitrant warts. Of the 18 patients who completed 3 months of treatment, 16 (89%) had either dramatic improvement or complete resolution. The treatment was well tolerated.

Cimetidine therapy for warts: a placebo-controlled, double-blind study. Yilmaz E, Alpsoy E, Basaran E. J Am Acad Dermatol 1996;34:1005–7.

In this randomized placebo-controlled, double blind study, 70 patients with multiple warts received either cimetidine 25–40 mg/kg daily or placebo for 3 months. Most patients had previously received conventional treatment for their warts and not responded. Of the 54 evaluable patients, the cure rate in the active and placebo group was similar (32 and 30.7%, respectively).

Another double blind placebo-controlled study showed a similar result. The authors, however, suggested a trend towards efficacy in younger patients (Rogers CJ, Gibney MD, Siegfried EC, et al. J Am Acad Dermatol 1999;41:123–7).

Comparison of combination of cimetidine and levamisole with cimetidine alone in the treatment of recalcitrant warts. Parsad D, Saini R, Negi KS. Aust J Dermatol 1999; 40:93–5.

In this double blind study, 48 patients were randomized to have either high-dose cimetidine alone or in combination with levamisole for 12 weeks. The dose of levamisole was 150 mg on two consecutive days per week. In the levamisole plus cimetidine group, 15 (71%) patients were cured compared to eight (38%) in the cimetidine-only group. In the levamisole group, mild side effects were recorded in four patients; however, severe nausea led to withdrawal from the study in two patients.

Verrucae treated by levamisole. Amer M, Tosson Z, Soliman A, et al. Int J Dermatol 1991;30:738–40.

A double blind placebo-controlled study of oral levamisole given at a dose of 5 mg/kg on three consecutive days every 2 weeks for up to 5 months in 40 patients with viral warts. In the active treatment group 12 (60%) patients showed complete resolution compared to one patient (5%) in the control group.

Another placebo-controlled study of 49 patients with common warts (Schou M, Helin P. Acta Derm Venereol 1977;57:449–54) treated with a similar regimen of levamisole failed to show any significant effect.

Oral zinc sulphate in the treatment of recalcitrant viral warts: randomized placebo-controlled clinical trial. Al-Gurairi FT, Al-Waiz M, Sharquie KE. Br J Dermatol 2002;146:423–31.

Forty patients with recalcitrant warts were treated with oral zinc sulphate at a dose of 10 mg/kg daily up to a maximum of 600 mg daily for up to 2 months. Almost all patients who completed the study (20 of 23) responded with complete clearance of the warts. None in the placebo group responded. All patients suffered with nausea, but not severe enough to discontinue treatment. It was perhaps relevant that all patients with warts had a significantly lower serum zinc level (mean 62.5 µg/100 ml ± 10.72) than that of a matched healthy population (mean 87.8 µg/100 ml ± 10.06).

Treatment of extensive warts with etretinate: a clinical trial of 20 children. Gelmetti C, Cerri D, Schiuma AA, Menni S. Pediatr Derm 1987;4 :254–8

This was an open study of 20 children (mean age 8.5 years) with resistant common warts (11), plane warts (two), plantar warts (one), genital warts (three), and mixed (three). A dose of 1 mg/kg daily was given for a maximum of 3 months. Sixteen children were cleared of their warts and were free of warts at review after 12 months. The other four children had a significant improvement in their warts. None of the children stopped treatment because of side effects, while one child had transient alopecia, which recovered after discontinuation of treatment.

Etretinate is no longer available, but its active metabolite, acitretin, is equally effective at lower doses for other indications such as psoriasis.

Effects of hypnotic, placebo, and salicylic acid treatments on wart regression. Spanos NP, Williams V, Gwynn MI. Psychosom Med 1990;52:109–14.

Patients were randomized to undergo hypnotic suggestion, topical SA, placebo, or no treatment for 6 weeks. Six of ten patients in the hypnotic group lost one or more wart, compared to four of the remaining 30 patients.

Anecdotal reports
Refractory human papillomavirus-associated oral warts treated topically with 1–3% cidofovir solutions in human immunodeficiency virus type 1-infected patients. Husk R, Zouboulis CC, Sander-Bahr C, et al. Br J Dermatol 2005; 152:590–1.

Intravenous cidofovir for recalcitrant verruca vulgaris in the setting of HIV. Hivnor C, Shepard JW, Shapiro MS, Vittorio CC. Arch Dermatol 2004;140:13–4.

Large plantar wart caused by human papillomavirus-66 and resolution by topical cidofovir therapy. Davis MD, Gostout BS, McGovern RM, et al. J Am Acad Dermatol 2000;43:340–3.

Topical vitamin D3 derivatives for recalcitrant warts in three immunocompromised patients. Egawa K, Ono T. Br J Dermatol 2004;150:374–6.

Topical maxacalcitol under occlusion was effective in three patients with resistant warts who suffered with HTLV-1 infection, SLE and Crohn's.

Plantar wart treatment with combination imiquimod and salicylic acid pads. Tucker SB, Ali A, Ransdell BL. J Drugs Dermatol 2003;2:124–6

There are a few reports of imiquimod combined with salicylic acid being effective in resistant warts by presumably allowing the imiquimod to penetrate more effectively into the wart.

Evidence levels **A** Double-blind study **B** Clinical trial ≥ 20 subjects **C** Clinical trial < 20 subjects **D** Series ≥ 5 subjects **E** Anecdotal case reports

Vitiligo

Suhail M Hadi, James M Spencer

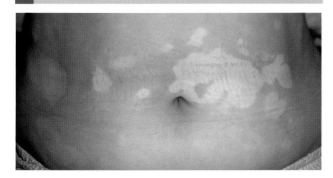

Vitiligo is an acquired idiopathic hypomelanotic disorder in which localized areas are devoid of melanocytes, resulting in depigmented macules which are often symmetrically distributed. The disease has 1–2% worldwide prevalence without predilection for age, sex, or race. Vitiligo can be quite psychologically and socially distressing, and in some cultures results in affected individuals being ostracized. Because of lack of melanin pigment, there is an increased risk of sunburn and a theoretic increased risk of skin cancer within the amelanotic areas, and there is association with ocular abnormalities, especially iritis.

There are multiple hypotheses to explain the etiology of vitiligo: autoimmune, autocytotoxic, neural, and hereditary. The autoimmune theory is supported by the association with a number of autoimmune diseases – thyroid disease, diabetes mellitus, Addison's disease, and pernicious anemia – the finding of organ-specific autoantibodies and circulating melanocyte autoantibodies, and, in addition, evidence of cellular immunity by immunohistologic study of perilesional skin and T-cell analysis of peripheral blood.

MANAGEMENT STRATEGY

The substantial disfigurement associated with vitiligo can cause serious emotional stress for the patient, which necessitates treatment. Sun protection of the vitiliginous areas with sunblocks is important because of increased vulnerability to the effects of ultraviolet light. Cosmetic improvement can be achieved by camouflage products and self-tanning dyes.

Although vitiligo is a notoriously challenging disease to treat, there are several options. More than one treatment modality should be tried for many months before a patient is deemed resistant to therapy.

Associated autoimmune disease should be looked for. Recommended blood tests include thyroid studies, antinuclear antibodies (ANA) and screening for other organ-specific autoantibodies, fasting blood glucose levels, and complete blood count with indices for pernicious anemia.

Treatment options include topical corticosteroids and topical low-dose 8-methoxypsoralen (8-MOP) (0.1%) with UVA for small, localized patches. For widespread disease, systemic therapy with 8-MOP, 5-MOP, 4,5,8-trimethyl-psoralen or a combination of these, along with sunlight or artificial UVA, may be beneficial. If patients do not achieve

visible repigmentation after 25–30 sessions with a given psoralen, an alternative therapy should be sought. Topical and systemic PUVA therapy may require 100–300 treatment sessions to achieve complete repigmentation. Narrowband UVB radiation and 5-MOP with UVA, have been shown to be effective alternatives to conventional PUVA, with fewer phototoxic effects. L-phenylalanine, khellin with UVA, and pseudocatalase with UVA are other alternative treatments that may be beneficial for some patients. Topical calcipotriene has been used in combination with topical corticosteroids, with narrowband UVB, and with PUVA, with some success. The most recent effective and approved therapy for vitiligo is the 308-nm excimer laser with or without topical calcineurin antagonists (tacrolimus and pimecrolimus). The pattern of repigmentation differs with different treatment modalities; it can be perifollicular, marginal, or diffuse.

For patients with refractory segmental or localized disease, thin split-thickness and suction blister epidermal grafting have been reported to be the most effective transplantation methods. Single hair grafting is effective for eyelid and eyebrow disease. Other surgical methods are autologous non-cultured melanocyte–keratinocyte cell transplantation and cultured pure melanocyte suspension.

Cosmetic tattooing is used for localized stable vitiligo, especially of the mucosal type.

Patients with extensive disease (>50% body area) who desire permanent matching of skin color but for whom repigmentation is not possible can be depigmented with 20% monobenzyl ether of hydroquinone, two times daily for 9–12 months. The results are excellent but irreversible. For vitiligo universalis, treatment with topical 4-methoxyphenol and the Q-switched ruby laser has been effective.

SPECIFIC INVESTIGATIONS

- ANA
- Complete blood count with indices
- Fasting blood glucose
- Thyroid-stimulating hormone (TSH)
- Immunohistopathology of skin

Incidence and significance of organ-specific autoimmune disorders (clinical, latent or only autoantibodies) in patients with vitiligo. Betterle C, Caretto A, DeZio A, et al. Dermatologica 1985;171:419–23.

Compared with controls matched for sex, age, and race, vitiligo patients had an increased frequency of clinical autoimmune diseases of the thyroid (7.5%), stomach (0.8%), parathyroid (1%), and adrenal gland (1.3%).

Clinical and immunological studies in vitiligo in the United Arab Emirates. Galadari I, Bener A, Hadi S, Lestringant GG. Allerg Immunol (Paris) 1997;29:297–9.

Sixty-five patients with vitiligo were evaluated. A positive family history of vitiligo was found in 19% of patients. An association with other autoimmune diseases was found in 6% of patients.

Autoimmune diseases in vitiligo: do anti-nuclear antibodies (ANA) decrease thyroid volume? Zettinig G, Tanew A, Fischer G, et al. Clin Exp Immunol 2003;131:347–54.

In this study, 106 patients with vitiligo and 38 controls were evaluated. Autoimmune thyroiditis (AT) was significantly more frequent in vitiligo (21% vs 3%). Vitiligo may precede AT by 4–35 years. Vitiligo patients with elevated ANA had significantly smaller thyroid volume compared to those with normal ANA. No statistically significant association with HLA was found in vitiligo patients.

Inflammatory changes in vitiligo: stage I and II depigmentation. Sharquie KE, Mehenna SH, Naji AA, Al-Azzawi H. Am J Dermatopathol 2004;26:108–12.

Epon-embedded sections from 25 patients with vitiligo and 11 normal volunteers were studied. Focal spongiosis was found in 48% of vitiligo patients (marginal areas and stage 1 vitiligo). Epidermal mononuclear cell infiltrate was found in 80% of both marginal skin and stage I vitiligo. The number of inflammatory cells was more than in stage II vitiligo and uninvolved skin. Thus, the authors concluded that vitiligo is an inflammatory disease and the epidermal lymphocytic infiltrate is most likely the primary immunologic event.

New insights into the pathogenesis of vitiligo: imbalance of epidermal cytokines at sites of lesions. Moretti S, Spallanzani A, Amato L, et al. Pigment Cell Res 2002;15: 87–92.

In vitiligo the expression of epidermal cytokines may be modified compared with normal skin. Fifteen patients with active non-segmental vitiligo were evaluated. Compared with perilesional, nonlesional, and healthy skin, in vitiligo skin there was significantly lower expression of keratinocyte-derived cytokines with stimulatory activity on melanocytes, e.g. granulocyte–monocyte colony-stimulating factor, and significantly higher expression of keratinocyte-derived cytokines with inhibitory activity on melanocytes, e.g. interleukin-6 and tumor necrosis factor α.

The majority of patients with vitiligo do not have an accompanying systemic disease, but directed medical history and blood tests are helpful to identify high-risk individuals who require further evaluation.

FIRST LINE THERAPIES

■ Topical corticosteroids	A
■ Topical photochemotherapy	B
■ Systemic photochemotherapy	B
■ Narrowband UVB	B
■ 308-nm excimer laser	B
■ Topical tacrolimus or pimecrolimus	B
■ Topical tacrolimus plus 308-nm excimer laser	A
■ Narrowband UVB microphototherapy	B
■ Topical calcipotriene and narrowband UVB	C
■ Monochromatic excimer light	B

A double-blind randomized trial of 0.1% tacrolimus vs 0.05% clobetasol for the treatment of childhood vitiligo. Lepe V, Moncada B, Castanedo-Cazares JP, et al. Arch Dermatol 2003;139:581–5.

Twenty patients with vitiligo were treated for 2 months. Ninety percent of patients experienced some repigmentation. The mean percentage of repigmentation was 49.3% for clobetasol and 41.3% for tacrolimus. The authors concluded that tacrolimus is almost as effective as clobetasol and is better for sensitive areas (eyelids) because, unlike clobetasol, it does not cause skin atrophy.

Ophthalmologic examination should be performed after starting topical corticosteroids on the eyelids.

Treatment of vitiligo with UV-B radiation vs topical psoralen plus UV-A. Westerhof W, Nieuweboer-Krobotova L. Arch Dermatol 1997;133:1525–8.

Patients with extensive vitiligo were treated with topical PUVA for 4 months (n = 28) or 311-nm UVB radiation for 4 months (n = 78). Forty-six percent of patients treated with topical PUVA and 67% of patients treated with the 311-nm UVB showed repigmentation. The authors concluded that narrowband UVB is as efficient as topical PUVA but with fewer adverse effects.

PUVA treatment of vitiligo: a retrospective study of Turkish patients. Sahin S, Hindioglu U, Karaduman A. Int J Dermatol 1999;38:542–5.

Thirty-three patients were treated with systemic PUVA. Overall, 85% showed some improvement; 36% achieved 51–75% repigmentation, and 18% achieved greater than 75% repigmentation. The best results were on the face and trunk.

Skin cancers associated with photochemotherapy have been reported, but are extremely rare in patients with vitiligo.

Treatment of vitiligo vulgaris with narrow band UVB (311 nm) for one year and the effect of addition of folic acid and vitamin B12. Tjioe M, Gerritsen MJ, Juhlin L, van de Kerkhof PC. Acta Derm Venereol 2002;82:369–72.

Twenty-seven patients with vitiligo were treated three times a week for 1 year. Successful repigmentation was achieved in 92% of patients. Co-treatment with vitamin B12 and folic acid did not improve the outcome.

Treatment of vitiligo with the 308-nm excimer laser: a pilot study. Spencer JM, Nossa R, Ajmeri J. J Am Acad Dermatol 2002;46:727–31.

Twenty-nine patches from 18 patients with vitiligo were treated three times a week for a maximum of 12 treatments. Some repigmentation was achieved in 57% of patches that had received at least six treatments and in 82% of patches that had undergone all 12 sessions.

The use of the 308-nm excimer laser for the treatment of vitiligo. Hadi SM, Spencer JM, Lebwohl M. Dermatol Surg 2004;30:983–6.

Thirty-two patients with vitiligo were treated with the excimer laser for 30 sessions, or 75% pigmentation, whichever occurred first. Overall, 55 spots were treated: 53% had ≥75% pigmentation, and 34% had ≥50% pigmentation. Facial lesions responded best, with 72% achieving ≥75% pigmentation, and 76% achieving ≥50% pigmentation.

Treatment of vitiligo by 308-nm excimer laser: an evaluation of variables affecting treatment response. Ostovari N, Passeron T, Zakaria W, et al. Lasers Surg Med 2004;35: 152–6.

Thirty-five patients were treated twice a week for a maximum of 24 sessions. Repigmentation occurred in 88.5% of the plaques; 27% of the plaques achieved 75% repigmentation. UV-sensitive areas of the body (face, neck, and trunk) tended to respond much better than UV-resistant areas (bony prominences, extremities): 57% versus 16% achieved 75% repigmentation, respectively.

The excimer laser, emitting light at 308 nm, has recently become available as a new form of phototherapy. The UV light emitted from this laser is in the UVB range and is in the form of laser light. It is possible that the light–tissue interaction is different when the light is given in the form of laser light as compared to conventional incoherent light, and may produce a superior result. In clinical trials of the phototherapy of psoriasis, this laser has achieved dramatically faster responses than is possible with conventional phototherapy.

Tacrolimus ointment promotes repigmentation of vitiligo in children: a review of 57 cases. Silverberg NB, Lin P, Travis L, et al. J Am Acad Dermatol 2004;51:760–6.

Fifty-seven pediatric patients with vitiligo were treated with topical tacrolimus for at least 3 months. Tacrolimus was effective for childhood vitiligo, especially on the head and neck (89% response rate). Sixty-three percent of patients with lesions on the extremities responded.

Combined excimer laser and topical tacrolimus for the treatment of vitiligo: a pilot study. Kawalek AZ, Spencer JM, Phelps RG. Dermatol Surg 2004;30:130–5.

Twenty-four patches from eight patients with vitiligo (elbows, knees) were treated with the excimer laser three times a week for 24 sessions or 10 weeks. In addition, topical tacrolimus 0.1% ointment and placebo were applied to randomized patches twice daily throughout the trial. Fifty percent of patches treated with combination excimer laser and tacrolimus achieved a successful response (75% pigmentation) compared with 20% for the placebo group.

Narrow-band UV-B micro-phototherapy: a new treatment for vitiligo. Menchini G, Tsoureli-Nikita E, Hercogova J. J Eur Acad Dermatol Venereol 2003;17:171–7.

A total of 734 patients with vitiligo (segmental and non-segmental) underwent a mean of 24 sessions of focused beam narrowband UVB (microphototherapy – Bioskin) over 12 months. Approximately 70% achieved normal pigmentation on more than 75% of the treated areas.

Topical calcipotriene and narrowband ultraviolet B in the treatment of vitiligo. Kullavanijaya P, Lim HW. Photodermatol Photoimmunol Photomed 2004;20:248–51.

Twenty patients with symmetrical vitiligo were treated with narrowband UVB three times per week; in addition, calcipotriene ointment was applied to lesions on one side of the body. Nine of 17 patients who completed the study achieved appreciably better pigmentation on the UVB plus calcipotriene side.

Monochromatic excimer light 308 nm in the treatment of vitiligo: a pilot study. Leone G, Iacovelli P, Paro Vidolin A, Picardo M. J Eur Acad Dermatol Venereol 2003;17:531–7.

Thirty-seven patients with vitiligo (acrofacial, focal, segmental, generalized) were treated twice weekly for a maximum of 6 months. Ninety-five percent of patients showed signs of pigmentation within the first eight sessions. Excellent pigmentation was achieved in 18 patients and good pigmentation in 16 patients. Compared with the 308-nm excimer laser, this modality can treat larger areas within shorter time.

Vitiligo treated by psoralens, a long-term follow-up study of the permanency of repigmentation. Kenney JA Jr. Arch Dermatol 1971;103:475–80.

Twenty-one psoralen-treated vitiligo patients who had obtained satisfactory repigmentation were located and examined. In the 10–14 years without treatment group, 12 patients had 25 areas with 100% or greater retention. In the 3–9 years without treatment group, nine patients had 18 areas with 100% or greater retention. The repigmentation can therefore be regarded as permanent.

SECOND LINE THERAPIES

■ Intralesional steroids	B
■ 5-MOP	E

Vitiligo and intralesional steroids. Vasistha LK, Singh G. Indian J Med Res 1979;69:308–11.

Twenty-five patients were treated with 10 mg/mL triamcinolone acetonide weekly for 8 weeks. There was no significant difference in the steroid versus water treated control group with respect to pigmentation. Atrophy, telangiectasia, infection, and intradermal hemorrhage were some of the side effects, therefore this treatment is not recommended.

5-Methoxypsoralen. A review of its effects in psoriasis and vitiligo. McNeely W, Goak KL. Drugs 1998;56:667–90.

Treatment with oral 5-MOP (not available in the USA) and oral 8-MOP resulted in similar lesion clearance rates. Patients treated with 5-MOP often required a greater total UV exposure than 8-MOP recipients. Short-term cutaneous and gastrointestinal side effects were markedly less with 5-MOP, although the long-term tolerability of this treatment has not yet been established.

THIRD LINE THERAPIES

■ Monobenzyl ether of hydroquinone (MBEHQ)	C
■ L-Phenylalanine and UVA	B
■ Khellin and UVA (KUVA)	B
■ Pseudocatalase and UVA	B
■ Topical fluorouracil	B
■ Surgical grafting	B
■ Dermabrasion and thin split-thickness skin graft	D
■ Ruby laser	C
■ Levamisole	B
■ Cosmetic tattooing	B

Monobenzyl ether of hydroquinone. Moser D, Parrish J, Fitzpatrick T. Br J Dermatol 1977;97:669–79.

Of 18 patients treated with MBEHQ therapy twice daily over a 1-year period, eight achieved complete depigmentation, three had marked but not complete depigmentation, and the remaining seven had either poor or no depigmentation. The depigmentation is permanent. Major side effects are erythema, pruritus, contact dermatitis, and complete and irreversible depigmentation at the application sites and also at remote sites.

L-Phenylalanine and UVA irradiation in the treatment of vitiligo. Siddiqui AH, Stolk LML, Bhaggoe R, et al. Dermatology 1994;188:215–18.

Response to L-phenylalanine (L-Phe) plus UVA irradiation was positive. An increased L-Phe dose resulted in increased L-Phe plasma levels but not in improved clinical results.

Treatment of vitiligo with khellin and ultraviolet A. Ortel B, Tanew A, Honigsmann H. J Am Acad Dermatol 1988;18: 693–701.

Thirty-eight patients were treated three times weekly with khellin, a furanochromone, together with UVA irradiation. In patients who received 100–200 treatments, 41% achieved more than 70% repigmentation. This success rate is comparable to the rate obtained with psoralens. The major advantage of khellin is that it does not induce skin phototoxicity with UVA. Seven patients experienced a mild elevation of liver transaminases and their treatments were discontinued. With proper instruction and regular monitoring of patients, khellin photochemotherapy can be considered safe with natural sunlight, or as a home treatment with artificial UVA.

Treatment of vitiligo with a topical application of pseudo-catalase and calcium in combination with short-term UVB exposure: a case study on 33 patients. Schallreuter KU, Wood JM, Lemke KR, Levenig C. Dermatology 1995;190: 223–9.

Thirty-three patients were treated with pseudocatalase and calcium chloride twice daily and with total body UVB exposure twice weekly 1 h after application of the cream. A mean treatment duration of 15.3 months resulted in excellent repigmentation on the face and dorsum of the hands in 90% of patients, 90–100% repigmentation in all cases of focal vitiligo, and partial but slow response in segmental vitiligo. The cream was well tolerated and without side effects, except for one patient who developed contact sensitivity to para-aminobenzoic acid ester.

Topically administered fluorouracil in vitiligo. Tsuji T, Hamada T. Arch Dermatol 1983;119:722–7.

Following an epidermal abrasion on day 1, 5% fluorouracil cream applied daily under occlusive dressings resulted in complete or almost complete repigmentation in 64% of patients. No systemic toxicity was observed.

A systematic review of autologous transplantation methods in vitiligo. Njoo MD, Westerhof W, Bos JD, Bossuyt PM. Arch Dermatol 1998;134:1543–9.

Sixty-three studies were analyzed: 16 on minigrafting, 13 on split-thickness grafting, 15 on grafting of epidermal blisters, 17 on grafting of cultured melanocytes, and two on grafting of non-cultured epidermal suspension. The highest mean success rates were achieved with split-skin grafting and epidermal blister grafting. No controlled trials were included. No conclusion could be made about the effectiveness of culturing techniques because of the small sample sizes studied.

A good review article.

Comparison of melanocytes transplantation methods for the treatment of vitiligo. Czajkowski R. Dermatol Surg 2004;30:1400–5.

Twenty patients were treated: 10 of 10 patients treated with suction blister graft and 6 of 10 patients treated with cultured autologous melanocytes transplantation achieved successful repigmentation.

Treatment of vitiligo by transplantation of cultured pure melanocyte suspension: analysis of 120 cases. Chen YF, Yang PY, Hu DN, et al. J Am Acad Dermatol 2004;51:68–74.

A total of 120 patients were treated with transplantation of autologous cultured pure melanocyte suspension after CO_2 laser abrasion. Overall, 90–100% coverage was achieved in 84% of patients with stable localized vitiligo and in 54% of patients with stable generalized vitiligo, while only 14% of patients with active generalized vitiligo achieved good repigmentation.

Vitiligo: repigmentation with dermabrasion and thin split-thickness skin graft. Agrawal K, Agrawal A. Dermatol Surg 1995;21:295–300.

A case series of 21 patients with 32 localized, stable, and refractory vitiligo patches treated by dermabrasion and thin split-thickness skin graft were assessed. The graft take was 100% in 27 patches and 90–95% in the remaining five. One hundred percent repigmentation was achieved in 22 patches and 90–95% in 10. Satisfactory color was achieved in an average of 6.3 months and complications were minor.

Unfortunately, the authors do not qualify the graft appearance with respect to texture and contour.

Autologous epidermal grafting with PUVA-irradiated donor skin for the treatment of vitiligo. Lee AY, Jang JH. Int J Dermatol 1998;37:551–4.

PUVA-irradiated donor sites resulted in an increased number of melanocytes and improved clinical outcome.

Single hair grafting for the treatment of vitiligo. Na GY, Seo SK, Choi SK. J Am Acad Dermatol 1998;38:580–4.

Fourteen of 17 patients with localized/segmental vitiligo and one of four patients with generalized vitiligo achieved perifollicular pigmentation. Single hair grafting is especially effective for small vitiliginous areas and on hairy parts of the skin such as eyelids and eyebrows.

Depigmentation therapy in vitiligo universalis with topical 4-methoxyphenol and the Q-switched ruby laser. Njoo MD, Vodegel RM, Westerhof W. J Am Acad Dermatol 2000;42:760–9.

Eleven of 16 patients treated with 4-methoxyphenol (4-MP) cream twice daily achieved total depigmentation within 6–24 months. Four of the patients had recurrences after a treatment-free period of between 2 and 36 months. Four of the five patients who did not respond to 4-MP were subsequently successfully treated with the Q-switched ruby (QSR) laser. Nine of 13 patients treated between two and 10 times with QSR laser therapy achieved total depigmentation. Three of the four unresponsive patients had successful depigmentation with the 4-MP cream.

Effect of prolonged treatment with levamisole on vitiligo with limited and slow-spreading disease. Pasricha JS, Khera V. Int J Dermatol 1994;33:584–7.

Levamisole (an immune modulator) was given as a 150-mg oral dose on two consecutive days every week for 4–48 months in 64 patients with limited and slow-spreading vitiligo. Levamisole alone was given to 14 patients, 38 patients were also treated with fluocinolone acetonide acetate ointment once daily, and 12 patients with topical 0.05% clobetasol propionate. In 34 of 36 patients with active disease, progression stopped within 2–4 months. Repigmentation was seen in 9 of 14 treated with levamisole only,

Evidence levels **A** Double-blind study **B** Clinical trial ≥ 20 subjects **C** Clinical trial < 20 subjects **D** Series ≥ 5 subjects **E** Anecdotal case reports

in 33 of 38 treated with levamisole and flucinolone, and in all 12 patients treated with levamisole and clobetasol propionate. Minimal side effects were reported, except in two cases with severe vomiting.

Evaluation of cosmetic tattooing in localized stable vitiligo. Mahajan BB, Garg G, Gupta RR. J Dermatol 2002;29: 726–30.

Thirty patients with localized, stable vitiligo – 19 with skin lesions, nine with mucosal lesions, and two with both skin and mucosal lesions – were treated and followed up for 6 months. Color matching was considered excellent in 23 cases (76.7%). Excellent results were achieved in all mucosal patches.

Vulvodynia

Neda Ashourian, Ginat Mirowski

Vulvodynia is a multifactorial group of physical and clinical conditions that present as altered sensory function in the vulva despite a normal clinical exam. Pain is localized to the vulva and/or the vulvar vestibule. Vulvodynia is subcategorized into vulvar vestibulitis syndrome and dysesthetic vulvodynia. In vulvar vestibulitis, altered sensation is restricted to the vestibules and is elicited by touch; in dysesthetic vulvodynia, the discomfort is more generalized and unprovoked. While debate continues over the proper use of this terminology, the International Society for the Study of Vulvar Disease defines vulvodynia as 'chronic vulvar discomfort, characterized by the patient's complaint of burning, stinging, irritation, or rawness'.

The differential diagnosis of vulvodynia includes a number of neurologic conditions including postherpetic neuralgia, and pudendal nerve entrapment. Infections (e.g. *Candida albicans*) and dermatoses (including contact dermatitis) are common culprits. Less clearly defined causes include immune-mediated inflammation and oxalate crystalluria. Other etiologies include referred pain from interstitial cystitis or from the gastrointestinal tract, as in patients with irritable bowel syndrome. Vulvodynia in some women has followed laser therapy for genital warts or malignancy removal. This chapter will focus on strategies for the management of vulvodynia.

MANAGEMENT STRATEGY

Vulvodynia describes a group of symptoms, not necessarily a specific disorder. Thus the mainstay of management strategy should focus on arriving at the correct etiology and ruling out other causes of vulvar irritation and vulvitis. Symptomatic relief is a priority. In addition to the physical discomfort associated with vulvodynia, patients also find vulvodynia psychologically distressing and socially embarrassing. The goal of treatment is to offer relief from the sensory discomfort.

Once essential vulvodynia is diagnosed, appropriate treatment may be instituted. The mainstay in treatment is the use of low-dose antidepressant regimens with *amitriptyline, imipramine* and *desipramine*, and anticonvulsants such as *gabapentin*. Relief may not be immediate and the patient should be advised to undergo an adequate course of therapy before determining treatment failure. Surgical interventions should be reserved for treatment of refractory cases. Complications include wound infection, uneven healing, Bartholin's duct stenosis with cyst formation, and recurrence or worsening of symptoms.

SPECIFIC INVESTIGATIONS

- Clinical visual and manual examination
- Direct smear of vaginal secretions to rule out *Trichomonas vaginalis*
- Whiff test for bacterial vaginosis
- Direct mycology to rule out fungi or infestations
- Tape test for pinworms (if perirectal pruritus is present)
- Papanicolaou smear
- Microbiologic testing of secretions for bacteria and fungi
- Viral studies
- Blood glucose
- Colposcopy
- Biopsy
- Trial of hormone replacement therapy
- Patch testing
- Evaluation for the presence of primary or concomitant psychiatric disorders

International Society for the Study of Vulvar Disease Taskforce. Burning vulvar syndrome: report of the ISSVD taskforce. J Reprod Med 1984;29:457.

FIRST LINE THERAPIES

■ Low-dose antidepressants	B
■ Anticonvulsants such as gabapentin	C
■ Topical lidocaine	B

Dysesthetic ('essential') vulvodynia. McKay M. J Reprod Med 1993;38:9–13.

Low-dose amitriptyline, starting at 10 mg daily and increasing to a maximum of 75 mg daily, in conjunction with 5% lidocaine gel is recommended as the treatment of choice for vulvodynia.

Amitriptyline vs. placebo for treatment of vulvodynia: a prospective study. Abstract presented at the Biennial Meeting of the American Society for Colposcopy and Cervical Pathology. Scottsdale, AZ. March, 1998.

Prospective, placebo-controlled trial that reported limited treatment success of amitriptyline for the treatment of vulvodynia.

Response to treatment in dysaesthetic vulvodynia. Munday PE, McKay M. J Obstet Gynaecol 2001;21:610–13.

Thirty two women were treated with a tricyclic antidepressant drug and behavioral interventions: a complete response was recorded in 47% after 6 months.

Gabapentin therapy for vulvodynia. Ben-David B, Friedman M. Anesth Analg 1999;89:1459.

A study to evaluate the effectiveness of gabapentin for the treatment of essential vulvodynia in 17 patients suffering from vulvar pain and deemed to lack dermatoses, infections, or other gynecologic or systemic causes including atrophy. Among the 17 patients, who ranged from 26 to 82 years of age, 12 were postmenopausal. Twelve had failed prior treatment with amitriptyline. Fourteen (82%) had either partial or complete relief with gabapentin. Seven had complete relief and seven had significant relief. Three patients failed to respond to gabapentin. Symptomatic relief occurred at between 2 and 4 weeks from the onset of treatment. No cases of late failure of therapy were reported and four patients were able to terminate treatment without recurrence of their symptoms.

Overnight 5% lidocaine ointment for treatment of vulvar vestibulitis. Zolnoun DA, Hartmann KE, Steege JF. Obstet Gynecol 2003;102:84–7.

Sixty one women with vulvar vestibulitis were instructed to place a cotton ball coated with 5% lidocaine ointment in the vestibule and apply the ointment to the affected areas nightly for an average of 7 weeks; 57% reported a 50% or greater reduction in pain with intercourse. Nearly two-thirds of the women who were unable to have intercourse prior to treatment reported the ability to have intercourse after treatment.

SECOND LINE THERAPIES

■ Urinary oxalate reduction therapy	B
■ Nitroglycerin cream	B
■ Acupuncture	C
■ Electromyographic biofeedback	B

Urinary oxalate excretion and its role in vulvar pain syndrome. Baggish MS, Sze EH, Johnson R. Am J Obstet Gynecol 1997;177:507–11.

In 130 consecutive patients with vulvar pain syndrome and 23 volunteers without symptoms, urinary oxalates were found to be nonspecific irritants that appeared to aggravate vulvodynia, but the role of oxalates in the etiology of vulvodynia was not confirmed.

A pilot study of the use of a low oxalate diet in the treatment of vulval vestibulitis. Poole G, Ravenhill PE, Munday S. J Obstet Gynaecol 1999;19:271–2.

Six (37%) of sixteen women responded to a low oxalate diet.

Acupuncture for vulvodynia. Powell J, Wojnarowska F. J Roy Soc Med 1999;92:579–81.

Twelve patients with vulvodynia were treated weekly with acupuncture. Monitoring included a questionnaire and a visual analogue scale for pain. Half had treatment for the first 5 weeks only, the other half for the second 5 weeks only. Two patients reported themselves cured and three reported improvement. Four were slightly better. Three reported no effect at all.

Acupuncture for the treatment of vulvar vestibulitis: a pilot study. Danielsson I, Sjoberg I, Ostman C. Acta Obstet Gynecol Scand 2001;80:437–41.

Fourteen young women with vulvar vestibulitis were enrolled in the study and 13 fulfilled the acupuncture treatment a total of ten times. For evaluation, quality of life (QOL) assessments were made before starting the treatment and then at 1 week and at 3 months after it was completed. The treatment was well tolerated and the QOL measurements were all significantly higher after both the last acupuncture and 3 months later compared to before the treatment was started.

Treatment of vulvar vestibulitis syndrome with electromyographic biofeedback of pelvic floor musculature. Glazer HI, Rodke G, Swencionis C, et al. J Reprod Med 1995;40:283–90.

Thirty three women were provided with portable electromyographic (EMG) biofeedback devices and encouraged to perform pelvic floor muscle rehabilitation exercises daily. After an average of 16 weeks, subjective reports of pain decreased 83%. Twenty two of the 28 patients who had abstained from intercourse for more than 1 year prior to

treatment resumed intercourse by the end of the treatment period. Pain relief was maintained at 6 month follow-up.

Treating vulvar vestibulitis with electromyographic biofeedback of pelvic floor musculature. McKay E, Kaufman RH, Doctor U, et al. J Reprod Med 2001;46:337–42.

Twenty nine patients performed biofeedback-assisted pelvic floor muscle rehabilitation exercises; 20 of the 29 women (69%) became sexually active and 24 (83%) reported negligible or mild pain. Five of the 29 did not show any significant improvement.

Safety and efficacy of topical nitroglycerin for treatment of vulvar pain in women with vulvodynia: a pilot study. Walsh KE, Berman JR, Berman LA, Vierregger K. J Gend Specif Med 2002 ;5:21–7.

Thirty four women were treated with 0.2% nitroglycerin cream applied directly to the skin of the affected area at least three times per week 5–10 min prior to sexual relations. Nearly all the patients reported a significant improvement in pain.

THIRD LINE THERAPIES

■ Surgery	D
■ Psychotherapy	E
■ Hypnosis	E
■ Interferon	B
■ Botulinum toxin A	E
■ Spinal cord stimulator	E
■ Flashlamp excited dye laser	C

Pudendal canal syndrome as a cause of vulvodynia and its treatment by pudendal nerve decompression. Shafik A. Eur J Obstet Gynecol Reprod Biol 1998;80:215–20.

Eleven women with vulvodynia ranging in age from 28 to 53 years had significant increase of the pudendal nerve terminal motor latency, and motor and sensory changes suggested a pudendal canal syndrome. Pudendal nerve block, as a diagnostic and therapeutic test, effected temporary pain relief. Pudendal nerve decompression was performed via a fasciotomy to release the pudendal nerve in the ischiorectal fossa. Vulvar pain disappeared in nine of the 11 patients. Stress urinary incontinence was relieved in four of six patients, anal reflex normalized in five of seven women, and vulvar and perineal hypoesthesia in four of six.

Interferon therapy for condylomatous vulvitis. Horowitz BJ. Obstet Gynecol 1989;73:446–8.

Thirty patients with vulvar vestibulitis syndrome underwent colposcopy; human papillomavirus (HPV) infection was found on biopsy in 17 patients. All patients received interferon-α-2b recombinant intradermal injections into the vestibule three times weekly for 4 weeks. Of the HPV-positive women, 15 (88%) responded with complete resolution of vulvar pain. Five women reported flu-like symptoms as a result of the injections. Patients without evidence of HPV failed to respond to interferon therapy. Studies by other authors have demonstrated efficacy with intramuscular interferon in HPV-positive patients with vulvodynia.

A randomized comparison of group cognitive–behavioral therapy, surface electromyographic biofeedback, and vestibulectomy in the treatment of dyspareunia resulting

from vulvar vestibulitis. Bergeron S, Binik YM, Khalife S, et al. Pain 2001;91:297–306.

Seventy eight women were randomly assigned to a 12-week trial of group cognitive behavioral therapy (CBT), EMG biofeedback, or vestibulectomy. After 6 months, completers of the study had statistically significant reductions on pain measures regardless of treatment assignment; the vestibulectomy group was slightly more successful than the two other groups.

Behavioral approach with or without surgical intervention to the vulvar vestibulitis syndrome: a prospective randomized and non-randomized study. Weijmar Schultz WC, Gianotten WL, van der Meijden WI, et al. J Psychosom Obstet Gynaecol 1996;17:143–8.

Forty eight women were either randomized or given a choice between CBT or vestibulectomy followed by CBT. Both interventions were beneficial to most women. The difference in outcome between the two different treatments was not statistically significant.

Botulinum toxin A for vulvodynia: a case report. Gunter J, Brewer A, Tawfik O. J Pain 2004;5:238–40.

A 22-year-old woman with severe vulvar pain extending beyond the boundaries of the vestibule received a 10 U of botulinum toxin A injection into the muscles of the perineal body at two sites. Four weeks after the injection, the area of pain was reduced in size and confined to the vestibule only. A vestibulectomy was therefore performed 5 weeks after injection. Three years later, the patient remained pain free.

Spinal cord stimulation for intractable vulvar pain. A case report. Whiteside JL, Walters MD, Mekhail N. J Reprod Med 2003;48:821–3.

A 21-year-old woman failed to respond to a partial vulvar vestibulectomy with Bartholin gland excision, but had temporary relief following bilateral hypogastric plexus blocks. A permanent spinal cord stimulator was implanted, with sustained symptom relief.

The surgical treatment of vulvar vestibulitis syndrome: a follow-up study. Bergeron S, Bouchard C, Fortier M, et al. J Sex Marital Ther 1997;23:317–25.

The postoperative follow-up ranged from 1.1 to 10 years, with a mean of 3.3 years. Vestibulectomy yielded a positive outcome for 63.2% of the participants and moderate to no improvement for the other 36.8%. The surgery was linked to a significant increase in intercourse frequency for the entire sample and to an increase in oral and manual stimulation for the women with successful surgical outcomes.

Vestibulectomy for vulvar vestibulitis. Gaunt G, Good A, Stanhope CR. J Reprod Med 2003;48:591–5.

A retrospective chart review of 42 patients postvestibulectomy at the Mayo Clinic from 1992 to 2001. Thirty-eight of 42 patients (90%) had a significant improvement in their symptoms.

Hypnotherapy as a treatment for vulvar vestibulitis syndrome: a case report. Kandyba K, Binik YM. J Sex Marital Ther 2003;29:237–42.

A 26-year-old woman received twelve sessions of psychotherapy, of which eight were devoted to hypnosis. Treatment was successful and she remained pain free at 12-month follow-up.

Flashlamp-excited dye laser therapy of idiopathic vulvodynia is safe and efficacious. Reid R, Omoto KH, Precop SL, et al. Am J Obstet Gynecol 1995;172:1684–96; discussion 1696–701.

The authors report on 168 women with treatment-refractory vulvovaginal pain who were treated with flashlamp-excited dye laser photothermolysis. Only 50 patients (less than one-third) failed to report improvement with flashlamp-excited dye laser treatment. Microsurgical Bartholin gland removal was then performed, with subsequent improvement in over 80% of the subjects.

Xanthomas

Lucile E White, Marcelo G Horenstein, Christopher R Shea

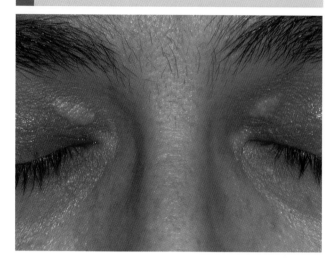

Xanthomas are flat, yellow plaques or nodules consisting of abnormal lipid deposition. Clinically, xanthomas can be classified as eruptive, tuberoeruptive, tuberous, tendinous, or plane. Plane xanthomas are the most common and include xanthelasma palpebrarum, xanthoma striatum palmaris, and intertriginous xanthomas.

MANAGEMENT STRATEGY

Xanthomas may be idiopathic or a sign of underlying hyperlipidemia. *Diagnosing and treating the underlying disease* is necessary to not only decrease the size of the xanthomas, but also prevent the risks of atherosclerosis associated with lipoprotein disorders. Treatment of the hyperlipidemia initially consists of *diet and lipid-lowering agents* such as statins, fibrates, bile-acid binding resins, probucol, or nicotinic acid. The lipid-lowering effects of these agents have been well documented, but few studies mention the efficacy of these drugs at resolving xanthomas, limiting an evidence-based evaluation of what would appear to be a rational management approach. It would appear that eruptive xanthomas usually resolve within weeks of initiating systemic treatment, tuberous xanthomas usually resolve after months, but tendinous xanthomas take years to resolve or may persist indefinitely. *Surgery or locally destructive modalities* can be used for idiopathic or unresponsive xanthomas.

SPECIFIC INVESTIGATIONS

- Serum lipid panel of cholesterol, triglycerides, VLDL, LDL, and HDL
- Gas–liquid and high-performance liquid chromatography to diagnose sitosterolemia
- Capillary gas chromatography of urine to diagnose cerebrotendinous xanthomatosis
- Serum protein electrophoresis, immunoelectrophoresis, or immunofixation to detect M proteins

Excluding an underlying condition is essential in the management of most clinical forms of xanthomas. Eruptive xanthomas typically occur in the setting of hypertriglyceridemia. Hypertriglyceridemia can be the result of lipoprotein lipase deficiency, familial hyperlipoproteinemia, or secondary causes such as diabetes mellitus, alcohol ingestion, or exogenous estrogens. Tuberoeruptive and tuberous xanthomas can be considered to represent parts of a spectrum and are seen most commonly in the setting of familial dysbetalipoproteinemia. Tuberous xanthomas may also be a presentation of homozygous familial hypercholesterolemia, cerebrotendinous xanthomatosis, or sitosterolemia. Patients with sitosterolemia and cerebrotendinous xanthomatosis may have normal serum lipid panels; it may therefore be indicated to refer them to an academic center where liquid chromatography for plant sterols or urinary gas chromatography can be performed. Tendinous xanthomas can also be seen with cerebrotendinous xanthomatosis, sitosterolemia, or more commonly, heterozygous familial hypercholesterolemia. Certain xanthomas are diagnostic for an inherited hyperlipidemia: xanthoma striatum palmaris for familial dysbetalipoproteinemia and intertriginous xanthomas for homozygous familial hypercholesterolemia. With these clinical presentations, a serum lipid panel should still be ordered to confirm these diagnoses. Xanthelasma palpebrarum, a type of plane xanthoma, has a less definite association with hyperlipidemia with levels of total cholesterol elevated in only about half of those affected. Less commonly, plane xanthomas can signal a monoclonal gammopathy. In this situation, the differential diagnosis of necrobiotic xanthogranuloma with paraproteinemia, a condition usually associated with lymphoproliferative disorders, should be considered.

Serum lipid and lipoprotein profiles in patients with xanthomas. Hata Y, Shigematsu H, Tsushima M, et al. Jpn Circ J 1981;45:1236–41.

Dermal, subcutaneous, and tendon xanthomas: diagnostic markers for specific lipoprotein disorders. Cruz PD, East C, Bergstresser PR. J Am Acad Dermatol 1988;19:95–111.

Normocholesterolemic xanthomatosis. Parker F. Arch Dermatol 1986;122:1253–6.

Sitosterolaemia and xanthomatosis in a child. Cheng WF, Yuen YP, Chow CB, et al. Hong Kong Med J 2003;9: 206–9.

Capillary gas chromatography of urine samples in diagnosing cerebrotendinous xanthomatosis. Bouwes Bavinck JN, Vermeer BJ, Gevers Leuen JA, et al. Arch Dermatol 1986; 122:1269–72.

Serum lipoproteins and cholesterol metabolism in xanthelasma. Epstein NN, Rosenman RH, Gofman JW. Arch Dermatol 1952;65:70–81.

The pathogenesis and clinical significance of xanthelasma palpebrarum. Bergman R. J Am Acad Dermatol 1994;30: 236–42.

Monoclonal gammopathies and skin disorders. Daoud MS, Lust JA, Kyle RA, Pittelkow MR. J Am Acad Dermatol 1999;40:507–38.

FIRST LINE THERAPIES

■ Low-fat diet and systemic lipid-lowering therapy – statins, bile-acid binding resins, fibrates, and/or nicotinic acid	B

Opposite effects on serum cholesteryl ester transfer protein levels between long-term treatments with pravastatin and probucol in patients with primary hypercholesterolemia. Inazu A, Koizumi J, Kajinami K, et al. Atherosclerosis 1999;145:405–13.

This prospective study examined whether pravastatin or probucol was better at regressing tendon xanthomas and xanthelasma in patients with primary hypercholesterolemia. In both the pravastatin and probucol groups, xanthelasma regressed in two of four patients. Achilles tendon xanthoma regressed in four of five patients treated with pravastatin and two of five patients on probucol.

Drug treatment of lipid disorders. Knopp RH. N Engl J Med 1999;341:498–511.

This review of managing lipid disorders does not mention specific efficacy for xanthomas.

A comparative study of the therapeutic effect of probucol and pravastatin on xanthelasma. Fujita M, Shirai K. J Dermatol 1996;23:598–602.

Fifty four patients were treated with probucol or pravastatin. Xanthelasma regressed in 13 of 36 patients treated with probucol and one of 18 patients treated with pravastatin. Total cholesterol levels decreased in both treatment groups, while HDL cholesterol decreased only in those treated with probucol.

Effects of probucol on xanthomata regression in familial hypercholesterolemia. Yamamoto A, Matsuzawa Y, Yokoyama S, et al. Am J Cardiol 1986;57:H29–35.

This study examined 51 patients with familial hypercholesterolemia, including eight homozygotes. Patients were treated with combinations of probucol, cholestyramine, clofibrate, and compactin. The sizes of Achilles tendon xanthomas were decreased in all patients who received probucol. Probucol possibly reduces the size of HDL particles, increasing reverse cholesterol transport.

Use of combined diet and colestipol in long-term (7–7½ years) treatment of patients with type II hyperlipoproteinemia. Kuo PT, Kiyoshi H, Kostis JB, Moreyra AE. Circulation 1979;59:199–212.

Twenty one patients with atherosclerosis and cutaneous, tendinous, or corneal xanthomas were followed for up to 7½ years. Patients were placed on a low-fat, low-cholesterol diet and colestipol, a bile-acid binding resin. This regimen caused tendinous xanthomas to disappear in two of 11 patients and improve in nine of 11 patients. Xanthelasma disappeared in two of four patients and improved in two of four patients.

SECOND LINE THERAPIES

■ Surgery	B
■ CO$_2$ laser	B
■ Erbium:YAG laser	C
■ Pulsed dye laser	B
■ Argon laser	B

Treatment of xanthelasma by excision with secondary intention healing. Eedy DJ. Clin Exp Dermatol 1996;21:273–5.

Xanthelasmas were removed in 28 patients by scissor excision. After 18 months, two patients, one with hypercholesterolemia and one with primary biliary cirrhosis, had recurrence. One patient developed scarring. No ectropion developed.

Xanthelasma: follow-up on results after surgical excision. Mendelson BC, Masson JK. Plast Reconstr Surg 1976;58:535–8.

Surgical excision of xanthelasma was performed in 100 patients. Of patients who were having their lesions treated for the first time, 26/68 (38%) recurred. Factors that predicted recurrence were systemic hyperlipidemia, involvement of all four eyelids, and a previous history of recurrent xanthelasma.

Xanthelasma palpebrarum. Parkes ML, Waller TS. Laryngoscope 1984;94:1238–40.

Parkes and Waller review several different methods of excision, suggesting that routine blepharoplasty with staged excisions achieves the best results.

Xanthelasma palpebrarum: treatment with the ultrapulsed CO$_2$ laser. Raulin C, Schoenermark MP, Werner S, Greve B. Lasers Surg Med 1999;24:122–7.

Ultrapulsed CO$_2$ laser delivers high energy in short pulses and reduces the risk of scarring and hyperpigmentation seen with continuous mode CO$_2$ lasers. Twenty three patients with 52 xanthelasmas were treated. All xanthelasmas were removed completely. One patient experienced mild erythema for 4 months, but no permanent hyperpigmentation or ectropion developed. Three patients had recurrent lesions at an average follow-up time of 10 months.

Xanthelasma palpebrarum: treatment with the erbium:YAG laser. Borelli C, Kaudewitz P. Lasers Surg Med 2001;29:260–4.

Fifteen patients with 33 xanthelasmas were treated with an erbium:YAG laser at settings between of 300 mJ, 2 Hz for a 2 mm spot size and 1200 mJ, 6 Hz for a 10 mm spot size. All xanthelasmas were removed completely. Postoperative erythema resolved within 2 weeks. No scarring or ectropion developed. No lesions recurred over a 7–12-month follow-up period.

Treatment of diffuse plane xanthoma of the face with erbium:YAG laser. Lorenz S, Hohenleutner S, Hohenleutner U, Landthaler M. Arch Dermatol 2001;137:1413–5.

A patient presented with diffuse plane xanthomas of her entire face and neck. Erbium:YAG laser partially cleared the xanthomas. Two months later, a second treatment was performed for the persistent lesions. The treated lesions did not recur over a 12-month follow-up. Because of the risk of scarring, her neck and earlobe region were not treated.

Treatment of xanthelasma palpebrarum with argon laser photocoagulation. Basar E, Oguz H, Oxdemir H, et al. Int Ophthalmol 2004;25:9–11.

Twenty four patients with 40 xanthelasmas were treated with an argon laser at settings of 500 μm, 0.1–0.2 s, and 900 mW. Complete removal of all lesions occurred with one to four sessions at intervals of 2–3 weeks. Six lesions recurred over 8–12 months and required re-treatment. Erythema persisted for 1 month in eight lesions. Hyper-pigmentation occurred in one patient and persisted for 3 months, while hypopigmentation occurred in two lesions. No bleeding, infections, or ectropion occurred

Histopathological study of xanthelasma palpebrarum after pulsed dye laser. Soliman M. J Eur Acad Dermatol Venereol 2004;18(suppl):19–33.

Twenty six patients were treated with fluences ranging from 6.5 to 8 J/cm^2, a spot size of 5 mm, and a pulse width of 450 ms. All patients experienced very good to excellent clinical improvement with one to three treatments at 3–4 week intervals.

THIRD LINE THERAPIES

■ Di- or trichloracetic acid	C
■ Cryotherapy	E

Treatment of xanthelasma palpebrarum with bichloracetic acid. Haygood LJ, Bennett JD, Brodell RT. Dermatol Surg 1998;24:1027–31.

Of 13 patients with 25 lesions, ten patients had complete clearing with bichloracetic acid application. Five lesions recurred and required a second treatment to achieve complete resolution. No infections, scars, or complications were reported.

Cryotherapy may be effective for eyelid xanthoma. Hawk JL. Clin Exp Dermatol 2000;25:351.

One patient was treated with liquid nitrogen applied for 0.5–1 s. Treatment was carefully limited to only the yellow areas. Previous treatment with trichloroacetic acid had been unsuccessful.

Xeroderma pigmentosum

W Clark Lambert, Claude E Gagna, Santiago A Centurión

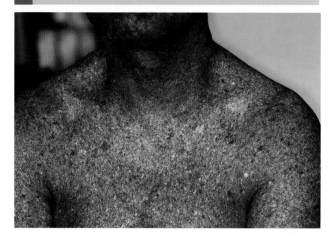

Xeroderma pigmentosum (XP) is a rare, autosomal recessive, inherited disease characterized by markedly increased sensitivity to UV radiation. In the natural environment, this hypersensitivity, particularly to the shorter wavelengths of UV found in sunlight, leads to profound premature solar aging effects in sun-exposed areas of the skin, lips, eyes, and anterior oral cavity, including the tongue. These changes are quite strikingly limited to sun-exposed areas, with almost total sparing of habitually covered areas and, usually, a sharp line of demarcation between them. Some patients also develop a progressive neurological component, unrelated to sun exposure, which varies from mild high-frequency nerve deafness to severe, life-threatening disease. Moriz Kaposi, in 1870, coined the name xeroderma (the second term, pigmentosum, was added 12 years later) to describe the very characteristic dry, dyspigmented skin that is the first permanent cutaneous change observed in these patients. All of the changes seen in photoaging, with the notable exception of solar elastosis, are visible at a very early age, often in early childhood. Later, sun-induced neoplasms – including actinic (solar) keratoses, keratoacanthomas, squamous cell carcinomas, basal cell carcinomas, and melanomas – appear, often in large numbers. Much less commonly, superficial soft tissue neoplasms, particularly angiosarcomas, may also appear. The overall distribution of these neoplasms mimics that seen in the general population, but the genetic alterations tend to differ, with, for example, mutations in the p53 tumor suppressor gene occurring earlier and more frequently in skin neoplasms in XP patients. These neoplasms characteristically occur much earlier in life and in much larger numbers in patients with XP.

MANAGEMENT STRATEGY

Although the diagnosis is usually straightforward, it is often made more difficult by the great heterogeneity in severity as well as in features, such as neurodegeneration, of the disease. There are at least eight complementation groups (i.e. genetic subtypes), each associated with at least one different defective gene, and there are also marked differences depending on the specific mutation within each gene. Most groups are associated with a defect in one of the 40 or so proteins that mediate nucleotide excision repair, the principal mechanism by which UV-induced adducts in cellular DNA, particularly cyclobutane pyrimidine–pyrimidine dimers and 6-4 pyrimidine–pyrimidone photoproducts, are repaired in skin cells. These groups are labeled XPA–XPG. A subset of cases, in the variant group (XPV), is instead defective in a DNA polymerase, polymerase η (eta), that synthesizes DNA past these adducts, and is therefore said to take part in 'trans-lesional synthesis'. This allows more 'error prone' polymerases, such as polymerase ζ (zeta), to carry out this function, producing errors in DNA replication leading to mutations. The expense associated with determining the complementation group means that this subtyping has not been carried out in many cases. This should change now that more sophisticated molecular studies have become available and are performed following initial testing of patients' fibroblasts for decreased survival and decreased DNA repair – 'unscheduled' DNA synthesis (UDS) – in response to UV irradiation (see below).

The diagnosis is made by recognizing the characteristic dry, dyspigmented skin, sun sensitivity, and especially (when manifest) the presence of cancerous and precancerous skin lesions in sun-exposed areas arising at an early age, often in childhood. Other photosensitive disorders can usually be distinguished from XP on clinical grounds, especially if the diagnosis is aided by specific laboratory tests. For example, the sun-sensitive porphyrias show characteristic skin biopsy changes and chemical changes in blood, urine, and/or feces, but no skin tumors. The nevoid basal cell carcinoma syndrome shows basal cell but not squamous cell carcinomas and extensive palmar pits and jaw cysts, but not the skin changes characteristic of XP. Differentiation from the Rothmund–Thomson syndrome may be challenging, but sun sensitivity is less severe and tumors are not seen in this poikilodermatous condition. Fanconi anemia also shows dyspigmentation but no atrophy, less sun sensitivity, and no tumors; skeletal anomalies, especially of the thumbs, are often present. Dyskeratosis congenita shows dyspigmentation, but it and the ichthyoses show ichthyotic changes, and there are characteristic alterations on biopsy. Bloom syndrome shows telangiectasias, especially on the conjunctivae, but no tumors. Cockayne syndrome shows severe neurological abnormalities without skin neoplasms. The newly described UV sun-sensitivity syndrome shows sun sensitivity but few to no skin changes and no tumors.

In individual cases, skin tumors may be predominantly squamous cell and basal carcinomas or may consist almost entirely of melanomas. The basis for this phenomenon is unknown, although it is known that patients in the variant (XPV) complementation group are particularly prone to develop melanomas. These melanomas may be histologically different and clinically less aggressive then those occurring in normal individuals. Lesions on the lips, tongue, and anterior oral cavity are mostly keratoses and squamous cell carcinomas. Eye lesions include conjunctivitis, pingueculae, entropions, and ectropions.

In extremely rare situations, XP may coexist with the even rarer Cockayne syndrome or UV-sensitive trichothiodystrophy.

Avoidance of sun exposure, combined with *surgical treatment* of precancerous and cancerous cutaneous, ocular, and oral lesions as they arise, is the mainstay of treatment of XP. Both must be pursued vigorously if the patient is to survive beyond childhood, and both impose a major burden on the patient's family and physicians. There are a number of special considerations, as follows.

Avoidance of sun exposure is usually difficult, often prohibitively so for the patient's family. The sun sensitivity of these patients is usually extreme. In early childhood they may sunburn with very little sun exposure, and the parents may even be accused of child abuse. As the child grows older, extreme measures may be necessary for protection from the sun at home. The damage is cumulative, and measures sufficient to protect the child from sunburn may be insufficient to prevent skin cancers and eye damage later. Children may or may not cry or otherwise express pain when exposed to sunlight. UV-protective goggles are necessary as well as complete coverage when outdoors in sunlight.

When these children enter school, special arrangements must be made to keep them away from sunlight. This is often less difficult than one might suppose, and many schools – especially in the USA, where they are required by federal law to provide a safe environment – are frequently very cooperative. These children must be kept away from windows when indoors and be thoroughly covered when outdoors. Special arrangements need to be made for events, such as fire drills, in which it is necessary for the buildings to be evacuated. Other children and even adults need to be educated about the disease, and be reassured that it is not contagious. Most indoor lighting is not a threat, even if it is fluorescent, provided that the patient is not directly exposed to the fluorescent bulbs (i.e. provided that there is the usual plastic plate between the naked bulbs and the area they are illuminating). An important exception is mercury arc lamps used in street lighting and in some open spaces such as gymnasiums. Indoor use of such lamps is illegal in many states, but they are sometimes used in spite of this. Their distinctive bluish color usually makes them easily identifiable. When possible, scanning the environment with a UVB and/or UVA meter can be very helpful; however, these meters are expensive, require expertise to use, and easily go out of calibration.

Since cells in the variant (XPV) complementation group of XP are sensitive to caffeine, showing defective DNA lesion bypass synthesis when it is present, it may be prudent for XP patients in this group, or who have not been typed for complementation group, to avoid dietary caffeine. It is found in non-decaffeinated coffee, tea, cola-type sodas, and many chocolate-flavored items, such as candy bars. We are not aware of a recorded example of a patient with XP having clinical hypersensitivity to caffeine, however, and this precaution may be unnecessary. We also advise XP patients to avoid smoking as well as second-hand tobacco smoke, and they should avoid toxic fumes and exposure to carcinogens whenever possible.

The sacrifices required to protect an XP patient from these hazards may overwhelm the resources a family can or may choose to provide. It is not inappropriate for a family to decide that they will only go so far to protect the XP patient, lest they ruin the quality of life for the unaffected family members in a vain attempt to protect the member or members with XP. This is a decision only they can make, and there are no correct or incorrect answers. They should be protected from overzealous third parties who may choose to intervene, especially without providing meaningful support. They should especially be warned against opportunistic purveyors of expensive 'space suits', sometimes supported by dubious 'foundations', which cost thousands of dollars but provide no more protection, or even less protection, than ordinary clothing with a close enough weave to block most sunlight exposure. Although there are legitimate vendors of sun-protective clothing, no protective garb should ever cost more than about $200.

It is important that the family understand the prognosis, and this itself may be challenging. Since in the early stages XP patients often do not appear very ill, parents may doubt the validity of the prognosis or even the diagnosis. At this stage they are very vulnerable to practitioners of 'alternative medicine', and are often lost to follow-up, only to return years later much the worse for their 'alternative care', both financially and medically. Thus, counseling must be done with great sensitivity, and some medical practitioner, social worker, or volunteer needs to make a major personal commitment to the family for the XP patient to survive to adulthood in most cases. If they do reach adulthood, however, XP patients are often able to cope surprisingly well on their own, at least for the short term, except for the need for extensive outpatient medical care.

For assistance regarding these aspects of XP management, the patient and family should be directed to the XP Society, Poughkeepsie, NY (email: <xps@xps.org>).

Surgical management of XP is very challenging. One must be aware that, depending on the frequency with which new tumors arise in an individual patient, it will be necessary to excise tumors again and again in the same fields as the patient ages. Often hundreds or even thousands of cancers must be removed from the sun-exposed skin of these patients. It must also be kept in mind that, even with the best of care, many of these patients will probably eventually succumb to metastatic skin cancer, with others succumbing to the severe, progressive neurological disease that occurs in some XP patients. Thus, one does not have the luxury of excising skin cancers, even melanomas, with the wide margins used in otherwise normal persons. To do so will often cause the patient to undergo massive morbidity when other cancers are removed from the same fields later, and the wider margins will not protect the patient from metastatic cancer arising from other sites. Accordingly, the risk–benefit considerations of surgical margins are drastically different in severely affected XP patients than in otherwise normal individuals. In patients in whom it is anticipated that numerous tumors will arise, the margins should be quite narrow, with frequent follow-up and re-excision as needed. Mohs' chemosurgery may be extremely valuable in these patients, but the surgeries required may be so numerous that this is impractical. Each patient must be managed individually. In patients in whom fewer tumors are expected, the management plan may be modified accordingly. Thus, some XP patients should be managed similarly to normal persons. Patients must be followed, if possible, at frequent intervals by a dermatologist, an ophthalmologist, and an oral surgeon, as well as, less frequently, by a neurologist, depending upon the frequency with which tumors arise, the presence and severity of neurological disease, and logistical factors.

Topical 5-fluorouracil (Efudex®) to eliminate skin cancers in the developmental stage may be a very useful modality. The inflammatory reaction to this agent may be marked, and compliance is strained in these XP patients, but the results are quite good. In other patients there is no such reaction, but the results are nonetheless quite satisfactory. Although the skin may improve both clinically and histologically, however, cancers may continue to arise, due to the cumulative effect of lifelong UV radiation exposure, so that continued careful follow-up to detect and remove these tumors must be done.

Topical imiquimod cream has been reported to be of benefit in a number of patients, producing clinical improvement in sun-exposed skin. As is the case for topical 5-fluorouracil, however, cancers may continue to arise. If they are well enough tolerated, both imiquimod and 5-fluorouracil may be used. These are applied twice daily, once daily, or three times per week, depending on the level of inflammation induced (alternating morning and night or every other day if both are administered).

If metastatic disease develops, there are anecdotal reports of good results from single lesion excisions, even of pulmonary lesions. Often, melanocytic malignancies have better than expected prognoses in these patients, especially in patients in whom they are multiple. However, the eventual prognosis is guarded, with death from metastatic disease the rule. These patients also have a slightly increased incidence of internal cancers, especially brain tumors. In underdeveloped countries, where surgical management is less readily available, death usually occurs due to sepsis from an untreated skin cancer.

In some complementation groups (especially XPA, XPD, and XPG), neurological complications, independent of sun exposure, develop and are progressive. These are usually mild, involving most commonly high-frequency hearing loss. More severe neurological deficiency is usually apparent quite early in the course of the disease; it is also progressive. The term De Sanctis–Cacchione syndrome should be reserved only for patients with very severe neurological disease. Some patients become blind, more in consequence of loss of their eyes due to sun-induced eye lesions and surgery for skin lesions than because of any neurological deficiency. It may be prudent to prepare patients for this eventuality while they are still sighted and can more easily learn Braille and other skills. There are rare reports of life-threatening vocal cord paralysis, sometimes exacerbated by anesthesia, in XP patients.

Kraemer and his associates have championed the use of *retinoids* in high doses to control the rate of development of skin cancer, especially nonmelanocytic skin cancer, in patients with XP. Under physiologic conditions, retinoic acid acts to modulate gene expression mechanisms so as to control the normal rate of cellular differentiation in the skin and elsewhere. Artificial retinoids, especially in non-physiologic doses, can suppress the premature keratinization seen in squamous carcinogenesis and increase the responsiveness of the premalignant cells to normal growth and differentiation control mechanisms. They may also enhance immune responsiveness to these neoplasms. Oral administration of *isotretinoin* (13-*cis*-retinoic acid) by Kraemer et al. and others, including one of the authors (WCL), has indeed led to at least a two-thirds diminution in the rates of development of skin cancers in XP patients. When administered episodically, the drug also has the effect of causing tumors to arise in crops; these can be synchronized with surgical intervention, simplifying treatment in patients who can be seen only at intervals in particular clinics due to logistical factors. The doses recommended by Kraemer et al. are as follows:

- High dose: 2.0 mg/kg body weight daily.
- Intermediate dose: 1.0 mg/kg body weight daily.
- Low dose: 0.5 mg/kg body weight daily.

Although good results have been obtained with these doses of isotretinoin, its use, especially in children, has been sharply limited by attendant side effects, particularly bone abnormalities, mucocutaneous toxic effects, and abnormal triglyceride levels and liver function tests. Thus, high-dose therapy should be avoided if possible. In some reports, this drug has been combined with topical imiquimod or topical 5-fluorouracil, with good results.

There are a small number of reports of *resurfacing* chronically sun-damaged skin in patients with XP. Techniques have included full-thickness grafting, dermabrasion, and use of chemical peels. A small number of patients have undergone CO_2 laser resurfacing under general anesthesia, with apparent clinical benefit. Although long-term follow-up to date has been limited, these modalities may prove to be valuable treatment options in selected patients with XP.

Yarosh and his associates have obtained preliminary success in correcting the sun sensitivity of epidermal cells of XP patients by introducing a *bacterial DNA repair enzyme* into them, using a topically applied cream containing the enzyme within artificial microcells. The enzyme, endonuclease V of bacteriophage T4, acts only on pyrimidine dimers, having no effect on 6-4 photoproducts. However, it is highly efficient; unlike mammalian endonucleases, it does not have to undergo a complex interaction with chromatin proteins in order to cleave its substrate. This enzyme does not appear to enter dermal cells, nor does it reverse mutagenic events that have already occurred in any of these cells. Clinical trials have produced promising results, but have now been suspended due to regulatory issues, and this treatment modality is not currently available.

Sarasin and his associates have successfully introduced the human *XPC* gene into skin cells of patients in the XPC complementation group. Using a retrovirus as vector, both keratinocytes and skin fibroblasts have been corrected, and have been shown to have normal phenotypes following UV exposure in a sophisticated tissue culture assay. However, this system must undergo significant further development before it can be tested clinically, and there is currently no gene therapy available for any complementation group of XP.

SPECIFIC INVESTIGATIONS

- Fibroblast culture test (UDS test)
- Examination and biopsy for skin cancers

DNA repair-deficient diseases, xeroderma pigmentosum, Cockayne syndrome and trichothiodystrophy. Lehmann AR. Biochimie 2003;85:1101–11.

Common pathways for ultraviolet skin carcinogenesis in the repair and replication defective groups of xeroderma pigmentosum. Cleaver JE. J Dermatol Sci 2000;23:1–11.

Rare diseases provide rare insights into DNA repair pathways, TFIIH, aging and cancer. Bohr VA, Sander M, Kraemer KH. DNA Repair 2005;4:293–302.

Xeroderma pigmentosum and other disorders of DNA and chromosomal instability. Lambert WC, Kuo H-R, Lambert MW. Curr Opin Dermatol 1997;4:76–93.

Evidence levels A Double-blind study B Clinical trial ≥ 20 subjects C Clinical trial < 20 subjects D Series ≥ 5 subjects E Anecdotal case reports

These are general reviews in which the complex biology of XP and related disorders, such as Cockayne syndrome and sun-sensitive cases of trichothiodystrophy, is discussed.

Fibroblast culture tests (tests of cell survival following UV irradiation and the UDS test) will soon be available (at the Genomic Instability and Mutagenesis Laboratory, UMDNJ, Newark, NJ – recently relocated from the Armed Forces Institute of Pathology, Washington, DC, under a contractural arrangement with the National Cancer Institute, N.I.H.) to confirm the diagnosis of XP, but they are relatively expensive and may be unnecessary to establish the diagnosis in well-developed cases. On the other hand, it is invaluable, sometimes essential, in early cases to establish the diagnosis so that sun protection can be provided before irreversible photodamage to exposed tissues accumulates to reach unacceptable levels. Either the UDS test or cell survival studies, or both, in patients' cells, following UV exposure, should be done whenever possible on clinically sun-sensitive children and in siblings of XP patients. Molecular studies that can follow these tests now make specific complementation group assignment as well as specific mutation identification within reach, information which is rapidly becoming more useful in management of these patients as well as prenatal diagnosis. Contact this laboratory at gimutlab@umdnj.edu or by contacting one of us (WCL) at lamberwc@umdnj.edu.

Genomic structure, chromosomal localization and identification of mutations in the xeroderma pigmentosum variant (XPV) gene. Yuasa M, Masutani C, Eki T, Hanaoka F. Oncogene 2000;19:4721–8.

This paper reviews the 'trans-lesional synthesis' defect found and characterized in cells of XP variant patients.

The role of sunlight and DNA repair in melanoma and non-melanoma skin cancer: the xeroderma pigmentosum paradigm. Kraemer KH, Lee M-M, Andrews AD, Lambert WC. Arch Dermatol 1994;130:1018–21.

Questionnaires completed by physicians on 132 patients with XP were reviewed by the Xeroderma Pigmentosum Registry (KHK, ADA, and WCL). The sites at which melanomas and nonmelanoma skin cancers arose were found to be similar to those in the general US population, but to differ from each other.

This refuted earlier papers, based on literature reviews, which had found a different result.

FIRST LINE THERAPIES

■ Avoidance of sun exposure	E
■ Surgical excisions (see above)	E
■ Topical 5-fluorouracil (5%)	C
■ Topical imiquimod (5%)	E

Xeroderma pigmentosum. Lambert WC, Kuo H-R, Lambert MW. In: Chu AC, Edelson RA, eds. Malignant Tumors of the Skin. London: Chapman & Hall; 1999:497–522.

This is a general review of XP in which therapy and management issues are discussed.

Topical 5-fluorouracil to treat multiple or unresectable facial squamous cell carcinomas in xeroderma pigmentosum [Letter]. Hamouda B, Jamila Z, Najet R, et al. J Am Acad Dermatol 2001;44:1054. *See also* [Therapeutic results of 5-fluorouracil in multiple and irresectable facial carcinoma

secondary to xeroderma pigmentosum]. Boussen H, Zwik J, Mili-Boussen I, et al. Therapie 2001;56:751–4. In French.

Ten patients were treated in this Middle Eastern study (12 patients in the French article). Most showed varying degrees of clinical improvement, but 'deeper' or better-established tumors continued to arise.

Therapeutic response of a brother and sister with xeroderma pigmentosum to imiquimod 5% cream. Weisberg NK, Varghese M. Dermatol Surg 2002;28:518–23.

Two siblings with XP were treated with 5% imiquimod cream 'as frequently as tolerated'. The brother was treated twice daily, with little inflammation or dryness; the sister experienced extensive inflammation. Both patients showed clinical improvement and reduction in new tumor development. However, new tumors continued to arise in both patients.

The treatment of basal cell skin carcinomas in two sisters with xeroderma pigmentosum. Roseeuw D. Clin Exp Dermatol 2003;28(suppl 1):30–2.

Two sisters with XP were treated with imiquimod 5% cream, three times per week. Both experienced inflammation, but clearance of basal cell carcinomas was observed.

Excellent response of basal cell carcinomas and pigmentary characteristics in xeroderma pigmentosum to imiquimod 5% cream. Nagore E, Sevila A, Sanmartin O, et al. Br J Dermatol 2003;149:858–61.

A 19-year-old woman with XP was treated with imiquimod 5% cream, with improvement in clinical appearance and disappearance of very small basal cell carcinomas.

The treatment of basal cell carcinomas in a patient with xeroderma pigmentosum with a combination of 5% cream and oral acitretin. Giannotti B, Vanzi L, Difonzo EM, Pimpinelli N. Clin Exp Dermatol 2003;28(suppl 1):33–5.

A 15-year-old boy with XP was treated with imiquimod 5% cream three times per week, in combination with oral acitretin 20 mg daily. There were no adverse effects; all tumors resolved after 6 months of treatment.

SECOND LINE THERAPIES

■ Retinoid therapy	A

Prevention of skin cancer in xeroderma pigmentosum with the use of oral isotretinoin. Kraemer KH, Di Giovanna JJ, Mochell AN, et al. N Engl J Med 1988;318:1633–7.

This is the original paper in which use of oral retinoid therapy to diminish the rate of onset of skin cancers in XP patients was reported. Five XP patients with multiple squamous cell and basal cell carcinomas were treated with isotretinoin 2.0 mg/kg daily for 1 year. The rate of tumor development markedly diminished during treatment but returned to pretreatment levels after the drug was withdrawn. The dosage used was subsequently found to be associated with levels of toxicity inappropriate for many patients.

Oral isotretinoin prevention of skin cancer in xeroderma pigmentosum: individual variation in dose response [Abstract]. Kraemer KH, Di Giovanna JJ, Peck GL. J Invest Dermatol 1990;94:544.

Lower doses of oral isotretinoin, as given in the text, are recommended for some patients with XP, to limit side effects of the drug. However, the lower doses were found to be less effective.

Effect of isotretinoin therapy on natural killer cell activity in patients with xeroderma pigmentosum. Anolik JH, Di Giovanna JJ, Gaspari AA. Br J Dermatol 1998;138:236–41.

Decreased natural killer lymphocyte (NK cell) activity was found in three XP patients treated with oral isotretinoin at a dose of 1.0 mg/kg daily but not in three XP patients treated with 0.5 mg/kg daily of the drug. Two control XP patients showed no difference in NK cell function.

Cancer prevention in xeroderma pigmentosum variant. Somos S, Farkas B, Schneider I. Anticancer Res 1999; 19:2195–200.

This paper reports a favorable cancer prevention effect in an XPV patient, a 29-year-old female, treated with oral isotretinoin 2.0 mg/kg daily.

THIRD LINE THERAPIES

■ Resurfacing	E
■ Introduction of DNA repair enzymes into keratinocytes (not currently available)	A
■ Gene therapy (not yet tested in humans)	

Facial resurfacing in xeroderma pigmentosum with chemical peeling. Wee SY, Ahn DS. Plast Reconstr Surg 1999;103: 1464–7.

Results of treating two patients with XP using chemical peels of two different types are reported. Multiple peels with trichloroacetic acid were used in both patients, and a single peel with phenol was used in one of them, who was more severely affected. Favorable results are shown, with photographs. The results appear to support the authors' contention that chemical peels are superior to some other resurfacing techniques in management of XP patients with moderate sun damage. The authors also point out the ability to reapply the chemical peels, as indicated, at a later time as an advantage of this treatment modality.

Resurfacing the dorsum of the hand in a patient with xeroderma pigmentosum. Sonmez Ergun S. J Dermatol Surg 2003;29:782–4.

The advantages and disadvantages of full-thickness resurfacing of sun-damaged skin in XP are discussed.

Treatment should be individualized regarding patient and anatomic region. Full-thickness resurfacing of the face may not be warranted, because of regrowth of tumors around orifices and limited cosmetic result.

Deficiencies in chromatin associated DNA repair mechanisms in human genetic diseases. Lambert MW, Lambert WC. Progr Nucl Acids Res Molec Biol 1999;64:257–310.

Some of the complexities of DNA repair enzymes defective in XP and their interactions with chromatin are discussed. Bacterial enzymes, such as T4 endonuclease V, which are used in current gene therapy protocols (see below) bypass these complex interactions and act directly on human cellular DNA in vivo.

Effect of topically applied T4 endonuclease V in liposomes on skin cancer in xeroderma pigmentosum: a randomised study. Yarosh DB, Klein J, O'Connor A, et al. Lancet 2001;357:926–9.

In this prospective, multicenter, double-blind study, patients with XP were randomly assigned to topical treatment with T4 endonuclease V in a liposome delivery vehicle (T4N5 liposome lotion) or a placebo liposome lotion, to be applied daily for 1 year. The 20 patients treated with T4N5 liposome lotion had a marked reduction in the rate of development of actinic keratoses and basal cell carcinomas on sun-exposed areas compared with the eight patients treated with placebo lotion.

Topical enzyme therapy for skin diseases? Kraemer KH, DiGiovanna JJ. J Am Acad Dermatol 2002;46:463–6.

This is a review discussing multiple aspects of correction of DNA repair defects in the skin of XP patients by introducing corrective enzymes.

Genetic correction of DNA repair-deficient/cancer prone seroderma pigmentosum group C keratinocytes. Arnaudeau-Begard C, Brellier F, Chevallier-Lagente O, et al. Hum Gene Ther 2003;14:983–6.

The authors' systems for introducing a normal *XPC* gene into XPC keratinocytes and fibroblasts using a retrovirus vector and for reconstructing and testing skin in vitro are described.

Xeroderma pigmentosum: from symptoms and genetics to gene specific skin therapy. Magnaldo T, Sarasin A. Cells Tissues Organs 2004;177:189–98.

The authors review the current status of gene therapy for XP.

Xerosis

Ian Coulson

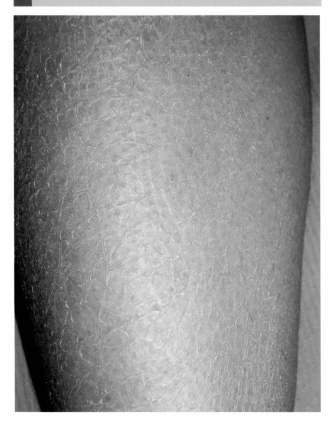

Xerosis is a term used to describe a skin condition where there is a rough dry textural feel to the skin, accompanied by fine scaling and sometimes fine fissuring. Increasing xerosis is usually accompanied by increasing itch. It is a description, not a diagnosis – it may result from a combination of environmental conditions (low humidity, degreasing of the skin by excessive bathing soap or detergent use), genetic disorders of keratinization (ichthyoses), Down syndrome, atopic eczema, endocrine disease states (hypothyroidism), and a host of underlying disease states such as chronic renal failure, liver disease, malnutrition, anorexia nervosa, essential fatty acid deficiency, Sjögren's syndrome, HIV infection, lymphoma, and carcinomatosis. It is more common in the elderly. Drugs are occasionally implicated.

MANAGEMENT STRATEGY

Initial evaluation should seek to distinguish simple xerosis from a genetic ichthyosis (see page 295) although the management of both conditions is similar. Family history, distribution, and morphology will help. A history of weight loss, dietary history, and body mass index may give clues towards an underlying metabolic or malabsorptive disorder. Dry eyes and mouth may indicate underlying Sjögren's syndrome. History and clinical examination should seek symptoms and signs of hypothyroidism and chronic renal disease. Drug use and sexual contact history may reveal HIV infection.

Xerosis is an almost universal accompaniment of atopic eczema, and seems to be a distinct entity from ichthyosis vulgaris.

The anchors of therapy for xerosis after any underlying disorders (if possible) are corrected are *improvement of the humidity* in the patient's environment, *avoidance of exacerbating factors* such as soap and detergents, and the use of *emollients or humectants*.

Low environmental humidity both at home and work will exacerbate xerosis of any cause. Arid air is a problem in air conditioned homes, offices, and vehicles. Hot dry air directed to the lower legs during the winter in the front of automobiles is a common cause of lower leg xerosis. In the home or workplace, humidifiers can be fitted over radiators; alternatively placing wet towels over them will increase air humidity.

Soaps and detergents degrease the skin, reduce epidermal thickness, and increase scale and itch, so are best avoided, and light emollient cleansers are suggested in their place. Bathing in tepid water is often preferred by patients, and patting the skin dry will produce less scale and dryness than vigorous toweling.

Emollients (that simply produce an impervious film over the epidermis and prevent 'transpiration') and humectants (such as lactic acid, urea, or glycerine that hold water in the epidermis osmotically) are the mainstays of therapy. For the most common type of xerosis, few good comparative studies exist, which is surprising because they are the most frequently used dermatological products! They should be used liberally and as frequently as possible; emollients are particularly valuable after bathing or showering to hold water in the epidermis. Light emollients for use in the shower or bath may be preferred to *bath oils* by some. Choice of emollient is entirely personal to the patient – a pack with small amounts of a variety of products for home trial or a self-selection 'tub tray' for the clinic is likely to enhance compliance.

Agents containing *α-hydroxy acids (AHAs)* may offer some advantages over conventional paraffin-based emollients, but this may be at the expense of irritation in some people. Low-concentration *salicylic acid* may help reduce scale in more severe xerosis, but it is essential to remember that systemic absorption and salicylism can occur.

Topical retinoids have only been used in the more severe ichthyoses and are too irritating for use in xerosis. Systemic therapies have little part to play in most patients.

SPECIFIC INVESTIGATIONS

- ■ Thyroid function tests
- ■ Renal function tests
- ■ Consider tests for Sjögren's syndrome, HIV infection, malignancy, and malabsorption, if clinically indicated
- ■ Drug history

Sjögren's syndrome: a retrospective review of the cutaneous features of 93 patients by the Italian Group of Immunodermatology. Bernacchi E, Amato L, Parodi A, et al. Clin Exp Rheumatol 2004;22:55–62.

Over half of 93 patients with Sjögren's syndrome had xerosis and its presence correlated with the presence of SSA and SSB antibodies.

HIV-associated pruritus: etiology and management. Singh F, Rudikoff D. Am J Clin Dermatol 2003;4:177–88.

Xerosis is one of the more common causes of itch in HIV infection and AIDS.

Xerosis from lithium carbonate. Hoxtell E, Dahl MV. Arch Dermatol 1975;111:1073–4.

Litt's Drug Eruption Reference Manual, 10th edn. (Jerome Z Litt, ed. London and New York: Taylor and Francis; 2004) lists in excess of 150 drugs (from acebutolol to zonisamide!) that have been implicated in causing xerosis. Cimetidine, protease inhibitors, and nicotinamide are perhaps the best known.

FIRST LINE THERAPIES

■ Soap avoidance	A
■ Humidification	C
■ Emollients	B
■ Bath oils	B

How useful are soap substitutes? Berth-Jones J, Graham-Brown RAC. J Dermatol Treat 1992;3:9–11.

Thirty eight subjects with atopic dermatitis, psoriasis, or senile xerosis were treated with emulsifying ointment BP or Wash E45® as soap substitutes. Dryness and itching improved in both treatment groups. Wash E45® was considered more effective as a cleanser.

The effect of washing on the thickness of the stratum corneum in normal and atopic individuals. White MI, McEwan Jenkinson D, Lloyd DH. Br J Dermatol 1987; 116:525–30.

A histological study confirming that stratum corneum thickness was reduced by washing with soap in both normal and atopic individuals. The stratum corneum was thinner in the atopic individuals than controls at baseline and was almost completely removed in the atopics by the use of soap.

The value of oil baths for adjuvant basic therapy of inflammatory dermatoses with dry, barrier-disrupted skin. Melnik B, Braun-Falco O. Hautarzt 1996;47:665–72.

The use of oil baths with emollients is an integral and indispensable constituent of maintenance therapy in dry skin conditions, atopic eczema, and inflammatory dermatoses.

A new technique for evaluating bath oil in the treatment of dry skin. Stanfield JW, Levy J, Kyriakopoulos AA, Waldman PM. Cutis 1981;28:458–60.

A comparative study confirming bath oils are superior to soap in lower leg xerosis in the elderly.

SECOND LINE THERAPIES

■ Urea-containing creams	B
■ Lactic acid-containing creams	B
■ Ammonium lactate creams	A
■ AHA creams	B
■ Thyroxine cream	D

A double-blind comparison of two creams containing urea as the active ingredient. Assessment of efficacy and side effects by non-invasive techniques and a clinical scoring scheme. Serup J. Acta Derm Venereol Suppl (Stockh) 1992;177:34–43.

A comparison of 3% and 10% urea cream showed that both were effective at reducing scale, dryness, and laboratory parameters (transepidermal water loss and colorimetric changes). The 10% cream was better at restoring the skin's water barrier function.

Clinical evaluation of 40% urea and 12% ammonium lactate in the treatment of xerosis. Ademola J, Frazier C, Kim SJ, et al. Am J Clin Dermatol 2002;3:217–22.

A double blind study comparing 40% urea cream with 12% ammonium lactate cream showing superiority of the urea cream. Flexural irritation was a problem.

Many urea-containing products contain lower concentrations than used in this study.

A controlled two-center study of lactate 12 percent lotion and a petrolatum-based creme in patients with xerosis. Wehr R, Krochmal L, Bagatell F, Ragsdale W. Cutis 1986; 37:205–7

Lactate 12% lotion was significantly more effective than a petrolatum-based cream in reducing the severity of xerosis during treatment and post-treatment phases.

Comparative efficacy of 12% ammonium lactate lotion and 5% lactic acid lotion in the treatment of moderate to severe xerosis. Rogers RS III, Callen J, Wehr R, Krochmal L. J Am Acad Dermatol 1989;21:714–16.

This comparative study of twice daily application of 5% lactic acid vs 12% ammonium lactate lotion showed superiority of 12% ammonium lactate in reducing the severity of xerosis.

A double-blind clinical trial comparing the efficacy and safety of pure lanolin versus ammonium lactate 12% cream for the treatment of moderate to severe foot xerosis. Jennings MB, Alfieri DM, Parker ER et al. Cutis 2003;71:78–82.

A study showing equivalence of a petrolatum compound and 12% ammonium lactate cream for foot xerosis.

An evaluation of the effect of an alpha hydroxy acid-blend skin cream in the cosmetic improvement of symptoms of moderate to severe xerosis, epidermolytic hyperkeratosis, and ichthyosis. Kempers S, Katz HI, Wildnauer R, Green B. Cutis 1998;61:347–50.

Twenty subjects completed a course of treatment with either regular or extra-strength AHA-blend cream on a test site compared with a currently marketed, non-AHA moisturizing lotion on a control site. Improvements were significant compared to baseline and compared to sites treated with the control lotion, but the AHA cream did cause some local mild to moderate adverse effects; all subjects were able to continue using the test product for the duration of the study.

Xerosis in hypothyroidism: a potential role for the use of topical thyroid hormone in euthyroid patients. Heymann WR, Gans EH, Manders SM, et al. Med Hypotheses 2001;57:736–9.

Euthyroid patients with xerosis were treated with an emollient to one leg and the same base with 7.5 µg/g thyroxine and the same concentration of tri-iodothyronine. In 20 of 24 patients control and thyroid hormone treated sides showed similar improvement. The authors hypothesize on a mechanism whereby thyroxine topically should help xerosis and propose further studies to optimize delivery and concentration.

Evidence levels **A** Double-blind study **B** Clinical trial ≥ 20 subjects **C** Clinical trial < 20 subjects **D** Series ≥ 5 subjects **E** Anecdotal case reports

Yellow nail syndrome

Robert Baran

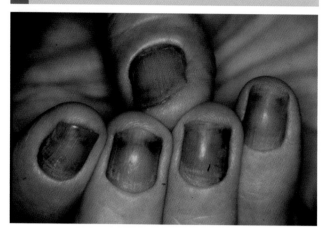

The yellow nail syndrome (YNS) is an uncommon disorder of unknown etiology characterized by the triad of yellow nails, lymphedema, and respiratory tract involvement. This term was originally used to describe the association of slow-growing yellow nails with primary lymphedema. Pleural effusion was later recognized to be an additional sign of the syndrome. Since then, other respiratory conditions such as bronchiectasis, sinusitis, bronchitis, and chronic respiratory infections have been associated with the disorder. Although all three signs that classically characterize the triad of YNS do not occur in every patient, the presence of typical nail changes should be considered an absolute requirement for the diagnosis.

MANAGEMENT STRATEGY

Although YNS may resolve spontaneously, treatment is usually demanded by patients for the management of the nails. They are unsightly, hard, and slow growing.

Underlying diseases such as respiratory disorders, malignancy, infections, immunologic and hematologic abnormalities, endocrine, connective tissue and renal abnormalities, and miscellaneous disorders including penicillamine therapy should be sought. Treatment of any concomitant disorder is mandatory, but does not always bring resolution of YNS, and cure of the nail is not always accompanied by disappearance of the other signs.

SPECIFIC INVESTIGATIONS

- Rule out nail fungal infection or pseudomonal infection
- Complete blood count
- Urinalysis, proteinuria
- Immunoelectrophoresis
- Thyroid stimulating hormone
- Waaler-Rose test for serum rheumatoid factors
- Chemistry profile with blood creatinine
- Sinus and chest radiography
- Ear, nose, and throat, and pulmonary investigations
- Liver enzymes, alkaline phosphatases

Yellow nail syndrome in rheumatoid arthritis: report of three cases. Mattingly PC, Bossingham DH. Ann Rheum Dis. 1979;38:475–8.

Several other reports have associated YNS with both rheumatoid disease and therapies given for rheumatoid arthritis.

There are anecdotal reports of YNS with tuberculosis, solid carcinomas, and lymphomas.

FIRST LINE THERAPIES

■ α-Tocopherol	D
■ Itraconazole or fluconazole	C
■ Treatment of the concomitant disorder	E

Yellow nail syndrome. Response to vitamin E. Ayres S, Mihan R. Arch Dermatol 1973;108:267–8.

Vitamin E at dosages ranging from 600 to 1200 IU daily can induce complete clearing of the nail changes.

The new oral antifungal drugs in the treatment of the yellow nail syndrome. Baran R. Br J Dermatol 2002;147: 189–91.

Itraconazole pulse therapy or, better, fluconazole combined with vitamin E produce a positive effect on nail growth.

Syndrome des ongles jaunes associé à une polyarthrite rhumatoide. Régression sous chrysothérapie. Launey D, Hebbar M, Louyot J, et al. Rev Med Interne 1997;18:494–6.

In a patient with YNS associated with rheumatoid arthritis, the nail abnormalities completely regressed after gold therapy for arthritis.

Yellow nail syndrome resolution following treatment of pulmonary tuberculosis. Pang SM. Int J Dermatol 1993;32: 605–6.

Treatment of pulmonary tuberculosis cured a patient with YNS.

Yellow nail syndrome. Possible association with malignancy. Guin JD, Elleman JH. Arch Dermatol 1979;115:734–5.

Treatment of associated malignancy may improve the YNS.

SECOND LINE THERAPIES

■ Intradermal triamcinolone injections in the proximal nail matrix	C
■ Topical vitamin E	E

Intradermal triamcinolone acetonide injection in the yellow nail syndrome. Abell E, Samman PD. Trans St Johns Hosp Dermatol Soc 1973;59:114–16.

Complete recovery of normal nail growth in five of ten cases of YNS has followed injection of triamcinolone acetonide to the posterior nail fold of affected finger nails using a needleless injector.

Successful use of topical vitamin E solution in the treatment of nail changes in yellow nail syndrome. Williams BC, Buffham R, du Vivier A. Arch Dermatol 1991;127:1023–8.

Topical vitamin E solution in dimethyl sulfoxide has been shown to be successful in the treatment of nail changes in YNS.

THIRD LINE THERAPIES

■ Oral zinc supplementation	E
■ Dietary treatment	E
■ Octreotide	E

Yellow nail syndrome cured by zinc supplementation. Arroyo JF, Cohen ML. Clin Exp Dermatol 1992;18:62–4.

Total resolution of yellow nails and lymphedema was observed following oral zinc supplementation for 2 years.

Yellow nail syndrome in a 10-year-old girl. Gocmen A, Kucukosmanoglu O, Kiper N, et al. Turk J Pediatr 1997;39: 105–9

Low-fat diet supplemented with medium chain triglycerides brought moderate improvement for lymphedema of the lower extremities.

Dietary treatment of chylous ascites in yellow nail syndrome. Tan WC. Gut 1989;30:1622–3

Dietary restriction of fat and supplements of medium chain triglycerides were successful.

Successful octreotide treatment of chylous pleural effusion and lymphedema in the yellow nail syndrome. Makrilakis K, Pavlatos S, Giannikopoulos G, et al. Ann Intern Med 2004;141:246–7.

Octreotide, a somatostatin analogue, was effective in a classical case of YNS with yellow nails, lymphedema of the lower extremities, and recurrent chylous pleural effusion.

Index

Note to Index: where synonyms are indexed, the preferred names follow in parentheses